# ADVANCED ANESTHESIA
# REVIEW

# ADVANCED ANESTHESIA REVIEW

EDITED BY
*Alaa Abd-Elsayed*

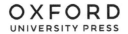

# OXFORD
## UNIVERSITY PRESS

Oxford University Press is a department of the University of Oxford. It furthers the University's objective of excellence in research, scholarship, and education by publishing worldwide. Oxford is a registered trade mark of Oxford University Press in the UK and certain other countries.

Published in the United States of America by Oxford University Press
198 Madison Avenue, New York, NY 10016, United States of America.

Library of Congress Cataloging-in-Publication Data
Names: Abd-Elsayed, Alaa, editor.
Title: Advanced anesthesia review / [edited by] Alaa Abd-Elsayed.
Other titles: Advanced anesthesia review (Abd-Elsayed)
Description: New York, NY : Oxford University Press, [2023] |
Includes bibliographical references and index.
Identifiers: LCCN 2021039926 (print) | LCCN 2021039927 (ebook) |
ISBN 9780197584521 (paperback) | ISBN 9780197584545 (epub) |
ISBN 9780197584552 (OxMed)
Subjects: MESH: Anesthesia | Handbook
Classification: LCC RD81 (print) | LCC RD81 (ebook) | NLM WO 231 |
DDC 617.9/6—dc23
LC record available at https://lccn.loc.gov/2021039926
LC ebook record available at https://lccn.loc.gov/2021039927

DOI: 10.1093/med/9780197584521.001.0001

Printed by Marquis, Canada

*To my parents, my wife, and my two beautiful kids, Maro and George*

# CONTENTS

# PREFACE

The American Board of Anesthesiology (ABA) recently published a revised curriculum outline to address the relatively new board examination structure (basic and advanced written exams). Unfortunately, most of the textbooks in the current market were developed in accordance with the old curriculum and examination structure (only one written exam). This book is a highly needed review source for all examinees to be exposed to the latest advanced examination content.

This book was developed by having short chapters on each item in the ABA outline and includes high-yield points in each chapter. We did our best to include all the board-relevant and testable information in each chapter.

Our authors come from the most prestigious institutes in the country and put forth significant time and effort in the writing of each chapter. In addition, we also authored another book for the basic examination using the same strategy, which provides the needed basic knowledge related to the clinical topics addressed in this book.

You will find several concepts and principles repeated in different sections and in relation to different organ systems.

This intentionally placed repetition allows for high-yield information to be learned from different angles, as written by different authors, and in relation to different clinical contexts. So, I highly recommend not skipping the few similar topics when they show up in various different chapters of the book.

As you prepare for your advanced ABA examination, know that you have already gained the clinical experience needed to become an anesthesiologist. This test is just needed to confirm your level of knowledge. Learning is an ongoing experience during your training and thereafter. Reading this book and practicing questions will help you solidify the clinical expertise you gained across your training and will help you pass your exam.

I would like to thank the publisher for supporting this large project and all my colleagues who contributed to this book.

Alaa Abd-Elsayed, MD, MPH, FASA
Anesthesiology, University of Wisconsin, School of
Medicine and Public Health, Madison, Wisconsin

# CONTRIBUTORS

**Rany T. Abdallah, MD, PhD, MBA**
Center for Interventional Pain and Spine
Milford, DE, USA

**Mena Abdelmalak, MD, MBF**
Department of Anesthesiology, Perioperative, and Pain
    Medicine
Icahn School of Medicine at Mount Sinai
New York, NY, USA

**Alaa Abd-Elsayed, MD, MPH, FASA**
Associate Professor of Anesthesiology
Medical Director, UW Health Pain Services
University of Wisconsin School of Medicine and Public
    Health
Madison, Wisconsin, USA

**Soozan S. Abouhassan, MD, FASA**
Assistant Professor, Division Chief General Anesthesia
University Hospitals Cleveland Medical Center
Cleveland, OH, USA

**Christine Acho, DO**
Department of Anesthesiology Critical Care
University of Michigan
Ann Arbor, MI, USA

**Jonathan Adams, MD**
Department of Anesthesiology
Allegheny Health Network
Pittsburgh, PA, USA

**Deepak Agarwal, MBBS, MD**
Staff Anesthesiologist
Department of Anesthesiology
HSHS St. John's Hospital
Springfield, IL, USA

**Andaleeb A. Ahmed, MBBS, MPH**
Clinical Assistant Professor
Department of Anesthesiology
Tufts University School of Medicine
Lahey Hospital and Medical Center
Burlington, MA, USA

**Muhammad Fayyaz Ahmed, MBBS, MD**
Assistant Professor
Department of Clinical Anesthesiology
Lewis Katz School of Medicine
Temple University
Philadelphia, PA, USA

**Rohit Aiyer, MD**
Assistant Professor - Staff Physician
Department of Anesthesiology, Pain Management, and
    Perioperative Medicine
Henry Ford Health System
Detroit, MI, USA

**Abayomi Akintorin, MD**
Cook County Health Systems
Chicago, IL, USA

**Thomas Alberto, MD**
Department of Anesthesia and Pain Management
Cook County Health and Hospital Systems
Chicago, IL, USA

**Erica Alcibiade, DO**
Department of Anesthesiology
University of Cincinnati
Cincinnati, OH, USA

**Anthony Alexander, MBBS**
Department of Anesthesiology
Cook County Health and Hospital Systems
University of Cincinnati College of Medicine
Chicago, IL, USA

**Caroline Alhaddadin, MBBS**
Department of Anesthesia and Pediatric
University Hospitals/ Case Western Reserve University
Cleveland, OH, USA

**Piotr Al-Jindi, MD**
Anesthesiology Program Director
Department of Anesthesiology and Pain Management
Cook County Health
Chicago, IL, USA

**Kenan Alkhalili, MD**
Department of Anesthesia
Cook County Health and Hospital Systems
Chicago, IL, USA

**Yamah Amiri, MBBS**
Department of Anesthesia and Critical Care
University of Chicago
Chicago, IL, USA

**Ben Aquino, MD**
Assistant Professor
Department of Anesthesiology
Northwestern University
Chicago, IL, USA

**Lovkesh L. Arora, MBBS, MD, FASA**
Clinical Associate Professor
Department of Anesthesiology
University of Iowa Health Care
Iowa City, IA, USA

**Ami Attali, DO**
Division Chief Obstetrical High Risk Anesthesiology,
Medical Director High Risk Obstetrical Optimization Clinics
Department of Anesthesiology, Pain Management, and
    Perioperative Medicine
Henry Ford Health System
Detroit, MI, USA

**Subramanya Bandi, MD**
Department of Anesthesiology
Allegheny Health Network
Pittsburgh, PA, USA

**Jarrod Bang, MD**
Adult Cardiothoracic Anesthesia
Department of Anesthesia
University of Iowa
Iowa City, IA, USA

**Jason Bang, MD**
Department of Anesthesia and Pain Management
Cook County Health and Hospital Systems
Chicago, IL, USA

**Natalie R. Barnett, MD**
Icahn School of Medicine
New York, NY, USA

**Frank Barrack, MD**
Allegheny Health Network Anesthesia Residency
Pittsburgh, PA, USA

**Mariam Batakji, MD**
Pediatric Anesthesiology
Department of Pediatric Anesthesiology
Medical College of Wisconsin
Milwakee, WI, USA

**David Bennett, MD**
Department of Anesthesiology and Perioperative Medicine
University Hospitals
Cleveland, OH, USA

**Maura C. Berkelhamer, MD**
Director, Pediatric Perioperative Medicine
Assistant Professor of Anesthesiology and Pediatrics
Department of Anesthesiology and Perioperative Medicine
University Hospital Case Medical Center
Rainbow Babies and Children's Hospital
Cleveland, OH, USA

**Kristin Bevil, MS**
Assistant Professor
Department of Anesthesiology
University of Wisconsin School of Medicine and Public
    Health
Madison, WI, USA

**Anuschka Bhatia, MD**
Icahn School of Medicine at Mount Sinai
New York, NY, USA

**Callan Bialorucki, MD**
Department of Anesthesiology
The Ohio State University Wexner Medical Center
Columbus, OH, USA

**Scott Blaine, DO**
Department of Anesthesiology
University of Wisconsin School of Medicine and Public
    Health
Madison, WI, USA

**Joshua F. Bolanos, MD**
Department of Anesthesiology
Beth Israel Lahey Health
Burlington, MA, USA

**Elaine A. Boydston, MD**
Assistance Clinical Professor
Department of Anesthesiology and Perioperative Medicine
University of California Los Angeles
Los Angeles, CA, USA

**Lydia C. Boyette, DO, MBA, CA-1, PGY-2**
Department of Anesthesiology
University of Central Florida
Orlando, FL, USA

**Phillip G. Boysen, MD, MBA**
Professor
Department of Anesthesiology
University of Mississippi Medical Center
Jackson, MI, USA

**Katrina Brakoniecki, MD, MSc**
Regional Anesthesia and Acute Pain
Department of Anesthesiology
Saint Francis Hospital and Medical Center
Hartford, CT, USA

**Jordan Brewer, MD**
Department of Anesthesiology
University of Florida College of Medicine
Gainesville, FL, USA

**Heather Brosnan, MD**
Department of Anesthesiology
Westchester Medical Center/New York Medical College
Valhalla, NY, USA

**Anna-Kaye Brown, DO**
Department of Anesthesiology
Lewis Katz School of Medicine at Temple University
Pittsburgh, PA, USA

**Eric Brzozowski, MD**
Department of Anesthesiology and Perioperative Medicine
University Hospitals Cleveland Medical Center
Cleveland, OH, USA

**Timothy T. Bui, MD**
Department of Anesthesiology and Perioperative Medicine
University of California, Los Angeles
Los Angeles, CA, USA

**Melissa Anne Burger, MD**
Assistant Professor
Department of Anesthesiology and Surgery
University of Florida College of Medicine
Gainesville, FL, USA

**Garrett W. Burnett, MD**
Assistant Professor
Department of Anesthesiology, Perioperative, and Pain
    Medicine
Icahn School of Medicine at Mount Sinai
New York, NY, USA

**Jeffrey W. Cannon, MD**
Department of Anesthesiology and Perioperative Medicine
University Hospitals/Case Western Reserve University
Cleveland, OH, USA

**Dominic S. Carollo, MD**
Senior Staff Anesthesiologist and Senior Lecturer
Department of Anesthesiology and Perioperative Medicine
Ochsner Healthcare System
New Orleans, LA, USA

**J. P. Cata**
Anesthesiology and Surgical Oncology Research Group
Houston, TX, USA

**Michael Chang, MD**
Department of Anesthesiology
Westchester Medical Center
Valhalla, NY, USA

**Katya H. Chiong, MD, FASA**
Assistant Professor and Senior Attending Physician
Department of Anesthesiology and Perioperative Medicine
University Hospitals Cleveland Medical Center/Case Western
    Reserve University School of Medicine
Cleveland, OH, USA

**Heather Christopherson, MD**
Department of Anesthesiology
University of Central Florida/HCA GME Consortium,
    Orlando
Ocala Health, Florida
Ocala, FL, USA

**Alex Y. Chung, MD**
Anesthesiologist
Department of Anesthesia
Cincinnati Children Hospital Medical Center
Cincinnati, OH, USA

**Kevin W. Chung, MD**
Anesthesiologist
Department of Anesthesiology, Perioperative and Pain
    Medicine
Icahn School of Medicine at Mount Sinai
New York, NY, USA

**Alexandra N. Cole, MD**
Department of Anesthesia
Lahey Hospital and Medical Center
Burlington, MA, USA

**Gabriel M. Coleman, BSc**
Physician
Philadelphia College of Osteopathic Medicine
Philadelphia, PA, USA

**M. Anthony Cometa, MD**
Clinical Assistant Professor
Department of Anesthesiology
University of Florida
Gainesville, FL, USA

**Jay Conhaim, MD**
Department of Anesthesiology
University of Cincinnati Medical Center
Cincinnati, OH, USA

**Matthew T. Connolly, MD**
Cardiologist
Orthopaedic Hospital of Wisconsin-Glendale, USA

**Dillon B. Coplai, MD**
Department of Anesthesia
Lahey Clinic
Burlington, MA, USA

**Daniel Cormican, MD**
Attending Anesthesiologist and Intensivist
Department of Anesthesiology
Allegheny Health Network
Pittsburgh, PA, USA

**Elyse M. Cornett, PhD**
Assistant Professor and Director of Research
Department of Anesthesiology
LSU Health Shreveport
Shreveport, LA, USA

**Adi Cosic, DO**
Department of Anesthesiology
University Hospitals Cleveland Medical Center
Cleveland, OH, USA

**Derek Brady Covington, MD**
Department of Anesthesiology
University of Florida College of Medicine
Gainesville, FL, USA

**Dane Coyne, MD**
Assistant Professor of Anesthesiology
Department of Anesthesia and Perioperative Medicine
University Hospitals
Cleveland, OH, USA

**Ettore Crimi, MD**
Associate Professor - Program Director Anesthesiology
    Residency Program
Department of Anesthesiology
University of Central Florida
Orlando, FL, USA

**Caitlin N. Curcuru, MD**
Department of Anesthesia and Critical Care
The University of Chicago
Chicago, IL, USA

**Timothy Cutler, DO**
Department of Family Medicine
Firelands Regional Medical Center
Sandusky, OH, USA

**Al-Awwab Mohammad Dabaliz, MD, MBBS**
Department of Anesthesiology and Perioperative Medicine
University Hospitals Cleveland Medical Center
Cleveland, OH, USA

**Allison K. Dalton, MD**
Associate Professor, Director of Anesthesia Critical Care
Associate Chairman of Education
Department of Anesthesia and Critical Care
University of Chicago
Chicago, IL, USA

**Evan Davidson, MD**
Department of Anesthesiology
University of Central Florida/HCA GME Consortium,
    Orlando
Ocala Health Florida
Ocala, FL, USA

**Mark Dearden, MD, MPH**
Assistant Professor
Department of Anesthesiology
University of Cincinnati
Cincinnati, OH, USA

**Virgilio de Gala, MD**
Anesthesiologist
Department of Anesthesiology
Westchester Medical Center
Valhalla, NY, USA

**Daniel Denis, DO**
Department of Anesthesia and Perioperative Care
Rutgers–New Jersey Medical School
Newark, NJ, USA

**Suhas Devangam, MD**
Department of Anesthesiology
University of Cincinnati Medical Center
Cincinnati, OH, USA

**Christina D. Diaz, MD, FASA, FAAP**
Professor
Department of Anesthesiology
Medical College of Medicine/ Children's Wisconsin
Milwaukee, WI, USA

**Tara Doherty, DO**
Pediatric Anesthesiology
New York Medical College Maria Fareri Children's
    Hospital
Westchester Medical Center
New York, NY, USA

**Nupur Dua, MBBS, MD**
Department of Anesthesiology
University of Minnesota
Minneapolis, MN, USA

**Jeffery James Eapen, MD**
Department of Anesthesiology and Pain Management
Cook County Health Systems
Chicago, IL, USA

**Brent Earls, MD**
Anesthesiology
Department of Anesthesiology
Johns Hopkins University
Baltimore, MD, USA

**Maxim S. Eckmann, MD**
University of the Incarnate Word School of Medicine
San Antonio TX, USA
Vice Chairman, Clinical Research
Department of Anesthesiology
UT Health
San Antonio, TX, USA

**Nikki Eden, DO**
Cook County Health Systems
Chicago, IL, USA

**Narbeh Edjiu, MD**
Department of Anesthesiology
Allegheny Health Network
Pittsburgh, PA, USA

**Nwadiogo Ejiogu, MD**
OB Anesthesia
St. Luke's and Mount Sinai West Hospitals
New York, NY, USA

**Steven Ethier, DO**
Staff Anesthesiologist
Department of Anesthesiology
William Beaumont Hospital
Royal Oak, MI, USA

**Christopher O. Fadumiye, MD**
Assistant Professor
Department of Anesthesiology
Medical College of Wisconsin
Milwaukee, WI, USA

**Mohamed Fayed, MD, MSc**
Department of Anesthesiology
Henry Ford Health system
Detroit, MI, USA

**Diana Feinstein, DO**
Assistant Professor
Lewis Katz School of Medicine
Temple University
Philadelphia, PA, USA

**Kris Ferguson, MD**
Clinical Assistant Professor of Medical School Regional
    Campuses, Medical College of Wisconsin
Department of Interventional Pain Management
Aspirus Health System
Antigo, WI, USA

**Karim Fikry, MD**
Clinical Assistant Professor
Department of Anesthesia
Lahey Hospital and Medical Center
Burlington, MA, USA

**James Flaherty, MD**
Assistant Professor
Department of Anesthesiology
University of Minnesota
Minneapolis, MN, USA

**Timothy F. Flanagan, MD**
Clinical Associate
Department of Anesthesiology
Beth Israel Lahey Health
Burlington, MA, USA

**Timothy Ford, MD**
Department of Anesthesiology
University of Wisconsin at Madison
Madison, WI, USA

**Patrick Forrest, MD**
Senior Staff Physician
Department of Anesthesiology
Henry Ford Health System
Detroit, MI, USA

**Tiffany Frazee, MD**
Assistant Professor and Division Chief
Department of Pediatric Anesthesiology
Rainbow Babies and Children's Hospital
Cleveland, OH, USA

**Anthony Fritzler, MD, FASA**
Anesthesiologist
Department of Anesthesiology and Pain Medicine
Akron Children's Hospital
Akron, OH, USA

**Ilana R. Fromer, MD**
Assistant Professor
Department of Anesthesiology
University of Minnesota

**Elie Geara, MD**
Rainbow Babies and Children's Hospital
University Hospitals Cleveland Medical Center
Cleveland, OH, USA

**Alina Genis, MD**
Department of Anesthesiology
NYMC at Westchester Medical Center
Valhalla, NY, USA

**Shelley George, MD**
Department of Anesthesiology
Clinical Assistant Professor (Adjunct), Anesthesiology
Temple University, Lewis Katz School of Medicine,
    Pennsylvania, USA

**Mary Ghaly, MD**
Assistant Professor
Department of Anesthesiology and Perioperative Medicine
University Hospitals Cleveland Medical Center
Cleveland, OH, USA

**Priyanka Ghosh, MD**
Remedy Medical Group
San Francisco, CA, USA

**Christina Gibson, DO**
Allegheny Health Network
Pittsburgh, PA, USA

**Christopher Giordano, MD**
Department of Anesthesiology
University of Florida College of Medicine
Gainesville, FL, USA

**Brook Girma, MD**
Department of Anesthesiology
Louisiana State University School of Medicine
Shreveport, LA, USA

**Feodor J. Gloss, DO**
Cook County Health and Hospitals System
Chicago, IL, USA

**Vicko Gluncic, MD, PhD**
Department Chair and System Chair for Anesthesia - Sinai
    Health System
Department of Anesthesiology
Mount Sinai Hospital - Sinai Health System
Chicago, IL, USA

**Maria Gorneva, MD**
Cook County Health and Hospitals System
Chicago, IL, USA

**Ravi K. Grandhi, MD, MBA**
Medical Director
Department of Anesthesiology
Nazareth Hospital
Philadelphia, PA, USA

**Thomas Graul, DO**
Assistant Professor
Department of Anesthesiology
The Ohio State University
Columbus, OH, USA

**Ellyn Gray, MD**
Department of Anesthesia
University of Iowa Carver College of Medicine
Iowa City, IA, USA

**Matthew Gunst, MD**
Department of Anesthesiology
University of Florida College of Medicine
Gainesville, FL, USA

**Jayakar Guruswamy, MBBS, MD**
Assistant Professor
Department of Anesthesiology, Pain Management, and
    Perioperative Medicine
Henry Ford Health System
Detroit, MI, USA

**Howard B. Gutstein, MD**
Vice Chair, Research
Academic Officer
Anesthesiology Institute
Allegheny Health Network
Pittsburgh, PA, USA

**Chike Gwam, MBBS**
Associate Professor
Department of Anesthesiology
Cook County Health and Hospitals System
Chicago, IL, USA

**Michael J. Gyorfi, MD**
Department of Anesthesiology
The University of Wisconsin
Madison, WI, USA

**Florian Hackl, MD**
Clinical Assistant Professor in Anesthesiology
Department of Anesthesia
Lahey Hospital and Medical Center
Burlington, MA, USA

**Joseph Salama Hanna, MD**
Anesthesiology/Pain Medicine Staff, Clinical Assistant
    Professor Wayne State University School of Medicine
Department of Anesthesiology, Pain Management and
    Perioperative Medicine
Henry Ford Health System
Detroit, MI, USA

**Rewais B. Hanna, MD**
Department of Anesthesiology
University of Wisconsin School of Medicine and Public Health
Madison, WI, USA

**Alain Harb, MD**
Pediatric Anesthesia
Department of Anesthesiology and Perioperative Medicine
University Hospitals Cleveland Medical Center
Cleveland, OH, USA

**Brian Harris, MD**
Department of Sleep Medicine
UCLA
Los Angeles, CA, USA

**Ellen Hauck, DO, PhD**
Professor
Department of Anesthesiology
Temple University
Philadelphia, PA, USA

**Lacey Haugen, DO**
Cardiothoracic
Department of Cardiothoracic Anesthesia
Cleveland Clinic Main Campus
Cleveland, OH, US

**Elizabeth Haynes, MD**
Department of Anesthesiology
The Ohio State University
Columbus, OH, USA

**Afshin Heidari, MD**
Anesthesiologist and Interventional Pain
Department of Anesthesiology and Pain Medicine
Advocate Illinois Masonic Medical Center
Chicago, IL, USA

**Mada Helou, MD**
Assistant Professor of Anesthesiology, Program Director for
    Anesthesiology
Department of Anesthesiology and Preoperative Medicine
University Hospitals Cleveland Medical Center
Cleveland, OH, USA

**Sarah Helwege, DO**
Visiting Professor
Department of Anesthesiology
University of Iowa Hospitals and Clinics
Iowa City, IA, USA

**Bryan J. Hierlmeier, MD**
Associate Professor
Department of Anesthesiology
University of Mississippi Medical Center
Jackson, MS, USA

**Cassandra Hoffmann, MD**
Assistant Professor, Director Pediatric Regional Anesthesia
Department of Anesthesiology and Perioperative Medicine
University Hospitals Cleveland Medical Center, Rainbow
    Babies and Children's Hospital
Cleveland, OH, USA

**Cassian Horoszczak, MD**
Department of Anesthesiology
University at Buffalo
Buffalo, NY, USA

**Balazs Horvath, MD, FASA**
Associate Professor
Department of Anesthesiology
University of Minnesota
Minneapolis, MN, USA

**Meghan C. Hughes, MD, MPH**
Department of Family Medicine
Aspirus Hospital
Wausau, WI, USA

**Kevin Hui, MD**
Department of Anesthesiology
Westchester Medical Center
Valhalla, NY, US

**Nasir Hussain, MD, MSc**
Department of Anesthesiology
The Ohio State University
Wexner Medical Center
Columbus, OH, USA

**Peter Huynh, MD**

**Benjamin M. Hyers, MD**
Department of Anesthesiology, Perioperative and
    Pain Medicine
Icahn School of Medicine at Mount Sinai Hospital
New York, NY, USA

**Bilga Iana, MD**
Department of Anesthesia and Pain Management
Cook County Health and Hospital System
Chicago, IL, USA

**Rowaa Ibrahim, MD**
Department of Anesthesiology, Pain Management, and
    Perioperative Medicine
Henry Ford Health Systems
Detroit, MI, USA

**Mary J. Im, MD, MPH**
Clinical Assistant Professor
Department of Anesthesiology, Perioperative, and
    Pain Medicine
Stanford University School of Medicine
Stanford, CA, USA

**Shuchi Jain, DO**
Department of Anesthesiology
Henry Ford Health System
Detroit, MI, USA

**Dominika James, MD**
Associate Professor of Anesthesiology and Pain Medicine
Department of Anesthesiology
University of North Carolina at Chapel Hill
Chapel Hill, NC, USA

**Tatiana Jamroz, MD**
Section Head, Cardiac Division
Department of Anesthesiology
Cleveland Clinic Florida
Weston, FL, USA

**Jai Jani, BMedSci, BMBS**
Assistant Professor
Department of Anesthesia and Pain Management
Advocate Illinois Masonic Medical Center
Chicago, IL, USA

**Robert H. Jenkinson, MD**
Assistant Professor
Department of Anesthesiology
University of Utah
Salt Lake City, UT, USA

**Theodore Jeske, DO**
Department of Anesthesiology
Advocate Illinois Masonic Medical Center
Chicago, IL, USA

**Federico Jimenez-Ruiz, MD**
Department of Anesthesiology
University of Minnesota
Minneapolis, MN, USA

**Courtney R. Jones, MD**
Assistant Professor
Department of Anesthesiology
University of Cincinnati
Cincinnati, OH, USA

**Todd Everett Jones, MD**
Department of Anesthesiology
Division of Cardiothoracic Anesthesia
University of Florida College of Medicine
Gainesville, FL, USA

**Claire Joseph, DO**
Attending Anesthesiologist
Department of Anesthesiology, Perioperative Medicine
    and Pain Management; Division of Cardiac
    Anesthesia
Maimonides Medical Center
Brooklyn, New York, USA

**Maryam Jowza, MD**
Associate Professor
Department of Anesthesiology
University of North Carolina at Chapel Hill
Chapel Hill, NC, USA

**David Jury, MD, MS**
Staff Intensivist and Anesthesiologist, Clinical Assistant
    Professor, CCLCM
Department of Intensive Care and Resuscitation, Anesthesia
    Institute
Cleveland Clinic
Cleveland, OH, USA

**Jacob Justinger, MD**
Department of Anesthesiology and Perioperative Medicine
University Hospitals Cleveland Medical Center/ Case
    Western Reserve University
Cleveland, OH, USA

**Ihab Kamel, MD, MEHP, FASA**
Professor, Vice Chair for Education
Department of Anesthesiology
Temple University
Philadelphia, PA, USA

**Katarina Kapisoda, MD**
Department of Anesthesiology
University of Central Florida/HCA GME Consortium,
    Orlando
Ocala Health Florida
Ocala, FL, USA

**Daniel Gonzalez Kapp, PharmD, BCOP, BCPS**
UW Health
Madison, WI, USA

**Rami Edward Karroum, MD**
Staff Anesthesiologist, Clinical Assistant Professor
Department of Pediatric Anesthesia
Akron Children's Hospital
Akron, OH, USA

**Michael Kaufman, MD, FASA**
Assistant Clinical Professor and Interim Chair, Director of
    Transplant Anesthesia
Department of Anesthesiology and Interventional Pain
    Management
Lahey Hospital and Medical Center
Burlington, MA, USA

**Alan D. Kaye, MD, PhD**
Provost, Vice Chancellor of Academic Affairs, Chief
    Academic Officer, Professor, Director
Anesthesiology and Pharmacology, Toxicology, and
    Neurosciences
Louisiana State University Health Sciences Center
Shreveport, LA, USA

**Ashley Kelley, MD**
Assistant Professor
Department of Pediatric Anesthesiology
Westchester Medical Center
Valhalla, NY, USA

**Sahel Keshavarzi, MD**
Anesthesiologist
Department of Anesthesiology
Advocate Illinois Masonic Medical Center
Chicago, IL, USA

**John K. Kim, MD**
Attending Anesthesiologist
Department of Anesthesiology
North Shore University Hospital
Manhasset, NY, USA

**Roy Kim, MD**
Assistant Professor
Department of Anesthesiology and Pain Medicine
University of Wisconsin
Madison, WI, USA

**Jonathan W. Klein, DO, FAOCA, DAOBA**
Pediatric and Congenital Cardiac Anesthesiologist
Department of Anesthesia and Pain Medicine
Akron Children's Hospital
Akron, OH, USA
Vice-Chairman of the American Osteopathic Board of
    Anesthesiology
Adjunct Clinical Assistant Professor of Anesthesiology
Ohio University Heritage College of Osteopathic Medicine
Clinical Assistant Professor of Surgery, NEOMED
Department of Anesthesia and Pain Medicine

**Lisa Klesius, MD**
Assistant Professor
Department of Anesthesiology
University of Wisconsin Hospital and Clinics
Madison, WI, USA

**Benjamin Kloesel, MD, MSBS**
Assistant Professor
Department of Anesthesiology
University of Minnesota
Minneapolis, MN, USA

**Nebojsa Nick Knezevic, MD, PhD**
Vice Chair for Research and Education
Department of Anesthesiology Pain Management
Advocate Illinois Masonic Medical Center
Chicago, IL, USA

**Steven Knoblock, CRNA**
Nurse Anesthetist
Department of Anesthesia
Henry Ford Health System
Detroit, MI, USA

**Ryan Krebs, DO**
Henry Ford Health System
Detroit, MI, USA

**Elizabeth Kremen, MBBS**
Department of Anesthesiology
Advocate Illinois Masonic Medical Center
Chicago, IL, USA

**Dinesh J. Kurian, MD, MBA**
Assistant Professor
Department of Anesthesia and Critical Care
University of Chicago
Chicago, IL, USA

**Donnie Laborde, DC, FACO**
American Heart Association Instructor
Shreveport, LA, USA

**Kelsey E. Lacourrege, BS, MD, MPH**
School of Medicine
Louisiana State University School of Medicine in
    New Orleans
New Orleans, LA, USA

**Peter Lampert, MD**
Department of Anesthesiology
University of Wisconsin School of Medicine and
    Public Health
Madison, WI, USA

**Elizabeth Lange, MD**
Assistant Professor
Department of Anesthesiology
Northwestern University Feinberg School of Medicine
Chicago, IL, USA

**Dustin Latimer, MD**
Department of Internal Medicine
LSU Health Shreveport
Baton Rouge, LA, USA

**Itamar Latin, MD**
Clinical Assistant Professor
Department of Anesthesiology
Western Michigan University
Kalamazoo, MI, USA

**Alina Lazar, MD**
Assistant Professor
Department of Anesthesia and Critical Care
University of Chicago
Chicago, IL, USA

**Evan E. Lebovitz, MD, MBA**
Assistant Professor
Department of Anesthesiology and Perioperative Medicine
University of Pittsburgh Medical Center
Pittsburgh, PA, USA

**Albert Lee, MD**
Anesthesiology Critical Care Medicine Physician
Department of Anesthesiology and Perioperative Medicine
UCLA
Los Angeles, CA, USA

**Ethan H. Leer, MD**
Assistant Professor
Department of Anesthesiology
Westchester Medical Center
Valhalla, New York, USA

**Gretchen A. Lemmink, MD**
Assistant Professor of Anesthesiology and Critical Care
    Medicine
Department of Anesthesiology
University of Cincinnati College of Medicine
Cincinnati, OH, USA

**Richard Lennertz, MD, PhD**
Assistant Professor
Department of Anesthesiology
University of Wisconsin—Madison
Madison, WI, USA

**James Leonardi, MD**
Department of Anesthesiology
Allegheny Health Network
Pittsburgh, PA, USA

**Adam Lepkowsky, MD**
Department of Anesthesia and Perioperative Medicine
University Hospitals Cleveland Medical Center/Case Western
    Reserve University
Cleveland, OH, USA

**Lora B. Levin, MD**
Chief, Obstetric Anesthesia
Department of Anesthesiology and Perioperative Medicine
University Hospitals Cleveland Medical Center
Cleveland, OH, USA

**Samuel Linares, MD**
Department of Anesthesiology and Pain Management
Cook County Health Systems
Chicago, IL, USA

**Zhe Ma, MD**
Department of Anesthesiology, Perioperative and
    Pain Medicine
Icahn School of Medicine at Mount Sinai Hospital
New York, NY, USA

**Sarah Maben, MD**
Staff Intensivist and Anesthesiologist
Department of Anesthesiology
Lahey Hospital and Medical Center
Burlington, MA, USA

**Sohail K. Mahboobi, MD, FASA**
Assistant Clinical Professor
Department of Anesthesiology and Interventional Pain
    Management
Lahey Hospital and Medical Center
Burlington, MA, USA

**Ashok Kumar, MD**
Anesthesiologist
Department of Anesthesiology
University at Buffalo
Buffalo, NY, USA

**Mollie K. Lagrew, MD**
Department of Internal Medicine
University of Florida College of Medicine
Gainesville, FL, USA

**Neisaliz Marrero-Figueroa, MD**
Department of Anesthesiology
University of Central Florida/HCA GME Consortium, Orlando
Ocala Health, FL, USA

**Hannah Masters, MD**
Anesthesiology
Medical College of Wisconsin Affiliated Hospitals
Milwaukee, WI, USA

**David Matteson, MD, MS**
Allegheny Health Network
Pittsburgh, PA, USA

**John Mattimore, MD**
Staff Anesthesiologist
Department of Anesthesiology and Interventional Pain
    Management
Lahey Hospital and Medical Center
Burlington, MA, USA

**Kim Mauer, MD**
Anesthesiology
Department of Anesthesiology
Oregon Health and Science University
Portland, OR, USA

**Joseph J. McComb, DO, MBA**
Vice Chair, Quality and Performance Improvement
Department of Anesthesiology
Temple University School of Medicine
Philadelphia, PA, USA

**Matthew McConnell, MD**
Department of Anesthesiology
Allegheny General Hospital
Allegheny Health Network
Pittsburgh, PA, USA

**Megan Rodgers McCormick, DO**
Physician, Pediatric Anesthesiologist
Department of Anesthesiology and Perioperative Medicine
Rainbow Babies and Children's Hospital
Cleveland, OH, USA

**Lauren McGinty, PharmD, BCOP**
Clinical Hematology and Oncology Pharmacist
Department of Pharmacy
UW Health—University Hospital
Madison, WI, USA

**Roneisha McLendon, MD, MS**
Obstetric Anesthesiologist, Associate Program Director
Department of Anesthesiology
Ochsner Health
New Orleans, LA, USA

**Michelle McMaster, BSN, MD**
Associate Professor
Department of Anesthesiology
Lewis Katz School of Medicine
Philadelphia, PA, USA

**Connor McNamara, MD, MS**
Assistant Professor, Critical Care Anesthesiology; Program
    Director, Critical Care Anesthesiology
Department of Anesthesiology and Perioperative Medicine
University Hospitals Cleveland Medical Center
Cleveland, OH, USA

**Maggie W. Mechlin, MD**
Assistant Professor
Department of Anesthesiology
University of Cincinnati College of Medicine
Cincinnati, OH, USA

**Justin Merkow, MD**
Assistant Professor
Department of Anesthesia
University of Colorado
Denver, CO, USA

**Daniella Miele, DO**
Adjunct Assistant Professor
Department of Anesthesiology
Temple University Hospital
Philadelphia, PA, USA

**Steven Minear, MD**
Associate Professor
Department of Anesthesia
Cleveland Clinic Florida
Reston, FL, USA

**Asif Neil Mohammed, MD**
Assistant Professor
Department of Anesthesiology
University of Miami
Coral Gables, FL, USA

**Sarah Money, MD**
Associate Professor
Department of Pain Division
Henry Ford Health System
Detroiy, MI, USA

**Gina Montone, MD**
Department of Anesthesiology
Allegheny Health Network
Pittsburgh, PA, USA

**Benjamin B. G. Mori, MD**
Department of Anesthesia
Cool County Health
Chicago, IL, USA

**Michael Morkos, MD**
Department of Anesthesiology
Allegheny Health Network
Pittsburgh, PA, USA

**Anna Moskal**
Department of Anesthesiology
Advocate Illinois Masonic Medical Center
Chicago, IL, USA

**Maria E. Munoz-Allen, MD**
Associate Professor Clinical Anesthesia
Department of Anesthesiology
Temple University Hospital
Philadelphia, PA, USA

**Rotem Naftalovich, MD, MBA**
Assistant Professor, Head of Neurosurgical Anesthesia
Department of Anesthesiology
Rutgers, New Jersey Medical School
Newark, NJ, USA

**Ruzanna Nalbandyan, MD**
Anesthesiologist
Department of Anesthesiology
Grand Strand Medical Center
Myrtle Beach, SC, USA

**Syed Sohaib Nasim, MD**
Department of Anesthesiology
Cleveland Clinic Florida
Weston, FL, USA

**Ned F. Nasr, MD**
Vice Chairman
Department of Anesthesiology and Pain Management
Cook County Health and Hospital Systems
Chicago, IL, USA

**Harsh Nathani, MBChB**
Cook County Health Systems
Chicago, IL, USA

**Ryan Nazemian, MD, PhD**
PhD candidate in Clinical Translational Science
    program
Anesthesiology and Preoperative Medicine
University Hospitals Cleveland Medical Center/Case
    Western Reserve University
Case Western Reserve University
Cleveland, OH, USA

**Greta Nemergut, PharmD**
Clinical Pharmacist
UW Health Department of Pharmacy
University of Wisconsin Hospital and Clinics
Madison, WI, USA

**Patrick Newman, MD**
Assistant Professor
Department of Anesthesiology
University of Mississippi Medical Center
Jackson, MI, USA

**Wendy Nguyen, MD, M Ed**
Assistant Professor
Department of Anesthesiology
University of Minnesota Medical School
Minneapolis, MN, USA

**Peter Nielson, MD**
Clinical Associate
Department of Anesthesiology
Lahey Hospital and Medical Center
Burlington, MA, USA

**Edward Noguera, MD**
Lahey Clinic
Anesthesiologist/Intensivist
Medical Director SICU/CVICU
Cleveland Clinic Florida
Weston, FL, USA

**Bryan Noorda, MD**
Anesthesia Residency
Allegheny Health Network
Pittsburgh, PA, USA

**Adambeke Nwozuzu, MD, MHS**
Department of Anesthesiology
University of Central Florida/HCA GME Consortium,
    Orlando
Ocala Health, Florida
Ocala, FL, USA

**Devin O'Conor, MD**
Department of Anesthesiology
Icahn School of Medicine at Mount Sinai Hospital
New York, NY, USA

**Justin L. O'Farrell, BS**
School of Medicine
University of the Incarnate Word School of Osteopathic
    Medicine
San Antonio, TX, USA

**Shelley Ohliger, MD**
Assistant Professor
Department of Anesthesiology
University Hospitals/Rainbow Babies & Children's Hospital
Cleveland, OH, USA

**Barbara Orlando, MD, PhD**
OB Anesthesia Attending
St. Luke's and Mount Sinai West Hospitals
New York, NY, USA

**Feroz Osmani, MD**
Icahn School of Medicine at Mount Sinai Hospital
New York, NY, USA

**Robert M. Owen, MD**
Icahn School of Medicine at Mount Sinai Hospital
New York, NY, USA

**Peter Papapetrou, MD**
Physician
Department of Anesthesiology and Interventional
    Pain Management
Altru Health System
Grand Forks, ND, USA

**Helen Pappas, MD, FASA**
Assistant Professor
Department of Anesthesiology
Northwestern University Feinberg School of Medicine
Chicago, IL, USA

**Marisa Pappas, MD**
Cardiac Anesthesiologist
Department of Anesthesiology
VA
New Orleans, LA, USA

**Daniel Ramirez Parga, MD**
Department of Anesthesiology
Children's Hospital at Montefiore
Bronx, NY, USA

**Snigdha Parikh, DO**
Department of Anesthesiology, Pain Management, and
    Perioperative Medicine
Henry Ford Health System
Detroit, MI, USA

**Nicholas M. Parker, PharmD, RPh, CNSC**
Clinical Pharmacist
Surgery and Surgical Nutrition Support
UW Health
Madison, WI, USA

**Nimesh Patel, MD, BSc (Hons)**
Department of Anesthesiology, Pain Management and
    Perioperative Medicine
Henry Ford Health System
Detroit,MI, USA

**Priyanka H. Patel, DO**
Department of Anesthesiology
Allegheny General Hospital
Allegheny Health Network
Pittsburgh, PA, USA

**Ravi Patel, MD**
Department of Anesthesiology
University of Miami Hospital and Jackson Memorial
    Hospital
Miami, FL, USA

**Elisha Peterson, MD, FAAP, FASA**
Assistant Professor
Division of Anesthesiology, Pain, and Perioperative Medicine
Children's National Hospital
Washington, DC, USA

**Andrew Pfaff, MD**
Physician
Department of Anesthesiology
Ascension St. Vincent
Evansville,IN, USA

**Bethany Potere, MD, MSc**
Department of Anesthesiology
Ohio State University
Columbus, Ohio, USA

**Amit Prabhakar, MD, MS**
Assistant Professor
Department of Anesthesiology
Division of Critical Care
Emory University School of Medicine
Atlanta, GA, USA

**Monica Prasad, B.S in Biochemical Engineering**
Medical Doctor
Wayne State University School of Medicine
Detroit, MI, USA

**Keth Pride, MD**
Associate Professor
Department of Anesthesiology, Chronic Pain
University of Wisconsin hospital and clinics
Madison, WI, USA

**Sangini Punia, MBBS**
Clinical Assistant Professor
Department of Anesthesia
University of Iowa Health Care
Carver College of Medicine
Iowa City, IA, USA

**Nawal E. Ragheb-Mueller, DO, PhD, MPH, FASA**
Attending Physician
Department of Anesthesiology and Pain Medicine
Cook County Hospital and Health Systems
Chicago, IL, USA

**Abed Rahman, MD**
Cook County Health and Hospitals System
Chicago, IL, USA

**Syed A. Rahman, MD**
Department of Anesthesiology and Pain management
John H Stroger hospital of Cook County Health Systems
Chicago, IL, USA

**Shobana Rajan, MD**
Anesthesiology Institute
Allegheny Health Network
Pittsburgh, PA, USA

**Maria F. Ramirez, MD**
Assistant Professor
Department of Anesthesiology and Perioperative Medicine
The University of Texas MD Anderson Cancer Center
Houston, TX, USA

**Adnan Raslan, MD**
Department of Anesthesiology
Emory University School of Medicine
Atlanta, GA, USA

**Harsh Rawal, MD**
Academic Hospitalist
Department of Internal Medicine
University of Connecticut
Hartford, CT, USA

**Dmitry Roberman, DO**
Anesthesiologist
Department of Anesthesiology
Temple University Health System
Philadelphia, PA, USA

**Hess Robertson, MD**
Assistant Professor
Department of Anesthesiology
University of Mississippi Medical School
Jackson, MS, USA

**Marc Rodrigue, DO**
Department of Anesthesiology
Allegheny Health Network
Pittsburgh, PA, USA

**Evgeny Romanov, MD**
Lahey Clinic
Burlington, MA, USA

**Vincent Roth, MD**
Department of Anesthesiology
University of Southern California
Los Angeles, CA, USA

**Alexander Rothkrug, MD**
Clinical Associate
Department of Anesthesiology and Interventional
    Pain Medicine
Lahey Hospital and Medical Center
Burlington, MA, USA

**Miguel Rovira, MD**
Department of Anesthesiology
University of Florida
Gainesville, FL, USA

**Kasia Rubin, MD, MBA**
Associate Professor
Department of Anesthesiology
Cleveland Clinic Lerner College of Medicine of Case Western
    Reserve University
Cleveland, OH, USA

**Anesh Rugnath, MD**
Associate Professor
Department of Anesthesiology
University of Mississippi Medical Center
Jackson, MS, USA

**Timothy Rushmer, MD**
Department of Anesthesiology
University of Wisconsin School of Medicine and
    Public Health
Madison, WI, USA

**Ramsey Saad, MD**
Anesthesiology
Department of Anesthesiology
Henry Ford Health System
Detroit, MI, USA

**Samiya L. Saklayen, MD**
Assistant Professor
Department of Anesthesiology
The Ohio State University
Columbus, OH, USA

**Wael Ali Sakr Esa, MD, PhD, MBA, FASA**
Section Head Orthopedic Anesthesia
Department of General Anesthesia
Cleveland Clinic Foundation
Cleveland, OH, USA

**Irim Salik, MD**
Associate Professor of Anesthesiology/ Associate
    Program Director
Department of Anesthesiology
Westchester Medical Center
Valhalla, NY, USA

**Sabrina S. Sam, MD**
Cook County Health Systems
Chicago, IL, USA

**Binoy Samuel, MD**
Department of Anesthesia and Pain Management
Cook County Health and Hospital Systems
Chicago, IL, USA

**Joseph Sanders, MD**
Program Director Adult Cardiothoracic Anesthesiology
Department of Anesthesiology
Henry Ford Health System
Detroit, MI, USA

**Lisgelia Santana, MD, FAAP**
Director of Pediatric Pain Management
Pediatric Anesthesiologist
Department of Anesthesiology
Nemours Children's Hospital
Associate Professor
University of Central Florida College of Medicine
Orlando, FL, USA

**Syena Sarrafpour, MD**
Beth Israel Deaconess Medical Center
Department of Anesthesia, Critical Care, and Pain Medicine
Harvard Medical School
Boston, MA, USA

**James Schiffenhaus, MD**
Department of Anesthesiology
Rutgers, New Jersey, Medical School
Newark, NJ, USA

**Elizabeth Scholzen, MD, MHA**
Department of Anesthesiology
University of Wisconsin Hospital and Clinics
Madison, WI, USA

**Kristopher M. Schroeder, MD, FASA**
Professor
Department of Anesthesiology
University of Wisconsin School of Medicine and Public Health
Madison, WI, USA

**Nathan Schulman, MD**
Assistant Clinical Professor
UCLA Department of Anesthesiology and Perioperative
    Medicine
Los Angeles, CA, USA

**Courtney L. Scott, MD**
UCLA Department of Anesthesiology and Perioperative
    Medicine
David Geffen School of Medicine at UCLA
Los Angeles, CA, USA

**Nitin Sekhri, MD**
Medical Director of Pain Management
Department of Anesthesiology
Westchester Medical Center
Valhalla, NY, USA

**Breethaa Janani Selvamani, MBBS**
Department of Anesthesia
University of Iowa Hospitals
Iowa City, IA, USA

**Anuj A. Shah, MD, DO**
Department of Physical Medicine and Rehabilitation
Rehabilitation Institute of Michigan (Detroit Medical Center)
Detroit, MI, USA

**Jarna Shah, MD**
Assistant Professor
Department of Anesthesiology
University of Arkansas for Medical Sciences
Little Rock, AR, USA

**Manan Nimish Shah, MD**
Anesthesiologist
Department of Anesthesia and Perioperative Care
Rutgers University
Newark, NJ, USA

**Nimit K. Shah, MBBS, FRCA, FCARCSI, DA, DNB, EDAIC, EDRA**
Department of Anesthesiology
Cook County Health and Hospitals System
Chicago, IL, USA

**Sadiq S. Shaik, MD**
Assistant Anesthesiology Professor
University of Central Florida College of Medicine
Pediatric Anesthesiologist
Nemours Children's Hospital
Orlando, FL, USA

**Victoria Shapiro, DO**
Clinical Assistant Professor
Department of Anesthesiology
Westchester Medical Center
Valhalla, NY, USA

**Archit Sharma, MD, MBA,FASA**
Associate Professor
Department of Anesthesia
University of Iowa Hospitals Carver College of Medicine
Iowa City, IA, USA

**Balram Sharma, MD**
Assistant Professor
Department of Anesthesiology
Lahey Hospital and Medical Center
Burlington, MA, USA

**Surangama Sharma, MD**
Clinical Assistant Professor
Department of Anesthesia
University of Iowa Health Care
Iowa City, IA, USA

**Peter Shehata, DO, MA**
Department of Anesthesiology
Cleveland Clinic Foundation
Cleveland, OH, USA

**Suleman Sheikh, DO**
Department of Anesthesiology
University at Buffalo
Buffalo, NY, USA

**John S. Shin, MD**
Assistant Clinical Professor
Department of Anesthesiology and Perioperative
    Medicine
David Geffen School of Medicine at UCLA
Los Angeles, CA, USA

**Mo Shirur, MD**
Department of Anesthesiology, Perioperative and
    Pain Medicine
Icahn School of Medicine at Mount Sinai
New York, NY, USA

**Shahla Siddiqui, MD, DABA, MSc, FCCM**
Department of Anesthesia, Critical Care, and
    Pain Medicine
Beth Israel Deaconess Medical Center
Harvard Medical School
Boston, MA, USA

**Brett Simmons, MD, MS**
Allegheny Health Network
Pittsburgh, PA, USA

**Jamie W. Sinton, MD**
Assistant Professor
Department of Anesthesiology, Perioperative and
    Pain Medicine
Baylor College of Medicine
Houston, TX, USA

**Eellan Sivanesan, MD**
Assistant Professor
Department of Anesthesiology and Critical Care Medicine
Johns Hopkins University - School of Medicine
Baltimore, MD, USA

**Sarah C. Smith, MD**
Assistant Professor
Department of Anesthesiology
Westchester Medical Center
New York Medical College
Valhalla, NY, USA

**Iwan Sofjan, MD**
Assistant Professor
Department of Anesthesiology
Westchester Medical Center
Valhalla, NY, USA

**Mahad Sohail**
Department of Anesthesiology and Critical Care Medicine
Beth Israel Deaconess Medical Center
Boston, MA, USA

**Jacqueline Sohn, DO**
Department of Anesthesiology and Perioperative Medicine
University Hospitals Cleveland Medical Center
Cleveland, OH, USA

**Kevin Spencer, MD**
Anesthesiologist
Henry Ford Health System

**Christina Stachur, MD, MPH**
Assistant Professor
Department of Anesthesiology and Perioperative Medicine
University Hospitals Cleveland Medical Center
Cleveland, OH, USA

**Scott Stayner, MD, PhD**
Surgery Center Medical Director
Department of Pain Medicine
Nura Pain Clinics
Minneapolis, MN, USA

**Mark L. Stram, MD**
Clinical Assistant Professor
Department of Anesthesiology
University of Wisconsin School of Medicine and
    Public Health
Madison, WI, USA

**Charlotte Streetzel**
Department of Anesthesiology
University of Florida College of Medicine
Gainesville, FL, USA

**Felipe F. Suero, MD, FASA**
Assistant Professor
Department of Anesthesia
Temple-North Campus (FCCC/JEANES H.), TEMPLE
Philadelphia, PA, USA

**Kim Sung, MD**
Physician, Cardiothoracic Anesthesiologist
Department of Anesthesia
University of Iowa Hospitals and Clinic
Iowa City, IA, USA

**Erika Taco, MD**
Department of Anesthesiology
Henry Ford Health System
Detroit, MI, US

**Racha Tadros, MD, MSc**
Department of Anesthesiology
The Ohio State University
Wexner Medical Center
Columbus, OH, USA

**Colby B. Tanner, MD**
Assistant Clinical Professor
Department of Anesthesiology and Perioperative Medicine
UCLA Health
Los Angeles, CA, USA

**Pritee Tarwade, MD**
Mayo Clinic
Department of Anesthesiology–Critical Care
Rochester, MN, USA

**Camila Teixeira, MD**
Clinical Researcher
Department of Anesthesiology
Cleveland Clinic Florida
Weston, FL, USA

**Richard Tennant**
Department of Anesthesiology
University of Wisconsin School of Medicine and
    Public Health
Madison, WI, USA

**Jordan Thompson, MD**
Department of Anesthesiology
University of Florida College of Medicine
Gainesville, FL, USA

**Dillon Tinevez, MD**
Department of Anesthesiology
Advocate Illinois Masonic Medical Center
Chicago, IL, USA

**Gabriella Tom Williams, MD**
Department of Anesthesiology
University of Florida
Gainesville, FL, USA

**Kenneth S. Toth, MD**
Cook County Health and Hospital Systems
Chicago, IL, USA

**Jay Trusheim, MD**
Department of Anesthesia
Ochsner Health System
New Orleans, LA, USA

**Mitchell H. Tsai, MD, MMM, FASA, FAACD**
Professor
Department of Anesthesiology
Department of Orthopaedics and Rehabilitation (by courtesy)
Department of Surgery (by courtesy)
University of Vermont Larner College of Medicine
Burlington, VT, USA

**Luis Tueme, MD**
Assistant Professor
Department of Anesthesiology
UT Health and Science Center at San Antonio
San Antonio, IL, USA

**Anna Tzonkov, MD**
Attending Anesthesiologist
Department of Anesthesiology
Cook County Health
Chicago, IL, USA

**James Urness, MD**
Department of Anesthesiology
Henry Ford Hospital
Detroit, MI, USA

**Ifomachukwu Uzodinma, MD**
Anesthesiologist and Pain Medicine Physician
Department of Anesthesiology and Pain Management
Cook County Health and Hospital Systems
Chicago, IL, USA

**Karel T. S. Valenta, MD**
Department of Anesthesiology and Pain Management
Cook County Health and Hospital Systems
Chicago, IL, USA

**Bharathram Vasudevan, MBBS, MD**
Department of Anesthesiology
Cook County Health and Hospital Systems
Chicago, IL, USA

**Kevin E. Vorenkamp, MD, FASA**
Chief, Division of Pain Medicine
Department of Anesthesiology
Duke University
Durham, NC, USA

**Anureet Walia, MD**
Assistant Professor
Department of Anesthesia
University of Iowa Hospitals and Clinics Carver College of
    Medicine
Iowa City, Iowa, USA

**Matt Warth, BS**
Georgia State University
Lawrenceville, GA, USA

**Cassandra Wasson, DO**
Anesthesiology
Medical College of Wisconsin
Milwaukee, WI, USA

**Stacey Watt, MD, MBA, FASA**
Clinical Professor and Anesthesiology Residency Program
    Director
Department of Anesthesiology
University at Buffalo
Buffalo, NY, USA

**Tristan E. Weaver, MD**
Assistant Professor
Department of Anesthesiology
The Ohio State University
Wexner Medical Center
Columbus, OH, USA

**Corinne K. Wong, MD**
Department of Anesthesiology
United Anesthesia Services
Bryn Mawr, PA, USA

**Caylynn Yao, MD**
Department of Anesthesiology
MedStar Georgetown University Hospital
Washington, DC, USA

**Peter Yi, MD, MSEd**
Assistant Professor
Department of Anesthesiology and Critical Care
Duke University
Durham, NC, USA

**Joshua D. Younger, MD**
Associate Chief, Division of Obstetric Anesthesia
Department of Anesthesiology, Pain Management, and
    Perioperative Medicine
Henry Ford Health System
Detroit, MI, USA

**Christine S. Zaky, MS**
M.D. Candidate
Stritch School of Medicine, Loyola University Chicago
Westlake, OH, USA
Department of Biological Sciences
University of Pittsburgh
Pittsburgh, PA, USA

**Sherif Zaky, MD, MSc, PhD**
Associate Professor and Medical Director
Department of Anesthesiology and Pain Management
Ohio University- Firelands Health System
Westlake, OH, USA

**Eric P. Zhou, MD**
Department of Anesthesiology, Critical Care and Pain Medicine
Boston Children's Hospital, Harvard Medical School
Boston, MA, USA

**Steven Zhou, BA, MD**
Clinical Instructor House Staff
Department of Anesthesiology
The Ohio State University
Columbus, OH, USA

# Part 1

# MONITORING METHODS

# 1.

# VASCULAR PRESSURES

*Amit Prabhakar and Adnan Raslan*

## INTRODUCTION

The most common vascular pressures include arterial blood pressure, central venous pressure (CVP), pulmonary pressures, and left ventricular end-diastolic pressure (LVEDP). This chapter reviews the fundamentals of these aforementioned vascular pressures and the clinical relevance of each.

## ARTERIAL BLOOD PRESSURE

Fluctuations in blood pressure can result in systemic malperfusion and subsequently result in end-organ damage. Arterial blood pressure measurements are the foundation of systemic blood pressure calculations and can be derived by either noninvasive or invasive methods. It is imperative for clinicians practicing in the perioperative space to understand the intricacies of the different measuring techniques. Intermittent noninvasive blood pressure monitoring is done by inflating a pneumatic cuff, which first occludes arterial blood flow and then slowly deflates until blood flow resumes.[1]

Noninvasive techniques are most commonly performed via the automated oscillometric method; however, the manual auscultatory method may still be used in certain clinical situations. The manual auscultatory method involves auscultation of the Korotkoff sounds as the pneumatic cuff is deflated to distinguish both the systolic and diastolic blood pressures. The automated oscillometric method involves a computer that analyzes the oscillations of the artery as the cuff is deflated. Rapidly increasing oscillations represent the systolic blood pressure, while the diastolic blood pressure is represented by rapidly decreasing oscillations.[1,2] The mean arterial pressure (MAP) is identified as the point of maximum oscillations. The most common sites for noninvasive blood pressure monitoring include the arms and legs. Normal systolic and diastolic blood pressure ranges are 120–140 and 60–80 mm Hg, respectively.

Clinical scenarios in which there are significant perturbations in arterial pressure warrant invasive blood pressure monitoring in order to help increase accuracy and prevent end-organ damage. Invasive monitoring involves arterial cannulation with a catheter, which is then connected to a fluid-filled and pressurized tubing system. The catheter senses the dynamic changes in blood flow. This mechanical energy is then converted into an electrical signal, which is then displayed as a waveform on a monitor.[1]

## CENTRAL VENOUS PRESSURE

Central venous pressure is an invasive vascular pressure measured most commonly by cannulation of the subclavian vein, internal jugular vein, or femoral vein. CVP is used to measure right atrial pressure and approximate right heart function. The ideal catheter position is at the cavoatrial junction. The catheter is connected to a pressurized, fluid-filled system that converts the mechanical energy from dynamic blood flow to an electrical impulse. This impulse is then converted to a tracing displayed on a monitor. As seen in Figure 1.1, the CVP waveform is broken down into three positive deflections (a, c, and v waves) and two negative slopes (x and y descents). The waves correspond with atrial contraction, tricuspid valve closure, and right atrial filling, respectively. The x descent corresponds to atrial relaxation, and the y descent corresponds to early ventricular filling with diastolic relaxation. The normal range of CVP is between 0 and 10 mm Hg and ideally measured at the level of the tricuspid valve.

## PULMONARY ARTERY PRESSURE

Pulmonary artery pressure (PAP) is an invasive measurement that is most commonly facilitated by central venous cannulation with a catheter in the pulmonary artery. Similar to systemic arterial blood pressure, PAP includes both systolic and diastolic components predicated by the different stages of cardiac contraction. A normal value for systolic PAP is 15–25 mm Hg, and the normal diastolic PAP is 8–12 mm

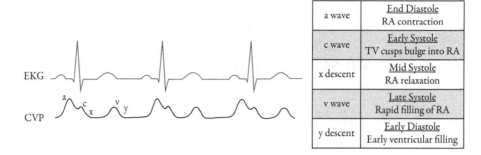

| a wave | End Diastole<br>RA contraction |
| c wave | Early Systole<br>TV cusps bulge into RA |
| x descent | Mid Systole<br>RA relaxation |
| v wave | Late Systole<br>Rapid filling of RA |
| y descent | Early Diastole<br>Early ventricular filling |

**Figure 1.1** Central venous pressure tracing and interpretation. RA, right atrium; TV, tricuspid valve.

Hg. The placement of a pulmonary artery catheter (PAC) is facilitated by an inflatable balloon and also has several orifices to facilitate blood draws. PACs are most often used to guide intravascular resuscitation and facilitate serial hemodynamic monitoring throughout the perioperative period for major vascular or cardiothoracic surgeries.

## PULMONARY CAPILLARY WEDGE PRESSURE

Pulmonary capillary wedge pressure (PCWP), also known as pulmonary artery occlusion pressure, is used as an indirect measurement of left atrial pressure. It is measured by advancing a PAC into the distal pulmonary vasculature and inflating the balloon at the end of the catheter, thus occluding vascular flow. The lack of forward pulmonary blood flow allows for left atrial pressure calculations. PCWP can be used to characterize the severity of left-sided cardiac function and differentiate potentially confounding cardiopulmonary pathologies. A normal PCWP ranges between 6 and 12 mm Hg.[3] In a patient with a right-to-left shunt, it is better to use $CO_2$ to inflate the balloon as it is safer if the balloon ruptures. For accurate measurement, the PAC should be placed in zone 3.

## LEFT VENTRICULAR END-DIASTOLIC PRESSURE

Left ventricular end-diastolic pressure is the pressure in the left ventricle at the end of diastole immediately before contraction. This invasive measurement is most commonly obtained during cardiac catheterization. LVEDP measurement is dependent on both intravascular volume status and left ventricular compliance. Thus, it is a helpful marker to identify and quantitate the severity of left ventricular systolic or diastolic dysfunction. LVEDP, left ventricle ejection fraction, and systemic blood pressure are among the strongest predictors of morbidity and mortality in regard to ischemic heart disease, cardiac surgery, and left heart catheterization.[4]

## ANESTHETIC CONSIDERATIONS

### ARTERIAL PRESSURES

The accuracy of noninvasive arterial measurements may be limited by certain clinical features, such as prior lymph node dissection, presence of preexisting vascular access, patient movement, significant atherosclerotic disease, and body habitus.[2] It is imperative that the appropriate cuff size is used to ensure accuracy. A cuff that is either too small or too large can result in an overestimation or underestimation, respectively. Potential complications of noninvasive arterial measurements include neuropathic pressure injury, paresthesia, compartment syndrome, and thrombophlebitis.[2]

Invasive arterial blood pressure measurement via an arterial line allows for continuous blood pressure monitoring during longer surgeries with the potential for significant hemodynamic fluctuations. The most common sites for cannulation include the radial, brachial, axillary, and femoral arteries. Complications associated with invasive arterial lines include infection, distal ischemia, nerve injury, hematoma formation, vasospasm, and thrombosis.[5] An Allen test can be used prior to radial artery cannulation to assess the adequacy of collateral circulation in the hand; however, there are conflicting views on its ability to reliably predict ischemic injury.

### CENTRAL VENOUS PRESSURE

Elevations in CVP can be seen in patients with heart failure due to poor contractility, tricuspid regurgitation, and pulmonary artery stenosis. These pathologies lead to poor forward flow and venous congestion. Decreases in CVP can occur in the setting of decreased venous return, such as hypovolemia or vasodilation.

### PULMONARY ARTERY PRESSURE

A number of disease processes can affect pulmonary circulation and lead to increases in the pulmonary vascular pressures, ultimately affecting the function of the right ventricle, including pulmonary hypertension and right-sided myocardial infarction. Severe or sustained increases in these pressures can lead to eventual right heart failure. Pulmonary circulation monitoring, with regard to heart failure treatment, has become a target of therapy as elevated pulmonary artery pressures have been shown to be associated with an adverse prognosis for patients with right heart failure.[3] The main contraindications of pulmonary artery catheterization include right-sided endocarditis, tumors or masses of the right heart, and significant tricuspid or pulmonary valve disorders.

## REFERENCES

1. Saugel B, et al. Measurement of blood pressure. *Best Pract Res Clin Anaesthesiol.* 2014;28:309–322.
2. Alpert BS, et al. Oscillometric blood pressure: a review for clinicians. *J Am Soc Hypertens.* 2014;8(12):930–938.
3. Nair R, Lamaa N. Pulmonary capillary wedge pressure. In: StatPearls. Treasure Island, FL: StatPearls Publishing; April 26, 2021. https://www.ncbi.nlm.nih.gov/books/NBK557748/
4. Li YY, et al. Predictors of inpatient outcomes in hospitalized patients after left heart catheterization. *Am J Cardiol.* 2009;103(4):486–490.
5. Gu WJ, et al. Ultrasound guidance facilitates radial artery catheterization: a meta-analysis with trial sequential analysis of randomized controlled trials. *Chest.* 2016;149(1):166–179.

# 2.

# BRAIN AND SPINAL CORD FUNCTION

*Vicko Gluncic*

- The cerebral cortex is a thin, gray coating of the hemispheres. The coordinated activity of cortical neurons is the physiological substrate of higher brain functions, such as cognition and consciousness.
- Motor and somatosensory cortex are located in the frontal and parietal lobes (respectively) and are organized somatotopically. The visual cortex is in the occipital lobe. Both frontal cerebral lobes are involved in inhibition of inappropriate behavior, motivation, judgment, and working memory. Some functions are lateralized; the dominant hemisphere (usually the left) controls the language via the inferior frontal lobe (Broca's area) and temporal lobe (Wernicke's area). The nondominant hemisphere mediates attention and visual and spatial analyses (parietal lobe).
- Arousal is mainly mediated by the reticular activating system, a network of neurons located in the brainstem, with numerous projections to thalamus and hypothalamus, which are then connected to the cortex. The arousal system can be affected by lesions to the brain, drugs (anesthetics), and metabolic abnormalities.[1]

- The effects and the depth of general anesthesia can be assessed by evaluation of processed electroencephalography (EEG) signals.[2]
  - Bispectral analysis (BIS) is based on the relationship between delta and theta waves and is expressed as the bispectral index (range 0–100; 0 is complete absence of cerebral function, 100 indicates normal activity).
  - Entropy combines the analyses of irregularity in EEG signals (increased brain concentration of an anesthetic is mirrored by a decrease in irregularities) with frontal electromyographic activity.
  - Evoked potentials monitor a response in specific brain areas when a sensory stimulation is applied to a peripheral nerve. Most anesthetic agents lead to an increase in latency and a reduction in the amplitude of those responses.
- Cerebral blood flow (CBF) depends on the cerebral perfusion pressure (CPP) and the cerebral vascular resistance (CVR) (CBF = CPP/CVR).[3] The skull has a fixed volume containing brain, blood, and cerebrospinal fluid (CSF), hence CPP is the mean arterial pressure (MAP) minus the intracranial

pressure (ICP) (normal values: MAP 90 mm Hg, ICP < 15 mm Hg).

- The average CBF rate is 50 mL/100 g/min and is higher in the gray (~70 mL/100 g/min) than in the white matter (~20 mL/100 g/min).
- The cerebral metabolic rate for oxygen describes the rate of oxygen consumption (~3 mL/100 g/min).
- The CBF is tightly controlled by autoregulation via metabolic, myogenic, and neurogenic mechanisms. It remains constant for the MAP between 50 and 150 mm Hg (the "autoregulatory range").
- Within physiologic range, the CBF depends (almost) linearly on the arterial $CO_2$ tension ($PaCO_2$): For each 1 mm Hg change in $PaCO_2$, the CBF changes by 3% of the baseline. However, $O_2$ has a very mild effect on CBF, except at abnormally low levels.[4]
- Cerebrospinal fluid provides mechanical protection and buoyancy, ensures a constant chemical environment, and is involved in regulation of ICP and central control of respiration (via chemoreceptors). The volume of CSF is about 150 mL, with a daily production of 500 mL (or 3 mL/min). The CSF pressure of an adult, measured at the lumbar puncture with the patient on his or her side, is 100–180 mm $H_2O$ (8–15 mm Hg). A routine lumbar puncture removes about 10 mL of CSF, but up to 40 mL can be safely harvested.
- One source of CSF is the choroid plexus, a vascular structure located in the ventricles. In addition, there is influx from the brain interstitial fluid, mediated by water channels.[5] CSF circulates through the entire ventricular system, flows into the subarachnoid space, and is reabsorbed into the venous circulation of the dural sinus via arachnoid granulations.
- The central nervous system (CNS) parenchyma is separated from the blood by the blood-brain barrier (BBB). The BBB exists at the level of the microvasculature and is composed of endothelial cells connected by tight junctions. Endothelial cells produce a basement membrane, which encloses pericytes. Finally, astrocytes are in contact with the microvasculature via their endfeet and lay down the parenchymal basement membrane.
- The BBB can be freely crossed by highly lipid-soluble molecules (passive transport), such as $CO_2$, $O_2$, steroids, and inhalational anesthetics.
- There are active transport systems that allow water-soluble molecules (e.g., D-glucose, lactate, cholin, and insulin) to cross the BBB.
- The spinal cord is a column of the CNS extending from the level of the foramen magnum to the lower border of the first lumber (L1) vertebra (adult) or L3 (newborn). It has five levels, with a total of 31–32 pairs of spinal nerves. A spinal nerve has a ventral (motor fibers) and dorsal root (sensory fibers).

- The gray matter forms the core of the spinal cord and has the following projections: dorsal, ventral, and lateral horns. The white matter is organized into three columns/funiculi (dorsal, lateral, and ventral), containing ascending and descending tracts.
- The following are the most important ascending tracts:
  - *Dorsal columns.* Dorsal columns (medial lemniscus pathways) mediate tactile discrimination, vibration sense, form recognition, and conscious proprioception. First-order neurons are located in dorsal root ganglia. They give raise to gracile fasciculus (lower extremity), cuneate fasciculus (upper extremity), and collaterals (spinal reflexes). Second-order neurons are located in gracile and cuneate nuclei; their axons decussate and form the medial lemniscus. Third-order neurons are located in the thalamus and project to the somatosensory cortex.
  - *Spinothalamic tracts.* The lateral spinothalamic tract mediates sensations of pain and temperature. First-order neurons are in the dorsal root ganglia. Second-order neurons are in the dorsal horn; their axons are in the ventral commissure and ascend to the thalamus. Third-order neurons project from the thalamus to the somatosensory cortex. The anterior spinothalamic tract is organized similarly, but conveys sensory information on crude touch and pressure.
- The following are the most important descending tracts:
  - The lateral corticospinal tract mediates voluntary motor activity. It originates in the motoric areas of the cerebral cortex and runs in medullary pyramids. About 90% of the fibers decussate as the lateral corticospinal tract. The lateral corticospinal tract runs in the lateral funiculus and synapses along the length of the spinal cord.
  - The Hypothalamospinal tract projects without interruption from the hypothalamus to the ciliospinal center of the lateral column.

## REFERENCES

1. Benghanem S, et al. Brainstem dysfunction in critically ill patients. *Crit Care.* 2020;24(1):5.
2. Nunes RR, et al. Intraoperative neurophysiological monitoring in neuroanesthesia. *Curr Opin Anaesthesiol.* 2018;31(5):532–538.
3. Madhok DY, et al. Overview of neurovascular physiology. *Curr Neurol Neurosci Rep.* 2018;18(12):99.
4. Hoiland RL, et al. Regulation of the cerebral circulation by arterial carbon dioxide. *Compr Physiol.* 2019;9(3):1101–1154.
5. Nakada T, Kwee IL. Fluid dynamics inside the brain barrier: current concept of interstitial flow, glymphatic flow, and cerebrospinal fluid circulation in the brain. *Neuroscientist.* 2019;25(2):155–166.

# 3.

# MIXED VENOUS OXYGEN SATURATION

*Heather Christopherson and Ettore Crimi*

## INTRODUCTION

Mixed venous oxygen saturation ($SvO_2$) is the percentage of oxygenated hemoglobin in the blood returning to the right side of the heart. $SvO_2$ reflects the balance between oxygen delivery and oxygen consumed by tissues. It is useful to assess the adequacy of tissue perfusion and oxygenation and to identify global tissue hypoxia during the perioperative period and in critically ill patients.[1]

## SVO$_2$ MONITORING AND PHYSIOLOGY

Measurement of $SvO_2$ occurs in the proximal pulmonary artery (PA), where blood is a mixture of venous blood from the superior and inferior vena, coronary sinus, and Thebesian veins. $SvO_2$ can be measured intermittently via an oximeter from blood samples obtained from the distal port of the PA catheter. Alternatively, it can be measured continuously by catheters that use infrared oximetry. The continuous methods are costly and require daily recalibration because of signal drift. Central venous oxygen saturation ($ScvO_2$) has been used as a surrogate for $SvO_2$. $ScvO_2$ is obtained from a central venous line and reflects the percentage of oxygenated hemoglobin of blood in the superior vena cava only. A significant difference exists between these two values. $SvO_2$ reflects the balance of the oxygen delivery and consumption of the entire body, while $ScvO_2$ reflects variation of this balance in the upper body. The $ScvO_2$ value is 2%–5% less than $SvO_2$ in healthy patients due to the high oxygen content of venous blood from the kidneys. The $ScvO_2$ value is 5% to 18% higher than the $SvO_2$ in patients with shock due to the redistribution of blood toward cerebral and coronary circulations at the expense of mesenteric, splenic, and renal circulations.[2,3]

The $SvO_2$ reflects the balance between the oxygen delivered and the oxygen consumed. Oxygen delivery ($DO_2$) is calculated as

$$DO_2 = CO \times CaO_2$$

where CO is cardiac output and $CaO_2$ is the arterial $O_2$ content. The normal DO is 1000 mL/min (normal range 700–1400 mL/min).

Oxygen consumption ($VO_2$) is calculated by the Fick equation as

$$VO_2 = (CaO_2 - CvO_2) \times CO$$

where CO is cardiac output, $CaO_2$ is the arterial $O_2$ content, and $CvO_2$ is the mixed venous oxygen content. Normal $VO_2$ is 250 mL/min (normal range 180–280 mL/min).

If 1000 mL/min of oxygenated blood is delivered to the tissues and 250 mL/min of oxygen is consumed, normally 750 mL/min (or 75%) of the oxygenated blood return to the right side of the heart and represent a venous oxygen reserve. If oxygen delivery decreases, either increased cardiac output or oxygen extraction will compensate to maintain aerobic metabolism. A value of mixed $SvO_2$ less than 50% is associated with cellular hypoxia, development of anaerobic metabolism, and lactic acidosis.

The $SvO_2$, can be calculated from the Fick equation as

$$SvO_2 = SaO_2 - (VO_2/CO \times 1.39 \times Hgb)$$

where $SvO_2$ is mixed venous oxygen saturation, $SaO_2$ is arterial oxygen saturation, $VO_2$ is oxygen consumption, CO is cardiac output, and Hb is hemoglobin concentration. The normal $SvO_2$ is 65%–75%, which corresponds to a mixed venous oxygen tension ($PvO_2$) of 35–45 mm Hg. A 1 mm Hg change in $PvO_2$ causes 2% changes in $SvO_2$.

The four main determinants of $SvO_2$ are cardiac output, hemoglobin concentration, arterial oxygen saturation, and oxygen consumption (Table 3.1). A change in $SvO_2$ identifies a global change in oxygen delivery/consumption balance. To identify which determinants have changed, $SvO_2$ monitoring has to be combined with clinical evaluation and monitoring of other hemodynamic and respiratory parameters. $SvO_2$ is a global value and does not necessarily identify local ischemia in single organs.[3]

*Table 3.1* FACTORS THAT AFFECT SVO2

| | | MIXED VENOUS OXYGEN SATURATION | | | |
|---|---|---|---|---|---|
| LOW (<65%) | FACTORS | DIFFERENTIAL | HIGH (>75%) | FACTORS | DIFFERENTIAL |
| | ↓SaO2 | Low FiO$_2$ | | ↑SaO2 | Oxygen Therapy<br>PA catheter distal migration |
| | ↓Hb | Hemorrhage | | ↑Hb | Blood Transfusion |
| | ↓CO | Heart failure | | ↑CO | Inotropic agents, Cirrhosis |
| | ↑VO2 | Thyroid storm | | ↓VO2 | General anesthesia |
| | | Pain | | | Hypothermia |
| | | Shivering | | | Hypothyroidism |

CO, cardiac output; Hb, hemoglobin; SaO2, arterial oxygen saturation; VO2, venous oxygen consumption.

A drop in SvO$_2$ can be the result of a decrease in cardiac output, hemoglobin concentration, or arterial oxygen saturation or an increase in oxygen consumption. Clinicians can use changes in SvO$_2$ to identify imbalances in oxygen delivery and consumption and guide their therapeutic strategy.[3,4] A decrease in SvO$_2$ due to a low SaO$_2$ secondary to respiratory failure will prompt an increase of the fraction of inspired oxygen (FiO$_2$) and/or positive end-expiratory pressure. Alternatively, if the decreased SvO$_2$ is due to reduced cardiac output from heart failure, inotropic support could be initiated and titrated to desired effect. If decreased SvO$_2$ is due to blood loss, as commonly seen in the operating room or trauma bay, the clinician will initiate a transfusion protocol. Examples of increased oxygen consumption leading to reduced SvO$_2$ often seen in the perioperative setting include pain, shivering, and less commonly malignant hyperthermia and thyroid storm.

An increased SvO$_2$ value has a broader differential, and under most circumstances is less ominous than a decreased value. Commonly, a false elevation is the result of distal migration of the PA catheter into the pulmonary capillary blood, where the oxygen saturation is 100%. Repositioning the PA catheter into the proper location can normalize the SvO$_2$. Other common causes are high cardiac output, acquired or congenital peripheral shunts, low states of peripheral oxygen uptake, and left-to-right cardiac shunts.

Hepatic cirrhosis is a disease associated with increased SvO$_2$ values due to both an increased cardiac output and the acquired shunting of blood secondary to hepatic congestion. Arterial-venous shunts (cardiac shunts, arterial-venous fistula) allow a more arterial blood to bypass the capillary system, leading to mixing with the venous circulation before returning to the heart without undergoing oxygen extraction. A decreased oxygen consumption as observed with hypothermia, general anesthesia, and hypothyroidism will increase the SvO$_2$ value. SvO$_2$ measurement has been used extensively during the perioperative period (e.g., vascular and cardiac surgery) and in several critical diseases (e.g., heart failure, sepsis, traumatic and hemorrhagic shock, patients on extracorporeal membrane oxygenation).

## REFERENCES

1. Havashi MS, et al. Venous oximetry, In: Layon AJ, ed. Civetta, Taylor, & Kirby's Critical Care Medicine. 5th ed. Philadelphia, PA: Wolters Kluwer; 2018:228–247.
2. Gutierrez G. Central and mixed venous O$_2$ Saturation. *Turk J Anaesthesiol Reanim.* 2020;48:2–10.
3. Shepherd S, et al. Role of central and mixed venous oxygen saturation measurement in perioperative care. *Anesthesiology.* 2009 Sep;111:649–656.
4. Walley KR. Use of central venous oxygen saturation to guide therapy. *Am J Respir Crit Care Med.* 2011 Sep 1;184(5):514–520.

# 4.

# CARDIAC OUTPUT

*Adambeke Nwozuzu and Ettore Crimi*

## INTRODUCTION

Cardiac output (CO) can be defined as the volume of blood pumped out of the ventricle with each heartbeat. It is dependent on the stroke volume (SV) and the heart rate (HR):

$$CO = SV \times HR$$

In a resting state, the normal adult CO ranges between 4.0 and 8.0 L/min. The cardiac index is derived from the CO and body surface area and ranges between 2.5 and 4.2 L/min/m$^2$.

Invasive methods to monitor CO include pulmonary artery thermodilution, transpulmonary thermodilution, dye densitometry, and lithium dilution. Minimally invasive methods are esophageal Doppler and pulse wave analysis by an arterial catheter. Noninvasive methods are echocardiography, transthoracic bioimpedance, and noninvasive pulse wave analysis.[1,2]

## FICK METHOD

According to the Fick equation, CO can be calculated as

$$CO = VO_2 / (CaO_2 - CvO_2)$$

where $VO_2$ is the oxygen consumption, $CaO_2$ is the arterial content of oxygen, and $CvO_2$ is the mixed venous content of oxygen. Limitations with the Fick method include sampling errors and difficulty obtaining continuous measurements. An indirect method to calculate CO uses partial $CO_2$ rebreathing, where $CO_2$, measured by capnography, replaces $VO_2$.[3]

## INDICATOR DILUTION METHODS

### THERMODILUTION CARDIAC OUTPUT

Thermodilution monitoring is the gold standard technique. It is performed by injecting a known temperature and volume of cold saline through the proximal port of a pulmonary artery catheter (PAC) into the right atrium. As the blood flows across the pulmonary artery, the change in temperature is recorded by a thermistor located at the tip of the PAC. A thermodilution curve is generated, where temperature is plotted by a function of time (Figure 4.1). The change in temperature is inversely proportional to the CO. The CO is calculated based on the Stewart-Hamilton equation, where CO equals the amount of the indicator divided by the area under the thermodilution curve. Limitations of this technique include operator technique, fluctuations of blood temperature, intracardiac shunting, and tricuspid and pulmonic valve regurgitation.[1,3]

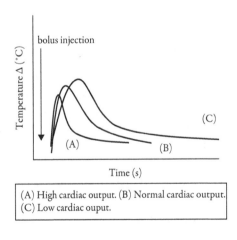

(A) High cardiac output. (B) Normal cardiac output. (C) Low cardiac ouput.

**Figure 4.1** Comparisons in cardiac output thermodilution curves.

## OTHER DILUTION TECHNIQUES

Transpulmonary thermodilution estimates CO from the left side of the heart and requires a central venous catheter (CVC) and cannulation of a major artery. A cold saline bolus is injected through the CVC, and the change in temperature is recorded via an arterial catheter thermistor. Alternatively, dye dilutions can also be used to estimate CO. The dye densitometry technique is used to measure the arterial concentration of indocyanine green (ICG). A bolus of ICG is administered intravenously and detected within the arterial systemic circulation. The area under the dye curve estimates the CO. With low CO, dye dilution techniques tend to be accurate because it is not readily absorbed in the tissues; therefore, the downstream concentration of the dye is easily detectable. Lithium dilution involves injection of small boluses of lithium through a venous catheter. The concentration of lithium is measured over time via an arterial catheter equipped with a lithium-sensitive electrode. Nondepolarizing neuromuscular blockades can potentially cross-react with the lithium sensor and lead to an overestimation of CO.[1,4]

## ALTERNATIVE METHODS

### ESOPHAGEAL DOPPLER

The Doppler technique uses an esophageal probe to calculate the velocity of blood in the descending thoracic aorta. The CO is calculated using the velocity-time interval (VTI), HR, and cross-sectional area of the aorta (CSA). The CSA is based on the age, height, and weight or directly measured with the transducer. To calculate the VTI, the angle of incidence between the ultrasound beam and blood flow should be close to zero; an angle of incidence closer to 90 will yield unreliable and inaccurate values.[4]

### ECHOCARDIOGRAPHY

A combination of two-dimensional (2-D) ultrasound (US) and pulsed-wave Doppler measurements are used to calculate SV and CO by measuring the left ventricular outflow tract (LVOT) cross-sectional area and the VTI, respectively.[5] SV is calculated as

$$SV = \text{cross-sectional area (CSA)} \times VTI$$

where CSA is calculated as

$$CSA = (\text{LVOT Diameter})^2 \times 0.785$$

The CO is calculated by multiplying the SV by the HR. The LVOT diameter is measured from the parasternal long-axis view with transthoracic echocardiography (TTE) or the

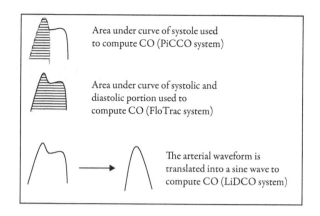

**Figure 4.2** Different analyses used from arterial waveforms to compute CO.

midesophageal long-axis view with transesophageal echocardiography (TEE). The VTI is measured from the apical five-chamber view with TTE or the deep-trans gastric view with TEE. Inaccurate CO values result from any error in LVOT measurement.

### PULSE WAVE ANALYSIS

Arterial pulse wave analysis uses the contour of the arterial waveform via an arterial catheter or a noninvasive finger cuff to determine the vascular compliance and systemic vascular resistance and estimate SV and CO (Figure 4.2). Current available methods can be noninvasive (EV1000) or invasive (Flo-Trac; PiCCO [Pulse Index Continuous Cardiac Output] and LiDCO [Lithum Dilution Cardiac Output]) and require calibration to improve accuracy (PiCCO and LiDCO).[4]

The EV1000 and Flo-Trac system use a mathematical model to compute CO. PiCCO and LiDCO systems use a combination of transpulmonary thermodilution and pulse contour analysis. The PiCCO system requires a CVC and a femoral arterial catheter; after a cold saline bolus injection, it estimates the SV using the area under the systolic portion of the arterial waveform to compute CO (see Figure 4.2). The LiDCO system requires a CVC and a radial or brachial artery and uses lithium thermodilution. The arterial waveform is translated to a sine wave, referred to as a lithium washout curve, to compute CO.

### THORACIC BIOIMPEDANCE

Thoracic bioimpedance uses plethysmography to measure CO. A low-amplitude, high-frequency electrical current is applied to electrodes that are placed at the lateral aspects of the neck and chest. These electrodes detect the electrocardiographic signal that is used for the timing of recorded measurements. The electrical current preferentially travels down the thorax through the path of least resistance, the aorta. During a cardiac cycle, as blood is ejected through the aorta, the impedance (or resistance) is measured over a time interval. The SV is derived by changes in the size and volume of the aorta in systole, and subsequently a CO is computed. Obesity, pleural effusions, electrical interference, arrhythmias, and low hematocrit can all affect the bioimpedance.[4]

## REFERENCES

1. Kobe J, et al. Cardiac output monitoring: technology and choice. *Ann Card Anaesth.* 2019;22:6–17.

2. Saugel B, Vincent JL. Cardiac output monitoring: how to choose the optimal method for the individual patient. *Curr Opin Crit Care.* 2018;24:165–172.
3. Mittnacht AJC, et al. Monitoring of the heart and vascular system. In: Kaplan JA, ed. *Kaplan's Cardiac Anesthesia.* 7th ed. Elsevier; 2017:390–426.
4. Sangkum L, et al. Minimally invasive or noninvasive cardiac output measurement: an update. *J Anesth.* 2016;30:461–480.
5. Quiñones MA, et al. Doppler Quantification Task Force of the Nomenclature and Standards Committee of the American Society of Echocardiography. Recommendations for quantification of Doppler echocardiography: a report from the Doppler Quantification Task Force of the Nomenclature and Standards Committee of the American Society of Echocardiography. *J Am Soc Echocardiogr.* 2002;15:167–184.

# 5.

# COAGULATION MONITORS

*Christopher Giordano and Gabriella Tom Williams*

## CONVENTIONAL COAGULATION ASSAYS: PT/INR, PTT, AND ACT

The cascade model of coagulation is based on in vitro testing of the theoretically isolated extrinsic and intrinsic pathways (Figure 5.1). Prothrombin time (PT) focuses on the extrinsic pathway by measuring the time for plasma to form a fibrin clot in the presence of thromboplastin.[1] The use of thromboplastin does not consider that thrombin may be inhibited in vivo by protein C, protein S, or antithrombin III, which are anticoagulants that balance coagulation with fibrinolysis.[2] Similar to other in vitro assays, these testing techniques focus solely on procoagulant activity despite the understanding that hemostasis relies on an equilibrium between procoagulant and anticoagulant factors.[1,2] A shift between these two counterbalancing forces alters the coagulation profile. Despite these limitations, the focus of PT on procoagulants does not impede its use in evaluating anticoagulant therapies, which target specific procoagulant factors.[2] As a method of standardizing PT, the World Health Organization developed the international

normalized ratio (INR), which allows for the universal comparison of laboratory values in monitoring warfarin therapy.

The counterpart to PT is partial thromboplastin time (PTT), which uses partial thromboplastin, free of tissue factor, to assess the intrinsic pathway of coagulation.[1] PTT assay addresses factor (VIII, IX, XI, XII) deficiencies that contribute to clinical coagulopathies, and it measures the effect of anticoagulant agents, such as unfractionated heparin and direct thrombin inhibitors. A similar metric to PTT is the activating clotting time (ACT), a rapid point-of-care test that indirectly measures large-dose heparin activity in the presence of a kaolin or Celite activator.[1] At high blood concentrations of unfractionated heparin (>1 IU/mL), ACT provides a more precise evaluation than PTT.[3] The utility of ACT is most apparent during cardiac and vascular procedures, where its speed and efficiency in the operating room guide real-time therapeutic heparin titration and monitoring. Prolonged ACT can be caused by hemodilution, hypothermia, thrombocytopenia, and platelet dysfunction.

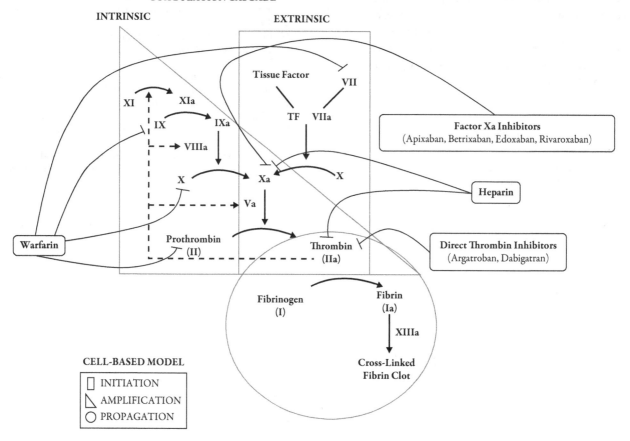

COAGULATION CASCADE

**Figure 5.1** Overlap of the coagulation cascade where the intrinsic, extrinsic, and common pathways represent the foundation and the cell-based model highlights the synchronous initiation, amplification, and propagation that occurs leading to hemostasis. Common anticoagulants are represented with their site of inhibition.

## VISCOELASTIC HEMOSTATIC ASSAYS: TEG, ROTEM, AND SEER

An older approach to coagulation monitoring that has resurfaced in the last few decades is viscoelastic testing, which better captures the entire in vivo hemostasis profile. These tests highlight the dynamics of coagulation without introducing artificial activating substances or environments as occurs with PT/INR, PTT, and ACT. Viscoelastic testing focuses on analyzing properties of clot timing, strength, and durability. Thromboelastography (TEG) uses an oscillating cylinder with a fixed sensory pin immersed in whole blood.[4] The formation of a clot results in torque on a pin that is measured via an optical sensor.[4] The strength of the clot is visualized on a graph analyzing properties of the platelet-fibrin interactions and the eventual fibrinolysis through five main parameters: reaction time (R), K value, alpha angle, maximum amplitude (MA), and lysis at 30 minutes (LY30). R corresponds to coagulation factor (enzyme) activity, while the K value quantifies the speed of clot formation.[1] The alpha angle reflects increasing thrombin generation and fibrin accumulation. The summation of R, K, and alpha angle represents initial coagulation

and quantifies the time to clot formation. The MA of the graph depicts the maximum clot strength determined by fibrin-platelet interactions.[1] After the MA, fibrinolysis is evaluated via the LY30, which is the percentage of the MA reduction after 30 minutes (Figure 5.2). Alterations in the length or angle of each parameter represent an underlying cause of coagulopathy that guides specific blood component therapy.

Rotational thromboelastometry (ROTEM) constructs a similar graph from an oscillating pin that measures resistance in a fixed container.[4] As opposed to an oscillating cylinder described in TEG, a pin oscillation provides the graph with alternative nomenclature and measured variables. In short, the parameters include clotting time, alpha angle, clot formation time, maximum clot firmness, and clot lysis. Differences in mechanics and measured parameters used in each method limit the comparability of the two. Focusing the evaluation on specific blood component deficits that alter the parameters of the graphs provides clinical insight into which coagulation therapy will best treat a patient's coagulopathy: platelets, fibrinogen, or enzymes.

Because platelet-fibrin interactions are tightly coupled, it is difficult for TEG and ROTEM to differentiate which

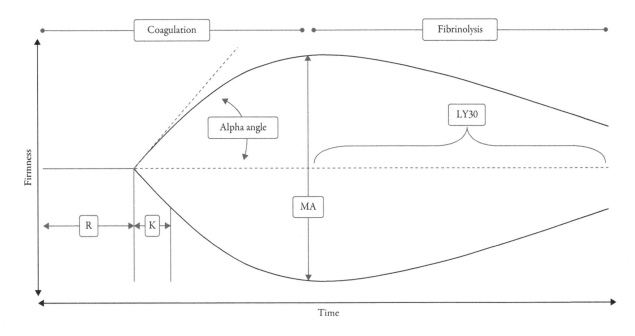

| VARIABLE | MEASUREMENT | ABNORMALITY | GRAPH | TREATMETNT |
|---|---|---|---|---|
| **Reaction Time (R)** | Coagulation factor activity and time to clot onset | Elevated R: Factor deficiency | | FFP, PCC, isolated factor concentrates |
| **Alpha angle** | Speed of fibrin accumulation and cross-linking | Decreased alpha angle: Hypofibrinogenemia | | Cryoprecipitate, Recombinant fibrinogen |
| **Max Amplitude (MA)** | Maximum clot strength | Decreased MA: Thrombocytopenia | | Platelets |
| **Lysis at 30 mins (LY30)** | Percentage MA reduction at 30 minutes | Decreased MA + increased LY30: Fibrinolysis | | TXA, Aminocaproic acids |

FFP: fresh-frozen plasma, PCC: prothrombin complex concentrate, TXA: tranexamic acid

**Figure 5.2** Two-dimensional graph constructed from thromboelastography representing platelet fibrin interactions and eventual fibrinolysis. The graph identifies each of the five parameters, and the table provides examples of abnormalities and blood replacement products utilized to restore hemostasis.

of the two components may be contributing more to a coagulopathy. Platelet function assays provide a focused assessment of platelet aggregation and can identify platelet inhibition due to congenital or acquired platelet disorders.[1] A survivable hematocrit and baseline platelet and fibrinogen counts are fundamental to these assays; deficits in either will prolong these parameters and interfere with coagulation.

Novel advancements in ultrasound have furthered the understanding of the evolution of clotting mechanisms. Sonic estimation of elasticity via resonance (SEER) uses whole blood in a rigid wall chamber with an ultrasound probe. High-energy ultrasound waves induce a shear wave repeatedly on a naturally evolving blood clot as clot formation occurs.[4] Low-energy ultrasound measures the displacement as the clot forms and lyses. A waveform is constructed that coincides with clot stiffness and durability. The shear modulus represents the combination of activated platelets and the fibrin network's ability to withstand mechanical disruptions that occur under in vivo interactions.[4]

## ANESTHETIC CONSIDERATIONS

Hemostasis point-of-care assays are more readily used in the operating room to guide therapeutic decision-making. ACT has proved to be a necessity during cardiopulmonary bypass surgeries and vascular procedures.[2] Its rapid ability to evaluate heparin activity at high blood concentrations allows it to serve as a key indicator for intraoperative and postoperative heparin and subsequent protamine titration.[3] Due to the complexity of these procedures and the physiologic effect of surgery on coagulation (e.g., fibrinolysis, platelet function/consumption, hypothermia, hemodilution, cardiopulmonary bypass), ACT-guided heparin therapy occurs at regular intervals and continues after surgery to ensure appropriate hemostasis.

Viscoelastic testing can efficiently analyze whole-blood clotting and lysis in real time, which can guide the selection of blood component therapy. TEG provides quantitative and qualitative data that determine which component deficit is interfering with appropriate coagulation based on the parameter affected. In a patient with an elevated R time, an enzymatic factor deficiency is the most likely defect, requiring fresh frozen plasma therapy.[5] An increase in K value or a decrease in the alpha angle is influenced by fibrinogen deficiency and can be remedied with cryoprecipitate.[5] A decrease in MA suggests aberrant platelet or fibrin interactions via thrombocytopenia/platelet dysfunction or hypofibrinogenemia/dysfibrinogenemia; a quantitative platelet count or functional fibrinogen assay can further elucidate the condition. In the event of a platelet disorder from end-stage renal disease, transfusion of platelets or DDAVP (desmopressin) can be given. If the etiology is dysfibrinogenemia, the K value could similarly be decreased, and cryoprecipitate could ameliorate the condition. Hyperfibrinolysis may cause an increased LY30, in which case antifibrinolytic therapy such as tranexamic acid or aminocaproic will attenuate clot lysis[5] (Figure 5.2).

## REFERENCES

1. Slaughter TF. Patient blood management: coagulation. In: Miller RD, et al. Miller's *Anesthesia*. 8th ed. Elsevier; 2014:1868–1880.
2. Tripodi A, Mannucci PM. The coagulopathy of chronic liver disease. *N Eng J Med*. 2011;365(2):147–156.
3. Prisco D, Paniccia R. Point-of-care testing of hemostasis in cardiac surgery. *Thromb J*. 2003;1(1):1.
4. Corey FS, Walker WF. Sonic estimation of elasticity via resonance: a new method of assessing hemostasis. *Ann Biomed Eng*. 2015;44(5):1405–1424.
5. Olson JC. Thromboelastography-guided blood product use before invasive procedures in cirrhosis with severe coagulopathy: a randomized controlled trial. *Clin Liver Dis (Hoboken)*. 2019;13(4): 102–105. doi:10.1002/cld.749

# 6.

# ULTRASOUND-GUIDED PLACEMENT OF VASCULAR CATHETERS

*Harsh Rawal and Rany T. Abdallah*

## INTRODUCTION

Placement of catheters by ultrasound (US) has gained increasing popularity in the last decade. A key reason is the safety associated with real -time visualization and significantly reduced number and severity of complications. Traditionally, catheter placement has been done with anatomical landmarks. However, that cannot be applied to patients who do not fit the "normal anatomy" criteria.

Additionally, vascular thrombosis, which cannot be recognized without US visualization, could act as a hindrance in the placement of these catheters, especially central venous catheters (CVCs).

A small linear probe (5–15 MHz) is used in identifying the superficial skin structures up to 20–50 mm under the skin. US can be used in both static and real-time modes. Usually for catheter placement, the short axis with out-of-plane view is preferred. The short-axis view demonstrates the needle as only an echogenic point, which may or may not be the tip of the needle. When using the long-axis view, the entire length of the needle can be visualized, which additionally gives a sense of the depth of the needle. This view can help prevent distant wall punctures.[1]

The following are indications for placement of CVCs[2]:

1. Monitoring central venous pressure
2. Emergency resuscitation
3. Hemodialysis (using hemodialysis catheter)
4. Delivery of critical medication
5. Pulmonary artery catheterization

Contraindications:

1. Thrombosis of the vessel
2. Uncooperative patient
3. Coagulopathy (low platelets, high international normalized ratio, high activated partial thromboplastin time)
4. Skin infection over the site of insertion

Techniques for placing different types of vascular catheters:

1. Explain the procedure to the patient, including potential complications; obtain written consent; and look for contraindications.
2. Equipment:
   Sterile gloves, gown, cap, mask, face shield
   Skin prep and drape towels
   Lidocaine, sterile gauze
   Syringes: Non–Luer lock
   Saline flushes, scalpel, catheter dilators, needle, guide wire, sutures, needle driver, biopatch, skin dressing

Internal jugular (IJ) catheter placement: In the absence of contraindications, place the patient in a 10°–15° Trendelenburg position. This helps to engorge the vein and prevent air embolism. Generally, the right IJ is preferred as it is a more direct approach to the superior vena cava (SVC).

The probe is placed at the site of needle insertion. Artery and vein are identified on US as shown in Figures 6.1A and 6.1B. The vein is usually compressible and more

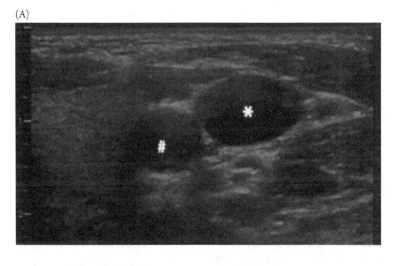

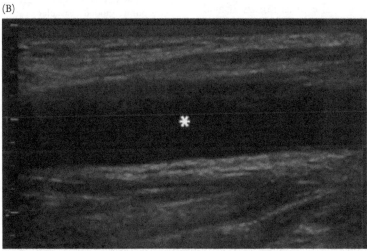

**Figure 6.1** Ultrasound view of the right internal jugular vein (*) in short-axis (A) and long-axis (B) views and its relation to the carotid artery (#).

lateral compared to the carotid artery, which is pulsatile and noncompressible.

Prepare the area by scrubbing the site with chlorhexidine. Drape the site. Flush the lumen of the central line catheter with saline or heparin. Prepare the US probe with a long sterile sleeve.

Prepare the insertion site by infiltrating 1% lidocaine using a 25-gauge needle to minimize pain. Puncture the skin at the apex of the triangle at the medial head of the sternocleidomastoid muscle. Continue to aim toward the ipsilateral nipple at a 45° angle. Typically, the vein is accessed at 0.5 inch or 1.3 cm. Using US, follow the shadow of the needle. When the IJ is entered, a flash of venous blood is obtained. Maintain a steady position of the needle to confirm dark, nonpulsatile flow.

Once the needle is in the vein, deploy the guide wire. It is important to watch the monitor to look for signs of arrhythmias. Withdraw the needle, leaving the wire in place.

Confirm the position of the guide wire using US in both short-axis and long-axis views (Figure 6.1A and 6.1B). Incise the skin by making a stab wound using a scalpel at the site of insertion. Advance the dilator 1–2 cm. Use 4 by 4 gauze to minimize blood loss.

Advance the catheter over the guide wire. The tip should lie at the junction of SVC and Right atrium (RA). Remove the wire. Check for blood return in all ports. Flush all ports, cap the hub, and secure the line. Apply a sterile dressing. Obtain a chest x-ray to confirm line placement. Confirm the absence of pneumothorax or hemothorax. Dispose sharps in an appropriate sharps container.[2]

*Dialysis catheter placement*: similar in approach to the IJ catheter placement, the dialysis catheter is larger than the regular IJ catheter. The dialysis catheters are available in diameters of 8–13.5 French and varying lengths (9–50 cm).[3] The dialysis catheters are further classified into tunneled and nontunneled and double versus triple lumen. Tunneled catheters are usually larger, around 15.5–16 French. They can be used for about 3 weeks.[3] The third lumen, if available, can be used for medication delivery.[3]

Femoral venous catheters: Indications and contraindications are similar as mentioned above. Femoral venous catheters, if left in place, have higher chances of thrombosis and infection compared to subclavian catheters. Rates for subclavian line–related infections were 1.2/1000 days, and there were rates of 4.5/1000 days with femoral lines. Similarly rates of thrombosis were 1.9% and 21.5%, respectively.[4]

The basic process of femoral line insertion remains the same as for IJ or subclavian insertion using the Seldinger technique and selection of the appropriate catheter based on the indication for the procedure. Using US guidance, the structures can be identified as the vein is more medial than the artery.

*Subclavian catheters*: The subclavian vein runs under the middle third of the clavicle, and the artery runs posterior and superior to it. Place the probe just proximal to the insertion site; identify the vein by compressibility. After adequate local anesthesia, the needle is inserted at the site at a 30° angle to the skin, and the direction of the needle for this particular procedure is toward the sternal notch, with the needle tracking just beneath the clavicle. The rest of the process, including US confirmation and catheter insertion, is similar to that of IJ insertion.

## ULTRASOUND USE IN CLINICAL PRACTICE FOR VASCULAR CATHETER PLACEMENT

A survey among 2000 senior anesthesiologists in the United Kingdom revealed that only 27% used US as their first-choice approach for CVC placement via the IJ. The surface landmark technique was used by 50%, and 30% used carotid palpation as their preferred choice.[5] In the United States, a 2016 survey revealed more frequent use depending on the site, with 31% for subclavian, 80% for IJ, and 45% for femoral vein (FV). Among emergency room physicians, the use of US for CVC placement has been upward of 80%. Over time, there has been a steady increase in the use of US for these procedures given the increasing evidence of safety and accuracy associated with visualization.

## REFERENCES

1. Troianos CA, et al. Special articles: guidelines for performing ultrasound guided vascular cannulation: recommendations of the American Society of Echocardiography and the Society of Cardiovascular Anesthesiologists. *Anesth Analg.* 2012;114:46–72.
2. Graham A, et al. Central venous catheterization. *N Engl J Med* 2007;356:e21.
3. Bander SJ, et al. Central catheters for acute and chronic hemodialysis access. In: Post TW, ed. *UpToDate*. UpToDate; 2021.
4. McGee DC, Gould MK. Preventing complications of central venous catheterization *N Engl J Med.* 2003;348:1123–1133.
5. McGrattan T, et al. A survey of the use of ultrasound guidance in internal jugular venous cannulation. *Anaesthesia.* 2008;63: 1222–1225.

# 7.

# POINT-OF-CARE ULTRASOUND (POCUS)

*Harsh Rawal and Rany T. Abdallah*

## INTRODUCTION

Point-of-care ultrasound (POCUS) has been evolving as a valid and reliable tool in diagnosis and clinical decision-making and as a timely intervention modality for patient care. Over the past five decades, ultrasound has evolved, making it a very handy, cost-effective, and accurate bedside tool for clinical diagnosis.[1] The use of POCUS has been steadily expanding to heart examination in acute decompensated situations and hemodynamic compromise and evaluation of preoperative surgical patients. Moreover, lung examination using ultrasound has proven superior to physical examination in diagnosis of conditions like pulmonary edema, pleural effusions, and even pneumonias.[2] This use of ultrasound (US) has helped clinicians distinguish between heart and lung examinations. Table 7.1 summarizes the different findings of POCUS examination in different types of shock.

## POCUS AND DIFFERENT ORGAN SYSTEMS

### CARDIAC EXAMINATION

Goal-directed echo is different from a standard detailed exploratory echocardiogram in that the main aim would be to identify acute hemodynamic and cardiac compromise.

Focused examination includes a problem-oriented, goal-directed, time-sensitive, simplified, and easily repeatable modality performed by clinicians at bedside (Figure 7.1). There is a difference between limited examination and focused examination; focused examination refers to a narrow, specific question and scope of expertise.[3] Findings from focused examination do not replace a complete thorough echocardiogram. The suggested targets for focused cardiac examination are as follows:

1. Pericardial effusion and tamponade physiology
2. Assessment of volume status
3. Gross assessment of left ventricular (LV) systolic function
4. Assessment of volume status
5. Occasionally, intracardiac masses depending on their size

### Views and Areas of Interest

Ideal standard views for focused examination:

1. Subcostal four chamber view: The advantages of a subcostal view are that there is no bone or lung obstruction to the view. It is effective if it is difficult to reposition the patient on the left side. To obtain the subcostal view, place the transducer under the

*Table 7.1* POCUS FINDINGS IN DIFFERENT TYPES OF SHOCK

|  | DISTRIBUTIVE | CARDIOGENIC | HYPOVOLEMIC | OBSTRUCTIVE |
|---|---|---|---|---|
| Cardiac Findings | Spectrum from hyperdynamic to decreased left ventricular function | Decreased left ventricular function | Hyperdynamic | Dilated right ventricle or pericardial effusion |
| Inferior Vena Cava Findings | Range from collapsible to dilated | Noncollapsible | Collapsible | Noncollapsible |
| Lung Findings | Negative | B lines present | Negative | Focal or negative |
| Abdominal Findings | Negative | Negative | Evaluate for hemorrhage | Negative |

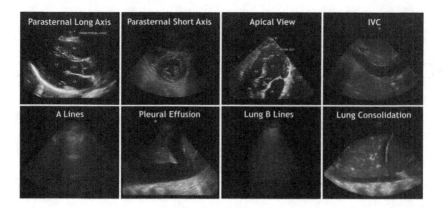

**Figure 7.1** POCUS Cardiac examination demonstrating different views on transthoracic echo (TTE) and corresponding structures visualized. (Amer Johri, MD, MSc, FRCPC, FASE, Clinician Scientist, KGHRI, Associate Professor, Echocardiography and Founder & Director, Cardiovascular Imaging Network, Salwa Nihal, MSc, and Julia Herr, MSc, Queen's University, Kingston, Ontario, Canada)

xiphoid and a little to the right of the sternum, with the transducer marked to the left with the plane directed upward and to the left shoulder. Structures visualized include all four chambers.

2. Subcostal inferior vena cava: The preferred way to obtain this view is to start with the four-chamber view and then rotate the transducer counterclockwise and then to the right. The subcostal view shows the vena cava in long axis. In addition, it shows the hepatic veins and sometimes the SVC.

3. Parasternal long axis: Structures visualized are the anterior-to-posterior right ventricle RV, interventricular septum, LV, inferolateral wall of LV, aortic valve, mitral valve, and pericardium.

4. Parasternal short axis: The structures visualized are RV, right atrium (RA), aortic valve, interatrial septum, left atrium (LA), RV outflow tract, and pulmonary artery.

5. Apical four chamber: Structures visualized are all four chambers (LA, LV, RA, RV) and both interatrial and ventricular septum.

## Limitations

1. Limited accuracy for determining pericardial constriction, pulmonary hypertension, and diastolic dysfunction since there is no spectral Doppler

2. Focus cannot accurately quantify valvular regurgitation or stenosis but can see gross valvular abnormalities

3. May miss aortic dissection, LV aneurysm, LV thrombus, valvular vegetations and occasionally even loculated effusions

## LUNG EXAMINATION

Point-of-care US has gained increasing usability with lung examinations in the last decade and has been a helpful alternative to traditional radiography.[4] At the bedside, POCUS can sometimes be helpful in differentiating pathologies that cannot be diagnosed using traditional US.[4]

## Indications and areas of interest

1. Focused Assessment with Sonography for Trauma (FAST) examination includes the extended form of FAST (EFAST) pneumothorax, hemothorax, rib fractures, hematomas

2. Pneumonia

3. Empyema

4. Chronic obstructive pulmonary disease

5. Pulmonary embolism

6. Acute respiratory distress syndrome

## Technique

Usually the FAST examination uses the outside-to-inside approach, beginning from the thoracic wall (subcutaneous tissue, musculature, ribs) to the inferior border of the diaphragm, spleen, liver, and heart and its major vessels. Normally, the parietal and visceral pleural appear as a single hyperechoic line underneath the skin and subcutaneous tissue roughly about 1 cm from the skin margin. The pleural line is usually dynamic, but in the case of a pneumothorax, lung sliding is disrupted, and the pleural line appears static. Fluid collection in the thoracic pleural cavity will produce an anechoic or hypoechoic layer between the pleural layers. US has demonstrated higher sensitivity in detecting pleural effusions with even fluid amounts as low as 5–20 mL. Infectious conditions change the echogenicity of the parenchyma, making it more echogenic compared to the nonechogenic normal lung. Additionally, air bronchograms may be visualized as well, pointing toward a consolidation. These US findings combined with the history and laboratory diagnostics prove to be helpful in arriving at a quick diagnosis.

## Indications

1. Intussusception
2. Appendicitis
3. Undifferentiated acute abdominal pain
4. Free fluid
5. Intraperitoneal air
6. Acute diverticulitis
7. Colonic tumors

## Technique

A linear probe is best to examine an area of interest. For example, to examine the colon, place in the transverse position in the right lower quadrant. From anterior to posterior, the following structures should be visualized: the rectus muscle, the iliac vessels, the psoas muscle, and the iliac crest. In case of obstruction of the view, use graded compression to move bowel air out of the way to better see the anatomy. Transverse and longitudinal orientations should both be used to examine the intestines. The probe is moved to follow the structures of interest.

Trained personnel can detect as little as 10 mL free fluid using an US. The pelvic, hepatorenal, and perisplenic areas are usually dependent areas that start accumulating fluid. Trendelenburg and reverse Trendelenburg positions help move the fluid. Bedside US can also help in diagnostic and therapeutic paracentesis for free fluid in the abdomen. US can diagnose fluid; however, it will not be able to tell the difference between serous, hematogenous, or purulent composition of the fluid.

## REFERENCES

1. Cid X, et al. Impact of point-of-care ultrasound on the hospital length of stay for internal medicine inpatients with cardiopulmonary diagnosis at admission: study protocol of a randomized controlled trial—the IMFCU-1 (Internal Medicine Focused Clinical Ultrasound) study. *Trials.* 2020;21(1):53.
2. Xirouchaki N, et al. Lung ultrasound in critically ill patients: comparison with bedside chest radiography. *Intensive Care Med.* 2011;37(9):1488–1493.
3. Spencer KT, et al. Focused cardiac ultrasound: recommendations from the American Society of Echocardiography. *J Am Soc Echocardiogr.* 2013;26(6):567–581.
4. Taylor A, et al. Thoracic and lung ultrasound. In: *StatPearls.* Treasure Island, FL: StatPearls Publishing; August 13, 2020. https://www.ncbi.nlm.nih.gov/books/NBK500013

# 8.

# ASA MONITORING STANDARDS

*Nikki Eden and Shobana Rajan*

## INTRODUCTION

The American Society of Anesthesiologists (ASA) set four key monitoring parameters required at a minimum for all anesthesia care conducted in the United States: oxygenation, ventilation, circulation, and temperature.[1] These include the use of pulse oximetry, oxygen concentration, capnography, end-tidal $CO_2$, electrocardiography (ECG), blood pressure, heart rate, temperature, and audible alarms associated with each. These apply to all general, regional, and monitored anesthesia care and are to be conducted by qualified anesthesia personnel for the entirety of the anesthetic procedure.[2]

## BASIC MONITORING STANDARDS

Oxygenation, ventilation, circulation, and temperature are the four clinical factors that drive the need for monitoring during anesthesia, regardless of the type or complexity of anesthesia required (Table 8.1). Prior to the development of

**Table 8.1** ASA MONITORING STANDARDS TO BE USED DURING ALL GENERAL, REGIONAL, AND MONITORED ANESTHESIA CARE

| FUNCTION | PHYSICAL SIGNS | MONITOR | EQUIPMENT ALARMS |
|---|---|---|---|
| Oxygenation | Color of skin and mucous membranes | Pulse oximetry, inhaled oxygen concentration | Low-oxygen saturation, concentration |
| Ventilation | Breath sounds, chest rise and fall | Capnography, EtCO$_2$, ventilator alarms | Disconnect alarm, tidal volume measurement, EtCO$_2$ limit alarms |
| Circulation | Pulse palpation, chest auscultation | ECG, blood pressure, pulse rate | ECG, blood pressure cuff, pulse oximeter |
| Temperature | Skin | Temperature sensor | Low-temperature alarm |

EtCO$_2$, end-tidal CO$_2$.

*Standards for Basic Anesthetic Monitoring.* American Society of Anesthesiologists; 2015. Printed with permission.[1]

monitoring standards, standards of care varied widely and often relied heavily on clinical acumen instead of true data.

## OXYGENATION

Oxygenation is the ability of the body to adequately deliver oxygen to the tissues.

### Pulse Oximetry

Pulse oximetry is a measure of the arterial oxygen saturation at any given time. This is normally measured by a probe on a patient's finger; however, the earlobe or toe may also be used. The pulse oximeter uses two wavelengths of light (660-nm red light for oxyhemoglobin and 940-nm infrared light for deoxyhemoglobin) to determine absorbance of the light transmitted through the tissue during regular blood flow.[3] Absorbances are measured during both the pulsatile, or systolic, phase and the nonpulsatile, or diastolic, baseline phase. The difference in absorbance between the phases represents the addition of oxygen within the blood and equates to the arterial oxygen saturation.

In healthy patients, we expect the SpO$_2$ (oxygen saturation as measured by pulse oximetry) to be in the high 90% range. In a patient with known lung abnormalities such as chronic obstructive pulmonary disease or asthma, SpO$_2$ may be lower due to the inability to completely oxygenate the blood secondary to damaged alveoli or poor perfusion. A target SpO$_2$ should be individualized to each patient based on known comorbidities. Still, a low SpO$_2$ alarm is mandatory during anesthesia.

There are a number of different factors that can affect pulse oximetry that the anesthesiologist should be wary of to avoid improperly diagnosing hypoxemia. The most commonly seen disruptions come from wearing of nail polish on the finger where the pulse oximetry probe is placed. The color of the polish can interfere with the absorbance of light and give incorrectly low readings. Continually, improper placement of the probe so that it is not securely attached to the tissue or those with low blood flow states such as peripheral vascular disease may also cause inaccurate readings. Conversely, the presence of carbon monoxide in the blood converts hemoglobin to carboxyhemoglobin, which absorbs a high level of red light and can falsely elevate the SpO$_2$, even though the patient may be truly hypoxemic.

### Inhaled Oxygen Concentration

Analyzers within the ventilators determine the delivered concentrations of oxygen, inhaled anesthetics, air, and nitrous oxide to the patient to ensure there is no hypoxic gas mixture. A safety alarm measuring low oxygen concentrations must always be on. Conversely, the oxygen analyzer will also help guide the overuse of oxygen at inappropriately high levels.

## VENTILATION

Ventilation describes the ability to adequately deliver oxygen to the patient and in return the patient excretes carbon dioxide.

### Capnography

Capnography measures the waveform produced by carbon dioxide during all phases of breathing (Figure 8.1). Phase 1 shows the inspiratory baseline, measuring the vital capacity that the patient is able to inhale. Next, the upstroke is the beginning of exhalation, with the expiratory plateau coming at the end of exhalation. This plateau is useful for demonstrating underlying lung diseases. For example, a steep sloping plateau can represent obstructive lung disease as the patient has difficulty fully exhaling. Finally, phase 4 marks the end of exhalation and the transition to the next inspiratory breath.[4]

Capnography is useful for confirming correct placement of endotracheal tubes, especially distinguishing placement in the trachea versus esophagus. Capnography can also be

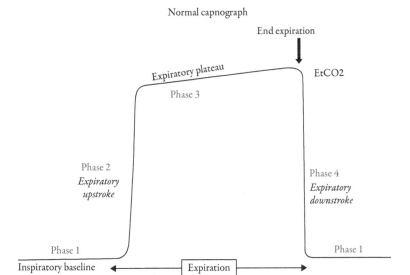

Normal capnograph

End expiration

Expiratory plateau

EtCO2

Phase 3

Phase 2
*Expiratory upstroke*

Phase 4
*Expiratory downstroke*

Phase 1

Phase 1

Inspiratory baseline

Expiration

**Figure 8.1** Capnography tracing depicting carbon dioxide levels during mechanical ventilation in a healthy patient. Reprinted with permission from Springer, Data Interpretation in Anesthesia: Capnography I by Raghuvender G, Raj TD, ed, 2017.

helpful in the evaluation of shunting, dead space, and pulmonary pathology.[4]

## End-Tidal CO$_2$

The normal range of end-tidal CO$_2$ is between 35 and 45 mm Hg. A number of factors can alter the concentration of CO$_2$ and can give important clues concerning underlying physiologic changes during the anesthesia. Increases in CO$_2$ can be due to hypoventilation, rebreathing, iatrogenic addition of CO$_2$ such as during laparoscopy, or conditions leading to increased CO$_2$ production, such as sepsis, fever, or malignant hyperthermia. Decreases in CO$_2$ can be seen with hyperventilation, low cardiac output/cardiac arrest, pulmonary embolism, hypothermia, and endobronchial intubation or inadvertent extubation. This is important because intubation of the esophagus will create a nearly flat line instead of the proper waveform due to there being no carbon dioxide excreted and is one of the quickest indicators of unsuccessful tracheal intubation.[2] All of the different causes of CO$_2$ changes can be assessed through carefully looking at the capnography waveform shape and size in addition to all vitals to obtain a better picture of the patient.

## CIRCULATION

Circulation describes both the function of the heart and the dynamic peripheral vasculature.

### Electrocardiography

Prior to the induction of anesthesia, ECG leads are placed on the patient to monitor cardiac function through cardiac rhythm in multiple ECG leads. This will also give the heart rate, which can be compared to the pulse oximetry heart rate to ensure correct monitoring. Normally, five leads are placed on the patient in their corresponding anatomical position, both upper extremities and lower extremities and one chest lead in the V1 or V5 position. This provides good detection ability for ischemia, dysrhythmias, and tachyarrhythmias, with upward of 75% of ischemic episodes detectable with the use of this arrangement. Adding a second chest lead, such as V4, increases the sensitivity of the ECG for detection of ischemia to 90%.[5]

An alarm should be set to detect bradycardia and tachycardia. While some monitors can detect ST segment elevations or depressions, visual monitoring by the anesthesiologist is essential so an acute cardiac event is not missed. Comparison of printed rhythm strips at baseline and during an incident can be extremely useful. In addition, ECG filtering can be used to remove artifact, which will distort the true picture. These include low-pass filters to remove high-frequency interference and high-pass filters to remove low-frequency interference.[3,5]

### Arterial Blood Pressure Monitoring

Most commonly, an inflatable automatic blood pressure cuff is used for blood pressure monitoring during anesthesia. If there is significant cardiopulmonary pathology or a need for tight blood pressure control, invasive arterial blood pressure monitoring may be indicated. The usual site chosen for direct cannulation is the radial artery due to ease of access, but may also be placed in the femoral, brachial, or axillary arteries. An Allen test is an easy way to determine patency of the ulnar artery, which is crucial if the radial artery is cannulated, thus diminishing blood flow to the hand.

Common issues with arterial line monitoring include improper zeroing and placement of the transducer, artifact due to harmonic resonance within the tubing ("whipping"), and catheter kinking or malpositioning causing dampening of the waveform. For every 15 cm in height the transducer is moved up or down, there is a corresponding change of 10 mm Hg in the blood pressure reading.[3] Placing the transducer higher than necessary leads to falsely low readings and vice versa.

## TEMPERATURE

Numerous factors cause decreases in body temperature during anesthetic procedures. The patient is often exposed to the room in order to access the site needed for surgery; large surgical incisions allow for evaporation; inhaled anesthetics create reduced thermoregulation; and anesthetics have vasodilatory properties. In the first hour after anesthetic induction, core temperature can drop up to 1.5°C, and as the case is prolonged, the temperature may continue to decrease. Even mild hypothermia can lead to significant postoperative complications like hypoxia, hypocapnia, infection, and delayed wound healing; therefore, it is important to avoid.[1]

Conversely, increasing temperature during a case can be a cause for concern as well. It may be due to simple overaggressive warming with forced air or potentially something worse, like the beginning signs of sepsis, drug reaction, or malignant hyperthermia. If worried for a pathologic process, check for other signs to correlate, including tachycardia, hypotension, increasing $CO_2$, or flushing of the patient. Whatever the cause, increased temperature can lead to increased metabolism, provoking excessive oxygen consumption, especially in the myocardium.

To maintain precise temperature monitoring throughout the anesthesia, a temperature probe should be placed as close to the core as functionally able. For routine cases, an esophageal temperature probe will suffice. Skin, rectal, and axillary temperatures are a poor substitute.

## REFERENCES

1. American Society of Anesthesiologists, Committee on Standards and Practice Parameters. Standards for basic anesthetic monitoring. 2015. https://www.asahq.org/standards-and-guidelines/standards-for-basic-anesthetic-monitoring

2. Noncardiovascular monitoring. In: Butterworth JF IV, et al., eds. *Morgan & Mikhail's Clinical Anesthesiology*. 6th ed. New York, NY: McGraw-Hill; 2018: Chap. 6. http://accessmedicine.mhmedical.com/content.aspx?bookid=2444&sectionid=189635630

3. Connor CW, Conley CM. Commonly used monitoring techniques. In: Barash P, et al., eds. *Clinical Anesthesia*. 8th ed. Philadelphia, PA: Lippincott Williams and Wilkins; 2017:184–186.

4. Raghuvender G. Capnography I. In: Raj TD, ed. *Data Interpretation in Anesthesia*. Switzerland: Springer; 2017:36.

5. De Silva A. Anesthetic monitoring. In: Stoetling RK, Miller RD, ed. *Basics of Anesthesia*. 5th ed. Philadelphia, PA: Elsevier; 2007:307–310.

# Part 2

# VENTILATORS

# 9.

# CONTINUOUS POSITIVE AIRWAY PRESSURE AND POSITIVE END-EXPIRATORY PRESSURE

*Breethaa Janani Selvamani and Archit Sharma*

## INTRODUCTION

Continuous positive airway pressure (CPAP) is the application of positive pressure to the airway throughout the respiratory cycle in a spontaneously breathing patient. Positive end-expiratory pressure (PEEP) is defined as a residual pressure above atmospheric maintained at the airway opening at the end of expiration.[1] PEEP can be applied to both mechanically ventilated and spontaneously breathing patients. Though CPAP incorporates PEEP, both terms are not synonymous and cannot be used interchangeably. Both CPAP and PEEP reduce the work of breathing and improve oxygenation by increasing functional residual capacity (FRC).

## INITIATING CPAP/PEEP THERAPY

Atelectasis is a shrunken airless state resulting from partial or complete collapse of alveoli. This leads to a decrease in FRC, increased intrapulmonary shunt, and hypoxemia. Factors promoting atelectasis include general anesthesia, higher inspired oxygen concentration, mechanical ventilation, shallow breathing, blockage of airway, surfactant deficiency, and acute respiratory distress syndrome (ARDS). The goals of CPAP/PEEP therapy are to recruit alveoli, increase FRC, and enhance tissue oxygenation. CPAP/PEEP can be applied to the airway either noninvasively through a face mask or nasal cannula or invasively using an endotracheal or tracheostomy tube.

## PHYSIOLOGICAL EFFECTS OF CPAP/PEEP

### PULMONARY EFFECTS

Therapy with CPAP/PEEP increases transpulmonary pressure, expands collapsed alveoli, and thereby increases FRC. The resultant increase in lung volume may increase lung compliance and decrease the work of breathing. The dead space (Vd) may be reduced if ventilation perfusion mismatch is reduced. However, when excessive CPAP/PEEP is applied, Vd may increase due to distension of airways, overexpansion of alveoli, and redistribution of perfusion.

### CARDIOVASCULAR EFFECTS

Use of CPAP/PEEP increases the intrathoracic pressure by increasing the transpulmonary pressure, which may have undesirable cardiovascular effects. Venous return decreases due to increased intrathoracic pressure, which in turn results in decreased cardiac output. PEEP may also induce ventricular dysfunction, primarily due to increased intrathoracic pressure.[2] CPAP/PEEP increases pulmonary vascular resistance and right ventricular afterload, which may cause leftward shift of the interventricular septum and reduction of left ventricular compliance.[3]

### RENAL EFFECTS

Positive end-expiratory pressure causes a reduction in renal blood flow due to both increased inferior vena cava pressure and reduced cardiac output. Consequently, urine output and sodium excretion decrease. PEEP also increases antidiuretic hormone secretion from action on sinoaortic baroreceptors.

**Optimum PEEP:** PEEP should be set at an appropriate level to maintain alveolar patency while avoiding overdistention as well as collapse during expiration. Repeated collapse and reexpansion of alveoli are associated with ventilator-associated lung injury. PEEP can be set at a minimum (3 to 5 cm $H_2O$) to preserve FRC, which is also called physiological PEEP or therapeutic PEEP (>5 cm $H_2O$), which is used to treat refractory hypoxemia. Higher levels of therapeutic PEEP are employed in patients with ARDS, where it is beneficial but often associated with cardiopulmonary complications. The term *optimum PEEP* was first coined in 1975 by Suter et al.[4] The PEEP level is considered optimal when there are maximal beneficial effects (increase in FRC, static compliance, decreased shunting, and oxygen delivery) and fewest cardiopulmonary side effects (barotrauma, volutrauma, decreased venous return, and decreased cardiac output). The optimum PEEP has since been redefined and is currently considered as the PEEP level at which static compliance is the highest.

**Clinical Application:** ARDS is a prime example in which PEEP remains an effective means of improving oxygenation. PEEP should be instituted early in ARDS to maintain the lung open. It has a protective effect against lung damage by avoiding alveolar edema, bronchial damage, and atelectrauma induced by repeated opening and closure of alveoli.[5] Some of the other indications for PEEP therapy include recurrent atelectasis with low FRC, reduced lung compliance, bilateral infiltrates on chest x-ray, refractory hypoxemia, pneumonia, and cardiogenic pulmonary edema. A minimum PEEP (physiological PEEP) is indicated in all patients undergoing general anesthesia with endotracheal intubation as FRC is invariably reduced. The indications for CPAP therapy are similar to PEEP therapy except that patients breathe spontaneously and provide the work of breathing at all times during CPAP.

**Risks and Concerns:** CPAP/PEEP is concerning if it is applied in a patient with an untreated significant pneumothorax or a tension pneumothorax since this can be made worse. Relative contraindications include untreated hypovolemia, raised intracranial pressure, recent lung surgery, and unilateral lung diseases like bronchopleural fistula.

**Complications:** The complications of CPAP/PEEP are related to the amount of positive pressure applied and include barotrauma, pneumothorax, pneumomediastinum, pneumopericardium, subcutaneous emphysema, decreased cardiac output, and raised intracranial pressure. PEEP may contribute to ventilator-associated lung injury by overdistention and increased airway pressures. CPAP/PEEP can aggravate hypoxemia in patients with unilateral lung diseases by redistributing blood from ventilated areas of the lung. PEEP can aggravate hypoxemia by increasing pulmonary vascular resistance, thereby promoting extrapulmonary right-to-left shunting in neonates. This is especially true for neonates with cyanotic congenital heart disease.

**Weaning From CPAP/PEEP:** The exact duration of CPAP/PEEP therapy required for patients with acute lung injury or ARDS is variable. Patients should be able to maintain adequate oxygenation on an inspired oxygen concentration of less than 0.50 and be hemodynamically stable and nonseptic before weaning from CPAP/PEEP is attempted.

**Bilevel Positive Airway Pressure (BiPAP):** BiPAP is a form of noninvasive ventilation therapy in which both an inspiratory positive airway pressure (IPAP) and an expiratory positive airway pressure (EPAP) are independently titrated and set. The EPAP essentially functions as a PEEP and overcomes atelectasis and upper airway occlusion and aids in improving the oxygenation of the patient. IPAP is the extra amount of pressure support that the patient receives on top of the EPAP for an inspiratory effort; hence, this works to augment the ventilation and increases the removal of $CO_2$. BiPAP is an effective strategy to decrease the work of breathing as it aids an inspiratory effort (IPAP) and prevents airway collapse (EPAP). The "delta" between the EPAP and IPAP decides the ventilatory support that is provided to the patient; the bigger this difference, the more the ventilatory support. BiPAP can be an effective strategy in obesity-hypoventilation syndrome and chronic obstructive pulmonary disease exacerbation, where a larger tidal volume will help in removing extra $CO_2$.

## ANESTHETIC CONSIDERATIONS

### PREOPERATIVE

Therapy with CPAP is commonly used in patients with obstructive sleep apnea (OSA). Thorough history and physical examination should help identify patients with reduced FRC and at risk of desaturation during anesthesia. Face mask CPAP by providing a pneumatic splint helps to prevent pharyngeal obstruction and increase FRC. CPAP/PEEP therapy is invaluable in assisting with preoxygenation of these patients before induction of anesthesia.

### INTRAOPERATIVE

Atelectasis is inevitable in the supine anesthetized patient, and PEEP should be applied to prevent this. PEEP should be titrated based on a patient's oxygenation. Intraoperatively, CPAP is valuable for spontaneously breathing patients to maintain adequate minute ventilation and normocapnia.

### POSTOPERATIVE

Mask CPAP can be applied postoperatively to prevent atelectasis and improve oxygenation. It is especially valuable in patients with OSA and patients who had undergone upper abdominal surgery. The effectiveness of CPAP is similar to the use of a recruitment maneuver in postoperative patients.

## REFERENCES

1. American College of Chest Physicians. Society of Thoracic Surgeons. Pulmonary terms and symbols: a report of the ACCP-STS Joint Committee on Pulmonary Nomenclature. *Chest*. 1975;67:583–593.
2. Pick RA, et al. The cardiovascular effects of positive end-expiratory pressure. *Chest*. 1982;82:345–350.
3. Jardin F, et al. Influence of positive end-expiratory pressure on left ventricular performance. *N Engl J Med*. 1981;304:387–392.
4. Suter PM, et al. Optimum end-expiratory airway pressure in patients with acute pulmonary failure. *N Engl J Med*. 1975;292:284–289.
5. Brower RG, et al.; National Heart, Lung, and Blood Institute ARDS Clinical Trials Network. Higher versus lower positive end-expiratory pressures in patients with the acute respiratory distress syndrome. *N Engl J Med*. 2004;352:327–336.

# 10.

# NEBULIZERS, HUMIDIFIERS, DRUG DELIVERY SYSTEMS

*Nasir Hussain and Alaa Abd-Elsayed*

## INTRODUCTION

Common anesthetic medications in particular can be delivered through a variety of mechanisms, including the traditional vaporizer, nebulizers, and humidifiers.

## VAPORIZERS

Commonly used volatile anesthetic gases, including isoflurane, desflurane, and sevoflurane, require vaporization prior to being delivered to the patient. Each vaporizer is agent specific and has a concentration dial that permits adjustment of anesthetic gas delivery. For safety, the interlocking system prevents the concurrent use of multiple vaporizers. The basic mechanism of a vaporizer revolves on the fact that volatile anesthetics in a closed container exist in both the gaseous and liquid phases at room temperature; the exception to this is desflurane, which, due to its low boiling point, is pressurized in its vaporizer. With a rise in temperature, more liquid particles transition to the gaseous phase, and vapor pressure increases.[1] This gas then becomes entrained in the carrier fresh gas flow, which is inhaled to the patient. Common vaporizers are discussed next.

## VARIABLE BYPASS VAPORIZER

The basic premise of the variable bypass vaporizers relies on the splitting ratio,[1] wherein a percentage of fresh gas flow passes through the vaporizer containing liquid anesthetic and the remainder goes through a bypass that does not make any contact with the volatile anesthetic. These vaporizers are agent specific and temperature corrected; as a result, they deliver a constant concentration of volatile anesthetic regardless of temperature or flow changes. The temperature compensation is accomplished through the presence of a bimetallic strip that bends in response to temperature changes; the direction of bending then determines the quantity of gas flowing through the vaporizer.[1] As a result of this, even altering the gas flow does not significantly affect the concentration of volatile anesthetic delivered; however, two exceptions exist. At high gas flows (>15 L/min), lower than expected concentrations are delivered, and at low gas flows (<250 mL/min), higher than expected concentrations are delivered. This is due to the rapid passing of gas at high flows, which reduces agent absorption time and an abundance of time for agent absorption at very low gas flows. Common examples of these vaporizers include the Drager Vapor 19.n and Datex-Ohmeda Tec 7 (Figure 10.1).[1]

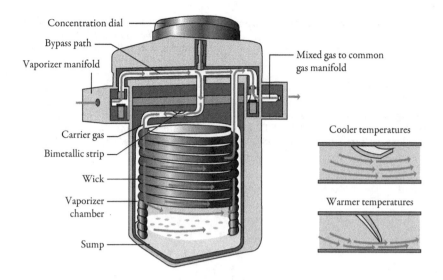

**Figure 10.1** Path of fresh gas flow in a variable bypass vaporizer. Reprinted with permission from Springer, Data Interpretation in Anesthesia: Capnography I by Raghuvender G, Raj TD, ed, 2017.

Of note, although modern vaporizers are agent specific and have keyed fillers, it still may be possible to inadvertently fill vaporizers with the incorrect anesthetic. For instance, incorrectly filling an isoflurane vaporizer with sevoflurane will lead to less anesthetic vapor released, secondary to the lower vapor pressure of sevoflurane. Also important is the prevention tilting of older vaporizers (i.e., Tec 4, Tec 5, and Drager Vapor 19.n), which would lead to an excess amount of anesthetic delivered.[1]

### MEASURED FLOW VAPORIZER

Unlike variable bypass vaporizers, measured flow vaporizers (i.e., Tec 6, D vapor, and Sigma Alpha) work by direct absorption of the anesthetic vapor to the fresh gas flow (i.e., no splitting).[2] The most commonly encountered volatile anesthetic agent that utilizes this is desflurane. Desflurane is unique in that it has a very high vapor pressure at sea level and would otherwise boil at room temperature. As a result, its unique vaporizer is electrically heated to 39°C, which creates a vapor pressure of 2 atm.[1] Thus, whatever concentration is dialed is delivered to the patient (i.e., concentration calibrated); however, these vaporizers do not compensate for altitude changes (as seen with variable bypass vaporizers). As a result, the concentration may need to be increased at high elevations due to the decreased partial pressure of desflurane.

### NEBULIZERS

In contrast to vaporizers, nebulizers produce an aerosol of droplets that become suspended in gas; they do not inherently vaporize liquids. Several types of nebulizers exist,

including jet, spinning disk, and ultrasonic.[3] Jet nebulizers are the more commonly used devices and work by using compressed air (high pressure) to generate a fine mist. On the other hand, spinning disk nebulizers use centrifugal forces on a rotating disk to break down liquid into droplets. Finally, the newer ultrasonic nebulizers use high-frequency transducers that vibrate in order to produce a fine mist. The use of ultrasonic nebulizers is limited due to the transfer of heat to the medication of interest. It is important to note that these devices are considered as an example of an active humidifier since they require a liquid supply.

### HUMIDIFIERS

#### BUBBLE HUMIDIFIERS

The bubble humidifiers devices work by "bubbling" gas flow through a liquid reservoir.[3] The bubbles then absorb the liquid vapor as they pass through the reservoir. This mechanism is relatively inefficient at heating the inspired gas but can be combined with heated humidifiers to increase efficiency. Due to the presence of a reservoir, these are also considered an example of an active humidifier.

#### HEATED HUMIDIFIERS

Unlike bubble humidifiers, heated humidifiers actively heat and evaporate a reservoir of water into vapor, which is then taken up by the fresh gas as it passes through the humidification chamber.[3] Often used in the critical care unit, a heating humidifier is also contained within the breathing apparatus in order to conserve temperature throughout the tubing. Due to a reservoir being present and being battery powered, these are also considered an example of an active humidifier.

## NONVOLATILE GAS DELIVERY

The most commonly used nonvolatile gas for anesthesiology is nitrous oxide, which has a high vapor pressure and low boiling point.[2,4] As a result, it is in gaseous form at room temperature and is directly administered in its gaseous state.

## REFERENCES

1. Butterworth JF IV, et al. The anesthesia workstation. In: Butterworth JF IV, et al., eds. Morgan & Mikhail's Clinical Anesthesiology. 6th ed. New York, NY: McGraw-Hill Education; 2018: Chap. 4.
2. Chakravarti S, Basu S. Modern anaesthesia vapourisers. *Indian J Anaesth*. 2013;57:464–471.
3. McNulty G, Eyre L. Humidification in anaesthesia and critical care. *BJA Education*. 2015;15:131–135.
4. Covarrubias M, et al. Mechanistic insights into the modulation of voltage-gated ion channels by inhalational anesthetics. *Biophys J*. 2015;109:2003–2011.

# 11.

# ELECTRICAL, FIRE, AND EXPLOSION HAZARDS

*Suleman Sheikh and Stacey Watt*

## SURGICAL FIRES AND EXPLOSIVE SAFETY IN THE OPERATING ROOM

### INTRODUCTION

The term *surgical fires* is used to describe fires that occur on the patient's body surface or internal organ.[1,2] More specifically, the term *airway fires* denotes flames in the patient's airway or external respiratory devices. High-risk procedures are considered those with enriched oxygen, most commonly localized in the head, neck, and upper trunk regions.[1] In the operating room (OR), these three components are considered to be provided by the patient (ignition), surgeon (heat), and anesthesiologist (oxygen), respectively (Figure 11.1).[2]

### IGNITION SOURCES

Ignition sources include direct patient-related factors and indirect patient-related factors. Direct patient-related sources include body parts with increased flammability (hair, skin, gastrointestinal tract gases). Precautions include hair removal, application of nonflammable gel, and decreasing fermented gases (e.g., methane and hydrogen) in the colon by preoperatively administering bowel preparations. Indirect patient-related sources include drapes, sponges, gauze, sterile preparations, endotracheal tubes, nasal cannulas, wires, and endoscopes. Precautions include applying drapes to prevent pockets that allow pooled oxygen, saline-soaking sponges and gauzes, and allowing volatile sterile preparations time to dry.[2] Airway devices are difficult to take precaution against as they are necessary during procedures; however, when appropriate the use of metal tubes or a nonflammable laryngeal tube may be helpful.[3,4]

### HEAT SOURCES

Heat-related sources provided by the surgeon are cautery devices, including the laser, Bovie, and fiber-optic light; cord drills/high-speed burrs; and defibrillators. Laser beams transmit energy of specific wavelengths that is absorbed by the tissue. Shorter lasers transmit higher energy, which thus increases the risk of fires or explosions when in contact with endotracheal tubes, drapes, and sponges. Notably, laser light can be reflected by equipment in the OR. Thus, it is important to monitor the path of a laser as laser contact

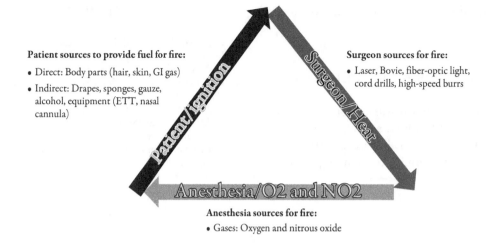

Patient sources to provide fuel for fire:
• Direct: Body parts (hair, skin, GI gas)
• Indirect: Drapes, sponges, gauze, alcohol, equipment (ETT, nasal cannula)

Surgeon sources for fire:
• Laser, Bovie, fiber-optic light, cord drills, high-speed burrs

Anesthesia sources for fire:
• Gases: Oxygen and nitrous oxide

Figure 11.1 Risks in the operating room. ETT, endotracheal tube; GI, gastrointestinal.

could be made with the eyes. Induced pneumothorax after laryngeal surgery has also been reported.[5]

## OXYGEN AND NITROUS OXIDE

Room air is composed of 78% nitrogen and 21% oxygen. It is important to note a threshold as low as 16% oxygen concentration is needed to spontaneously combust patient-related fuel sources. Preprocedural factors to be considered include patient selection and if a nasal cannula or air blender would suffice. If increased oxygen is required, the delivery of the lowest fraction of inspired oxygen necessary (goal maximum 30% $O_2$) is important. Securing the airway properly can prevent the escape of oxygen into the atmosphere. In high-risk procedures, temporarily decreasing $O_2$ delivery and negating the use of nitrous oxide and using a cuffed tracheal tube filled with saline as opposed to air are beneficial.[2]

## MANAGEMENT

In the event an OR fire does occur, management equipment includes sterile saline, $CO_2$ fire extinguisher, rigid laryngoscopes, extra drapes, and backup external respiratory devices/tubes that can be used to replace the airway circuit. With an airway fire, management includes removal of the tracheal tube and cessation of all gases, removal of direct/indirect patient-related sources from the airway, followed by pouring saline into the airway. For nonairway fires, management includes stopping the flow of all gases, removal of all patient-related sources, and extinguishing all items on fire with saline or water or covering the flames. If the fire is not extinguished despite these actions, using a fire extinguisher followed by activation of the fire alarm, evacuation, and OR door closure are appropriate. If the fire is extinguished by the initial management steps, then airway ventilation should be reestablished/maintained and the airway examined for inhalation injury.[2]

## ELECTRICAL SAFETY IN THE OPERATING ROOM

### INTRODUCTION

An electric shock occurs when a current passes through the body that comes in contact with the electrical circuit loop system. The effect depends on the impedance and strength of the current. The strength of the current is measured as a macroshock (milliamperes) or microshock (microamperes). Macroshocks cause respiratory paralysis, prolonged muscular contraction, and ventricular fibrillation. Microshocks occur in patients with an external conduit in direct contact with the body. Therefore, such patients are more susceptible because microshocks can lead to cardiac dysarrthymias. Modern day electrical engineering has minimized the risk of electrical shock in the OR through the concepts of grounding and isolation transformers.[3]

### PREVENTION: GROUNDING, ISOLATION TRANSFORMERS

The concept of grounding can be applied to both electrical power and equipment. In electrical power, the term *grounding* refers to an electrical supply that has a "hot" wire that delivers the voltage (~120 V) and a "neutral" wire that connects to the ground (0 V), providing a current through a closed loop. When an individual contacts the current and acts as the connection to the ground, they complete this circuit and receive a shock. Contrastingly, ungrounded electrical power has no connection to the earth. Electrical equipment is generally ungrounded or grounded. In the OR, electrical equipment is grounded, and the electrical power is ungrounded. This minimizes the risk of electrical shock by preventing a person in contact with the circuit acting as the closed-loop connection to the ground. This ungrounded electrical power supplying grounded electrical equipment is done through an isolation transformer. With an isolation transformer, there is a gap or indirect connection in power from the ground, making it ungrounded. This prevents macroshocks in the OR.[3]

## REFERENCES

1. Bruley ME, et al. Surgical fires: decreasing incidence relies on continued prevention efforts. *Pa Patient Saf Advis.* 2018;15(2):1–12.

2. Apfelbaum JL. Task Force on Operating Room Fires. Practice advisory for the prevention and management of operating room fires: an updated report by the American Society of Anesthesiologists Task Force on Operating Room Fires. *Anesthesiology.* 2013;118(2):271–290.

3. Ehrenwerth J. Electrical and fire safety. In: Barash PG, et al., eds. *Clinical Anesthesia.* 8th ed. Wolters Kluwer; 2017:109–140.

4. Jones TS, et al. Operating room fires. *Anesthesiology.* 2019;130(3):492–501.

5. Levin PR, et al. The burned patient, laser surgery and operating room fires. In: Duke J, Keech B, eds. *Anesthesia Secrets.* 5th ed. Saunders/Elsevier; 2016:330–339.

# Part 3

# ANESTHESIA PROCEDURES, METHODS, AND TECHNIQUES

# Part 4

# 12.

# CONTROLLED HYPOTENSION

*Anthony Alexander and Feodor J. Gloss*

## INTRODUCTION

Controlled hypotension is the deliberate reduction of arterial blood pressure during the conduct of anesthesia. This technique is useful in various types of surgical procedures, including neurosurgical, aneurysm, middle ear, endoscopic sinus, orthognathic, urologic, and orthopedic procedures. In these surgeries, the use of controlled hypotension aims to reduce operative blood loss and improve visibility in the surgical field.[1]

## TARGET BLOOD PRESSURE

While there are normal blood pressures for patient groups based on age, the definition of hypotension is not absolute. Allowable hypotension must take the patient's baseline blood pressure and associated comorbidities into account. Sources define target blood pressure as a reduction of systolic blood pressure to 80–90 mm Hg, mean arterial pressure (MAP) to 50–65 mm Hg, or a 30% reduction of MAP from baseline.[2] Even at these low blood pressures, adequate perfusion to vital organs is maintained by organ microcirculatory autoregulation.

## BENEFITS OF CONTROLLED HYPOTENSION

Improving the quality of the operative field and reducing perioperative blood loss are the two main benefits for controlled hypotension. The quality of the operative field is a difficult endpoint to quantify objectively, and as such, high-quality evidence proving this as a benefit is lacking. However, the studies that do exist demonstrated improved operative field quality in tympanoplasty, mandibular osteotomy, and endoscopic sinus surgery.[2,3] There are also studies that showed that controlled hypotension also reduced intraoperative blood loss.[2] This decreases the need for allogenic transfusion and potentially the attendant risks of transfusion-associated lung injury, hemolytic and nonhemolytic transfusion reactions, infection, and other complications.

## RISKS OF CONTROLLED HYPOTENSION

Hypotension of any etiology carries with it the concern for end-organ hypoperfusion. Early studies that focused on the effects of controlled hypotension on the myocardial, renal, hepatic, splanchnic, and cerebral microcirculations failed to demonstrate increased morbidity.[3,4] At the same time, it is intuitive that patients with conditions that place them at increased risk for ischemia secondary to prolonged hypotension are less suitable candidates for this technique. Thorough preoperative evaluation enables the provider to perform a complete risk-benefit assessment and to modify the technique based the patient's particular risk for ischemic complications.

**Possible Contraindications to Controlled Hypotension:** The contraindications to controlled hypotension include cerebrovascular disease, ischemic heart disease, severe valvular heart disease, renal vascular disease, peripheral vascular disease, and hepatic dysfunction.

## INTRAOPERATIVE MONITORING

Close monitoring of arterial blood pressure is essential to reduce the risk of complications from end-organ hypoperfusion. This may be achieved by the placement of an arterial catheter to provide beat-to-beat blood pressure monitoring. The arterial catheter also serves the secondary function of allowing blood draws to monitor for metabolic acidosis and elevated lactate, which are evidence of poor tissue perfusion.[5] Attention should be paid to the position of the transducer in patients in head-up positions. The transducer in those cases should be leveled at the tragus, which corresponds to the level of the Circle of Willis, to avoid inadvertently low cerebral perfusion pressures.

## METHODS OF ACHIEVING CONTROLLED HYPOTENSION

### PHYSICAL AND VENTILATORY METHODS

In surgeries of the head and neck, a reverse Trendelenburg position may be used to reduce venous pressure at the surgical site, thereby reducing bleeding. Reverse Trendelenburg position also causes venous pooling in the lower extremities, reducing venous return, cardiac output, and blood pressure. By causing hypocapnia and vasoconstriction, hyperventilation is another technique that may reduce blood flow to the surgical field.

### PHARMACOLOGICAL METHODS

#### Neuraxial Anesthesia

Spinal and epidural anesthesia induce sympathetic blockade. This causes peripheral vasodilation, reduced venous return, and hypotension. This technique is limited to use in abdominal and lower extremity procedures. As an additional limitation, the amount of hypotension produced can be difficult to control and may require starting a low-dose epinephrine infusion.[3]

#### Volatile Anesthetics

Inhalational anesthetics such as isoflurane, desflurane, and sevoflurane produce peripheral vasodilation but only mild hypotension at clinical doses. Adjuvant hypotensive agents are therefore required to produce adequate hypotension while reducing the risk of toxicity from higher doses of inhalational agents.[4]

#### Remifentanil

Remifentanil is a potent μ-opioid analgesic with established use in total intravenous anesthesia. It has a rapid onset and short elimination half-life. An adverse effect of remifentanil is hypotension, which can be used in combination with propofol and sevoflurane to produce effective controlled hypotension. This combination is as effective as nitroprusside and esmolol[2] without the added risk of a potent hypotensive agent. Use of other opioids, such as sufentanil and alfentanil, is less ideal due to their longer context-sensitive half-times.

### Calcium Channel Blockers

Nicardipine is a dihydropyridine calcium antagonist that inhibits the entry of calcium into vascular smooth muscle cells, causing vasodilation. Diltiazem has also been used as an adjunct in spine surgery and achieves hypotension by negative chromotropic and dromotropic effects.

### Vasodilators

Sodium nitroprusside produces rapid and reversible venous and arterial dilation. The mechanism is through increased nitric oxide production, which induces guanylate cyclase activity, leading to the production of cyclic guanosine monophosphate (cGMP). It has hemodynamic disadvantages, including reflex tachycardia via the baroreceptor mechanism, myocardial ischemia, and rebound hypertension. Tachycardia may be blunted with adjunctive use of a β-blocker such as esmolol.[1] Prolonged and high-dose infusions may produce tachyphylaxis and cyanide toxicity. Raised intracranial pressure, increased shunt fractions, and platelet dysfunction are also known complications. Nitroglycerin is a less-potent option that primarily causes dilation of the venous capacitance vessels, decreased venous return, and proportionally decreased cardiac output. Unlike nitroprusside, it has no toxic metabolites, but doses greater than 5 mg/kg/d may produce methemoglobinemia.

### β-Blockers

Esmolol is the most useful drug in the β-blocker class. It is a short-acting, cardioselective β-blocker that reduces cardiac output by reducing heart rate. Reduction in plasma renin activity and catecholamine levels also results in decreased blood pressure. Esmolol may be used alone or in combination with other hypotensive agents at a dose of $100–330$ μg/kg/min. Use of labetalol is limited by its slower onset and time to peak concentration.

## REFERENCES

1. Barak M, et al. Hypotensive anesthesia versus normotensive anesthesia during major maxillofacial surgery: a review of the literature. *Scientific World Journal*. 2015;2015:480728.
2. Choi W, Samman N. Risks and benefits of deliberate hypotension in anaesthesia: a systematic review. *Int J Oral Maxillofac Surg*. 2008;48:687–703.
3. Degoute C-S Controlled hypotension: a guide to drug choice. *Drugs*. 2007;67(7):1053–1076.
4. Degoute C-S, et al. Remifentanil and controlled hypotension; comparison with nitroprusside or esmolol during tympanoplasty. *Can J Anesth*. 2001;48(1):20–27.
5. Dutton RP. Controlled hypotension for spinal surgery. *Eur Spine J*. 2004;13(suppl 1):66–71.

# 13.

# HYPERBARIC MEDICINE
## INDICATIONS FOR AND APPLICATION OF HYPERBARIC OXYGEN THERAPY

*Derek Brady Covington and Christopher Giordano*

## INTRODUCTION

Hyperbaric oxygen therapy (HBOT) is the medical use of oxygen at higher than atmospheric pressures. HBOT occurs in two different types of chambers: monoplace and multiplace. Monoplace chambers are pressurized with oxygen, treat a single patient at one time, and are relatively small in size and mobile. Multiplace chambers are pressurized with air (while the patients receive oxygen via face mask, endotracheal tube, or hood); treat multiple patients (or critically injured patients requiring ventilation or intravenous medications via infusion pumps); and are relatively large in size and nonmobile. Notably, an inside tender called a hyperbaric technician, or healthcare provider trained in hyperbaric medicine, accompanies patients into multiplace chambers, while no tender is inside a monoplace chamber. Thus, if a patient requires emergent medical attention, the treatment session in a monoplace chamber must be aborted, while a treatment session in a multiplace chamber may continue depending on the judgment of the supervising physician. Treatments can vary from 2 hours to more than 6 hours depending on the treatment indication.

## MECHANISMS

Along with the hyperoxygenation that occurs when increased pressure dissolves additional oxygen into the plasma, HBOT induces several additional therapies via alternative mechanisms of action.

The following underlying mechanisms are involved in the treatment effects of HBOT[1]:

1. Hyperoxygenation
2. Vasoconstriction
3. Angiogenesis
4. Fibroblast proliferation
5. Antibiotic synergy
6. Increased erythrocyte deformability
7. Reduced leukocyte adherence to vascular tissue and reduced postischemic vasoconstriction
8. Reduced lipid peroxidation following carbon monoxide poisoning
9. Limited postischemic reductions in adenosine triphosphate (ATP) production and decreased lactate accumulation in ischemic tissue

## INDICATIONS

There are 14 indications for HBOT supported by the Undersea and Hyperbaric Medicine Society (UHMS) and reimbursed by the Centers for Medicare and Medicaid Services (CMS).[2] The most commonly encountered indications that may require the aid of an anesthesiologist are severe decompression sickness, arterial gas embolism (AGE), carbon monoxide poisoning, intracranial abscess, and severe anemia. The 14 conditions are as follows[2]:

1. Acute traumatic peripheral ischemia
2. Crush injuries and suturing of severed limbs (acute)
3. Acute peripheral arterial insufficiency
4. Compromised skin grafts (acute)
5. Osteoradionecrosis
6. Soft tissue radionecrosis
7. Gas gangrene (acute)
8. Progressive necrotizing infections
9. Chronic refractory osteomyelitis
10. Chronic nonhealing wounds (diabetic and nondiabetic ulcers)
11. Carbon monoxide poisoning
12. Decompression sickness
13. Gas embolism
14. Idiopathic sudden sensorineural hearing loss

## CONTRAINDICATIONS AND COMPLICATIONS

The only contraindication to HBOT is an untreated pneumothorax because increased pressurization could exacerbate a pneumothorax as well as evolve it into a tension pneumothorax. Asthma and chronic obstructive pulmonary disease are relative contraindications and should be assessed with a thorough history and physical examination, as well as imaging studies such as a chest radiograph.

The most common complication secondary to HBOT is middle ear barotrauma or the inability to equalize the middle ear space with resultant otalgia. Although an oxygen-induced seizure may manifest secondary to central nervous system toxicity, these are exceedingly rare and often benign. The precise mechanism of hyperoxic seizures remains unclear; however, it appears to involve focal depolarization of oxygen toxicity trigger nuclei, which are subcortical areas of the brain with significant redox signaling mechanisms.[3] Simply decreasing the partial pressure of oxygen will abate the seizure, and once the patient is oriented, treatment can resume.

## CLINICAL APPLICATIONS

When treating a mechanically ventilated patient, it is imperative to consider the volume of the endotracheal cuff. In accordance with Boyle's law, as pressure increases, volume decreases. Thus, on pressurization of the chamber (also known as the descent phase), gas must be added to the endotracheal tube cuff to maintain an adequate seal on the tracheal mucosa. On depressurization (or the ascent phase), gas must be removed from the endotracheal tube cuff to prevent excessive expansion and damage to the trachea. The use of a manometer while adding or removing gas from the endotracheal tube facilitates the maintenance of proper cuff volume and subsequent seal. Boyle's law also explains the etiology of ear pain secondary to inadequate middle ear equalization and pressure on the tympanic membrane from ambient pressure exposure.

Arterial gas embolisms occur in aquatic environments; commercial construction zones, such as tunneling projects; and occasionally as medical complications at normobaric pressure. Iatrogenic AGEs may stem from neurological surgeries, such as sitting craniotomies or spinal surgeries that can compromise bridging veins during surgical dissections, laparoscopic surgeries, and endoscopies. They can also occur during the administration of intravenous fluids or blood products, especially when administered with pressure bags. These patients may develop rapid, severe neurologic signs and should be treated with HBOT as soon as possible. Although HBOT was traditionally thought of as "shrinking" the size of these gas bubbles and minimizing downstream blood flow obstruction, more recent evidence suggests that the majority of gases are rapidly removed from the bloodstream. Subsequent HBOT minimizes the inflammation secondary to vascular endothelial disruption and edema.

If critically injured patients require HBOT, it is imperative that ventilators, syringe pumps, and all other medical devices are safe for hyperbaric oxygen. Often, these devices feature brushless motors to reduce the risk of spark; the manufacturer has certified them as safe for hyperbarics.

## REFERENCES

1. Gill AL, Bell CAN. Hyperbaric oxygen: its uses, mechanisms of action and outcomes. *QJM*. 2004;97:385–395.
2. Moon R, ed. *Hyperbaric Oxygen Therapy Indications*. 14th ed. Best Publishing; 2018.
3. Ciarlone GE, et al. CNS function and dysfunction during exposure to hyperbaric oxygen in operational and clinical settings. *Redox Biol*. 2019;27:101159.

# 14.

# HIGH-ALTITUDE ANESTHESIA

*Mark Dearden*

## INTRODUCTION

Issues related to high-altitude anesthesia fall into two categories: physiologic effects and issues related to the function of anesthesia equipment. As altitude increases, several environmental factors exert effects. These may include colder temperatures, increased ultraviolet light, and the remoteness and isolation of austere environments. But, the most critical factor is hypoxia. Total pressure exerted by the atmosphere (barometric pressure, $P_B$) is the sum of the combined pressure of all constituent gases and amounts to approximately 760 mm Hg at sea level. Oxygen makes up approximately 21% of atmospheric gas, with nitrogen making up most of the rest. The $PO_2$ of oxygen at sea level is about 159 mm Hg. With rising altitudes, atmospheric pressure drops and with it the content of atmospheric gas. The proportion of oxygen within the mixture remains constant. However, because the $P_B$ is lower, the $PO_2$ along with the partial pressures of other gases drop proportionally. At 8000 feet, the $PO_2$ is 120 mm Hg, and at top of Mount Everest (29,000 ft) it drops to about 33% of sea-level values (Figure 14.1).[1-3] Hypobaric hypoxia has deleterious and possibly fatal effects on human physiology. Compensatory physiologic changes should be recognized and understood. Likewise, some anesthesia equipment will malfunction at altitude if not appropriately compensated.

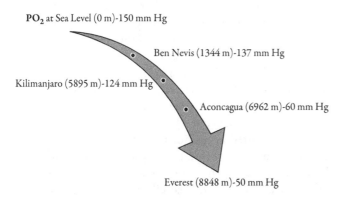

$PO_2$ at Sea Level (0 m)-150 mm Hg

Ben Nevis (1344 m)-137 mm Hg

Kilimanjaro (5895 m)-124 mm Hg

Aconcagua (6962 m)-60 mm Hg

Everest (8848 m)-50 mm Hg

**Figure 14.1** $PO_2$ changes with altitude.

## CLINICAL FEATURES

Because the body requires oxygen to metabolize, shortages cause significant morbidity and stimulate compensatory mechanisms. With acute exposure, peripheral arterial chemoreceptors (normally suppressed by central $CO_2$ receptors) detect low oxygen levels and stimulate responses within the cardiovascular, respiratory, renal, and hematopoietic systems. Acutely, sympathetic stimulation causes increased heart rate and increasing cardiac output. Vasodilation, which is seen at altitude, is antagonized by increased sympathetic tone, resulting in increased blood pressure (BP), which can persist for several weeks. Over the first several days, hematopoiesis increases, raising hemoglobin. However, increased oxygen-carrying capacity may be offset by increased blood viscosity and result in little improvement in tissue oxygenation. Increased blood cell count and a nearly 20% drop in plasma volume account for the higher viscosity. Reduced $PaO_2$ at the peripheral chemoreceptors also produces ventilatory changes. There is a rapid increase in minute ventilation, leading to an increased $PAO_2$ and decreased $PaCO_2$ (see Figure 14.2). Hypocapnia causes a left shift in the oxygen-hemoglobin dissociation curve, aiding $O_2$ loading in the lungs but limiting unloading at the tissues. This shift is opposed by an increase in 2,3-diphosphoglycerate (2,3-DPG) that occurs over several days. Respiratory alkalosis is partially compensated by renal excretion of bicarbonate.[1-3]

## DIAGNOSIS

Altitude illness can present in several ways and should be ruled out prior to settling on other diagnoses with similar presentations. Acute mountain sickness (AMS) usually onsets between 4 and 12 hours after ascent. It is characterized by headache, nausea, anorexia, fatigue, sleep disturbance, and dizziness. Susceptibility is independent of physical fitness. Proposed etiologies include brain swelling caused by increased cerebral blood flow combined with changes to blood-brain barrier permeability.[1] The most severe form of

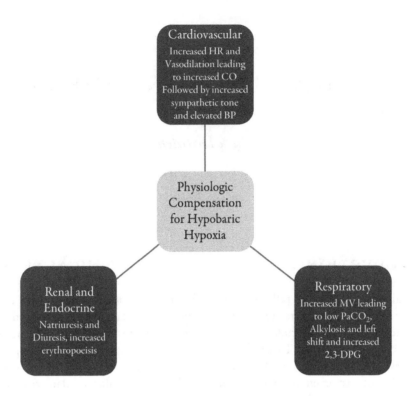

**Figure 14.2** Compensation for hypoxia. CO, cardiac output; HR, heart rate; PaCO$_2$, arterial partial pressure of carbon dioxide.

AMS is high-altitude cerebral edema (HACE). It can be differentiated from AMS by the presence of ataxia, confusion, altered consciousness, or psychiatric symptoms. On magnetic resonance imaging, HACE shows not only cerebral edema, but also microhemorrhages. HACE is life threatening. High-altitude pulmonary edema (HAPE) is noncardiogenic pulmonary edema with an incidence that rises with elevation and faster ascent. Exertional dyspnea and dry cough are hallmarks. The cough may become productive of pink frothy sputum. Radiography shows patchy edema. Unless the patient is descended, HAPE can also be fatal.

## ANESTHETIC CONSIDERATIONS

### PREOPERATIVE

The most effective treatment for all types of AMS is descent from altitude. Strong consideration should be given to delaying any surgery that is not life or limb sparing until the patient can be moved to a lower elevation. Increased ventilatory drive is an important compensatory mechanism, and premedications that decrease ventilatory drive should be used with caution. Ketamine seems to be an appropriate medication given both its minimal respiratory depression and minimal interference with pharyngeal and laryngeal reflexes. Supplemental O$_2$ in the preoperative period is beneficial for compensating for atmospheric changes. Gastric emptying is delayed at altitude, and a rapid-sequence induction is appropriate if general anesthesia is planned.

### INTRAOPERATIVE

Higher than typical levels of inspired O$_2$ should be maintained throughout the intra- and postoperative period. It has been suggested that at 5000 feet the fraction of inspired oxygen should be at least 30% and 40% at 10,000 feet.[2] The issue may be further complicated by uncalibrated flowmeters. Spinning bobbin flowmeters rely on gas density, which is altered at altitude. Variations in flow may reach up to 20% at 10,000 feet.

As total P$_B$ decreases, the anesthetic power of nitrous oxide wanes to roughly 50% at 5000 feet and becomes almost insignificant at 10,000.[2] Anesthetic gas partial pressure (mm Hg), rather than concentration, correlates with anesthetic effects. Modern standard vaporizers are agent specific, temperature compensated, and variable bypass (isoflurane, sevoflurane, enflurane). Their design ensures partial pressures are unaffected by altitude, resulting in unchanged gas delivery. For example, if the atmospheric pressure is half its sea-level value (380 vs. 760 mm Hg), the same number of anesthetic gas molecules will create a higher concentration of anesthetic gas vapor in the vaporizing chamber. However, the partial pressure remains unchanged. A vaporizer that put out 2% isoflurane, for example, now puts out 4%, but the partial pressure (i.e., the dose measured in millimeters of mercury) is the same (2% × 760 mm Hg = 15.2 mm Hg = 4% × 380 mm Hg). Therefore, no compensation is needed. The dial reading will be inaccurate, but the gas effect will be preserved as if it were accurate.

A desflurane vaporizer is different. The pressure in the vaporizing chamber is held constant at 2 atm and is independent of ambient pressure. So, a vaporizer that produces 5% desflurane at sea level will also produce 5% desflurane at altitude—into less atmospheric pressure—reducing partial pressure and underdosing the patient. Close attention to depth of anesthesia is important when choosing a gas technique.

Total intravenous anesthesia with ketamine, propofol, or some combination is effective and is nearly unaffected by altitude.[4] Likewise, regional anesthesia shows few effects owing to elevation changes and is recommended for procedures involving the extremities.

## POSTOPERATIVE

Patients should be monitored closely in the postoperative period for worsening AMS and provided with adequate supplemental oxygen. Delayed recovery from general anesthesia has been reported and may be difficult to distinguish from central nervous system signs of worsening AMS.[4] Aeromedical evacuation is becoming more common. Air-filled spaces will expand with the rapid ascent experienced during takeoff. Unvented pneumothorax, pneumoperitoneum, pneumocephalus, and bowel gas will all expand, possibly to dangerous levels. Air bubbles in intravenous lines and tracheal cuffs should also be monitored. Moving quickly from sea level to 18,000 feet will double the volume of trapped gas.[3]

## REFERENCES

1. Bartsch P, Swenson E. Acute high-altitude illness. *N Engl J Med.* 2013;368(24):2294–2302.
2. Bosco G, Comporesi E. Anesthesia at high altitude. In: Ehrenwerth J, et al., eds. *Anesthesia Equipment Principles and Applications.* 2nd ed. Elsevier; 2013;570–580.
3. Cumpstey AF, et al. Clinical care in extreme environments: physiology at high altitude and in space. In: Gropper MA, ed. *Miller's Anesthesia.* 9th ed. Elsevier; 2019:2313–2337.
4. Xu R, et al. Total intravenous anesthesia produces outcomes superior to those with combined intravenous–inhalation anesthesia for laparoscopic gynecological surgery at high altitude. *J Int Med Res.* 2017;45(I):246–253.

# Part 4

# NERVOUS SYSTEM

# 15.

# CENTRAL AND PERIPHERAL NERVOUS SYSTEMS

*Syed Sohaib Nasim and Steven Minear*

## INTRODUCTION

The brain is organized into the cerebrum, diencephalon, brainstem, and cerebellum. The corpus callosum connects the left and right cerebrum.[1] The cerebral cortex has four lobes: frontal, parietal, temporal, and occipital.[1-4] The lateral sulcus separates the temporal lobe from the parietal and frontal lobes. The central sulcus divides the frontal and parietal lobes. The occipital lobe is posterior, and the parieto-occipital sulcus separates the parietal and temporal lobes.[4]

The temporal lobe performs primary auditory and somatosensation. The primary somatosensory cortex processes touch, pressure, pain, vibration, movement, and position. The frontal lobe processes motor information.[4] The primary motor cortex sends signals to the spinal cord for skeletal muscle movement. The frontal lobe also contains Broca's area, typically on the left, and is responsible for language. The prefrontal lobe is a cognitive center of the brain.[4]

Subcortical nuclei coordinate cortical processes. The amygdala and hippocampus modulate long-term memory. The basal nuclei include the caudate, putamen, and globus pallidus.[4] The globus pallidus contains two pathways: the direct and indirect, which disinhibits or does not excite the thalamus, respectively. The substantia nigra pars compacta produces dopamine, activating the direct and inhibiting the indirect pathway.[2,4]

The diencephalon is located beneath the cerebrum, forming the wall of the third ventricle. It consists of thalamus (relays information to and from the cerebral cortex) and hypothalamus (regulates body temperature).[1,4] The brainstem is composed of midbrain and hindbrain (pons and medulla). It is located in the ventral surface of the forebrain, connects the brain and spinal cord, and acts as a coordination center. The midbrain coordinates visual, auditory, and somatosensory information, while the pons serves as a bridge to the cerebellum.[1,4] Passing through the center of the midbrain is the cerebral aqueduct, forming the tectum and tegmentum. The tectum contains four colliculi, inferior colliculus, and superior colliculus. The inferior colliculus relays auditory signals to the thalamus. The superior colliculus is responsible for combining sensory signals, and it orients eyes to sound or touch. The tegmentum contains nuclei that communicate with the cranial nerves.[1]

The pons connects the brainstem to the cerebellum; is responsible for receiving information from the sensory system, brain, spinal cord; and regulates motor movements.[1,4] The medulla is responsible for processing information from cranial nerves. The reticular formation regulates sleep and wakefulness.[4]

Cerebral blood flow (CBF) is composed of anterior circulation from the carotid arteries and posterior circulation from the vertebral arteries, which combine to form the basilar artery.[2] The basilar artery connects with the internal carotid arteries to form the circle of Willis. The anterior and posterior communication arteries complete the loop. This circle generates branches: the anterior, middle, and posterior cerebral arteries. Superficial cortical veins drain into dural sinuses, which drain into the internal jugular veins.[2]

Autoregulation of CBF is well developed. In normal adults, cerebral blood flow is about 50 mL per 100 g of brain tissue per minute, assuming the cerebral perfusion pressure (CPP) is between 60 and 160 mm HG. If the CPP is outside this range, then CBF becomes dependent on mean arterial pressure. If the perfusion pressure falls below 60 mm Hg, cerebral ischemia often occurs.[2]

Cerebral blood flow is dependent on $PaCO_2$: For every 1 mm Hg increase in $PaCO_2$, CBF increases 1–2 mL/100 g/min for $PaCO_2$ levels greater than 25 mm Hg.[2] CBF does NOT change with changes in $PaO_2$ between 60 and 300 mm Hg. If the $PaO_2$ decreases below 60 mm Hg, there is a sharp increase in CBF due to cerebral vasodilation.[2]

## CEREBRAL METABOLIC RATE

The cerebral metabolic rate increases with neuronal activity. The increase in brain metabolism increases CBF, known as flow-metabolism coupling. Mechanistically, glutamate is released, which results in synthesis of nitric oxide, leading to vasodilation.[2]

## CEREBROSPINAL FLUID

Cerebrospinal fluid (CSF) is produced by choroid plexuses in the lateral and fourth ventricles, provides a cushion, and serves as an excretion pathway. The adult makes 150 mL/d of CSF, and it is absorbed in the arachnoid villi. The fluid consists of 15 to 45 mg/dL protein and 50–80 mg/dL glucose. A normal CSF pressure is 100–180 mm $H_2O$ lying on the side and 200–300 mm $H_2O$ sitting.[2]

Acute system respiratory acidosis does not immediately affect the CSF because hydrogen ions are excluded by the blood-brain barrier (BBB).[3] With rapid changes in $PaCO_2$, the CBF changes; however, it is not sustained, and CBF returns to normal over 6–8 hours.[3] Over this time, the CSF extrudes bicarbonate and returns to normal levels. With hyperventilation, a decrease in $PaCO_2$ results in an increase in CSF pH, while CBF decreases. However, both CSF pH and CBF return to normal in 8 to 12 hours.[3]

## BLOOD-BRAIN BARRIER

In the brain, the endothelial cells contain tight junctions and form the BBB. The BBB maintains homeostasis and allows specific molecules to pass.[2] Due to lipid solubility, lipophilic compounds pass through more easily than hydrophilic compounds. Glucose and amino acids enter endothelial cells via transporters, while proteins use receptor-mediated processes to cross the BBB. The BBB can be disrupted by stroke, infections, metabolic disorders, demyelination, degenerative disease, trauma, and some tumors.[2]

## THE SPINAL CORD

The spinal cord extends from the medulla to the lumbar region, with sensory axons entering posteriorly (ascending tracts) in the vertebral column and motor axons entering anteriorly (descending tracts) in the vertebral column.[5] The ascending tracts carry information for tactile (spinotectal), vibration (dorsal column), pain (lateral spinothalamic), and pressure (ventral spinothalamic). The descending tracts carry information for posture, balance, and tone from different areas. The spinal cord itself terminates as the cauda equine.[5]

The spinal arc reflex is controlled by the spinal cord and ends at the peripheral effector. The reflexes are either monosynaptic or polysynaptic.[5] Monosynaptic reflexes are found in musculoskeletal reflexes: biceps brachii (C5, C6); triceps brachii (C6, C7, C8); brachoradialis (C5, C6, C7); quadriceps femoris (L2, L3, L4); and triceps surae (S1, S2).[5] Alternatively, polysynaptic reflexes have one or more interneurons involved. An example is the withdrawal reflex that moves away multiple muscle groups when touching a hot pan.[5]

## REFERENCES

1. Ludwig PE, et al. Neuroanatomy, central nervous system (CNS). In: *StatPearls*. Treasure Island, FL: StatPearls Publishing; August 10, 2020.
2. Miller RD, ed. *Miller's Anesthesia*. 8th ed. Philadelphia, PA: Churchill/Livingstone; 2015:387–419.
3. Miller RD. *Miller's Anesthesia*. 8th ed. Philadelphia, PA: Churchill/Livingstone; 2015:2158–2196.
4. Thau L, et al. Anatomy, central nervous system. In: *StatPearls*. Treasure Island, FL: StatPearls Publishing; May 24, 2020.
5. Harrow-Mortelliti M, et al. Physiology, spinal cord. In: *StatPearls*. Treasure Island, FL: StatPearls Publishing; April 5, 2020.

# 16.

# DRUG METABOLISM

*Theodore Jeske and Nebojsa Nick Knezevic*

## INTRODUCTION

Every time your patient receives a drug, a complex process occurs. ADME (absorption, distribution, metabolism, and excretion) of a particular drug will provide vital information for the treatment of your patients.[1]

## LIVER

Metabolism (or biotransformation) is most often dependent on the liver. *Bioavailability* represents the fraction of the dose of active drug that reaches the systemic circulation and is dependent on *first-pass metabolism* in the liver. This occurs when a drug is enterally-administered, relying on the absorption from the gastrointestinal tract (via the portal vein) to the liver. For parenterally-administered drugs, this process does not occur, and bioavailability is often considered to be 1, or 100%. Regardless of the administration route, metabolism in the liver is often vital.

In general, metabolism in the liver transforms an active drug (nonpolar) into inactive drug/metabolites (more polar), which are more easily excreted via the kidneys. There are exceptions to this general course (e.g., prodrug activation and production of certain active toxic metabolites via the liver). For example, enalapril requires hepatic biotransformation to an active metabolite, enalaprilat. An example of toxic metabolite production via hepatic biotransformation exists with acetaminophen's toxic metabolite N-acetyl-*p*-benzoquinone imine (NAPQI), which requires conjugation with reduced glutathione to be inactivated.

## TWO PHASES OF METABOLISM IN THE LIVER

### Phase 1: Microsomal Oxidation of Drugs (Main Route for Most Drugs)

Microsomes from the liver's smooth endoplasmic reticulum contain a family of enzymes consisting of mixed-function oxidases or cytochrome P450 (CYP450) isozymes, which can oxidize a variety of drugs.

Examples of reactions catalyzed by the mixed-function oxidases (CYPs) include side-chain oxidation, hydroxylation, N-oxidation, sulfoxidation, and N-dealkylation. Ultimately, the goal is to deactivate most drugs to a more polar and easily excretable form.

**CYP Induction/Inhibition:** Furthermore, currently active or coadministered drugs may have induction or inhibiting properties on CYP450 enzymes (most notably CYP3A4 and CYP2D6). For example, if your patient is taking a drug that inhibits CYP2D6 (e.g., paroxetine, fluoxetine, quinidine, etc.), which is needed for metabolism of a drug that you are about to administer (e.g., β-blocker such as metoprolol), this may result in toxic buildup of the mentioned drug (in this example, a dangerous bradycardia if dosing was improperly adjusted).

**Single-Nucleotide Polymorphisms:** Single-nucleotide polymorphisms (SNPs) can also play a role in both phase 1 and phase 2 reactions, resulting in a more rapid or slower metabolism depending on your patient's genetic profile.

Several SNPs may occur in select patients for CYP2D6, often resulting in reduced functionality and producing either a lack of therapeutic effect (e.g., codeine to morphine) or toxic buildup at normal doses (e.g., venlafaxine, tricyclic antidepressants, β-blockers). Conversely, ultrarapid CYP2D6 metabolizers may have a shorter duration of action of various drugs or excessive production of active metabolites (e.g., codeine to morphine).

A common SNP occurs with *N*-acetyltransferase 2 (*NAT2*), which is an enzyme involved in phase 2 metabolism. Slow metabolizers with a less functional NAT2 experience a toxic buildup of drugs metabolized via this pathway (e.g., hydralazine, isoniazid, procaine amides, and various sulfa drugs).

### Phase 2: Conjugation Reactions

Conjugation reactions in phase 2 involve the coupling of drugs or metabolites to small polar molecules. Examples of

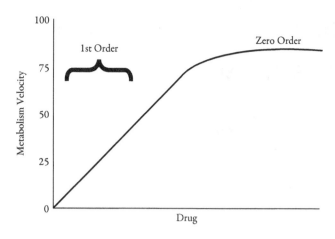

Figure 16.1

phase 2 conjugation reactions include glucuronide conjugation, sulfate conjugation, and *N*-acetylation.

## KINETICS OF DRUG METABOLISM

### FIRST-ORDER KINETICS (*SATURABLE* ELIMINATION KINETICS): LINEAR

With first-order metabolism, a constant *fraction* of the drug is eliminated per unit time, and the actual amount eliminated is dependent on the drug's plasma concentration. The $t_{1/2}$ *is constant* in first-order kinetics: There is a constant fraction of drug eliminated per unit time; more drug present results in more drug eliminated since 50% is metabolized per half-life.

A *linear* relationship exists in first-order kinetics between clearance and plasma drug concentration as well as between dosing rate and steady-state drug concentration. For example, when the dose is doubled, plasma drug concentration at steady state will double because the metabolism also doubles. Plasma drug concentration directly drives the rate of metabolism.

Most drugs initially undergo first-order metabolism; however, first order has *saturable* elimination kinetics (Figure 16.1). For any drug undergoing first-order metabolism, if a high enough drug concentration is present, transporters and enzymes involved in this process will become saturated, and metabolism then relies on zero-order kinetics.

### ZERO-ORDER KINETICS (CAPACITY-LIMITED ELIMINATION KINETICS): NONLINEAR

With zero-order kinetics, the rate of metabolism is constant and does not depend on the concentration of the drug present. A constant *amount* of drug is eliminated per unit of time, with *zero* regard for the drug's plasma concentration. The fraction of drug eliminated (and $t_{1/2}$) is variable, whereas the amount eliminated is constant.

Thus, there is a *nonlinear* relationship between drug clearance and plasma drug concentration. For example, when the dose is increased by 20%, plasma drug concentration may increase by 100%. This is because the same amount of drug is eliminated per unit time regardless of plasma concentration. Therefore, $t_{1/2}$ *is not constant*: A constant *amount* of drug is eliminated per unit time regardless of drug concentration; however, the *fraction* eliminated is variable.

Zero-order kinetics is usually only relevant for certain drugs at therapeutic concentrations (e.g., phenytoin, high-dose aspirin, and ethanol typically undergo zero-order metabolism). However, at high enough concentrations, any drug that typically undergoes first-order kinetics will exhibit saturation of drug-metabolizing enzymes and/or transporters, and will switch to zero order (Figure 16.2).

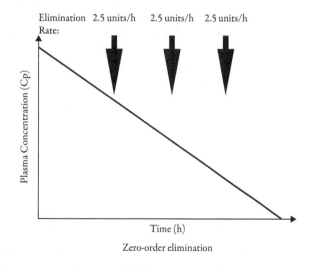

Zero-order elimination

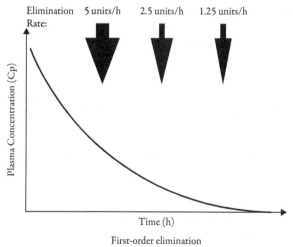

First-order elimination

Figure 16.2

## DRUG DOSING: SPECIAL CONSIDERATIONS IN ANESTHESIOLOGY

There are special considerations for drug dosing in anesthesiology[2]:

- When considering the two main classes of local anesthetics, it is important to remember that with amino*esters,* metabolism depends only on plasma esterases, whereas for amino*amides,* metabolism depends on the liver for biotransformation.
- For patients with either liver disease or kidney disease, the maintenance dose must be decreased, as reduced clearance ability warrants smaller doses that should be administered at longer intervals.
- For liver disease, a loading dose usually needs to be increased because patients tend to have an increased Vd (volume of distribution) due to *decreased albumin* production.
- For kidney disease patients, no change in loading dose is required; see the following formula:

$$\text{Loading Dose} = TC \times Vd \quad \text{Maintenance Dose} = TC \times CLp$$

TC, target concentration of drug at steady state; Vd, volume of distribution; and CLp, drug clearance from the plasma.

## REFERENCES

1. Correia MA. Drug biotransformation. In: Katzung BG, ed. *Katzung & Trevor Basic and Clinical Pharmacology.* 14th ed. McGraw-Hill Education; 2017: Chap. 4.
2. Kim TK. Basic principles of pharmacology. In: Gropper MA, et al., eds. *Miller's Anesthesia.* 9th ed. Elsevier; 2019: Chap. 24fs.

# 17.

# INTRACRANIAL PRESSURE

*John S. Shin and Timothy T. Bui*

## INTRODUCTION

Intracranial pressure (ICP) exerts a direct effect on cerebral perfusion pressure (CPP) as CPP is equal to the difference between the mean arterial pressure and the ICP. Thus, maintaining normal ICP is essential to ensuring adequate cerebral perfusion. Given that the skull volume is fixed, intracranial volume is then the main determinant of ICP.[1]

The four intracranial components that determine intracranial volume and by extension ICP are cells, intracellular and extracellular fluid, cerebrospinal fluid (CSF), and blood. The brain, comprising cells and the surrounding intracellular and extracellular fluid, makes up 80% of intracranial volume.[2] CSF and blood make up the other 8% and 12%, respectively.

The compliance of this system allows for small increases in volume without increasing ICP.[1] CSF can flow down the foramen magnum into the intrathecal space to decrease ICP, while cerebral vasoconstriction decreases the blood flow and volume to the brain.[1,3] After these compensatory mechanisms are exhausted, ICP increases exponentially with even small increases in intracerebral volume. The brain and fluid volumes are more or less fixed and require surgical and/or pharmacological intervention to decrease significantly.

Normal ICP is less than 10 mm Hg; a prolonged increase in ICP greater than 15 mm Hg can lead to irreversible ischemia by decreasing CPP.[2] Additionally, the increased pressure within a fixed volume can cause the brain to herniate across the meninges, downward through the foramen magnum, or through a craniotomy site if the skull is open.

## ANESTHETIC CONSIDERATIONS

### PREOPERATIVE

Preoperative evaluation is paramount to detecting symptoms associated with increased ICP. Symptoms such as headache, nausea/vomiting, altered mental status, somnolence, neck rigidity, or papilledema are potential clinical manifestations of increased ICP.[1]

Radiological findings of increased ICP include midline shift, obliteration of the basal cisterns, loss of sulci, ventricular enlargement or effacement, and parenchymal edema.[1]

Administration of steroids beginning 48–72 hours before surgery can reduce the edema and blood-brain barrier permeability associated with tumors.[1]

### INTRAOPERATIVE

Intraoperatively, ICP can be decreased by manipulating the four intracranial volume compartments as detailed in Table 17.1. With regard to the cells comprising the brain, surgical resection of the cells is the main method to directly decrease cellular volume.[1]

The second compartment, intracellular and extracellular fluid, can be decreased by diuretics. Loop and osmotic diuretics decrease ICP by decreasing intracellular and extracellular fluid, as well as triggering a reduction in CSF production.[1] Osmotic diuretics such as mannitol are commonly used as they are extremely effective at reducing extracellular fluid. However, if the blood-brain barrier is not intact, hyperosmolar components can cross and worsen intraparenchymal cerebral swelling.[1,2]

Third, CSF can be removed to alleviate increased ICP by either ventriculostomy or lumbar puncture.

Last and most significantly, cerebral blood flow (CBF) can be modulated to decrease the volume of intracranial blood. This can be done via venous or arterial systems. Cerebral venodilation leads to increased blood volume and thus increased ICP. Venous drainage can be maximized by positioning (neutral, heads-up posture avoiding extreme flexion or extension, avoidance of circumferential neck collars), as well as minimizing elevated intrathoracic pressure that decreases venous return (positive end-expiratory pressure, coughing).[1] General anesthesia with paralysis prevents coughing and the associated increased intrathoracic pressure.[1]

Arterial vasodilation occurs due to increased $PaCO_2$, which directly increases CBF. This vasodilation can be particularly damaging if patients have preexisting ischemic regions of the brain as a "steal" phenomenon may occur. With a steal, ischemic regions of the brain already receiving maximal blood flow from regional vasodilation receive less blood flow due to global vasodilation, shunting blood to other nonischemic regions.[2]

Hyperventilation decreases vasodilation and CBF by decreasing $PaCO_2$. ICP is maximally reduced at $PaCO_2$ 25–30 mm Hg; $PaCO_2$ less than 25 leads to no further reduction.[1] This reduction of ICP is temporary as the respiratory alkalosis corrects within 6–18 hours.[1] Caution should be exercised to avoid overhyperventilating as the resulting hypocapnia can lead to cerebral vasoconstriction severe enough to cause ischemia.

Hypoxemia at $PaO_2$ levels less than 50–60 mm Hg also increases CBF and ICP. However, there is little to no change as long as the $PaO_2$ remains greater than 60 mm Hg.[1]

A second method of decreasing CBF and by extension ICP is to decrease the cerebral metabolic rate of oxygen ($CMRO_2$). This can be achieved by hypothermia, as well as with anesthetics. Hypothermia directly reduces $CMRO_2$; cerebral metabolism decreases by 5% per 1°C drop in body temperature.[1] All volatile and intravenous anesthetics (other than nitrous oxide and ketamine) also reduce $CMRO_2$.[2] However, anesthetics also decrease mean arterial pressure, so a balance must be found to maintain the CPP. Of the intravenous anesthetics, ketamine alone increases CBF. Inhaled volatile anesthetics disrupt coupling between cerebral vasodilation and $CMRO_2$ by causing dose-dependent cerebral vasodilation while decreasing $CMRO_2$. On the other hand, nitrous oxide both directly vasodilates and increases $CMRO_2$.[1]

*Table 17.1* METHODS FOR DECREASING INTRACRANIAL PRESSURE BY INTRACRANIAL COMPONENT

| CELLS | FLUID | CSF | BLOOD |
|---|---|---|---|
| Surgical removal | Diuretics (loop or osmotic) | Drainage via ventriculostomy, lumbar puncture | Improve venous drainage (positioning, minimize intrathoracic pressure) |
| | Steroids | | Decrease CBF (hyperventilation, hypothermia, anesthetics) |

Perioperative complications such as seizures also increase $CMRO_2$ and CBF, leading to an increase in ICP.[1]

## REFERENCES

1. Patel PM, et al. Cerebral physiology and the effects of anesthetic drugs. In: Miller RD, ed. *Miller's Anesthesia*. 8th ed. Philadelphia, PA: Elsevier/Saunders; 2015:387–422.

2. Morgan GE, et al. *Morgan & Mikhail's Clinical Anesthesiology*. 6th ed. (Butterworth JF, Mackey DC, Wasnick JD, eds.). New York: McGraw-Hill Education; 2018.

3. Matsumoto M, Sakabe T. Effects of anesthetic agents and other drugs on cerebral blood flow, metabolism, and intracranial pressure. In: Cottrell JE, Patel P, eds. *Cottrell and Patel's Neuroanesthesia*. 6th ed. Edinburgh: Elsevier; 2017:74–90.

# 18.

# BRAIN VOLUME

*John S. Shin and Timothy T. Bui*

## INTRODUCTION

Brain volume consists of cells, intracellular and extracellular fluid, and blood within vasculature. Brain volume and cerebrospinal fluid comprise the total intracranial volume and thus determine intracranial pressure (ICP) since the skull is a fixed volume.[1] The brain (cells, intracellular and extracellular fluid) makes up 80% of intracranial volume, with blood contributing an additional 12%, for a total contribution of 92% of intracranial volume (Figure 18.1). Cerebrospinal fluid makes up the last 8%.[2] Neurons only account for roughly half of brain volume, with the remainder comprising glial cells and fluid/blood.[3] Brain volume can be modulated by a change in cell number/size, intra- or extracellular fluid, hemorrhage, or cerebral blood flow from vasodilation/vasoconstriction.[2]

An increase in brain volume beyond the compliance of the system can lead to elevated ICP and irreversible ischemia by decreasing cerebral perfusion. Symptoms of elevated ICP include nausea/vomiting, altered mental status, somnolence, neck rigidity, and papilledema.[1]

Rapid decreases in brain volume can also have severe consequences. This occurs most commonly in the setting of hypernatremia, which draws water out of the brain cells via an increased osmotic gradient. This leads to a rapid decrease in brain volume and potentially ruptured cerebral veins, causing focal intracerebral or subarachnoid hemorrhage.[2]

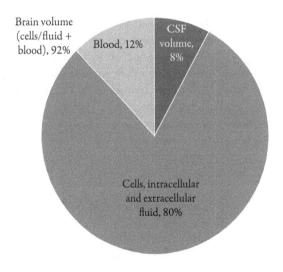

**Figure 18.1** Components of intracranial volume. Adapted from Reference 2.

Disruption in the blood-brain barrier can have significant impacts on brain volume. This disruption can occur secondary to severe hypertension, tumors, trauma, strokes, infection, hypercapnia, hypoxia, and/or sustained seizure activity.[1]

## ANESTHETIC CONSIDERATIONS

### PREOPERATIVE

Symptoms of elevated ICP as mentioned should be noted during preoperative evaluation. Patients may additionally need airway protection if they are unable to protect their airway due to a decreased Glasgow Coma Scale score and/or altered mental status.

If the elevated ICP is secondary to a brain tumor, administration of preoperative steroids beginning 48–72 hours prior to surgery can reduce edema and reduce the permeability of the blood-brain barrier.[1]

### INTRAOPERATIVE

Increased brain volume can be rapidly reduced by resecting the cellular mass, modulating the intra- or extracellular fluid, or affecting blood flow to the brain.[1] All of these measures can treat elevated ICP.

Brain water content can be rapidly reduced by diuresis. Mannitol is an osmotic diuretic that is most commonly given as a 1.0 g/kg infusion over 10–15 minutes.[1] Mannitol does not normally cross the blood-brain barrier, which allows for establishment of an osmotic gradient that pulls fluid out of the cells into the intravascular space.[1,2] This leads to a decrease in brain intracellular fluid content and brain volume. Mannitol is often used in combination with a loop diuretic such as furosemide, which maintains the osmotic gradient set up by mannitol by removing the fluid drawn out from the intravascular space.[1]

Blood flow to the brain is the most significant and varied approach for influencing brain volume.[1] Methods for decreasing cerebral blood flow include positioning to maximize venous drainage (head elevated, neck in neutral position); minimizing intrathoracic pressure (low positive end-expiratory pressure [PEEP]); hyperventilating; inducing mild hypothermia; and administering intravenous

---

**Box 18.1 MANAGEMENT OF INCREASED BRAIN VOLUME**

Preoperative
- Steroids if tumor present

Intraoperative
- Positioning: head elevated, neck in neutral position

Medications
- Diuresis (mannitol, furosemide)
- Intravenous anesthetics

Ventilation:
- Low intrathoracic pressure (low PEEP)
- Hyperventilation

Temperature
- Hypothermia if possible

Adapted from Reference 3.

---

anesthetics rather than inhaled agents.[1,3] A summary of the various methods to decrease brain volume can be found in Box 18.1. This is further detailed in Chapter 17, Intracranial Pressure.

### POSTOPERATIVE

Many of the same concepts intraoperatively can be applied to the postoperative setting as well. If patients are resistant to diuresis with mannitol, hypertonic saline is frequently used, particularly in the intensive care unit.[1]

Since hypothermia promotes a decreased cerebral metabolic rate and consequently decreased cerebral blood flow, prevention of postoperative hyperthermia is important to avoid increases in cerebral blood flow.[3]

### REFERENCES

1. Patel PM, et al. Cerebral physiology and the effects of anesthetic drugs. In: Miller RD, ed. *Miller's Anesthesia*. 8th ed. Philadelphia, PA: Elsevier/Saunders; 2015:387–422.
2. Morgan GE, et al. *Morgan & Mikhail's Clinical Anesthesiology*. 6th ed. (Butterworth JF, Mackey DC, Wasnick JD, eds.). New York: McGraw-Hill Education; 2018.
3. Matsumoto M, Sakabe T. Effects of anesthetic agents and other drugs on cerebral blood flow, metabolism, and intracranial pressure. In: Cottrell JE, Patel P, eds. *Cottrell and Patel's Neuroanesthesia*. 6th ed. Edinburgh: Elsevier; 2017:74–90.

# 19.

## INCREASED INTRACRANIAL PRESSURE AND HERNIATION

*Syed Sohaib Nasim and Steven Minear*

### INTRODUCTION

A normal human brain weighs 1400 g and contains 75 mL of cerebrospinal fluid (CSF) and 75 mL of blood. The cranium absorbs 100–150 mL of additional fluid before the intracranial pressure (ICP) begins to rise.[1] The rise in ICP occurs with the exhaustion of compensatory mechanisms, leading to herniation.[1]

### BRAIN HERNIATION

Brain herniation is a life-threatening event that occurs when the ICP increases and leads to brain protrusion through the openings in the cranium.[1,2] Symptoms of increased ICP and herniation include headache, weakness, loss of consciousness, elevated blood pressure, pupillary dilation, cardiac and respiratory arrest, and loss of brainstem reflexes.[2] The symptoms depend on the specific part of the brain that herniates, compressing local structures and causing particular symptoms. The etiology of increased ICP and herniation are[2,3]

1. Tumor
2. Infections
3. Hematoma (subdural, epidural, intracerebral hemorrhage)
4. Trauma
5. Cerebrospinal fluid volume (choroid plexus tumor, obstructive and nonobstructive hydrocephalus)
6. Encephalopathy[2,3]

There are six types of brain herniation based on the structure where the brain tissue herniates (Figure 19.1):

1. Subfalcine herniation: The cingulate gyrus herniates under the falx cerebri due to a mass or hematoma in the cerebral hemisphere. This results in compression of the anterior cerebral artery, causing infarction and leg paralysis on the contralateral side.[2,4]

2. Transtentorial central herniation (downward): A type of transtentorial herniation in which both temporal lobes and the diencephalon herniate through the tentorium. Central herniation can be ascending or descending depending on the location of the tumor; however, descending herniation is more common.[2,4] This causes damage to the midbrain, which presents as fixed (mitotic) pupils and decerebrate posturing. If the brainstem is involved, it could lead to respiratory arrest. The herniation could also lead to stretching of the basilar artery, leading to tearing and bleeding, known as Duret hemorrhage. The pituitary stalk can also be compressed as a complication, leading to diabetes insipidus.[2,4]

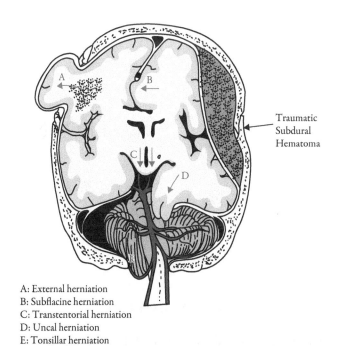

Traumatic Subdural Hematoma

A: External herniation
B: Subflacine herniation
C: Transtentorial herniation
D: Uncal herniation
E: Tonsillar herniation

**Figure 19.1** Source: Decker, R. Pearson-Shaver AL. Uncal herniation. In: StatPerals [Internet]. Treasure Island (FL): StatPearls Publishing; 2020.

3. Transentorial upward herniation: A less common type of herniation in which an infratentorial mass pushes the brainstem upward through the tentorial. This also causes compression of the third ventricle, leading to hydrocephalus.[2-4] Further herniation leads to compression of the superior cerebellar arteries, presenting with occipital headache, nausea, and vomiting in the early stages. In the later stages, there are breathing difficulties and loss of brainstem reflexes. If the mass is located in the posterior fossa, it presents as a cerebellar hemorrhage, causing ataxia and dysarthria.[2-4]

4. Transentorial uncal herniation: Another subtype of transtentorial herniation where the medial temporal and the uncus herniate through the tentorium, which is formed by the skull and meninges dura matter. Often this is due to a mass that pushes the temporal lobe and leads to compression of the midbrain.[2,3] The uncus herniation causes compression of the third cranial nerve (unilateral dilated and fixed pupil, eye deviation) and posterior cerebral artery (causing contralateral homonymous hemianopia). If the herniation progresses, the upper part of the brainstem and thalamus can be compressed, leading to loss of consciousness, unequal pupillary size, and breathing problems.[2,3]

5. Cerebellar tonsillar herniation: An infratentorial mass (tumor or hemorrhage) causes increased pressure on the cerebellar tonsils and leads to herniation through the foramen magnum.[2-4] This compresses the brainstem and also occludes the CSF flow, presenting with headache, vomiting, and impaired consciousness (hydrocephalus). If not addressed immediately, medulla compression leads to sudden cardiac and respiratory arrest.[2-4]

6. Transcalvarial herniation: A type of herniation that results from a trauma or fracture in the skull. The brain herniates through the path of least resistance, causing stretching of brain structures. The cortical vessels can also get compressed as the brain herniates through the skull, leading to hemorrhage and infarction.[2,4]

## REFERENCES

1. Miller RD. *Miller's Anesthesia*. 8th ed. Chapter 70. Anesthesia for Neurologic Surgery. Drummond J, Patel P, Lemkuil B. Philadelphia, PA: Churchill/Livingstone; 2015:2158–2196.

2. Munakomi S, Das J. Brain herniation. In: *StatPearls*. Treasure Island, FL: StatPearls Publishing; 2020.

3. Kenneth M. Brain herniation. In: *Merck Manual Professional Version*. Whitehouse Station, NJ: Merck; 2020. https://www.merckmanuals.com/professional/neurologic-disorders/coma-and-impaired-consciousness/brain-herniation

4. Oropello JM et al. Head Injury. In: Hall JB, Schmidt GA, Kress JP. eds. *Principles of Critical Care, 4e*. McGraw-Hill; Accessed September 02, 2020. https://accessmedicine-mhmedical-com.ccfla.ohionet.org/content.aspx?bookid=1340&sectionid=80026986

# 20.

# ELECTROENCEPHALOGRAMS

*Rany T. Abdallah and Gabriel M. Coleman*

## INTRODUCTION

An electroencephalogram (EEG) is a device used to measure electrical activity in the brain by placing several pairs of electrodes at specific positions over the scalp. When an axon excites a neuron, a small, varying electrical field is generated that is picked up by the nearest electrode. Each pair of electrodes receives activity from different populations of neurons, which are transferred to a medium in a readable pattern. Distinct cortical areas will display similar electrical activity, which can be used to isolate and observe specific activity. There are five different electrical patterns whose frequencies correlate to levels of activity[1]:

- Gamma rhythms (30–80 Hz): Learning, forming of working memory
- Beta rhythms (12–30 Hz): Attentive, alert
- Alpha rhythms (8–12 Hz): Resting state
- Theta rhythms (4–8 Hz): Light sleep
- Delta rhythms (<4 Hz): Deep sleep

The amplitude on the resulting waves represents the strength of the pattern in microvolts. When trying to detect neuronal activity, an electrode will also capture other electrical signals in the general vicinity. Raw EEG data are difficult to read, with the multitude of "noise" coming from other sources, but they can be processed to represent more specific information useful to patient assessment and anesthetic practices. Unfortunately, this processing takes time, and to interpret live data, someone needs to be trained to read raw data.

## CLINICAL RELEVANCE

One of the more popular uses of EEG is to observe brain activity during sleep and diagnose sleep disorders.[2] The phases of sleep can be separated into non–rapid eye movement (NREM) and rapid eye movement (REM) sleep. In NREM sleep, there are four stages characterized by theta and delta waves progressing into deeper sleeping, ending in stage IV, which is considered to be the deepest sleep stage. The brain activity patterns during REM sleep are remarkably similar to those of an awake state, but after about 10 minutes of REM sleep, the body will typically cycle back through the four NREM sleep stages.[2]

*Insomnia* is a disorder in which a patient has an inability to fall asleep or sleep for an extended period of time. By comparing EEG signals during NREM and REM sleep between insomniacs and control individuals, it can be shown that insomniacs experience lower levels of NREM sleep waves, with an elevated level in beta waves.[2]

The EEGs are also commonly used to define and classify seizures that are common in patients with *epilepsy*. These seizures are caused by abnormal brain activity, which can be either localized to one area of the brain or generalized throughout, which can result in myriad abnormal sensory, motor, cognitive, and mood symptoms.

It has been shown that an increase in $CO_2$ causes vascular changes in the brain, and there is some evidence that it also affects neural tissue as well. In general, *hypercapnia* has deleterious effects and reduces metabolic activity in the brain. By using an EEG on patients subjected to normocapnia and hypercapnia conditions, it can be concluded that hypercapnia results in a low arousal state by an increase in lower frequencies, like theta and delta waves. Conversely, during hyperbaric oxygen exposure, specific cortical areas present with decreased delta waves and significantly increased alpha waves.

*Hypothermia* is a drop in body temperature below 35°C, and it can interrupt many homeostatic functions and decrease activity in the nervous system. In a clinical setting, mild therapeutic hypothermia (TH) can be used to treat comatose patients who have had a cardiac arrest by increasing the chance that their heart starts again. An EEG is then used to predict neurological activity after the patient has experienced both a lack of blood flow to the brain due to cardiac arrest and nervous system interruption due to TH. Patients with spontaneous patterns or epileptic-like spikes rarely recover from cardiac arrest and TH, while those with milder abnormal patterns show a higher survival rate on discharge.

*Brain death* is important to diagnose as early as possible to distinguish from severe brain damage for the possibility of organ transplantation and so that discontinuing life support can be considered. Even a patient with critical brain damage has a possibility of restoring some level of neuronal activity. There are multiple methods for diagnosing brain death after basic clinical criteria have been met, but using an EEG is not time or labor intensive.

## ANESTHETIC CONSIDERATIONS

Using an EEG in anesthetic capacities is helpful to determine the depth of a patient's consciousness since anesthetic chemicals with their own molecular targets can affect neural circuits differently.[3]

Propofol augments γ-aminobutyric acid (GABA) A receptor–mediated inhibition in the neocortex, thalamus, and brainstem. EEG changes during propofol induction are a rise in the appearance of slow wave oscillations (0.1–1 Hz). The appearance of delta oscillations corresponds with the patient's loss of responsiveness. An additional bolus can further slow oscillations or cause burst suppression.[3]

Ketamine induces general anesthesia by blocking *N*-methyl-d-aspartate (NMDA)–mediated receptor interactions, which in turn inhibits excitatory activity in the neocortex, hippocampus, and limbic system. Ketamine initially produces gamma (30-Hz to 40-Hz) oscillation in the frontal lobes, followed by rhythmic theta waves, and followed by periodic bursts of delta waves.

Inhaled anesthetics are as follows:

- Isoflurane: A burst suppression pattern typically occurs with isoflurane concentrations greater than 2% in $O_2$ or 1.5% in 70% $N_2O$.

- Desflurane: Burst suppression appears at a MAC of at least 1.25.
- Sevoflurane: Epileptiform activities are frequently noted with rapid inhalational induction with 7% to 8% sevoflurane and during steady anesthesia with higher than 1.5 MAC of sevoflurane in both adult and pediatric patients.

## REFERENCES

1. Constant I, Sabourdin N. The EEG signal: a window on the cortical brain activity. *Paediatr Anaesth*. 2012;22(6):539–552.
2. Marchant N, et al. How electroencephalography serves the anesthesiologist. *Clin EEG Neurosci*. 2014;45(1):22–32.
3. Fahy BG, Chau DF. The technology of processed electroencephalogram monitoring devices for assessment of depth of anesthesia. *Anesth Analg*. 2018;126(1):111–117.

# 21.

# EVOKED POTENTIALS
## LOOK AT EFFECT OF ALL AGENTS ON SSEPS AND WHICH IS MOST SENSITIVE AND MOST RESISTANT

*Timothy Ford and Alaa Abd-Elsayed*

## SENSORY EVOKED POTENTIALS

Sensory evoked potentials involve applying a current to a sensory nerve and measuring the response on the sensory cortex with a scalp electrode. Evaluation is performed by measuring the amplitude (which is the voltage measurement from the peak apex to the succeeding trough or a designated baseline). Latency is the time from stimulation to the specific peak. Examples of sensory evoked potentials that are monitored intraoperatively include auditory, visual, and somatosensory evoked potentials (SSEPs). Sensory evoked potentials are low in amplitude, and multiple responses are averaged and summated to produce a tracing and reduce background noise of baseline electrical activity of the brain.

## SOMATOSENSORY EVOKED POTENTIALS

Somatosensory evoked potentials are obtained by placement of subdermal electrodes adjacent to sensory peripheral nerves. Stimulation of these nerves produce an SSEP.

These electrodes are commonly placed to stimulate the median nerve, common peroneal nerve at the level of the knee, and the posterior tibial nerve at the ankle. Recording electrodes are placed on the scalp to measure the response. The anatomical pathway for the transmission of impulses occurs via the dorsal columns–medial lemniscus pathway: (1) Impulses originate at the peripheral nerves and are transmitted to the cell bodies of the dorsal root ganglia; (2) from there the impulses ascend through the dorsal columns of the spinal cord to the dorsal column nuclei at the cervical medullary junction; (3) at this point the impulses are transmitted through where second-order fibers decussate and travel to the thalamus through the medial lemniscus to the thalamus; and finally the impulses are transmitted via third-order fibers and continue from the thalamus to the frontoparietal sensory cortex. The response recorded at the scalp is the net result of the neuronal inputs through the spinal cord to the brain. Intraoperative changes in amplitudes or latencies indicate compromised sensory pathways. Significant events are defined as an amplitude loss of greater than 50% or latency increase greater than 10%. Given SSEPs measure only the sensory pathways, it is possible to have motor deficits after surgery with intact SSEPs. That is why it is important to monitor both in certain procedures.

## BRAINSTEM AUDITORY EVOKED POTENTIALS

Brainstem auditory evoked potentials (AEPs) are utilized in procedures that are associated with risks of injury to the vestibulocochlear nerve and the brainstem. Surgeries with increased risk to these structures include acoustic neuroma resection, cerebellar pontine angle tumors, and trigeminal nerve microvascular decompression. Neurosurgical procedures involving vascular or neoplastic lesions of the posterior fossa will utilize AEPs in conjunction with SSEPs. The most common type of AEPs utilized intraoperatively are brain auditory evoked responses (BAERs). This technique utilizes the placement of surface disk electrodes placed on both earlobes and the vertex. Responses are then recorded following a brief auditory stimulus delivered to one ear. The vestibulocochlear nuclei and pathways span the pons and medulla of the brainstem and thus serve as an assessment of brainstem function. Less common techniques used to measure AEPs include electrocochleography and direct auditory nerve action potential.

## VISUAL EVOKED POTENTIALS

Visual evoked potentials (VEPs) are a far less commonly used form of intraoperative monitoring due to high intraindividual variability because of their sensitivity to many parameters, resulting in unreliable results. They are typically generated by placing small goggles on the patient; the goggles contain light-emitting diodes, facilitating flash stimuli over closed eyelids. There is a single channel over the visual cortex that records the signal responses.

## MOTOR EVOKED POTENTIALS

Motor evoked potentials (MEPs) are used to monitor the motor tracts of the spinal cord, which differ with their location in the spinal cord and thus differ in their blood supply. These potentials are evoked by direct stimulation on the spinal cord or by transcranial stimulation of the motor cortex. With transcranial stimulation, the stimulating electrode is placed between the intermediolateral sulcus and the dentate ligament. Transcranial stimulation is typically produced by electric stimulation. Alternatively, magnetic induction is another means to carry out transcranial stimulation; however, it is more

*Table 21.1* ANESTHETIC EFFECTS ON EVOKED POTENTIALS

| EVOKED POTENTIAL | EFFECTS | |
| --- | --- | --- |
| SOMATOSENSORY EVOKED POTENTIALS (SSEPS) | LATENCY | AMPLITUDE |
| Isoflurane, enflurane, halothane, propofol, thiopental, fentanyl, sufentanyl, morphine, droperidol, diazepam, isovolemic hemodilution | ↑ | ↓ |
| Nitrous oxide | 0 | ↓ |
| Etomidate | ↑ | ↑ |
| Ketamine | ? | ↑ |
| Midazolam | 0 | ↓ |
| Muscle relaxants | 0 | 0 |
| • Hypothermia | ↑ | ↓ |
| • Hyperthermia, hypoxia, hypotension | 0 | ↓ |
| • Hypocarbia | ↑ | 0 |
| Brainstem auditory evoked responses (BAERs) | • More resistant to anesthetic influences<br>• Are subcortical and reproducible with all general anesthetics<br>• Affected by changes in temperature and carbon dioxide | |
| Visual evoked potentials (VEPs) | • Exquisitely sensitive to many central nervous system–active medications, including nitrous oxide and volatile anesthetics | |
| Motor evoked potentials (MEPs) | • Volatile anesthetics, barbiturates, and benzodiazepines suppress MEPs in a dose-dependent manner<br>• Propofol causes a dose-dependent suppression of MEPs but less so than volatile anesthetics<br>• Muscle relaxants should be avoided in the case of myogenic MEPs | |

sensitive to anesthetics, making electrical stimulation the preferred method of transcranial stimulation. On stimulation, the impulses extend down the lateral corticospinal and anterior corticospinal tract. The response can be recorded over the spinal cord in the case of spinal MEPs or over muscles in the case of myogenic MEPs. Myogenic MEPs are less invasive and more sensitive to ischemia compared to spinal MEPs and thus are most commonly utilized intraoperatively.

## MORPHOLOGY OF EVOKED POTENTIALS AND EFFECTS OF ISCHEMIA

The response of evoked potentials is measured on a plot of voltage versus time. Common changes in evoked potentials that indicate neural injury include decreases in amplitude or an increase in latency compared to baseline potentials.

## ANESTHETIC EFFECTS ON EVOKED POTENTIALS

While evoked potentials are a validated method of assessing neurologic functional intensity in patients under general anesthesia, there are important anesthetic strategies that must be implemented to reduce confounding the clinical utility of evoked potentials (Table 21.1). Etomidate and ketamine increase amplitudes, so they have been used to enhance SSEP recordings in patients with preexisting pathologies that made it impossible to obtain reproducible recordings.

## REFERENCES

1. Koht A, et al. Neuromonitoring in surgery and anesthesia. In: Post T, ed. *UpToDate*. Waltham, MA: UpToDate; 2020. www.update.com
2. Barash PG, et al. *Clinical anesthesia*. 8th ed. Wolters Kluwer Health; 2017:2499–2503.
3. Hayashi H, Kawaguchi M. Intraoperative monitoring of flash visual evoked potential under general anesthesia. *Korean J Anesthesiol*. 2017;70(2):127–135.

# Part 5

# REGIONAL ANESTHESIA

# 22.

# COMMON COMPLICATIONS OF LOCAL ANESTHETICS

*Rewais B. Hanna and Alaa Abd-Elsayed*

## INTRODUCTION

Local anesthetics (LAs) are weak bases (with pKa 7.5–9.5), and they exist in an ionized form at body pH. The uncharged base form of most agents is more lipid soluble and can rapidly reach the site of action, where it can then be ionized and work on sodium channels. These drugs work on $Na^+ K^+$ ATPase (adenosine triphosphatase). The administration of LAs decreases sodium inflow and thus diminishes the propagation of a pain stimulus through nervous fibers, avoiding depolarization.[1,2] Peripheral, neuraxial, and regional anesthesia all rely on the administration of LAs to reversibly disrupt the nerve signal to reduce preoperative or postoperative pain. These medications come in different forms, including topical, infiltrative, injectable, field block, or peripheral nerve block. Serum concentrations are highest in intravenous administration, followed by intercostal, caudal epidural, lumbar epidural, brachial plexus, and subcutaneous.[2] Generally, LAs are very safe when properly used. However, time- and dose-dependent local and systemic toxicity and hypersensitivity reactions are all risks with the administration of LAs.

## SYSTEMIC TOXICITY

The most feared complication of LA systemic toxicity is cardiac arrest and/or seizures. Recognizing LA toxicity is paramount for clinicians. Clinically, systemic toxicity presents as effects on the central nervous system (CNS) or cardiovascular systems. Classically, the first sign will be CNS activation, which progress from perioral paresthesia, facial paresthesia, disarthria, metallic taste, diplopia, and auditory disturbances to seizures. Cardiac activation may occur with a rise in blood pressure and tachycardia. There may also be signs of myocardial depression, prolonged conduction interval, bradycardia, hypotension, and heart failure. Last, signs of nervous system depression, such as respiratory depression, appear with lidocaine serum concentration higher than 15 µg/mL. Signs and symptoms of CNS toxicity commonly include convulsions, followed by coma and respiratory depression. Risk of toxicity increases with the following risk factors: extremes of age, cardiac disease, renal insufficiency, hepatic disease, and pregnancy.

## EXTREMES OF AGE

Infants under the age of 4 months are at highest risk due their lower levels of AAG and immature hepatic clearance. In these children, doses for repeat or continuous administration should be reduced by 15% from published standard adult dosages. On the other hand, elderly individuals similarly have impaired hepatic function, and LA doses should be reduced in these patients as well.

## ORGAN DYSFUNCTION

Those with underlying cardiac disease are also at increased risk for systemic toxicity with LA. This is due to the lack of perfusion of the kidneys and liver, impairing LA clearance and increasing serum concentration. Patients with end-stage hepatic disease should similarly have reduced LA dosage.

## PREGNANCY

Several factors increase the risk of LA toxicity in pregnant patients, including hormone imbalance, reduced levels of AAG, increased cardiac output, and lower pseudocholinesterase activity. The Food and Drug Administration recently issued a warning against the use of 0.75% bupivacaine for obstetrical anesthesia due to case reports of cardiac arrest with difficult resuscitation in those patients who received bupivacaine for epidural anesthesia. Generally, bupivacaine carries the greatest risk of direct cardiac toxicity.

## ALLERGIC HYPERSENSITIVITY REACTIONS

The first and most important step in reducing the risk of allergic reactions to LA is via thorough history taking. Often, patients will report allergic reactions from LAs; however, this may be from a syncopal/vasovagal episode during the injection process. It is important to differentiate between true allergic reactions and sympathetic or psychomotor stimulation. True allergic reactions account for less than 1% of unexpected complications of LA.[3] There are two types of allergic reactions to LA: contact dermatitis (delayed type IV hypersensitivity) or rarely generalized urticaria/anaphylaxis (rapid, type I hypersensitivity). Symptoms of contact dermatitis from LAs include delayed localized swelling, which is rarely dangerous. On the other hand, symptoms of a type I hypersensitivity reaction include localized eczematous and pruritic rash appearing within 72 hours at the site of administration. Rarely, vesiculation, blistering, or weeping may also occur. More rarely, type I allergic reactions to LAs may include pruritus, urticaria, bronchospasm, angioedema, rhinitis, laryngeal edema, and/or anaphylaxis within 1 hour of administration. In these situations, the potential offending agent should be stopped, and patients should have a patch test to confirm the diagnosis of LA allergy. These patients are highly unlikely to be allergic to another LA in a distinct chemical group. In general, if a patient has suspected allergic reactions to LAs, they can be referred to an allergist or dermatologist for skin testing and a subcutaneous challenge.

## ALLERGIES TO PABA

Local anesthetics are organized into two categories: ester and amide compounds. Due to a P-aminobenzoic acid (PABA) metabolite, allergic reactions are more common with esters. Patients who are allergic to esters should receive a preservative-free amide LA. On the other hand, amide compounds do not undergo this metabolism and are less likely to be the cause of allergic reactions. Last, diphenhydramine can be used as an alternative to ester and amide LAs in shorter procedures.

## ALLERGIES TO PRESERVATIVES IN LAS

The preservatives (methylparaben) or antioxidants (sulfites) are two substances within the solution of LAs. These two compounds are the most likely cause of allergic reactions to LAs. Methylparaben is included in an effort to prevent microbial growth, and sulfites prevent the oxidation of vasopressors.[1] Methylparaben has a similar structure to PABA, sulfonamide antibiotics, and ester-type LAs.

Other antioxidants include sodium metabisulfite, acetone sodium bisulfite, and ascorbic acid. Chelating agents such as disodium ethylenediaminetetraacetic acid (EDTA)

and stabilizers such as edetate calcium disodium are added to LAs. All those agents can cause allergic reactions with different severities. Sodium metabisulfite has neurotoxic potential.

## RECOMMENDATIONS

- A maximum dose of LA should be based on lean, rather than actual, body weight.
- The dose of LA should be reduced for patients who are at risk (e.g., pregnancy, uremia) for rapid uptake of LA from the injection site.
- The dose of LA should be reduced for patients with low levels of alpha-1-acid glycoprotein (e.g., neonates, pregnant patients), who are at risk for high concentrations of free LA after injection.
- The dose of LA should be reduced for patients who have increased neural sensitivity to LA (e.g., older adults, pregnant patients).
- The dose of LA for continuous or repeat administration should be reduced for patients at risk for reduced clearance of LA (e.g., renal, hepatic, or cardiac disease).
- Addition of epinephrine to LA solutions can slow the rate of absorption and reduce peak plasma levels and may act as a marker for intravascular injection. Epinephrine reduces the absorption of LA by 20% to 50%, depending on the site of injection and the LA.[4]

## IN CASE OF SUSPECTED TOXICITY

- Stop injection.
- Call for help, lipid toxicity kit, and cognitive aids.
- Arrange for possible cardiopulmonary bypass.
- Manage the airway.
- Suppress seizures; benzodiazepine are preferred.
- Manage arrhythmias and provide cardiovascular support.
- Initiate lipid rescue therapy using 20% lipid emulsion:
  - Bolus lipid emulsion over 2 to 3 minutes and begin infusion based on ideal body weight as follows:
    - ≤70 kg: 1.5 mL/kg IV followed by infusion at 0.25 mL/kg/min IV.
    - >70 kg: 100 mL IV followed by infusion of 200 to 250 mL IV over 15 to 20 minutes.
    - Repeat bolus once or twice and double infusion rate for persistent cardiovascular instability.
    - Continue infusion for at least 10 minutes after hemodynamic stability is achieved.
    - Maximum dose is approximately 12 mL/kg.[5]

## REFERENCES

1. Becker DE, Reed KL. Local anesthetics: review of pharmacological considerations. *Anesth Prog.* 2012;59(2):90–103.
2. Hogan QH. Pathophysiology of peripheral nerve injury during regional anesthesia. *Reg Anesth Pain Med.* 2008;33(5):435–441.
3. McCaughey W. Adverse effects of local anesthetics. *Drug Saf.* 1992;7(3):178–189.
4. Scott DB, et al. Factors affecting plasma levels of lignocaine and prilocaine. *Br J Anaesth.* 1972;44(10):1040.
5. Cave G, et al. Management of severe local anesthetic toxicity. AAGBI Safety Guideline. 2010.

# 23.

# PERIPHERAL AND AUTONOMIC NERVE BLOCKS

*James Flaherty and Federico Jimenez-Ruiz*

## INTRODUCTION

Peripheral and autonomic nerve blocks use targeted local anesthetic injections to prevent axonal signal transmission. Local anesthetics reversibly bind to the alpha subunit on the intracellular aspect of axonal sodium channels (Figure 23.1), halting action potential propagation and preventing signal transmission to the central nervous system. This results in anesthesia and/or analgesia.

Peripheral nerve blocks can be used to provide analgesia or as an alternative to general anesthesia. Peripheral nerve blocks improve pain control, decrease opioid consumption, and can decrease opioid-related adverse drug events. These benefits are balanced by the time and resource utilization required to perform the block. With the advent of ultrasound and subsequent development of plane blocks, the majority of anatomic locations are able to be blocked. However, the benefit of some peripheral nerve blocks are better established than others, and this benefit must be weighed against known side effects when deciding whether it is appropriate to provide regional anesthesia. In some situations, the benefit of peripheral nerve blocks may surpass the provision of analgesia, such as with their use to enhance regional blood flow for arteriovenous fistula creation.

Autonomic nerve blocks, targeting sympathetic fibers, are used in the treatment of chronic pain.

## CONTRAINDICATIONS

- Absolute: patient refusal, infection at puncture site
- Relative: Systemic infection, coagulopathy and/or anticoagulant use, preexisting neurologic disease

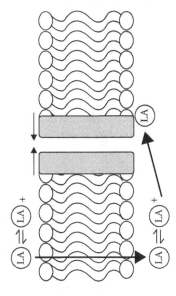

**Figure 23.1** The un-ionized form of local anesthetics (LA) traverse the lipid bilayer and must become protonated before attaching to the alpha subunit of the intracellular aspect of the sodium channel, inactivating the channel and preventing action potential propagation. Source: Decker, R. Pearson-Shaver AL. Uncal herniation. In: StatPerals [Internet]. Treasure Island (FL): StatPearls Publishing; 2020.

## TECHNIQUES

- Paresthesia: Based on the occurrence of a paresthesia with needle-to-nerve contact. It requires knowledge of anatomic landmarks to localize nerves and can be difficult to decipher perineural versus intraneural location of the needle. Anatomic variants may make this approach impossible.
- Peripheral nerve stimulation: Nerve localization is facilitated by electric current applied to the tip of a needle to stimulate nerves and cause muscles to contract. The negative terminal (cathode) should be applied to the needle. Higher energy current is applied initially to localize the nerve but should be reduced to 0.5 mA or less to ensure localization immediately adjacent to the nerve. A motor response generated below 0.2–0.5 mA may indicate intraneural needle placement.
- Ultrasound: This allows direct visualization of nerves and fascial planes. High-frequency ultrasound waves bounce off tissues, return to the ultrasound probe, and are processed to generate an image. Ultrasound guidance has expanded the use of regional anesthesia and has allowed for the identification of novel targets. New block techniques are relatively easily learned after achieving familiarity with ultrasound basics[1]:
  - Differences in acoustic impedance allow for the identification of structures. Nerves are more easily identified when surrounded by tissues with a different acoustic impedance (fat, fluid) compared with similar impedance (muscle)
  - The highest possible frequency transducer is used to optimize visualization of the target. Higher frequency probes produce better axial resolution. Frequency is limited by depth of penetration; deeper targets will require lower frequency transducers to be used as higher frequency waves are more rapidly attenuated.
  - In-plane imaging is generally used to visualize the entire trajectory of the needle, facilitating the avoidance of trauma to nerves and vascular structures.
  - Sliding is used to identify structures; tilting may improve visualization (anisotropy); compression will compress vascular structures and bring targets closer to the surface; rocking may improve needle visualization by decreasing the incident angle between ultrasound and needle; and rotation improves alignment of needle and ultrasound waves.
  - Doppler imaging uses frequency shifts to identify vascular structures; blue indicates flow away from the transducer, while red indicates flow toward the transducer.
  - Needle visualization is improved by minimizing refraction and reflection away from the probe by keeping the needle as perpendicular as possible to the ultrasound beam.

## CLINICAL ASSESSMENT

Success of a block can be monitored by assessing sensory and/or motor blockade in the expected distribution of the nerve targets. Additional methods of assessing block success include objective measures of vasodilation and skin temperature.

## COMPLICATIONS

- Nerve injury: The etiology of peripheral nerve injury includes mechanical trauma, chemical trauma, pressure injury, and ischemia. Rates of peripheral nerve injury have remained stable in the decades before and after the introduction of ultrasound to regional anesthesia. No one method of nerve localization is clearly superior with regard to the incidence of peripheral nerve injury. Rates of long-term injury range from two to four events for every 10,000 blocks performed. However, peripheral nerve blocks themselves may not represent an independent risk factor for perioperative nerve injury. Transient neuropathy, conversely, is relatively common after peripheral nerve blocks and is most common after interscalene block, with an incidence of 2.84%. Paresthesias may not correlate with risk of nerve injury. Nerve injury may be more common in patients with preexisting neurologic disease, the "double-crush" theory.[2]
- Bleeding: This can range from bruising to hemorrhage and is likely to be less consequential in superficial, compressible locations compared with deeper locations. It may lead to neurovascular compromise and nerve injury via ischemia. The American Society of Regional Anesthesia guidelines recommend holding prophylactic dose antithrombotic medications for two half-lives and treatment dose antithrombotic medications for five half-lives prior to block placement. These guidelines do not stratify by specific block type. Vascular puncture is less common with ultrasound assistance.
- Infection: In contemporary practice, the incidence of infectious complications of single-injection peripheral nerve blocks is exceedingly low, with no such events occurring in a large retrospective evaluation.[3] Catheter colonization is common, but consequential infection remains rare with continuous techniques. The risk of infection with continuous catheters increases with the duration that the catheter remains in situ, with an inflection point at 4 days.[4]
- Local anesthetic systemic toxicity (LAST) risk is roughly 1:1000. The incidence has declined since the

advent of ultrasound, potentially related to reduced volumes of local anesthetics used. The pattern of LAST has also shifted from an acute presentation within minutes of injection to a delayed presentation.

## SINGLE-INJECTION BLOCKS VERSUS CATHETERS

Continuous blocks improve pain control on postoperative days 0–2, decrease cumulative opioid use, and improve patient satisfaction when compared with single-injection blocks.[5] However, continuous catheters increase resource utilization. Regarding nerve localization technique, the likelihood of difficult or inaccurate catheter placement is decreased with ultrasound guidance.

## REFERENCES

1. Sites BD, et al. Artifacts and pitfall errors associated with ultrasound-guided regional anesthesia. Part I: understanding the basic principles of ultrasound physics and machine operations. *Reg Anesth Pain Med.* 2007;32(5):412–418.
2. Neal JM, et al. The second ASRA practice advisory on neurologic complications associated with regional anesthesia and pain medicine: executive summary 2015. *Reg Anesth Pain Med.* 2015;40(5):401–430.
3. Allakad H, et al. Infection related to ultrasound-guided single-injection peripheral nerve blockade: a decade of experience at Toronto Western hospital. *Reg Anesth Pain Med.* 2015;40(1):82–84.
4. Bomberg H, et al. Prolonged catheter use and infection in regional anesthesia. *Anesthesiology.* 2018;128(4):764–773.
5. Bingham AE, et al. Continuous peripheral nerve block compared with single-injection peripheral nerve block: a systemic review and meta-analysis of randomized controlled trials. *Reg Anesth Pain Med.* 2012;37(6):583–594.

# 24.

# AUTONOMIC NERVE BLOCKS

## STELLATE, CELIAC, AND LUMBAR SYMPATHETIC

*Steven Ethier and Keth Pride*

## INTRODUCTION

Autonomic nerve blocks (ANBs) work by blocking the transmission of action potentials along the neural network of the autonomic nervous system (ANS). The ANS is divided into the sympathetic nervous system (SNS) and the parasympathetic nervous system (PNS). The SNS has presynaptic cell bodies in the *T1-L2 lateral horn* of the spinal cord that reaches postsynaptic cell bodies and ganglia throughout the body. In general, these function to control blood pressure, temperature, and vascular flow. The PNS, on the other hand, derives innervation from the *cranial nerves (III, VII, IX, X)* and the *sacral nerves (S2-S4)*. These sacral nerves are also called the pelvic splanchnic nerves. The ganglia in the PNS are different from the SNS in that they are not continuous along the spinal column, but more discrete

and near the end-organ of interest. The sacral segments help control micturition, defecation, and sexual function.[1]

Some of these ganglia, which house the postganglionic cell bodies, are targets for ANBs. Some of the most common autonomic nerve blocks clinically include the stellate ganglion, celiac plexus, and lumbar plexus blocks, all of which are within the SNS.

Of these two systems, it is the SNS that is more commonly targeted for regional anesthesia. Using ultrasound or fluoroscopic guidance, local anesthetic with or without steroid is injected around the area of the relevant ganglia. When performed properly, blockade of these ganglia can result in *improved circulation* and pain relief, especially in patients with *vaso-occlusive disease* (i.e., Raynaud vasospasm, frostbite, angina). It can also provide relief of *visceral pain* (i.e., gastrointestinal cancers) and *neuropathic pain* (i.e., herpes zoster virus, diabetic neuropathy). Of note, sympathetic nerve blocks will *NOT* alleviate somatic pain (i.e., second-degree burns, incisional pain).[1]

For refractory pain, an ANB may be used as both a diagnostic and therapeutic modality after medical management has failed. The diagnostic block is more of a test of efficacy and aids in determining the cause of pain and its underlying pathology. For example, if the diagnostic block provides significant analgesia, then a therapeutic intervention (i.e., ablation vs. neurolysis) could be performed with a goal of longer lasting pain relief.[1]

## STELLATE GANGLION BLOCK

- *Definition*: Sympathetic ganglion formed by the fusion of the first thoracic ganglion (T1) and the inferior cervical ganglion.
- *Location*: Anterior to C7 transverse process (between C6 and C7), medial to scalene muscles, and lateral to trachea, esophagus, internal jugular vein, carotid artery, and the thyroid (Figure 24.1).
- *Technique*: The patient is placed in the supine position with head turned to the contralateral side, and a high-frequency linear ultrasound probe is placed midline transversely at the level of the cricoid cartilage. The probe is then slid laterally until the thyroid and carotid artery are appreciated, then inferiorly until the transverse process of C6 or C7 can be seen. The stellate ganglion can be blocked by approaching in an anteromedial direction, avoiding vascular structures, guiding the needle inferior to the carotid artery and medial to the longus colli muscle, and targeting the area just superficial to the transverse process of C6 or C7.
- *Clinical Relevance*: Used as a diagnostic and therapeutic modality for the *upper extremity* (complex regional pain syndrome [CRPS], phantom limb pain, neuropathic pain, atypical facial pain, and arterial vascular insufficiency of the upper extremity, angina, etc.) and trunk.
- *Complications*: Ipsilateral Horner syndrome (*expected*), vasovagal reaction, pneumothorax, brachial plexus palsy, hematoma, local anesthetic systemic toxicity (LAST), vertebral artery injection causing *seizure*, hemothorax, chylothorax, infection, intrathecal or epidural injection, hoarseness (recurrent laryngeal nerve), and phrenic nerve palsy.
- *Additional Pearls*: Could be blocked during a *brachial plexus block* (i.e., interscalene or supraclavicular block) incidentally, again resulting in Horner syndrome (*ptosis, miosis, anhidrosis* with or without enophthalmos and/or hyperemia of the eye).[2] Block success is associated with increased temperature in the ipsilateral upper extremity. At C7, the ganglion is bounded anteriorly with the pleural dome, vertebral artery, and carotid sheath, which is why it is preferred to do the block at the level of C6.

## CELIAC PLEXUS BLOCK

- *Definition*: The celiac plexus includes the celiac ganglia, the largest ganglia of the ANS, and the aorticorenal ganglia; is formed by the greater and lesser splanchnic nerves (*T5-T12*) and some fibers of the vagus nerve (SNS *and* PNS); overall the block decreases SNS greater than the PNS, leading to an overall *increase* in PNS activity; distribution is from the stomach to the midtransverse colon, including the gallbladder and *pancreas*.
- *Location*: Located *retroperitoneal* at T12-L1 between the aorta and inferior vena cava, surrounding the abdominal aorta near the crus of the diaphragm; typically, a posterior approach is performed just below *12th rib* (Figure 24.2).

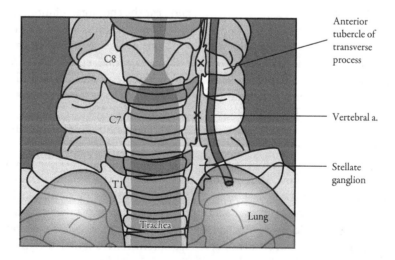

**Figure 24.1** Anatomy of the stellate ganglion. Source: Decker, R. Pearson-Shaver AL. Uncal herniation. In: StatPerals [Internet]. Treasure Island (FL): StatPearls Publishing; 2020.

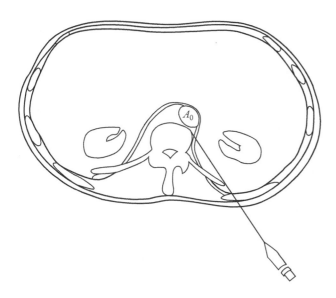

Figure 24.2 Schematic of the posterior approach for a celiac plexus block. Source: Decker, R. Pearson-Shaver AL. Uncal herniation. In: StatPerals [Internet]. Treasure Island (FL): StatPearls Publishing; 2020.

- *Technique (Double-Needle Retrocrural Approach)*: The patient is placed in a prone position on the fluoroscopy table. The fluoroscope is tilted craniocaudally until the superior end plate of L1 vertebral body (VB) is square, then tilted obliquely (25°–35°) to the ipsilateral side until the tip of the L1 transverse process is in line with the lateral aspect of the L1 VB. A needle is then inserted in this coaxial view, targeting the inferolateral aspect of this transverse process and advanced until contact is made with the lateral aspect of the L1 VB. The needle is then advanced in the lateral view carefully until the tip lies (1–2 mm) beyond the posterior aspect of the L1 VB or until pulsation emanating from the aorta and transmitted to the advancing needle is observed. Contrast is injected to confirm optimal and nonintravascular spread of medication. A test dose is administered, followed by local anesthetic with or without steroid. The same procedure is then repeated on the opposite side. Ultimately, the tip of the needle should be just posterior to the aorta on the left and to the posterolateral aspect of the aorta on the right.

- *Clinical Relevance*: Primarily used for *upper abdominal visceral* (i.e., *cancer) pain* as it receives innervation from the abdominal viscera; examples include pancreatic cancer, intractable pain related to chronic pancreatitis (a more controversial indication), and pain from prior radiation; can be performed under fluoroscopy or via endoscopic retrograde cholangiopancreatography.

- *Complications*: Most commonly *orthostatic hypotension* and *diarrhea*; others include intravascular injection/ LAST, hiccups, reactive pleurisy, aortic dissection, interscapular back pain, retroperitoneal hemorrhage, chylothorax; more rare complications are disruption of the *artery of Adamkiewicz* leading to paraplegia, epidural injection, and transient motor paralysis.[3]

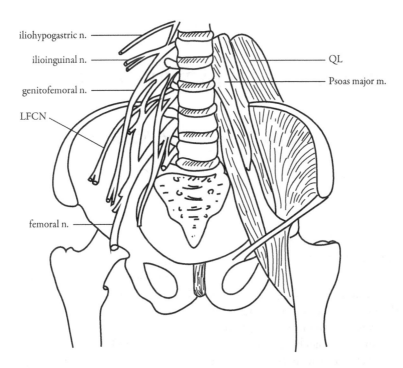

Figure 24.3 Anatomy of the lumbar plexus. Source: Decker, R. Pearson-Shaver AL. Uncal herniation. In: StatPerals [Internet]. Treasure Island (FL): StatPearls Publishing; 2020.

## LUMBAR SYMPATHETIC BLOCK

- *Definition*: The lumbar sympathetic ganglia comprises the *L1-L4* nerve roots with a contribution of T12 as well; branches include iliohypogastric (T12-L1), ilioinguinal (L1), genitofemoral nerve (L1-L2), lateral femoral cutaneous nerve (LFCN) (L2-L3), and femoral nerve (L2-L4); it spares the sciatic nerve (see Figure 24.3).
- *Location*: Anterolateral surface of L2-L4 vertebral bodies, *anteromedial to psoas muscle*; the patient typically is prone with the needle entry at L2 or L3, around 8 cm from the midline, going through the psoas muscle.
- *Technique*: The patient is placed in the prone position on the fluoroscopy table. The fluoroscope is tilted craniocaudally until the superior end plate of L3 VB is square, then tilted obliquely to the ipsilateral side until the tip of the L3 transverse process is in line with the lateral aspect of the L3 VB. A needle is then inserted in this coaxial view, targeting the superolateral aspect of this transverse process, and advanced until contact is made with the lateral aspect of the L3 VB. The needle is then walked off and advanced in the lateral view until the tip is 3–5 mm dorsal to the most ventral aspect of the L3 VB. Contrast is injected to confirm optimal and nonintravascular spread of medication. A test dose

is administered, followed by local anesthetic with or without steroid.
- *Clinical Relevance*: Indicated for *lower extremity pain* (CRPS, vaso-occlusive pain, neuropathic pain); can also alleviate intestinal and urinary visceral pain.
- *Complications*: *Genitofemoral nerve injury* (ejaculatory problems in males, especially if bilateral), LAST, intrathecal/epidural injection, perforation to surrounding structures (i.e., renal hematoma), orthostasis and hypotension from *lower extremity venous pooling*.
- *Additional Pearls*: The sciatic nerve is spared when blocking this plexus.[4,5]

## REFERENCES

1. Gibbons CH. Basics of autonomic nervous system function. *Handb Clin Neurol*. 2019;160:407–418.
2. Nader A, Benson HT. Peripheral sympathetic blocks. In: Raja SN, et al. *Essentials of Pain Medicine and Regional Anesthesia*. 2nd ed. London: Elsevier Churchill Livingstone; 2004:687–693.
3. Mercadante S, Nicosia F. Celiac plexus block: a reappraisal. *Reg Anesth Pain Med*. 1998;23:37–48.
4. Awad IT, Duggan EM. Posterior lumbar plexus block: anatomy, approaches, and techniques. *Reg Anesth Pain Med*. 2005;30:143–149.
5. Capdevila X, et al. Approaches to the lumbar plexus: success, risks, and outcome. *Reg Anesth Pain Med*. 2005;30:150–162.

# 25.

# PERIPHERAL NERVE BLOCKS (HEAD)

*Keth Pride and Scott Blaine*

## INTRODUCTION

Regional anesthesia for procedures involving the head can be easily achieved through the careful application of peripheral nerve blockade. Because the head has predictable surface and bony landmarks, blocks can easily be placed pre- and intraoperatively to provide both regional anesthesia and/or postoperative analgesia with minimal complications. As with all procedures, this should be discussed carefully and completely in the preoperative setting with both the patient and operating surgeon in order to promote open communication and adequate understanding of the proposed nerve block.

## RETROBULBAR AND PERIBULBAR BLOCKS

The retro- and peribulbar nerve blocks are usually employed to provide regional anesthesia for surgery involving the cornea, anterior chamber, and lens and have replaced general anesthesia for many procedures.

The retrobulbar block (intraconal) provides globe anesthesia and akinesia. It is a form of regional anesthetic used to provide sensory anesthesia to the cornea, uvea, and conjunctiva by blocking the ciliary nerves. In this technique, local anesthetic is injected into the area located behind the globe of the eye in the muscle cone known as the retrobulbar space. Successful blockade provides *akinesia* of the extraocular muscles by blocking cranial nerves II, III, and VI (and sometimes IV through local diffusion), which prevents movement of the globe.[1]

When compared to a peribulbar block, a retrobulbar block is *deeper* and uses less *volume*. It also does not anesthetize cranial nerve VII (facial nerve), allowing the patient to close the eye with the orbicularis oculi (CN VII) but not open it with the levator muscle (CN III).[1]

A peribulbar block (extraconal) is performed by injecting local anesthetic both above and below the orbit into the orbicularis oculi muscle. This provides blockade of the ciliary nerves, as well as CN III and VI, but does not block CN II. Although historically it was thought that the retrobulbar block held a greater chance for complications due to its deeper and more invasive nature, a Cochrane review performed in 2008 by Alhassan et al. found no significant differences in success rate or complications between peribulbar and retrobulbar blocks.[2]

Complications associated with these blocks include retrobulbar hemorrhage, central retinal artery occlusion, subconjunctival edema, penetration or perforation of the globe, central spread of local anesthetic, oculocardiac reflex, diplopia, and postoperative strabismus.[2]

Contraindications to both the peribulbar and retrobulbar blocks include procedures lasting more than 90–120 minutes, age less than 15, uncontrolled cough or tremors, disorientation or mental impairment, excessive anxiety or claustrophobia, language barrier or deafness, bleeding or coagulopathies, and a perforated globe.[2]

## TRIGEMINAL NERVE: SUPRAORBITAL, SUPRATROCHLEAR, INFRAORBITAL

The trigeminal nerve, the largest of the cranial nerves, provides sensory innervation to the majority of the face and jaw. Careful application of peripheral blockade not only can provide postoperative analgesia, but also can help in the management of chronic pain associated with the trigeminal nerve and its branches.

The frontal nerve, a branch of the V1 ophthalmic nerve, exits the orbit at the superior orbital fissure and divides into the supraorbital and supratrochlear nerves. These branches supply sensory innervation to the anterior scalp, forehead, the medial part of the upper eyelid, and the root of the nose. It is typically anesthetized for lower forehead and upper eyelid surgery, including laceration repair, craniotomies, frontal ventriculoperitoneal shunt placement, or local tumor, nevus, or dermoid cyst excision. Interestingly, surgery on one side of the forehead requires bilateral supratrochlear nerve blocks due to the overlapping distributions of the nerves.[3]

This block is achieved by finding the supraorbital foramen, located approximately 2 cm from the midline in adults, usually in the same sagittal plane as the pupil. A needle (often a 25-gauge intradermal needle in adults, 30 gauge in children) is introduced 0.5 cm under the inferior edge of the eyebrow and is directed medially and cephalad. With care not to penetrate the foramen, 1–2 mL of local anesthetic is then injected. In order to block the supratrochlear nerve, the top of the angle formed by the eyebrow and the nasal spine is palpated. The supratrochlear nerve can be blocked immediately following the supraorbital nerve block by directing the needle toward the midline about 1 cm and injecting an additional 1–2 mL of local anesthetic.[4] After the injection, it is recommended that firm pressure and light massage be applied to optimize anesthetic spread and prevent ecchymosis. Complications associated with these blocks are rare but may include hematoma, intravascular injection, and eye globe damage.

Infraorbital nerve block is most commonly used in the pediatric population undergoing cleft lip repair to provide early postoperative analgesia and help avoid opioids. Other main indications are endoscopic sinus surgery, rhinoplasty or nasal septal repair, and transsphenoidal hypophysectomy.[5] It can be achieved using an intraoral or extraoral approach. Regardless of the chosen technique, it is recommended to keep a finger on the infraorbital foramen throughout the procedure to prevent the penetration of the foramen, resulting in damage to the eyeball. Both approaches require a 25- or 27-gauge needle to inject 1–3 mL of local anesthetic targeting the space located between the infraorbital foramen and the ipsilateral nare.[3]

Complications include hematoma formation, persistent paresthesia of the upper lip, and penetration of the foramen, which may result in nerve damage or globe injury. The intraoral approach is not advised in neonates and small infants because of its proximity to the orbit.[3]

## GREATER AND LESSER OCCIPITAL NERVES

The greater occipital nerve (GON) provides sensory innervation to the majority of the posterior scalp from the external occipital protuberance to the vertex. The lesser occipital nerve (LON) is also a sensory cutaneous nerve that provides innervation to the upper part of the posterior earlobe and lateral posterior scalp. Applications for occipital nerve blocks include postoperative analgesia for posterior craniotomies, ventriculoperitoneal shunt surgery, as well as for diagnoses and treatment of various headache syndromes.

Located on a line drawn from the external occipital protuberance to the unilateral mastoid, the GON can be found approximately at one-third the distance from midline, just medial to the occipital artery. Direct palpation may elicit paresthesia across the distribution of the nerve. Using these landmarks, the GON can be blocked with a 25-gauge needle directed at 90° toward the occiput, advanced to the ostium, and withdrawn 1–2 mm. After aspiration, 1–3 mL of local anesthetic is injected. After injection, again, firm pressure and light massage should be applied to optimize anesthetic spread and promote hemostasis. Numbness across the posterior and top of the head is a sign of a successful block.[4]

The LON can be targeted approximately two-thirds from the midline along the same line formed by the external occipital protuberance and the ipsilateral mastoid using a similar technique and materials used to block the GON. Ultrasound guidance may also be employed as a confirmatory tool using the greater occipital artery as an additional landmark.[4]

Due to their relatively superficial course, there are only minimal complications associated with blockade of these nerves, the most common being intravascular injection of either the greater occipital or the vertebral artery.

## REFERENCES

1. Murray MJ, et al. *Faust's Anesthesiology Review.* Elsevier Saunders; 2015:292–293.
2. Alhassan MB, et al. Peribulbar versus retrobulbar anesthesia for cataract surgery. *Cochrane Database Syst Rev.* 2008;(3):CD004083.
3. Kandarian B, et al. Head and neck regional anesthesia techniques. *ASRA News.* 2017;17(4):38–44.
4. Benzon HT, et al. *Practical Management of Pain.* Elsevier; 2014: 706–709.
5. Sola C, et al. Nerve blocks of the face. https://www.nysora.com/techniques/head-and-neck-blocks/nerve-blocks-face; 2021.

# 26.

# PERIPHERAL NERVE BLOCKS (NECK)

*Scott Blaine and Keth Pride*

## INTRODUCTION

Peripheral blockade of nerves in the neck is most often used to facilitate awake endotracheal intubation for the patient with a difficult airway.[1] Although topicalization with minimal-to-moderate sedation is often sufficient to perform an awake intubation, one should be knowledgeable concerning alternative methods should the need arise. In addition to the nerves supplying the larynx and pharynx, there is also a rich cervical plexus of nerves that can be targeted when anesthesia of more superficial structures of the neck is desired.[2]

## CERVICAL PLEXUS

The cervical plexus is formed by the confluence of the anterior branches of the first four cervical nerves. This plexus emerges into the superficial tissues along the posterior border of the sternocleidomastoid (SCM). Both *deep* (as the spinal nerves exit the intervertebral foramen) and *superficial* (as terminal branches emerge along the posterior border of the SCM) blocks can be performed. Deep cervical plexus blockade necessitates entry into the prevertebral fascia, which encloses the spinal column and associated muscles. For this reason, it is associated with phrenic nerve paresis (C3-5).[3]

Surgeries in which a cervical plexus block can be employed for supplemental anesthesia include local skin lesion removal, lymph node dissection, excision of thyroglossal or branchial cleft cysts, carotid endarterectomy, and vascular access surgery.

Contraindications include conditions that might alter patient anatomy, such as previous radiation, surgery, or active infection in the region. In addition, deep cervical plexus block is relatively contraindicated in patients with preexisting pulmonary compromise as there is a notable risk of respiratory collapse from phrenic nerve paresis.

As mentioned, phrenic nerve palsy is the primary complication to consider when performing the deep cervical plexus block. One might reasonably decide to do a superficial cervical plexus block for a patient with underlying respiratory compromise to reduce the risk of phrenic nerve paresis.[3] Other complications include hematoma, dysphonia or dysphagia if local anesthetic (LA) spreads to involve CN IX and X, impairment of the baroreceptor reflex if LA is inadvertently injected into the carotid sheath, and spinal anesthesia if LA spreads to involve the spinal nerves as they exit the spinal cord.[2]

## GLOSSOPHARYNGEAL

The glossopharyngeal nerve arises from the brainstem, exits the skull through the jugular foramen, and courses caudally just anterolateral to the carotid artery. In the neck, it has several branches, of which the *lingual branch* can be easily accessed in the submucosa for blockade. This branch provides sensory information from the posterior third of the tongue and the vallecula, and it also serves as the afferent limb of the gag reflex.

Both intraoral and peristyloid approaches can be utilized to achieve desired anesthesia of the glossopharyngeal nerve. The *intraoral approach* is often easier to visualize as long as the patient has adequate mouth opening and there are no anatomical abnormalities prohibiting visualization of the tonsillar pillars. The glossopharyngeal nerve crosses over the posterior tonsillar pillar (or palatopharyngeal arch), entering the submucosa just medial to the anterior tonsillar pillar (ATP, or palatoglossal arch), where it terminates in the tongue.

With the patient's mouth open, the tongue can be retracted medially with a tongue depressor or the blade of a laryngoscope to expose the tonsillar pillars. The inferior border of the ATP should be identified as it connects to the tongue; 0.5 cm lateral to this conjunction is where LA can be injected. The same process should be repeated on the contralateral side.

The *peristyloid approach* uses the styloid process as the landmark for anesthetizing the glossopharyngeal nerve. The styloid process can be palpated at about the midway point between the mastoid process and the angle of the mandible. The block needle should be aimed directly at the styloid process until contact with the bone is made. At this point, the needle should be directed just posterior to the styloid process until contact with the bone is lost, at which point the LA should be injected.

Although the surface landmarks in this area of the neck may be more salient and more easily accessed than those in the mouth, extra care should be taken given the proximity of the carotid artery (deep and anterior to the glossopharyngeal). As always, aspiration prior to injection of LA should be performed. Complications for this block are relatively few, but include those shared by most blocks, including infection, bleeding, LA toxicity, and inadvertent intravascular injection.

## SUPERIOR LARYNGEAL

The superior laryngeal nerve arises from the vagus nerve at about the level of the hyoid bone. Here it splits into an *internal branch* (which dives through the thyrohyoid membrane) and an *external branch*. Together, these branches provide sensory innervation to the laryngeal muscles cephalad to the vocal cords.

To perform the block, the patient is positioned supine with as much neck extension as can be tolerated. Palpation of the greater horn of the hyoid (its most lateral point) is attempted. The block needle should be inserted in a trajectory aimed at the greater horn. Once contact is made, the needle is directed just inferior to this, and the LA is injected. This provides anesthesia to both internal and external branches of the superior laryngeal nerve.

In the event that the hyoid bone is difficult to palpate, the most lateral margin of the thyroid cartilage can also serve as a landmark.[1] The block needle can be directed at this landmark, and then the LA can be injected just superior to this. Ultrasound may also be useful in identifying the hyoid bone in obese patients whose hyoid bone or thyroid cartilage are not easily palpated.

Alternatively, an *internal approach* to anesthetizing the superior laryngeal nerve can be utilized. After penetrating the thyrohyoid membrane, the internal branch continues along the piriform recesses in the submucosa. Pledgets can be soaked in 4% lidocaine (concentration less than this may not be sufficient) and deposited in both recesses for 5–10 minutes to achieve adequate anesthesia. This obviously requires a cooperative patient whose oropharynx has already been topicalized in order to get the pledgets down into the piriform recesses.

## TRANSTRACHEAL (RECURRENT LARYNGEAL)

The recurrent laryngeal nerve branches off the vagus nerve and makes a U-turn in a cephalad direction, where it eventually provides sensory and motor innervation to the muscles of the glottis. Direct blockade of the recurrent laryngeal nerve is avoided because it can lead to significant airway compromise.[1]

In practice, the recurrent laryngeal nerve can be anesthetized by more of a topicalized route. A needle with an angiocath over it should be inserted through the cricothyroid membrane, with negative pressure applied to the plunger while advancing. As the needle enters the airway, bubbles in the syringe serve as confirmation of appropriate placement. At this point, the needle can be withdrawn, leaving the angiocath in place. Then, 4% lidocaine can be sprayed through the angiocath.[4] From this entry point, the LA injected will be deposited just below the vocal cords and should anesthetize the recurrent laryngeal nerve. Aside from temporary discomfort and coughing (which actually helps spread the LA), complications from this block are few.

## REFERENCES

1. Ahmad I. Regional and topical anesthesia for awake endotracheal intubation. https://www.nysora.com/techniques/head-and-neck-blocks/airway/regional-topical-anesthesia-awake-endotracheal-intubation/; 2021.
2. Jerry D, et al. Cervical plexus block—landmarks and nerve stimulator technique. https://www.nysora.com/techniques/head-and-neck-blocks/cervical/cervical-plexus-block/; 2021.
3. Kim J-S, et al. Cervical plexus bock. *Korean J Anesthesiol.* 2018;71(4):274–288.
4. Kandarian B, et al. Head and neck regional anesthesia techniques. *ASRA News.* 2017;17(4):38–44.

# 27.

# EXTREMITY NERVE BLOCKS

*James Flaherty and Federico Jimenez-Ruiz*

## INTRODUCTION

This chapter covers high-yield concepts for most peripheral nerve blocks.

## UPPER EXTREMITY

**Brachial Plexus blocks:** The brachial plexus is made up of spinal nerve roots C5-T1. The following are different techniques that allow blockade of the brachial plexus at different levels

- Interscalene block: Targets nerve roots C5, C6, C7. The inferior roots (C8-T1) are usually spared (ulnar sparing).
  - When performed with nerve stimulator, abdominal twitches correspond to phrenic nerve stimulation (needle is misplaced anteriorly).
  - Expect 100% ipsilateral phrenic nerve blockade due to anesthetic spread; it may lead to a 25% reduction of forced vital capacity.[1,2]
  - Blockade of ipsilateral recurrent laryngeal nerve may lead to ipsilateral vocal cord palsy, manifested by hoarseness. If bilateral recurrent laryngeal nerve blockade occurs, patients may present with complete airway obstruction.
- Supraclavicular block: Targets the trunks (superior, middle, and inferior).
  - This is referred to as the "spinal of the arm."
  - The most common complication is phrenic nerve blockade (40%–60%). Most serious complication: pneumothorax.[3]
- Infraclavicular block: This targets the cords (lateral, posterior, and medial) and carries the "highest risk for pneumothorax."
  - It is a suitable place for catheter-based brachial plexus analgesia.
  - It is associated with patient discomfort due to the needle traversing the pectoral fascia.
- Axillary block: Targets the branches (medial, ulnar, radial) and a complementary musculocutaneous nerve block is required for procedures using a tourniquet in the upper arm.
  - Relevant sonoanatomy: Three out of four major nerve branches to the arm are contained in the axillary nerve sheath. The radial nerve is the most posterior and

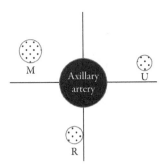

**Figure 27.1** Anatomical location of the median, ulnar and radial nerves in relation to the axillary artery.

closest to the humerus, observed at 6 o'clock relative to the axillary artery on ultrasound imaging. The median nerve is anterolateral and seen at 9 o'clock. The ulnar nerve is seen at 3 o'clock (Figure 27.1).

## DISTAL UPPER EXTREMITY BLOCKS

- Musculocutaneous nerve block (C5-C6): This nerve travels within the belly of the coracobrachialis muscles outside of the axillary nerve sheath.
- Ulnar nerve block (C8-T1): Proper blockade produces inability to adduct the thumb.
  - Can be blocked between the olecranon and the medial epicondyle of the humerus, where the ulnar nerve is not in direct contact with the ulnar artery.
- Radial nerve block (C5-T1): As a "field block" it requires more extensive infiltration.
  - This may be blocked at the elbow or at the anatomic snuffbox. Proper blockade leads to wrist drop.
- Median nerve block (C6-T1): The "fan technique" is recommended to increase the success rate of this block.
  - Insert the needle between the tendons of the palmaris longus and flexor carpi radialis.
  - Proper blockade leads to "hand of benediction."
- Wrist block: This block involves anesthesia of the median, ulnar, and radial nerves.
  - Need to block dorsal and ventral branches of radial and ulnar nerves.

## LOWER EXTREMITY

- Lumbar plexus: This is formed by the ventral rami of L1-L4 with a small contribution of subcostal nerve T12.
  - The lumbar plexus block reliably blocks the femoral, lateral femoral cutaneous, and obturator nerves. It spares the sciatic nerve. It provides anesthesia to the hip and anterolateral and medial aspects of the thigh and the saphenous nerve below the knee.
  - The use of ultrasound does not allow a reduction of the volume or dose of local anesthetics. Nerve

stimulation is frequently used to identify the right plane by eliciting stimulation of the roots (patellar twitch). Another approach is the psoas compartment block, in which a needle is placed 5 cm lateral to the midline at the L4 level; a needle is advanced to touch the transverse process of L5, then walked of superiorly and medially until quadriceps (femoral nerve) or adductor (obturator nerve) twitch is elicited.
  - Complications: The most serious complication is epidural spread, with risk of high neuraxial anesthesia block and hypotension. Other complications include spinal anesthesia and retroperitoneal/renal hematoma.
- Femoral nerve block: This nerve is formed by the posterior divisions of the ventral rami of L2-L4.
  - When using a nerve stimulator, contraction of the quadriceps indicates proper needle placement. If sartorius muscle contraction is observed, the needle needs to be moved deeper and laterally.
  - Relevant anatomical landmarks are the femoral crease, pubic tubercle, and femoral artery (medially). Major muscles supplied by the femoral nerve include the anterior compartment muscles: quadriceps, sartorius, and pectineus.
- Lateral femoral cutaneous nerve (LFCN) is formed by the L2-L3 nerve roots.
  - The LFCN provides sensory innervation to the anterolateral thigh extending toward the knee. This is a common site for donor skin grafting. Meralgia paresthetica is entrapment of the LFCN associated with burning pain over the nerve's distribution. The classic presentation is in pregnant women with prolonged labor while legs are in stirrups.
  - Relevant anatomical landmark is the anterior superior iliac spine. The entry point is 2 cm medial and 2 cm caudal to the anterior superior iliac spine. The needle is then moved in a fan-like pattern laterally and medially during anesthetic injection.
- Obturator nerve block: This nerve is formed by L2-L4.
  - The obturator nerve is a mixed nerve that provides innervation to the adductor muscles of the thigh and cutaneous innervation of the medial thigh in 30% of patients.
  - It is used for enhanced analgesia after major knee surgery, as treatment and/or diagnosis of adductor muscle spasm, and to block the obturator reflex in transurethral bladder tumor resections of the lateral bladder wall.[4]
  - Relevant ultrasound anatomical landmarks can be remembered by the mnemonic ALABAMa, which refers to structures from lateral to medial: AL, adductor longus; AB, adductor brevis; AM, adductor magnus.
- Adductor canal block: This technique blocks femoral nerve branches.

- This is used as an analgesic adjunct for knee surgery. The goal is to block the saphenous nerve (L3-L4), which is a terminal sensory branch of the femoral nerve providing innervation to the medial aspect of the leg and foot.
  - Contents of the adductor canal are the saphenous nerve, femoral artery, and femoral vein.
  - An adductor canal block provides non-inferior analgesia to a femoral nerve block while sparing quadriceps function, which may reduce the risk of falls.[5]
- Sciatic nerve block: This is formed by the ventral rami of L4-S3 and can be performed by several approaches: transgluteal, infragluteal, or popliteal.
  - Popliteal approach: This involves the relevant anatomy of the popliteal fossae: tendon of biceps femoris, lateral border of semimembranosus muscle, and heads of medial and lateral gastrocnemius muscles. Typically this is blocked at the point of bifurcation into the tibial and common peroneal nerves.
  - Infragluteal approach: This involves the greater trochanter of the femur, ischial tuberosity, and sciatic groove (target).
  - Ankle blocks: A successful ankle block involves blocking all five nerves of the foot. These may be blocked by landmark infiltration or under ultrasound guidance.
  - Sensory-only nerves are the superficial peroneal, saphenous, and sural nerves.
  - Motor and sensory nerves are the deep peroneal and posterior tibial nerves.

## REFERENCES

1. Urmey WF, et al. One hundred percent incidence of hemidiaphragmatic paresis associated with interscalene brachial plexus anesthesia as diagnosed by ultrasonography. *Anesth Analg.* 1991;72(4): 498–503.
2. Fujimura N, et al. Effect of hemidiaphragmatic paresis caused by interscalene brachial plexus block on breathing pattern, chest wall mechanics, and arterial blood gases. *Anesth Analg.* 1995;81(5):962–966.
3. Schubert A-K, et al. Interscalene versus supraclavicular plexus block for the prevention of postoperative pain after shoulder surgery: a systematic review and meta-analysis. *Eur J Anaesthesiol.* 2019;36(6):427–435.
4. Bolat D, et al. Impact of nerve stimulator-guided obturator nerve block on the short-term outcomes and complications of transurethral resection of bladder tumour: a prospective randomized controlled study. *Can Urol Assoc J.* 2015;9(11–12):E780–E784.
5. Karkhur Y, et al. A comparative analysis of femoral nerve block with adductor canal block following total knee arthroplasty: a systematic literature review. *J Anaesthesiol Clin Pharmacol.* 2018;34(4):433–438.

# 28.

# TRUNCAL NERVE BLOCKS

*Elizabeth Scholzen and Lisa Klesius*

## INTERCOSTAL NERVE BLOCKS

### INTRODUCTION

The intercostal nerves innervate the majority of the skin and muscles of the chest and upper abdomen. Today, intercostal nerve blocks (ICNBs) can be used for many surgeries, including breast surgery, thoracic surgery (both videoscopic and thoracotomy), or upper abdominal surgery. They can also be used in patients with traumatic rib fractures who may have contraindications to neuraxial analgesia.

### ANATOMY

Thoracic nerves exit through the intervertebral foramen and divide into the anterior rami, which continues to the sympathetic chain; the posterior rami, which provide innervation to the posterior paravertebral region; and the ventral ramus, which provide innervation anteriorly around the chest and abdominal wall. The ventral ramus continues as the intercostal nerve (ICN) and is the intended target of this nerve block. The ICN runs in the subcostal grove of the rib inferior to the intercostal vein and artery. The lateral cutaneous branch takes off at the midaxillary point, and the ICN continues anteriorly as the anterior cutaneous branch.[1]

### TECHNIQUE

The location of an ICNB can be variable but should be performed posterior to the midaxillary line to ensure the lateral cutaneous branch of the ICN is anesthetized. Most commonly, the block is performed at the angle of the rib where the rib is most superficial and easiest to palpate. To perform the block, a needle is inserted until the inferior aspect of the rib is contacted. The needle is then "walked off" the inferior border of the rib until the needle is advanced through the internal intercostal fascia, where 3–5 mL of local anesthetic is injected. The ICNB can be performed at various desired levels to block multiple ICNs (Figure 28.1).

### CONTRAINDICATIONS

Absolute contraindications are relatively rare and include patient refusal and local skin infection over the area of injection. Relative contraindications include current anticoagulation or disorders of coagulation. However, if the block is performed in a compressible area, such as the midaxillary line, the block is considered a superficial nerve block, and anticoagulation guidelines are less restrictive.

### COMPLICATIONS

Complications are relatively rare but can be severe. Complications include pneumothorax and local anesthetic systemic toxicity (LAST), particularly given the high uptake of local anesthetic in the intercostal region. Bleeding, infection, nerve damage, and unintentional intravascular injection are also possible. Finally, local anesthetic may track toward the paravertebral/epidural or intrathecal space, leading to complications such as hypotension or total spinal anesthetic, respectively.

## PARAVERTEBRAL NERVE BLOCK

### INTRODUCTION

The paravertebral block (PVB) anesthetizes multiple ventral rami as they exit the intervertebral foramen and provides unilateral or bilateral analgesia of the chest or abdomen, depending on the level of the block. This block is often used for thoracic and breast surgeries and can be used for either postoperative analgesia or primary surgical anesthesia.

### ANATOMY

The goal of the PVB is to block ventral rami at multiple sequential levels by injecting local anesthetic into the paravertebral space. The paravertebral space is bounded anteriorly by the parietal pleura, medially by the vertebral column, and posteriorly by the superior costotransverse ligament and transverse process of the vertebral body.

### TECHNIQUE

There are multiple techniques described for performing a PVB, including using a loss of resistance technique or ultrasound guidance. Either an in-plane or out-of-plane approach can be used depending on provider preference. The block is performed by injecting 10–12 mL of local anesthetic into the paravertebral space. The coverage of nerve

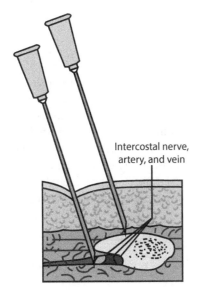

Intercostal nerve, artery, and vein

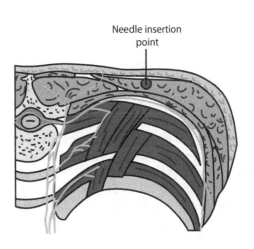

Needle insertion point

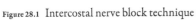

**Figure 28.1** Intercostal nerve block technique

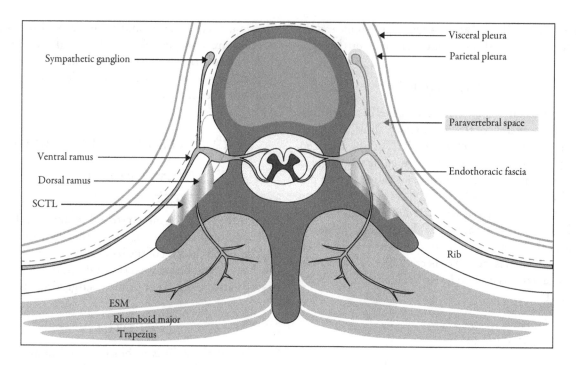

**Figure 28.2** Anatomy of the paravertebral space and surrounding structures

blockade depends on the level of local anesthetic injection and spread. Local anesthetic spread is usually seen one to two dermatomal levels above and below the injected level (Figure 28.2).

## CONTRAINDICATIONS

Absolute contraindications include patient refusal and infection over the injection site or in the paravertebral space. Relative contraindications include coagulation disorders or continuation of anticoagulation medications. The risks and benefits need to be evaluated for these patients before proceeding with a PVB. In addition, caution should be taken in patients with spinal abnormalities or previous thoracic surgery as there may be a higher risk of pleural puncture.

## COMPLICATIONS

The most feared complication of a PVB is the development of a pneumothorax after accidental pleural puncture. Pneumothorax may not be immediately evident, and any patient suspected of a pleural puncture should be examined with a chest x-ray or ultrasound to assess for pneumothorax. Hypotension due to spread of local anesthetic into the epidural space can also occur with PVBs. Similar to all nerve blocks, complications including bleeding, infection, nerve damage, or unintentional intravascular injection leading to LAST may occur.[2]

## ILIOINGUINAL NERVE BLOCK

### ANATOMY

The ilioinguinal nerve arises from the L1 spinal nerve root and innervates the skin over the upper medial thigh, anterior surface of the scrotum or labia majora, and mons pubis. This block can be used for analgesia or surgical anesthesia for inguinal hernia repair when paired with an iliohypogastric nerve block, which anesthetizes the inguinal crease and hypogastric region. The ilioinguinal and iliohypogastric nerves can be blocked as they travel between the transversus abdominus and internal oblique muscles, medial and superior to the anterior superior iliac spine (ASIS).

### TECHNIQUE

This block is typically performed using ultrasound guidance with the patient in the supine position. When the ultrasound transducer is placed medial to the ASIS pointing toward the umbilicus, the ilioinguinal nerve can be seen laying between the internal oblique and the transversus abdominus muscles. After the needle is advanced to the appropriate fascial plane, approximately 10 mL of local anesthetic is administered to anesthetize the nerve.[3]

### CONTRAINDICATIONS

Contraindications include patient refusal or infection over the injection site.

## COMPLICATIONS

The ilioinguinal block is considered a relatively safe block. Complications specific to the block include temporary femoral nerve block with accompanying quadriceps weakness (more common with a landmark-based approach given the larger anesthetic volume used), pelvic hematoma, and urinary retention. Other complications, common to all nerve blocks, include bleeding, infection, unintentional intravascular injection, and nerve damage.[4]

## GENITOFEMORAL NERVE BLOCK

The genitofemoral nerve provides additional innervation to the inguinal region, and its blockage can be combined with the ilioinguinal nerve block to provide additional anesthesia for inguinal hernia repair surgery. This nerve block can also be combined with the femoral nerve block to be used for primary surgical anesthesia for vein-stripping surgery in place of a spinal anesthetic.

### ANATOMY

The genitofemoral nerve arises from the L1 and L2 nerve roots of the lumbar plexus. The nerve divides into the genital branch (innervates the skin of scrotum/mons pubis) and the femoral branch (innervates the skin over the upper anterior thigh) when it reaches the inguinal ligament.[5]

### TECHNIQUE

Similar to the ilioinguinal block, the genitofemoral block is typically performed under ultrasound guidance with the patient in the supine position. The ultrasound probe is placed lateral to the pubic tubercle superior to the inguinal ligament until the spermatic cord is identified. The needle is then inserted adjacent to the spermatic cord and where local anesthetic is injected. Local anesthetic spread can be visualized surrounding the spermatic cord. More frequently, this nerve block is performed on the surgical field under direct visualization by the surgeon.[6]

### CONTRAINDICATIONS

Contraindications include patient refusal or infection over the injection site.

### COMPLICATIONS

Complications are relatively rare and include bleeding, infection, unintentional intravascular injection, and nerve damage.

### REFERENCES

1. Ho A, et al. Intercostal nerve block—landmarks and nerve stimulator technique. New York Society of Regional Anesthesia. https://www.nysora.com/regional-anesthesia-for-specific-surgical-procedures/thorax/intercostal-nerve-block/
2. Karmakar M, et al. Thoracic and lumbar paravertebral block—landmarks and nerve stimulator technique. New York Society of Regional Anesthesia. https://www.nysora.com/regional-anesthesia-for-specific-surgical-procedures/abdomen/thoracic-lumbar-paravertebral-block/
3. Truncal and cutaneous blocks. New York Society of Regional Anesthesia. https://www.nysora.com/techniques/truncal-and-cutaneous-blocks/truncal-and-cutaneous-blocks/
4. Larson S, et al. Femoral nerve paralysis following open inguinal hernia repair. *Am J Med Case Rep*. 2015;3(3):85–87.
5. Al-Alami A, et al. New approach of ultrasound-guided genitofemoral nerve block in addition to ilioinguinal/iliohypogastric nerve block for surgical anesthesia in two high risk patients: case report. *Open J Anesthesiol*. 2013;3:298–300.
6. Singh S, Vadera H. Ultrasound guided hernia blocks. *Anaesth Pain Intensive Care*. 2015;19(3):366–371.

# 29.

# SPINE-RELATED PROCEDURES

*Mary Ghaly and Sherif Zaky*

## INTRODUCTION

Neuroaxial anesthetic techniques not only provide means for anesthesia during surgery but also are commonly used for perioperative analgesia.

## PREOPERATIVE CONSIDERATIONS

The patient's interview should include specific history of anesthetic complications during epidural or spinal anesthesia, history of coagulopathy or any anticoagulant medications, and history of spine disorders or surgeries. Patients should have frequent monitoring of blood pressure and pulse oximetry during the procedure. Supplemental oxygen via nasal cannula or face mask with end-tidal $CO_2$ monitoring is recommended if sedation is provided. Patients should have an adequately functioning intravenous line prior to the procedure

### CONTRAINDICATIONS TO NEUROAXIAL BLOCKADE

- Absolute contraindications: Patient refusal, high intracranial pressure, infection at the site of injection, coagulopathy, severe stenotic valvular heart disease, and severe hypovolemia
- Relative contraindications: Uncooperative patient, preexisting neurological deficits, stenotic valvular heart disease and severe spinal deformity[1]

## EPIDURAL ANESTHESIA

### INDICATIONS

- Primary anesthetic for abdominal and lower extremity surgeries
- Postoperative pain control and in chronic pain conditions
- Labor analgesia

### COMPLICATIONS

- Intravascular injection, epidural hematoma, epidural abscess, nerve injury, and inadvertent dural puncture

### TECHNIQUES

#### Midline Approach

The patient is positioned in a sitting (or lateral) position (Figure 29.1). A horizontal line is drawn between the iliac crests (Tuffier's line) to indicate the L4-5 interspace. The patient's back is prepped and draped in a sterile fashion. A skin wheal is made in the midline with local anesthetic. A 17- or 18-gauge touhy needle is directed perpendicular to the coronal plane with a slight cephalad tilt and advanced

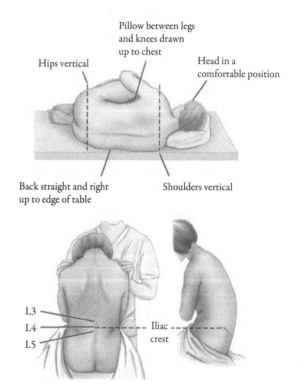

Pillow between legs and knees drawn up to chest

Hips vertical

Head in a comfortable position

Back straight and right up to edge of table

Shoulders vertical

L3
L4
L5

Iliac crest

Figure 29.1 Positioning for spinal and epidural anesthesia.

until an increase in resistance is felt. This should indicate contact with the supraspinous ligament, then continued advancement is made into the interspinous ligament. At that point, a syringe containing either preservative-free saline or air is attached, and the needle is advanced in an incremental or continuous fashion using the loss-of-resistance technique to identify the epidural space.[1] The thoracic vertebral interspaces between T3 and T9 are functionally unique because of the acute downward angle of the spinous processes. Blockade of these middle thoracic interspaces usually requires use of the paramedian approach.

## Paramedian Approach

A point approximately one-half inch lateral to the midline at the level of the inferior border of the spinous process is identified and infiltrated with a local anesthetic. An epidural needle is inserted and advanced perpendicular to the skin into the subcutaneous tissues. The needle is then redirected slightly medial and cephalad and advanced until lamina is contacted. The needle is "walked off" the lamina medially and cephalad employing a loss-of-resistance or hanging drop technique to identify the epidural space. In the paramedian approach, the epidural needle penetrates the paraspinous muscles, then enters the ligamentum flavum en route to the epidural space; the paramedian approach is lateral to the supraspinous and interspinous ligaments.

## CATHETER PLACEMENT AND TEST DOSE

Once the epidural space has been identified, a catheter is advanced into the epidural space, typically 3–5 cm past the needle tip (Figure 29.2). At this time, the catheter is aspirated in order to detect intrathecal or intravascular placement. After negative aspiration, a test dose of lidocaine with epinephrine can be administered. Intravascular injection of the test dose may produce a metallic taste in the mouth secondary to the lidocaine and a rapid increase in heart rate secondary to the epinephrine. Sudden motor blockade of the lower extremities indicates an intrathecal injection of local anesthetic.

## Transforaminal Approach

### Indications
The transforaminal approach is usually used to provide selective anterior epidural spread at a certain spinal nerve root in conditions such as lumbar radiculopathy.

### Complications
Direct trauma to the spinal cord and/or nerve roots, spinal cord ischemia, and infection in the epidural space.

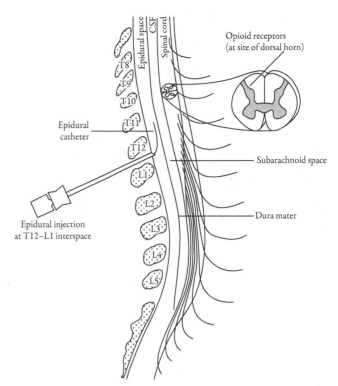

**Figure 29.2** Epidural catheter placement.

### Technique
In this technique, the patient is placed in the prone position on the fluoroscopy table. An oblique fluoroscopic view is usually utilized to identify the ipsilateral neural foramen. The skin is infiltrated at a point just inferior to the middle of the corresponding pedicle (chin of the Scotty dog). A 22-gauge blunt tip needle is then advanced until the tip impinges on bone over the pedicle, then redirected inferiorly into the targeted spinal foramen.[2] An anteroposterior fluoroscopic view is obtained to verify that the needle is not medial to the 6 o'clock position of the pedicle to avoid placement of the needle too deep. Then 0.2 to 0.4 mL of contrast is injected under fluoroscopic guidance. The contrast should be seen flowing proximally around the pedicle into the epidural space, distal along the nerve root sheath with no evidence of subdural, subarachnoid, or intravascular spread. A mixture of a preservative-free local anesthetics and steroid is then slowly injected through the needle.

## Caudal Approach

### Indications
The caudal approach is commonly used in pediatrics for postoperative pain control after surgeries such as inguinal hernia repair and hypospadias correction. It can be also used in chronic pain management for conditions such as postlaminectomy syndrome.

*Technique*

The sacral hiatus is the access point for the epidural space for this approach. The sacral hiatus is identified by palpating the two sacral cornu laterally and the coccyx inferiorly.

The patient is placed in the prone position. After prepping and draping the skin in a sterile fashion, the skin over the sacral hiatus is anesthetized. A 25-gauge needle is typically used. As the ligament is penetrated, a "pop" will be felt. Needle position is confirmed using an air acceptance test or with contrast dye spread if fluoroscopy is utilized. A local anesthetic is then slowly injected to the epidural space. Steroid might be added for treatment of chronic pain conditions.

## SPINAL (SUBARACHNOID) ANESTHESIA

The spinal cord ends at approximately L1-L2 in the majority of adults. Since there is a differential in the density of neural blockade depending on the fiber type, the sympathetic blockade is typically at least two dermatome levels higher than the sensory blockade, and the sensory blockade is two levels higher than the motor blockade. The small C-type nerve fibers responsible for temperature change are the first to be affected, so one can test the level of a spinal block within the first few minutes by wiping a wet alcohol pad over the patient's skin bilaterally.[1]

### INDICATIONS

Indications are surgical procedures involving the mid to lower abdomen, perineum, and lower extremities including total hip and knee replacements.

### COMPLICATIONS

1. Sudden and severe hypotension
2. Postdural puncture headache
3. Same as epidural anesthesia

### TECHNIQUE

This technique can be done using midline or paramedian approaches, similar to epidural anesthesia. The technique is very similar except that the needle is further advanced until it penetrates the dura, which is accompanied by a characteristic popping sensation. The stylet is then removed to confirm the return of cerebrospinal fluid into the hub of the needle. The local anesthetic can then be slowly injected through the needle, reconfirming the correct location by a second aspiration near the end of the injection. Once complete, the needle and syringe are withdrawn and removed from the patient's back.

## FACET JOINT INJECTION

Each facet joint receives innervation from the medial branch at the same level as well as the level above. The most commonly affected facet joints are L3-4, L4-5, and L5-S1 for the lumbar region and C3-4, C4-5, and C5-6 for the cervical region.

### INDICATIONS

Facet arthropathy.

### TECHNIQUES

#### Medial Branch Block Technique

Using fluoroscopy, the junction between the transverse process and the superior articular process at the level to be blocked is identified for the medial branch block technique. After preparation of the skin with antiseptic solution, a skin wheal of local anesthetic is raised. A 25-gauge, 3½-inch needle is inserted and directed toward the most superomedial point at which the transverse process joins the vertebra. After negative aspiration, 0.5 mL of local anesthetic with or without steroid is injected through the spinal needle.[3]

#### Intra-Articular Technique

In the intra-articular technique, a 25-gauge, 3½-inch needle is advanced in an oblique fluoroscopic view to enter the target joint. After negative aspiration, 0.1–0.2 mL of contrast medium is injected under fluoroscopy to confirm needle placement. After correct needle placement is confirmed, 0.3 mL of local anesthetic with or without steroid is slowly injected through the spinal needle.[4]

### ULTRASOUND-GUIDED NEURAXIAL PROCEDURES

Advantages of ultrasound guidance include identifying correct vertebral level, identifying midline, identifying depth of various structures (spinous processes, lamina, epidural and subarachnoid spaces); identifying the optimal interspace; and identifying anatomical abnormalities (scoliosis, prior laminectomy and instrumentation). A low-frequency curvilinear ultrasound probe (2–5 MHz) is often used.[5]

### REFERENCES

1. Mogan GE, Mikhael MS. Regional anesthesia and pain management: spinal, epidural and caudal blocks. In: *Clinical Anesthesiology*. 4th ed. Lange/McGraw; 2006:289–321.

2. Benzon HT. Selective nerve root blocks and transforaminal epidural steroid injections. In: *Essentials of Pain Medicine*. 3rd ed. Elsevier; 2011:314–317.
3. Waldman SD. Lumbar facet block: medial branch technique. In: *Atlas of Interventional Pain Management*. 4th ed. Philadelphia, PA: Saunders; 2016:1721–1729.
4. Waldman SD. Lumbar facet block: intra-articular technique. In: *Atlas of Interventional Pain Management*. 4th ed. Philadelphia, PA: Saunders; 2016:1777–1785.
5. Chin KJ, et al. Ultrasound imaging facilitates spinal anesthesia in adults with difficult surface anatomic landmarks. *Anesthesiology* 2011;115:94–101.

# 30.

# DIAGNOSIS AND MANAGEMENT OF LOCAL ANESTHETIC SYSTEMIC TOXICITY (LAST)

*Kristopher M. Schroeder and Andrew Pfaff*

## INTRODUCTION

Local anesthetic systemic toxicity (LAST) may be a serious and life-threatening event that follows the administration of local anesthetics. In the perioperative setting, these local anesthetics have generally been administered by the anesthesia team. However, local anesthetic may be administered in excess by the surgical team or other colleagues outside of the perioperative arena. In fact, half of all cases of LAST occur following the administration of local anesthetic by nonanesthesiologists.[1] While the use of ultrasound guidance may decrease the risk of LAST, the use of high-volume fascial plane techniques, the application of multiple regional anesthesia techniques, or peripheral nerve catheters may increase the risk of this outcome. In addition, liposome-encapsulated local anesthetic formulations are associated with a risk of LAST if communication is inadequate or if local anesthetic is used inappropriately. Regardless, a thorough understanding of the presenting signs/symptoms, management, and strategies to minimize the risk of LAST is critical to ensure that patients receive regional anesthesia in a safe manner.

Fortunately, the risk of LAST following regional anesthesia techniques is generally considered to be quite low (2–2.8/10,000 peripheral nerve blocks, 0.7–1.8/10,000 epidurals) and decreasing over time.[2,3] There are a number of potential risk factors that might influence this risk in an individual patient. Neonates/infants, the elderly, and pregnant women appear to be at elevated risk for the development of LAST. In addition, those patients with significant renal, cardiac, and hepatic disease may be considered to be at elevated risk. The site of injection likely influences the risk of LAST, with the risk higher with upper extremity blocks than with lower extremity blocks.[1,3] Intercostal, psoas compartment, and proximal sciatic blocks may also be associated with significant vascularity, which may increase the risk of systemic effects.[3] Fascial plane blocks and continuous catheter techniques likely represent risk factors for the development of LAST. Liposomal bupivacaine, tumescent local anesthesia (maximum tumescent lidocaine dose 45 mg/kg with liposuction and 28 mg/kg without liposuction), airway topicalization (maximum lidocaine dose for airway topicalization 9 mg/kg), and intravenous local anesthetic administration must be done carefully to reduce the risk of LAST.[1] See Table 30.1 for recommended maximum doses.

Symptoms of LAST can be varied and impact a variety of organ systems over a wide period of time. Immediate reactions generally result from injection into the circulatory system. Delayed reactions (>20 minutes following a bolus injection) may result from systemic absorption of local anesthetic. The central nervous system may display signs of excitation, including perioral paresthesia, metallic taste, dizziness, confusion, agitation, sensory and visual disturbances, muscle contractions, unconsciousness, seizures, coma, and respiratory arrest. The cardiovascular

|  | PLAIN MAXIMUM DOSE (MG/KG) | WITH EPINEPHRINE MAXIMUM DOSE (MG/KG) |
|---|---|---|
| Lidocaine | 5 | 7 |
| Mepivacaine | 5 | 7 |
| Bupivacaine | 2 | 3 |
| Levobupivacaine | 2 | 3 |
| Ropivacaine | 3 | 3 |

Adapted from Reference 2.

system may display signs of excitation (hypertension and tachycardia) or depression (bradycardia [asystole] and hypotension). Dysrhythmia presentation can be highly variable and may include bradyarrhythmias, asystole, narrow- and wide-complex tachyarrhythmias, ventricular ectopy, or ST segment changes[1] (Figure 30.1). Symptomology can be challenging, and only 16% of patients report precursor symptoms, 41% have no neurologic symptoms prior to cardiac pathology, and general anesthesia or deep sedation may complicate efforts at symptom monitoring.[4]

Reducing this risk of LAST can be accomplished via a variety of collaborative mechanisms. Communication is critical to ensuring that all parties are aware of the mass and type of local anesthetic administered and what additional local anesthetic might be further administered. This discussion may be appropriate prior to a time-out procedure before the regional anesthesia procedure and in the operating room prior to the surgical procedure. This information may also be included in a detailed "handoff" procedure from the block team to the nursing/surgical teams, electronic medical record orders/alerts, or physical reminders (i.e., bracelets) to alert other providers of administered local anesthetic. Continuous communication with the patient regarding symptoms of LAST may be helpful. Close attention to weight-based dosing and the use of lean versus actual body weight to calculate maximum doses should be standard practice (Table 30.1). The use of ultrasound guidance may be associated with a significant decrease in LAST (65% reduction) versus nerve stimulation. Slow and fractionated injections (3- to 5-mL aliquots) of local anesthetics should only occur following aspiration to assess for intravascular needle positioning. The addition of epinephrine to local anesthetic solutions may also assist in the detection of intravascular injections (heart rate increase $\geq$ 10, systolic blood pressure increase $\geq$ 15 mm Hg).[4] The utility of an epinephrine-containing "test" dose may be diminished in the elderly, sedated, and patients treated with $\beta$-blockers. Proper syringe labeling, the use of unique connectors, and proper monitoring/preparation should all help to decrease the risk of LAST development.[1] The risk of severe LAST events may also be reduced through the use of local anesthetics less likely to cause severe cardiovascular collapse (i.e., ropivacaine or levobupivacaine vs. standard racemic bupivacaine).[4]

Management of LAST is greatly dependent on symptoms, but outcomes are improved by early detection and treatment. Treatment may be facilitated by easy access to American Society of Regional Anesthesia and Pain Medicine (ASRA) treatment checklists and preassembled

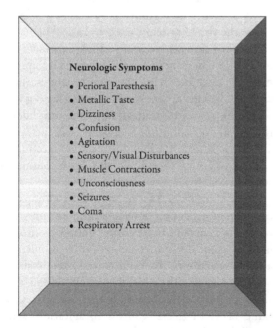

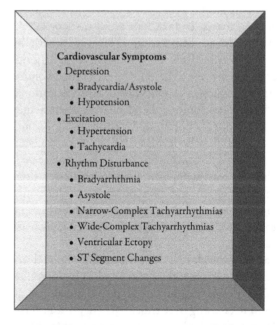

**Figure 30.1** Local anesthetic systemic toxicity symptoms.

LAST rescue kits. Early management should include cessation of local anesthetic administration and obtaining additional help. Supplemental oxygen should be administered and airway management with 100% oxygen should be considered if the patient is either unable to protect their own airway or there is concern regarding the development of hypoxia, hypercarbia, or acidosis. Hyperventilation causes decreased $PaCO_2$ (reduced seizure threshold), increased PH (decreased drug binding to proteins), and decreased incidence of seizures. Seizure activity should be terminated through the administration of benzodiazepines or small-dose propofol administration if there are no signs of cardiovascular compromise. Muscle relaxant administration should be considered if there are ongoing muscular contractions that might result in the development of metabolic acidosis.[1,5]

Intravenous lipid emulsion should be considered early in the course of any episode of LAST. In 2017, changes in the ASRA checklist for treatment of LAST simplified dosing by recommending a 100-mL bolus of 20% lipid emulsion in all patients greater than 70 kg (1.5 mL/kg in patients < 70 kg). Generally, a 200- to 250-mL infusion of lipid emulsion is then recommended over 15–20 minutes (0.25 mL/kg/min in patients < 70 kg). Boluses of lipid emulsion may be repeated in patients who remain unstable, with a maximum recommended dose of 12 mL/kg. If lipid emulsion therapy is required, assistance with case management can be found on the ASRA LAST™ smartphone app, and cases should be reported (http://lipidrescue.org).[5]

Following resolution of a LAST event, patients should be monitored for at least 4–6 hours following a cardiovascular event and 2 hours following a limited central nervous system event. In the event of cardiac arrest, advanced cardiac life support therapy should be initiated with reduced doses of epinephrine (≤1 μg/kg) and avoidance of vasopressin, calcium channel blockers, β-blockers or other local anesthetics. Amiodarone may be required in severe and treatment-unresponsive cases, cardiopulmonary bypass may be required and should be considered early.[3,5]

Other reactions to local anesthetics include

- Allergy: Methylparapan is a preservative in both amide and ester local anesthetics and can cause allergic reactions.
- Neural toxicity: Chloroprocaine in the presence of sodium bisulfite and low PH may cause neurotoxicity.
- Methemoglobinemia may occur with prilocaine.
- Cauda equina syndrome has been reported in the past with high concentrations of lidocaine when allowed to accumulate around the sacral nerve roots.

- Transient neurologic symptoms: Severe pain radiating down both legs has been reported most frequently with lidocaine.

## ANESTHETIC CONSIDERATIONS

### PREOPERATIVE CONSIDERATIONS

Prior to considering a regional anesthesia procedure, a LAST kit should be constructed that contains lipid emulsion; benzodiazepines and airway management equipment should also be immediately available. Intravenous access and standard American Society of Anesthesiologists monitors are mandatory. Supplemental oxygen should be administered in most cases.

### INTRAOPERATIVE CONSIDERATIONS

While sedation may be required to facilitate comfortable block placement, constant communication with the patient throughout block placement should be maintained to evaluate for the development of LAST symptoms. Ultrasound guidance should likely be considered in most cases to decrease the risk of intravascular injection. Epinephrine may be considered as an additive to increase the recognition of intravascular injections. Gentle syringe aspiration should occur prior to and intermittently during a fractionated local anesthetic injection.

### POSTOPERATIVE CONSIDERATIONS

Following regional anesthesia procedures, patients should be continuously monitored for the development of LAST symptoms.

### REFERENCES

1. Mörwald EE, et al. Incidence of local anesthetic systemic toxicity in orthopedic patients receiving peripheral nerve blocks. *Reg Anesth Pain Med*. 2017;42:442–445.
2. El-Boghdadly K, Chin KJ. Local anesthetic systemic toxicity: continuing professional development. *Can J Anesth*. 2016;63:330–349.
3. El-Boghdadly K, et al. Local anesthetic systemic toxicity: current perspectives. *Local Reg Anesth*. 2018;11:35–44.
4. Safety Committee of Japanese Society of Anesthesiologists. Practical guide for the management of systemic toxicity caused by local anesthetics. *J Anesth*. 2019;33:1–8.
5. Neal JM, et al. The American Society of Regional Anesthesia and Pain Medicine checklist for managing local anesthetic systemic toxicity. 2017 version. *Reg Anesth Pain Med*. 2018;43:150–153.

31.

# INTRAVENOUS LIPID EMULSION THERAPY AND THE AMERICAN SOCIETY OF REGIONAL ANESTHESIA CHECKLIST FOR LOCAL ANESTHETIC TOXICITY

*Kristopher M. Schroeder and Andrew Pfaff*

## INTRODUCTION

Identified as a promising resuscitation medication for local anesthetic systemic toxicity (LAST) in 1998, intravenous lipid emulsion (ILE) has become the cornerstone of therapy for patients with episodes of LAST and other intoxications.[1] The American Society of Regional Anesthesia and Pain Medicine (ASRA) convened its first conference on LAST in 2001, with updates in 2008 and 2017 as more translational studies were completed. Out of these practice advisories came a LAST checklist that provides the anesthesiologist with a rubric for the diagnosis, management, and monitoring of patients who have suspected or confirmed LAST.[1] While the practical aspects of advanced cardiac life support (ACLS), such as prompt chest compressions and advanced airway management, remain largely unchanged during resuscitation from LAST, the pharmacologic management of LAST differs from other cardiac arrest scenarios, primarily in that the mainstay of treatment is ILE.[1] ILE affects the distribution and metabolism of local anesthetics within the body in addition to providing direct positive cardiovascular effects.[1,2]

Previously described as a static "lipid sync," ILE acts more as a dynamic "shuttle" that redistributes local anesthetic from sites of toxicity to sites of storage or metabolism.[2] ILE partitions local anesthetic in a concentration-dependent manner inside liposomes. Lipophilic drugs (e.g., bupivacaine) appear to be bound more avidly than hydrophilic drugs (e.g., ropivacaine), suggesting that recovery from hydrophilic drug toxicity may be prolonged or less pronounced.[2] ILE redistributes the local anesthetic from the brain and heart, the sites of primary toxicity in LAST, to be metabolized by the liver or to be stored by the muscles and adipose tissue.[2] Secondarily, ILE appears to have cardiotonic and vasoactive effects, which has been studied both in the absence and in the presence of LAST. Both the bolus volume and direct effects of lipid given during resuscitation appear

to contribute to positive inotropy and lusitropy, perhaps due to the heart's preference for fatty acid as a preferred fuel source during aerobic conditions.[2] ILE directly raises blood pressure as well, although whether this is a direct effect of ILE or simply a reversal of local anesthetic-mediated vasodilation is unknown.[2] Additionally, some evidence exists that ILE may reduce the burden of ischemia-reperfusion injury that occurs after successful resuscitation from LAST.[2]

Intravenous lipid emulsion should be dosed at 1.5 mL/kg, up to 100 mL, as a rapid bolus over 2–3 minutes, followed by an infusion of 0.25 mL/kg/min (ideal body weight) over 15–20 minutes.[1,3] The bolus can be repeated twice if resuscitation is prolonged, where the total volume of ILE may approach 1 L. However, the total cumulative dose of ILE should be less than 12 mL/kg.[1,3] Epinephrine boluses should be reduced to 1 µg/kg or less as opposed to the typical 1-mg dose recommended in other ACLS scenarios. Vasopressin, β-blockers, calcium channel blockers, and other local anesthetics should not be given. In the event of seizures, benzodiazepines are preferred over propofol, particularly in hemodynamically unstable patients.[1,3,4] As resuscitation may be prolonged in patients with LAST, early notification of the cardiopulmonary bypass team may be warranted.[1,3] All of these recommendations can be found in the ASRA practice advisory, which is reproduced in part here and is available on the ASRA website or in the ASRA LAST™ smartphone application (Table 31.1).[3]

After an episode of LAST, patients should have critical care–level monitoring for a minimum of 2 hours after an isolated central nervous system event and 4–6 hours after a cardiovascular event.[1,3] Redistribution out of "sink" tissues such as muscle and adipose can cause cardiovascular depression to recur.[2] If the episode of LAST is short-lived without any cardiovascular instability, one can consider moving forward with the anesthetic after a monitoring period of 30 minutes.[1,3] If ILE is administered during an

**Table 31.1** DOSING OF INTRAVENOUS LIPID EMULSION AS DESCRIBED IN THE ASRA LAST CHECKLIST.[3]

| LIPID EMULSION 20% (PRECISE VOLUME AND FLOW RATE ARE NOT CRUCIAL) | |
| --- | --- |
| GREATER THAN 70 KG PATIENT | LESS THAN 70 KG PATIENT |
| Bolus 100 mL Lipid Emulsion 20% rapidly over 2–3 minutes Lipid emulsion infusion 200–250 mL over 15–20 minutes | Bolus 1.5 mL/kg Lipid Emulsion 20% rapidly over 2–3 minutes Lipid emulsion infusion ~0.25 mL/kg/min (ideal body weight) |
| If patient remains unstable: Re-bolus once or twice at the same dose and double infusion rate; be aware of dosing limit (12mL/kg) Total volume of lipid emulsion can approach 1 L in a prolonged resuscitation (e.g., > 30 minutes) | |

Source: ASRA, Copyright 2017.

episode of LAST, the event should be reported (http://www.lipidrescue.org).[4]

## ANESTHETIC CONSIDERATIONS

### PREOPERATIVE

Prior to performing a regional anesthetic, a preassembled LAST rescue kit should be available. ASRA recommends the kit contain, at a minimum, 1 L of ILE; several large syringes, needles, and intravenous tubing for ILE administration; and the ASRA LAST checklist to assist providers with patient management.[1,3] Alternatively, providers may also purchase the ASRA LAST smartphone application, which reproduces the ASRA LAST checklist in an interactive format. Additional standard resuscitation supplies, such as advanced airway equipment, code medications, and benzodiazepines for seizure management, should also be readily available. The ASRA Timeout™ smartphone application can be used to verify that all necessary resuscitation materials are available and that proper consideration of patient comorbidities, medication dosing, and procedure technique has occurred.

### INTRAOPERATIVE

The ASRA LAST checklist details several methods to decrease the risk of intravascular injection, thus decreasing the risk of LAST.[1,3] Incremental dosing of local anesthetics (e.g., 3- to 5-mL aliquots) using continuous ultrasonography is recommended to avoid vascular puncture and to reduce the total volume of local anesthetic required for a successful procedure.[1,3,5] Gentle aspiration of the syringe should occur prior to and intermittently during injection. A pharmacological marker of intravascular injection, such as epinephrine, should be considered when feasible.[1,3]

### POSTOPERATIVE

Patients should be continuously monitored for the development of LAST symptoms during and after a regional anesthetic.[1,3] While half of cases of LAST show symptoms within 1 minute after injection, in rare instances the development of LAST has been delayed as much as 30 minutes after the injection of local anesthetic.[5] If LAST does occur, patients should be monitored for a minimum of 2 hours after a central nervous system event and for 4–6 hours after a cardiovascular event.[1,3]

## REFERENCES

1. The third American Society of Regional Anesthesia and Pain Medicine practice advisory on local anesthetic systemic toxicity. Executive SUMMARY 2017. *Reg Anesth Pain Med.* 2018;43:113–123.
2. Fettiplace MR, Weinberg G. The mechanisms underlying lipid resuscitation therapy. *Reg Anesth Pain Med.* 2018;43:138–149.
3. Neal JM, et al. The American Society of Regional Anesthesia and Pain Medicine checklist for managing local anesthetic systemic toxicity. 2017 Version. *Reg Anesth Pain Med.* 2018;43:150–153.
4. El-Boghdadly K, et al. Local anesthetic systemic toxicity: current perspectives. *Local Reg Anesth.* 2018;11:35–44.
5. Safety Committee of Japanese Society of Anesthesiologists. Practical guide for the management of systemic toxicity caused by local anesthetics. *J Anesth.* 2019;33:1–8.

# ROLE OF REGIONAL ANESTHESIA IN ENHANCED RECOVERY PROTOCOLS

*Kristopher M. Schroeder and Andrew Pfaff*

## INTRODUCTION

### ENHANCED RECOVERY GENERAL CONSIDERATIONS

Enhanced recovery protocols following surgical procedures have become a tremendously popular and important topic for academicians to debate and for clinicians to attempt to implement. The etiology for this interest is likely multifactorial. Clearly, there is a desire to improve the delivery of patient care, decrease pain and opioid requirements, and generally improve perioperative outcomes. However, there are also a number of important logistical concerns that have driven the implementation of these protocols as they will ideally result in decreased revenue expenditures and duration/need for costly inpatient hospital admissions.

In the pursuit of these novel care pathways, efforts have now been made to collaboratively evaluate all aspects of the perioperative process to ascertain what care components can be optimized to improve patient care. There are a number of core tenants to enhanced recovery protocols that may be worthy of attention. Prehabilitation, strength training or physical therapy prior to surgical interventions may allow patients to present to surgery in an optimized physical condition that improves their ability to navigate the perioperative process. Optimizing adverse health conditions (smoking cessation, weight optimization, diabetes control, etc.) may further improve perioperative outcomes and reduce the incidence of adverse events, including surgical site infections. Core to any enhanced recovery pathway are efforts to improve patient education to alleviate patient anxiety, improve patient and family readiness, and create a framework to provide realistic perioperative outcomes for patients with regard to pain and strategies for pain management. Novel fasting guidelines have recognized that traditional advice to maintain nothing by mouth may be overly restrictive and result in patients presenting for surgery in a dehydrated and catabolic state. Careful attention is applied to intravenous fluid administration, and efforts are made to minimize overly aggressive efforts at volume resuscitation. Efforts are made in these protocols to expedite the recovery of gastrointestinal function via minimization of opioid administration, decreased utilization of nasogastric tubes, aggressive treatment/prophylaxis for nausea, and early feeding. Within these pathways, efforts are made to mobilize patients early and limit the development of weakness that develops from prolonged periods of immobilization while decreasing the development of deep venous thrombosis and atelectasis/pneumonia.[1]

### ENHANCED RECOVERY ANALGESIC CONSIDERATIONS

Core to the success of any perioperative enhanced recovery protocol are efforts to address the pain associated with surgical procedures and minimize the requirement for opioid analgesics. These efforts may certainly be complicated in patients with chronic opioid requirements or pain conditions. However, attention to pain and opioid administration may benefit patients through reductions in opioid-related side effects, decreased surgical stress responses, hastened return of bowel function, decreased length/requirement for hospital inpatient admissions, decreased chronic pain and opioid requirements, reductions in morbidity/mortality, and decreased healthcare costs.[2] Other potential benefits of regional anesthesia procedures as a component of an enhanced recovery pathway include improved mobility, decreased postoperative nausea and vomiting, and improved organ function.[2] Additionally, there is an increased understanding that acute pain and opioid requirements in the immediate postoperative setting may increase the risk of long-standing pain conditions and increase the risk of opioid abuse.[3,4]

The role of regional anesthesia in enhanced recovery protocols depends greatly on the planned surgical procedure, available equipment, and skill/training of the anesthesiologist. In addition, there are several patient-specific characteristics (coagulopathy, preexisting nerve injury, respiratory insufficiency, etc.) that may impact the ability to deliver a particular type of regional anesthesia. With any planned regional anesthesia procedure, consideration should be given to the impact that the procedure may have on the ability of the patient to safely ambulate, and consideration should be given to procedures less likely to result in significant motor weakness.

When considering surgical patients that might benefit from enhanced recovery protocols, the prototypical example are those patients presenting for colorectal surgery. In these patients, the increasing variety and indications of fascial plane blocks have facilitated the ability to minimize opioid administration, smoothly transition to oral analgesic administration, facilitate early postoperative ambulation and minimize the risk of urinary retention, and contraindications to venous thromboembolism prophylaxis administration (Box 32.1; Figure 32.1). While colorectal surgery is commonly associated with enhanced recovery pathways, cardiac, gynecology, breast, thoracic, urology, vascular, and orthopedic surgical procedures have also benefited from the implementation of enhanced recovery pathways that include regional anesthesia procedures. While traditional approaches to interventional pain management (i.e., epidural analgesia) continue to maintain a place in perioperative pain management, the diversity of cases that might benefit from enhanced recovery protocols, including regional anesthesia, benefits greatly from improvements in ultrasound technology and increased understanding of fascial plane anatomy and global skill with regional anesthesia. Unfortunately, clinical studies have yet to match enthusiasm for a number of fascial plane blocks, and further research is required to make definitive recommendations for the provision of fascial plane block analgesia.[1–3,5]

## ANESTHETIC CONSIDERATIONS

### PREOPERATIVE CONSIDERATIONS

When considering pain management as a component of enhanced recovery pathways, the preoperative arena represents a time period that might benefit from significant and thoughtful planning. In patients requiring chronic opioid agonist or agonist-antagonist therapy, collaboration with the patient's primary opioid prescriber will optimize the ability to adequately manage pain and minimize the risk of abuse in at-risk patients. A thorough conversation with the patient that establishes expected analgesic regimens and realistic pain goals may be beneficial. In general, activating regional anesthesia procedures in the preoperative arena will facilitate the ability to minimize intraoperative opioid requirements and potentially limit the development of opioid-induced hyperalgesia. Utilization of catheter-based techniques will facilitate the ability to continue any regional anesthesia–based technique into the postoperative period. In certain circumstances, the preoperative administration of multimodal analgesics (gabapentinoids, acetaminophen, nonsteroidal anti-inflammatory drugs [NSAIDs], methadone, dexamethasone) may serve as useful adjuncts.[1,3,4]

### INTRAOPERATIVE CONSIDERATIONS

During surgery, efforts should be made to limit opioid and other sedative administration to limit the development of opioid-induced hyperalgesia, limit the development of postoperative nausea and vomiting, and increase postoperative alertness. These efforts could include a reliance on regional anesthesia techniques for the provision of analgesia; the administration of nonopioid analgesics (i.e., ketamine, methadone, magnesium, acetaminophen, NSAIDS, lidocaine infusions, $\alpha_2$ agonists, etc.); and the use of other agents that might result in reduced opioid requirements (i.e., esmolol).

### POSTOPERATIVE CONSIDERATIONS

Following surgery, efforts should continue to be made to minimize opioid administration through the use of multimodal analgesics (gabapentinoids, acetaminophen, NSAIDs, ketamine, lidocaine infusions, etc.) and regional anesthesia techniques. Consideration should be given to the administration of nonmedicinal forms of pain management (i.e., transcutaneous electrical nerve stimulation unit, mindfulness, guided relaxation, massage, heat/cold administration, etc.). If opioids are required, efforts should be made to limit dose requirements and restrict administration to the oral route.

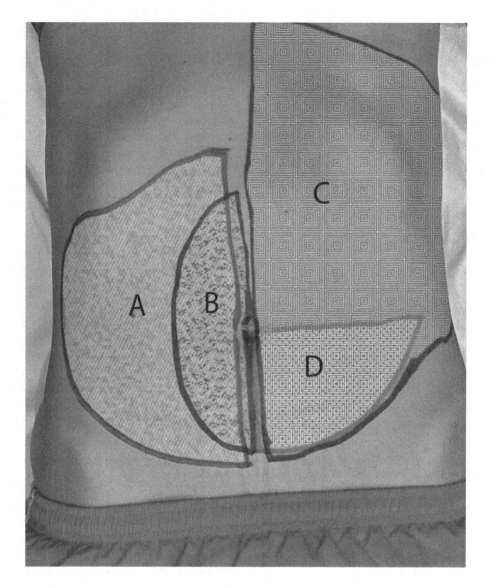

**Figure 32.1** Expected coverage of fascial plane blocks utilized for abdominal surgery: A, quadratus lumborum block; B, rectus sheath block; C, erector spinae block; D, transversus abdominis block.

## REFERENCES

1. Afonso AM, et al. Enhanced recovery programs in outpatient surgery. *Anesthesiol Clin.* 2019;37:225–238.
2. McIsaac DI, et al. Impact of including regional anaesthesia in enhanced recovery protocols: a scoping review. *Br J Anaesth.* 2015;115:ii46–ii56.
3. Beverly A, et al. Essential elements of multimodal analgesia in enhanced recovery after surgery (ERAS) guidelines. *Anesthesiol Clin.* 2017;35:e115–e143.
4. Echeverria-Villalobos M, et al. Enhanced recovery after surgery (ERAS). A perspective review of postoperative pain management under ERAS pathways and its role on opioid crisis in the United States. *Clin J Pain.* 2020;36:219–226.
5. Carli F, Clemente A. Regional anesthesia and enhanced recovery after surgery. *Minerva Anestesiol.* 2014;80:1229–1233.

# 33.

# INNERVATION OF PELVIC STRUCTURES

*Peter Yi and Kevin E. Vorenkamp*

## INTRODUCTION

The visceral organs in the pelvis include the bladder, ureters, rectum, and the male or female reproductive organs. In the female, these include the uterus, cervix, ovaries, and fallopian tubes, and in the male the ductus deferens, seminal glands, and prostate. The innervation of the pelvis is complex and can be confusing. Pelvic visceral organs receive autonomic, visceral, and somatic nerve input from multiple sources, including specific spinal nerves and a network of plexuses.

The pelvic organs are innervated by the autonomic nervous system, by both the sympathetic and parasympathetic components. The sympathetic nervous system arises from the thoracolumbar spine as the sympathetic chain, while the parasympathetic nervous system originates from the cranial-sacral spinal cord. In the sympathetic system, the preganglia are close to the spinal cord, while in the parasympathetic system, the preganglia are further from the spinal cord but in close proximity to the visceral organ. In general, sympathetic nerves cause muscle contraction and vasoconstriction, while the parasympathetic nerves have the opposite actions of muscle relaxation and vasodilation. For example, the parasympathetic nervous system causes relaxation of the urethral sphincter, facilitating urination when not in a "fight-or-flight" state.[1]

The sympathetic chain courses along the anterolateral border of the thoracic and lumbar vertebral bodies (T10-L2). From the sympathetic ganglion, gray communicating rami via *thoracolumbar splanchnic nerves* join the superior hypogastric plexus, then separate into a right and left hypogastric nerve before entering the inferior hypogastric plexus.[2] From the inferior hypogastric plexus, sympathetic nerves continue on to innervate the pelvic visceral organs. The sympathetic chain terminates at a single ganglion at the sacrum, known as the ganglion impar (ganglion of Walther). Sympathetic fibers from the ganglion impar, called *sacral splanchnic nerves*, course with somatic branches of sacral and coccygeal spinal nerves to innervate

the perineum and contribute visceral branches to the inferior hypogastric plexus.

The parasympathetic nerves arise from the sacral segments of the spine (S2-S4) and are also known as the *pelvic splanchnic nerves*. These nerves converge at the inferior hypogastric plexus with sympathetic nerves and course with these sympathetic nerves to various secondary plexuses of pelvic organs (i.e., vesicle plexus, prostate plexus, vaginal plexus, etc.). The nerves from the inferior hypogastric plexus therefore carry mixed sympathetic and parasympathetic nerves to provide opposite responses at the pelvic organs.

Visceral afferent fibers run along both sympathetic and parasympathetic nerves to various organs and are responsible for classic visceral symptoms of dull, achy, diffuse pain. The visceral innervation of the pelvic organs is complex and often difficult to elucidate due to phenomena known as viscerosomatic and viscerovisceral convergence, which is beyond the scope of this chapter.[3]

The terminal nerves of the *lumbar plexus* (Figure 33.1) include the iliohypogastric nerve, ilioinguinal nerve, genitofemoral nerve, lateral femoral cutaneous nerve, femoral nerve, and obturator nerve.[4] These somatic nerves carry purely motor, purely sensory, or both motor and sensory information. The *iliohypogastric nerve* supplies sensation to the inguinal region, lower abdomen, flank, and posterolateral gluteal skin in the pubic region. It has a motor component to parts of the abdominal wall. The *ilioinguinal nerve* supplies sensation to the anteromedial thigh, the base of the penis and anterior scrotum in males, and the mons pubis and labia majora in females. The ilioinguinal nerve provides motor supply to part of the psoas muscle. The femoral branch of the *genitofemoral nerve* innervates the anterior superior thigh, while the genital branch supplies the mons pubis and labia majora in the female and the penis and scrotum in the male. The genital branch provides motor innervation to the cremasteric muscle. The *lateral femoral cutaneous* nerve is purely sensory, supplying the lateral aspect of the thigh. The *femoral*

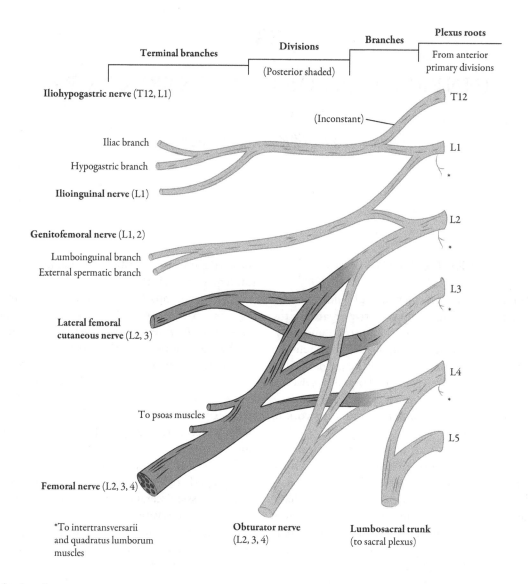

Iliohypogastric nerve (T12, L1)

(Inconstant)

T12

Iliac branch

L1

Hypogastric branch

Ilioinguinal nerve (L1)

*

Genitofemoral nerve (L1, 2)

L2

Lumboinguinal branch
External spermatic branch

*

Lateral femoral
cutaneous nerve (L2, 3)

L3

*

L4

To psoas muscles

*

L5

Femoral nerve (L2, 3, 4)

*To intertransversarii
and quadratus lumborum
muscles

Obturator nerve
(L2, 3, 4)

Lumbosacral trunk
(to sacral plexus)

Figure 33.1 The lumbar plexus.

*nerve* is the main nerve to the lower extremity from the lumbar plexus. It provides sensation to the anterior thigh and motor innervation to the quadricep muscles. The *obturator nerve* innervates the pelvic parietal peritoneum and the medial thigh and also supplies motor innervation to the adductor muscles of the thigh. Articular branches of both the femoral and obturator nerves provide sensory innervation to the hip joint and are established targets for hip joint radio-frequency ablation for chronic hip pain. The lumbosacral trunk from the lumbar plexus continues on to the sacral plexus.

The *sciatic nerve* is the major terminal nerve from the *sacral plexus* (see Figure 33.2).[4] Nerves innervating multiple muscles in the pelvis (superior/inferior gluteal muscles, quadratus femoris, obturator internus, etc.) also originate from the sacral plexus, as well as smaller nerves contributing to the lumbar and pudendal plexuses.

The *pudendal nerve* arises from S2–S4 in the *sacral and coccygeal plexuses* (see Figure 33.3).[4] The pudendal nerve is one of the major somatic nerves of the perineum. It innervates various muscles of the pelvic floor (e.g., the levator ani muscle, erectile muscles, urethral and anal sphincters) and supplies sensation to the perineum, perianal region, clitoris, and external genital organs of both sexes.

Innervation of the pelvic structures is complex and can be intimidating. Although this is a brief overview, the innervation of the pelvic organs can be organized into the basic divisions of the nervous system (autonomic, visceral, and somatic) to gain a better understanding of how the pelvis is innervated.

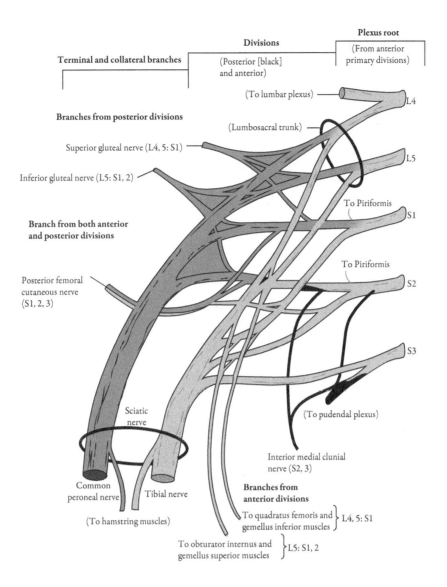

**Figure 33.2** The sacral plexus.

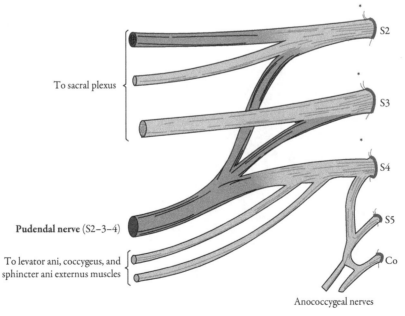

**Figure 33.3** Sacral and coccygeal plexus.

# REFERENCES

1. Westfall TC, et al. Neurotransmission: the autonomic and so-
matic motor nervous systems. In: Brunton LL, et al., eds. *Goodman
& Gilman's: The Pharmacological Basis of Therapeutics*. 13th ed.
McGraw-Hill; August 2020: Chap. 8.

2. Abouassaly R, et al. Pelvic innervation. In: Campbell-Walsh
Urology. Published online 2011:13–14.

3. Kibe H, et al. Pelvic and abdominal pain. In: Bajwa ZH, et al., eds.
*Principles and Practice of Pain Medicine*. 3rd ed. McGraw-Hill;
2017: Chap. 44. Accessed August 23, 2020.

4. Waxman SG. *Clinical Neuroanatomy*. 29th ed. McGraw-Hill
Education; 2020: Figure C-10, Figure C-12, Figure C-18, Appendix C.

# Part 6

# PHARMACOLOGY

# 34.

# GENERAL CONCEPTS IN PHARMACOLOGY

*Daniel Gonzalez Kapp*

## INTRODUCTION

Pharmacology is the basic science underlying the complex therapeutic actions of anesthetics. Primary areas of research in pharmacology include drug discovery, drug composition, pharmacokinetics, pharmacodynamics, and toxicology. Knowledge of a drug's pharmacology is fundamental to understating the potential therapeutic benefits and risks of the drug when used in clinical practice. Key chemistry-related concepts within pharmacology describing a drug's ability to distribute through the body and interact with its target include pH, pKa, and protein binding.[1]

## DRUG DISTRIBUTION

The ability of a drug to reach various targets within the body is dependent on its partition and distribution between compartments, mainly from the blood into the body tissues.

## PH

The acidity (or basicity) of a solution is described by its pH, a measure of the hydrogen ion concentration when in aqueous solution; the acidity of a solution is inversely correlated with pH, with more acidic solutions having a lower pH. Strong acids (and bases) are substances that exist in a completely ionized form when in solution.

## PKA

Most drugs used in practice are either weak acids or weak bases that, in contrast to strong acids or bases, exist in an equilibrium between the parent compound (i.e., un-ionized) and a dissociated ionic form (i.e., ionized).[2] Typically, a drug must pass through several barriers (e.g., blood-brain barrier) before reaching the intended target and may include passive diffusion across plasma membranes, dissolution or protein transport in the blood, and active transmembrane transport. In the case of passive transport across lipid

bilayers, only lipophilic compounds will easily pass through the membrane, while highly ionized compounds require a mechanism of active transport (e.g., transporter proteins); therefore, because weak acids (and bases) exist in an equilibrium between a lipophilic (i.e., un-ionized) and hydrophilic state (i.e., ionized), they are able to both cross lipid membranes and undergo dissolution in biologic solutions, the extent of which is dependent on the degree of ionization.[3] The pKa is the pH at which a compound exists in equal concentrations of ionized and un-ionized forms. The flux of a drug across a membrane therefore depends on the drug's pKa and the pH gradient across the membrane. The relative proportion of ionized to un-ionized forms of a drug can be derived from the Henderson-Hasselbalch equation (Figure 34.1).

$$\mathrm{pH} = \mathrm{p}K_\mathrm{a} + \log_{10}\left(\frac{[\text{Base}]}{[\text{Acid}]}\right)$$

**Figure 34.1** Henderson-Hasselbalch equation.

## PROTEIN BINDING

Drug transport through the body via plasma is facilitated in part by binding of the un-ionized drug to plasma proteins. While protein binding is beneficial to the drug distribution process, only unbound drug is able to freely move across membranes such as the blood-brain barrier. Therefore, drugs that are highly protein bound (>80%) are expected to have a very low concentration of unbound ionized (i.e., active) forms in the plasma, making the therapeutic action of these compounds highly sensitive to changes in plasma protein concentration or displacement by more highly bound drugs (Table 34.1).[4]

Furthermore, protein binding is influenced by the relative pH of the blood and plasma and therefore may be affected by physiologic states such as those caused by hyper- or hypoventilation. Albumin is the most common and abundant plasma protein involved in the transport of drugs,

**Table 34.1** PRIMARY FACTORS AFFECTING DRUG PROTEIN BINDING

| FACTOR | AFFECT | EXAMPLE |
|---|---|---|
| Drug-drug interactions | Displacement of one drug from plasma protein by another may lead to unpredictable dose-response relationship. | Nonsteroidal anti-inflammatory drugs can displace phenytoin from plasma binding sites, leading to toxic effects from phenytoin at otherwise normal doses. |
| Hypoalbuminemia | Highly protein-bound drugs will have an increase in free drug (i.e., active) concentration, potentially leading to an exaggerated drug response to otherwise normal doses. | Plasma albumin concentration is often decreased in the elderly, in neonates, and in the presence of malnutrition, liver, renal, or cardiac failure and malignancy. |

particularly those that are weak acids or neutral compounds. The drugs used in the clinical practice of anesthesiology, specifically the intravenously administered compounds that create the hypnotic aspect (unconsciousness) and the analgesic aspect (opiates) of an anesthetic, provide important insights into principles that can be applied to drug development in general. Additionally, research involving these drugs and their therapeutic applications has advanced some of the fundamental principles of pharmacokinetic and pharmacodynamic modeling. This chapter reviews several examples of anesthetic drugs used in clinical pharmacology and points out how they provide insights into methods of applying these modeling concepts to modern drug development in general (© 2008 American Society for Clinical Pharmacology and Therapeutics).[3] To a lesser extent, and for drugs that are weak bases, globulins (e.g., $\alpha_1$-acid glycoprotein) can also bind drugs in circulation.

## ANESTHETIC CONSIDERATIONS

### PREOPERATIVE

Preoperative assessment should include consideration of the chemistry-related factors affecting the transportation and distribution across body compartments of each anesthetic agent to be used. Example patient-specific conditions to evaluate include those affecting blood pH (e.g., hyperventilation), plasma protein binding (e.g., low albumin due to malnutrition), and the pH of local environments (e.g., low pH in tissue due to infection). Careful evaluation of potential drug-drug interactions between highly protein-bound drugs is required as any displacement of drug from plasma protein may exaggerate clinical effects.

### INTRAOPERATIVE

Patients should be monitored for aberrations of physiologic pH (i.e., acidosis or alkalosis) as changes in blood or tissue pH may lead to supra- or subtherapeutic drug action. Close monitoring for drug toxicity intraoperatively in those with underlying conditions affecting protein binding is required as unpredictable changes in active drug concentrations are possible.

### POSTOPERATIVE

Continued monitoring for and correction of acidosis or alkalosis is required. For highly protein-bound drugs, changes in plasma protein concentration postoperatively may lead to changes in total serum drug concentration; laboratory measurement of free drug concentration may be necessary.[5]

## REFERENCES

1. Johnson KB, Egan TD. Pharmacokinetics, biophase, and pharmacodynamics and the importance of simulation. In: Johnson KB, ed. *Clinical Pharmacology for Anesthesiology*. McGraw-Hill Education; 2015: Chap. 1. http://accessanesthesiology.mhmedical.com/content.aspx?aid=1103962917
2. Johnson KB, Egan TD. Principles of pharmacokinetics and pharmacodynamics: applied clinical pharmacology for the practitioner. In: Longnecker DE, et al, eds. *Anesthesiology*. 3rd ed. McGraw-Hill Education; 2017: Chap. 36. http://accessanesthesiology.mhmedical.com/content.aspx?aid=1144118152
3. Kern SE, Stanski DR. Pharmacokinetics and pharmacodynamics of intravenously administered anesthetic drugs: concepts and lessons for drug development. *Clin Pharmacol Ther*. 2008;84(1):153–157.
4. Shafer SL. The pharmacology of anesthetic drugs in elderly patients. *Anesthesiol Clin North Am*. 2000;18(1):1–29.
5. Roberts F, Freshwater-Turner D. Pharmacokinetics and anaesthesia. *Contin Educ Anaesth Crit Care Pain*. 2007;7(1):25–29.

# 35.

# PHARMACOGENETICS AND GENETIC FACTORS IN DRUG DOSE-RESPONSE RELATIONSHIPS

*Daniel Gonzalez Kapp*

## INTRODUCTION

Pharmacogenetics and pharmacogenomics are related areas of research aimed to determine the relationship between genotypic variation, including changes in gene expression, and variations in drug response seen across patient groups.[1] From a practical standpoint, identifying and understanding the genetic bases of variability in drug response due to changes in pharmacokinetics (e.g., drug absorption, distribution, metabolism, excretion) or pharmacodynamics (e.g., drug receptor up- or downregulation) are essential for the practitioner to fully anticipate, recognize, and mitigate potential drug toxicity or ineffectiveness. The ultimate goal of pharmacogenetics and pharmacogenomics is to personalize the therapeutics for an individual by leveraging the identification of phenotypic variation in drug response due to genetic mutations, polymorphisms, and gene expression to develop tailored.

## TERMINOLOGY

Historically, the term *pharmacogenetics* has referred to the pharmacokinetics-based investigation of specific genotypes, where a limited number of variants affect drug metabolism.[1] The term *pharmacogenomics* is a newer concept and refers to the population-based investigation of the complex gene expression patterns within the entirety of the genome and their effects on drug action, facilitated by recent advances in genomic analysis (e.g., DNA sequencing, multigene mapping).

## GENETIC FACTORS IN DRUG DOSE-RESPONSE RELATIONSHIPS

The principle concept of pharmacogenetics is genetic polymorphism, where a persistent genetic variation in an individual causes a phenotypic variant of the usual drug dose-response relationship.[2] These genetic variations can either be acquired (e.g., due to prior cytotoxic chemotherapy) or inherited (e.g., CYP2D6 enzyme polymorphisms). Genetic polymorphisms can lead to phenotypic variation in either drug efficacy (e.g., subtherapeutic effect due to higher drug metabolism) or predisposition to drug toxicity (e.g., narrow therapeutic window due to loss-of-function mutations in metabolizing enzymes).

The most common underlying variation in DNA sequence associated with genetic polymorphisms is a change in a single nucleotide (i.e., single-nucleotide polymorphism, SNP), occurring at frequencies of greater than 1% in the population.[3] An SNP arising from a substitution in the coding region of a gene can affect protein stability or substrate affinity through a change in amino acid sequence. Less obvious but of equal importance, SNPs in the noncoding region of a gene can alter regulatory regions (e.g., promoter sequence, intron position) important for gene expression or splicing. Beyond SNPs, other less common but generally more disruptive sequence changes include insertions or deletions of nucleotide(s) at loci required for drug metabolism (e.g., CYP enzymes) or drug receptor regulation.[4]

## GENETIC VARIABILITY OF DRUG METABOLISM: CYTOCHROME P450

The cytochrome P450 (CYP) pathway is critical for the metabolism of most drugs and xenobiotics. In humans, the most prominent subfamilies (and isoforms) involved with drug metabolism are CYP3A (e.g., CYP3A4), CYP2D (e.g., CYP2D6), CYP1A (e.g., CYP1A2), and CYP2C (e.g., CYP2C9, CYP2C19).[5] Phenotypic variation in the drug dose-response curve may arise from either a loss-of-function or gain-of-function mutation in a prominent CYP isoform. Whether these mutations lead to an increase or decrease in drug activity is dependent on the drug's chemical properties in vivo; drugs that are active as the parent compound will be inactivated at a slower rate, while prodrugs requiring metabolic transformation will have less therapeutic effect.

## ISOFORMS CYP2D6 AND CYP3A4

The CYP2D6 isoform is responsible for the metabolism of numerous pertinent drugs, including codeine, tramadol,

**Table 35.1** PERIOPERATIVE DRUGS AND GENETIC POLYMORPHISMS

| DRUG CLASS | EXAMPLE AGENTS | GENETIC BASIS OF VARIANTS | CLINICAL EFFECT |
|---|---|---|---|
| Analgesics | Codeine, tramadol, hydrocodone | CPY2D6 (prodrugs) | Reduced or increased drug effect |
| Analgesics | Fentanyl, alfentanil | CYP3A4 | Reduced drug effect |
| Anti-arrhythmics | Procainamide | N-Acetyltransferase 2 (NAT2) | Increased drug effect |
| Anticoagulants | Warfarin | CYP2C9 | Increased drug effect |
| Anticonvulsants | Phenytoin | CYP2C9 | Increased drug effect |
| β-Blockers | Metoprolol, carvedilol, propranolol, labetalol, and timolol | CPY2D6 | Reduced or increased drug effect |
| Calcium channel blockers | Diltiazem, verapamil | CYP3A4 | Reduced drug effect |
| Inhaled anesthetics | Desflurane, halothane, isoflurane | RYR1/CACNA1S | Increased risk of malignant hyperthermia |
| Neuromuscular blocking agents | Succinylcholine | Butyrylcholinesterase (BCHE) | Increased drug effect |

β-blockers, flecainide, propafenone, and diltiazem. There are 12 known mutations leading to a spectrum of CYP2D6 enzymatic activity, ranging from poor metabolizer (10% of population) to ultrarapid metabolizer (5%–7% of population) phenotypes. Reduced CYP2D6 metabolism of codeine, tramadol, and hydrocodone to their active metabolites leads to reduced analgesic effect and increased risk for toxicity. Both CYP2D6 and CYP3A4 are involved in the metabolism of oxycodone, methadone, and tramadol, while only CYP3A4 is responsible for fentanyl metabolism.

### CYP2C9

The CYP2C9 isoform is responsible for the metabolism of common analgesics (nonsteroidal anti-inflammatory drugs), anticoagulants (e.g., warfarin), and anticonvulsants (e.g., phenytoin). In the case of warfarin, low metabolizer phenotypes are highly sensitive to warfarin and therefore are at increased risk for bleeding events perioperatively and during chronic therapy (Table 35.1).

## ANESTHETIC CONSIDERATIONS

### PREOPERATIVE

Patients should be evaluated for pharmacogenetic variants that increase the risk for drug toxicity or that may alter the response to anesthetics. Notable drug classes associated with phenotypic variation include anticoagulants (e.g., warfarin [CYP2C9]), analgesics (e.g., hydrocodone [CYP2C9]), and β-blockers (CYP2D6).

### INTRAOPERATIVE

Intraoperative use of analgesics, anticonvulsants, and antiarrhythmics should be continuously monitored for unexpected drug responses or toxicity due to CYP isoform variants if not identified preoperatively (e.g., fentanyl [CYP3A4], phenytoin [CYP2C6], β-blockers [CPY2D6]).

### POSTOPERATIVE

In most cases, the effects of genetic variation on drug pharmacokinetics and pharmacodynamics will extend into the immediate postoperative period and will continue until drug discontinuation, requiring careful monitoring for toxicities. Pharmacogenetic evaluation of any new or modified therapies (e.g., warfarin [CYP2C9]) should occur during the discharge process to prevent adverse events (including subtherapeutic use) in the outpatient setting.

## REFERENCES

1. Roden DM, et al. Pharmacogenomics. *Lancet*. 2019;394(10197): 521–532.
2. National Institutes of Health. What is epigenetics? Genetics Home Reference. 2020. Accessed August 2, 2020. https://ghr.nlm.nih. gov/primer/genomicresearch/pharmacogenomics
3. Roden DM. Pharmacogenetics. In: Brunton LL, et al., eds. *Goodman & Gilman's: The Pharmacological Basis of Therapeutics*. 13 ed. McGraw-Hill Education; 2017: Chap. 7. http://accessanesthesiology. mhmedical.com/content.aspx?aid=1162533468
4. Saba R, et al. Pharmacogenomics in anesthesia. *Anesthesiol Clin*. 2017;35(2):285–294.
5. U.S. National Institute of General Medicine Sciences. Pharmacogenomics. 2020. Accessed September 2, 2020. https://www.nigms. nih.gov/education/fact-sheets/Pages/pharmacogenomics.aspx

# 36.

# MALIGNANT HYPERTHERMIA

*Peter Papapetrou and Kris Ferguson*

## INTRODUCTION

Malignant hyperthermia (MH) is a rare autosomal dominant skeletal muscle genetic disorder in humans that becomes evident when these individuals undergo general anesthesia; it can be fatal if unrecognized and untreated. When exposed to potent volatile inhalational anesthetics (halothane, sevoflurane, desflurane, isoflurane) or succinylcholine, a hypermetabolic response can result in affected individuals, resulting in hyperthermia, increased oxygen consumption, increased carbon dioxide production, muscle rigidity, hyperkalemia, and acidosis.[1] Diagnosis can be made by clinical presentation as well as through laboratory findings. Prompt treatment with dantrolene is required, followed by cooling the patient, as well as supportive therapy.

## PATHOPHYSIOLOGY

The hypermetabolic state that characterizes MH is caused by an uncontrolled release of intracellular $Ca^{2+}$ from the sarcoplasmic reticulum of skeletal muscle cells due to a defect in the ryanodine receptor $Ca^{2+}$ channel. When exposed to inhalational anesthetics or succinylcholine, the increased intracellular $Ca^{2+}$ causes abnormal skeletal muscle metabolism, which manifests as increased heat production, increased $O_2$ consumption, and increased $CO_2$ production.

## CLINICAL DIAGNOSIS

In a patient exposed to volatile anesthetics or succinylcholine who exhibits unexplained symptoms of a hypermetabolic state, MH needs to be included in the differential diagnosis. Suspicion should be high if the patient becomes tachycardic, tachypneic, cyanotic, and hyperthermic; and develops muscle rigidity or dysrhythmias. Suspicion should also be high if muscle rigidity occurs after an adequate dose of succinylcholine.[2] The earliest signs include increased end-tidal $CO_2$ (ETCO$_2$), tachycardia, and tachypnea. Arterial blood gases usually show metabolic/respiratory acidosis. A clinical grading scale, which is scored based on weighted elements of MH manifestations, was developed by Larach and colleagues.[3] Though the grading scale is not required to make the diagnosis of MH, it can be helpful for determining the likelihood of a patient having MH. The criteria used in the grading scale are shown in Table 36.1.

*Table 36.1* CLINICAL GRADING SCALE FOR MALIGNANT HYPERTHERMIA CRITERIA

| PROCESS | MANIFESTATION |
|---|---|
| Rigidity | a. Generalized muscle rigidity<br>b. Masseter muscle spasm followed by succinylcholine administration |
| Muscle breakdown | a. Elevated creatine kinase > 20,000 IU after anesthetic that included succinylcholine<br>b. Elevated creatine kinase > 10,000 IU after anesthetic without succinylcholine<br>c. Cola-colored urine in the perioperative period<br>d. Myoglobin in urine > 60 µg/L<br>e. Myoglobin in serum > 170 µg/L<br>f. Blood/plasma/serum $K^+$ > 6 mEq/L (in absence of renal failure) |
| Respiratory acidosis | a. PETCO$_2$ > 55 mm Hg with appropriately controlled ventilation<br>b. Arterial PaCO$_2$ > 60 mm Hg with appropriately controlled ventilation<br>c. PETCO$_2$ > 60 mm Hg with spontaneous ventilation<br>d. Arterial PaCO$_2$ > 65 mm Hg with spontaneous ventilation<br>e. Inappropriate hypercarbia (anesthesiologist's judgment)<br>f. Inappropriate tachypnea |
| Temperature increase | a. Inappropriately rapid increase in temperature<br>b. Inappropriately increased temperature > 38.8°C in the perioperative period |
| Cardiac involvement | a. Inappropriate sinus tachycardia<br>b. Ventricular tachycardia or ventricular fibrillation |

## LABORATORY DIAGNOSIS

The caffeine-halothane contracture test is considered the gold standard test to diagnose MH. It is an in vitro test where muscle fibers contract in the presence of either halothane or caffeine. The protocol of the test, developed by the North American Malignant Hyperthermia Group, has a sensitivity of 97% and a specificity of 78%, providing some level of confidence in determining the presence of MH.

## TREATMENT

Important initial steps when encountering an acute MH crisis is promptly recognizing the clinical symptoms and immediately discontinuing the triggering agent. Dantrolene should be administered in doses of 2.5 mg/kg as needed, up to a maximum of 10 mg/kg, until clinical symptoms improve. Currently, dantrolene is the only known drug to treat MH. Its mechanism of action is suspected to involve lowering cytoplasmic $Ca^{2+}$.[4] Once symptoms resolve, dantrolene should be continued at 1 mg/kg every 4–6 hours for at least 24 hours postepisode until creatine kinase (CK) decreases and signs of a hypermetabolic state are resolved. Close monitoring of clinical symptoms and laboratory values should occur for at least 48–72 hours postepisode in anticipation of possible recrudescence, which can occur in up to 20% of MH patients. Calcium channel blockers should not be given in the presence of dantrolene because myocardial depression has been demonstrated in animals.

Simultaneously during a crisis, the patient should be cooled through various mechanisms, which decreases oxygen consumption. Core cooling is much more efficacious than surface cooling and is accomplished with cold gastric, bladder, and rectal lavage. Groin and axilla ice packs can also be effective.

Furthermore, the patient should be hyperventilated, and dysrhythmias should be closely monitored and treated. Serum $K^+$ should be measured. Arterial blood gases should also be measured to evaluate the degree of metabolic acidosis, as well as to monitor the effectiveness of therapy and the progress in correcting a metabolic acidosis.

Consider antiarrhythmics, management of hyperkalemia with insulin and glucose, diuretics, and sodium bicarbonate.

## SUMMARY FOR MANAGEMENT OF A SUSPICIOUS EPISODE OF MALIGNANT HYPERTHERMIA CRISIS

1. Discontinue all volatile anesthetic agents and succinylcholine. Maintain anesthesia with total intravenous anesthesia (TIVA).
2. Increase minute ventilation to 10 L/min to flush out volatile anesthetic agents and to decrease $ETCO_2$. Administer 100% oxygen.
3. Inform the surgeon of MH suspicion in order to expedite or abort the procedure. Obtain assistance from the Malignant Hyperthermia Association of the United States Hotline (1-800-644-9737).
4. Administer dantrolene 2.5 mg/kg. Repeat dose until a decrease in $ETCO_2$, rigidity, or heart rate is observed.
5. Obtain blood gas analysis in order to evaluate if bicarbonate therapy is necessary. Place an arterial or central catheter for serial blood gas and CK measurements.
6. Cool the patient if hyperthermic. Decrease room temperature, surface cool with ice, and core cool with gastric, bladder, and rectal lavage.
7. Treat hyperkalemia with insulin and glucose. Monitor serum $K^+$ and glucose levels.

Measure CK baseline and monitor every 6 hours until CK plateaus.

## ANESTHETIC CONSIDERATIONS

### PREOPERATIVE

Preoperative assessment should include identifying patients with a suspected history of MH as well as their family members with known or suspected MH; CK might be elevated in some patients. In these patients, local or regional anesthesia should be used whenever possible, and there should be strict avoidance of triggers (potent volatile anesthetic agents and succinylcholine). Prepare the anesthesia machine by removing vaporizers, replacing rubber hoses and soda lime, then flush with high-flow air or oxygen (10 L/min) for 10 minutes.

### INTRAOPERATIVE

Patients who are MH susceptible should receive TIVA if a general anesthetic is required. In addition, an MH cart with necessarily medications and supplies to treat an MH crisis should be readily available. Should an MH crisis develop intraoperatively, follow the steps discussed previously. All susceptible patients should have core temperatures monitored if they are receiving a general anesthetic. Trismus or masseter muscle spasm following inhalation induction and succinylcholine is associated with approximately 50% incidence of MH.

### POSTOPERATIVE

Patients susceptible to MH who received a nontriggering anesthetic agent do not need additional monitoring in the postanesthesia care unit. In patients with an MH crisis, intensive care unit monitoring is necessary for at least 48–72 hours to ensure they do not experience a recrudescence of an MH crisis, which can be fatal and needs to be treated with the same urgency as the initial crisis. Potassium was reported to cause retriggering in a patient with MH.

## REFERENCES

1. Rosenberg H, et al. Malignant hyperthermia. *Orphanet J Rare Dis.* 2015;10:93.
2. Gronert G. *Anesthesiology.* 1980;53:395–423.
3. Larach MG, et al. A clinical grading scale to predict malignant hyperthermia susceptibility. *Anesthesiology.* 1994;80(4):771–779.
4. Longnecker DE, et al. Malignant hyperthermia. In: Anesthesiology. 2nd ed. McGraw-Hill: 2012:1491–1504.

# 37.

# BUTYRYLCHOLINESTERASE (PSEUDOCHOLINESTERASE) DEFICIENCY

*Brian Harris and Kris Ferguson*

## INTRODUCTION

Pseudocholinesterase (plasma cholinesterase, butylcholinesterase, PCHE) is a serine hydrolase responsible for the hydrolysis of exogenous esters in the body, such as succinylcholine, mivacurium, and ester-type local anesthetics.[1] It exists as an $\alpha_2$-globulin, typically as a tetramer; is produced in the liver; is found chiefly in not only the plasma and liver but also other major organs; and has a half-life of 8–12 days.[1]

## PATHOPHYSIOLOGY

Pseudocholinesterase deficiency becomes clinically relevant only when considering its function in terminating the action of medications administered to a patient. Patients have no detectable dysfunction or disease as a result of reduced or absent plasma levels of PCHE unless given a medication that causes a complication due to the failure of PCHE to hydrolyze the agent in question. It was originally defined because of discovering "succinylcholine apnea," which was an unexpectedly prolonged action of succinylcholine in an anesthetized patient, therefore causing prolonged apnea. Though prolonged apnea is the major clinical concern

resulting from PCHE deficiency, ester-linked anesthetics are metabolized by PCHE (as well as red cell esterases), and their metabolism may also be delayed. In one study, the metabolism of chloroprocaine was five times slower in homozygous atypical-cholinesterase patients versus controls.[1] There is a theoretical concern that cocaine (an ester-linked local anesthetic) toxicity may be exacerbated in patients with PCHE deficiency, though a specific study of this phenomenon is lacking.[2]

Pseudocholinesterase deficiency exists as either a homozygous or heterozygous expression of atypical PCHE due to a mutation in chromosome 3, a drug- or toxin-mediated reduction in PCHE (by consumption or reduction in production), or a disease-induced reduction in production. It should be noted that while the causes of PCHE deficiency are numerous and common, most fail to rise to clinical significance, as it requires an approximately 75% reduction in the activity of PCHE to produce a noticeable difference in the action of succinylcholine.[2] Heterozygotes, and even genotypes that include two atypical PCHEs, frequently result in enzymatic activity sufficient to avoid clinical notice. Similarly, disease states such as liver disease and malnutrition have to be relatively severe in many cases to produce a clinically significant PCHE deficiency. Even a reduction of 75% prolonged the activity of succinylcholine in one study from $3.0 \pm 0.15$ minutes to $8.6 \pm 0.7$ minutes, and clinically significant prolongation of succinylcholine (from all causes) only occurs in approximately 1/2500 patients.[3]

## SELECTED CAUSES OF PSEUDOCHOLINESTERASE DEFICIENCY

Selected causes of PCHE deficiency are given in the table that follows:

| Drug Mediated | Genetic | Disease/Other |
|---|---|---|
| Serotonin; steroids; procaine; pancuronium; hexafluronium; organophosphates; acetylcholinesterase inhibitors (neostigmine, pyridostigmine, edrophonium); chlorpromazine; monoamine oxidase inhibitors; nitrogen mustard; cyclophosphamide | ~40 variants of atypical, silent, or K/J/H plasma cholinesterase Homozygous atypical 1/3200 (dibucaine number [DN] 23–30, increased length of succinylcholine 4–8 hours) Heterozygous atypical 1/480 (DN 50–60, increased length of succinylcholine 50%–100%) Mixed atypical—rare | Liver disease, malnutrition, myxedema, sepsis, myocardial infarction, pregnancy, plasmapheresis, burn patients |

## GENETICS OF ATYPICAL PSEUDOCHOLINESTERASE

Atypical PCHEs exist as a mutation of the BCHE gene on chromosome 3 (at 3q26.1), typically due to a frame shift or substitution, and as such are passed along as an autosomal recessive inheritance pattern.[1] Over 40 variations are known to exist; atypical variants are unable to hydrolyze succinylcholine; silent variants produce no enzyme; and K, J, and H variants produce a normal enzyme at reduced levels. There also exist rare variants of the gene (as well as isoenzymes of PCHE) that have activity far more than the normal variant.

The most clinically significant cases for the anesthesiologists are the homozygous atypical, homozygous silent, or mixed atypical/silent variations; succinylcholine apnea can persist for 3–8 hours, or in some case reports, even longer. Heterozygous phenotypes can occasionally produce clinically significant succinylcholine apnea (approximately 1/500 cases of heterozygous BCHE), but the combination of a heterozygote phenotype with an acquired deficiency or drug-mediated reduction in PCHE can also result in significantly increased succinylcholine

apnea. An increased level of suspicion should exist when BCHE abnormalities are suspected or when one or more risk factor exists.[3]

As with many autosomal recessive diseases, there is some association between ethnic background and specific atypical/silent genotypes. South African blacks and Aleutian and Inuit peoples have a higher incidence of a silent genotype; people of Israeli descent tend have a higher incidence of atypical BCHE than Americans; and those with Huntington chorea have a higher incidence of the fluoride-resistant genotype. Most of the ongoing research into the BCHE gene, family inheritance, and atypical gene phenotypes is conducted by a few research units, such as Viby-Mogensen and the University of Michigan Department of Anesthesia.

In European populations, incidence of a normal genotype is estimated to be in excess of 96%; heterozygotes of any type are around 3%, and the most serious phenotype (any combination of silent/atypical/fluoride resistant) is estimated by Hanel and Viby-Mogensen to be about 0.061% in the Danish population.[1]

## ANESTHETIC CONSIDERATIONS

### PREOPERATIVE

Prevention of succinylcholine-induced apnea can potentially be achieved by a careful family history, testing in families known to have a history of the disorder, and a raised clinical suspicion of patients who have multiple severe factors for acquired PCHE deficiency. It may be wise to limit the use of ester local anesthetics in patients known to have or be at risk for the disorder. Bracelets are indicated for those who have homozygous deficiencies or a history of succinylcholine apnea.

The dibucaine number (DN) and fluoride number are clinical tests used to determine the reduced PCHE activity resulting from the addition of sodium fluoride or dibucaine to the patient's serum; higher numbers reflect a greater activity of PCHE. Qualitative deficiencies (DN, fluoride number) do not apply to acquired deficiencies of the enzyme. Diagnosis of a quantitative deficiency of PCHE may be obtained from a colorimetric assay using benzyl choline as a substrate and comparing the test assay to a control. If BCHE is discovered with appropriate testing, then by necessity avoid the offending drugs.[1]

### INTRAOPERATIVE

Symptoms typically do not manifest until after the surgery or the expected termination of action of anesthesia medications becomes delayed.

## POSTOPERATIVE

If BCHE is diagnosed, treatment of succinylcholine apnea is chiefly supportive; no reversal is indicated. Supportive care consists of mechanical ventilation and appropriate sedation until sufficient renal clearance of succinylcholine permits recovery of neuromuscular function. Some texts have noted that administration of plasma products, which likely contain functional PCHEs from the donor, may significantly shorten the duration of apnea. In almost all cases, the risk of transfusion would far outweigh the advantage of shortening the neuromuscular block by a few hours, and no such treatment is advocated.

## REFERENCES

1. Viby-Mogensen J. Correlation of succinylcholine duration of action with plasma cholinesterase activity in subjects with normal enzyme. *Anesthesiology.* 1980;53:517.
2. Faust RJ. Prolongation of succinylcholine effect. *Anesthesiol Rev.* 2002;57:137.
3. Barash, PG, et al. Clinical anesthesia. Malignant hyperthermia and other pharmacogenetic disorders. *Clin Anesth.* 2006;20:547–548.

# 38.

# PROLONGED QT SYNDROME

*Kris Ferguson and Peter Papapetrou*

## INTRODUCTION

Long QT syndrome (LQTS) is a life-threatening cardiac arrhythmia that can be inherited or acquired. Inherited LQTS syndrome is due to several mutations in various genes. There is also variable penetrance of the disorder, ranging from asymptomatic to lethal.[1] Presentation will range from asymptomatic electrocardiographic (ECG) findings to torsade de pointes and sudden death. Torsade de pointes is a form of polymorphic ventricular tachycardia with prolonged QT; it is treated with magnesium, and if this is not effective, then overdrive pacing. This is a disorder impacting younger individuals.[2] Without appropriate treatment, LQTS can be a lethal disorder. However, with early identification and treatment, outcomes are good. There are specific anesthetic considerations that can improve patient outcomes.

## EPIDEMIOLOGY

Prevalence of LQTS is difficult to determine as some patients will have normal QT intervals and many will be asymptomatic. Structurally, these patients have normal hearts. A diagnosis is based on ECG findings, symptoms, and genetics.[1] The QT interval varies with heart rate; thus the QTc is used and is calculated using Bazett's equation: QTc = QT/(square root of the RR interval where QT is the time from the start of the Q wave to the end of the T wave measured in seconds).[1] QTc varies with age, gender, activity level, and sympathetic activity. QTc greater than 450 increases risk, 460–480 is higher risk, and greater than 480 is a significant risk factor (Table 38.1).[1–3] A genetic diagnosis is difficult due to the variability in penetrance. A reasonable estimate at the disease prevalence is approximately 1/3000.

Less than 1 point, probability is low, 2–3 intermediate, greater than 4 points, probability is high.[1]

## GENETICS

Thus far, there are several long QT (LQT) genotypes, LQT 1–8, with LQT 1–3 the most common.[1] There are individuals with LQTS with no genetic findings. There are two clinical syndromes: Romano-Ward (RW) syndrome and Jervell Lange-Nielson (JLN) syndrome. RW is more common, is autosomal dominant, and does not involve hearing impairment. RW is associated with LQT 1–6. JLN is an autosomal

### Table 38.1 LQTS DIAGNOSTIC CRITERIA

| History of | |
|---|---|
| 1. Fainting with stress | 2 |
| 2. Fainting without stress | 1 |
| 3. Congenital deafness | 0.5 |
| **Family history** | |
| 1. Family members diagnosed with LQTS | 1 |
| 2. Unexplained sudden cardiac death in immediate family member < 30 | 0.5 |
| **ECG findings** | |
| 1. QTc > 480 ms | 3 |
| 460–480 ms | 2 |
| >450 ms in males | 1 |
| 2. Torsade de pointes | 2 |
| 3. T-wave alternans | 1 |
| 4. Notched T wave in 3 leads | 1 |
| 5. Low heart rate for age | 0.5 |

recessive cardioauditory syndrome associated with congenital deafness and associated with LQT1 and LQT5. LQT1 accounts for 42% of all congenital LQTS, LQT2 45%, and LQT3 5%. LQTS 1 and 2 are adrenergic dependent regarding torsade de pointes. Intense exercise, sudden noises, or the fight-or-flight response can trigger torsade. LQT2 are particularly sensitive to loud noises. LQT3 do not trigger with adrenergic stimulation but are triggered when at rest or sleeping.[1]

## PATHOPHYSIOLOGY

Long QT syndrome is a disorder of cardiac ion channels or induced by drugs or metabolic derangements (Table 38.2).[1–3] LQTS has a prolonged QT interval and abnormal T-wave morphology due to delayed repolarization and disordered repolarization. Aberrant depolarization and repolarization lead to syncope, seizure, and sudden cardiac death, typically caused by a polymorphic ventricular arrhythmia called torsade de pointes.

## ANESTHETIC CONSIDERATIONS

### PREOPERATIVE

Sympathetic stimulation should be kept to a minimum preoperatively. The temperature should be comfortable; try to minimize anxiety and avoid loud, startling noises. A multidisciplinary approach involving the surgeon, cardiology, and anesthesiologist would optimize the outcome. β-Blockers should be continued. If there is a pacemaker or defibrillator, it should be interrogated preoperatively. The pacemaker and implantable cardioverter-defibrillator should be put in asynchronous mode. Consider an external defibrillator/pacemaker placement in the preoperative setting. Consider midazolam to minimize the stress response. While ketamine has been safely used as a premedication in children, it may be best to avoid its use due to QT prolongation.[2,3] Ensure electrolytes are optimized prior to an elective case. Avoid hypokalemia, hypomagnesemia, and hypocalcemia and consider pretreating with magnesium 30 mg/kg as it blocks inward sodium and potassium currents. Strongly consider an arterial line and central venous access.

### Table 38.2 DRUGS THAT PROLONG THE QT INTERVAL

| CARDIAC | ANTIMICROBIALS | PSYCHOTROPICS | MISCELLANEOUS |
|---|---|---|---|
| Amiodarone | Clarithromycin | Chlorpromazine | Chlorpromazine |
| Bepridil | Erythromycin | Haloperidol | Cisapride |
| Disopyramide | Grepafloxacin | Mesoridazine | Domperidone |
| Dofetilide | Pentamidine | Pimozide | Droperidol |
| Ibutilide | Sparfloxacin | Thioridazine | Halofantrine |
| Procainamide | Azithromycin | Lithium | Haloperidol |
| Quinidine | Foscarnet | Quetiapine | Levomethadyl |
| Sotalol | Gatifloxacin | Risperidone | Mesoridazine |
| Flecainide | Levofloxacin | Venlafaxine | Methadone |
| Moexipril/hydrochlorothiazide | Moxifloxacin | Ziprasidone | Organophosphates |
| Nicardipine | Telithromycin | | Pimozide |
| Isradipine | | | Thioridazine |
| Dobutamine | | | Amantadine |
| Dopamine | | | Octreotide |
| Ephedrine | | | Ondansetron |
| Epinephrine | | | Salmeterol |
| Isoproterenol | | | Tacrolimus |
| Midodrine | | | Terfenadine |
| Norepinephrine | | | Tamoxifen |
| Phenylephrine | | | Tizanidine |

## INTRAOPERATIVE

Intraoperatively, thiopental has been safely used as an induction agent despite prolonging the QT interval. Propofol has minimal impact on the QT interval. Propofol has been shown to reverse QT prolongation caused by sevoflurane. Midazolam can be used as a preoperative anxiolytic and as an induction agent. While volatile anesthetics prolong the QT interval, halothane, enflurane, isoflurane, and sevoflurane have been safely used in LQTS.[3] It is reported nitrous oxide has been safely used. Halothane does sensitize the heart to catecholamines, so be cautious with its use. Avoid succinylcholine as it can cause bradycardia and potassium shifts and prolongs the QT. Vecuronium and atracurium have no impact on the QT interval. Pancuronium is best avoided as it has vagolytic effects. Neuromuscular reversal agents such as glycopyrrolate, neostigmine, or edrophonium all prolong the QT interval. Neostigmine and edrophonium cause bradycardia and should be avoided. Opioids have been used without ill effects. Fentanyl or morphine can blunt the sympathetic response to intubation. Use caution with droperidol as it does increase the QT interval; ondansetron possibly increases the QT interval, but this risk is balanced against the risk of postoperative vomiting. Regional anesthesia such as epidurals with local anesthetics and opioids should be considered, especially in obstetrics. For cesarean section, spinal anesthesia works well but avoid epinephrine.

## POSTOPERATIVE

Continuous monitoring of the QT interval in the postanesthesia unit is critical as effects of anesthesia are wearing off, and the sympathetic output may be increased due to postoperative pain or anxiety. Ensure a calm, quiet, and comfortable environment.

## REFERENCES

1. Schwartz PJ, et al. Long QT syndrome: from genetics to management. *Circ Arrhythm Electrophysiol.* 2012;5(4):868–877.
2. Kies SJ, et al. Anesthesia for patients with congenital long QT syndrome. *Anesthesiology.* 2005;102:204–210.
3. Whyte SD, et al. The safety of modern anesthesia for children with long QT syndrome. *Anesth Analg.* 2014;119(4):932–938.

# 39.

# RAPID METABOLIZERS

*Nicholas M. Parker*

## INTRODUCTION

Some enzymes responsible for drug metabolism are subject to significant genetic variation. While many genotypes result in worse enzyme function, a few alleles code for an "ultrametabolizer" phenotype.

## ENZYMES AND PREVALENCE

### CYP2D6

Enzymes in the family known as cytochrome P450 (CYP450) are involved in the metabolism of many drugs. One subtype of this enzyme, CYP2D6, is subject to extensive genetic polymorphism with clinically significant impacts on how certain drugs affect patients. Most variants of the gene for CYP2D6 produce enzymes with normal function, poor function, or no function at all. However, some patients carry duplicate copies of alleles with normal function, resulting in enzyme activity that is double, triple, or more compared to baseline.

The prevalence of ultrametabolizers in the population varies by race (Table 39.1).[1] This is significant because clinical trials may not adequately enroll non-White patients, so adverse effects or treatment failure caused by ultrametabolism may be underreported. Adverse effects or treatment failure in non-White patients may also be misattributed to cultural differences in how those patients describe symptoms, rather than true differences in pharmacological effect.

## CYP2C19

Another CYP450 enzyme with an ultrametabolizer variant is CYP2C19. The CYP2C19*17 allele causes increased expression of the gene, causing higher levels of enzyme activity than the wild type. As with CYP2D6, the prevalence of CYP2C19 ultrametabolizers varies by race (Table 39.1).[1]

## IDENTIFICATION OF ULTRAMETABOLIZERS

### GENETIC TESTING

The availability and clinical utility of genetic testing continues to grow. Several commercial laboratory tests are available, and patients may have genetic information from consumer kits they purchased themselves. Insurance coverage of genetic testing will vary and should be verified before ordering. Prospective genetic testing before starting a specific medication is currently rare, especially with regard to ultrametabolizers, but genetic screening may well become routine practice in coming years. Genetic testing may also be ordered to investigate the cause of adverse effects or treatment failure.

### ADVERSE EFFECTS

Patients reporting unexpectedly severe adverse reactions to certain drugs could be ultrametabolizers. Codeine, for example, is inactive until metabolized to morphine by CYP2D6.[1-3] An ultrametabolizer may experience sedation or respiratory depression from codeine even at the usual starting dose. Codeine is contraindicated in nursing mothers in case the infant is an ultrametabolizer—a well-tolerated dose of codeine in the mother could cause overdose in the infant.[2] Tramadol likewise has an active metabolite produced by CYP2D6, so an ultrametabolizer may have a prolonged or exaggerated response to this drug.[1-3]

### TREATMENT FAILURE

More commonly, ultrametabolizers will have a diminished response to certain drugs. For drugs that are titrated to a clinical effect or target blood concentration, the provider may note that unusually high doses are necessary; the highest tolerated dose may be inadequate to produce the intended therapeutic effect. Other drugs more commonly used at fixed doses may simply not work. While the cause of treatment failure may be complex, the ultrametabolizer phenotype should be considered in order to appropriately guide changes in drug therapy. For example, most proton pump inhibitors (PPIs) like pantoprazole are metabolized by some degree by CYP2C19.[2,3] Ultrametabolizers may need higher or more frequent doses of PPIs or may have a better response to histamine H2 antagonists such as famotidine.

## DRUG-DRUG-GENE INTERACTIONS

Ultrametabolizers are particularly susceptible to drug-drug interactions when the overexpressed enzyme is involved. The most dangerous scenario would be when a drug is titrated to a high dose due to rapid clearance by CYP2D6 or CYP2C19, then a second drug is started that inhibits the enzyme. This interaction could rapidly lead to toxic levels of the first drug since being an ultrametabolizer does not seem to protect against enzyme inhibition.[4] For example, voriconazole is metabolized primarily by CYP2C19 and is typically dosed to a target blood concentration. A CYP2C19 ultrametabolizer would be titrated to a high dose of voriconazole. If this patient then received a CYP2C19 inhibitor like cimetidine or fluoxetine, they may experience liver toxicity from excessive levels of voriconazole.[2-4]

*Table 39.1* PREVALENCE OF CYP2D6 AND CYP2C19 ULTRAMETABOLIZER ALLELES BY RACE

| ULTRAMETABOLIZER ALLELE | PREVALENCE BY RACE | | |
| --- | --- | --- | --- |
| | BLACK RACE | ASIAN RACE | WHITE RACE |
| CYP2D6*1xN | 1.5% | 0.28% | 0.8% |
| CYP2D6*2xN | 1.6% | 0.38% | 1.3% |
| CYP2C19*17 | 16% | 2.7% | 21% |

Reference: Katzung BG, ed. *Basic & Clinical Pharmacology*. 14th ed. McGraw-Hill; Accessed August 23, 2020. https://accessmedicine-mhmedical-com.ezproxy.library.wisc.edu/content.aspx?bookid=2249&sectionid=175220393

## EFFECTS ON SELECTED DRUGS

Important substrates of CYP2D6 and CYP2C19 are listed in Table 39.2.[2,3] In a known or suspected ultrametabolizer, these drugs may need to be administered at a higher dose or a different drug should be selected.

*Table 39.2* PARTIAL LIST OF DRUGS METABOLIZED BY CYP2D6 OR CYP2C19 THAT MAY BE PERTINENT TO ANESTHESIA[a]

| ENZYME | SELECTED SUBSTRATES |
| --- | --- |
| CYP2D6 | Cyclobenzaprine, methadone, carvedilol, clonidine, flecainide, lidocaine, metoprolol, propranolol, ranolazine, ondansetron, donepezil, amitriptyline, aripiprazole, atomoxetine, bupropion, clozapine, duloxetine, fluoxetine, haloperidol, mirtazapine, nortriptyline, olanzapine, quetiapine, risperidone, venlafaxine, dextromethorphan, tamsulosin, tolterodine. |
| | **Codeine is activated by CYP2D6 and should be avoided in ultrametabolizers.** |
| | **Tramadol, hydrocodone, and oxycodone have active metabolites produced by CYP2D6, which may require dose reduction or alternate therapy in ultrametabolizers.** |
| CYP2C19 | Methadone, cilostazol, labetolol, propranolol, verapamil, omeprazole, pantoprazole, ondansetron, voriconazole, clobazam, amitriptyline, citalopram, diazepam, sertraline, vortioxetine. |
| | **Clopidogrel is activated by CYP2C19, which has no clinical impact in ultrametabolizers.** |

[a]Ultrametabolizers may need different doses of these drugs or alternate therapy.

Reference: Pharmacogenomic associations tables. Mayo Clinic Laboratories. Updated April 2019. Accessed August 29, 2020. https://www.mayocliniclabs.com/it-mmfiles/Pharmacogenomic_Associations_Tables.pdf

## IMPLICATIONS FOR ANESTHESIA

### PREOPERATIVE

Review the patient's allergies and current medications. Review past laboratory results for genetic testing that impacts drug metabolism. Keep in mind that black patients are more likely to be CYP2D6 ultrametabolizers than are White or Asian patients.

### INTRAOPERATIVE

In known or suspected ultrametabolizers, avoid giving drugs metabolized by that enzyme (or be prepared to use higher doses). If a CYP2D6 or CYP2C19 substrate is less effective or wears off more quickly than usual, make note of this and consider switching to a different drug rather than increasing the dose.

### POSTOPERATIVE

If an unusual response to a drug was identified during surgery, update the patient's allergy list and consider referral for genetic testing.

### REFERENCES

1. Katzung BG, ed. *Basic & Clinical Pharmacology.* 14th ed. McGraw-Hill. Accessed August 23, 2020. https://accessmedicine-mhmedical-com.ezproxy.library.wisc.edu/content.aspx?bookid=2249&sectionid=175220393
2. Lexicomp. Wolters Kluwer; 2020. Accessed August 23, 2020. http://online.lexi.com
3. Mayo Clinic Laboratories. Pharmacogenomic associations tables. Updated April 2019. Accessed August 29, 2020. https://www.mayocliniclabs.com/it-mmfiles/Pharmacogenomic_Associations_Tables.pdf
4. Bahar MA, et al. Pharmacogenetics of drug–drug interaction and drug–drug–gene interaction: a systematic review on CYP2C9, CYP2C19 and CYP2D6. *Pharmacogenomics.* 2017;18(7):701–739.

# 40.

# ADDICTION

*Anuj A. Shah and Christine S. Zaky*

## INTRODUCTION

Addiction is a chronic physiological need for a habit-forming substance despite the harmful consequences. Addiction involves preoccupation and compulsion in seeking and taking the drug, the inability to control the frequency, duration, and intake of the drug, and the emergence of negative affect and maladaptive behavior. The drug addiction cycle includes three stages, shown in Figure 40.1.[1]

## PREVALENCE

It is estimated that about 7% of the American population meet the criteria for alcohol misuse or alcoholism. In fact, alcohol dependence in 2016 was shown to be the most prevalent substance use disorder globally, and cannabis and opioid use disorders were found to be the most common drug use disorders. Deaths from prescription opioid overdose have increased five-fold from 1999 to 2016, killing more than heroin and cocaine.[2]

## PATHOPHYSIOLOGY OF ADDICTION

The pathophysiology of addiction is based on a disorder that consists of three stages: preoccupation, negative affect, and intoxication. These stages can be identified as a cycle with elements that feed into one another, causing the pathological state of addiction. As an individual moves through the cycle, there is a change from positive reinforcement driving the motivation to negative reinforcement of the behavior, ultimately leading to addiction. Advancement through the cycle causes changes in brain circuitry, inducing neuroplastic changes and adjustments of critical neurotransmitters such as dopamine, γ-aminobutyric acid, glutamate, opioid peptides, acetylcholine, and serotonin.[1] Alterations in brain circuits occur, including areas such as the ventral tegmental area (VTA), cerebellum, nucleus accumbens, and amygdala.

The VTA is connected to the ventral striatum through the mesolimbic pathway. Because this pathway is predominantly dopaminergic, it is commonly referred to as the reward pathway. Research has shown the VTA, along with its dopaminergic neurons, having a predominant role in the response to drug abuse.[3] It is hypothesized that the constant release of dopamine due to drug abuse causes sensitization of the mesolimbic pathway, which, in turn, fuels the desire for more of the drug that caused the dopamine release. Increased stimuli resulting in enhanced neural connections describe long-term potentiation.[2] Long-term depression is the decreased responsiveness over time from neural stimuli.

## CLINICAL MANIFESTATIONS

### BEHAVIOR PATTERNS

The behavior of the addict involves occupation with thinking about and engaging in the addictive behavior. An active addict may demonstrate maladaptive behavior, such as[4]

- Prescription forgery
- Selling and stealing drugs
- Seeing multiple doctors and pharmacies to obtain drugs
- Risk-taking behavior, especially while abusing psychotropic drugs
- Signs of intoxication, such as impairment of physical, mental, and social skills

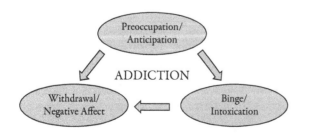

Figure 40.1 The drug addiction cycle outlining its three stages.

In addition, the addict often presents themselves in denial, creating an obstacle in treatment and often requiring group intervention.

## DIAGNOSIS AND TREATMENT

The first step of diagnosis requires acknowledgment of the disorder and a need for treatment. An addiction or rehabilitation specialist may assess the addiction, often requiring blood tests to assess if medical treatment is needed. Certain criteria for addiction from the *Diagnostic and Statistical Manual of Mental Disorders, Fifth Edition (DSM-5)* are employed in diagnosis.

Acute alcohol intoxications are treated with long-acting benzodiazepines like chlordiazepoxide or diazepam. Disulfiram will cause quick hangover-type symptoms to discourage the patient from further drinking. Disulfiram disrupts normal alcohol metabolism through irreversible inhibition of aldehyde dehydrogenase. Disulfiram is used for a patient who recently quit and is beginning abstinence, while acamprosate is used by a patient to become abstinent by decreasing initial withdrawal symptoms. To maintain abstinence, naltrexone is used to remove the sensation of pleasure seen with alcohol use.[2] Naltrexone acts by binding to opioid receptors in the brain and displacing any opioid drugs to suppress cravings.

Inpatient or outpatient substance use treatment programs should be made available to patients who are suspected to have opioid use disorder. For acute intoxications, naloxone should be used quickly to reverse the effects of the drug. The patient's vital signs should be monitored, and the patient should be given intravenous hydration and a repeat naloxone dose if necessary.[5] Naloxone has a high affinity for μ-opioid receptors, which allows the drug to be removed. However, patients at high risk for overdose should be given naloxone kits for at-home use.

Opioid withdrawal can be effectively managed with buprenorphine. Buprenorphine is a partial μ- and κ-antagonist, serving to prevent cravings and decrease withdrawal symptoms.[5] Another pharmacologic agent, methadone, a μ agonist, can be used to control opioid withdrawal symptoms and accomplish detoxification. Withdrawal symptoms are scaled using the Clinical Opioid Withdrawal Scale. Antidiarrheals can also be given to help with withdrawal symptoms along with intravenous hydration.[5] Clonidine can be used to provide relief of many opioid withdrawal symptoms, such as vomiting, diarrhea, abdominal cramps, sweating, anxiety, and tremor.

Pharmacological treatments have been the most effective when combined with group meetings, psychological support, and physician advice.[2] This helps to limit the progression of misuse to addiction in patients on that path. Early intervention has proven to be the most beneficial.

## REFERENCES

1. Herman MA, Roberto M. The addicted brain: understanding the neurophysiological mechanisms of addictive disorders. *Front Integr Neurosci*. 2015;9(18):1–2.
2. Fluyau D, Charlton TE. Addiction. In: *StatPearls*. Treasure Island, FL: StatPearls Publishing; July 10, 2020.
3. McMahon B, et al. Assessment of psychology of pain. In: *Wall and Melzack's Textbook of Pain*. 6th ed. Philadelphia, PA: Elsevier/Churchill Livingstone; 2013:353–354.
4. Prater CD, et al. Successful pain management for the recovering addicted patient. *Prim Care Companion J Clin Psychiatry*. 2002;4(4):125–131.
5. Azadfard M, et al. Opioid addiction. In: *StatPearls*. Treasure Island, FL: StatPearls Publishing; August 14, 2020.

# 41.

# ANESTHETIC IMPLICATIONS OF ADDICTION

*Brian Harris and Kris Ferguson*

## INTRODUCTION

Though estimates vary, approximately 10% of adults have admitted to the use of illicit drugs. Up to a third of Americans suffer from an alcohol-related medical problem, and some 200,000 deaths can be linked to the use of alcohol.[1] It is a certainty that many patients we see in everyday surgery, regardless of our practice demographics, will suffer from a substance abuse disorder. Given the wide range of anesthetic interactions, comorbid conditions, and increased postprocedure risks, it is imperative, now more than ever, that the practicing anesthesiologist be an expert in the recognition and management of this disease in the perioperative period.

## PREOPERATIVE EVALUATION

Anesthetic care for the patient with substance use disorder (SUD) begins with identification of the risk factors present based on the type, severity, and chronicity of the substance in question. We must then develop a collaborative anesthetic plan that considers the specific goals and values of the patient, is nonjudgmental, avoids stigmatization, and maintains patient safety as the highest priority.

A careful history and physical will employ a high index of suspicion, with the recognition of a wide variety of nonspecific but suggestive signs and symptoms, ranging from tremors, diaphoresis, and agitation to an atypical affect, odor of alcohol on the breath, poor dentition, abnormal pupils, or unusual skin lesions. A substance use history should be asked of all patients, emphasizing that our need to know deals exclusively with the consequences of proceeding with anesthesia/surgery with a substance in the patient's system. Your state's prescription monitoring system can reveal patterns of prescription that deviate from the norm.

Drug testing can confirm suspicions where a simple history of substance use may fail, particularly for patients who are acutely intoxicated or unable to give a reliable history.

It should be noted, however, that the reasons for false negatives (and false positives) are numerous. Windows for detections of some substances, like cocaine (benzoylecgonine) can be as short as 2 days, and a vast number of substances of abuse are either difficult to test for (like fentanyl) or not commonly known (kratom, tianeptine) and therefore missed; emerging drugs of abuse will always outpace our ability to test for them.[1] Not all patients will admit use, even when clinicians assure them of the confidentiality and medical necessity of these questions.

Where suspicion or evidence of substance abuse exists, additional testing should focus on the presence and severity of suspected diseases that are associated with the abused substance. Just as we obtain pulmonary function tests and listen thoroughly to the lungs of the patient with chronic obstructive pulmonary disease, so too should we obtain an electrocardiogram and focus on functional capacity for patients with a history of stimulant use, liver function tests for those with a history of heavy alcohol use, or testing for infectious diseases and endocarditis for the patient with a history of intravenous drug abuse.

## ANESTHESIA PLAN

If substance abuse is suspected or confirmed through history and physical or testing, it is often advisable to postpone elective procedures. When risks of delay outweigh the benefits of further workup or treatment, general considerations for reducing risk include the possibility of regional anesthesia (being aware that many forms of substance abuse can increase risk of peripheral neuropathy and hypotension), predicting the need for an increased level of care by avoiding the expectation of ambulatory surgery, and promoting the availability of supportive care for the patient in the postanesthesia care unit.[2] Clinicians should consider postponing elective procedures until a drug is out of the patient's system but consider risks of postponing procedure as well.

## ALCOHOL

A history of the patient's use of alcohol should be thorough and include date of last use, volume of use, presence of complications such as blackouts, delirium tremens, liver complications, coagulation history, other medications that have been prescribed, and if recent use has occurred. Other laboratory values, such as aspartase aminotransferase/alanine aminotransferase, γ-glutamyl transferase, international normalized ratio, bilirubin, as well as examination for hepatomegaly, and signs of portal hypertension can be useful in evaluating the degree of liver damage. Chronic alcoholics should also receive an evaluation of cardiovascular and neurological function.[2]

Patients who are acutely intoxicated, as with other drugs, should have procedures postponed in the case of elective surgeries. As alcohol itself results in numerous accidents that require surgical intervention, the acuity of the procedure does not make postponement advisable in many cases. Acutely intoxicated patients require a reduced dose of induction and maintenance medications (including a reduced Minimum Alveolar Concentration [MAC]) and may suffer prolonged awakening. They should be considered to have full stomachs, and their incidence of aspiration and other airway events is markedly elevated due to delayed gastric emptying, loss of tone in the lower esophageal sphincter, airway edema, and potentially loss of airway reflexes. Cardiopulmonary compromise, including possible prior aspiration, diminished ability to cough, hypotension, and reduced catecholamine response, are common.

Patients with chronic alcoholism should be optimized as much as possible preoperatively; in patients with active disease, this may include admission to an inpatient service and monitoring via a Clinical Institute Withdrawal Assessment (CIWA) protocol until issues such as deranged electrolytes, administration of thiamine, hydration, nutrition, and coagulation abnormalities can be addressed. Those with chronic alcoholism have an unpredictable response to the induction of anesthesia (can be markedly resistant to barbiturates or, if also acutely intoxicated, require a lower dose). They often require additional postoperative care, have a higher rate of prolonged hospitalization due to postoperative complications such as infection, delirium, ventilator-associated pneumonia, and other issues.

For patients with durable remission, considerations focus on chronic diseases they may have contracted while suffering alcohol use disorder (AUD) (as above), as well as preventing a relapse. Many may be taking medication-assisted treatment (MAT), such as acamprosate (no known anesthetic risk); disulfuram (risk of intraoperative hypotension and liver damage; decreased metabolism of anesthetic medications such as benzodiazepines; should be withheld 10 days prior to surgery); and naltrexone (see opioids). As patients with AUD are prone to having cross addiction, many have requests regarding which drugs should be avoided (e.g., benzodiazepines), and standard precautions minimizing opioid or other addiction medications, as well as enlisting the support of a sponsor or family member in their administration, are recommended.

## OPIOIDS

Perioperative management of the opioid-tolerant patient should include maintenance of the patient's tolerance throughout the surgery and postoperative period. MAT (Table 41.1) is common for patients who have sought treatment; management varies by type of MAT.[2] For those using illicit opioids or misusing prescribed opioids, efforts should be made to quantify the use in Morphine Milligram Equivalent(s) (MMEs) and prescribe sufficient opioids to avoid withdrawal. After surgery, these patients often exhibit an increased perception of pain; adjunct medications as well as a carefully titrated dose of opioids can be employed to treat postoperative pain. Partial opioid agonists are to be avoided as they may precipitate withdrawal.

Note that maintenance of anesthesia with remifentanil in the tolerant patient is not generally effective; volatile anesthetic or propofol is preferred for general anesthesia. Acutely intoxicated patients tend to require less anesthetic than those with chronic tolerance. Regional anesthetics in the appropriate circumstance can be beneficial and avoid difficult-to-control pain, but their baseline opioid must be maintained regardless.

*Table 41.1* PERIOPERATIVE MANAGEMENT OF MEDICATION-ASSISTED TREATMENT

| MEDICATION-ASSISTED TREATMENT | PERIOPERATIVE MANAGEMENT |
|---|---|
| Naltrexone: Noncompetitive opioid antagonist | Hold 72 hours prior to surgery (note: Vivitrol is 30-day depot form) |
| Buprenorphine: Partial opioid agonist/antagonist with "ceiling effect", long half-life | May continue if procedure does not involve planned use of opioids (regional, sedation only)<br>Opioids other than sufentanyl likely to be completely blocked by higher buprenorphine doses for up to 3 days after last dose<br>Consult with MAT prescriber for coordination; titrating to an opioid antagonist for maintenance prior to major surgery common |
| Methadone: Full opioid antagonist; long, variable half-life, and multiple metabolites | Generally, continue at preoperative dose and administer additional opioids during perisurgical period<br>Risk of prolonged QT<br>Additive effect with other opioids, sedative-hypnotics |

## BENZODIAZEPINES/BARBITURATES

As with alcohol, acute intoxication with sedatives is likely to reduce anesthetic requirements, while the opposite is true with chronic exposure. Barbiturate use, while uncommon, can profoundly increase cross-tolerance to a wide variety of drugs, anesthetic and otherwise, due to the induction of hepatic microsomal enzymes.[2] Careful monitoring of warfarin, digitalis, phenytoin, and volatile anesthetics in this context is recommended.

With either benzodiazepines or barbiturates, patients are at increased risk for withdrawal in the postanesthesia setting. Careful communication with postoperative care and floor nursing should include a CIWA protocol to prevent seizures. For the patient with chronic exposure to benzodiazepines, use extreme caution with flumazenil, which may cause acute withdrawal and seizures (no effect on barbiturates).

## COCAINE/AMPHETAMINES

Acute intoxication with cocaine or other amphetamines renders the patient vulnerable to myocardial ischemia during the perioperative period. The goal of the anesthetic should be control of the heart rate and avoiding the introduction of any additional unnecessary sympathetic stimulation.[2] Treatment for hypertension, tachycardia, or signs of cardiac ischemia (nitroglycerine, β-blockers, availability of interventional cardiologist) should be at hand, and careful five-lead monitoring for ischemia and arrhythmia is vital. Anesthetic gases may exacerbate cocaine's effect on the myocardium, increasing risks of arrhythmia.

Acutely intoxicated patients often require additional anesthesia and may have emergence delirium. Those with a history of recent chronic use may instead suffer catecholamine depletion or hypotension and may require direct sympathomimetics, as ephedrine may be ineffective.[2] Note that cocaine abuse (and its commonly associated adulterants) may result in thrombocytopenia, neutropenia, and deterioration/increased friability of nasal/airway tissue, potential confounders in both regional and general anesthesia planning.

## POSTOPERATIVE

In general, patients with a history of substance abuse require an elevated level of care postoperatively, are often inappropriate for ambulatory surgery centers, and require a raised level of suspicion for anesthetic complications. For many, pain and anxiety will be difficult to manage, and patients may benefit from an acute pain consult, if available. For those who are not in remission and are amenable, a chemical dependency consult or referral to an addiction specialist is indicated.[1]

Given the high likelihood that controlled substances may be misused by the patient with SUD or may represent a possibility of relapse for the patient in remission, they should be prescribed for the minimum possible interval and under supervision of a supportive party where possible. Nonaddictive substances, such as nonsteroidal anti-inflammatory drugs, acetaminophen, antispasmodics, $N$-methyl-D-aspartate receptor antagonists, local anesthetics, or nondrug alternatives can often be of use.

## REFERENCES

1. National Institute on Drug Abuse. Trends and statistics. https://www.drugabuse.gov/drug-topics/trends-statistics
2. Moran S, et al. Perioperative management in the patient with substance abuse. *Surg Clin North Am.* 2015;95:417–428.

# 42.

# ADDICTION VERSUS TOLERANCE

*Anuj A. Shah and Christine S. Zaky*

## INTRODUCTION

Substance abuse is the use of any illegal substance or the inappropriate use of controlled substances. Active addiction requires maladaptive behavior, such as compulsive and continued use of a drug despite demonstrated physiological, psychological, and social harm. Physical dependence is defined as "development of physical withdrawal syndrome following abrupt dose reduction." Importantly, the manifestation of physical dependence and tolerance does not indicate addiction in the patient. Tolerance is the decreasing pharmacological effect of a drug's properties, requiring more of the drug to elicit the same response.[1]

## OPIOID ADDICTION VERSUS TOLERANCE PHYSIOLOGY AND PHARMACOLOGY

Addiction involves changes in brain circuitry and activation of the reward pathway. Prefrontal cortex abnormalities in drug-addicted individuals have been shown to lead to favoring immediate reward over delayed but more favorable responses.[2,3]

Opioid tolerance, specifically, can be described as the decline in drug effect, resulting from drug-activated changes in receptor binding or mechanisms that limit the drug's effect on receptor-mediated signaling pathways, thereby changing the response of neural systems. Two theories of opioid tolerance are opioid receptor desensitization and downregulation.

The desensitization mechanism involves changes in the opioid receptor which is a G protein–coupled receptor (GPCR). Tolerance occurs when activation by opioids of enzymes such as GPCR kinases, β-arrestins, and adenylyl cyclase decouple the opioid receptor from the G protein or couple the opioid receptor to a nonanalgesic G protein.

The second mechanism involves the endocytosis of the opioid receptor, the mechanism that determines receptor density on the cellular membrane. The internalization of the receptor renders it nonfunctional and downregulated, allowing for the development of tolerance.[2]

## MANAGEMENT STRATEGIES

Physicians often use strategies such as opioid-sparing therapies and opioid rotation to treat opioid tolerance. Opioid-sparing therapies aim to minimize opioid dosage while providing for optimal pain relief. This can be achieved through adjuvant drug therapy, such as using anticonvulsants and antidepressants as well as using nondrug therapies such as exercise, cold, and heat. Opioid rotation uses a change of opioids while maintaining equianalgesic doses, taking advantage of incomplete cross-tolerance.[2]

To note, sometimes a higher dosage is required initially in therapy, not due to tolerance but to pseudotolerance, that is, to factors such as change in medications, increased physical exercise, and so on.

## ANESTHETIC IMPLICATIONS OF PATIENT ADDICTION

Patients will present for anesthesia and analgesia in a variety of stages, including acutely intoxicated, in withdrawal, or in stages of treatment and recovery. Patients suffering from addiction do not present an absolute contraindication to treatment with controlled substances, but precautions should be taken to avoid exposure and prevent relapse.[4] Working with an interdisciplinary healthcare team is critical.

### PREOPERATIVE AND PERIOPERATIVE MANAGEMENT AND EVALUATION

Preoperative and perioperative management and evaluation include[4]

- Currently prescribed medications, including medication-assisted treatment (methadone, naltrexone, buprenorphine)

*Table 42.1* PERIOPERATIVE MANAGEMENT ACCORDING TO THE ABUSED SUBSTANCE

| PERIOPERATIVE MANAGEMENT WITH SUBSTANCE ADDICTION | AIRWAY MANAGEMENT | INTRAOPERATIVE MANAGEMENT | POSTOPERATIVE MANAGEMENT |
|---|---|---|---|
| Alcohol | – Acutely intoxicated patient with full stomach<br>– ↑ Risk of aspiration<br>– ↑ Risk of acute respiratory distress syndrome<br>– Chronic alcoholic<br>– ↑ Risk for pneumonia | – Acute intoxication<br>  – Care with $O_2$ titration due to ↓ tolerance for hypoxia<br>– Patient with cirrhosis<br>  – ↑ Risk for bleeding | – Implement withdrawal prophylaxis using lorazepam, haloperidol, or clonidine<br>– ↑ Risk of wound infection due to immunosuppression |
| Benzodiazepines | – No airway concern outside of overdose<br>– Flumazenil used for overdose | –Not widely reported | – Continue treatment if on medication preoperatively<br>– Withdrawal symptoms: anxiety, poor sleep, tremors, and seizures<br>– Abuse<br>– Tapered dose withdrawal regimen |
| Cocaine | – Chronic nasal cocaine use<br>  – Caution with intubation due to septal destruction and soft palate necrosis<br>– Smoked crack cocaine<br>  – Can cause interstitial fibrosis, alveolar hemorrhage, and pulmonary hypertension | – Acute intoxication<br>  – Watch for hemodynamic instability<br>  – Avoid ketamine and halothane due to negative cardiac effects<br>– Chronic users<br>  – Normal anesthesia is relatively safe | – Withdrawal symptoms: anxiety, restlessness, tremors |
| Methamphetamine and amphetamines | – Poor oral hygiene and diet<br>  – Lead to damaged and loose teeth than can dislodge during intubation<br>– Inhaled methamphetamine<br>  – Pulmonary toxicity, ↓ number of alveolar sacs, pulmonary hypertension | – Continue prescription amphetamines to prevent hemodynamic instability<br>– Methamphetamines associated with cardiomyopathy<br>– Risk of hemodynamic compromise | – Withdrawal symptoms: increased sleeping, eating, and depression symptoms<br>– Psychosocial support |
| Heroin | – Several factors can compromise ventilation<br>– Overdose can cause pulmonary edema<br>– Chronic use can cause pulmonary hemorrhage due to hypoxia and granulomatous infiltration<br>– Delayed gastric emptying can cause aspiration | – Anesthesia and analgesia may be difficult especially in long-term users<br>– May have increased sensitivity to pain caused by opioid-induced hyperalgesia<br>– Opioids need to be continued to prevent withdrawal | – Withdrawal can begin within 6 to 18 hours<br>– High doses of narcotics may be needed to prevent or alleviate symptoms<br>– Epidural anesthesia alone can lead to withdrawal if oral or intravenous opioids are not also given<br>– Consider transitioning to a methadone maintenance program |
| Methadone | –Usually taken orally without much effect to airway | –Management similar to heroin | – Withdrawal can begin within 24 to 48 hours<br>– If used for pain control, caution should be taken because a small dose increase can cause toxicity<br>– Management similar to heroin |
| Prescription opioid | – Inhalation of crushed pills can cause septal or soft palate necrosis.<br>– Pulmonary talcosis can occur with injection of grounded pills | –Management similar to heroin | – Withdrawal symptoms dependent on formulation of drug<br>– Epidural bupivacaine has been shown to be effective in chronic morphine users<br>– Management similar to heroin |

*Table 42.1* CONTINUED

| PERIOPERATIVE MANAGEMENT WITH SUBSTANCE ADDICTION | AIRWAY MANAGEMENT | INTRAOPERATIVE MANAGEMENT | POSTOPERATIVE MANAGEMENT |
|---|---|---|---|
| Marijuana | – Airway effects are mild compared to nicotine cigarettes<br>– Long-term use can cause chronic cough and mild airflow obstruction | – Can increase the stimulatory effects of amphetamines and cocaine and the depressant effects of alcohol and benzodiazepines<br>– Low doses<br>– ↑ Sympathetic stimulation<br>– High dose inhibits sympathetic activity and have unopposed parasympathetics (bradycardia, hypotension) | – Withdrawal symptoms: anxiety, irritability, depressed mood, and lack of appetite<br>– Patients with chronic cough have increased risk of wound dehiscence<br>– Observe for stridor caused by upper airway edema |

Source: From Reference 5.

- Past anesthesia history
- Adherence to prescribed medications
- Substance(s) or prescription medications being abused
- Last time of substance use as well as triggers for use
- Dose, frequency, and route of administration of the substance
- The current level of pain (patient may overreport pain due to fear of being undertreated)
- Social support

Table 42.1 summarizes perioperative management in patients suffering from substance abuse.

## REFERENCES

1. Prater CD, et al. Successful pain management for the recovering addicted patient. *Prim Care Companion J Clin Psychiatry.* 2002;4(4):125–131.
2. Dupen A, et al. Mechanisms of opioid-induced tolerance and hyperalgesia. *Pain Manag Nurs.* 2007;8(3):113–121.
3. Koob GF, et al. Pathophysiology of addiction. *Psychiatry.* August 2008:354–378.
4. Vadivelu N, et al. Perioperative analgesia and challenges in the drug-addicted and drug-dependent patient. *Best Pract Res Clin Anaesthesiol.* 2014;28(1):91–101.
5. Moran S, et al. Perioperative management in the patient with substance abuse. *Surg Clin North Am.* 2015;95(2):417–428.

# 43.

# CNS DRUGS FOR NONANESTHETIC USE

*Nitin Sekhri and Kevin Hui*

## INTRODUCTION

The central nervous system (CNS) is a common target of drugs used by anesthesiologists in the perioperative period outside of anesthetizing patients. Despite being active in the CNS, these drugs can affect other organ systems, such as respiratory, gastrointestinal, and circulatory. Furthermore, they can also have potentially dangerous adverse effects, particularly in interaction with anesthetics.

## OPIOID AGONISTS

Opioids remain a common class of medication used for pain due their powerful analgesic properties, but have other effects, such as alterations of constipation, drowsiness, and respiratory depression. These effects are achieved through binding of opioid receptors $\mu$, $\delta$, and $\kappa$, which can be found throughout the body.[1,2] Agonism at these receptors leads to hyperpolarization of the neuron membrane, reducing neurotransmission of nociception.[1]

Opioids that bind strongly to $\mu$-opioid receptors are primarily responsible for respiratory depressive effects, which primarily causes a dose-dependent respiratory rate depression by its effects on the central respiratory centers.[2]

## ANESTHETIC CONSIDERATIONS

**Preoperative:** The chronic opioid amount is quantified by a unit of measurement through conversion to morphine milligram equivalents (MME). Opioid tolerance has two requirements: dose and time. The patient must be on more than 60 MME per day for more than 7 days.[3] If patients are on extended-release or long-acting opioids, effort must be made to give the patients the medication prior to surgery.

**Intraoperative:** Patients who are on chronic opioids will likely require higher doses of opioids intraoperatively. If the patient has a transdermal delivery system of an opioid, it should not be warmed as increased cutaneous circulation to the area can increase the amount of opioid delivered. Nonopioid analgesics should be maximized.

**Postoperative:** Controlling pain for patients on chronic opioids is difficult. All efforts must be made to maximize nonopioid analgesics. Continuing their home MME and adding more opioid will likely be needed.[3,4]

## OPIOID USE DISORDER AND MEDICATION-ASSISTED THERAPY

Three drugs are utilized for patients with opioid use disorder (OUD) to aid in their recovery and remission: buprenorphine (often with naloxone to help deter aberrant behavior), methadone, and naltrexone. Buprenorphine, given its low bioavailability, is administered via buccal, sublingual, subcutaneous, or subdermal (via an implant) routes, and providers need a special waiver in order to prescribe. Buprenorphine has a very high affinity for the $\mu$-receptor, higher than most traditional opioids used perioperatively. Methadone, for its use in OUD, is delivered orally, decreasing the euphoria associated with taking opioids and is only available through an opioid treatment program (OTP), unlike the other two options. Naltrexone, for OUD, is available in an intramuscular injection and oral formulation.

## ANESTHETIC CONSIDERATIONS

**Preoperative:** Methadone, a full $\mu$-agonist, should be continued when possible after confirming with an OTP. Methadone and buprenorphine may both prolong QTc;

evaluation with an electrocardiogram is warranted.[1-4] Both buprenorphine and naltrexone will either partially or completely block opioids from having their full effect.[1,4] Discussions with the prescriber about discontinuation of these medications should be considered, when possible.

**Intraoperative:** Patients who have had their buprenorphine and naltrexone continued preoperatively will likely have very high opioid requirements intraoperatively. Consequently, opioids may be of little effect and nonopioid analgesics may be needed as well as drugs to aid with the nociceptive sympathetic reflex.

**Postoperative:** Patients with OUD on medication-assisted therapy will likely have more uncontrolled pain postoperatively. Patients who are on methadone should have their medications continued and be prescribed additional opioids when possible. Patients who did not stop their buprenorphine or naltrexone preoperatively will have very high, variable opioid requirements postoperatively; with possible no effect of opioids.[4]

## A-$_2$-AGONISTS

The $\alpha_2$-agonists have an effect as a sedative and as a pain adjunct. Their function is derived from direct agonism of the $\alpha_2$-adrenoreceptor, which leads to analgesic, sympatholytic, and anxiolytic effects. Two common drugs used are clonidine and dexmedetomidine, with dexmedetomidine having higher binding specificity.[1,2] The onset of action with intravenous administration for both medications is rapid at less than 5 minutes, with clonidine having a slightly longer redistribution half-life of 10 minutes, while dexmedetomidine has a shorter half-life of 6 minutes.[1] Unlike opioid agonists, $\alpha_2$-agonists do not have respiratory depressive effects. Their use as pain adjuncts and sedatives also helps to limit overall opiate usage. However, hypotension and bradycardia are common adverse effects of these medications due to their inhibition of sympathetic response.

## ANESTHETIC CONSIDERATIONS

**Preoperative:** Evaluation of cardiovascular status would be important when considering use of $\alpha_2$-agonists.

**Intraoperative:** The use of $\alpha_2$-agonists preoperatively can greatly increase the risk of intraoperative severe hypotension, bradycardia, and cardiac arrest.[1,2]

**Postoperative:** These adjuncts can be incredibly useful in perioperative and postoperative pain management.[1,2]

## ANTIDEPRESSANT MEDICATIONS

Antidepressants are a group of medications aimed mainly toward treatment of depression and anxiety. They encompass a broad spectrum of medications, including tricyclic antidepressants (TCAs), monoamine oxidase inhibitors (MAOIs), selective serotonin reuptake inhibitors (SSRIs), and serotonin norepinephrine reuptake inhibitors (SNRIs).[5] This may lead to greater effects on both heart rate and blood pressure.[5] Many antidepressants utilize the P450 system for metabolism, particularly CYP3A4 and CYP2D6. TCAs can lower seizure threshold.

## ANESTHETIC CONSIDERATIONS

**Preoperative:** Electrocardiography is essential to identify an arrhythmia or abnormal intervals, particularly for patients on TCAs.

**Intraoperative:** SSRIs and SNRIs reduce platelet levels of serotonin, thus increasing risk of bleeding. TCAs can increase the risk of arrhythmias with volatile anesthetics and sympathetically active drugs. They can also increase the sympathetic effects of vasopressors. Directly acting sympathomimetic drugs should be used if a patient is on MAOIs, along with avoidance of meperidine and dextromethorphan given the risk of serotonin syndrome.[2,5]

**Postoperative:** Use of the opioid analgesics tramadol and codeine should be avoided, if possible, given that many antidepressants have activity at CYP2D6. Care should be taken when using any serotonergic drugs, particularly meperidine given the risk of serotonin syndrome. Monitoring for bleeding should be heightened, particularly if other platelet aggregating inhibitors are being used.

## REFERENCES

1. Johnson K. *Clinical Pharmacology for Anesthesiology*. New York, NY: McGraw-Hill Education Medical; 2015.
2. Gropper M, Miller R. *Miller's Anesthesia*. Philadelphia, PA: Elsevier; 2020.
3. Coluzzi F, et al. The challenge of perioperative pain management in opioid-tolerant patients. *Ther Clin Risk Manag*. 2017;13:1163–1173.
4. Harrison TK, et al. Perioperative considerations for the patient with opioid use disorder on buprenorphine, methadone, or naltrexone maintenance therapy. *Anesthesiol Clin*. 2018;36(3):345–359.
5. Saraghi M, et al. Anesthetic considerations for patients on antidepressant therapy—part I. *Anesth Prog*. (2017;64(4):253–261.

# 44.

# NONSTEROIDAL ANTI-INFLAMMATORY DRUGS (NSAIDS)

*Lauren McGinty*

## INTRODUCTION

Nonsteroidal anti-inflammatory drugs (NSAIDs) are widely used for a variety of indications based on their analgesic, anti-inflammatory, and antipyretic effects. Common indications for this class of medications include rheumatoid arthritis, osteoarthritis, ankylosing spondylitis, tendonitis, and bursitis. They can also be used for gout, dysmenorrhea, migraine, mild-to-moderate pain, and fever. Of note, while NSAIDs help relieve symptoms, they do not typically alter the underlying disease process. NSAIDs also do not tend to provide benefit for visceral or neuropathic pain.[1,2]

## MECHANISM OF ACTION

The NSAIDs primarily exert their effects through the reversible inhibition of cyclooxygenase (COX) (Figure 44.1). The two main isoforms of COX are COX-1, which is constitutively expressed in most tissues, and COX-2, which is constitutively expressed in a few areas but mainly functions as an inducible enzyme, with expression increasing in response to inflammatory stimuli. COX enzymes are involved in the transformation of arachidonic acid to prostaglandins, prostacyclin, and thromboxanes. These substances play important physiological roles that help explain both the efficacy

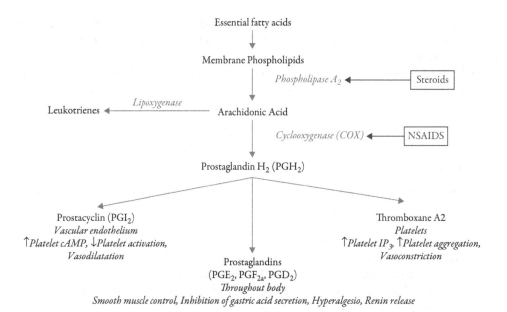

Essential fatty acids

Membrane Phospholipids

*Phospholipase $A_2$* ← Steroids

Leukotrienes ← *Lipoxygenase* ← Arachidonic Acid

*Cyclooxygenase (COX)* ← NSAIDS

Prostaglandin $H_2$ (PGH$_2$)

Prostacyclin (PGI$_2$)
*Vascular endothelium*
↑*Platelet cAMP,* ↓*Platelet activation,*
*Vasodilatation*

Thromboxane A2
*Platelets*
↑*Platelet IP$_3$,* ↑*Platelet aggregation,*
*Vasoconstriction*

Prostaglandins
(PGE$_2$, PGF$_{2a}$, PGD$_2$)
*Throughout body*
*Smooth muscle control, Inhibition of gastric acid secretion, Hyperalgesio, Renin release*

Figure 44.1

and toxicity of NSAIDs. For example, prostaglandins play a role in causing bronchodilation, maintaining renal perfusion through increased renal blood flow, and protecting the gastrointestinal (GI) tract by reducing acid secretion and increasing protective mucus production and blood flow. Prostaglandins also contribute to fever when they act in the hypothalamus and to inflammation, along with both peripheral and central sensitization. When it comes to platelet aggregation, thromboxane $A_2$ plays an essential role. Inhibition of COX not only interrupts these normal physiological roles but also effectively reduces pain, inflammation, and fever.[1–3]

Most NSAIDs are weak acids that are highly protein bound with good oral absorption, small volumes of distribution, and minimal first-pass metabolism. They are primarily hepatically metabolized and renally excreted. Due to significant variability in their half-lives, some NSAIDs only need to be taken once daily, while others may require dosing as frequent as every 4 hours.[1,2]

## COX SELECTIVITY

The majority of available NSAIDs are nonselective NSAIDs, meaning they inhibit both COX-1 and COX-2. However, in an effort to selectively target inflammation and minimize unwanted effects on the GI tract and platelets associated with COX-1 inhibition, COX-2–selective NSAIDs were developed. The only remaining commercially available COX-2–selective NSAID in the United States is celecoxib, as other agents have been removed from the market due to cardiovascular risk. While concerns have also been raised about celecoxib's cardiovascular adverse

effect profile compared to that of nonselective NSAIDs, the PRECISION trial demonstrated no significant differences in cardiovascular outcomes associated with ibuprofen, naproxen, and celecoxib.[4] Although not classified as COX-2–selective NSAIDs, certain nonselective agents, including diclofenac, meloxicam, nabumetone, and etodolac, also display a degree of COX-2 selectivity at lower doses.[1,3]

## ADVERSE EFFECTS AND PRECAUTIONS

The majority of available NSAIDs carry three black box warnings in common. The first warning states that these agents may increase the risk of serious cardiovascular thrombotic events, myocardial infarction, and stroke. Of note, this warning does not apply to aspirin. The second warning states that NSAIDs are contraindicated for the treatment of perioperative pain related to coronary artery bypass graft surgery. The final black box warning focuses on increased risk of serious GI adverse events, including bleeding, ulceration, and stomach or intestinal perforation.[5]

Additional NSAID adverse effects include acute kidney injury, hyperkalemia, nausea, heartburn, and dyspepsia. Patients may also experience sodium and fluid retention, hypertension, elevated transaminases, non-GI bleeding, and skin rashes. NSAIDs should be used with caution in patients with asthma due to risk for bronchospasm. Caution should also be taken for patients who are elderly or have certain GI disorders, hypertension, heart failure, kidney disease, hepatic dysfunction, or bleeding risks based on the side-effect profile of NSAIDs. Because of the variety and potential severity of NSAID-related toxicities,

*Table 44.1* NONSTEROIDAL ANTI-INFLAMMATORY DRUG CHARACTERISTICS

| DRUG | SYSTEMIC ROUTES OF ADMINISTRATION | SPECIAL PRECAUTIONS | OTHER |
|---|---|---|---|
| Aspirin | PO and rectal | Contraindicated in children with viral infections due to risk of Reye syndrome<br>Can cause tinnitus, which may be a sign of salicylate toxicity | Primarily used for antiplatelet effects; use for pain and inflammation has fallen out of favor<br>Unlike other NSAIDs, it irreversibly inhibits platelet COX and is not highly protein bound |
| Celecoxib | PO | Possible risk of allergic reaction in patients with a sulfonamide allergy<br>Major substrate of CYP2C9 | Little or no effect on platelet function |
| Diclofenac | PO | | Also available as an ophthalmic solution and a topical patch, gel, and solution |
| Diflunisal | PO | | Limited antipyretic efficacy |
| Etodolac | PO | | |
| Fenoprofen | PO | | |
| Flurbiprofen | PO | | Also available as an ophthalmic solution |
| Ibuprofen | PO and IV | May interfere with the antiplatelet actions of low-dose aspirin | Can be used in infants for closure of patent ductus arteriosus |
| Indomethacin | PO, IV, and rectal | Commonly causes headaches | Intravenous form can be used in infants for closure of patent ductus arteriosus |
| Ketoprofen | PO | | |
| Ketorolac | PO, IV, IM, and intranasal | Use of systemic therapy for > 5 days contraindicated due to severe adverse effects | Also available as an ophthalmic solution<br>Commonly used postoperatively<br>Limited anti-inflammatory effect |
| Meloxicam | PO and IV | | |
| Meclofenamate | PO | | |
| Mefenamic acid | PO | | |
| Nabumetone | PO | | |
| Naproxen | PO | May interfere with the antiplatelet actions of low-dose aspirin | |
| Oxaprozin | PO | | Not useful for fever or acute pain due to slow onset |
| Piroxicam | PO | Risk of serious dermatologic reactions | Not useful for fever or acute pain due to slow onset |
| Sulindac | PO | | |
| Tolmetin | PO | | |

IV, intravenous; PO, oral.

From References 1–3 and 5.

it is generally recommended that these medications be used at the lowest effective doses for the shortest possible durations. It is important to keep in mind that adequate analgesia can typically be achieved with much lower doses of NSAIDs than those needed for anti-inflammatory effects. Taking NSAIDs with food or milk and potentially with a concomitant H$_2$ blocker or proton pump inhibitor can also help minimize the GI adverse effects. Patients should be encouraged to maintain adequate hydration to help avoid renal toxicity as well.[1–3]

It is important to note that using nonselective NSAIDs, particularly ibuprofen and naproxen, in combination with low-dose aspirin may reduce the cardiovascular benefits of aspirin. The concurrent use of these medications forces aspirin to compete for its binding site on COX-1 and decreases the percentage of COX-1 it is able to irreversibly inhibit, therefore limiting its antiplatelet activity. If concurrent use of aspirin and another nonselective NSAID is unavoidable, it is recommended that doses be staggered appropriately to minimize the interaction.[5]

When it comes to procedures, most NSAIDs should be held for at least 3 days prior to surgery to prevent bleeding complications. One notable exception is aspirin, which should be held for a minimum of 7 days before surgery since aspirin's inhibition of platelet COX is irreversible, and the body needs time to produce new platelets that have not come into contact with aspirin.[1,5]

Additional information on specific NSAIDs, routes of administration, and unique features or precautions are outlined in Table 44.1.

## REFERENCES

1. Grosser T, et al. Pharmacotherapy of inflammation, fever, pain, and gout. In: Brunton LL, et al., eds. *Goodman & Gilman's: The Pharmacological Basis of Therapeutics.* 13th ed. New York, NY: McGraw-Hill; 2018.
2. Brenner GM, Stevens CW. Drugs for pain, inflammation, and arthritic disorders. In: *Brenner and Stevens' Pharmacology.* 5th ed. Philadelphia, PA: Elsevier; 2018.
3. Waller DG, Sampson AP. Nonsteroidal antiinflammatory drugs. In: Medical Pharmacology and Therapeutics. 5th ed. Philadelphia, PA: Elsevier; 2018: Chap. 29.
4. Nissen SE, et al. Cardiovascular safety of celecoxib, naproxen, or ibuprofen for arthritis. *N Engl J Med.* 2016;375(26):2519–2529.
5. Lexicomp Online. Lexi-drugs. Hudson, OH: Lexicomp; August 1, 2020.

# 45.

# ACETAMINOPHEN

*Ifomachukwu Uzodinma*

## INTRODUCTION

Acetaminophen is a para-aminophenol (APAP) derivative, it is one of the most common antipyretic and analgesic medications used around the world. Acetaminophen was first used in clinical medicine in the 1890s, later gaining widespread use in the United States in the 1950s.[1,2] APAP remains one of the most popular analgesic agents used commonly in the pediatric, adult, and geriatric populations.

## MECHANISM OF ACTION

The exact mechanisms of action for acetaminophen remain unclear; however, it has been grouped with nonsteroidal anti-inflammatory medications (NSAIDs) as they work via the inhibition of the cyclooxygenase (COX) pathways. It is postulated that APAP specifically inhibits the COX-3 pathway.[1] Acetaminophen acts on descending serotonergic pathways and inhibits nitric oxide production, which therefore leads to *N*-methyl-D-aspartate (NMDA) receptor antagonisms and decreased substance P within the spinal cord.[1,2] It is also postulated that acetaminophen plays a role on endogenous cannabinoid receptors, acting as an agonist providing analgesia; however, the exact mechanism is poorly understood.[1,2] Acetaminophen lacks the ability to block peripheral prostaglandin production and does not act on platelets like the other NSAIDs. APAP does not predispose individuals to the classic adverse effects that are seen with regular use of NSAIDs, such as increased bleeding risks, gastric ulcers, and renal insufficiencies.

## PHARMACODYNAMICS

Acetaminophen is effective for use in both acute and chronic pain as a mild analgesic and adjuvant medication. Acetaminophen, as well as other NSAIDS, is recommended as a first-line agent, prior to initiating any opioid medications. As an adjuvant, acetaminophen can decrease opioid requirements up to 30% and may be preferred over NSAIDs in individuals with gastrointestinal, hematologic, and renal diseases.[2] The combination of acetaminophen with other NSAIDs improves the efficacy of each agent.[1]

## PHARMACOKINETICS

Acetaminophen is administered intravenously, orally, or rectally. After oral administration, acetaminophen has high oral bioavailability at approximately 90%.[3,4] Rectal absorption has a more variable bioavailability, reaching levels of 50%–80%.[3] It reaches peak plasma concentration after 90 minutes. Plasma half-life is approximately 2–3 hours.[1,3,4]

## METABOLISM

Acetaminophen is primarily metabolized by the liver via glucuronidation, sulfation, and cytochrome P (CYP) 450 metabolism, specifically the isoforms CYP2A1, CYP2E1, and CYP3A4.[3] Metabolism occurs within zone 3 of the liver, which also happens to be the zone most susceptible to oxidative stress and hypoxia.[3] Toxic levels of acetaminophen may lead to centrilobular necrosis.[3]

Roughly 5%–15% of the acetaminophen that is consumed is metabolized to a toxic intermediate, known as N-acetyl-*p*-benzoquinone imine (NAPQI).[4] Under normal conditions and with availability of glutathione (GSG), NAPQI is conjugated to a nontoxic intermediate. The conjugative pathway may become overwhelmed primarily via two mechanisms: decreased GSH or increased NAPQI production. When GSH stores are diminished, NAPQI is actively charged and reacts with hepatocytes, creating free radicals, resulting in cytotoxicity and hepatocellular damage.[4]

## DOSING OF AND PRECAUTIONS FOR ACETAMINOPHEN

For healthy adults, the recommended daily dose limit is 3 g; dosing should not exceed more than 4 g within 24 hours.[4] Precaution should be taken in individuals with a history of alcohol abuse or preexisting liver disorders as this increases the risk of liver damage; dosing should be limited to 2 g per 24 hours in this population.[4] Acetaminophen toxicity is now one of the most common causes of acute liver failure in the United States; this is based on both intentional and unintentional overdose.[2–4] The specific signs and symptoms of liver toxicity reflect those of any illness that manifests with liver damage; this includes elevated prothrombin time, elevated international normalized ratio, jaundice, scleral icterus, and right upper quadrant abdominal pain.

## N-ACETYLCYSTEINE AND ACETAMINOPHEN TOXICITY

Potential treatment for acetaminophen toxicity is the early administration of N-acetylcysteine (NAC). If NAC is given within 12 hours of acetaminophen toxicity, outcomes have yielded decreased morbidity and mortality.[4] NAC is the immediate precursor to GSH; therefore supplemental administration increases GSH levels, thereby increasing the conversion of NAPQI to a nontoxic metabolite. NAC also acts to conjugate unmetabolized acetaminophen.[4]

## REFERENCES

1. Smith HS. Potential analgesic mechanisms of acetaminophen. *Pain Physician.* 2009;12:269–280. https://painphysicianjournal.com/current/pdf?article=MTE4NA%3D%3D&journal=47
2. Toussaint K, et al. What do we (not) know about how paracetamol (acetaminophen) works? *J Clin Pharm Ther.* 2010;35:617–638.
3. Ghanem CI, et al. Acetaminophen from liver to brain: new insights into drug pharmacological action and toxicity. *Pharmacol Res.* 2016;109:119–131.
4. Hodgman MJ, Garrard AR. A review of acetaminophen poisoning. *Crit Care Clin.* 2012;28(4):499–516.

# 46.

# $\alpha_2$-AGONISTS

*Nimit K. Shah and Piotr Al-Jindi*

## INTRODUCTION

$\alpha_2$-Adrenergic receptors are $G_i$-coupled G protein–adrenoceptors and mediate an inhibitory role. When norepinephrine (NE) binds to $\alpha_2$--receptors, adenylyl cyclase is inhibited, leading to decreased cyclic adenosine monophosphate (AMP). This causes hyperpolarization and reduced subsequent neural firing due to changes in K and Ca ion conductance. This leads to decreased NE release, which results in sympatholytic effects with sedation and analgesia. Thus, it acts as a negative-feedback control on sympathetic outflow (Figure 46.1).

## DEXMEDETOMIDINE

Dexmedetomidine (Precedex) has a high specificity and sensitivity for $\alpha_2$- compared to $\alpha_1$-- adrenoceptors ($\alpha_2$-/$\alpha_1$-selectivity ratio of 1620[1,2]). It binds to $\alpha_2$-adrenergic receptors, which inhibits adenylyl cyclase and decreases NE release from the adrenergic nerve terminals.

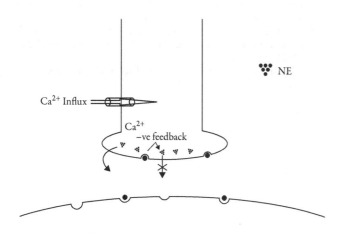

**Figure 46.1** $\alpha_2$-Adrenergic receptors.

## PHARMACOKINETICS

- Dexmedetomidine is a highly lipophilic drug undergoes rapid redistribution [half-life (T1/2a) of 6 minutes] and subsequent terminal elimination [half-life (T1/2b) of 2–3 hours].
- Dexmedetomidine has a very rapid onset and a short duration of action.
- It is highly protein bound (about 94%) in plasma.
- Extensive first-pass effects are observed after oral administration with a bioavailability (BA) of 16%. It is well absorbed through the intranasal (BA 65%), buccal mucosae (BA 82%), and intramuscular (BA 100%), routes.

### Metabolism and Excretion

- Dexmedetomidine is metabolized mainly in the liver to inactive metabolites, most of which are excreted in urine (95%).[2] Clearance is reduced in patients with severe hepatic impairment but not in patients with severe renal impairment,[1] although the sedative effect may be stronger due to reduced plasma protein binding.

## PHARMACODYNAMICS
### Circulation

- Dexmedetomidine causes reduction in both heart rate (HR) and blood pressure (BP) due to its sympatholytic effect.
- Usually, there is up to 15% reduction in HR, occasionally up to 30%, especially when a high dose is injected rapidly.
- Bradyarrhythmias can be detrimental in patients with heart block or cardiac diseases, elderly patients, hypovolemic patients, and patients on heart rate–slowing medications.

- Dexmedetomidine exhibits a biphasic response[2] when injected rapidly and in a high dose; there is an initial short, hypertensive phase and then subsequent hypotension. The initial hypertensive phase is due to first binding with $\alpha_{2B}$-receptors on the vascular smooth muscles, causing vasoconstriction. Subsequent hypotension is due to binding with $\alpha_{2A}$-receptors in the central nervous system (CNS), decreasing the sympathetic outflow.

## Respiration

- Dexmedetomidine exhibits sedation, which resembles endogenous sleep; the respiratory drive is maintained with no change in respiratory rate or tidal volume.

## Central Nervous System

- Dexmedetomidine presents arousable sedation.
- It induces sedation by decreasing the activity of adrenergic neurons in the locus ceruleus in the brainstem.
- It reduces MAC requirements for inhalational agents (anesthetic-sparing properties).
- Dexmedetomidine preserves both somatosensory evoked potentials and motor evoked potentials.
- Dexmedetomidine has no effect on intracranial pressure or cerebral perfusion pressures and produces a matched reduction in cerebral blood flow and cerebral metabolic rate.
- Dexmedetomidine analgesia (works at supraspinal and spinal levels) effects are on the central and spinal cord $\alpha_2$-receptors. There is hyperpolarization of interneurons and reduction of the release of pronociceptive transmitters such as substance P and glutamate.[1]

### SIDE EFFECTS AND TOXICITY

- Biphasic response
- Bradyarrhythmia and sinus arrest
- Hemodynamic instability, especially in elderly patients or patients with severe ventricular dysfunction (ejection fraction < 30%)
- Dry mouth and sedation[1]
- Rebound hypertension (abrupt withdrawal after prolonged use can result in a hypertensive crisis); not licensed for the use of infusion for more than 24 hours, so should be gradually tapered down

### INDICATIONS

- **Premedication:** Dexmedetomidine is used for anxiolysis, especially in pediatric patients.
- **MAC sedation.**
- **ICU sedation:** Dexmedetomidine is approved for infusions for up to 24 hours It reduces delirium as the sedation mimics natural sleep.
- **Procedural sedation[2]:** Dexmedetomidine is used for Magnetic resonance imaging; computed tomographic scans; awake fiber-optic intubation as it provides patency of the airway and maintains respiratory drive in addition to its antisialogogue effect; and neurosurgical procedures requiring perioperative active patient participation, including assessment of responses as it results in arousable sedation. It can be used in surgeries requiring neurophysiological monitoring.
- **Adjunct in general anesthesia:** Dexmedetomidine provides anxiolysis, sedation, analgesia, reduction in MAC requirements, an antishivering effect, and reduced postoperative emergence delirium.
- **Adjunct in neuraxial or peripheral nerve blocks:** Dexmedetomidine prolongs neuraxial and peripheral nerve blocks.
- **Treatment and prevention of emergence delirium[2]** are provided by dexmedetomidine.
- **Antishivering agent.**
- **Chronic pain treatment.**
- **Treatment of opioid, ethyl alcohol, nicotine withdrawal.**

### CLONIDINE

Clonidine belongs to the imidazoline group, with an $\alpha_2$-/$\alpha_2$-selectivity ratio of 200.[2] It has a similar mechanism of action as dexmedetomidine. Besides $\alpha_2$-receptors, it binds with imidazoline $I_1$ receptors in the CNS.

### PHARMACOKINETICS

- Clonidine is highly lipid soluble; it crosses the blood-brain barrier effectively.
- Clonidine is well absorbed orally, with a BA of 70% to 80%.
- Redistribution half-life is 20 minutes and terminal elimination half-life is 12 to 16 hours.
- Clonidine is only 20% protein bound.
- Clonidine is metabolized 50% in the liver, and the remaining 50% is excreted unchanged in the urine; the dose is reduced in both severe hepatic and renal impairment.

## PHARMACODYNAMICS

### Central Nervous System

- Clonidine sedative and analgesic effects have anesthetic and opioid-sparing properties.
- The MOA similar to dexmedetomidine.
- Clonidine reduces MAC by up to 50%.
- Clonidine mediates analgesia both centrally and peripherally; centrally, it is thought to act on $\alpha_2$-receptors in the substantia gelatinosa of the dorsal horn and by suppressing the release of substance P and glutamate. Peripherally it appears to block C fibers.
- When given neuraxially or perineurally concomitantly with local anesthetic, it prolongs the duration of the block.

### Circulation

- Clonidine decreases BP and HR, similar to dexmedetomidine.
- Clonidine has a biphasic response similar to dexmedetomidine due to the activation of peripheral postsynaptic $\alpha_{2B}$-receptors coupled with increasing activation of $\alpha_1$-receptors at higher doses.
- Clonidine causes rebound hypertension and tachycardia on sudden withdrawal, so infusions should be slowly titrated down.

### Respiration

- no clinically significant respiratory depression.

### Endocrine

- Clonidine obtunds the sympathoadrenal stress response to surgery.

## SIDE EFFECTS AND TOXICITY

The side effects and toxicity are similar to dexmedetomidine.

## INDICATIONS

- Clonidine is similar to dexmedetomidine, which is preferred.
- It is used as an antihypertensive agent.
- Intravenous clonidine has been shown to reduce the intensity of opioid-induced hyperalgesia.
- Clonidine is used as an adjunct in chronic cancer pain and neuropathic pain treatment.

## ANESTHETIC CONSIDERATIONS

### PREOPERATIVE

Patients on clonidine should have their clonidine continued day of surgery. Patients at high risk of perioperative myocardial infarction (MI) can have a clonidine patch the night before surgery, which has been shown to reduce the incidence of perioperative MI.[3] Both dexmedetomidine[4] and clonidine can be used for premedication for anxiolysis and for procedural sedation, especially in pediatric pts.

### INTRAOPERATIVE

Both dexmedetomidine and clonidine can be used as adjuncts to general anesthesia as they reduce MAC requirements, along with providing sedation, analgesia, anxiolysis, and hemodynamic stability. They can be used as an adjunct to local anesthesia in neuraxial or regional nerve blocks. Both can cause bradyarrhythmia.

### POSTOPERATIVE

Both dexmedetomidine and clonidine produce rebound hypertension if stopped abruptly; hence they should be gradually tapered down.

## REFERENCES

1. Vuyk J, et al. Intravenous anesthetics. In: Miller RD, ed. *Anesthesia*. 9th ed. Elsevier; 2020:670–675.
2. Giovannitti JA Jr, et al. Alpha-2 adrenergic receptor agonists: a review of current clinical applications. *Anesth Prog*. 2015;62:31–38.
3. Wallace AW, et al. Effect of clonidine on cardiovascular morbidity and mortality after noncardiac surgery. *Anesthesiology*. 2004;101:284–293.
4. Mahmoud M, Mason K. Dexmedetomidine: review, update, and future considerations of paediatric perioperative and periprocedural applications and limitations. Br J Anaesth. 2015;115:171–182.

# 47.

# TRANQUILIZERS

*Rohit Aiyer and Sarah Money*

## INTRODUCTION

Tranquilizers provide treatment of anxiety, tension, agitation, and aggression. They are broken down into two groups: major and minor tranquilizers. It should be noted that this terminology is somewhat dated as there are now more specific pharmacological subsets in each group. Major tranquilizers include antipsychotic medications, whereas minor tranquilizers include benzodiazepines.

## ANTIPSYCHOTICS (BUTYROPHENONES)

While historically known as major tranquilizers, today they are better known as antipsychotics. All antipsychotic agents target dopamine receptors for the clinical treatment of agitation, psychosis, and schizophrenia. However, it should be noted that antipsychotic medications all have varying levels of antagonist interaction with all the dopamine, histamine, and cholinergic receptors. Antipsychotic medications can be further broken down into two groups: first generation or typical antipsychotics and second generation or atypical antipsychotics.

The main distinguishing factor between the two generations is that first-generation antipsychotics all have high affinity for the dopamine $D_2$ receptor. Further studies have shown that $D_2$ receptor occupancy of 65%–70% is associated with antipsychotic effects. The side effects of the first-generation antipsychotic group are primarily neurological and associated with the extrapyramidal motor system. Extrapyramidal symptoms have been thought to correlate with $D_2$ receptor occupancy of 80% or greater as this includes clinical symptoms such as dystonia, akathisia, and tardive dyskinesia. Among the first-generation antipsychotics, there are three main subgroups: phenothiazines, butyrophenones, and thioxanthenes.[1]

One of the most widely used antipsychotics is haloperidol, which is a butyrophenone. Early research demonstrated haloperidol selectively blocks $D_2$ dopamine receptors. Furthermore, studies have shown that excess dopamine is present in patients with hyperactive or mixed-type delirium, particularly with regard to agitation, restlessness, irritability, distractibility, increased psychomotor activity, combativeness, and hyperalertness. As a result, dopamine antagonists such as haloperidol can mitigate and alleviate symptoms of delirium. It is also postulated that $D_2$ antagonists enhance acetylcholine release, which may be another mechanism by which delirium is controlled[2]

Haloperidol is the most commonly used pharmacological treatment in the intensive care unit to treat delirium.[2] Pharmacologically, haloperidol is the preferred antipsychotic due to its relatively low anticholinergic side-effect profile, few active metabolites, and low chance of sedation, compared to other first-generation antipsychotics.[3] It should be noted that haloperidol is generally indicated in only hyperactive (not hypoactive) delirium, and this medication should only be administered until the agitation has been alleviated and then discontinued.[2] For patients younger than 65, doses can range between 1 and 5 mg, depending on the level of agitation. Research has also shown that appropriate dosing with haloperidol for treatment of delirium is in the range of 0.25 to 0.50 mg per dose for geriatric patients. For patients who are severely agitated, 5 to 10 mg intravenously has been utilized in an inpatient hospital setting, however, electrocardiogram monitoring is reccomended as this administration route carries an elevated risk of QT prolongation. It should also be noted that haloperidol is not approved by the U.S. Food and Drug Administration (FDA) for treatment of agitation or delirium.[3] Nevertheless, despite this and the wide availability of various antipsychotic medications, due to its excellent clinical efficacy, haloperidol continues to be the pharmacological choice for treatment of agitation and delirium.

## BENZODIAZEPINES

Benzodiazepines' main FDA approved clinical indication is management of short term anxiety symptoms or anxiety disorders. When prescribing benzodiazepines, clinicians should be aware of the risks involved, which include dependence, tolerance, sedation, drug-drug interactions and potential for abuse. Pharmacologically, these drugs act as a positive allosteric modulation on the γ-aminobutyric acid (GABA) A receptor, which allows for the increased conductance of chloride ions. The benzodiazepines bind to an area created by α and γ subunits, which cause a structural change in the ligand-gated, chloride-selective GABA$_A$ receptor. As a result, this structural change in the receptor allows for chloride ions to travel through, causing hyperpolarization of the cell. Lipid solubility plays a role in the clinical response of benzodiazepines, the higher lipid solubility, the higher absorption rate, and the quicker onset compared to benzodiazepines with low lipid solubility.[4]

Benzodiazepines can be administered through several routes, which include oral, sublingual, intravenous, intranasal, or rectal. They are classified according to their elimination half-life: short acting (e.g., alprazolam) have a half-life between 1 and 12 hours, intermediate acting (e.g., lorazepam) have a half-life between 12 and 40 hours, and long acting (e.g., diazepam) have a half-life between 40 and 250 hours.[5] They can also be classified according to their potency, as low-potency medications include oxazepam and temazepam, whereas high-potency benzodiazepines include alprazolam, lorazepam, and clonazepam. This is related to the affinity of benzodiazepines to receptor binding, with lorazepam having less affinity than alprazolam but greater affinity than clonazepam[4]. For preoperative anxiety and sedation, midazolam is primarily used. For comparison, itit is much more potent than diazepam and very short acting. At physiologic pH, midazolam is extremely lipid soluble and therefore crosses the blood-brain barrier quickly, allowing for rapid onset of clinical response. It has a short half-life and is primarily metabolized by cytochrome P450 into the inactive metabolite 1-hydroxymidazolam. The recommended initial dosing of midazolam in a preoperative setting is 0.5–1 mg intravenously, and then to evaluate sedative effect before repeating another dose if clinically indicated.[4] It should be noted that a major adverse effect of benzodiazepines is delirium, which is commonly seen in the intensive care unit. This risk for delirium is even higher in the geriatric population and should be a consideration when selecting an anxiolytic medication if this is necessary.

## REFERENCES

1. Miyamoto S, et al. Treatments for schizophrenia: a critical review of pharmacology and mechanisms of action of antipsychotic drugs. *Mol Psychiatry.* 2005;10:79–104.
2. Latronico N. Haloperidol and delirium in the ICU: the finger pointing to the moon. *Intensive Care Med.* 2018;44:1346–1348.
3. Markowitz JD, Narasimhan M. Delirium and antipsychotics: a systematic review of epidemiology and somatic treatment options. *Psychiatry (Edgmont).* 2008;5(10):29–36.
4. Griffin CE 3rd, et al. Benzodiazepine pharmacology and central nervous system-mediated effects. *Oscher J.* 2013;13(2):214–223.
5. Fox C, et al., eds. Antianxiety agents. In: *Clinical Aspects of Pain Medicine and Interventional Pain Management: A Comprehensive Review.* Paducah, KY: ASIPP; 2011: 543–552.

# 48.

# ANTIDEPRESSANTS, ANTIPARKINSON DRUGS

*Dustin Latimer and Elyse M. Cornett*

## INTRODUCTION TO ANTIDEPRESSANTS

Antidepressants are some of the more commonly prescribed medication in America, with millions of individuals taking antidepressants for not only depression or anxiety, but also chronic pain, low energy, and other off-brand uses.[1] The class of drugs termed *antidepressants* include selective serotonin reuptake inhibitors (SSRIs), serotonin norepinephrine reuptake inhibitors (SNRIs), tricyclic antidepressants (TCAs), and monoamine oxidase inhibitors (MAOIs).

## SELECTIVE SEROTONIN REUPTAKE INHIBITORS

When a patient is taking an SSRI, it is important to be aware of notable drug interactions that SSRIs may have. SSRIs may cause cytochrome P450 (CYP) inhibition and synergistic effects with anticoagulants and potentially cause serotonin syndrome.[1] Fluoxetine and paroxetine are potent CYP inhibitors.[1] SSRIs reduce the level of platelets and can increase the risk of bleeding because platelets release serotonin, and there may be less serotonin for platelets to utilize in patients taking SSRIs.[1] SSRIs may also inhibit the metabolism of nonsteroidal anti-inflammatory drugs (NSAIDs), which consequently increases the level of NSAID within the bloodstream and increasing bleeding risk[1] Another bleeding risk may occur with an interaction between warfarin and SSRIs; both drugs are highly plasma protein–bound drugs, so there is a possibility of plasma protein–binding competition, and higher levels of SSRIs can outcompete the warfarin, which will increase the warfarin concentration in the bloodstream.[1]

## SEROTONIN NOREPINEPHRINE REUPTAKE INHIBITORS

Serotonin Norepinephrine Reuptake Inhibitors act as antidepressants primarily, but can also be used for fibromyalgia, symptom management of menopause, and general anxiety disorder. Duloxetine and venlafaxine are two of the most common SNRIs prescribed. SNRIs are slightly more selective for norepinephrine reuptake when compared to serotonin, and one side effect that should be monitored is the development of hypertension and tachycardia due to the activation of adrenergic agonists.[1] Venlafaxine is a weak inhibitor of CYP2D6, and duloxetine is a moderate inhibitor of CYP2D6.[1] CYP2D6 interactions are important in the postoperative period because of the metabolism of codeine and tramadol by CYP2D6; inhibition of CYP2D6 can decrease the level of prodrug being converted into the active analgesic metabolite.[1] Like SSRIs, SNRIs can increase the risk of bleeding because of the role serotonin plays with platelet count.[1]

## TRICYCLIC ANTIDEPRESSANTS

The TCAs are some of the older antidepressants that have fallen out of popular use for depression due to the side-effect profile, but they are still used in some patients, so it is pertinent to discuss them. TCAs act by inhibiting the reuptake of serotonin and norepinephrine. Amitriptyline, clomipramine, doxepin, imipramine, and trimipramine are all examples of tertiary amine TCAs. Desipramine, nortriptyline, and protriptyline are all examples of secondary amine TCAs. Tertiary amine TCAs have more serotonin reuptake inhibition, while secondary amine TCAs have more norepinephrine reuptake inhibition. TCAs have a long list of interactions with various CYP enzymes, which should be reviewed in patients taking TCAs.

## MONOAMINE OXIDASE INHIBITORS

Monoamine oxidase inhibitors are rarely used as antidepressants in modern times because of their side effects and interactions with other drugs and food, which can lead to serotonin syndrome. They work to increase stores of presynaptic norepinephrine. Isocarboxazid, phenelzine, selegiline, and tranylcypromine are examples of MAOIs. Foods containing high levels are tyramine, such as cured meat, aged cheese, and draft beer, should be avoided in patients taking MAOIs because this combination can cause dangerously high blood pressures.

## INTRODUCTION TO PARKINSON DISEASE AGENTS

Parkinson disease is a clinically diagnosed disease of the brain that is seen primarily in the older population. These patients have a loss of dopaminergic neurons in the substantia nigra, resulting in cogwheel rigidity, bradykinesia, and tremors. The primary treatment option for individuals suffering from Parkinson disease is pharmacological therapy to improve dopaminergic activity via dopamine levels or sensitivity of dopamine receptors. This section looks at the anesthetic considerations in patients with Parkinson disease and the pharmacological agents they are taking.

### L-DOPA AND DOPAMINE AGONISTS

Parkinson disease is pathological loss of dopamine because of the destruction of dopaminergic neurons, so the first-line treatment is replacing the lost dopamine to regain normal movement. This is done with L-DOPA, a prodrug that converts to dopamine within the brain, or with a dopamine agonist such as bromocriptine, pramipexole, and cabergoline.[2] L-DOPA has a half-life of about 1–3 hours, so patients are advised to take this medication as close to their surgery as possible and prioritize their L-DOPA medication postoperatively to ensure they do not miss their dose postoperatively.[2] L-DOPA can be administered perioperatively by a nasogastric tube if the surgery is particularly lengthy.[2] Patients taking

L-DOPA should avoid inhalant anesthetics such as halothane because of halothane's sensitization of the heart to catecholamines.[2]

## MONOAMINE OXIDASE INHIBITORS

Selegiline is a type B MAOI used to treat Parkinson disease by prolonging dopamine's action in the striatum and decreasing symptoms.[2] There is an extensive list of anesthetic agents that should be avoided in patients taking MAOIs, but selegiline is an MAOI-B type, which narrows the list of potential complications for anesthetic agents as it does not interact with as many agents as MAOI-A types do.[2] One of the few known anesthetic agent combinations that should be avoided is meperidine and selegiline; there have been reports of agitation, muscle rigidity, and hyperthermia in patients receiving both of these drugs.[2]

## OTHER ANESTHETIC CONSIDERATIONS IN PARKINSON PATIENTS

Parkinson disease patients must be monitored closely at a multisystem level during all aspects of surgery. Table 48.1 is an abbreviated chart of possible complications that have been reported in patients with Parkinson disease.

*Table 48.1* COMPLICATIONS ASSOCIATED WITH PARKINSON DISEASE

| Respiratory | Rigidity causing respiratory impairment<br>Bradykinesia or uncoordinated involuntary movements of respiratory muscles |
|---|---|
| Cardiovascular | Arrhythmias<br>Hypertension<br>Orthostatic hypotension<br>Autonomic dysfunction |
| Gastrointestinal | Susceptibility to reflux due to involuntary muscle spasms |
| Endocrine | In patients taking selegiline, possible abnormal glucose metabolism |
| Central nervous system | Tremor<br>Rigidity<br>Hallucinations<br>Akinesia<br>Speech impairment |

From Reference 2.

## REFERENCES

1. Saraghi M, et al. Anesthetic considerations for patients on antidepressant therapy-part I. *Anesth Prog.* 2017;64:253–261.
2. Nicholson G, et al. Parkinson's disease and anaesthesia. *Br J Anaesth.* 2002;89:904–916.

# 49.

# AROUSAL AGENTS

*Greta Nemergut*

## INTRODUCTION

Emergence from anesthesia is generally done by removing the anesthetic agents in a way that permits the patient to wake safely. However, there are times that emergence from anesthesia is delayed in patients, and reversal agents need to be used to arouse the patient to a wakeful state if the delay is due to prolonged drug effects. There are reversal agents for opioids, benzodiazepines, anticholinergic drugs, and neuromuscular blockers. These drugs and their actions and place in therapy are addressed (Table 49.1).

## NALOXONE

Opioids can contribute to delay in emergence due to their sedative effects, which are additive with other anesthetic agents. Additionally, patients have varying sensitivity to

**Table 49.1 SUMMARY OF REVERSAL AGENTS AND DOSE**

| DRUG CLASS | REVERSAL AGENT | DOSE/INTERVAL | MAXIMUM DOSE |
|---|---|---|---|
| Opioids | Naloxone | 40 μg IV every 2 to 5 minutes | 10 μg/kg or 200 μg |
| Benzodiazepines | Flumazenil | 0.2 mg IV over 30 seconds to 1 minute | 1 mg |
| Anticholinergics | Physostigmine | 0.5 mg to 1 mg IV over 5 to 10 minutes | 2 mg |
| NMBA | Neostigmine | 0.03 mg/kg to 0.07 mg/kg IV over 1 minute | Dosed to effect; given with glycopyrrolate 10 μg/kg to prevent bradycardia |
| NMBA (rocuronium and vecuronium) | Sugammadex | 2 mg/kg to 4 mg/kg IV slow IV push | Single dose is given |

Adapted from References 1–3.

opioids, which can contribute to delayed emergence and can be related to age or metabolism. Naloxone, an opioid antagonist, can be given if sedation is thought to be related to opioid therapy. It is typically dosed at a 40-μg injection and can be given every 2 to 5 minutes, with a maximum dose suggested of 10 μg/kg or 200 μg total.[1,2] The half-life of the drug is only 1 to 1.5 hours, so it may be less than the opioid it is reversing, so repeat doses may be needed.[1] The dose will depend on several factors, including how much opioid the patient received and the weight of the patient.

## FLUMAZENIL

As with opioids, the sedative effects and respiratory depressive effects of benzodiazepines are also additive with other agents. Flumazenil is a reversal agent for benzodiazepines that can be used if the benzodiazepine is thought to be the cause of the oversedation and delayed awakening. It acts by competitively inhibiting the γ-aminobutyric acid (GABA)/benzodiazepine receptor complex, specifically the benzodiazepine receptor site.[3] Flumazenil is dosed at 0.2 mg IV given over 30 seconds. The dose can be repeated, if needed, to a maximum dose of 1 mg.[1,3] Since the benzodiazepine being reversed can have longer action than flumazenil, patients should be monitored for recurrence of sedation. If this occurs, flumazenil can be repeated, but no more than 3 mg should be given within an hour.[1]

## PHYSOSTIGMINE

Physostigmine reverses anticholinergic effects. An anticholinergic overdose generally presents as mydriasis, hypothermia, redness, and/or anhidrosis. Physostigmine can be

used at doses of 0.5 to 2 mg slow IV push, but electrocardiogram monitoring should occur to detect bradycardia, and patients should be observed for seizure activity or bronchospasm.[1] Physostigmine is lipid soluble and can cross the blood-brain barrier.

## NEOSTIGMINE

Neostigmine is an acetylcholinesterase inhibitor that can be used as a reversal agent for nondepolarizing neuromuscular blocking agents (NMBAs).[3] It is dosed at 0.03 mg/kg to 0.07 mg/kg and administered as an intravenous push over 1 minute. The lower 0.03 mg/kg dose is recommended when using as a reversal agent for NMBAs with shorter half-lives, such as rocuronium, and the higher 0.07 mg/kg dose is recommend for use in reversing NMBAs with longer half-lives, including vecuronium and pancuronium.[1-3] Neostigmine should always be administered with an anticholinergic agent, such as glycopyrrolate, to lessen the risk of bradycardia that accompanies the use of this drug.[1,3] The dose of glycopyrrolate is 10 μg/kg. Neostigmine, pysidostigmine, and edrophonium are not lipid soluble (unlike physostigmine) so they do not cross the gastrointestinal tract or the blood-brain barrier. It is important to notice that even with a normal train of four, up to 70% of the postjunctional receptors may be occupied by non-depolarizing muscle relaxants (NDMRs).

## SUGAMMADEX

Sugammadex is a modified γ-cyclodextrin that binds selectively to NMBAs, forming a complex with rocuronium and vecuronium in plasma, and that reduces the amount of NMBA that is available to bind at nicotinic receptors and exert their action.[3] The drug is generally dosed at 2 mg/kg (for moderate blocks) to 4 mg/kg (for deep blocks) as a single intravenous dose.[1,3] If immediate reversal of rocuronium is needed, a dose of 16 mg/kg of sugammadex can be given within 3 minutes after giving a single dose of rocuronium of 1.2 mg/kg.[3]

## ANESTHETIC CONSIDERATIONS

### PREOPERATIVE

Preoperative risks factors for prolonged effects of anesthetics include drug interactions with preoperative prescription drugs, as well as recreational drug and alcohol. A complete drug history needs to be taken and assessed. Also, hepatic and renal function can result in prolonged drug effects, as well as weight and age of the patient.[1]

### INTRAOPERATIVE

Central nervous system effects of different anesthetic agents are synergistic, like benzodiazepine and opioids, and need to be considered when administering the drugs. Medications that primarily work on GABA receptors, like midazolam and propofol, tend to produce synergy when given with agents that work on other receptors.[1]

### POSTOPERATIVE

Patients need to be assessed for continued action of the reversal agents as well as potential side effects that the drugs can cause. Since naloxone and flumazenil have a shorter half-life than some of the drugs they are reversing, sedation may reoccur, and subsequent doses of the reversal agents may need administered. Physostigmine has a risk of bradycardia, and monitoring is needed. Neostigmine for reversal of NMBAs requires use of glycopyrrolate to lessen the risk of bradycardia, and heart rate should be monitored.

## REFERENCES

1. Pai SL. Delayed emergence and emergence delirium in adults. In: Holt NF, ed. *UpToDate*. Waltham, MA: UpToDate. Accessed September 1, 2020. https://www.uptodate.com/contents/dela yed-emergence-and-emergence-delirium-in-adults?search=dela yed%20emergence%20and%20emergence%20delirium&source= search_result&selectedTitle=1~145&usage_type=default&displ ay_rank=1
2. Desikan SR. Delayed emergence. In: Fleisher LA, Rosenbaum SH, ed. Complications in Anesthesia. 3rd ed. Elsevier; 2018:535–538.
3. Lexicomp Online. *Lexi-Drugs Online*. UpToDate; 2September 1, 2020.

# 50.

# ANTIEMETICS

*Jeffery James Eapen and Jason Bang*

## INTRODUCTION

Antiemetics are a category of medications aimed at antagonizing the neurotransmitter receptors known to be involved in the physiology of nausea and vomiting. Postoperative nausea and vomiting (PONV) has a 20%–30% occurrence overall and is rated by many patients as more concerning than postoperative pain.[1,2] These medications are classed based on the primary receptor they target, which include 5-HT$_3$ (5-hydroxytryptamine, serotonin), dopamine 2 receptor, histamine 1 receptor, and neurokinin 1 receptor. The physiology behind nausea and vomiting is thought to be centrally mediated, involving the chemoreceptor trigger zone in the area postrema and the nucleus of the tractus solitarius in the brainstem; each of these locations contains the receptors on which antiemetics act.[1]

## 5-HT₃ ANTAGONISTS

Serotonin is usually released from the enterochromaffin cells, which stimulates the chemoreceptor trigger zone of the area postrema, subsequently activating the vomiting center. Ondansetron is a synthetic carbazole that binds and antagonizes 5-HT₃ receptors centrally and peripherally. Side effects include headache, constipation, flushing, bradycardia, and QT prolongation. There are no considerations for renal impairment, but due to its hepatic metabolism, dosage adjustments should be made in hepatic impairment.[1]

## DOPAMINE ANTAGONISTS

Metoclopramide (Reglan) acts at the chemoreceptor trigger zone of the area postrema by antagonizing dopamine receptors. It also acts as a prokinetic peripherally, resulting in increased gastric emptying and esophageal sphincter tone.[1] Metoclopramide can cross the blood-brain barrier, allowing for potential side effects of extrapyramidal effects, particularly in patients with Parkinson disease. Of note, when used at the dose of 10 mg, the medication has been shown to have no clinically relevant antiemetic effect. When the dose of 20 mg or greater was used, it was shown to be as effective as other antiemetics.[3,4]

Droperidol is a butyrophenone class of antidopaminergic agent that works at the chemoreceptor trigger zone of the area postrema. Its use has fallen out of favor due to cases of QT interval prolongation, an important consideration that should be assessed prior to use.

Phenothiazines such as prochlorperazine (Compazine) and promethazine (Phenergan) are a class of antidopaminergic agents that also have anticholinergic and antihistaminic blocking effects at the chemoreceptor trigger zone and are useful in the treatment of nausea and vomiting. Side effects include acute dystonia, tardive dyskinesia, dry mouth, urinary retention, tachycardia, and drowsiness.[1]

Domperidone (Motilium) is an antidopaminergic agent that is used in the management of nausea and vomiting associated with migraines. The drug antagonizes peripheral dopamine 2 and 3 receptors. Of note, the medication can result in increased prolactin levels due to blocking of dopamine receptors in the anterior pituitary, resulting in galactorrhea as a side effect. Domperidone is also a medication that can prolong the QT interval, which can precipitate sudden cardiac death.

## ANTICHOLINERGIC

Scopolamine is an anticholinergic medication used in the management of PONV and motion sickness. It acts on muscarinic receptors on the vestibular nuclei that contribute to motion sickness as well as the receptors on the chemoreceptor trigger zone that activate the vomiting center.[1]

## ANTIHISTAMINE

Cyclizine is a piperazine derivative used to treat motion sickness, radiotherapy-induced emesis, PONV, and opioid-induced emesis. It works as a histamine 1 receptor antagonist, which is primarily present centrally in the vomiting center. Side effects include tachycardia, drowsiness, blurred vision, and pain on injection.[1]

## NEUROKININ 1 ANTAGONIST

Aprepitant is a neurokinin 1 receptor antagonist that functions to prevent the binding of substance P (agonist of the receptor) at the nucleus of the tractus solitarius in the brainstem.[3] This class of medication is usually reserved for cases of refractory PONV as its common medical use is in chemotherapy-induced nausea and vomiting. This medication must be used with caution in patients taking warfarin as it can significantly decrease the international normalized ratio.

## MISCELLANEOUS

Dexamethasone is an antiemetic corticosteroid that is used in the treatment of PONV. Proposed mechanisms of action in regard to antiemetic effects are reductions in the release of arachidonic acid or reduced permeability of the blood-brain barrier. Propofol is an intravenous anesthetic agent that is used for rescue therapy of refractory PONV at subhypnotic doses of 10–20 mg. It has been proven that total intravenous anesthesia using propofol infusion dramatically decreases the risk of PONV maintenance of anesthesia through volatile anesthetics.[1]

## ANESTHETIC CONSIDERATIONS

The risk factors for PONV include female gender, nonsmoker, history of motion sickness, and postoperative opioid use. The incidence based respectively on the number of risk factors are as follows: 1%–21%, 2%–39%, 3%–61%, and 4%–78%.[1]

## REFERENCES

1. Lyons S. Ballisat B. Antiemetic drugs: pharmacology and an overview of their clinical use. Update. *Anaesthesia*. 2016;31:42.

2. Apfel CC, et al. Who is at risk for postdischarge nausea and vomiting after ambulatory surgery? *Anesthesiology*. 2012;117(3): 475–486.

3. George E, et al. Neurokinin-1 and novel serotonin antagonists for postoperative and postdischarge nausea and vomiting. *Curr Opin Anaesthesiol*. 2010;23(6):714–721.

4. Wallenborn J, et al. Prevention of postoperative nausea and vomiting by metoclopramide combined with dexamethasone: randomized double blind multicentre trial. *BMJ*. 2006;333:324.

# 51.

# ANTIASPIRATION MEDICATIONS

*Nimit K. Shah and Abed Rahman*

## INTRODUCTION

Pulmonary aspiration is one of the most common causes of airway-related mortality. It is defined as inhalation of oropharyngeal or gastric contents into the respiratory tract.[1,2] Inhalation of solid material can lead to physical obstruction, whereas acidity of the fluid will lead to pneumonitis.[2] Our normal physiologic mechanisms to prevent aspiration include our upper and lower esophageal sphincters and laryngeal reflexes, which are abolished with the use of medication to induce general anesthesia. The consequences of aspiration can range from benign to fatal. Every effort should be made to recognize the risk of aspiration and prevent it from occurrence. It has been long thought that a gastric fluid volume of 0.4 mL/kg (25 mL/70 kg) and pH of less than 2.5 were risk factors for significant aspiration sequelae.[3] Recent data have shown these surrogate endpoints for aspiration risk should not be used, but instead patient, surgical, and anesthetic risk factors should be considered for pharmacological prophylaxis.[4]

## ANESTHETIC CONSIDERATIONS

Three main factors that need to be considered to accurately assess the aspiration risk in a patient are patient, surgical, and anesthetic factors, as listed in Table 51.1.

### PREOPERATIVE

Patients at higher risk of aspiration should be identified before surgery. The risk factors are patient, surgical, and anesthetic risk factors. Patients with inadequate nothing by mouth (nil per os, NPO) status and/or those presenting for emergency/trauma surgery; patients presenting with bowel obstruction; patients with diabetic neuropathy, hiatus hernia, gastroesophageal reflux disease, prior bowel surgeries; patients on opioids; pregnant patients; morbidly obese patients; patients who are obtunded; and patients under the influence of alcohol are at high risk of aspiration under anesthesia. Patients undergoing laparoscopic, abdominal, or thoracotomy surgery; patients in lithotomy or Trendelenburg position intraoperatively; or

**Table 51.1 ASSESSMENT OF ASPIRATION RISK**

| PATIENT FACTORS | SURGICAL FACTORS | ANESTHETIC FACTORS |
|---|---|---|
| Full stomach<br>– Inadequate fasting status<br>– Trauma/emergency surgery<br>– Bowel obstruction | Positioning<br>– Lithotomy<br>– Trendelenburg | Light anesthesia |
| Delayed gastric emptying<br>– Uncontrolled diabetes<br>– Recent opioid consumption | Type of surgery<br>– Laparoscopic<br>– Abdominal<br>– Thoracotomy | Supraglottic airways |
| Anatomy<br>– Hiatal hernia<br>– Gastroesophageal reflux<br>– Pregnancy<br>– Morbid obesity | Length of surgery > 2 hours | Positive pressure ventilation |
| Prior surgeries on the gastrointestinal tract | | Difficult airway |

patients undergoing surgeries of more than 2 hours duration are also at risk of aspiration. Patients with a difficult airway on examination, patients planned for supraglottic airway, and patients requiring PPV are also at risk of aspiration. All these patients should ideally have an adequate fasting status. The fasting guidelines[5] are given in Table 51.2.

If the patients do not have an adequate fasting status or are at risk of aspiration, antiaspiration medications should be administered preoperatively. These medications may exert their effect by increasing the pH or decreasing the volume of gastric fluids or increasing gastric motility. Table 51.3 shows the various agents that can be used as well as their own individual characteristics. Particulate antacids include aluminum hydroxide, calcium carbonate,

**Table 51.2 FASTING GUIDELINES**

| INGESTED MATERIAL | MINIMUM FASTING PERIOD |
|---|---|
| Clear liquids | 2 hour |
| Breast milk | 4 hour |
| Infant formula | 6 hour |
| Nonhuman formula | 6 hour |
| Light meal | 6 hour |
| Fatty meal | 8 hour |

magnesium oxide, and sodium bicarbonate. Aspiration of antacid particles can cause as much damage as acidic aspirate. Sodium citrate (Bicitra) is a nonparticulate antacid that is effective in raising gastric fluid pH in both elective and emergency surgical patients if given within 15 to 60 minutes before induction of anesthesia. It has the fastest onset of action of 30 minutes, and its effects last for 1 hour. Thus, an additional agent such as a proton pump inhibitor or a histamine 2 receptor antagonist should be added in combination. The onset of the last two classes is between 1 and 2 hours, and their effects can last between 3 and 6 hours depending on the specific agent used.

Histamine receptor antagonists are associated with sinus bradycardia and atrioventricular block, hepatotoxicity, and neuropsychiatric complications. Proton pump inhibitors are mainly metabolized in the liver by the cytochrome P450 system and can delay elimination of diazepam, phenytoin, and warfarin. Hepatotoxicity and leukopenia has also been reported. Metoclopramide increases the lower esophageal sphincter pressure, speeds gastric emptying time, and has antiemetic properties. It has no direct effect on gastric fluid pH. Prokinetic agents that can increase gastric motility may have some benefit in patients with underlying neuropathy but should be used with caution in patients with a history of bowel obstruction or risk factors for developing extrapyramidal symptoms

## INTRAOPERATIVE

General anesthesia should be avoided if possible in patients with a high risk of aspiration and regional anesthesia or neuraxial blockade should be considered. If general anesthesia is necessary, rapid sequence induction with cricoid pressure should be performed. Use of cricoid pressure is contentious as it may decrease the lower esophageal sphincter tone, and it can make direct laryngoscopy difficult. Trendelenburg or lithotomy position should be avoided. High doses of opioids and N20 should be avoided. Dexamethasone 8 mg IV may be given soon after induction as it is shown to prevent postoperative nausea and vomiting and hence perioperative aspiration. Ondansetron 4 mg IV may also be given toward the end.

## POSTOPERATIVE

Patients should be extubated awake and preferably in the lateral position or with the head upright or own position.

*Table 51.3* ANTIASPIRATION MEDICATIONS

| DRUG CLASS | DOSE | ONSET | DURATION OF ACTION | MECHANISM OF ACTION | SIDE EFFECTS |
|---|---|---|---|---|---|
| Proton pump inhibitors<br>  Omeprazole<br>  Pantoprazole<br>  Lansoprazole | 20 mg by mouth<br>20 mg by mouth or intravenous<br>15 mg by mouth | 1 hour<br>1 hour<br>2 hours | 5–6 hours<br>24 hours<br>5–6 hours | Increases pH and decreases gastric volume | VAP (ventilator-associated pneumonia) |
| H₂ blockers<br>  Cimetidine<br>  Famotidine<br>  Ranitidine | 300 mg intravenous/ by mouth<br>20 mg intravenous<br>150 mg by mouth<br>50 mg intravenous | 2 hours<br>2 hours<br>3 hours<br>1 hour | 10 hours<br>10–12 hours<br>15 hours | Increases pH and decreases gastric volume | VAP<br>Cimetidine:<br>Gynecomastia; inhibits CYP450; crosses blood-brain barrier, causing neurological symptoms, hypotension, bradycardia, bronchoconstriction, impotence, neutropenia, and thrombocytopenia |
| Nonparticulate antacids<br>  Sodium citrate (Bicitra) | 15–30 mL | 30 minutes | 1 hour | Increase PH, increase gastric motility, increases lower esophageal sphincter tone, neutralizes gastric acidity | |
| Prokinetic agents<br>  Metoclopramide<br>  Erythromycin | 10 mg intravenous or oral | 1–3 minutes intravenous<br>30–60 minutes oral | 8 hours | Increases gastric motility | Extrapyramidal symptoms |

# REFERENCES

1. Agnew NM, et al. Gastroesophageal reflux and tracheal aspiration in the thoracotomy position: should ranitidine premedication be routine? *Anesth Analg.* 2002;95:1645–1649. https://journals.lww.com/anesthesia-analgesia/Fulltext/2002/12000/Gastroesophageal_Reflux_and_Tracheal_Aspiration_in.31.aspx

2. Aspiration prevention and prophylaxis: preoperative considerations. February 28, 2015. https://clinicalgate.com/aspiration-prevention-and-prophylaxis-preoperative-considerations/

3. Roberts RB, Shirley MA. Reducing the risk of acid aspiration during cesarean section. *Anesth Analg.* 1974;53:859–868.

4. Schreiner MS. Gastric fluid volume: is it really a risk factor for pulmonary aspiration? *Anesth Analg.* 1998;87(4):754–756.

5. Practice guidelines for preoperative fasting and the use of pharmacologic agents to reduce the risk of pulmonary aspiration: application to healthy patients undergoing elective procedures: an updated report by the American Society of Anesthesiologists Task Force on Preoperative Fasting and the Use of Pharmacologic Agents to Reduce the Risk of Pulmonary Aspiration. *Anesthesiology.* 2017;126:376–393.

# 52.

# CHRONIC OPIOID DEPENDENCE AND THERAPY

*Nicholas M. Parker*

## INTRODUCTION

Many medications used in anesthesia carry significant risk for addiction, abuse, and dependence due to their potent effects on the central nervous system. While nonopioids like benzodiazepines and ketamine can be misused, opioid abuse is more deadly and pervasive and is the focus of this chapter. Addiction is a psychiatric condition defined by continued use of a drug for a nonmedical purpose in the face of negative consequences. Opioid use disorder (OUD) affects at least 2 million people in the United States, and drug overdose is now responsible for over 100,000 deaths *every year*.[1] Treatment of OUD involves counseling and support in addition to one of several medications (known as medication-assisted therapy or MAT).[2]

## MEDICATION-ASSISTED THERAPY

### NALTREXONE

Naltrexone is an opioid antagonist and is used to prevent euphoria if an opioid is used. Naltrexone can be taken orally or given as a long-acting injection (Vivitrol). No special privileges are needed to prescribe either form of naltrexone.[2] Opioid abstinence is needed prior to starting naltrexone to avoid causing rapid withdrawal.[3,4]

### BUPRENORPHINE

Buprenorphine is a partial opioid agonist/antagonist that helps patients with OUD avoid withdrawal while also blunting the effects of other opioids if used.[2] Many physicians and other providers can prescribe buprenorphine for opioid maintenance after meeting specific requirements set by the USs Substance Abuse and Mental Health Services Administration (SAMHSA).[2] Buprenorphine is usually formulated with naloxone, an opioid antagonist, to deter illicit intravenous administration (e.g., Suboxone).[5] Because buprenorphine is a partial agonist/antagonist of opioid receptors, it can trigger withdrawal symptoms if given soon after other opioids.[3–5] Wait at least 24 hours after the last dose of opioid analgesics to start or restart buprenorphine; however, if opioid withdrawal symptoms occur sooner than 24 hours, buprenorphine can be initiated when those symptoms begin.

## METHADONE

Methadone is a full opioid agonist that may also be used to maintain patients with OUD to avoid withdrawal symptoms that could prompt the patient to seek illicit opioids. In the outpatient setting, methadone may be prescribed for OUD only through a certified opioid treatment program (OTP) regulated by SAMHSA.[2] Inpatient, methadone may be used to prevent withdrawal in two situations: if patients receive methadone from an OTP, their usual dose may be continued as an inpatient; otherwise, methadone may be initiated in a patient admitted for reasons other than OUD if withdrawal would complicate their medical care.[2]

## OVERDOSE PREVENTION TOOLS

### NALOXONE

Naloxone (Narcan) should also be made available to any patient with OUD, taking high doses of opioids for pain, or potentially in a position to help someone with OUD. This opioid antagonist is used as a rescue medication to treat known or suspected opioid overdose.[5] In the community, naloxone is available as a nasal spray or as a talking autoinjector. It is crucial to remember that naloxone has a short duration of action (about 20–30 minutes), so repeated dosing of naloxone may be necessary to prevent recurrent respiratory depression.[5]

## PRESCRIPTION DRUG MONITORING PROGRAMS

Prescription drug monitoring programs (PDMPs) are important tools that can decrease the risk of opioid overdose or misuse by identifying patients who have recently received opioid prescriptions from other providers, have previously reported lost prescriptions, or have had previous overdose events. Providers prescribing opioids for any reason should review the patient's profile on their state's PDMP before sending the prescription.

## IMPLICATIONS FOR ANESTHESIA

### PREOPERATIVE

Identify patients taking medications for OUD. Develop a patient-specific plan for pain control while minimizing the risk of relapse or overdose. For non-urgent surgeries, oral naltrexone should be stopped 1 week prior to surgery and the surgery should be at least 4 weeks after the last dose of intramuscular naltrexone (Vivitrol®).[3-5] Buprenorphine may be held, reduced, or continued in the days leading up to surgery. The appropriate plan must be individualized and depends on the patient's risk of relapse, the dose of buprenorphine being used, and the amount of pain expected after the surgery.[3-5] Methadone should be continued throughout the preoperative period.[3-5]

### INTRAOPERATIVE

Patients with residual naltrexone or buprenorphine activity at the time of surgery may have significantly higher opioid dose requirements to attain adequate analgesia.[3,4] Consider use of nonopioid agents such as ketamine and/or plan for using higher doses of opioids intraoperatively. Methadone will not impede the effect of other opioids used intraoperatively, but patients taking methadone may be profoundly opioid tolerant and therefore may also require higher doses of opioid analgesics or benefit from nonopioid agents. Methadone also causes significant QTc prolongation, which can lead to torsade de pointes.[5] Monitor the patient's heart rhythm during surgery, avoid other QTc-prolonging agents if possible, and maintain high-normal serum levels of potassium and magnesium.

### POSTOPERATIVE

Naltrexone should not be restarted until the patient has been opioid free for at least 1 week.[3-5] If complete clearance of opioids is uncertain, a test dose of naloxone (e.g., 0.1 mg) may be given; if no withdrawal symptoms are induced, naltrexone may safely be restarted. If the naloxone does cause withdrawal, it at least will be short-lived, and the patient should wait several more days before using naltrexone.[5] Patients initially requiring high doses of opioids due to residual naltrexone or buprenorphine will become gradually more sensitive to opioids as the naltrexone or buprenorphine wears off. Avoid scheduled or long-acting opioids and ensure standard doses of opioid analgesics remain available to the patient. For example, order oxycodone 5–20 mg every 3 hours as needed rather than 15–20 mg every 3 hours as needed. Patients who have been weaned off methadone during a hospital stay must *not* be instructed to resume their usual methadone dose at discharge as this carries a high risk of overdose. The patient should work with their OTP to retitrate the dose. Under no circumstances can methadone be prescribed for OUD at hospital discharge; ensure the patient will be able to present to their OTP in a reasonable time frame after discharge.[2] Keep in mind that OTPs may have limited weekend hours. Prevent opioid overdose for all patients by prescribing naloxone and limiting prescriptions for opioids.

## REFERENCES

1. Ahmad FB, et al. Provisional drug overdose death counts. National Center for Health Statistics. 2020. https://www.cdc.gov/nchs/nvss/vsrr/drug-overdose-data.htm
2. Medication Assisted Treatment. Substance Abuse and Mental Health Services Administration, United States Department of Health and Human Services. https://www.samhsa.gov/medication-assisted-treatment
3. Bryson EO. The perioperative management of patients maintained on medications used to manage opioid addiction. *Curr Opin Anaesthesiol*. 2014;27(3):359–364.
4. Shah S, et al. Analgesic management of acute pain in the opioid-tolerant patient. *Curr Opin Anaesthesiol*. 2015;28(4):398–402.
5. Lexicomp. Wolters Kluwer; 2020. Accessed August 23, 2020. http://online.lexi.com

# 53.

# SYMPATHETIC NERVOUS SYSTEM
## ANATOMY, DRUGS, RECEPTORS, AND TRANSMITTERS

*Shelley George*

## ANATOMY

The preganglionic myelinated nerves of the sympathetic nervous system originate from cell bodies in the gray matter of the lateral horn of the spinal cord. The nerves then travel in three main routes: the sympathetic ganglia or sweat glands, the adrenal medulla, or the prevertebral ganglia.

1. The preganglionic fiber may travel to the ganglia, which lie in the sympathetic chain, and then continues to travel from the ganglia through the postganglionic fiber to the target organ. The postganglionic fibers are unmyelinated, long, and travel far throughout the body.[1]
2. The nerve impulse may travel a second path directly to the adrenal medulla. Preganglionic fibers that leave the central nervous system (CNS) and travel directly to the adrenal medulla and release ACh (nicotinic). The adrenal medulla then releases norepinephrine and epinephrine from the chromaffin cells.[1]
3. A third pathway that the impulse may travel is to synapse with unpaired prevertebral ganglia, such as the celiac and superior and inferior mesenteric ganglia.[1]
   a. Nerve fibers that follow the first pathway are able to travel directly to the closest ganglia or cephalad or caudad to higher or lower ganglia in the sympathetic chain. From the ganglia, the unmyelinated postganglionic fibers travel to the effector organ.
   b. Other unmyelinated postganglionic nerve fibers travel from the ganglion to the sweat glands. The neurotransmitter released is acetylcholine (ACh), which activates muscarinic cholinergic receptors.

## NEUROTRANSMITTERS

Acetylcholine is the neurotransmitter that is released from all preganglionic sympathetic fibers. It activates nicotine cholinergic receptors in the sympathetic ganglion and adrenal medulla. The neurotransmitters released from the postganglionic fibers include norepinephrine (NE), epinephrine (Epi), and dopamine (DA), and these fibers act on adrenergic receptors, although NE is more extensively released and understood.[1,2]

### SYNTHESIS OF NOREPINEPHRINE

Norepinephrine is synthesized in the postganglionic nerve terminal. First, tyrosine is transported to the axoplasm and converted to dopa. Cytoplasmic enzymes then convert dopa to DA, which subsequently travels to storage vesicles. In the storage vesicles, DA is converted to NE. NE is finally released when intracellular calcium increases after an action potential is received at the nerve terminal. The action of NE is terminated in two ways:

1. Active reuptake into the presynaptic terminal (primary)[1,2]
2. Metabolism by monoamine oxidase or catechol-O-methyl-transferase after reuptake into neuronal cells[1,2]

## RECEPTORS

The NE, Epi, and DA bind to adrenergic receptors on the target organ and blood vessels. These adrenergic receptors are classified according to their response to the neurotransmitter and include α, β, and dopaminergic. The dopaminergic receptors are only activated by dopamine.

These classes are further broken down into subtypes which help decipher their action: 1, $\alpha_2$, $\beta_{1,2,3}$, and $DA_{1,2}$.

## Table 53.1 COMMON ACTIONS ASSOCIATED WITH EACH RECEPTOR

| TARGET ORGAN | RECEPTOR ON ORGAN | ACTION |
|---|---|---|
| CNS | $\alpha_2$ | Sedation |
| Eyes | $\alpha_1$ | Mydriasis |
| Lungs | $\alpha_1$ | Bronchoconstriction |
| | $\beta_2$ | Bronchodilation |
| Heart | $\alpha_1$ | Decreased heart rate and contractility |
| | $\beta_1$ | |
| | $DA_1$ | Increased heart rate, conduction, and contractility Vasodilation |
| Blood vessels | $\alpha_1$ | Vasoconstriction (leads to increased peripheral vascular resistance, afterload, and blood pressure) |
| | $\beta_2$ | Vasodilation |
| Gut | $\alpha_1$ | Sphincter contraction |
| | $\beta_2$ | Relaxation |
| | $DA_1$ | Vasodilation |
| Genitourinary | $\alpha_1$ | Sphincter contraction |
| | $\beta_2$ | Bladder relaxation |
| | $\beta_3$ | Bladder relaxation |
| | $DA_1$ | Vasodilation |
| Uterus | $\alpha_1$ | Contraction |
| | $\beta_2$ | Relaxation |
| Smooth muscle | $\alpha_2$ | Vasoconstriction |
| | $\beta_2$ | Relaxation |
| Fat | $\alpha_1$ | Inhibits lipolysis |
| | $\beta_3$ | Lipolysis |
| Pancreas | $\alpha_1$ | Inhibits insulin secretion |
| | $\beta_2$ | Insulin secretion |
| Liver | $\beta_2$ | Gluconeogenesis and Glycogenolysis |

The adrenergic receptors are coupled with G proteins that either stimulate or inhibit adenylyl cyclase to increase or decrease cyclic adenosine monophosphate. Each receptor then generates a specific function in the target organ. Often α- and β-receptors will work opposite each other (Table 53.1).

If the $\alpha_2$-receptors are located presynaptically, it inhibits adenylyl cyclase and intracellular calcium, creating a negative-feedback loop.

The $\beta_2$-receptors activate the uptake of potassium into the cells.

**Agonists:** Compounds that bind the receptor to produce its action are called agonists (Table 53.2).[1,2]

## Table 53.2 COMMON AGONISTS AND THE RECEPTORS THEY ACTIVATE[A]

| AGONIST | RECEPTOR EFFECT |
|---|---|
| Phenylephrine | Marked $\alpha_1 > \alpha_2$ |
| Clonidine | Moderate $\alpha_2 > \alpha_1$ |
| Dexmedetomidine | Marked $\alpha_2 > \alpha_1$ ($\alpha_2$ effect greater than clonidine) |
| Norepinephrine | $\alpha_1 = \alpha_2 = \beta_1$ (all moderate) |
| Dobutamine | Marked $\beta_1$ |
| Epinephrine | Marked $\beta_1 > \beta_2 = \alpha_1 = \alpha_2$ |
| Ephedrine (indirect acting) | $\alpha_1 = \beta_1 > \beta_2$ |
| Terbutaline | Marked $_2$ |
| Dopamine | Marked $DA_1 = DA_2 > \alpha_1 = \alpha_2 = \beta_1 > \beta_2$ |
| Fenoldapam | Marked $DA_1$ |

[A]Agonists do not activate each receptor equally.[2]

**Antagonists:** Substances that bind the receptor to inhibit their action are considered agonists (Table 53.3).[1,2]

# ANESTHETIC CONSIDERATIONS FOR AUTONOMIC NEUROPATHY/DYSFUNCTION

## PREOPERATIVELY

Look for signs and symptoms preoperatively, such as postural hypotension, resting tachycardia, gastroparesis, erectile dysfunction, or urinary incontinence.[3]

## Table 53.3 COMMON ANTAGONISTS AND THE RECEPTORS THEY INHIBIT

| RECEPTOR | ANTAGONIST |
|---|---|
| $\alpha_1$ and $\alpha_2$ | Phenoxybenzamine ($\alpha_1 > \alpha_2$; irreversible) Phentolamine (reversible) Tolazoline |
| $\alpha_1$ | Prazosin Terazosin, doxazosin, trimazosin |
| $\alpha_2$ | Yohimbine |
| $\beta_1$ and $\beta_2$ | Propranolol, carvedilol timolol, nadolol, pindolol sotalol, labetalol ($\beta_1 = \beta_2$) Labetalol and carvedilol (also $\alpha_1$ antagonist) |
| $\beta_1$ | Metoprolol, atenolol, esmolol, acebutolol |

A patient should be monitored closely intraoperatively especially if he or she has resting tachycardia or prolonged QTc on the electrocardiogram (ECG). The patient may have a larger decrease in heart rate and blood pressure than normally seen in patients without autonomic dysfunction and may require high doses of vasopressor on induction. Volatile anesthetics will cause severe hypotension due to loss of compensatory mechanisms. Positive pressure ventilation can decrease cardiac output and worsen hypotension.

An invasive arterial line or central line may be necessary to monitor the patient.

This patient is more susceptible to severe intraoperative hypothermia, and the practitioner must be vigilant in monitoring the temperature.

Neuraxial anesthesia can cause such severe hypotension that may be associated with cardiac or cerebral injury.

Postoperatively, the patient should be placed on supplemental oxygen as they are prone to silent myocardial infarctions, and supplemental medications may be needed to augment blood pressure and heart rate in the postanesthesia care unit. A five-lead ECG should be monitored closely for changes, and a 12-lead ECG should be monitored if the vitals are unstable.

## REFERENCES

1. Grecu L. The autonomic nervous system anatomy and physiology. In: Barash G, et al., eds. Clinical Anesthesia. 7th ed. Philadelphia, PA: Lippincott Williams & Wilkins; 2017:333–360.
2. Butterworth JF IV, et al., eds. *Morgan & Mikhail's Clinical Anesthesiology*. 6th ed. McGraw-Hill; 2018.
3. Bankenahally R, Krovvidi H. Autonomic nervous system: anatomy, physiology, and relevance in anaesthesia and critical care medicine. *BJA Educ.* 2016;16(11):381–387.

# 54.

# PARASYMPATHETIC NERVOUS SYSTEM
## ANATOMY, TRANSMITTERS, RECEPTORS, DRUGS

*Maria E. Munoz-Allen*

## PARASYMPATHETIC NERVOUS SYSTEM ANATOMY

The parasympathetic nervous system (PSNS) arises from cranial nerves III (midbrain), VII, IX, and X (medulla oblongata) and from sacral segments of the spinal cord.[1] The ganglia of the PSNS are located very near or within the innervated organ, which makes its responses more focused and less widespread and robust.[1]

*Acetylcholine* is the neurotransmitter (pre- and postsynaptic) for the PSNS.[2]

### ACTIONS

**Eye:** Fibers from the Edinger-Westphal nucleus of the oculomotor nerve course in the midbrain to synapse in the ciliary ganglion. This causes miosis by contraction of the iris sphincter and contraction of the ciliary muscle for near vision.

**Salivary Glands:** Fibers from the lacrimatory nucleus to the facial nerve synapse to the ganglia of the submaxillary or sublingual glands and the sphenopalatine ganglion. Fibers from the glossopharyngeal nerve synapse in the otic ganglion. The postganglionic fibers innervate the mucous, salivary, and lacrimal glands. The vagus nerve is the most important of the parasympathetic (PS) nerves. The preganglionic fibers are long, and as with the other PS nerves do not synapse until they arrive at small ganglia at the thoracic or abdominal viscera. The PS nerves synapse have a 1:1 ratio of nerve to effector cell; however, the vagal innervation of the Auerbach plexus may connect 1 nerve fiber to 8000 cells.

**Heart:** Decrease heart rate, decrease conduction velocity, and decrease contraction.

**Lungs:** Bronchial constriction, increase secretions.

**Stomach, Small Intestine, Proximal Colon:** Increase tone and motility; increase secretions, nausea, and vomiting.

**Pancreas:** Increase insulin secretion.

**Sacral Segment:** S2-S4; pelvic splanchnic nerves synapse in terminal ganglia at the rectum and genitourinary organs.

**Bladder:** Sphincter relaxation, detrusor contraction.

**Bowel:** Fecal incontinence.

The overall response of the PSNS stimulation is more localized than the sympathetic reaction. Activation of the PS system helps to conserve energy and maintain organ function essential for maintenance of life.[1]

## TRANSMITTERS: ACETYLCHOLINE

Acetylcholine (ACh) is the neurotransmitter for the PSNS, part of the sympathetic nervous system, some neurons in the central nervous system (CNS), and somatic nerves innervating skeletal muscle.

Acetylcholine is not recycled but constantly synthesized in the presynaptic terminal by acetylation of choline by acetyl coenzyme A in a process catalyzed by choline acetyltransferase. ACh is quickly hydrolyzed by plasma cholinesterases found in neurons at the neuromuscular junction.

## RECEPTORS

*Cholinergic receptors* are subdivided into two major subgroups based on the affinity for the alkaloids nicotine and muscarine.

**Nicotinic receptors:** Nicotine stimulates the autonomic ganglia and skeletal muscle receptors.

**Muscarinic receptors:** Muscarine activates end-organ effector cells in bronchial smooth muscle, salivary glands, and the sinoatrial node.

Acetylcholine stimulates both subgroups of receptors.

**Agonist of acetylcholine receptors:** One of the few agonists in use, carbachol (topical or intraocular) constricts the pupil for long-term treatment of wide-angle glaucoma. It is better tolerated than the ophthalmic anticholinesterase agents.

## MUSCARINIC ANTAGONISTS: ANTICHOLINERGIC

Muscarinic antagonists (anticholinergics) compete with ACh for access to receptors and antagonize muscarinic agonists, including at noninnervated muscarinic receptors.[2] They may enhance sympathetic activity.

## DRUGS

**Atropine:** This is a tertiary amine that crosses the blood-brain barrier (BBB) and causes CNS stimulation; it has a mild antisialagogue effect and causes a moderate increase in heart rate (HR). It has a short duration. The adult dose is 0.5 mg to a maximum of 3 mg; at a very small dose (less than 0.4 mg) it may cause paradoxical bradycardia.

**Glycopyrrolate:** This is a quaternary amine that does not cross the BBB, does not have CNS effects, has a moderate antisialagogue effect, and causes a mild increase in HR. It has a long duration; intramuscularly it is a better antisialagogue and has a negligent cardiovascular effect.

**Scopolamine:** This is a tertiary amine that crosses the BBB, impairs memory, and has sedative effects; it has no effect to a mild effect on HR. It has a short duration. It can be clinically useful in trauma cases when anesthetic agents are relatively contraindicated due to hypotension. It is also used for prevention of motion sickness.

**Cholinesterase inhibitors:** The cholinesterase inhibitors produce sustained systemic cholinergic agonism by preventing the breakdown of ACh, thus increasing its availability at the synaptic cleft. They are used in the treatment of certain arrhythmias and myasthenia gravis and to reverse neuromuscular blockade.

**Neostigmine:** Neostigmine is a carbamate; it does not cross the BBB. The maximum dose is 0.08 mg/kg, up to 5 mg in adults. The effects are apparent in 5–10 minutes and last over an hour. Full recovery depends on the nondepolarizing agent used and the intensity of the blockade. Pediatric and elderly patients may be more sensitive to its effects.

When reversing nondepolarizing muscle relaxants, concomitant administration of anticholinergic agents minimizes muscarinic side effects.

Glycopyrrolate 0.2 mg per 1 mg of neostigmine has a similar time of onset and is preferred to 0.4 mg atropine per 1 mg of neostigmine, which results in more tachycardia.

Neostigmine may cross the placenta and cause fetal bradycardia. Atropine should be used in this scenario.

**Pyridostigmine:** Pyridostigmine is a carbamate similar to neostigmine with an onset of action of 10–15 minutes and a longer duration of about 2 hours. Administration should include glycopyrrolate 0.05 mg per 1 mg pyridostigmine or atropine 0.1 mg per 1 mg of pyridostigmine to prevent bradycardia. Glycopyrrolate is preferred over atropine.

**Edrophonium:** Edrophonium lacks a carbamate group

and has limited liposolubility due to a quaternary ammonium group. Edrophonium has the fastest onset of action and the shortest duration; it is much less potent than neostigmine. The dose is 0.5–1 mg/kg. It should be paired with atropine to prevent bradycardia, with 0.014 mg of atropine per 1 mg of edrophonium. If glycopyrrolate is used, it should be given several minutes prior to edrophonium: 0.007 mg of glycopyrrolate per 1 mg of edrophonium.

**Physostigmine:** Physostigmine is a tertiary amine with a carbamate group; it is lipid soluble and crosses the BBB. The CNS penetration limits its use as a reversal agent but makes it useful for the treatment of central anticholinergic toxicity caused by atropine or scopolamine. It may be effective at a dose of 0.04 mg/kg in preventing postoperative shivering.

At recommended doses, it is unlikely to cause bradycardia but atropine or glycopyrrolate should be available. Glycopyrrolate will not reverse CNS effects. Physostigmine is completely metabolized by plasma esterases, so renal excretion is not a consideration.

## REFERENCES

1  Glick D. The autonomic nervous system. In: Miller R, ed. *Miller's Anesthesia.* 7th ed. Philadelphia, PA: Elsevier, Churchill, Livingstone; 2010:261–298.
2  Cholinesterase inhibitors. In: Butterworth JF IV, et al., eds. *Morgan & Mikhail's Clinical Anesthesiology.* 6th ed. McGraw-Hill; 2016:221–227.
3  Grecu L. Central and autonomic nervous system. In: Barash G, et al., eds. *Clinical Anesthesia Fundamentals.* Wolters Kluwer; 2015:72–80.

# Part 7

# CENTRAL NERVOUS SYSTEM

# 55.

# ANATOMY OF THE NERVOUS SYSTEM

*Timothy Cutler and Sherif Zaky*

## INTRODUCTION

Nociception, from the Latin "noci" (harm or injury), is the neural response to a noxious stimulus. This cascade ends in one experiencing pain, which the International Association for the Study of Pain defines as "an unpleasant sensory and emotional experience associated with actual or potential tissue damage." The normal physiology of nociception involves a series of three neurons, which perform four processes: transduction, transmission, modulation, and perception.

## TRANSDUCTION

During transduction, sensory nerve endings transform potentially harmful stimuli into electrical activity. The afferent fibers that sense thermal, mechanical, and chemical tissue damage are called nociceptors. Nociceptors are mostly the free endings of Aδ and C fibers and are responsible for pain transduction. There are also specialized nociceptive

structures like Pacinian corpuscles, which play a lesser role. Peripheral nerve fibers are classified based on myelination, diameter, and rate of conduction (Table 55.1).

There are several types of nociceptors, which respond to different stimuli, including *mechanoreceptors* (pinches or pricks), *silent nociceptors* (inflammation), and *polymodal nociceptors* (excessive temperature, pressure, and pain-producing alogens). Alogens are produced by tissue damage and include substance P, bradykinin, histamine, serotonin, $H^+$, $K^+$, prostaglandins, and adenosine triphosphate (ATP).[1] Polymodal mechano-heat nociceptors are the dominant type of nociceptors.

## TRANSMISSION

After nociceptor activation, three neurons communicate in series to transmit a peripheral signal to the cerebral cortex. These neurons communicate via synapses where neurotransmitters provide inhibitory or excitatory signals from one neuron to another. These neurotransmitters often work in combination

*Table 55.1* CLASSIFICATION OF PERIPHERAL NERVE FIBERS

| FIBER GROUP | MYELINATION | DIAMETER (MM) | CONDUCTION | FUNCTION |
| --- | --- | --- | --- | --- |
| Aα | Yes | 12–20 | 70–120 | - Motor nerves<br>- Proprioception |
| Aß | Yes | 5–12 | 30–70 | - Light touch<br>- Pressure |
| Aγ | Yes | 3–6 | 15–30 | - Skeletal muscle tone<br>- Proprioception |
| Aδ | Yes | 2–5 | 12–30 | - Fast pain<br>- Touch<br>- Temperature |
| B | Yes | <3 | 3–15 | - Preganglionic autonomic fibers |
| C | No | 0.5–1.5 | 0.5–2.6 | - Slow pain<br>- Touch<br>- Temperature<br>- Postganglionic autonomic fibers |

**Table 55.2  MAJOR NEUROTRANSMITTERS INVOLVED IN PAIN PATHWAY**

| EXCITATORY NEUROTRANSMITTERS | RECEPTOR | INHIBITORY NEUROTRANSMITTERS | RECEPTOR |
| --- | --- | --- | --- |
| Glutamate | NMDA, AMPA, kainate | GABA | $GABA_A$, $GABA_B$ |
| Aspartate | NMDA, AMPA, kainate | Glycine | Glycine |
| Substance P | $NK_1$ | Serotonin | $5\text{-}HT_1$ ($5\text{-}HT_3$) |
| Adenosine triphosphate | $P_1$, $P_2$ | Norepinephrine | $\alpha_2$ |
| CGRP | | ß-Endorphins | $\mu$, $\delta$, K |
| Vasoactive intestinal peptide | | Enkephalins | $\mu$, $\delta$, K |
| Cholecystokinin | | Acetylcholine | Muscarinic |

AMPA, α-amino-3-hydroxy-5-methyl-4-isoxazole propionic acid; GABA, γ-aminobutyric acid; NK, neuromedin K; NMDA, N-methyl-D-aspartate.

to create complex signaling (Table 55.2). Substance P and calcitonin gene–related peptides (CGRP) are the most important neurotransmitters involved. Specifically, substance P functions to excite interneurons and second-order neurons while also sensitizing nociceptors, stimulating mast cell degranulation, and prompting serotonin release from platelets. Further, its vasodilatory effects aid in leukocyte chemotaxis and production of inflammation.

## FIRST-ORDER NEURONS

Located in the dorsal root ganglia, a first-order neuron has a single axon that bifurcates to both innervate peripheral tissues and synapse with a second-order neuron in the dorsal horn. Afferent fibers segregate in the spinal cord into medial (large, myelinated) and lateral (small, unmyelinated) fibers. These afferent fibers often ascend several segments via the Lissauer tract before synapsing with a second-order neuron in the ipsilateral dorsal horn (Figure 55.1).[1]

## SECOND-ORDER NEURONS

The gray matter of the spinal cord is divided into 10 laminae. The dorsal horn is made of the first six laminae, and this is the site of all afferent neural activity, making it the principal site of pain modulation, with multiple ascending and descending pain pathways present. Nociceptive C fibers synapse with second-order neurons in laminae I and II, with some synapsing in lamina V. Aδ fibers also synapse with neurons in lamina I and V, with fewer synapsing in lamina X (Figure 55.2).[2]

Second-order neurons are either nociceptive-specific or wide-dynamic-range (WDR) neurons. WDR neurons are more prevalent and have a larger receptive-specific field than nociceptive-specific neurons. Nociceptive-specific neurons are silent at baseline, responding only when a noxious stimulus is detected. WDR neurons are more prevalent, have a larger receptive field, and also receive nonnoxious stimuli from Aß, Aδ, and C fibers.

## SPINOTHALAMIC TRACT

The spinothalamic tract (STT) is the major pain pathway. It is located in the anterolateral portion of the white matter of the spinal cord, but the cell bodies of the neurons that make up the STT are located in laminae I, V, and VII (Figure 55.3). These second-order neurons project their axons upward in the dorsal column several segments before crossing the midline to ascend the STT on the contralateral side. Second-order neurons then synapse with third-order neurons in the thalamus.

The STT is divided into lateral (neospinothalamic) and medial/ventral (palaeospinothalamic) tracts. The lateral portion communicates mostly with the ventral posterolateral nucleus of the thalamus and transmits discriminatory information like location and intensity of pain, whereas the medial portion communicates with the medial thalamus and is responsible for the autonomic or unpleasant emotion perception of pain.[3]

## ALTERNATE PAIN PATHWAYS

While the STT is the main pain pathway of the spinal cord, there are alternative pathways hat play a lesser but important role in transmission of pain (Figure 55.3).

- *Spinoreticular tract:* Mediates arousal and autonomic response to pain.

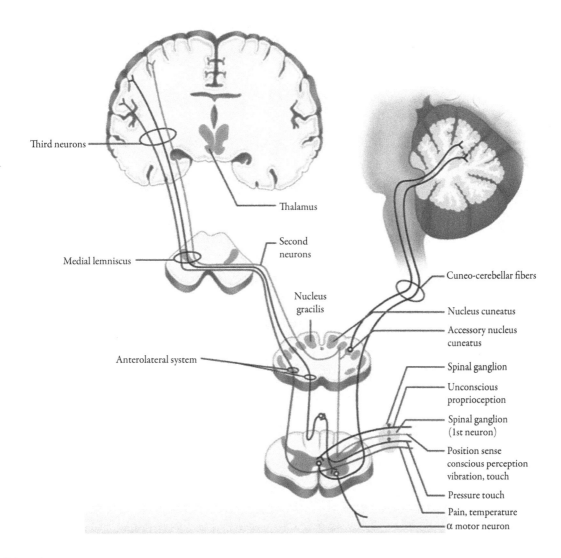

Figure 55.1 Pain pathways.

Third neurons

Thalamus

Medial lemniscus

Second neurons

Nucleus gracilis

Anterolateral system

Cuneo-cerebellar fibers

Nucleus cuneatus

Accessory nucleus cuneatus

Spinal ganglion

Unconscious proprioception

Spinal ganglion (1st neuron)

Position sense conscious perception vibration, touch

Pressure touch

Pain, temperature

α motor neuron

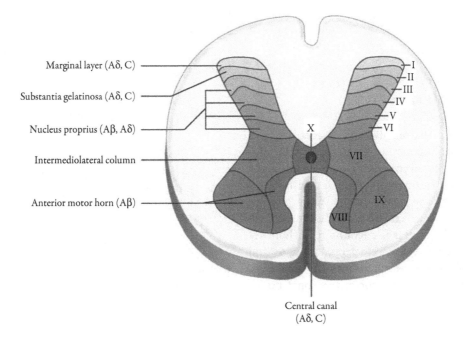

Figure 55.2 Rexed laminae of spinal cord.

Marginal layer (Aδ, C)

Substantia gelatinosa (Aδ, C)

Nucleus proprius (Aβ, Aδ)

Intermediolateral column

Anterior motor horn (Aβ)

I
II
III
IV
V
VI
X
VII
IX
VIII

Central canal (Aδ, C)

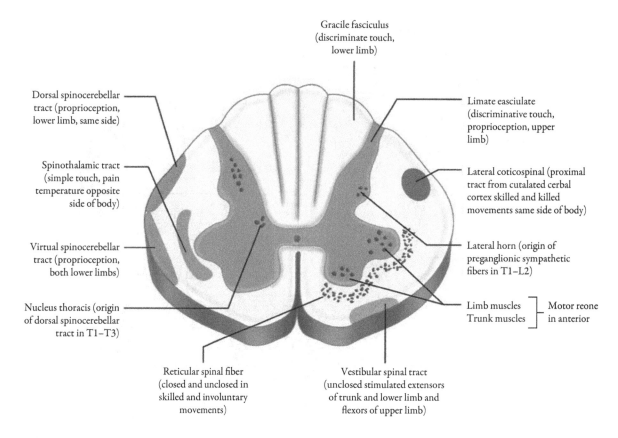

**Figure 55.3** Spinothalamic tract and other pain pathways.

- *Spinomesencephalic tract:* Activates descending antinociceptive pathways via periaqueductal gray matter.
- *Spinohypothalamic and spinotelencephalic tracts:* Activate hypothalamus to elicit emotional behavior.
- *Spinocervical:* Ascends ipsilaterally to the lateral cervical nucleus, which transmits signal to the contralateral thalamus.

## SYMPATHETIC AND MOTOR INTEGRATION

Afferent activity from the somatic and visceral nervous systems functions in conjunction with the skeletal and sympathetic systems in several locations, including the spinal cord and brain. In the spinal cord, motor neurons from the dorsal horn synapse directly with afferent neurons and provide a mechanism for reflex muscle activity when a painful stimulus is encountered. There are also synapses between nociceptive afferent neurons and neurons in the intermediolateral column (sympathetic system) that reflexively control vasoconstriction, smooth muscle contraction, and catecholamine release (local and medullary).[4]

## THIRD-ORDER NEURONS

Located in the thalamus, third-order neurons transmit signals through the internal capsule into the somatosensory areas in the post–central gyrus and also through the corona radiata into the superior sylvian fissure.

## REFERENCES

1. Katz N, Ferrante FM. Nociception. In: Ferrante FM, Vaded Boncouer TR, eds. *Postoperative Pain Management.* 1st ed. New York, NY: Churchill Livingstone; 1993: Chap. 2, 74.
2. Bonica JJ. Anatomic and physiologic basis of nociception and pain. In: Bonica JJ, ed. *The Management of Pain.* 2nd ed. Philadelphia, PA: Lea and Febiger; 1990:128.
3. Fields HL. Central nervous system mechanisms for control of pain transmission. In: Fields HL, ed. Pain. New York, NY: McGraw-Hill; 1987:99.
4. Warfield CA. *Principles and Practice of Pain Management.* New York, NY: McGraw-Hill; 1993:315.

# 56.

# NEUROLOGICAL DISORDERS

*Maryam Jowza and Dominika James*

## INTRODUCTION

Neurological diseases are a heterogeneous group of disorders with varying etiologies. In this chapter, we focus on the specific congenital and neurodegenerative disorders listed in Table 56.1 and explore anesthetic implications of each.

## TUBEROUS SCLEROSIS

Tuberous sclerosis (TS) is an autosomal dominant disease whose features include mental retardation, seizures, and facial angiofibroma. The key pathology of this disorder is growth of benign hamartomatous lesions and malformations in organs.[1,2] Affected organs include the brain (cortical tubers, giant cell astrocytoma); heart (cardiac rhabdomyosarcoma); and kidneys (angiomyolipoma). Patients may have nodular tumors in the oral cavity, including larynx. There is an association with Wolf-Parkinson-White (WPW) syndrome.[2]

### ANESTHETIC CONSIDERATIONS

#### Preoperative

Preoperatively, assess for affected organ systems with attention to the brain, heart, and kidney. Patients may present with seizure disorder or mental handicap. Further examination of the upper airway can yield abnormalities.

#### Intraoperative

Intraoperatively, response to anesthetics is not altered in patients with TS.

## NEUROFIBROMATOSIS

Neurofibromatosis (NF) is an autosomal dominant disorder with variable expression of mesodermal and ectodermal tissue.[1,3] It is further categorized into two subtypes based on clinical and genetic differences: NF type 1 and NF type 2. NF 1 is the more common subtype and is also known as von Recklinghausen disease. Differentiation of the two subtypes is beyond the scope of this chapter.

Neurofibromatosis, while variable in clinical features and severity, is progressive and can affect all systems. Clinical features include café-au-lait spots (flat areas of skin hyperpigmentation), which are present in most individuals. NF usually involves the skin but can occur in deeper structures, such as nerve roots, viscera, and blood vessels. While histologically benign, the presence of neurofibromas in specific tissues can cause functional changes and therefore pose a problem. For example, neurofibromas on nerve roots can cause pain and weakness, or neurofibromas around airway structures may cause airway compromise. A minority of patients with NF may also develop intracranial tumors, including acoustic neuromas, as well as spinal cord tumors. Kyphoscoliosis may appear later in life. Patients may also have intellectual delay and seizure disorder. Pheochromocytomas, albeit rare, occur with increase in frequency in patients with NF than the general population, with frequency estimated to be around 1%.[3]

### ANESTHETIC CONSIDERATIONS

#### Preoperative

Preoperative considerations revolve around clinical manifestations. For example, in patients with intracranial tumors, consideration for intracranial pressure is important. Airway examination should evaluate for airway patency. Cervical spine mobility should be assessed especially for patients with kyphoscoliosis. For patients with seizure disorder, antiepileptic drugs should be continued on the day of surgery.

#### Intraoperative

Intraoperatively, care should be taken with positioning as it relates to the cervical spine. Patients who have laryngeal neurofibromas may pose a special challenge for

*Table 56.1* SUMMARY OF NEUROLOGIC DISEASES COVERED IN THIS CHAPTER

| NEUROLOGIC CONDITION | PATHOGENESIS | SYMPTOMS SIGNS | TREATMENT | ANESTHETIC IMPLICATION |
|---|---|---|---|---|
| Tuberous Sclerosis | Autosomal Dominant | Seizures, mental retardation, angiofibromas, oral lesions | AED's, surgical removal of tumors | Difficult airway<br>Intraoperative seizure<br>Cardiac dysrhythmias (WPW Syndrome)<br>Impaired renal function |
| Neurofibromatosis | Autosomal Dominant | Café au lait spots, neurofibromas, seizures, intellectual handicap, kyphoscoliosis, CNS and spinal cord tumors, pheochromocytoma | AED's<br>Surgical removal<br>Scoliosis repair | Increased sensitivity to NMBD<br>Care with regional anesthesia |
| Parkinson's Disease | Dopaminergic fiber depletion in basal ganglia leading to enhanced extrapyramidal motor symptoms and exaggerated cholinergic activity | Rigidity, akinesia, resting tremor, shuffling gait, lack of facial expression, cognitive deficits, depression. | Dopamine replacement<br>Levodopa + carbidopa<br>Other<br>Amantadine<br>Selegiline (MAOI)<br>Anticholinergic drugs<br>Benztropine<br>Procyclidine<br>Trihexyphenid<br>Orphenadrine<br>Biperiden<br>Surgical<br>DBS | Hemodynamic instability<br>Dysrhythmias<br>Hypersensitivity to catecholamines (use direct vasopressors)<br>Must continue perioperative dopamine replacement to avoid muscle rigidity and ventilatory compromise, and risk of neuroleptic malignant like syndrome<br>Avoidance of:<br>-alfentanil (dystonic reaction)<br>- antidopaminergic medications: Droperidol, Haloperidol Metoclopromide Phenothiazines<br>Diphenhydramine, cyclizine and ondansetron are OK<br>If DBS in place avoid electrocautery |
| Alzheimer's Disease | Early onset (<60yo) genetic - autosomal dominant<br>Late onset (>60yo) degenerative | Cognitive impairment, apraxia, confusion, aphasia | Cholinesterase inhibitors<br>Donepezil<br>Rivastigmine<br>Galantamine<br>Memantine | Limitation of sedatives and hypnotics<br>Adequate pain control<br>Continuation of AD medications |

WPW, Wolf Parkinson White; AED, Antiepileptic Drugs; NMBD Neuromuscular Blocking Drugs; MAOI, Monoamine oxidase inhibitors; DBS, Deep Brain Stimulator; CSF, Cerebral Spinal Fluid; EMP, Evoked Motor Potentials; MRI, Magnetic Resonance Imaging.

intubation. Response to depolarizing muscle relaxants may be altered; some patients may display an increase in sensitivity, and others may demonstrate resistance. Response to nondepolarizing muscle relaxants can be exaggerated.

Regional anesthesia is not contraindicated, and successful and safe use of both peripheral nerve blocks and neuraxial anesthesia has been described.

## PARKINSON DISEASE

Parkinson disease (PD) is a neurodegenerative brain disorder of unknown etiology associated with degeneration and loss of dopaminergic neurons at the basal ganglia, leading to extrapyramidal symptoms. Clinically, patients can have muscle rigidity, akinesia, gait abnormality, and "pill-rolling" resting tremor.[1] Other manifestations include cognitive disorder leading to dementia, depression, swallowing difficulties, and ventilatory problems. Treatment focuses on replacement of dopamine and a decrease in the unopposed acetylcholine effects. Dopaminergic replacement is most often provided by administration of the dopamine precursor levodopa in combination with carbidopa to avoid peripheral conversion of levodopa to dopamine as this could lead to unintended elevation in heart rate and cardiac contractility. Anticholinergic medications used in treatment of mild PD antagonize unopposed acetylcholine effects at the level of basal ganglia. Other medications used for treatment of PD include the antiviral agent amantadine (unknown mode of action) and selegiline (monoamine oxidase inhibitor [MAOI] type B), which works by inhibiting breakdown of dopamine at the level of the central nervous system (CNS).[1,4]

## ANESTHETIC CONSIDERATION

### Preoperative

Missing dopaminergic medication perioperatively may lead to severe perioperative complications. Interruption of therapy for more than 6 hours can lead to an intraoperative increase in muscle rigidity and difficult ventilation, increased risk for aspiration, and overall increase in perioperative morbidity and mortality.

### Intraoperative

Therapeutic administration of dopamine, however, is not devoid of side effects. Levodopa is a dopamine precursor, so it may have systemic dopaminergic affects, leading to cardiac irritability and hemodynamic changes. Chronic depletion of catecholamine stores can lead to orthostatic hypotension. Direct-acting vasopressors are recommended for treatment of hypotension.[4]

To avoid external CNS conversion of levodopa to dopamine, levodopa is administered in combination with carbidopa (dopa carboxylase inhibitor). Levodopa may also be associated with preoperative nausea and vomiting, which in combination with PD-associated esophageal dysmotility, may lead to aspiration. MAOIs may be used in order to reduce dopamine degradation in the CNS. Nonselective MAOIs (except selegiline, which is selective MAOI B) may increase risk of intraoperative hypertensive crises, and concurrent use of certain anesthetic agents should be avoided in patients on nonselective MAOIs (meperidine, tramadol, tapentadol, methadone, pentazocine, methylene blue) as it can lead to serotonin toxicity. Alfentanil should also be avoided as it may lead to a severe dystonic reaction. Succinylcholine use is not contraindicated in PD.[4]

### Postoperative

The opioid medications listed above should be avoided in PD patients on MAOI therapy. While addressing postoperative nausea or delirium, medications with antidopaminergic properties should be avoided (droperidol, haloperidol, metoclopromide, phenothiazines). Ondansetron can be safely used. Postoperative treatment with dopaminergic medications should be continued in avoidance of rigidity and as such pulmonary complications (impaired ventilation, aspiration risk).

## ALZHEIMER DISEASE

Alzheimer disease (AD) is the most common cause of dementia (60%–80% of dementia cases) and the sixth leading cause of death in the United States. AD most often affects the elderly (>65 years old), but some patients may suffer an age-independent, genetically influenced, early-onset form of the disease.[1,5] AD is a chronic neurodegenerative disease characterized by progressive cognitive deficiencies associated with symptoms of memory loss, behavioral changes, aphasia (speech difficulties), agnosia (inability to recognize things), and apraxia (inability to perform purposeful movements/actions), which ultimately lead to impairment of daily life function. There is no cure for AD, but the symptoms may be modulated by use of anticholinesterase inhibitors (medications preventing synaptic acetylcholine degradation: donepezil, rivastigmine, galantamine) and memantine, which is involved in glutamate activity regulation. Acetylcholine and glutamate are the neurotransmitters involved in forming and processing memories, learning, as well as information retrieval and processing. Some of the associated side effects can include headache, dizziness, nausea, vomiting, anorexia, and change in bowel habits.[4]

## ANESTHETIC CONSIDERATION

### Preoperative

Anticholinergic medication should be continued preoperatively. Sedatives and hypnotics should be avoided.

### Intraoperative

Intraoperatively, patients with advanced stages of AD may suffer from significant confusion and may be poorly cooperative; however, patients who are able to participate may benefit from regional and neuraxial anesthesia. Regional anesthesia offers the benefit of decreasing the risk of anesthetic and sedative exposure postoperative delirium. Conversely, AD patients may find difficulty tolerating regional anesthesia, sedation, or monitored anesthesia care, necessitating implementation of a general anesthetic. Choice of anesthetic technique should thus be based on the patient's comorbidities and the degree of dementia. Caution should be taken when administering paralytics to patients on anticholinesterase inhibitors, as they may experience resistance to neuromuscular blocking drugs and prolongation of effects with succinylcholine.

## Postoperative

Postoperatively, focus should be placed on limiting exposure to sedative medications while formulating an adequate analgesic plan. Regional analgesia may be preferred when trying to restrict use of opioid analgesics. Nonpharmacological therapy, such as assurance of proper circadian cycle, frequent interactions with caregivers, and access to family members, is equally important to minimize delirium risk.

## REFERENCES

1. Pasternak JJ, Lanier WL. Diseases affecting the brain. In: Hines RL, Marschall KE, ed. *Stoelting's Anesthesia and Coexisting Disease*. 5th ed. Philadelphia, PA: Elsevier; 2008:199–237.
2. Lee JJ, et al. Anaesthesia and tuberous sclerosis. *Br J Anaesth*. 1994;73(3):421–425.
3. Hirsch NP, et al. Neurofibromatosis: clinical presentations and anesthetic implications. *Br J Anaesth*. 2001;86(4):555–564.
4. Brennan KA, Genever RW. Managing Parkinson's disease during surgery. *Br J Anaesth*. 2010;341:c5718.

# 57.

# MUSCULOSKELETAL SYSTEM

*Sarah Money and Rohit Aiyer*

## INTRODUCTION

The musculoskeletal system provides body structure, organ protection, hematopoiesis, and facilitation of movement. Muscle fibers can be classified as skeletal, cardiac, or smooth, and for purposes of this discussion, we focus on skeletal muscle. The musculoskeletal system is a core component of functional capacity, strength, and endurance. The communication circuit between the brain and skeletal muscle involves synaptic relays from the cerebral cortex, to interneurons within the thalamus, to the ventral horn of the spinal cord, along the motor neuron via a peripheral nerve, and finally to the skeletal muscle fiber. The motor neuron is a myelinated efferent nerve called an alpha ($\alpha$) motor neuron, transmitting signals at high speed to the skeletal muscle via the neuromuscular junction. This results in intentional movement. Alternatively, a myotactic or stretch reflex is a signal originating in a muscle, such as a knee jerk reflex, which then transmits in the afferent direction to the spinal cord. This then results in an efferent response back to the muscle without ascending to the brain.[1] A reflex, by definition, is unintentional and unconsciously mediated, and in a fully intact musculoskeletal system, both intentional movement and reflexes will be present. Musculoskeletal function depends on coordination of relaxed and active muscle tone to retain posture, balance, and movement. During muscle contraction, there is a transient rise in intracellular calcium with subsequent activation of actin and myosin. As the body grows older, changes occur in the musculoskeletal system, and this can manifest as decreased mobility and gait speed, slowed or absent reflexes, increased falls, increased rates of fractures, and hospitalizations.[2]

## NEUROMUSCULAR TRANSMISSION

Motor nerves innervate and control skeletal muscle. A motor unit is defined as a single motor neuron and all of the skeletal muscle fibers it innervates; when a motor unit fires a signal, the innervated muscle fibers contract. The ratio of motor neuron to skeletal muscle varies depending on the muscle function. For example, extraocular muscles requiring fine control have only a few muscle fibers to one motor neuron, while larger muscles may have thousands of muscle fibers innervated by a single motor neuron. A motor pool describes the group of motor neurons that innervate an entire muscle.

In order to contract, a muscle cell must be activated. Voluntary movements are dictated by the motor cortex, located in the frontal lobe. The premotor cortex and the supplementary motor cortex coordinate to generate a plan for movement, which is then executed by the primary motor cortex via descending pathways. Like the sensory cortex, the motor cortex is somatotopically organized in a motor homunculus, and each cerebral hemisphere controls the contralateral body.

The signal for movement travels from the motor cortex via descending motor pathways known as pyramidal and extrapyramidal tracts. Extrapyramidal tracts facilitate and inhibit muscle contraction in order to allow for balance and coordinated movement. The pyramidal tract consists of two distinct pathways: the corticobulbar and the corticospinal tracts. The corticobulbar, also known as the corticonuclear tract, carries efferent motor signals to the face, head, and neck, descending through the corona radiata to the brainstem, and terminating on the motor nuclei of cranial nerves (CNs; considered to be lower motor neurons) at the level of the midbrain, pons, and medulla. The motor component of the trigeminal nerve (CN V) innervates muscles of mastication; the motor component of the facial nerve (CN VII) innervates muscles of the upper and lower face; the glossopharyngeal nerve (CN IX) innervates muscles of the pharynx and larynx; and the spinal accessory nerve (CN XI) innervates the sternocleidomastoid and trapezius muscles.

The corticospinal tract conveys efferent motor signals through the spinal cord to muscles of the trunk and limbs. The signal descends from the motor cortex through the corona radiata to the medulla, where most of the fibers decussate and form the lateral corticospinal tract. The lateral spinothalamic tract descends down the spinal cord, where it synapses with lower motor neurons within gray matter in the anterior horn, exits the spine as ventral roots, which form peripheral nerves, and eventually innervates muscles of the upper and lower limbs.

Fibers that do not decussate in the medulla continue as the anterior corticospinal tract, descending to the spinal level of innervation, where they decussate and cross to the contralateral side to synapse on lower motor neurons in the anterior horn of the spinal cord. At this anatomical location these nerves exit the spine as the ventral root and form peripheral nerves to then innervate muscles of the trunk.[3]

Signal is propagated along nerves across synapses from the motor cortex to the neuromuscular junction, where acetylcholine (ACh) is released. Skeletal muscle cells are normally at rest and require depolarization via ACh receptor activation to initiate an action potential and muscle contraction. Once ACh is released, it is quickly degraded by acetylcholinesterases found in the synapse to allow for repolarization and subsequent repeat muscle contraction. The neuromuscular junction is exposed to the extracellular space, and while narrow (about 50 nm), it is the site of activity for agents used in neuromuscular blockade. Nondepolarizing muscle relaxants act at the neuromuscular junction by competitively inhibiting postsynaptic ACh receptors, thereby inhibiting muscle contraction. Succinylcholine binds to the postsynaptic ACh receptor to maintain continuous muscle depolarization and muscle paralysis.[4]

Muscles contract in an organized way, referred to as recruitment, or the size principle. This principle dictates that, initially, only a small amount of force is necessary and thus only a few muscle fibers are required. Therefore, small motor units innervating a few muscle fibers have the lowest threshold for activation, and these are recruited first during muscle contraction. However, as a task becomes more strenuous, more muscle fibers and force are needed, so larger motor units with a higher threshold of activation are recruited last. This system allows for the perfect amount of muscle recruitment and force for each task. However, as the body ages, this system begins to degrade. Sarcopenia (muscle loss) and osteopenia (bone loss) start at around age 30, but there is a sharp decline at age 60. This, combined with age-related hormonal changes, results in a decline in strength, endurance, function, and metabolism. Some of these changes can be overcome with exercise and conditioning.[5]

## REFERENCES

1. Karlet M. Musculoskeletal system anatomy, physiology, pathophysiology, and anesthesia management. *Nurse Anesth*. 36:760–781.e4.
2. Frontera W. Physiologic changes of the musculoskeletal system with aging: a brief review. *Phys Med Rehabil Clin N Am*. 2017;28:705–711.
3. Vanderah T. Overview of motor systems. In: *Nolte's Essentials of the Human Brain*. 2nd ed. Elsevier; 2010:118–123.
4. Brull S, Meistelman C. Pharmacology of neuromuscular blocking agents. In: *Miller's Anesthesia*. 27, 792–831.e8.
5. Bonewald L. Use it or lose it to age: a review of bone and muscle communication. *Bone*. 2019;120:212–218.

# 58.

# EPILEPSY

*Maryam Jowza and Dominika James*

## INTRODUCTION

Seizures are often related to other underlying conditions, such as trauma, tumor, or metabolic abnormality, with a 10% risk of lifetime occurrence.[1–3] In comparison, epilepsy is a congenital condition affecting approximately 1% of the population and involving recurrent seizure disorder. Epilepsy is most common at extremes of age and in those with structural brain abnormalities. Seizures can be classified as "focal" if the seizure arises from one hemisphere or "generalized" if the seizure arises from both hemispheres. Seizures are considered as "simple" when no loss of consciousness is involved and "complex" with loss of consciousness.[1]

Seizures can arise as a result of dysfunctional paroxysmal neuronal discharge resulting from dysregulation of neuronal circuits and imbalance between excitatory and inhibitory central nervous system (CNS) modulatory centers.[2] Although the precise mechanism leading to seizures is not known, seizures can be congenital, caused by structural CNS abnormality (tumor, scar), or associated with transient metabolic dysregulation, such as hypoglycemia, hyponatremia, medication toxicity or withdrawal (withdrawal of medications that inhibit neuronal transmission, e.g., as benzodiazepines or antiepileptic drugs [AEDs] may lead to unopposed neuronal excitation, leading to seizure).

## THERAPEUTIC OPTIONS

As epilepsy is thought to be due to an imbalance between excitatory and inhibitory neuronal activity, AEDs act by either increasing inhibitor neurotransmitter activity (γ-aminobutyric acid [GABA]), decreasing excitatory neurotransmitter activity (glutamate, aspartate) or reducing inward voltage-gated positive currents (sodium channels, calcium channels). Partial seizures are treated with carbamazepine, valproate, or phenytoin. For generalized seizures, medications such as barbiturates, gabapentin, or lamotrigine are used.[1] Phenytoin, barbiturates, and carbamazepine cause hepatic enzyme induction. AEDs are also associated with dose-dependent toxicity. Phenytoin may cause intraoperative hypotension and dysrhythmias, and valproate is associated with liver toxicity and increased bleeding).

Surgical options for treatment of refractory epilepsy include left vagal nerve stimulator implantation (right vagus nerve is not recommended due to significant cardiac innervation) or seizure site surgical resection (most often temporal lobectomy).[2]

The most favorite candidates for surgical resection are patients with complex partial seizures, unilateral temporal lobe focus, normal intelligence quotient, motivation, no diffuse brain damage, seizures that were uncontrolled by medications, and a seizure focus that is resectable without causing major neurologic damage.

Status epilepticus is defined as 30 minutes or more of continuous seizure activity without complete recovery or with incomplete recovery of consciousness.[3] This is a medical emergency as it can lead to cerebral damage and can be fatal. In the event of status epilepticus, one should secure the airway, ventilate the patient with oxygen, and monitor and support the cardiovascular function with establishment of intravascular access and administration of seizure-suppressing medications. Intubation should be performed using a short-acting muscle relaxant, such as succinylcholine or mivacurium, as continuous monitoring of tonic activity is essential for evaluating the efficacy of treatment. Use of thiopental or propofol is preferred over other sedatives due to their transient seizure-suppressing effects. Benzodiazepines remain the first-line therapy for status epilepticus, followed by fosphenytoin, levetiracetam, or valproate if the seizure is not resolved. Alternatively, use of intravenous phenobarbital may be considered.

## ANESTHETIC CONSIDERATIONS

Many of the antiepileptic medications tend to alter the pharmacokinetics and pharmacodynamics of anesthetic drugs by enzyme function alterations, such as enzyme induction or inhibition (Table 58.1). In turn, some anesthetic agents are known to affect the seizure threshold and may induce an intraoperative epileptic event. As such, these interactions

*Table 58.1* SUMMARY OF COMMONLY USED AEDS, SIDE EFFECTS, AND ANESTHETIC CONSIDERATIONS

| MEDICATION | SIDE EFFECTS | ANESTHETIC CONSIDERATIONS | ISOENZYME | EFFECT |
|---|---|---|---|---|
| Phenytoin | Gingival hyperplasia<br>Hirsutism<br>Aplastic anemia<br>SJS<br>D, C, S | Dysrhythmias<br>Hypotension | Induction CYP3A4<br>Induction CYP2C19 | Accelerated metabolism of benzodiazepines, buprenorphine, meperidine, methadone, and fentanyl<br>Resistance to NMBDs<br>Accelerated metabolism of diazepam |
| Fosphenytoin (better side-effect profile than phenytoin) | D, C, S | | No effect | |
| Valproic acid | Hepatic failure<br>Pancreatitis<br>D, C, S | Increased surgical bleeding<br>Thrombocytopenia | Induction CYP2C19<br>Inhibition CYP2D6 | Resistance to NMBDs<br>Accelerated metabolism of diazepam<br>Decreased methadone elimination |
| Carbamazepine | Diplopia<br>Agranulocytosis<br>SJS<br>D, C, S | Resistance to NMBDs<br>Hyponatremia | Induction CYP3A4<br>Induction CYP2C19 | Accelerated metabolism of benzodiazepines, buprenorphine, meperidine, methadone, and fentanyl<br>Resistance to NMBDs<br>Accelerated metabolism of diazepam |
| Oxycarbazepine | Hypersensitivity, rash<br>D, C, S | Hyponatremia | | |
| Phenobarbital | Withdrawal syndrome/ addiction<br>D, C, S | Hypotension (venous pooling and negative ionotropic effects)<br>CNS depression | Induction CYP3A4<br>Induction CYP2B6 | Accelerated metabolism of benzodiazepines, buprenorphine, meperidine, methadone, and fentanyl<br>Enhanced methadone metabolism |
| Lamotrigine | SJS, diplopia<br>Insomnia, D, C, S | | No effect | |
| Topiramate | Weight loss, nephrolithiasis<br>D, C, S | Renally excreted 65%<br>Metabolic acidosis | No effect | |
| Gabapentin | Weight gain, D, C, S | Renally excreted 100% | No effect | |
| Levetiracetam | D, C, S | Renally excreted 100% | No effect | |

C, confusion; D, dizziness; S-sedation; SJS, Stevens-Johnson syndrome.

must be taken into consideration when establishing the anesthetic plan.

## ANESTHETIC CONSIDERATION

### PREOPERATIVE

It is important to determine preoperatively if the patient has a known diagnosis of epilepsy or if they are experiencing new onset seizures. Those with a new onset of symptoms require an evaluation to determine the etiology of the seizures. As seizures can be caused by a variety of issues, including trauma, medication toxicity or withdrawal, fevers, tumors, or metabolic abnormalities, it is best that the presence of such conditions be determined prior to an anesthetic.[3] In the review of medical history, it is also important to determine the degree of control of seizures, triggers (fasting, sleep deprivation), and other comorbidities. The patient should continue to use anticonvulsants on the day of surgery.

### INTRAOPERATIVE

The main considerations intraoperatively when providing anesthetic care to patients with epilepsy include

- the ability of anesthetic agents to change (inhibit or potentiate) seizure activity; and
- the interaction of anesthetics with AEDs.

Therapeutics used to treat seizure disorder can have an impact on anesthetic agents in the perioperative period. Many of the agents can impact metabolism by the cytochrome P450 system, generally causing induction of the system, which leads to resistance to some anesthetics, opioids, and neuromuscular blockers. Table 58.1 is a summary of

**Table 58.2** PROCONVULSANT AND ANTICONVULSANT PROPERTIES OF ANESTHETICS

| MEDICATION | CONVULSANT/ ANTICONVULSANT? | NOTES |
|---|---|---|
| Benzodiazepines | Anticonvulsant | Potentiates GABA$_A$<br>Commonly used to treat acute seizures<br>First line in status epilepticus |
| Propofol | Anticonvulsant | Alternative to benzodiazepine in status epilepticus |
| Etomidate | Proconvulsant at usual dose, anticonvulsant at high dose | Avoid in epilepsy |
| Dexmedetomidine | No effect | |
| Barbiturates | Anticonvulsant | With exception of methohexital |
| Morphine | No effect when given intravenously | Reports of tonic/clonic movements when used epidurally, but safe intravenously |
| Fentanyl, alfentanil, remifentanil, sufentanil | Proconvulsant | Avoid high doses or rapid administration—reports of tonic/clonic movements |
| Nitrous oxide | No effect | Excitatory effects on central nervous system but does not induce seizures at doses used clinically |
| Halothane | Anticonvulsant | |
| Isoflurane | Anticonvulsant | |
| Desflurane | Anticonvulsant | Has been administered in the treatment of status asthmaticus |
| Sevoflurane | Dose dependent | Avoid > 1.5 MAC in epileptic patients and in the presence of hypocapnia |
| Ketamine | Proconvulsant | |
| Anticholinesterases | No effect | |
| Anticholinergics | No effect | |

NMBD, neuromuscular blocking drugs; MAC, minimal alveolar concentration.

Adapted from Bajwa SJ, Jindal R. Epilepsy and nonepilepsy surgery: Recent advancements in anesthesia management. *Anesth Essays Res*. 2013;7(1):10–17. doi:10.4103/0259-1162.1139

commonly used AEDs, their side effects and interactions with anesthetics, and their effect on enzymes.

Some anesthetic agents can have proconvulsant properties. For example, methohexital, alfentanil, and remifentanil can lower the seizure threshold. Agents such as benzodiazepines, propofol, and thiopental lower the seizure threshold. Table 58.2 summarizes medications and their known effects on seizures.

In order to avoid reduction of the seizure threshold intraoperatively, hypoxia, hypotension, hypocapnia, and hyponatremia should be avoided. Regional anesthesia can be employed safely in an epileptic patient.[4,5]

## POSTOPERATIVE

Patients should resume AED treatment as soon as possible postoperatively. If multiple doses may be missed, medications should be administered using either the oral route if possible or the intravenous route. Phenytoin, sodium valproate, and levetiracetam are available in intravenous form with oral and intravenous doses equivalent.[3] Patients with preexisting poorly controlled epilepsy are at highest risk for a seizure in the postoperative period and will require special attention and timely administration of AEDs.

## REFERENCES

1. Glauser T, et al. Evidence-based guideline: treatment of convulsive status epilepticus in children and adults: report of the Guideline Committee of the American Epilepsy Society. *Epilepsy Curr.* 2016;16(1):48–61.
2. Maranhão MV, et al. Epilepsy and anesthesia. *Rev Bras Anestesiol.* 2011;61(2):232–236.
3. Bajwa SJ, Jindal R. Epilepsy and nonepilepsy surgery: recent advancements in anesthesia management. *Anesth Essays Res.* 2013;7(1):10–17.
4. Perks A, et al. Anaesthesia and epilepsy. *Br J Anaesth.* 2012;108(4): 562–571.
5. Kofke WA. Anesthetic management of the patient with epilepsy or prior seizures. *Curr Opin Anaesthesiol.* 2010;23(3):391–399. doi:10.1097/ACO.0b013e328339250b

# 59.

# COMA
## DIAGNOSIS AND MANAGEMENT

*Hess Robertson and Philip G. Boysen*

## INTRODUCTION

Coma is defined as a state of profound unconsciousness caused by disease, injury, or poison. A medical description would also include a patient that cannot be awakened, fails to respond to painful stimuli (or light and sound), and does not initiate voluntary actions. The comatose patient also lacks a normal sleep-wake cycle. Interestingly, this definition would include patients under general anesthesia since the anesthetized, narcotized, and usually paralyzed patient falls within this scope.

There are two overriding principles that apply to the comatose patient.[1] The first is that coma is a true medical emergency, endorsed by the statement that "time is brain." The second principle follows from the first principle. Time management in this emergency situation does not allow for the usual sequence of history, physical examination, and laboratory test and imaging acquisition; diagnosis and management must be going on all at the same time, in parallel and not sequential fashion. Although a comatose patient cannot provide a history, emergency medical personnel, friends, and family might be available to give a history that points to cause.[2]

## DIFFERENTIAL DIAGNOSE OF COMA

Causes of coma can be categorized as follows:

- Neurological: involving a structural injury to the cerebral hemisphere or brainstem or compression of the brainstem from an extrinsic cause.
- Metabolic: caused by an acute metabolic or endocrine disorder (e.g. hypoglycemia)
- Diffuse physiological brain dysfunction due to intoxication with ethanol, drug overdose, seizure disorder, or hypothermia
- Psychiatric: meaning a functional rather than an organic cause; progression to this diagnosis only appropriate after other pathology has been ruled out[3]

The clinical examination of the unconscious includes response or nonresponse to verbal, tactile, and painful stimuli and whether or not the patient can follow simple commands. Assessment of cranial nerve function can be revealing. Pupillary examination can point to a specific cause. Small pupils (<2 mm) can be due to opioid intoxication or a pontine lesion. Midsize pupils (4–6 mm) that do not respond to light suggest a midbrain lesion. Dilated pupils (>8 mm) may be due to drugs (amphetamines or cocaine) or damage to the oculomotor nerve. A unilateral fixed pupil suggests damage to the third cranial nerve. Fundoscopy might reveal papilledema, seen in patients with hypertensive crisis or subarachnoid hemorrhage.

Generalized physical examination, especially the sense of smell of the examiner, can suggest hepatic encephalopathy, organophosphate poisoning, or ethanol (but be aware that this may be masking other injuries). Examine for injection sites, either subcutaneous or intravenous. Assess breathing pattern. Cheyne-Stokes breathing can occur with many underlying pathologies not related to the comatose state. Ataxic breathing, or Biot respiration, apnea interspersed with rapid shallow breathing, points to a pontine lesion. Central neurogenic hyperventilation, a rate of about 25 breaths per minute with very deep breaths points to a lesion in the pons or midbrain.[4]

A point-of-care glucose test should be done immediately. The serum urea nitrogen (BUN), calcium, liver function tests, coagulation profile (including thromboelastography if available), toxicology screen (acetaminophen and salicylates especially), electrocardiogram (ECG), chest x-ray (CXR), and arterial blood gas analysis (including a test for carbon monoxide) should follow as soon as possible. Urgent imaging of the brain is indicated and may show subarachnoid hemorrhage, subdural hematoma, ischemic stroke, tumor, or hydrocephalus, if present. Vasogenic edema bilaterally of the parietal-occipital lobes is associated with a reversible syndrome when blood pressure is controlled.

## AN ALGORITHM FOR INITIAL MANAGEMENT

There is an algorithm for initial management[5]:

- Assess airway, breathing, circulation (ABC); intubate the patient if apneic; immobilize the cervical spine in the trauma patient.
- Calculate the Glasgow Coma Score: Check blood glucose, treat hypoglycemia. Check pupil size and reactivity, treat with intravenous naloxone if opioid overdose is suspected.
- Take available history from bystanders while performing physical examination and while colleagues obtain blood specimens and order an ECG, CXR, urine for analysis, and arterial blood for analysis.
- Treat an evident cause for coma. There is a low threshold for computed tomographic (CT) scan of the head. Perform electroencephalography if there is suspicion of nonconvulsive status epilepticus with seizure activity in absence of motor signs.

- Initiate supportive therapy and specific therapy as indicated or suspected. Arrange for transfer to the intensive care unit as appropriate. Specific therapy is related to the diagnosis, including hypoglycemia, opioid toxicity (suspected or proven), benzodiazepine overdose, severe hyponatremia, hypercalcemia, and toxicity due to methanol, lithium, salicylate, or ethylene glycol. Hemodialysis may be indicated.
- If bacterial meningitis is suspected, begin empirical antibiotics and perform a lumbar puncture. If viral encephalitis is suspected, intravenous acyclovir should be given as soon as possible.

## PROGNOSIS OF COMA

Outcome and prognosis are determined by the underlying cause and rapidity of response to remediate the cause. Reversing a coma is more likely with an unremarkable brain CT and no focal neurologic findings on examination. Prolonged coma leads to a poor prognosis, but the early assessment of coma does not usually provide for an estimate of prognosis.

## GLASGOW COMA SCALE

| Eye opening | Movement | Verbal |
| --- | --- | --- |
| 4 spontaneous | 6 obeys commands | 5 oriented |
| 3 to speech | 5 localizes to pain | 4 confused |
| 2 to pain | 4 withdraws to pain | 3 inappropriate words |
| 1 none | 3 abnormal flexion + pain | 2 incomprehensible sounds |
| | 2 extensor response +pain | 1 none |
| | 1 – no response | |

The lowest score is 3 and is associated with poor prognosis, whatever the cause of coma.

Since the anesthetized, narcotized, and ventilated patient under anesthesia is essentially in an induced coma, the issues of monitoring, positioning, padding, and turning apply equally in a patient who presents in a comatose state.

## REFERENCES

1. Wijdicks EFM. Coma. *Pract Neurol.* 2010;10:51–60.
2. O'Callaghan P. Transient loss of consciousness. *Medicine.* 2012;40:427–430.
3. Horsting M, et al. The etiology and outcome of non-traumatic coma in critical care: a systematic review. *BMJ Anesthesiol.* 2015;15:65–74.
4. Edlow JA, et al. Diagnosis of reversible causes of coma. *Lancet.* 2014;384:2064–2076.
5. Cooksley T, Holland M. The unconscious patient. *Medicine.* 2013;41:146–160.

# 60.

# THERAPEUTIC BARBITURATE COMA

*Syed A. Rahman*

## INTRODUCTION

Neurons are particularly susceptible to ischemic injury, and pharmacological protection with appropriate monitoring may be employed to "rest" the brain before or during a regional disruption in nutrient flow.[1] Barbiturate coma is used for neuroprotection during focal cerebral ischemia and to treat intractable intracranial hypertension. Burst suppression with anesthetic agents (including barbiturates, propofol, and isoflurane) results in a large reduction in the cerebral metabolic rate of oxygen ($CMRO_2$) and hence their use in cases of brain ischemia and cerebrovascular surgery.[2]

## MECHANISM OF BURST SUPPRESSION EFFECT

Pharmacological agents used for burst suppression decrease the cerebral metabolic rate of oxygen significantly (about 50%), and this was thought to be the primary mechanism conferring neuroprotective benefit from periods of ischemia. Neuroprotective properties of anesthetic agents are now believed to result from various effects, including depression of cerebral metabolic rate and cerebral blood flow, antiseizure properties, and hypnotic activity. It is suggested that neuroprotective benefits may also be conferred by their antioxidant activity and γ-aminobutyric acid (GABA) ergic activity.[2] Maximum reductions in cerebral metabolism and cerebral blood flow occur with a burst suppression pattern on electroencephalography (EEG).[3]

Drug-induced inverse steal is another suggested mechanism that involves a reduction in cerebral metabolism, up to burst suppression, with agents that preserve flow-metabolism coupling, resulting in reduction of perfusion to well-perfused areas and a redistribution of blood flow to ischemic areas.[1]

## INDICATIONS

- Refractory status epilepticus.
- Intractable intracranial hypertension: Barbiturate coma could be used as a potential salvage therapy after failure of first-line therapies, including hyperventilation, head elevation, and osmotic therapy/diuretics. This includes patients with traumatic brain injury or intractable intracranial pressure (ICP) elevation following vascular procedures like arteriovenous malformation resection, extracranial-intracranial bypass, aneurysmorrhaphy, and significant bleeding due to ruptured aneurysms.[2,3]
- Procedures involving focal cerebral ischemia: Barbiturates have a neuroprotective role in procedures involving focal cerebral ischemia, but not global ischemia.[2] Barbiturates increase blood flow to ischemic areas of cortex and possibly reduce the size of cerebral infarction. This applies to neurosurgical procedures like carotid endarterectomy, cerebral aneurysm surgery with prolonged use of a temporary clip, cerebral bypass surgery with prolonged vascular clamping, or cardiac/aortic surgery with cerebral blood ischemia.

## ANESTHETIC AGENTS AND DOSING REGIMENS

Barbiturates, propofol, etomidate, and isoflurane have been used to achieve pharmacological burst suppression.

Optimal dosing is unknown, and there is a lack of high-quality evidence to guide drug therapy. A loading dose followed by a maintenance infusion is often used. Burst suppression on EEG is widely accepted as a standard endpoint for cerebral neuroprotection, and dosing regimens should utilize the lowest dose necessary to achieve EEG burst suppression.[2]

## BARBITURATES

Among the currently available anesthetic agents, barbiturates have the greatest potential neuroprotective benefit. These drugs are more effective when administered prior to the onset of an ischemic or pathological event. Barbiturates appear to be most effective in focal ischemia and not global ischemia. Pentobarbital and thiopental are the most used among barbiturates.

Pentobarbital has a half-life of about 30 hours and is often administered as a loading dose of 3–10 mg/kg followed by an intravenous (IV) infusion of 1–2 mg/kg/h to achieve burst suppression. Given its half-life, monitoring of pentobarbital blood levels and maintaining a blood level of 25–40 mg/mL shortens the recovery time.

Thiopental, with a quicker onset of action and a shorter half-life of 3–8 hours, is likely a barbiturate of choice for immediate effect. Often, a dose of 3–5 mg/kg IV is administered to attain blood levels of 10–30 mg/mL and achieves up to a 10-minute burst suppression.

- High-dose thiopental is effective in focal ischemia with a suggested initial loading dose of 25–50 mg/kg followed by an infusion to achieve a plasma concentration of 10–50 mg/L.
- A low initial dose followed by an infusion is used in intractable intracranial hypertension. An initial dose of 1–3 mg/kg is followed by intravenous infusion of 0.06–0.2 mg/kg/min.
- A low-dose bolus for short-term neuroprotection is typically a dose of 4 mg/kg administered over 3 minutes. It produces around 6 minutes of burst suppression.

Phenobarbital has a prolonged half-life of 80–120 hours and hence is not commonly used as a neuroprotective agent.

Because of high-dose barbiturate therapy for barbiturate coma, appropriate assessment of neurological condition and physical examination may not be possible for several days. Therefore, barbiturate coma is reserved for patients at high risk of ischemia and clear potential benefit.

## PROPOFOL

The neurometabolic changes from propofol anesthesia are similar to the homogeneous depression of cerebral metabolic rate seen with barbiturates. Propofol can be discontinued intraoperatively (when used during surgical procedures) after full restoration of cerebral blood flow and may possibly allow anesthetic emergence and extubation by the completion of the surgical procedure.

## ETOMIDATE

Etomidate was suggested as an alternative to barbiturates for burst suppression in view of its clinically favorable hemodynamic profile. However, concern about adrenocortical suppression and a lack of significant protective effects in subsequent studies has limited its use.

## ISOFLURANE

Isoflurane is a potent inhibitor of cerebral metabolic rate, and at clinically useful concentrations < 2 Minimum alveolar concentration can suppress brain electric activity as much to produce isoelectric EEG.

## MONITORING OF BARBITURATE COMA

Plasma levels of pharmacological agents have not been accurately shown to correlate with therapeutic benefit; hence, EEG monitoring is recommended. Burst suppression on EEG is widely accepted as a standard endpoint.

Invasive cardiopulmonary monitoring with arterial blood pressure is often required since barbiturate therapy decreases blood pressure in up to one in four treated patients, and this could offset the benefit of lowering ICP on cerebral perfusion pressure.[4] Frequent blood gas chemistries may be needed to monitor for dyskalemia and other adverse effects.

## ANESTHETIC CONSIDERATIONS

### PREOPERATIVE

A preoperative assessment of the patient's underlying medical problems and baseline neurological status is important. Barbiturates are contraindicated in patients with acute intermittent porphyria, and other pharmacological agents would have to be employed for therapeutic coma.

### INTRAOPERATIVE

Invasive cardiopulmonary monitoring with an arterial line, central venous access, and pulmonary artery catheter may be required to monitor and maintain hemodynamics intraoperatively. Depression of cardiac output and arrythmias from bolus dosing of anesthetic agents often requires fluid optimization and vasopressor infusion. EEG monitoring is the standard endpoint and is required intraoperatively for inducing therapeutic barbiturate coma.

### POSTOPERATIVE

Delayed emergence and difficulty in evaluating postoperative neurological status occurs with the high doses of anesthetic medications administered. This may require critical care unit admission and continued postoperative ventilation. Difficulty in evaluating postoperative neurological status from high doses of intraoperative anesthetic agents (to induce therapeutic coma) may warrant the use of neurophysiologic and imaging studies to identify adverse neurological events.

## REFERENCES

1. Sreedhar R, Gadhinglajkar S. Pharmacological neuroprotection. *Indian J Anaesth.* 2003;47:8–22.
2. Ellens NR, et al. The use of barbiturate-induced coma during cerebrovascular neurosurgery procedures: a review of the literature. *Brain Circ.* 2015;1:140–145.
3. Brain Trauma Foundation et al. Guidelines for the management of severe traumatic brain injury. VIII. Intracranial pressure thresholds. *J Neurotrauma.* 2007;24(suppl 1:S55–S58.
4. Roberts I. Barbiturates for acute traumatic brain injury. *Cochrane Database Syst Rev.* 2000;(2):CD000033.

# 61.

# DRUG INTOXICATION

*Sarah C. Smith*

## INTRODUCTION

In the emergent setting, anesthesiologists frequently encounter patients in an altered state of consciousness that may indicate acute drug intoxication, from either deliberate ingestion or secondary to poisoning. Taking steps to identify the substance to which the patient was exposed is essential.

## DRUGS OF ABUSE

### ETHANOL AND BENZODIAZEPINES

Ethanol and benzodiazepines both produce their sedating and anxiolytic effects by potentiating the action of γ-aminobutyric acid (GABA) in the central nervous system (CNS), but there are effects on other neurotransmitters as well, including elevated dopamine levels. High doses may result in profound respiratory depression, especially if ingested in combination with other agents. Ethanol is the most frequently abused drug worldwide and often contributes to accidents as it causes postural instability, poor judgment, and impaired reflexes. The unpleasant effects of ethanol intoxication are largely due to its metabolite, acetaldehyde. Acute intoxication with these agents may be accidental or deliberate in the case of attempted suicide or criminal poisoning. Rohypnol, for example, is a benzodiazepine that has

been used to induce anterograde amnesia and incapacity in sexual assault victims. While acute ethanol or benzodiazepine intoxication reduces the minimum alveolar concentration (MAC) of inhalational anesthetics, chronic use does the opposite while also causing cross-tolerance to opiates and anesthetics.[1]

## OPIATES

Acute opiate intoxication results in euphoria, sedation, miosis, and respiratory depression that may be life threatening. Aspiration and negative-pressure pulmonary edema are possible due to inability to protect the airway. The opiate antagonist naloxone should be administered with caution as it precipitates a rapid withdrawal syndrome characterized by tachycardia, hypertension, agitation, and nausea, which can be managed with clonidine and supportive measures. Chronic opiate abusers often suffer from a variety of other ailments, including infections linked to intravenous administration. Hyperalgesia and resistance to analgesics can make pain management difficult.[2]

## COCAINE AND METHAMPHETAMINE

Cocaine is extracted from *Erythroxylan coca* leaves and is available as a hydrochloride powder or in its alkalinized form as crack cocaine, both of which inhibit the uptake of norepinephrine, serotonin, and dopamine. Methamphetamine is a synthetic agent that causes similar euphoria, hyperarousal, and agitation by causing presynaptic release of the same excitatory neurotransmitters. Intoxication with both agents causes hypertension, tachycardia, and constriction of blood vessels, potentially resulting in myocardial infarction, ischemic stroke, aortic dissection, or aneurysm rupture. Serotonin syndrome is also possible. Chronic use may result in left ventricular hypertrophy and, ultimately, congestive heart failure. Anesthetic concerns include extreme hemodynamic instability, manifesting as either ephedrine-resistant hypotension or profound hypertension upon intubation. Hypertension can be managed with vasodilators, while β-agonists should be used with caution because of the resulting unopposed α-agonism.[1]

## MARIJUANA

Marijuana may increase the sedating effects of ethanol, benzodiazepines, or opiates, while it enhances the excitatory effects of cocaine or methamphetamine. Low doses may cause tachycardia and increased cardiac output, while higher toxic doses may cause bradycardia and hypotension, which can be exacerbated with the induction of anesthesia. Chronic users will have an increased MAC and exhibit cross-tolerance to opiates and anesthetics. Heavy smokers of marijuana may also have emphysema or reactive airway disease.[2]

## OTHER DRUGS OF ABUSE

Lysergic acid diethylamide (LSD) causes hallucinations by interfering with serotonin reuptake in the CNS. Phencyclidine (PCP) similarly inhibits CNS catecholamine reuptake in addition to other mechanisms, resulting in agitation, hallucinations, hypertension, and tachycardia. Either of these agents may precipitate the serotonin syndrome, as may 3,4-methyenedioxy-methamphetamine (MDMA) or "ecstasy," which has also been associated with seizures due to excess water intake and hypernatremia. Intoxication secondary to the inhalation of common household chemicals such as solvents, paint, and gasoline may present as CNS depression secondary to hypoxia, and persistent arrhythmias are also common.[1]

## CARBON MONOXIDE

Incomplete combustion of organic material results in the formation of carbon monoxide, which binds hemoglobin over 200 times more avidly than oxygen. Sources of exposure include fires and malfunctioning or poorly ventilated heating equipment. Initial symptoms are confusion, headaches, and fatigue, but severe poisoning can lead to somnolence, cardiovascular collapse, and death. While pulse oximetry will appear normal, an elevated carboxyhemoglobin level on co-oximetry is diagnostic. Treatment involves 100% oxygen therapy and hyperbaric oxygen therapy if severe. Because cyanide can be released from the burning of certain household items, residential fire victims should also be investigated for this form of toxicity and treated with hydroxycobalamin and sodium thiosulfate.[3]

## INSECTICIDES AND NERVE AGENTS

Many insecticides contain carbamates and organophosphates, both of which inhibit acetylcholinesterase, resulting in accumulation of acetylcholine at autonomic synapses and in neuromuscular junctions. Patients, who are usually agricultural workers, may be exposed by accidental or intentional ingestion or inhalation or via the skin.[4] Volatile organophosphates such as sarin, cyclosarin, soman, and tabun may also be used in chemical warfare, resulting in the rapid onset of severe symptoms. Another nerve agent, VX, is less volatile but may persist in the environment for longer periods of time and cause secondary contamination, presenting a significant risk for healthcare workers treating victims of this agent.[5]

Insecticide and nerve agent intoxication results in both muscarinic and nicotinic effects, manifesting as cholinergic crisis. Muscarinic signs include miosis, blurred vision, bronchoconstriction, coughing, salivation, rhinorrhea, lacrimation, sweating, nausea and vomiting, and abdominal cramping. Nicotinic effects include muscle fasciculations and weakness, tachycardia, mydriasis, and hyperglycemia. Toxicity victims will also exhibit CNS symptoms of ataxia, tremor, confusion, agitation, and fatigue, which may progress to life-threatening somnolence and respiratory depression. Emergence of symptoms can vary from a few minutes to a few days following exposure depending on the specific agent, route of exposure, and dose. Laboratory studies for erythrocyte acetylcholinesterase and plasma butyrylcholinesterase are diagnostic, and treatment includes the administration of pralidoxime, atropine, benzodiazepines, and supportive care.[4,5]

## ANESTHETIC CONSIDERATIONS

### PREOPERATIVE

It is important to tailor the anesthetic plan preoperatively to the agent causing intoxication. Signs of toxicity and anesthetic concerns for the major drugs of abuse are summarized in Table 61.1. If the patient is unconscious, other signs and symptoms of the source of intoxication should be investigated and appropriate laboratory studies pursued. If a patient presents for elective surgery with signs suggesting acute intoxication, postponement should be strongly considered.

*Table 61.1* DRUG INTOXICATION AND RELATED ANESTHETIC CONCERNS

| DRUG OF ABUSE | |
|---|---|
| Ethanol | **Mechanism of Action**<br>**Increased GABA-ergic activity**<br>**Signs of Toxicity**<br>*CNS:* euphoria, disinhibition, impaired judgment, reduced coordination, nystagmus, ataxia, slurred speech, amnesia, respiratory depression, loss of consciousness<br>*Cardiovascular:* tachycardia, vasodilation, "holiday heart" (atrial or ventricular arrhythmias)<br>*Gastrointestinal:* nausea and vomiting<br>*Metabolic:* hypoglycemia, lactic acidosis, hypomagnesemia, hypoalbuminemia, hypophosphatemia, hypocalcemia<br>**Anesthetic Concerns**<br>*Acute Intoxication:* hypotension on induction, decreased MAC, reduced ability to protect airway, potential arrhythmias<br>*Chronic Abuse:* increased MAC, cross-tolerance to anesthetics/opiates, hepatic dysfunction, potential life-threatening withdrawal syndrome |
| Benzodiazepines | **Mechanism of Action**<br>**Increased GABA-ergic activity**<br>**Signs of Toxicity**<br>*CNS:* euphoria, disinhibition, impaired judgment, reduced coordination, nystagmus, ataxia, slurred speech, amnesia, respiratory depression, loss of consciousness<br>**Anesthetic Concerns**<br>*Acute Intoxication:* hypotension on induction, decreased MAC, reduced ability to protect airway<br>*Chronic Abuse:* increased MAC, cross-tolerance to anesthetics/opiates, potential life-threatening withdrawal syndrome |
| Opiates | **Mechanism of Action**<br>Activation of $\mu$-, $\delta$-, and $\kappa$-opioid receptors<br>**Signs of Toxicity**<br>*CNS:* euphoria, sedation, respiratory depression, somnolence, potential serotonin syndrome<br>**Anesthetic Concerns**<br>*Acute Intoxication:* hypotension on induction, decreased MAC, reduced ability to protect airway<br>*Chronic Abuse:* increased MAC, cross-tolerance to anesthetics, severe withdrawal syndrome, hyperalgesia, blood-borne infections |
| Cocaine | **Mechanism of Action**<br>Decreased synaptic reuptake of norepinephrine, serotonin, dopamine<br>**Signs of Toxicity**<br>*CNS:* euphoria, agitation, impaired judgment, insomnia, potential serotonin syndrome<br>*Cardiovascular:* hypertension, tachycardia, vasoconstriction<br>*Pulmonary:* reactive/edematous airways if smoked<br>**Anesthetic Concerns**<br>*Acute Intoxication:* profound hemodynamic instability (severe hypo- or hypertension possible), end-organ ischemia (myocardial infarction [MI], stroke, renal dysfunction)<br>*Chronic Abuse:* possible left ventricular hypertrophy/congestive heart failure (LVH/CHF), renal dysfunction |
| Methamphetamine | **Mechanism of Action**<br>Increased presynaptic release of norepinephrine, serotonin, and dopamine<br>**Signs of Toxicity**<br>*CNS:* euphoria, agitation, impaired judgment, insomnia, potential serotonin syndrome<br>*Cardiovascular:* hypertension, tachycardia, vasoconstriction<br>*Pulmonary:* reactive/edematous<br>**Anesthetic Concerns**<br>*Acute Intoxication:* profound hemodynamic instability (severe hypo- or hypertension possible), end-organ ischemia (MI, stroke, renal dysfunction)<br>*Chronic Abuse:* possible LVH/CHF, renal dysfunction |
| Marijuana | **Mechanism of Action**<br>Cannabinoid receptor activation, increased CNS levels of dopamine, other less well-elucidated mechanisms<br>**Signs of Toxicity**<br>*CNS:* euphoria, sedation, impaired judgment, anxiety<br>*Cardiovascular:* tachycardia and increased cardiac output (low doses), hypotension (high doses)<br>*Pulmonary:* reactive/edematous airways if smoked<br>**Anesthetic Concerns**<br>*Acute Intoxication:* possible decreased MAC, hypotension on induction, reactive airway<br>*Chronic Abuse:* cross-tolerance with opiates/anesthetics, increased MAC, possible underlying emphysema or chronic obstructive pulmonary disease |

*(continued)*

*Table 61.1* CONTINUED

**DRUG OF ABUSE**

| | |
|---|---|
| LSD | **Mechanism of Action**<br>Activation and modulation of serotonin receptors<br>**Signs of Toxicity**<br>*CNS:* hallucinations, euphoria, distorted sense of time, anxiety, fear, depression, mydriasis, possible serotonin syndrome<br>*Cardiovascular:* tachycardia (mild)<br>*Metabolic:* hypoglycemia (mild)<br>**Anesthetic Concerns**<br>*Acute Intoxication:* unpredictable response to opiates/anesthetics<br>*Chronic Abuse:* limited effects |
| PCP | **Mechanism of Action**<br>NMDA receptor antagonist, dopamine 2 receptor agonist, prevents reuptake of dopamine, nicotinic acetylcholine receptor inhibitor<br>**Signs of Toxicity**<br>*CNS:* dissociation, agitation, slurred speech, mydriasis, nystagmus, poor coordination, hallucinations, sedation (high doses), seizures, possible serotonin syndrome<br>*Cardiovascular:* tachycardia, hypertension, hyperthermia<br>**Anesthetic Concerns**<br>*Acute Intoxication:* unpredictable response to opiates/anesthetics, hemodynamic instability (hypo- or hypertension possible)<br>*Chronic Use:* unpredictable response to opiates/anesthetics |
| MDMA | **Mechanism of Action**<br>Decreased synaptic reuptake of serotonin, norepinephrine, and dopamine<br>**Signs of Toxicity**<br>*CNS:* euphoria, restlessness, increased sociability, insomnia, hallucinations, possible serotonin syndrome<br>*Cardiovascular:* tachycardia, hypertension, vasoconstriction, arrhythmias<br>*Hepatic:* acute hepatic failure possible<br>*Metabolic:* hyperthermia, hyponatremia<br>**Anesthetic Concerns**<br>*Acute Intoxication:* unpredictable response to opiates/anesthetics, possible rhabdomyolysis, thermal dysregulation, hyponatremia due to excess water consumption<br>*Chronic Abuse:* unpredictable response to opiates/anesthetics |
| Inhalants | **Mechanism of Action**<br>Complex and multifactorial<br>**Signs of Toxicity**<br>*CNS:* agitation, disorientation, confusion, sedation, somnolence, respiratory depression<br>*Cardiovascular:* severe arrhythmias possible<br>*Pulmonary:* reactive/edematous airways<br>**Anesthetic Concerns**<br>*Acute Intoxication:* unpredictable response to opiates/anesthetics, acid-base abnormalities possible, reactive airways, potential hypotension on induction<br>*Chronic Abuse:* unpredictable response to opiates/anesthetics |

## INTRAOPERATIVE

Anesthetic agents should be carefully titrated to effect intraoperatively, particularly if the cause of the intoxication is unknown as many toxins alter MAC. Many forms of intoxication contribute to hemodynamic instability, and this may be particularly challenging during induction, and invasive monitoring should be strongly considered.

## POSTOPERATIVE

Patients may require a continuation of mechanical ventilation postoperatively until their level of consciousness returns to baseline. Ongoing effects of the intoxication or poisoning may necessitate an intensive care unit admission. Pain management in patients with substance abuse disorders can be particularly challenging due to hyperalgesia, coexisting withdrawal syndrome, or cross-tolerance to analgesics.

## REFERENCES

1. Beaulieu P. Anesthetic implications of recreational drug use. *Can J Anaesth.* 2017;64(12):1236–1264.
2. Hernandez M, et al. Anesthetic management of the illicit-substance-using patient. *Curr Opin Anaesthesiol.* 2005;18(3):315–324.
3. Wu PE, Juurlink DN. Carbon monoxide poisoning. *CMAJ.* 2014;186(8):611.
4. Vale A, Lotti M. Organophosphorus and carbamate insecticide poisoning. *Handb Clin Neurol.* 2015;131:149–168.
5. Chang A, et al. Nerve agent incidents and public health preparedness. *Ann Intern Med.* 2019;170(1):59–61.

# 62.

# PARAPLEGIA, QUADRIPLEGIA, SPINAL SHOCK, AUTONOMIC HYPERREFLEXIA, ACUTE SPINAL CORD INJURY

*Peter Papapetrou and Kris Ferguson*

## INTRODUCTION

The dramatic decrease in mortality of spinal cord injury patients over the last several decades is owed to improvements in treatment of renal and respiratory failure.[1] With increased survival in these patients, there is an increased number of spinal cord injury patients presenting for elective surgery. They carry unique cardiovascular, airway, and respiratory anesthetic considerations.

## SPINAL SHOCK/ACUTE SPINAL CORD INJURY

### CARDIOVASCULAR CHANGES

The initial result of a spinal cord injury is a brief and intense autonomic discharge from descending sympathetic nerves, leading to severe hypertension and arrhythmias. This is accompanied by afterload increases and potentially left ventricular failure. After a few minutes, the phenomenon of spinal shock ensues, which is caused by sudden loss of sympathetic discharge. Spinal shock is characterized by hypotension and bradycardia, primarily from reduced preload and vasodilation, with vagal parasympathetic discharge being unopposed. In addition, skeletal muscle flaccidity and loss of reflexes are also observed in spinal shock patients. With unopposed vagal tone, there is a risk of severe bradycardia and even asystole with tracheal intubation or tracheal suctioning in these patients. This phase of spinal shock can last a few days, but may last up to 6–8 weeks. At the end of this phase, there is a gradual return of neuronal connections distal to the site of injury and a return of sympathetic efferent discharge. Muscle tone and reflexes also return at the end of this phase.

## RESPIRATORY CHANGES

Patients with C1 or C2 spinal cord lesions are immediately apneic due to diaphragmatic paralysis. C3 or C4 lesions usually have the same result, though diaphragmatic function is sometimes spared. A patient with a C6 lesion is able to maintain their own ventilation as diaphragmatic innervation is spared. Intercostal function is lost with lower cervical lesions, but this is compensated by an increase in accessory muscle strength. Patients may have an inadequate cough and inability to clear secretions and thus may be prone to aspiration of gastric contents. In quadriplegics, vital capacity is reduced to 30% of normal, with some increase over the course of the first 6 months. Additionally, expiratory reserve volume and forced expiratory volume is significantly reduced.

## GASTROINTESTINAL CHANGES

Paralytic ileus can be observed in spinal cord injury patients, which can affect diaphragmatic excursion and result in decreased functional reserve capacity. These patients are at an increased aspiration risk during induction of anesthesia as they have delayed gastric emptying and gastric distension.

## METABOLIC CHANGES

Metabolically, denervation of muscle results in an increased number of nicotinic receptors. This results in a much larger area of muscle membrane that responds to a succinylcholine-induced hyperkalemic response. This exaggerated hyperkalemic response can be observed anywhere from 3 days to 6 months from the time of injury and can result in ventricular fibrillation and cardiac arrest. Bone resorption can occur in patients with prolonged paralysis, resulting in hypercalcemia. Patients with impaired respiratory function may have respiratory acidosis with or without compensatory alkalosis.

## AUTONOMIC HYPERREFLEXIA

The most important implication of spinal cord lesions to the anesthesiologist is autonomic dysreflexia. First described in 1917, it is characterized by an exaggerated sympathetic response to certain stimuli below the level of the spinal cord lesion. The incidence of autonomic hyperreflexia is related to the level of the lesion, with 85% of autonomic hyperreflexia episodes occurring in patients with lesions higher than T7. It is caused by a massively inappropriate sympathetic response to a stimulus due to loss of descending inhibitory reflexes, as shown in Figure 62.1. The most common clinical symptom is hypertension, resulting in reflexive bradycardia, as well as headache and sweating. Less commonly seen are nausea, anxiety, and pupillary changes. The hypertensive episode is severe, with systolic pressure above 260 mm Hg and diastolic pressures of 170–220 mm Hg being reported. The hypertensive emergency can lead to retinal and intracranial hemorrhages, seizures, myocardial infarction, coma, and death. Removing the stimulus is the first step in management. If there is no improvement in hypertension, rapid onset antihypertensive medications such as phentolamine should be given.

## QUADRIPLEGIA

Total blood volume in quadriplegics is reduced, with some studies indicating it can be reduced to 60 mL/kg. Lung volumes are significantly reduced in quadriplegics, which can be as low as 30% of normal. Effective coughing is impaired in many quadriplegics, and to compensate, quadriplegics can achieve coughing by contracting the clavicular portion of the pectoralis major, which may cause airway compression. Due to their impaired ability to cough as well as development of increased secretions through loss of neuronal control of bronchial secretions, quadriplegics have a higher tendency to develop atelectasis. Ability to thermoregulate is reduced, with overall body temperature being reduced in quadriplegics. They also have delayed gastric emptying, with studies showing a five-fold increase in gastric emptying time compared to controls. Quadriplegic patients have a reduced sympathetic response to hypotension caused by positive-pressure ventilation, which creates a greater decrease in blood pressure.

## ANESTHETIC CONSIDERATIONS

### PREOPERATIVE

Whenever possible, regional anesthesia should be used in spinal cord injury patients. Spinal anesthesia prevents autonomic hyperreflexia and avoids airway manipulation as well as the increased risks of general anesthesia. If general anesthesia is required, special precautions need to be taken in patients with cervical spine disease. Intubating these patients using fiber-optic laryngoscopy is superior in order to limit cervical spine motion.[2] It is also important to take into account timing of their spinal cord injury. Anywhere from 3 days to 6 months postinjury, a patient can have an exaggerated hyperkalemic response to depolarizing muscle relaxants such as succinylcholine, which is attributed to an increased number of nicotinic

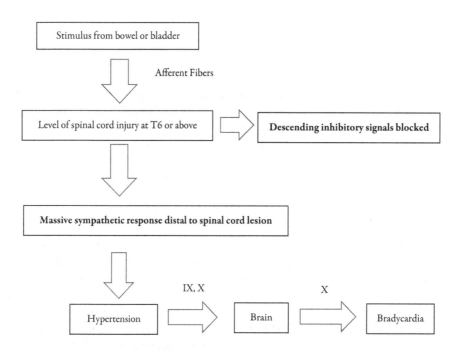

**Figure 62.1** Autonomic hyperreflexia in a spinal cord injury patient.

receptors from denervated muscle. The result may lead to ventricular fibrillation and cardiac arrest.

## INTRAOPERATIVE

Due to reduced lean tissue mass and lower blood volume, these patients have a smaller volume of distribution and thus higher sensitivity to intravenous induction agents intraoperatively. During induction, atropine can help prevent bradycardia during intubation of spinal shock patients. In patients with cervical spine lesions, hypercapnia and hypoxia can be common if a patient breathes spontaneously during general anesthesia. Positive pressure ventilation, however, causes a greater blood pressure decrease in quadriplegic patients.

## POSTOPERATIVE

Thermoregulation is greatly impaired in spinal cord injury patients. Close monitoring of body temperature is important postoperatively, as their ability to generate heat after surgery is significantly decreased. Respiratory function also needs to be closely monitored after surgery.

## REFERENCES

1. Hambly PR, Martin B. Anaesthesia for chronic spinal cord lesions. *Anaesthesia.* 1998;53:273–289.
2. Avitsian R, Farag E. Neuroanesthesia. In: Longnecker DE, et al., eds. *Anesthesiology,* 2nd ed. McGraw-Hill; 2012. Chap. 51, p. 894.

# 63.

# AIRWAY MANAGEMENT IN CERVICAL SPINE DISEASE

*Balram Sharma and Evgeny Romanov*

## INTRODUCTION

There are many causes of cervical spine instability. They can be classified as acute and chronic, with trauma accounting for the majority of acute cases. Despite advances made in the diagnosis and management of this disorder, it still remains a devastating event, often leading to permanent disability.[1,2] Causes of chronic spine instability include inflammatory diseases (rheumatoid arthritis, ankylosing spondylitis); congenital collagenous disorders (syndromes: Ehlers-Danlos, Down); and recent head, neck, or dental surgery.

## ANESTHETIC CONSIDERATIONS

### PREOPERATIVE MANAGEMENT

### Immobilization and Initial Assessment

One should assume that an injury to the cervical spine has occurred in all blunt trauma patients until proven otherwise. Routine spinal immobilization is recommended in most cases, except penetrating cervical spine injury.[3] Before transport of the patient, a hard cervical collar must be applied. A focused neurologic examination is necessary for all patients who may have a cervical spinal disorder. Particular attention should be payed to sensory and motor deficits, as well as signs of bowel and bladder incontinence or retention.

Manual in-line stabilization (MILS) (Figure 63.1) during airway management is the standard of care in patients with an acute cervical spine injury. This maneuver helps to keep the cervical spine immobile during intubation after the patient is delivered to an acute care facility. With this maneuver, an assistant grabs the patient's mastoid process with their fingertips, with the occiput in the palms of the hands. For tracheal intubation, the anterior part of the hard cervical collar should be removed. Intubations with a complete cervical collar in place may result in greater spinal subluxation. An assistant should provide enough strength to counter forces applied during laryngoscopy to keep the head and neck in the neutral position, without applying traction.[1]

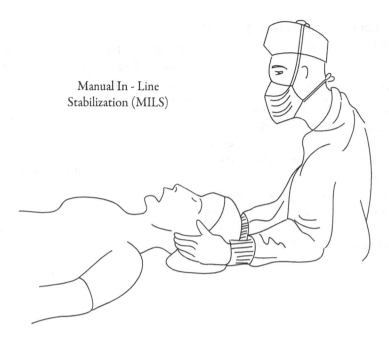

Manual In - Line
Stabilization (MILS)

**Figure 63.1** Manual in-line stabilization (MILS).

## Airway Management

The key to successful airway management in cervical spine instability is *avoidance of excessive movement of the head and neck* to prevent any further damage to the spinal cord. No technique for airway management has been shown to be superior to others for prevention of neurologic deterioration in the patient with cervical spine disease. However, videolaryngoscopic and flexible scope intubation (Figure 63.2) provide a better view with minimal motion of the cervical spine. Direct laryngoscopy with MILS can still be used but may result in greater pressure on the anterior tongue to achieve a similar view and thus more movement.[1] Cricothyroidotomy can be used as a last resort in patients with severely distorted airway anatomy. The advantages and disadvantages of various methods

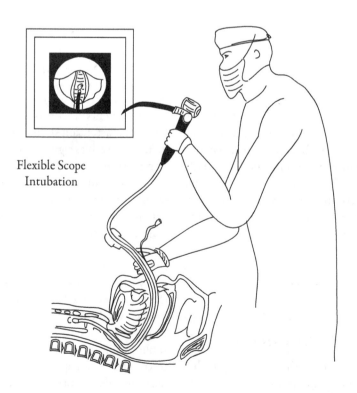

Flexible Scope
Intubation

**Figure 63.2** Flexible scope intubation.

**Table 63.1** ADVANTAGES AND DISADVANTAGES OF DIFFERENT AIRWAY ACCESS TECHNIQUES

| METHOD | ADVANTAGES | DISADVANTAGES |
| --- | --- | --- |
| Direct laryngoscopy with MILS | • Easily available | • Poor view with immobilized neck results in greater pressure on the tongue, the spine. and the unstable segment, with potential displacement of unstable fragment[4] |
| Videolaryngoscopy | • Provides better view[4]<br>• Does not increase the risk of anterior neck movement compared to direct laryngoscopy[4] | • Not always available |
| Flexible scope intubation | • Minimal movement of the neck<br>• Spontaneous ventilation is maintained until the airway is secured<br>• Positioning of the patient awake<br>• Maintenance of protective reflexes<br>• Ability to assess the neurologic status after intubation[1,4,5] | • Blood or secretions in the airway can make flexible scope intubation difficult<br>• Long preparation time<br>• Difficulty in their use in comatose, uncooperative, or anesthetized patients<br>• Coughing and gagging may cause movement of cervical spine[1,4,5] |
| Translaryngeal (retrograde) intubation | • Causes almost no neck movement | • Blood or secretions in the airway, long preparation time, and difficulty in their use in comatose, uncooperative, or anesthetized patients |
| Cricothyroidotomy | • Allows airway access with significant distortion of upper airway anatomy | • Long preparation time<br>• High risk of complications, including bleeding, incorrect placement, pneumothorax, esophageal or mediastinal perforation |

allowing airway access with cervical spine injury are outlined in Table 63.1.

### Flexible Scope Intubation Technique

Flexible scope intubation can be performed in either an awake patient with effective topical airway analgesia or in the patient after induction of anesthesia. An antisialagogue (glycopyrrolate, 0.2 mg IV) should be administered at least 15 minutes prior to the procedure. Topical anesthesia can be achieved with direct application of lidocaine. In most cases, the oral approach can be used. It starts with the placement of a bite block or intubating oral airway, followed by suctioning of the oropharynx. The endotracheal tube is placed into the intubating airway to a depth of 5 cm or is loaded directly onto and secured to the handle of the lubricated flexible intubating scope (FIS). The FIS is oriented so that the tip can be moved up and down in the midline and is inserted without a bend at the tip along the midline of the oropharynx (or into the endotracheal tube [ETT] if in the oral airway). The larynx should be visible in the midline; the FIS is passed through the vocal cords to the carina. The ETT is advanced over the FIS to 22 cm for women or 24 cm for men. The FIS is withdrawn, and the ETT position is confirmed in the usual manner.[5]

## INTRAOPERATIVE MANAGEMENT

### INDUCTION OF ANESTHESIA

Patients with acute spinal cord injury are at significant risk for hypotension during induction as a result of sympathetic denervation exacerbated by induction agents. Because traumatic spinal cord injury is often accompanied by other injuries, hypovolemia secondary to hemorrhagic shock can further worsen the hypotension.

Thus, the dose of induction agents in these patients should be reduced. Glycopyrrolate or atropine is commonly administered for bradycardic patients. Succinylcholine use should be avoided in all trauma patients 48 hours after the injury due to risk of life-threatening hyperkalemia.[1]

### MAINTENANCE

All patients with acute spinal cord injury require initial volume resuscitation with intravenous crystalloid, with the addition of colloid and blood products as necessary. Volume overload should be avoided to prevent pulmonary and spinal cord edema. Vasopressors with inotropic and chronotropic properties in addition to vasopressors (i.e., dopamine, norepinephrine, epinephrine) are often required.[1]

## EMERGENCE

Patients with a severe cervical spinal cord injury are most often left intubated at the end of surgical procedures, with the expectation that they will require assisted ventilation and possibly tracheostomy in the acute period after injury.[1]

## POSTOPERATIVE MANAGEMENT

The plan for postoperative care of patients with acute spinal cord injury depends on the level of injury, associated injuries, the intraoperative course, and the need for immediate postoperative neurologic assessment. Many patients with severe cervical cord injuries remain intubated and require mechanical ventilation and intensive care.[1]

## REFERENCES

1. Mathews L, et al. eds. *Anesthesia for Adults With Acute Spinal Cord Injury*. Retrieved August 14, 2020.
2. Hansebout R, et al., eds. *Acute Traumatic Spinal Cord Injury*. Retrieved August 10, 2020.
3. Raja A, ed. *Initial Management of Trauma in Adults*. Retrieved August 9, 2020.
4. Barash PG, et al., eds. *Clinical Anesthesia*. 8th ed. Wolters Kluwer; 2017.
5. Hagberg C, et al. Flexible scope intubation for anesthesia. In: Crowley M, ed. *UpToDate*. 2020. Retrieved August 16, 2020.

# 64.

# TETANUS

*Patrick Forrest*

## INTRODUCTION

Tetanus describes a bacterial infection by *Clostridium tetani*, an obligatory anaerobic gram-positive bacillus. Spores, which can be present in soil or feces, may enter the body through a laceration or other wound.[1] Proliferation only occurs in poorly oxygenated tissue and causes a localized infection with production of two toxins: tetanospasmin and tetanolysin, the former causing systemic symptoms and the latter causing local tissue damage that optimizes continued bacterial proliferation. Tetanus cannot be transmitted person to person. Tetanospasmin enters the bloodstream with eventual spread to the nervous system via the motor end plates, cell bodies, and eventually the presynaptic terminals. Although all neurons are affected, most affected are the inhibitory pathways that control the release of glycine in the spinal cord and γ-aminobutyric acid (GABA) in the brain.[2] Vaccination against tetanus is the only true preventive measure. Developed in 1923, the vaccine consists of a nontoxic derivative of the toxin that causes production of antitoxic antibodies in the body.[1] Vaccination begins at 2 to 3 months of age and consists of four subsequent injections that are spaced out over time. Immunity begins after the second injection.[2] Adults should receive a booster injection every 10 years for continuing immunity.

## CLINICAL FEATURES

Tetanus can produce both local and generalized infection depending on toxin loads. The first symptoms of generalized tetanus are typically neck stiffness, odynophagia, and masseter spasm (i.e., trismus or lockjaw).[2] Patients may develop risus sardonicus, a classic clenched-teeth facial expression. Progression to total body rigidity and muscle spasms usually occurs cranially with caudal spread. Spasms triggered by external stimuli such as sound and touch can be strong enough to produce fractures and tendon avulsions. Life-threatening complications include respiratory distress due to muscle dysfunction and autonomic instability.

Infants can be infected if mothers do not have adequate antibody titers during pregnancy, and this accounts for the majority of deaths due to tetanus. Neonatal tetanus presents most commonly during the first week of life and is characterized by inability to feed, vomiting, and convulsions.[2] These symptoms can mimic meningitis and sepsis on first inspection.

With the advent of mechanical ventilation, autonomic dysfunction due to tetanus became more apparent. Both sympathetic and parasympathetic systems can be affected. Labile hypertension, pyrexia, tachycardia, and significant vasoconstriction are caused by increased circulating levels of norepinephrine and, to a certain extent, epinephrine from blockade of inhibitory neurons. Parasympathetic overtones can produce the opposite effects: severe hypotension, decreased vascular tone, and bradycardia leading to sudden cardiac arrest.[1] Diagnosis of tetanus is made clinically and is not based on cultures as the positivity rate can be less than 50%.

## MANAGEMENT

Tetanus is treated with human antitetanus immunoglobulin (HTI). However, this only addresses circulating toxin and not the damage done to the central nervous system by already bound toxin.[3] Localized infection is eliminated by debridement of the affected tissues and antibiotics such as metronidazole and penicillin G with metronidazole being preferred due to less microbial resistance and side effects.

Rigidity, muscle spasm, and autonomic dysfunction can be controlled with various agents. Classically, patients were intubated, sedated, and relaxed with paralytic agents. However, this requires high levels of medical care and can lead to prolonged ventilation with subsequent risk of complication, such as ventilator-associated pneumonia and tracheal stenosis. Medications commonly used to mitigate rigidity and muscle spasms include benzodiazepines such as diazepam, magnesium sulfate via continuous intravenous infusion, and, to a lesser extent, intrathecal baclofen and dantrolene.[3] Treatment of autonomic dysfunction includes α- and β-blockers, opioids, and $α_2$-agonists. Pure β-blockers should not be used as sole agents as they can cause acute congestive heart failure from increases in systemic vascular resistance.[1] Morphine can help replace endogenous opioids that have been depleted, while clonidine and dexmedetomidine work centrally causing sedation and vasodilation. Muscle spasms resolve within 1 to 3 weeks,

with complete recovery at roughly 6 weeks without further complications.

## ANESTHETIC CONSIDERATIONS

### PREOPERATIVE

Patients with acute tetanus infection may present to the operating room (OR) for surgical wound debridement. Patients should be optimized in regard to hemodynamic stability and initial treatment initiated with HTI and antibiotics prior to presenting to the OR. Pertinent information in the preoperative assessment includes airway examination given possible trismus and respiratory status as chest wall rigidity may be present. A basic metabolic panel, complete blood cell count, and lactate level may be helpful to determine the severity of the disease. Premedication with a benzodiazepine and opioid may be warranted.

### INTRAOPERATIVE

The literature is sparse in regard to anesthetic agents intraoperatively. A case report from India demonstrated successful use of propofol and vecuronium for induction of anesthesia, with sevoflurane and nitrous oxide for maintenance of anesthesia.[4] Other agents used during the procedure included fentanyl and midazolam for premedication. The patient had been optimized in the hospital for 4 days prior to surgery with HTI, diazepam, phenobarbitone, and metronidazole.

Nondepolarizing muscle relaxants vecuronium, rocuronium, and atracurium have all been used in patients with tetanus. Pancuronium should be avoided due to its possible sympathetic effects. Care should be taken when using depolarizing agents such as succinylcholine as they may precipitate hyperkalemic arrest and further the risk of rhabdomyolysis. Rapid sequence induction should be considered due to risk of aspiration from gastrointestinal stasis and increased abdominal pressures in generalized tetanus. Volatile anesthetics may help with hemodynamic stability by enhancing postsynaptic inhibitory pathways while dampening sympathetic pathways (exception possibly being desflurane).[5] Esmolol, labetalol, clonidine, magnesium sulfate, and dexmedetomidine are commonly used perioperative medications that can aid in controlling any autonomic dysfunction.[3] Spinal anesthesia has also been used successfully for lower extremity debridement cases.[4]

### POSTOPERATIVE

Rigidity and muscle spasms may reoccur following the end of anesthesia. Care should be taken to ensure the patient has a patent airway with adequate tidal volumes and minimal signs of autonomic instability. Transfer to an intensive care unit can be optimal for increased observation or ventilatory support if needed.

## REFERENCES

1. Lipman J. Tetanus. In: Bersten AD, ed. *Oh's Intensive Care Manual*. 8th ed. Elsevier; 2019:692–696.
2. Cook TM, et al. Tetanus: a review of the literature. *Br J Anaesth*. 2001;87(3):477–487.
3. Rodrigo C, et al. Pharmacological management of tetanus: an evidence-based review. *Crit Care*. 2014;18(2):217.
4. Mahajan R, et al. General anesthesia in tetanus patient undergoing emergency surgery: a challenge for anesthesiologist. *Anesth Essays Res*. 2014;8(1):96–98.
5. Firth PG, et al. Airway management of tetanus after the Haitian earthquake: new aspects of old observations. *Anesth Analg*. 2011;113(3):545–547.

# 65.

# POSITIONING AND ANESTHESIA IN SITTING POSITION

*Sohail K. Mahboobi and Alexander Rothkrug*

## INTRODUCTION

Positions can cause physiological changes in the body by altering hemodynamics, respiratory mechanics, and compression effects.

## SUPINE

In the supine position, a patient lies flat on their back, with their arms at the sides or abducted. The functional residual capacity (FRC) and compliance are reduced due to cephalad movement of abdominal contents.[1] Adding positive end-expiratory pressure may mitigate these effects. Pregnant and obese patients may experience hypotension from compression of the inferior vena cava (IVC) against vertebral bodies. In others, the supine position allows greater venous return and higher cardiac output.

Ulnar nerve injury is the most common nerve injury and occurs more in males. The ulnar nerve passes through a groove superficial to the medial epicondyle of the humerus. Pronation or extension of the arm can compress the nerve within the groove. Slightly flexing and supinating the forearm relieves this tension. It is advisable to abduct the arms less than 90°, keep the hands pronated, and the head and neck neutral. The occiput, sacrum, and heels are prone to compression ischemia.[2]

## REVERSE TRENDELENBURG

In the reverse Trendelenburg position, the patient lies supine with an upward incline angle. The FRC and lung compliance increase. Hemodynamically, patients experience hypotension, and a cuff on the upper extremity may show higher blood pressure than seen at the brain. A benefit of reverse Trendelenburg is reduced passive regurgitation.

## TRENDELENBURG

The Trendelenburg position is characterized by the patient lying supine at a decline, greater than 15° head down. The FRC is reduced, leading to atelectasis and ventilation-perfusion (V/Q) mismatch. The cephalad movement of the diaphragm decreases compliance. The endotracheal tube may migrate endobronchial. In prolonged steep Trendelenburg, facial or laryngeal edema may occur, and a cuff leak test prior to extubation should be considered. Rise in intracranial pressure (ICP) and intraocular pressure and passive regurgitation are other risks associated with this position.

## LITHOTOMY

In lithotomy, the patient lies supine with both legs elevated and supported by surgical stirrups. The endotracheal tube may shift to stimulate the carina. Both legs should simultaneously be placed into the stirrups to avoid stretch injury. Lithotomy promotes central venous return and higher preload and cardiac output, which can be problematic in heart failure.

There are several risks of peripheral nerve injury, for example, the common peroneal nerve passes superficially over the fibular head, the saphenous nerve passes over the medial condyle of the tibia, the femoral nerve passes under the inguinal ligament, and stretch injury to the sciatic and obturator nerve occurs from excessive hip external rotation or flexion. Venous thromboembolism can occur secondary to obstruction of drainage.

The risk of compartment syndrome is higher and may present with lower extremity or calf pain out of proportion to clinical findings. Paresthesia and pain with passive toe extension are late signs. For procedures greater than 4 hours in length, the legs may intermittently be lowered to relieve compartmental pressure. The major risk factors include hypotension, hypovolemia, prolonged procedures (>4 hours), and the degree of leg elevation.[3]

## LATERAL POSITION

The lateral position is commonly used during thoracic, hip, and shoulder cases. It is crucial to secure the airway prior to positioning. In this position, contrary to awake state, the dependent lung may see greater perfusion but poorer ventilation, resulting in V/Q mismatch and hypoxemia.

The head and neck should remain in a neutral position to avoid brachial plexus injury. Often, axillary rolls are placed to prevent lower arm compression; however, if these are placed directly into the axilla they can cause brachial plexus injury. Padding between the legs is used to prevent common peroneal and saphenous nerve injury. The greatest number of ocular injuries occurs in the lateral position.

## PRONE

The prone position is used during intracranial and spine surgery. Ischemic optic neuropathy, retinal ischemia, and postoperative visual loss have been reported in this position. Frequent eye checks, though helpful, can predispose the patient to injury. It is helpful in hypoxic patients given the increased FRC and improved V/Q matching (hence

used in managing acute respiratory distress syndrome).[4] Pressure can be relieved from the abdomen to prevent IVC compression.

## SITTING/BEACH CHAIR

Seated or beach chair positioning is used in posterior fossa, posterior cervical spine, and shoulder surgeries.[5] This position improves venous and cerebrospinal fluid drainage, lowering ICP. Keeping the head and neck neutral and not overly flexed avoids the risk of spinal cord ischemia. Compression of the tongue can lead to airway obstruction. In awake patients, baroreceptor reflexes are responsible for an increase in systemic vascular resistance, blood pressure, and cardiac output; however, under anesthesia, this reflex is hypoactive. Venous pooling may present with resistant hypotension, and it is advisable to keep mean arterial pressure greater than 70 mm Hg or within 25% of the patient's baseline to avoid cerebral hypoperfusion. If using invasive monitoring, the transducer should be placed at the level of the tragus or circle of Willis.

Air emboli are more prevalent in this position, especially during craniotomy. Subatmospheric venous pressure is created by the dura and bone holding veins open. Dural sinuses are noncollapsible. Early detection of small air emboli (<10 mL) is made by TEE or precordial Doppler. The transesophageal echocardiography (TEE) probe itself can compress the tongue and cause edema and airway obstruction. Moderate size emboli (10–50 mL) may be noticed clinically by a decrease in end-tidal $CO_2$, tachycardia, and hypertension. Large emboli (>50 mL) usually present as tachycardia, arrhythmia, hypotension, right ventricular failure, and arrest. If an air embolism is suspected, flush the surgical field to avoid further air entrainment, increase $FiO_2$ (fraction of inspired oxygen) to 100%, treat hypotension with fluids and pressors, and treat any arrhythmia. It may also help to place the patient in the left lateral Trendelenburg position. Aspiration of air from a central line can be attempted but does not always work. Patients with patent foramen ovale or right-to-left shunts are at increased risk of paradoxical air emboli.

## REFERENCES

1. David K, et al. Patient positioning in anaesthesia. *Cont Educ Anaesth Crit Care Pain*. 2004;4(5):160–163.
2. Sawyer RJ, et al. Peripheral nerve injuries associated with anaesthesia. *Anaesthesia*. 2000;55(10):980–991.
3. MacIntyre PA. Compartment syndrome following prolonged positioning in the lithotomy position. *Anaesthesia*. 1996;51:511.
4. Kallet RH. A comprehensive review of prone position in ARDS. *Respir Care*. 2015;60:1660–1687.
5. Rains DD, et al. Pathomechanisms and complications related to patient positioning and anesthesia during shoulder arthroscopy. *Arthroscopy*. 2011;27(4):532–541.

# 66.

# AIR EMBOLISM

*Samuel Linares and Ned F. Nasr*

## INTRODUCTION

A vascular air embolism (VAE) occurs when any source of gas or air from the environment is trapped in the vasculature, causing a blockage in the circulatory system (venous much more common). The air entrainment is secondary to a pressure gradient between the venous opening and the level of the heart. Classically, the semisitting craniotomy is the surgical procedure associated with VAE; however, air embolism should be considered in any procedure where the surgical site is above the heart. It is difficult to determine the real incidence of air embolism as multiple subclinical cases are unnoticed; the overall incidence is unclear as the sensitivity of the detection device is fundamental to diagnose each case.[1,2]

## PATHOPHYSIOLOGY

Pathophysiologically, the two factors determining the morbidity and mortality are the volume of air trapped and the rate of accumulation. The lethal volume in adults has been described as 200 to 300 mL or 3–5 mL/kg. If the amount of air is small (<0.5 mL/kg), then what is observed is a reduction of end-tidal $CO_2$ ($ETCO_2$), oxygen desaturation, and altered mental status; moderate amounts (0.5–2 mL/kg) can present with shortness of breath, hypotension, pulmonary hypertension, and cerebral ischemia; large amounts (>2 mL/kg) present with right-side heart failure and cardiogenic shock. The rate of accumulation is a crucial factor; if the trapping is slow, the heart may be able to tolerate and manage over a prolonged period. Some of the complications associated with VAE include hypoxemia, and once the air embolus enters the pulmonary vasculature, there is an increase in the sympathetic response and associated vasoconstriction; this will lead to ventilation-perfusion mismatch, increased physiologic dead space, hypoxemia, and increased $PaCO_2$. The air trapped within the circulation activates endothelial mediators, which induce damage, reduce lung compliance, and increase airway resistance.[3]

## CLINICAL MANIFESTATIONS

Signs and symptoms can be divided into cardiovascular, pulmonary, and neurological. The clinical presentation is similar to other cardiac and pulmonary diseases, and the differential diagnosis is broad; VAE should be differentiated from acute coronary syndrome, cardiogenic shock, and pulmonary embolism. The most common cardiovascular signs and symptoms include arrhythmias and hypotension; if the air amount is significant, then there may be right-side heart failure, increased central venous pressure, and cardiogenic shock. Pulmonary clinical presentation includes shortness of breath, rales, wheezing, decreased $ETCO_2$, and oxygen saturation. The signs and symptoms in the central nervous system will develop depending on one of two possible mechanisms: associated with cardiovascular collapse secondary to outlet obstruction, heart failure or myocardial infarction; or associated with cerebral air embolism in patients with foramen ovale (paradoxical air embolism).

## TREATMENT

The main goals in treatment are to prevent further air entry, reduction of air entrained, and hemodynamic support. The first step in the treatment consists of alerting the surgical team; the surgeon should wax the skull edges (during neurosurgery), as well flood the surgical field to identify and occlude the possible access. The patient should be repositioned immediately to remove the gradient that exists between the surgical site and the heart; the Durant maneuver (partial left lateral decubitus) and Trendelenburg position have been described to aid in the removal of an airlock. This will prevent the passage of air from the right side of the heart with the aim of avoid right heart outlet obstruction. Bilateral jugular vein compression can be attempted with the aim to increase intracranial venous pressure and reduce the amount of air entering. Nitrous oxide should be stopped, as it can worsen and enlarge the air embolus.[1-3]

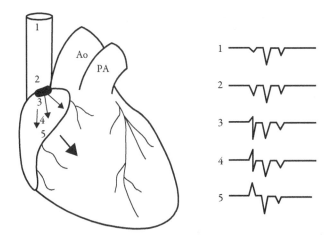

Figure 66.1 correspond to: Electrocardiographic changes during central catheter placement. A catheter located 2 cm distal to the superior vena cava-right atrial junction can be used to aspirate air located in the right atrium.

If a central venous line is in place, it can be used to aspirate the air located in the right atrium. The catheter should be positioned 2 cm distal to the superior vena cava–right atrial junction with position confirmed by either radiological or ultrasonography means or by use of an electrocardiogram (Figure 66.1). Unfortunately, this approach is not always successful. Multilumen catheters have shown success rates as low as 6% to 16%. Other devices, such as the multiorifice catheter (Cook Critical Care), have a success rate as high as 30% to 60%. Finally, hemodynamic support is fundamental and vasopressors can be started; the management goals should aim to optimize myocardial perfusion and provide inotropic support. Some authors recommend dobutamine as the best choice as increased cardiac function and decreased pulmonary vascular resistance have been seen.[1]

## ANESTHETIC CONSIDERATIONS

### PREOPERATIVE

Preoperatively, identify high-risk procedures and patients. In neurosurgical cases, if plausible, the traditional sitting position should be avoided, considering alternative positioning such as the prone or park bench position as these can reduce the risk of VAE. Leg rising and flex option in the operating table will increase the right atrial pressure and prevent the negative pressure gradient from the surgical site to the right heart. Studies have shown that prophylactic lidocaine can reduce brain edema associated with gas embolism in the brain. Benefits have also been associated with the use of heparin when administered before air embolization. Other prophylactic treatments, such as steroids or the use of positive end-expiratory pressure remain controversial, and most authors do not recommend it.

### INTRAOPERATIVE

Consider VAE immediately intraoperatively if the patient exhibits unexplained hypotension or decrease in $ETCO_2$. Patients undergoing insertion or removal of central venous catheters who report dyspnea or patients undergoing cesarean delivery who have sustained hypotension should alert the provider to this complication. Invasive and noninvasive methods have been developed to detect VAE; these have different sensitivity and limitations.[1,4,5]

Among the noninvasive methods, precordial Doppler ultrasound is the most sensitive; the probe should be placed over the third or fourth intercostal space in the right parasternal side. The major limitations are the difficulty of use in morbidly obese patients and the sounds of artifacts associated with the electrocautery use. The transesophageal

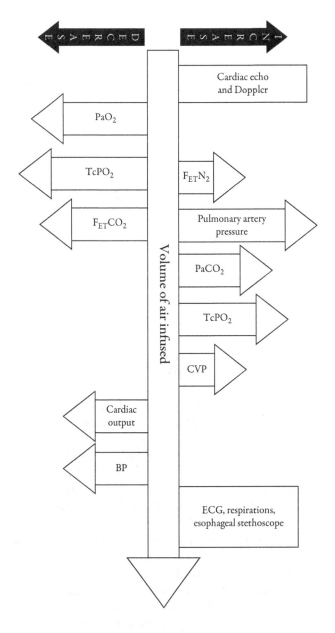

Figure 66.2 correspond to: Diagnostic methods sensitivity.

echocardiography is the most sensitive method, and paradoxical air embolism from the right to the left side heart.

End-tidal carbon dioxide and end-tidal nitrogen gas (ETN2) are noninvasive methods. A change of 2 mm Hg of $ETCO_2$ can indicate VAE; unfortunately, this method lacks specificity and can be difficult to assess in the setting of hypotension. A change in ETN2 of 0.04% can be detected; this usually happens 30–90 seconds before the $ETCO_2$ changes. The main limitations are the low availability and that this method is not useful if nitrous oxide is used. Other less sensitive methods include oxygen saturation, direct visualization, esophageal stethoscope, and electrocardiogram[1] (Figure 66.2).

## POSTOPERATIVE

Patients should continue care in the intensive care unit to ensure hemodynamic stability. If not diagnosed in the intraoperative period, changes in the sensorium during the recovery in the postoperative period should be suspicious of previous air embolism and associated cerebral ischemia.

## REFERENCES

1. Mirski MA, et al. Diagnosis and treatment of vascular air embolism. *Anesthesiology.* 2007;106(1):164–177.
2. Brull SJ, Prielipp RC. Vascular air embolism: a silent hazard to patient safety. *J Crit Care.* 2017;42:255–263.
3. Shaikh N, Ummunisa F. Acute management of vascular air embolism. *J Emerg Trauma Shock.* 2009;2(3):180–185.
4. Abcejo AS, et al. Urgent repositioning after venous air embolism during intracranial surgery in the seated position: a case series. *J Neurosurg Anesthesiol.* 2019;31(4):413–421.
5. McCarthy CJ, et al. Air embolism: diagnosis, clinical management and outcomes. *Diagnostics (Basel).* 2017;7(1):5.

# 67.

# CEREBRAL PROTECTION

*Roy Kim and Alaa Abd-Elsayed*

## INTRODUCTION

Researchers have been studying how to reduce perioperative brain injury for over 60 years.[1] Initially, we understood that ischemic or hypoxic insult was a result of metabolic demands outpacing the supply of nutrients (primarily oxygen). Although this does occur, research has demonstrated that this injury to brain tissue can stimulate active responses in the brain that can persist well after the substrate delivery has been restored to baseline levels. These responses include up regulation of transcription factors that can promote apoptosis, inhibition of protein synthesis, and neurogenesis.[2] Therefore, the idea of cerebral protection can extend further than simply altering the balance of supply and demand.

Cerebral metabolism can be divided into functional and cellular integrity components. The functional component involves about 60% of neuronal oxygen use and can be assessed by an electroencephalogram (EEG). The cellular integrity component consists of the remaining 40% and involves the oxygen utilized for protein synthesis and various other activities aimed toward maintaining cellular integrity. Anesthetic agents and hypothermia are two common strategies used to reduce oxygen consumption by the brain; increasing cerebral perfusion pressure (CPP) and oxygen delivery while depressing cerebral oxygen demand is a simplistic way to optimize cerebral protection.[3]

## ANESTHETIC CONSIDERATIONS

### PREOPERATIVE

It is important to determine the presence of any preoperative brain insult by completing a thorough physical examination. Any signs of acute brain injury from a stroke should be immediately involve a stroke specialist as the chance of reversibility is directly correlated with time since insult. Any chronic weakness or neuropathy should be noted to assess for any changes from baseline during the postoperative period. If there is any concern regarding possible acute brain injury, any elective surgeries should be postponed until a thorough evaluation can be carried out.

## INTRAOPERATIVE

Intraoperatively, important considerations if perioperative ischemic insult is likely include managing blood glucose levels, avoiding hyperthermia, establishing normocapnia, resisting use of steroids, and optimizing hemoglobin-oxygen saturation.[2] Regulation of anesthetic and physiologic parameters are discussed in material that follows.

### Temperature

Hypothermia effectively reduces both the functional and cellular integrity components of cerebral metabolism.[3] Studies have demonstrated deep hypothermia (18°C–22°C) is highly protective of cerebral tissue, and mild hypothermia (32°C–35°C) as seen in adults who survive out-of-hospital cardiac arrests also has beneficial cerebral protective effects.[3] Hyperthermia should absolutely be avoided since it increases cerebral metabolism and can worsen ischemic injury.

### Cerebral Perfusion Pressure, $O_2$, $CO_2$, Glucose Metabolism

The CPP is defined as mean arterial pressure minus intracranial pressure (CPP = MAP − ICP). In normal conditions, cerebral blood flow is autoregulated in a general range of 50–150 mm Hg. With chronic hypertension, this range can be shifted to the right. In general, CPP should be kept in a range of 60–70 mm Hg if clinically feasible.[3]

Producing hypocapnia via hyperventilation can lead to cerebral vasoconstriction, lowering cerebral blood flow and potentially worsening ischemic injury. Oxygen levels should be restored if ischemic injury has occurred; however, supranormal levels of oxygen in tissue can paradoxically lead to additional damage via free radical formation. High glucose levels during an ischemic condition can lead to intracellular acidosis, potentially exacerbating injury and worsening outcomes.[2]

### Anesthetic Agents

**Volatile Anesthetics**—Modern inhaled volatile anesthetics produce significant EEG suppression at clinically tolerated doses with rapid reversibility.[2] Although no human trials have been conducted with volatiles, animal studies have demonstrated protection from both focal and global ischemia, with sevoflurane showing long-term protection in one experimental model.[4]

**Other Anesthetics**—Barbiturates have been considered to be the "gold standard" for neuroprotective anesthetic agents (especially in focal ischemia), although their properties are supported by a single human study involving cardiopulmonary bypass patients. It is believed a dose-dependent reduction in the cerebral metabolic rate is the primary mechanism for cerebral protection.[3] Downsides of barbiturates are the long duration of action and potential cardiovascular instability.[2,3] Propofol has been shown to be neuroprotective in animal studies, but this has not been shown in humans.[3] Etomidate and lidocaine potentially could help lower the cerebral metabolic rate, but their efficacy has yet to be proven.

**Steroids:** Evidence for steroids is weak in terms of neuroprotection. Steroids such as dexamethasone can reduce swelling and edema in brain tissue, but its actual benefit for outcome is lacking.[2] In animal models, the increased glucose concentration that can result from steroid administration can potentially exacerbate injury from global ischemia.[5]

**Glucose Levels:** Hyperglycemia was proposed to cause harm to the brain, especially during time of ischemia.

## POSTOPERATIVE

Postoperatively, patients should be taken to an intensive care unit for monitoring and be followed by a neurologist if there are any concerns regarding neurological injury. A physical examination should be performed during the immediate postoperative phase to assess for new neurological deficits. The same considerations as above to manage a perioperative ischemic injury should continue to be utilized.

## REFERENCES

1. Bigelow WG, et al. Hypothermia; its possible role in cardiac surgery: an investigation of factors governing survival in dogs at low body temperatures. *Ann Surg.* 1950;132:849–866.
2. Fukuda S, Warner DS. Cerebral protection. *Br J Anaesth.* 2007; 99(1):10–17.
3. Grady RE. Neuroanesthesia: cerebral protection. In: Murray M, ed. Faust's Anesthesiology Review. Elsevier; 2015:307–309.
4. Pape M, et al. The long-term effect of sevoflurane on neuronal cell damage and expression of apoptotic factors after cerebral ischemia and reperfusion in rats. *Anesth Analg.* 2006;103:173–179.
5. Wass CT, et al. Insulin treatment of corticosteroid-associated hyperglycemia and its effect on outcome after forebrain ischemia in rats. *Anesthesiology.* 1996;84:644–651.

# 68.

# INTRACRANIAL ANEURYSMS AND ARTERIOVENOUS MALFORMATION

*Kenan Alkhalili and Ned F. Nasr*

## EPIDEMIOLOGY

The prevalence of intracranial saccular aneurysms is estimated to be 3%–5% irrespective of geographical location or ethnicity. The most frequent location for the aneurysms is the anterior communicating artery (35%); followed by the internal carotid artery (30%, including the carotid artery itself, the posterior communicating artery, and the ophthalmic artery); the middle cerebral artery (22%); and in the posterior circulation most commonly the basilar artery tip.[1]

The probability of rupture is mostly related to the size of the aneurysm. According to the International Study of Unruptured Intracranial Aneurysms, for patients with no history of subarachnoid hemorrhage (SAH) and aneurysms less than 7 mm in diameter, there were no ruptures among aneurysms in the anterior circulation, and the risk was 2.5% per year in those with aneurysms in the posterior circulation or posterior communicating artery. The risk of rupture increases in patients with a history of SAH, to 1.5% per year in the anterior circulation and 3.4% per year in the posterior circulation. History of SAH was not a predictor of rupture for aneurysms greater than 7 mm, and rupture risks were higher with larger aneurysms.[2]

Intracranial arteriovenous malformations (AVMs) occur and about 0.1% of the population, with the most common location supratentorial.[1] AVMs are estimated to cause 1%–2% of all strokes and are more commonly seen in younger population. The most common presentation of AVMs is intracranial hemorrhage, present in 40% to 60%, mostly intraparenchymal.

## PATHOPHYSIOLOGY

The pathophysiology of intracranial aneurysm is multifactorial and includes hemodynamic factors, lipid accumulation, arteriosclerosis, and smoking, as well as genetic predisposition.

The angioarchitecture of brain AVMs is composed of a central vascular nidus that is a conglomerate of arteries and veins without an intervening capillary network. Similarly, AVMs have multifactorial etiology, apparently both genetic mutation and angiogenic stimulation. AVMs can be symptomatic in three different ways: if they bleed; they are epileptogenic; and they have a "steal phenomenon," which is thought to be secondary to normal brain parenchyma relative ischemia, as blood bypasses the normal capillary bed.

## ANESTHESIA CONSIDERATIONS

### PREOPERATIVE

Preoperative assessment of modifiable and nonmodifiable risk factors of aneurysms/AVM rupture is important. Risk factors for an aneurysmal SAH include female sex, African American ethnicity, first-degree relative with SAH, low high-density lipoprotein cholesterol level, hypertension, obesity, alcohol abuse, and tobacco use.

Once the diagnosis of SAH is made, prompt treatment is recommended as the risk of rebleeding is highest within the first 12 hours of initial rupture. General recommendation for systolic blood pressure following rupture and prior to intervention is less than 160 mm Hg because of the risk of rebleeding, using a titratable drip such as nicardipine to control the systolic blood pressure is recommended.

### Management of Intracranial Aneurysm/AVMs

Cerebral aneurysm treatment can be performed through craniotomy and aneurysm clipping or endovascularly. The endovascular repair involves either coil embolization or flow-diverting techniques.

The management of AVMs is individualized based on a patient's age and medical comorbidities, as well as the natural history of the AVM dictated by its size, location, and venous drainage pattern. Interventional treatment is usually reserved for those with a history of rupture due to increased risk of rebleeding. In the ARUBA trial, the rate of symptomatic stroke and death was lower in the medical treatment group compared with the interventional group (10% vs. 31%).[3]

## Intracranial Aneurysm Rupture

Aneurysm rupture is a devastating event. Medical and neurological complications include elevated intracranial pressure, interventricular hemorrhage with subsequent hydrocephalus, seizures, hyponatremia, and delayed cerebral ischemia as a result of vasospasm.

To reduce the risk of rebleeding, intervention as early as feasible preferably, within 24 hours, is crucial. However, in patients who present within the vasospasm timeframe (typically 4 to 14 days), the timing of intervention remains controversial. The morbidity and mortality of ruptured aneurysms can be prognosticated by different radiological (modified Fisher grade) and clinical (Hunt and Hess classification) tools.

## Hunt and Hess Classification

Grade I: mild headache or nuchal rigidity

Grade II: moderate-to-severe headache, nuchal rigidity, cranial nerve palsy

Grade III: drowsiness, confusion, or mild focal deficit

Grade IV: stupor, hemiparesis, early decerebrate rigidity, vegetative disturbances

Grade V: deep coma, decerebrate rigidity, moribund

## INTRAOPERATIVE

Electrocardiographic changes are common with SAH and include ST segment changes, T-wave inversion, and prolonged QT interval with U waves. The anesthetic goal in the treatment of cerebral aneurysms and SAH is a balancing act of maintaining adequate cerebral perfusion pressure to prevent ischemia, while also controlling excessively high blood pressures to prevent aneurysmal rupture and further bleeding. Intraoperative aneurysm rupture can be catastrophic, and immediate intervention is critical (Figure 68.1). Placement of an arterial line preinduction enables tight hemodynamic control.

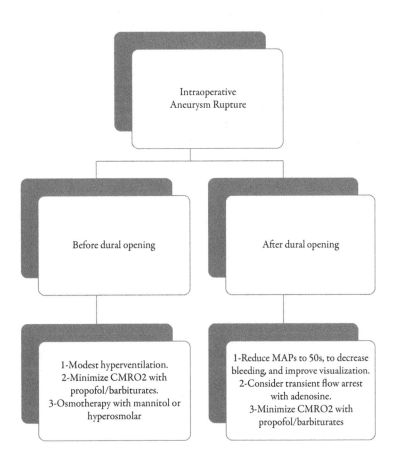

**Figure 68.1** Intraoperative aneurysm rupture management.

Generally, anesthetic considerations are the same for both the open and endovascular cerebral aneurysm obliteration. The need for brain relaxation is greater in clipping compared to coiling procedures.

Avoidance of movement is paramount and might necessitate general anesthesia in endovascular aneurysm surgery.

Intracranial pressure monitoring is beneficial for anesthesia induction. The external ventricular drain (EVD) can facilitate cerebrospinal fluid drainage for the purpose of reducing ICP for achieving brain relaxation. Monitoring cerebral function via cortical somatosensory evoked potentials and brainstem auditory evoked potentials can guide the application of temporary clipping (to facilitate dissection) and subsequent blood pressure adjustment if ischemia is detected. Alternately, temporary circulatory arrest with intravenous adenosine may be used to achieve the same goal. Hyperthermia should be avoided in brain surgeries. Therapeutic hypothermia (32°C–34°C), on the other hand, has not demonstrated beneficial long- or short-term neurologic outcomes in patient undergoing temporary clipping according to the Intraoperative Hypothermia for Aneurysm Surgery Trial.[4]

## CRITICAL CARE AND POSTOPERATIVE CONSIDERATIONS

Consideration of risk factors, hemodynamic stability, and close clinical monitoring during the vasospasm timeframe is of paramount importance. Vasospasm occurs in approximately 30% of patients with aneurysmal SAH.[5] To date it is unclear whether the type of treatment, surgical versus endovascular, affects the degree of vasospasm.

Conventionally, triple H therapy (hypertension, hemodilution, hypervolemia) has been proposed for prevention/treatment of vasospasm; however subsequent studies revealed that hypervolemia was not beneficial and might be harmful. Calcium channel blockers, in particular nimodipine, has been reported to reduce the risk of delayed cerebral ischemia.

The first line of management is hemodynamic augmentation by induced hypertension with vasopressors such as phenylephrine and norepinephrine, with subsequent assessment of clinical response. In the event of refractory medical treatment, a cerebral angiogram with intra-arterial administration of vasodilators such as nicardipine or verapamil, as well as balloon angioplasty for focal larger artery vasospasm, has been reported as effective treatment.

## REFERENCES

1. Brown RD Jr, et al. Unruptured intracranial aneurysms and arteriovenous malformations: frequency of intracranial hemorrhage and relationship of lesions. *J Neurosurg.* 1990;73(6):859–863.
2. Thompson BG, et al. Guidelines for the management of patients with unruptured intracranial aneurysms: a guideline for healthcare professionals from the American Heart Association/American Stroke Association. *Stroke.* 2015;46(8):2368–2400.
3. Mohr JP, et al. Medical management with or without interventional therapy for unruptured brain arteriovenous malformations (ARUBA): a multicentre, non-blinded, randomised trial. *Lancet.* 2014;383(9917):614–621.
4. Hindman BJ, et al. No association between intraoperative hypothermia or supplemental protective drug and neurologic outcomes in patients undergoing temporary clipping during cerebral aneurysm surgery: findings from the Intraoperative Hypothermia for Aneurysm Surgery Trial. *Anesthesiology.* 2010;112(1):86–101.
5. Suarez JI. Diagnosis and management of subarachnoid hemorrhage. *Continuum (Minneap Minn).* 2015;21(5 Neurocritical Care):1263–1287.

# INTERVENTIONAL NEURORADIOLOGY

*Kenan Alkhalili and Ned F. Nasr*

## INTRODUCTION

Interventional radiology is defined as the delivery of minimally invasive, targeted treatments, performed using imaging for guidance.

## ANESTHESIA CONSIDERATIONS

### PREOPERATIVE

Neurological assessment of the patient should be documented prior to the procedure, with specific attention the underlying pathology, Glasgow Coma Scale, and any prior deficits.

It is important to identify patients who may have contrast allergies or who are at high risk for contrast-induced nephropathy. Recent studies estimated all adverse reactions to iodinated contrast media range from 1% to 12%, with severe reactions comprising only 0.01% to 0.2% of total reactions.[1] Notation of preoperative hemodynamics is also important as hypertension and underlying neurovascular disease may alter the autoregulatory window to higher values. Hematological status is also pertinent due to the extensive use of antiplatelets/anticoagulation during interventional procedures.

### INTRAOPERATIVE

#### Choice of Anesthetic Technique

Both general anesthesia (GA) and sedation are used routinely in interventional radiology (IR) procedures; preference varies by center, case type, and surgeon.

#### General Anesthesia

General anesthesia goals revolve on patient maintaining immobility, improving fluoroscopic imaging quality, and facilitating safe device deployment. GA techniques should aim to maintain cerebral perfusion pressure, avoid extreme alteration of blood pressure, and enable rapid emergence for neurological assessment. A laryngeal mask airway may be used in some cases to avoid hemodynamic unpredictability with endotracheal intubation and extubation; however, the need to provide stillness and breath holds necessitates endotracheal intubation and neuromuscular blockade.

Total intravenous anesthesia (TIVA) or mixed anesthesia can be used. Patients seldom require 1.0 MAC (minimum alveolar concentration), as stimulation is minimal. Nitrous oxide is best avoided in angiography cases as it increases the risk of air emboli. Remifentanil on the other hand facilitates a smooth emergence without coughing or residual effects.

Ideally, all of these patients require urinary catheterization, as contrast dyes act as a diuretic.

#### Conscious Sedation

Pros of conscious sedation (CS) include the ability to perform intraoperative neurological testing and avoidance of the hemodynamic instability. Drawbacks of CS include lack of airway control, increased aspiration risk, and patient movement. Propofol and dexmedetomidine are frequently used for sedation in IR patients. Dexmedetomidine offers the advantage of decreased depressant effects on respiration and level of consciousness.

### ANESTHESIA FOR SPECIFIC INTERVENTIONAL NEURORADIOLOGY CASES

#### Endovascular Aneurysm Intervention

The goal endovascular aneurysm intervention is to optimize cerebral blood flow (CBF) while keeping intracranial pressure (ICP) under control. Propofol TIVA reduces CBF, ICP, and metabolic demand but often at the cost of a slower emergence compared with volatile agents. However, any volatile agent may result in increased CBF, cerebral blood volume, and ICP in patients with poor intracranial compliance. It is advised to use less than 1 MAC volatile agent as it limits significant cerebral hyperemia while maintaining the constrictive response to hypocapnia.

Additionally, ICP control can largely be accomplished with intermittent cerebrospinal fluid drainage from ventriculostomy tube.

## Anesthesia for Acute Ischemic Stroke

The endovascular treatment of acute ischemic stroke has advanced significantly, with notable transition from intra-arterial chemical thrombolysis to mechanical thrombectomy.[2] Techniques include stent retrievers, thrombus aspiration, and angioplasty. While the type of anesthesia is controversial, maintaining hypertension (systolic blood pressure [SBP] target 140 to 180 mm Hg) and preventing patient motion are the priorities. Postoperative SBP goal is usually dictated by the Thrombolysis in Cerebral Infarction scale.[3] Of note, GA is favored over CS in basilar artery manipulation cases due to the risk of loss of respiratory and consciousness control in this vascular territory.

## Cerebral Vasospasm Therapy

Cerebral vasospasm therapy typically occurs 4–14 days after the aneurysmal subarachnoid hemorrhage (SAH), with a peak incidence between 6 and 10 days. About 70% of SAH patients will demonstrate angiographic evidence of vasospasm; however, only 40% will have clinical symptoms.[4] For patients who are refractory to medical therapy, urgent endovascular intervention is performed and may often require more than one procedure. INR treatment options consist of vasodilator infusion as well as angioplasty. The usual SBP goal is 160 to 200 mm Hg range unless the patient's aneurysm remains unsecured.

### OTHER ANESTHESIA CONSIDERATIONS AND CHALLENGES

**Remote IR Suite Location:** Angiography suites are often remote from the main operating theater complex and easily available emergency support. Anesthetists should familiarize themselves with this isolated environment, the available equipment, and the procedure being undertaken and should ensure appropriate support is available.

**Anticoagulation:** Baseline activated clotting time (ACT) is obtained (normal range 90–130 seconds), and administration of intravenous heparin (70–100 U/kg) is often required to prevent vessel occlusion. The goal is to maintain a target of two to three times the baseline ACT. Aspirin and clopidogrel may also be required. Patients should be closely monitored for postprocedural bleeding.

**INR Complications Can Be Catastrophic:** In INR complications, which can be catastrophic, the anesthesiologist must (1) immediately ensure a secure airway and (2) assess whether the crisis is ischemic versus hemorrhagic.

Deliberate hypertension should be considered in case of ischemic complications, and a mean blood pressure increase of up to 40% above baseline may be pharmacologically induced in an attempt to increase CBF through collaterals. Meanwhile, the interventionist attempts to alleviate the occlusion through the aforementioned techniques. Deliberate hypotension while maintaining cerebral perfusion pressure greater than 60 is preserved for hemorrhagic complications. Other interventions include anticoagulation/antiplatelet reversal, ventriculostomy placement, and hyperosmolar therapy.

All patients are at risk of developing acute contrast-induced nephropathy. Risk factors include diabetes mellitus, high dose of contrast, volume depletion, coadministration of nephrotoxic medications, and preexisting renal disease. Limiting the dose of contrast agent and optimal hydration reduce the risk of acute kidney injury.

**Radiation Exposure:** Radiation exposure should be as low as reasonably achievable. All personnel working in the room should wear protective lead aprons and thyroid shields throughout the procedure.

## POSTOPERATIVE

Patients should be cared for in a high-dependency unit unless their neurological condition dictates admission to intensive care. Patients should remain supine until the femoral sheath is removed.

Maintenance of hydration is important as there can be a large osmotic diuresis due to hyperosmolar contrast used during the procedure. Continuous neurological observation should be made to identify any new neurological deficit and appropriate intervention undertaken.

## REFERENCES

1. Bottinor W, al. Adverse reactions to iodinated contrast media. *Int J Angiol*. 2013;22(3):149–154.
2. Alkhalili K, et al. Endovascular intervention for acute ischemic stroke in light of recent trials. *Sci World J*. 2014;2014:429549.
3. Pikija S, al. Higher blood pressure during endovascular thrombectomy in anterior circulation stroke is associated with better outcomes. *J Stroke*. 2018;20(3):373–384.
4. Dabus G, Nogueira RG. Current options for the management of aneurysmal subarachnoid hemorrhage-induced cerebral vasospasm: a comprehensive review of the literature. *Interv Neurol*. 2013;2(1):30–51.

# 70.

# PITUITARY ADENOMAS

*Benjamin B. G. Mori and Ned F. Nasr*

## INTRODUCTION

Pituitary adenomas are benign tumors of the pituitary gland, representing 10%–20% of intracranial neoplasms. Most adenomas (65%–70%) secrete an excess amount of hormone, including prolactin, growth hormone (GH), corticotropin (ACTH, adrenocorticotropin hormone), thyroid-stimulating hormone (TSH), while the remainder are clinically nonfunctioning and may result in hormone hyposecretion due to compression of the gland. Roughly half are classified as microadenomas (<1 cm) and are often found incidentally on head imaging. Macroademonas (≥1 cm) are the most common cause of hypopituitarism.[1]

## CLINICAL FEATURES

Pituitary adenomas can be asymptomatic, presenting with neurological symptoms related to mass effect and/or clinical features of pituitary hormone over- or undersecretion.[1] Nonfunctional adenomas usually present with altered vision (e.g., bitemporal hemianopsia, reduced visual acuity) due to compression of the optic chiasm. Other mass effect symptoms include headache, diplopia, cerebral spinal fluid (CSF) rhinorrhea, and Parinaud syndrome (i.e., paralysis of upward conjugate gaze). Compression of the gland itself can result in a constellation of symptoms relating to pituitary hormone deficiencies. The most common pituitary hormone deficiencies are of gonadotropins, resulting in hypogonadism.[1,2]

Functional adenomas often present with signs related to supraphysiologic levels of pituitary hormone(s). Thyrotroph adenomas, due to an oversecretion of TSH, result in hyperthyroidism. ACTH-secreting corticotroph adenomas result in Cushing disease. Hyperprolactinemia from lactotroph adenomas can lead to hypogonadism. Somatotroph adenomas can cause acromegaly due to increased GH secretion.[2]

## DIAGNOSIS

When a sellar mass is suspected, radiographic and laboratory testing is indicated. Magnetic resonance imaging (MRI) with gadolinium is the best imaging modality.[1] Laboratory-based evaluation of the hypothalamic-pituitary axis should be conducted whenever a pituitary mass is recognized.[1,2] Hormone hypersecretion can only be caused by adenomas, in contrast to hyperplasia, craniopharyngiomas, or carcinomas. Consequently, hormone hypersecretion identifies the mass as an adenoma and delineates its cell type composition.[2] Serum levels of prolactin, insulinlike growth factor 1 (IGF-1), ACTH, and 24-hour urinary free cortisol level should be measured. LH, FSH, thyroxine, and TSH levels should be tested when functional gonadotroph/thyrotroph adenomas are suspected.[1] Evaluation of hormone deficiency should be undertaken in all patients with macroadenomas.[1,2]

## TREATMENT

The transsphenoidal pituitary resection (TPR) is the mainstay of treatment for most adenomas. After surgery, patients should be monitored regularly, via serial MRI and hormonally, for tumor recurrence. Lifelong management of hormone deficiencies is often required. Radiation therapy is typically reserved for patients with residual tissue after surgery.[1] Medical therapy is used as adjunct therapy after a failed TPR.[2]

## ANESTHETIC CONSIDERATIONS

### PREOPERATIVE

Central hypothyroidism should be treated with levothyroxine preoperatively, and those patients with secondary adrenal insufficiency may require preoperative

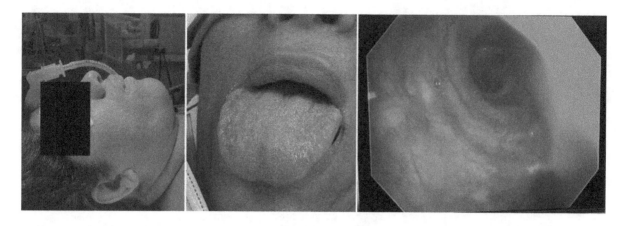

**Figure 70.1** The image on the left shows the coarse facial features and prognathic jaw of an acromegalic patient. The center image shows macroglossia, a feature characteristic of acromegaly. The image on the far right shows hypertrophy of laryngeal soft tissue and engorged tracheal vasculature, which may result in difficulty with laryngoscopy and intubation in these patients. Note that the tumor can cause palsies of cranial nerves III, IV, and VI (Figure 70.2).

stress dose steroids. Preoperative complete blood count (CBC) and blood typing with antibody screening should be obtained. Although significant bleeding is rare with TPR, there is the potential for catastrophic hemorrhage with cavernous sinus or carotid artery injury. In some cases, an anesthesiologist may place a lumbar CSF drain to improve surgical exposure and/or reduce CSF pressure.[3]

Patients with acromegaly are predisposed to both cardiomyopathy and obstructive sleep apnea (OSA). Preoperative electrocardiography and echocardiography are important tools for evaluating these patients. For those with OSA, sedative premedication should not be administered routinely.[3]

Difficult intubation incidence is reported to be between 10% and 30% in acromegalic patients, and Mallampati grade may not be predictive of the interior airway. Excess GH/IGF-1 stimulates hypertrophy of pharyngeal and laryngeal soft tissue, as demonstrated in Figure 70.1. Figure 70.2 shows the pituitary anatomy. Imaging and indirect laryngoscopy can used to better assess the airway preoperatively.

Contingency airway management plans should be made so, in case one plan fails, the alternative plan can be executed rapidly. In most cases, a flexible bronchoscope or a videolaryngoscope should be used. An awake fiber-optic intubation is a good strategy in a cooperative patient.[3]

### INTRAOPERATIVE

General anesthesia is required for all TPRs. The procedure is often performed endoscopically in a head-up position, with all its associated complications, including poor airway access, bleeding into the pharynx, and venous air embolism. Head extension during positioning can result in inadvertent endotracheal cuff herniation/extubation, and tissue enlargement in acromegaly can increase the risk of position-related neuropathies.[3]

The standard American Society of Anesthesiologists' monitors should be used. An arterial line is usually acceptable; however, many acromegalic patients have

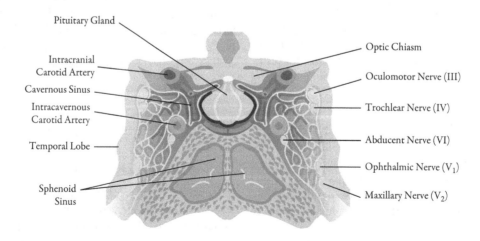

**Figure 70.2** Anatomy of the pituitary gland.

compromised collateral circulation between the radial and ulnar arteries secondary to soft tissue overgrowth around the wrist.[3] Cannulation of the dorsalis pedis artery or femoral artery may be a better alternative.

A variety of techniques can be used for induction and maintenance of anesthesia. Epinephrine-containing solutions are often applied to the nasal mucosa before incision to minimize bleeding, which can result in significant hypertension and arrhythmias. Generally, TPR is not particularly stimulating, except for during Mayfield pinning and drilling of the sphenoid bone. During these steps, transient deepening of anesthesia may be required. The procedure involves delicate dissection, where patient movement can result in cavernous sinus or internal carotid artery injury.[4] In the event of severe hemorrhage, conversion to open craniotomy may be needed.[4]

Intraoperative MRI may be used to achieve near-complete resection. If MRI confirms sufficient resection, the patient should be immediately awakened to facilitate a rapid neurologic examination. Emergence should, however, be smooth enough to avoid coughing, straining, and hypertension. At the end of surgery, the throat pack should be removed and the oropharynx suctioned for accumulated blood. The physiologic response to extubation can be mitigated with intravenous lidocaine, opioids, or a no-touch technique on awakening.[4]

## POSTOPERATIVE

Transsphenoidal pituitary resection is associated with low-to-moderate postoperative pain. Preoperative acetaminophen in conjunction with small doses of intraoperative opioids is usually sufficient. A multimodal postoperative nausea and vomiting prophylaxis strategy should be used. Postoperative retching/vomiting can increase venous pressure, cause epistaxis, disrupt the surgical wound, and increase the risk of CSF leak and meningitis.[4] Patients with acromegaly are at increased risk for postoperative airway obstruction and OSA.[3] Patients should be closely monitored in the postoperative period and judicious use of opioids and other respiratory depressant agents should be exercised.[4]

Disorders of sodium balance are common, usually occurring between postoperative days 5 to 9.[5] The syndrome

*Table 70.1* COMPARING AND CONTRASTING THE CLINICAL PRESENTATIONS OF CSW AND SIADH

|  | CSW | SIADH |
|---|---|---|
| Volume status | Hypovolemia | Euvolemia/hypervolemia |
| Serum Na concentration | ↓ | ↓ |
| Urine Na concentration | ↑ | ↑ |
| Urine output | ↑ | Normal |
| Pathophysiology | ↑Na and water secretion | Water retention due to ↑ antidiuretic hormone |
| Management | Fluid and sodium supplementation | Fluid restriction |

Watch for any cranial nerve palsies related to surgery (Figure 70.2).

Source: Table adapted from Oh JY, Shin JI. Syndrome of inappropriate antidiuretic hormone secretion and cerebral/renal salt wasting syndrome: similarities and differences. Front Pediatr. 2015;2:146.

of inappropriate antidiuretic hormone secretion (SIADH) is the primary cause of hyponatremia following TPR, followed by cerebral/renal salt wasting syndrome (CSW) and overadministration of desmopressin. See Table 70.1 comparing and contrasting the presentation of SIADH and CSW. SIADH accounts for about 90% of cases of severe hyponatremia (Na < 125 mEq/L) following surgery.[5]

## REFERENCES

1. Molitch ME. Diagnosis and treatment of pituitary adenomas: a review. *JAMA*. 2017;317(5):516–524.
2. Varlamov EV, et al. Functioning pituitary adenomas—current treatment options and emerging medical therapies. *Eur Endocrinol*. 2019;15(1):30–40.
3. Nemergut EC, Zuo Z. Airway management in patients with pituitary disease: a review of 746 patients. *J Neurosurg Anesthesiol*. 2006;18:73.
4. Bajwa SS, Bajwa SK. Anesthesia and intensive care implications for pituitary surgery: recent trends and advancements. *Indian J Endocrinol Metab*. 2011; 15(suppl 3): S224–S232.
5. Barber SM, et al. Incidence, etiology and outcomes of hyponatremia after transsphenoidal surgery: experience with 344 consecutive patients at a single tertiary center. *J Clin Med*. 2014; 3(4):1199–1219.

# 71.

# FLUID MANAGEMENT IN NEUROSURGERY

*Rotem Naftalovich and Daniel Denis*

## FLUID PHYSIOLOGY

Starling's law, $dV/dt = Kf((Pc - Pt) - \sigma(\pi c - \pi t))$, states that there are four principle forces regulating fluid exchange through the *capillaries*.[1] The intravascular hydrostatic pressure (Pc) and the interstitial oncotic pressure ($\pi t$) draw water from the intravascular space into the interstitial space, whereas the intravascular oncotic pressure ($\pi c$) and interstitial hydrostatic pressure (Pt) draw water from the interstitial space into the intravascular space. In actuality, the mechanism of edema formation is shaped by the absorbent gel nature of the interstitium, which causes it to capture water. This captured gel water does not contribute to lowering the osmotic pressure in the interstitium since the osmotic pressure does not easily change until the gel is saturated by water movement.[1]

In the peripheral tissues, water, oxygen, carbon dioxide, and low molecular weight (LMW) solutes such as electrolytes and sugars move freely across the capillary membrane. Therefore, no **osmotic gradient** is able to be established, and the administration of crystalloid solutions will not affect net movement of water to a significant degree. The administration of high molecular weight (HMW) colloids, such as albumin and hetastarch, can create an oncotic gradient that will drive fluid movement as per the **Starling equation**.[2]

In the central nervous system, the blood-brain barrier (BBB) is composed of endothelial cells with tight junctions approximately 1/10th the size of those in peripheral tissues. While water, oxygen, and carbon dioxide are able to freely move across the BBB, both LMW and HMW molecules are unable to do so. As a result, an osmotic gradient exists between the intravascular space and the interstitial space, which is a more predominant consideration with respect to water movement across an intact BBB.[2] Cerebral injury or inflammation may disrupt the BBB and allow passage of both LMW and HMW solutes.

## FLUID MANAGEMENT GOALS

Recall that cerebral perfusion pressure (CPP) is the difference between the mean arteriolar pressure (MAP) and the intracranial pressure (ICP). The goal of optimal fluid management in the neurosurgical patient is **euvolemia**, to minimize cerebral edema while preserving CPP and intravascular volume.[3] The traditional teaching of fluid management in neuroanesthesia was "keeping the patient dry" to reduce cerebral edema.[3] However, significant fluid restriction and hypotension can lead to increased ICP.[4] Intravenous fluids should be given to sufficiently maintain cardiac output and should not be withheld in the presence of cardiovascular instability. This may be guided by goal-directed fluid management, including pulse pressure variation and esophageal Doppler.

## CRYSTALLOIDS

A **crystalloid** is any solution that does not contain any HMW product and has an oncotic pressure of 0. Crystalloids can be made hypo-osmolar, hyperosmolar, or iso-osmolar by the addition of electrolytes or LMW solutes (Table 71.1).

Hypo-osmolar crystalloids have an osmolarity less than human plasma (<285 mOsm/L) and are typically avoided in the neurosurgical patient. Due to the BBB and the osmotic gradient, hypo-osmolar solutions will create the preferential movement of water from the intravascular space into the interstitial space and worsen cerebral edema.

Hyperosmolar crystalloids have an osmolarity greater than human plasma (>285 mOsm/L) and create an osmotic gradient favoring water movement from the interstitial space into the vasculature. They include mannitol and hypertonic saline. These can be used to treat cerebral edema via a decrease in cerebral water content and subsequently a decrease in ICP. Rapid correction of hyponatremia, greater than 0.5 mEq/L/h, can result in central pontine myelinolysis and should be avoided.

Iso-osmolar crystalloids have an osmolarity approaching human plasma (~285 mOsm/L) and therefore do not create significant osmotic gradients between the intervascular and interstitial space. These are the mainstay of volume repletion and maintenance fluid in the neurosurgical patient.

*Table 71.1* COMPARISON OF COMMON CRYSTALLOIDS AND COLLOIDS

| FLUID | OSMOLARITY (MOSM/L) | ONCOTIC PRESSURE (MM HG) | NA+ | CL- | CA2+ | K+ | DEXTROSE | OTHER |
|---|---|---|---|---|---|---|---|---|
| 0.9% saline | 308 | 0 | 154 | 154 | — | — | — | — |
| 3% saline | 1026 | 0 | 513 | 513 | — | — | — | — |
| 0.45% saline | 154 | 0 | 77 | 77 | — | — | — | — |
| Lactated Ringers (LR) | 273 | 0 | 130 | 109 | 3 | 4 | – | Lactate 28 |
| D5 LR | 525 | 0 | 130 | 109 | 3 | 4 | 50 g/100 mL | Lactate 28 |
| D5 0.45% saline | 406 | 0 | 77 | 77 | — | — | 50 g/100 mL | — |
| Plasmalyte | 294 | 0 | 140 | 98 | 3 | 5 | — | Acetate 27, gluconate 23 |
| 20% mannitol | 1098 | 0 | — | — | — | — | — | Mannitol 20 g/100 mL |
| Hetastarch 6% | 310 | 31 | 154 | 154 | — | — | — | Hetastarch 6 g/100 mL |
| Albumin 5% | 290 | 19 | 130–160 | 130–160 | — | — | — | Albumin 50 |

Excessive administration of 0.9% normal saline can lead to hyperchloremic metabolic acidosis and renal dysfunction.

Mannitol is a six-carbon sugar alcohol and is the most common hyperosmolar crystalloid given to neurosurgical patients (dose **0.25–1 g/kg**) to decrease cerebral swelling and improve surgical exposure.[2] Mannitol is relatively contraindicated in patients with congestive heart failure since the sudden increase in intravascular volume may be poorly tolerated. It is also contraindicated in patients with end-stage renal disease. Mannitol can cause hyponatremia and hyperkalemia. Its administration usually leads to a transient increase in blood pressure from the initial increased intravascular volume, which is then followed by a decrease in blood pressure from diuresis. A similar diuresis can also occur with excessive hyperglycemia.

Glucose-containing solutions are typically avoided in neurosurgical patients as hyperglycemia worsens cerebral recovery, leading to worse neurological outcomes in traumatic brain injury (TBI), subarachnoid hemorrhage (SAH), intracerebral hemorrhage, and ischemic stroke.[3] Glucose is also rapidly metabolized and in the process leaves free water which contributes to worsening cerebral edema.

## COLLOIDS

A **colloid** is a solution that contains HMW components (molecular weight > 30,000 Daltons) that do not cross capillary membranes or the BBB and have an effective oncotic pressure. They provide a greater degree of intravascular volume expansion. Hetastarches and dextran are associated with coagulopathies and have grown out of favor. Human albumin has not been widely studied in the neurosurgical population. In the disrupted BBB, there is a theoretical risk of colloid extravasation into the interstitial space with worsening of cerebral edema.

## SPECIFIC CLINICAL SCENARIOS

Patients with TBI often present with concomitant subdural or epidural hemorrhage. Because the cranium is a fixed cavity, even small increases in blood volume cause rapid increases in ICP and decreased CPP. The goal of fluid management should be to preserve MAP while decreasing ICP.[3] Active bleeding should be replaced with equal ratios of red blood cells to fresh frozen plasma to platelets. Albumin is typically avoided in TBI patients as studies have shown increased mortality when compared to crystalloid resuscitation.[5] There is concern that albumin can pass a compromised BBB, as can occur with TBI, and thereby have a reversed effect than intended.

Subarachnoid hemorrhage is frequently complicated by cerebral vasospasm, leading to ischemia. Treatment consists of nimodipine (likely more for neuroprotection) and "triple H" therapy—hypervolemia, hypertension, and hemodilution. The idea is to improve perfusion pressure and cerebral blood flow to ischemic regions. Efficacy of the traditional triple H therapy has been questioned due to hypervolemia-related side effects of pulmonary edema, myocardial ischemia (from increased afterload), and hyponatremia.[3] Patients refractory to medical management can undergo balloon angioplasty and direct intra-arterial injection of verapamil.

## REFERENCES

1. Iijima T. Complexity of blood volume control system and its implications in perioperative fluid management. *J Anesth.* 2009;23(4): 534–542.
2. Vagnerova K, Rusa R. Fluid management during craniotomy. In Cottrell JE, Patel P (eds.) *Cottrell and Patel's Neuroanesthesia.* Edinburgh, Scotland: Elsevier; 2017:152–165.
3. Bebawy J, Pasternak J. Anesthesia for neurosurgery. In Barash PG, et al. (eds.) *Clinical Anesthesia.* Philadelphia, PA: Wolters Kluwer; 2017:1015–1017.
4. Tommasino C. Fluids and the neurosurgical patient. *Anesthesiol Clin North Am.* 2002:20(2):329–346.
5. SAFE Study Investigators. Saline or albumin for fluid resuscitation in patients with traumatic brain injury. *N Engl J Med.* 2007:357(9), 874–884.

# 72.

# SPINAL FLUID DRAINAGE

*Deepak Agarwal and Lovkesh L. Arora*

## INTRODUCTION

Spinal fluid drainage is a procedure with growing evidence especially for thoracoabdominal aorta aneurysm or dissection surgery due to the neuroprotection it offers when combined with other neuroprotective techniques. It has also been used successfully in other pathological conditions, such as for the control of intracranial hypertension, aneurysmal subarachnoid hemorrhage; for its predictive value in shunting normal pressure hydrocephalus (NPH); for management of cerebrospinal fluid (CSF) leak; for intraoperative brain relaxation; and even for the management of bacterial meningitis and ventriculitis when used early in the course of treatment. Spinal fluid drainage comes with its own set of contraindications and complications that should be considered when making the decision to place them.

## INDICATIONS

**Neuroprotection for Thoracoabdominal Aorta Surgery:** Intrathecal CSF pressure monitoring with CSF drainage is frequently employed to maintain low CSF pressure (i.e., 8 to 10 mm Hg) to achieve optimal spinal cord protection. The rationale for CSF drainage involves decreasing pressure in the subarachnoid space to reduce resistance to blood flow through the collateral network of small vessels within the spinal canal, thereby improving perfusion to the spinal cord. Spinal Cord Perfusion Pressure (SCPP) = Mean arterial pressure (MAP) − Cerebrospinal fluid Pressure (CSFP or central venous pressure [CVP; whichever is greater]).[1]

**Prevention of Cerebral Vasospasm After Aneurysmal Subarachnoid Hemorrhage:** Cerebral vasospasm (CVS) continues to be A major complication after aneurysmal subarachnoid hemorrhage. Subarachnoid blood and its degradation products mostly contribute to CVS. Lumbar drainage of CSF is thought to promote circulation of newly produced CSF and blood cells from the ventricles through the subarachnoid space and prevent stasis of blood cells within the subarachnoid cistern, hence reducing the risk of vasospasm. Although it's use for this indication is still controversial as there is no conclusive evidence with existing data.[2]

**Control of Intracranial Hypertension:** In cases of uncontrolled intracranial hypertension, an intracranial or lumbar drain may be placed to remove CSF and monitor intracranial pressure. The choice to do either is based on feasibility of placement and, in the case of lumbar drain, brain imaging showing communication for CSF circulation. Although controversial, there have been studies showing promising results. There is definitely a need for randomized clinical trials concerning this indication.

**Predictive Value in Shunting Normal Pressure Hydrocephalus:** NPH refers to a condition of pathologically enlarged ventricular size with normal opening pressures on lumbar puncture. In patients with clinical and magnetic resonance imaging features suggestive of NPH, some institutions use either a one-time lumbar tap test or an indwelling lumbar drain trial to help identify patients likely to respond to shunt placement. The sensitivity and specificity of these tests are uncertain. Clinical improvement after continuous CSF drainage for a period of 3–5 days is a sensitive predictor for patients who might respond well to shunting with a high positive predictive value but a low negative predictive value with a high rate of false negatives.[3]

**Management of CSF leak:** CSF rhinorrhea can result from skull or nasal fractures, intracranial surgery, and inferior extension of sellar masses. Also, not extensively studied but has been tried as an in-between procedure for patient's not responding to conservative management strategies (bed rest, elevation of head, sinus precautions, prophylactic antibiotics) and in whom we want to avoid a surgical repair.

## THE PROCEDURE

The procedure for spinal fluid drainage is similar to the placement of a spinal anesthetic and can be performed in the sitting or the lateral decubitus position. Fluoroscopy can also be used to help place the catheter. A 20-gauge needle is used for a one-time spinal tap, but a bigger 14-gauge needle is used to access the intrathecal space to place the spinal drain catheter. The amount of catheter left in the intrathecal space varies between institutions and providers and can range from 12 to 20 cm. The midline approach is preferred to avoid hitting the epidural veins, which tend to run in the paramedian position. The catheter should be fixed meticulously, and strict sterile technique should be used during placement.[1]

## COMPLICATIONS

The complications can be divided into complications related to needle insertion, complications associated with the presence of an indwelling catheter in the intrathecal space, and complications associated with spinal fluid drainage.

**Complications Related to Needle Insertion:** Direct spinal cord or nerve root injuries occur from needle placement (avoided/minimized by insertion below the lower limit of the spinal cord L3/L4, L4/L5) or subsequent neuraxial hematoma (avoided/minimized by ensuring appropriate time gap between blood thinner use/administration and placement of catheter, decreasing placement attempts).

**Complications Associated With the Presence of an Indwelling Catheter in the Intrathecal Space:** Meningitis (avoided/minimized using sterile placement technique, including sterile technique while management of the drain) is associated with the presence of the indwelling catheter in the intrathecal space.

**Complications Associated With Spinal Fluid Drainage:** Symptomatic intracranial hypotension could present with a headache, cranial nerve palsy (most commonly abducens), and intracranial hemorrhage due to traction and resulting tear in bridging veins. The recommended maximum drainage is 10 mL/h.

## CONTRAINDICATIONS

The only absolute contraindication to spinal fluid drainage would be patient refusal. Caution should be used when making the decision to place a lumbar drain in the following conditions:

- Thrombocytopenia or other bleeding diathesis, including ongoing anticoagulant therapy (follow American Society of Regional Anesthesia and Pain Medicine guidelines)
- Suspected spinal epidural abscess or infection of the skin at the site of needle entry due to fear of seeding the intrathecal space and causing meningitis
- Noncommunicating hydrocephalus
- In the presence of large intracranial mass lesions

## REFERENCES

1. Christine AF, et al. Lumbar cerebrospinal fluid drainage for thoracoabdominal aortic surgery. *Anesth Analg.* 2010;111(1):46–58.
2. Li G, et al. Some cool considerations of external lumbar drainage during its widespread application in neurosurgical practice: a long way to go. *Chin Neurosurg J.* 2016;2:14.
3. Chen IH, et al. Effectiveness of shunting in patients with normal pressure hydrocephalus predicted by temporary, controlled-resistance, continuous lumbar drainage: a pilot study. *J Neurol Neurosurg Psychiatry.* 1994;57(11):1430.

# 73.

# STEREOTACTIC AND GAMMA-KNIFE TECHNIQUES, DEEP BRAIN STIMULATOR PLACEMENT, INTRAOPERATIVE WAKE-UP TECHNIQUES

*Roy Kim and Alaa Abd-Elsayed*

## STEREOTACTIC AND GAMMA-KNIFE TECHNIQUES

Stereotactic radiosurgery is most often done by means of gamma knife, and this technique of using highly focused radiation beams to selectively ablate localized lesions of the brain has advanced greatly since first conducted in 1958. This technique has the advantage of avoiding nearby healthy tissue to a greater extent than traditional methods. The gamma knife is suitable for treatment of deep and surgically inaccessible intracranial lesions; this technique can also be used to treat pain syndromes (trigeminal neuralgia), arteriovenous malformations, and other functional disorders.

Gamma knife radiosurgery involves application of a stereotactic head frame, followed by imaging (usually computed tomography or magnetic resonance imaging) of the head to define the lesions. Using the data from the images, radiation oncologists finalize a treatment protocol by calculating the brain lesion in three dimensions. Radiation beams are then positioned stereotactically, and the radiation dose is delivered. Since this is minimally invasive and does not involve a surgical incision, use of the gamma knife is considered relatively safe and does not require a significant hospital stay. However, common complications include headaches, nausea/vomiting, delayed seizures, and minor bleeding.[1]

## ANESTHETIC CONSIDERATIONS

A typical stereotactic radiosurgery procedure can take six to ten hours and can take place in a remote location due to the special equipment required, often posing special challenges for the anesthesiologist. The primary anesthetic goal is to avoid patient movement during the treatment, and general anesthesia is the preferred technique. Generally, for adults and older children, utilizing local anesthetic alone is sufficient during placement of the stereotactic frame.

Occasionally, if an endotracheal intubation is performed, inadvertent extubation is a risk during application of the head frame. Preoperative evaluation should document baseline neurological status, and the goal after the procedure is a quick wake-up to assess postoperative neurological status. The remaining challenges include common out-of–operating room issues, such as equipment failure, adequate supply of portable oxygen, availability of emergency equipment, and availability of staff if an emergency arises.[1]

## DEEP BRAIN STIMULATOR PLACEMENT

Deep brain stimulation (DBS) was first introduced in the late 1980s and is electrode implantation surgery into specific areas of the basal ganglia, often performed for Parkinson's disease. DBS is reversible, adjustable, and able to be safely placed bilaterally; it has been increasingly used for intractable epilepsy, chronic pain, and other movement disorders. DBS incorporates four components: intracranial electrodes (placed surgically inside brain), a plastic ring and cap seated onto a burr hole to fix the electrodes in place, an extension cable, and a pulse generator (often implanted into the chest or abdomen).

Deep brain stimulation surgery is best performed by an experienced neurosurgeon who has expertise in stereotactic and functional neurosurgery. There is typically coordination with a team of providers, including a neurologist, neuropsychologist, and neurophysiologist. The entire procedure can be completed on the same day or in a two-stage procedure (internalization of electrodes and generator on different days, typically a couple of days or up to 2 weeks after the first procedure). Electrode placement is often tested intraoperatively to ensure correct placement, and radiologic confirmation is performed postoperatively to check the final position of the leads and to rule out hemorrhage and pneumocephalus.[2] Patient noncompliance, debilitating medical conditions, dementia, and extensive brain atrophy are contraindications for DBS surgery.[3]

## ANESTHETIC CONSIDERATIONS

Anesthetic considerations include assessing and documenting any neurological findings and evaluating comorbidities prior to the surgery. Discuss medications used as some medications can affect intraoperative mapping. Careful patient selection is important, as greater than 30% failure rate has been seen due to inappropriate indications for surgery. A thorough airway assessment is important, and the patient should be assessed for ability to cooperate during the awake part of the surgery.

Propofol is the most commonly used anesthetic drug for sedation and general anesthesia during DBS insertion.[2] Benzodiazepines, opioids, and other sedative medications are ideally avoided as they interfere with cooperation during surgery and interpretation of tremor preoperatively.

Most medical centers have developed their own "optimal" regimen for anesthesia during DBS placement, which ranges from local anesthesia, monitored anesthesia care, and general anesthesia using an asleep-awake-asleep technique. Most centers will avoid general anesthesia since an awake technique carries advantages during the mapping phase, but general anesthesia may be required in certain patient populations (those with severe sleep apnea, uncontrolled anxiety, etc.).

Placement of DBS has the potential for adverse outcomes during the perioperative period. One study found intraprocedure complications occurred in 12%–16% of patients, with intracranial hemorrhage and seizure the two most common neurological complications.[2] Seizures have been reported to occur in 0.5%–4.5% of patients, often during stimulation testing; these are generally focal and self-limited. With any nonsecure airway technique, airway compromise is an important consideration, especially with a stereotactic head frame making airway access limited in an emergent situation. One study showed intraoperative respiratory complications occurring in 1.6%–2.2% of patients. Other common events include hypertension (due to patient distress or poor perioperative control) and less frequently venous air embolism (higher risk of semisitting position and occurs during creation of burr hole).[2]

## INTRAOPERATIVE WAKE-UP TECHNIQUES

The intraoperative wake-up test is one of several monitoring methods used to evaluate brain and/or spinal cord function during general anesthesia; it is still considered the gold standard for assessing spinal cord function during spinal surgery. To apply intraoperative wake-up tests, the anesthetic regimen must enable rapid patient recovery, an immediate neurological examination, and adequate postoperative amnesia. Patient compliance is key, and understanding the risks of waking up a patient during a surgical case can help prevent and reduce complications.

The anesthesia provider must recognize that complications of intraoperative wake-up are often due to significant patient movement. This can lead to injury to the patient, extubation, and dislodgement of monitors or lines. Although awareness is possible, it is not considered an adverse event and is fortunately a rare occurrence. All these risks should be discussed with the patient prior to the surgery, and the patient should understand that the wake-up period is very brief.[4]

There are various techniques that have been described to facilitate quick patient recovery. Muscle relaxation should be avoided after intubation to allow the patient to respond quickly to commands and assess motor function. Various techniques include propofol or dexmedetomidine infusion with or without a short-acting opioid such as remifentanil or sufentanil; utilizing a fast-acting volatile agent such as desflurane has also been described in the literature. One study demonstrated that the anesthetic regimen with desflurane and remifentanil allowed faster awakening during and after spinal surgery compared with a total intravenous anesthetic technique utilizing propofol and remifentanil.[4] Regardless of which technique is utilized, the anesthesiologist should have a goal of fast emergence and immediate neurological evaluation, all while preventing potential complications from a wake-up test such as patient injury, extubation, and patient recall. Working together with the surgeon will help facilitate this portion of the surgery and optimize outcomes.

## REFERENCES

1. Berg RJ, et al. Anesthetic considerations for gamma knife stereotactic radiosurgery in patients with intracranial lesions. *Contemp Neurosurg.* 2011;33(6):4.
2. Chakrabarti R, et al. Anesthetic challenges for deep brain stimulation: a systematic approach. *N Am J Med Sci.* 2014;6(8):359–369.
3. Deiner S, Hagen J. Parkinson's disease and deep brain stimulator placement. *Anesthesiology Clin.* 2009;27:391–415.
4. Grottke O, et al. Intraoperative wake-up test and postoperative emergence in patients undergoing spinal surgery: a comparison of intravenous and inhaled anesthetic techniques using short-acting anesthetics. *Anesth Analg.* 2004;99(5):1521–1527.

# 74.

# VENTRICULOSTOMY

*Roy Kim and Alaa Abd-Elsayed*

## INTRODUCTION

Conventional shunt surgery for patients with noncommunicating hydrocephalus has been replaced by endoscopic third ventriculostomy (ETV), as it is faster, simpler, and avoids major brain retraction or dissection.[1–3] Endoscopic procedures are also becoming more frequent in the pediatric population.[4] Due to its unique surgical technique, ETV can cause various perioperative complications, with reported rates ranging from 5% to 30% and operative mortality between 0% and 1%.[3]

Endoscopic third ventriculostomy involves establishing a connection between the third ventricle and prepontine subarachnoid space, allowing the flow of cerebrospinal fluid (CSF) to bypass the aqueduct. A ventriculoscope is inserted

into a frontal burr hole to the right of midline to gain access to the third ventricle. The surgery is generally carried out with the patient in supine or semisitting position, which will minimize loss of CSF and provide optimal views for the surgeon (Figure 74.1A and 74.1B).[2]

## ANESTHETIC CONSIDERATIONS

### PREOPERATIVE

Any electrolyte imbalances or hypovolemia should be corrected prior to surgery. A full history and physical should be conducted to note any neurological deficits prior to surgery, including a ophthalmic examination.[3] Generally, the

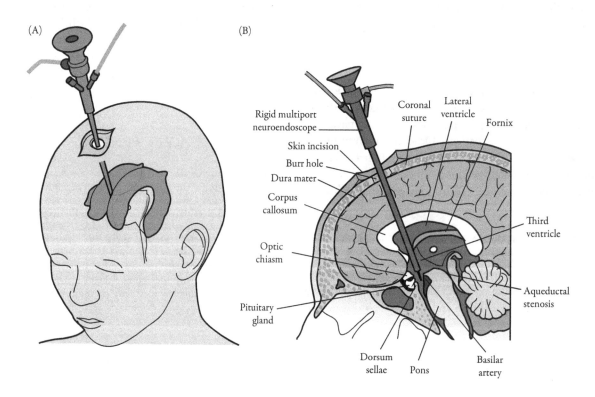

**Figure 74.1** (A) and (B) Surgical technique for ventriculostomy.

neurosurgery team will want to conduct a rapid postoperative neurological assessment and therefore avoiding long-acting anesthetics or sedatives is ideal.[2]

## INTRAOPERATIVE

Routine anesthesia monitoring intraoperatively is generally adequate for this approximately 20- to 120-minute surgical procedure.[1] Some authors recommend invasive blood pressure monitoring via arterial catheter for all patients, and some advocate for intracranial pressure (ICP) monitoring, but both are debatable.[2] Inhalational agents and intravenous anesthesia have both been successfully utilized as maintenance strategies for this surgical procedure; muscle relaxation should be maintained during the surgical period. Although volatile agents will increase cerebral blood flow, utilizing less than one minimum alveolar concentration will not increase cerebral blood flow significantly and is not contraindicated.[5] Nitrous oxide use is not recommended as it can potentially expand ventricular air bubbles and exacerbate a possible venous air embolism.[2]

Complications intraoperatively most often include tachycardia and hypertension, with some patients demonstrating bradycardia. Quickly alerting the surgeon most often can resolve these transient complications as it is due to surgical stimulation or traction on the brain. Minor bleeding is relatively common but easy to control; very rarely, major bleeding can occur that can obscure the endoscope, in which case hemodynamics should be optimized while the surgeon attempts to control the bleeding.[3] Delayed awakening after ETV is also reported as high as 15%, attributed largely to high pressure levels from entrapped air leading to pneumocephalus.[3] The goals for intraoperative management include complete muscle relaxation, cardiovascular stability, and rapid awakening to quickly assess neurological status after the procedure.[2]

## POSTOPERATIVE

Monitoring of complications is key, and, luckily, fatal complications described in literature are rare.[2] Patients may experience electrolyte imbalances (most often hyperkalemia and hypernatremia) and CSF leakage in the postoperative period, both of which should be closely monitored and optimized. Retinal hemorrhages due to sudden increases in ICP have also been reported and should be evaluated if there was any ICP concerns.[3] In addition, a variety of neurological complications such as cranial nerve palsy, convulsions, and memory loss have all been described and should be closely monitored during this period.[2]

## REFERENCES

1. El-Dawlatly A, et al. Anesthesia for third ventriculostomy. *Middle East J Anaesthesiol.* 2008;19:847–858.
2. Rajesh MC. Anesthesia for endoscopic third ventriculostomy in children. *Anesth Essays Res.* 2017;11(1):7–9.
3. Kawsar KA, et al. Avoidance and management of perioperative complications of endoscopic third ventriculostomy: the Dhaka experience. *J Neurosurg.* 2015;123:1414–1419.
4. Gorayeb RP, et al. Endoscopic third ventriculostomy in children younger than 1 year of age. *J Neurosurg.* 2004;100(5 suppl):427–429.
5. Krane EJ, et al. Anaesthesia for pediatric neurosurgery. In: Smith RM, et al., eds. *Smith's Anaesthesia for Infants and Children.* 7th ed. Philadelphia, PA: Mosby; 2006:651–684.

# 75.

# AWAKE CRANIOTOMY

*John S. Shin and Timothy T. Bui*

## INTRODUCTION

Awake craniotomy is a surgical technique that allows for patient participation in functional testing of eloquent cortical tissue in real time intraoperatively. This is typically indicated when the tissue to be resected is near eloquent areas of the brain, which allows for more extensive resection of tumor or ictal foci while also minimizing the resection of eloquent tissue, and it provides the potential for better outcomes. The extent of excision of axial and intracranial brain tumors (gross total resection vs. subtotal resection) has been associated with improved overall and progression-free survival, seizure control, and morbidity. Awake craniotomy allows for maximization of gross total resection and minimization of neurologic deficit by additional testing that would be otherwise unavailable. Awake craniotomy with intraoperative cortical mapping is now the standard of care for intracranial tumor resections in eloquent brain regions.[1,2] It is not only noninferior to general anesthesia but also has been associated with decreased surgery time, postoperative nausea and vomiting, and length of stay.[3]

## ANESTHETIC CONSIDERATIONS

### PREOPERATIVE

Preoperative evaluation must include assessment of the patient's anxiety, claustrophobia, risk of aspiration, and thorough evaluation of the airway (including risk of obstruction and likelihood of difficult mask ventilation or intubation). Patients are often surprised to learn that craniotomies can be performed awake, but patient participation is usually well tolerated.[2] Patients should be counseled regarding what to expect during the preoperative assessment in order to adequately prepare for the upcoming surgery.[1,2] On the morning of surgery, nonpharmacological approaches to anxiolysis are preferred in order to minimize any effect during the intraoperative awake testing phase.

### INTRAOPERATIVE

The two most common techniques for awake craniotomy are asleep-awake-asleep (AAA) and monitored anesthesia care (MAC). Both approaches allow for sedation and analgesia during the craniotomy, alertness during intraoperative testing, and sedation during closure.

Patient positioning is typically in the lateral or semilateral position. The patient must be in a comfortable position with appropriate padding of all pressure points. In addition, the surgical drapes should be secured upward and away from the patient's face as much as possible to ensure full access to the airway so that the patient and anesthesiologist are able to see each other during the awake testing phase.

Prior to pinning and incision, pain control is predominantly achieved by a scalp block with local anesthesia. This involves blocking the auriculotemporal, zygomaticotemporal, supraorbital, supratrochlear, lesser occipital, and/or greater occipital nerves via bupivacaine or ropivacaine.[3] Local anesthesia can also be administered by local infiltration of the surgical and Mayfield clamp pin sites.[2]

Awake craniotomies via the AAA technique involve general anesthesia during the initial asleep phase, using either total intravenous anesthesia or volatile anesthetic. The phases of the AAA approach and their surgical correlates are listed in Table 75.1. During the asleep phase, infusions of propofol, dexmedetomidine, and opioid (most commonly remifentanil given its rapid clearance) have been described with similar patient satisfaction.[3] Propofol and remifentanil have been the standard approach given its efficiency and reliability. Halogenated inhalational anesthetics are also used but may be suboptimal given the potential for increased intracranial pressure and higher risk of postoperative nausea and vomiting.[1] With regard to airway management, supraglottic airways are now preferred over endotracheal tubes by many as they minimize coughing or gagging on awakening, while still allowing for controlled ventilation.[2] After pinning, scalp incision, bone flap removal, and dural opening, patients are then awakened from general anesthesia to participate in brain mapping and cognitive testing (Table 75.1).[3] Surgical resection occurs while

**Table 75.1 SURGICAL STEPS DURING ASLEEP-AWAKE-ASLEEP CRANIOTOMY**

| | |
|---|---|
| Asleep | Mayfield clamp pinning, scalp incision, bone flap removal, dural opening |
| Awake | Brain mapping and functional testing of motor, sensory, cognitive, and speech function; tumor/ictal foci resection |
| Asleep | Closure of dura, calvarium, scalp |

patients perform cognitive tasks to allow for maximal resection with minimal neurologic deficits. Once complete, patients are sedated once more with the medications mentioned above for closure of the dura, calvarium, and scalp. The airway may or may not be resecured during this final asleep phase.

An alternative approach to awake craniotomy is MAC. Propofol and remifentanil are again the standard approach for MAC, but recent data suggest that dexmedetomidine as an alternative is noninferior and may lead to lower respiratory and hemodynamic complications. Typically, the patient is kept breathing spontaneously, requiring an optimal sedation level where the patient is drowsy but easily arousable. MAC allows for lower doses of sedative drugs than AAA, has no sharp transitions from asleep to awake, and minimizes the possibility of hypoactive and hyperactive delirium on emergence, which can affect brain mapping reliability. Given the decreased medication requirement, MAC also allows for less opioid and vasoactive medications.

Both AAA and MAC have been demonstrated to have equal efficacy in terms of brain mapping and surgical outcomes, but MAC has been demonstrated to potentially lead to shorter surgery duration and length of stay. Conversely, AAA theoretically provides more comfort for both the patient and the surgeon, as well as decreased movement, pain, and recall. Controlled ventilation also protects against hypoventilation and allows for hyperventilation if brain swelling occurs.[1]

## POSTOPERATIVE

Postoperative routine monitoring should be continued.

## CLINICAL CONSIDERATIONS

The most prominent complications with awake craniotomies are intraoperative seizures, with incidences ranging widely from 2.9% to 54%.[1,3] Intraoperative seizures are most often due to electrical cortical stimulation and can frequently be treated by cessation of stimulation or irrigation with ice cold crystalloid.[2] Propofol or benzodiazepines can also be utilized as necessary. The leading risk factor is a history of preoperative seizures.[3]

Airway compromise is also a consideration but is usually resolved by noninvasive maneuvers such as jaw lift and/or supplemental oxygen.[2] The rate of conversion to general anesthesia is as low as 2%.[3]

Overall, awake craniotomy should be considered the standard of care for resection of brain tumors and seizure foci in eloquent areas, with growing utility in other surgeries, such as resection of arteriovenous malformations.[2]

## REFERENCES

1. Kulikov A, Lubnin A. Anesthesia for awake craniotomy. *Curr Opin Anaesthesiol*. 2018;31(5):506–510.
2. Sewell D, Smith M. Awake craniotomy: anesthetic considerations based on outcome evidence. *Curr Opin Anaesthesiol*. 2019;32(5):546–552.
3. Emory L, Schubert A. Awake craniotomy, epilepsy, minimally invasive and robotic surgery. In: Cottrell JE, Patel P, eds. *Cottrell and Patel's Neuroanesthesia*. 6th ed. Edinburgh, Scotland: Elsevier; 2017:298–316.

# 76.

# POSTOPERATIVE VISUAL LOSS

*Camila Teixeira and Steven Minear*

## INTRODUCTION

The "Practice Advisory for Perioperative Visual Loss Associated With Spine Surgery" elaborated by the American Society of Anesthesiologists (ASA) Task Force has defined perioperative visual loss as a "permanent impairment or total loss of sight associated with a spine procedure during which general anesthesia is administered" (p. 274).[1] Postoperative visual loss (POVL) is a rare event that has a deep impact on the quality of life of patients undergoing surgical procedures, especially spine surgeries. Every effort must be taken by anesthesiology and surgical teams to prevent this catastrophic complication.

## ETIOLOGY

Postoperative visual loss has a multifactorial etiology. Any segment of the visual system can be involved, from the cornea to the occipital lobe. However, the most common site of permanent injury is the optic nerve, which is often related to ischemic optic neuropathy (ION).[2] Vision loss after neurosurgical procedures is most often reported in spine surgery and radical neck dissection. POVL occurring after nonocular surgery with general anesthesia typically results from anterior ischemic optic neuropathy (AION), posterior ischemic optic neuropathy (PION), central retinal artery occlusion (CRAO), or cortical blindness.[3]

- Ischemic optic neuropathy
  - Anterior ION: Surgical and patient characteristics can influence the perfusion pressure to the optic nerve head (ONH). Patients with smoking status and microvascular diseases, like hypertension, atherosclerosis, or diabetes, can present with poor autoregulation of blood flow to the ONH. Intraoperative factors that reduce the mean arterial pressure below the autoregulatory threshold may also precipitate AION in susceptible patients.[4] In addition, prone position can increase the intraocular pressure, leading to an intraocular perfusion pressure imbalance.
  - Posterior ION: This typically affects the posterior branch of the optic nerve, between the orbital apex and the entry of the central retinal artery.[5] PION is the most common cause of POVL and is positively correlated with severe hypotension, significant blood loss, and prolonged surgical times.
- Central retinal artery occlusion: The head positioning can lead to orbital congestion and consequently to CRAO. This mechanism of POVL is usually followed by signs of congestion, such as periorbital edema and/or ecchymosis. Some cases of CRAO have also been attributed to globe external compression from head positioning. Modifying the type of headrest of patients in prone positioning can reduce the risk of this complication.
- Cortical blindness: Visual loss after neurosurgery can also be associated with occipital or parietal lobe infarction. Typically, cortical blindness is a result of profound and sustained hypotension leading to an infarction in areas of the visual cortex. Alternatively, reports have associated air or particulate emboli with cortical blindness after cervical osteotomy.

## RISK FACTORS

Vascular risk factors, such as chronic hypertension, cardiac dysfunction, and renal and vascular disease, all increase the risk of POVL. The Task Force on POVL believes that the risk of ION could also be increased in patients where long surgical times, substantial blood loss, or both are expected.

## ANESTHETIC CONSIDERATIONS

According to the practice advisory of ASA Task Force on Perioperative Visual Loss Associated With Spine Surgery the following perioperative considerations should be taken into account concerning high-risk patients:

- Preoperative: Consider informing patients concerning the risk of POVL when prolonged procedures, substantial blood loss, or both are anticipated.
- Intraoperative: Intraoperative risk factors should be managed, such as
  - Blood pressure management: Systemic blood pressure should be monitored continually in high-risk patients.
  - Management of intraoperative fluids: Central venous pressure monitoring should be considered in high-risk patients. Colloids should be considered along with crystalloids in patients with substantial blood loss.
  - Management of anemia: Hemoglobin should be maintained at a minimum of 9.4 g/dL and hematocrit at 28%, and these values should be monitored.
  - Patient positioning: Direct pressure to the eye should be avoided to reduce the risk of CRAO or retinal ischemia in spine surgery patients in the prone position. When feasible, the head should be in a neutral forward position above the level of the heart.
  - Staging of surgical procedures: Special attention should be given to staging neurosurgical procedures with anticipated prolonged time length. Task force members considered procedures as "prolonged" after 6.5 hours.
- Postoperative considerations: For high-risk patients, the vision should be assessed when the patient becomes alert. If POVL is suspected, an ophthalmologist should be contacted to determine its cause. In order to rule out intracranial causes of visual loss, magnetic resonance imaging should be considered. Prompt anatomical and etiologic diagnosis is key to guide proper management and assess prognosis. Consider osmotic diuretics and high-dose steroids in the first 48 hours following ischemic optic neuropathy.

## REFERENCES

1. American Society of Anesthesiologists Task Force on Perioperative Visual Loss. Practice advisory for perioperative visual loss associated with spine surgery: an updated report by the American Society of Anesthesiologists Task Force on Visual Loss. *Anesthesiology*. 2012;116:274–285.
2. Lee LA, et al. The American Society of Anesthesiologists postoperative visual loss registry: analysis of 93 spine surgery cases with postoperative visual loss. *Anesthesiology*. 2006;105:652–659.
3. Gilbert ME. Postoperative visual loss: a review of the current literature. *Neuro-Ophthalmology*. 2008;32:194–199.
4. Hayreh SS. Anterior ischemic optic neuropathy. *Clin Neurosci*. 1997;4:383–417.
5. Sadda SR, et al. Clinical spectrum of posterior ischemic optic neuropathy. *Am J Ophthalmol*. 2001;132:743–750.

# 77.

# HYPOTHERMIA

*Jarrod Bang and Archit Sharma*

## INTRODUCTION

A complication attributed to typical mild intraoperative hypothermia is prolonged duration of postanesthetic recovery.[1]

Heat is transferred, and thus lost, by four mechanisms: radiation, convection, conduction, and evaporation. Under normal conditions, radiation is the most influential in an anesthetized patient, followed by convection. Temperature monitoring is an American Society of Anesthesiologists standard monitor for all types of anesthesia. There are multiple locations to measure body temperature in patients. Core temperature monitoring sites include the tympanic, esophageal, nasopharyngeal, pulmonary artery, rectal, and bladder. Each method has its own contraindications and possible complications, including misinterpretation. Skin temperature is another possible method, but this method has been shown to have inconsistent correlation to core temperatures due to variable degrees of peripheral vasoconstriction. Rectal temperature monitoring has been shown to be less reliable due to a slowed response to changes in core temperature. Bladder temperature is a reliable as long as urine output is maintained.

## THERMOREGULATION

Normothermia is maintained in the awake patient by several regulatory mechanisms, including shivering, vasoconstriction, vasodilation, sweating, and behavioral regulation (putting on warm clothing). These mechanisms are triggered by input from the hypothalamus, other brain centers, spinal cord, abdominothoracic tissues, and skin surface, with the hypothalamus interpreting these inputs. Temperature is tightly maintained under normal circumstances, with hypothermia being defined as a core temperature less than 36°C. Under general anesthesia, regulatory mechanisms for hyperthermia are increased, and mechanisms for hypothermia are greatly reduced. The net effect of these changes is a significant widening of the range of core body temperature of the anesthetized patient for which no regulatory response is triggered.

Three phases of changes in core temperature under anesthesia typically occur. In the initial phase, core body temperature mixes with the peripheral body compartments due to vasodilating effects of most anesthetics. The second phase of core temperature change is due to the decreased body heat production combined with increased heat loss due to surgical exposure and vasodilation. The third phase is a new steady state under anesthesia where the patient's body temperature finds a steady state due to equilibration of heat generation and heat loss.

## ADVERSE EFFECTS OF HYPOTHERMIA

**Increased Hospital/PACU Time:** Lenhardt et al. demonstrated that maintaining core normothermia decreases the duration of postanesthetic recovery and, hence, reduces costs of care.[2]

**Increase in Blood Loss/Transfusion:** Schmied et al. demonstrated that maintenance of intraoperative normothermia reduces blood loss and allogeneic blood requirements in patients undergoing total hip arthroplasty.[3]

**Increased Cardiac Morbidity:** Frank et al. demonstrated that in patients with cardiac risk factors who are undergoing noncardiac surgery the perioperative maintenance of normothermia is associated with a reduced incidence of morbid cardiac events and ventricular tachycardia. This was not due to shivering, and possibly due to arrhythmias and hypertensive response to stress of cold.[4]

Normothermia was associated with a 55% reduction in cardiac risk.

**Increased Infection Risk: Kurz** et al. showed that hypothermia may delay healing and predispose patients to wound infections. Maintaining normothermia likely decreases infectious complications in patients undergoing colorectal resection and shortens their hospitalizations.[5]

**Increased Anesthetic Potency:** Hypothermia increases anesthetic potency, decreases drug metabolisms, decreases minimum alveolar concentration 15% for every 1.0°C.

**Prevention of Hypothermia:** The various degrees of interactions that happen with the patient's thermoregulation can be divided into preoperative, intraoperative, and postoperative phases, which create avenues for the anesthesiologist to intervene and prevent hypothermia.

## ANESTHETIC CONSIDERATIONS

### PREOPERATIVE

Preoperative temperatures and interventions can have a large impact on intraoperative temperature. The most effective preoperative intervention to prevent hypothermia is prewarming patients peripherally, most commonly with a forced-air warmer. This intervention decreases the initial drop in patient temperature with induction of anesthesia and mixing of the peripheral and core body temperatures. Trauma patients can often experience hypothermia prior to entering the operating theater due to full-body exposure to identify injuries and large-volume fluid/blood product administration.

### INTRAOPERATIVE

Intraoperative interventions to avoid hypothermia are mostly aimed at optimizing heat exchange by radiation and convection. One method of preventing hypothermia is increased operating room ambient temperature. However, the temperatures to obtain maximal benefit from this method would create an environment that is suboptimal for the operating physicians. This is most effectively used in the patients most vulnerable to hypothermia: infants. Alternatively, a forced-air warmer can be used to heat the air surrounding the patient to create a microsphere of warm air. Warming of fluids has not been shown to be an exceptionally beneficial method of warming a hypothermic patient, but it is useful in mitigating the decrease in temperature caused by large-volume fluid resuscitation, especially if the fluids were previously refrigerated, such as blood products.

### POSTOPERATIVE

Shivering in the postoperative period is not only uncomfortable but also can be dangerous to the patient. Shivering causes increased systemic vascular resistance and significantly increased oxygen demand. In critical cardiovascular patients, this could introduce significant risk, including the possibility of tipping the ratio of oxygen demand to oxygen supply of a patient with coronary artery disease, resulting in demand coronary ischemia. Forced-air warming has been shown to be poorly effective in resolution of postoperative shivering as it is unable to quickly warm the patient due to vasoconstriction of the periphery to conserve heat. Medications such as meperidine have been shown to be effective in treating postoperative shivering due to unclear mechanisms.

## REFERENCE

1. Hines R, et al. Complications occurring in the postanesthesia care unit: a survey. *Anesth Analg.* 1992;74(4):503–509.
2. Lenhardt R, et al. Mild intraoperative hypothermia prolongs postanesthetic recovery. *Anesthesiology.* 1997;87(6):1318–1323.
3. Schmied H, et al. Mild hypothermia increases blood loss and transfusion requirements during total hip arthroplasty. *Lancet.* 1996;347(8997):289–292.
4. Frank SM, et al. Perioperative maintenance of normothermia reduces the incidence of morbid cardiac events: a randomized clinical trial. *JAMA.* 1997;277(14):1127–1134.
5. Kurz A, et al. Perioperative normothermia to reduce the incidence of surgical-wound infection and shorten hospitalization. *N Engl J Med.* 1996;334(19):1209–1216.

# 78.

# MONITORED ANESTHESIA CARE AND SEDATION

*Nikki Eden and Shobana Rajan*

## INTRODUCTION

The American Society of Anesthesiologists (ASA) defines monitored anesthesia care (MAC) as "a specific anesthesia service performed by a qualified anesthesia provider, for a diagnostic or therapeutic procedure"[1] (p. 438). With this, all aspects of anesthesia care are provided by the anesthesia provider, including a preprocedural assessment, intraoperative management, and postprocedural follow-up care.[1]

Table 78.1 depicts the different levels of sedation that a patient may experience depending on the complexity of the case and the necessity for deeper levels of sedation. These levels represent a spectrum; thus, they are not independent of one another.

Under certain circumstances, minimal ("conscious") or moderate sedation, in which a non–anesthesia provider both performs a procedure and manages the sedation, can be performed. In this circumstance, sedative medications are generally protocolized and limited so that the patient will maintain purposeful responsiveness and spontaneous respiration.[2]

## ASA GUIDELINES FOR SEDATION

Only physicians and other practitioners who are qualified by education, training, and licensure to administer deep sedation or general anesthesia may do so. Individual hospitals may mandate certain criteria to perform such sedation, and those guidelines must be followed in addition to the ASA guidelines.[2] Any physician who administers or supervises deep sedation or general anesthesia must be solely dedicated to that task and cannot be the provider performing the procedure, regardless of the type of procedure.[3]

## SEDATION GUIDELINES FOR NONANESTHESIOLOGISTS

Per the ASA:

The non-anesthesiologist physician will have satisfactorily completed a formal training program in the safe administration of sedative and analgesic

*Table 78.1* DEPTHS OF ANESTHESIA AND ASSOCIATED PHYSIOLOGIC FACTORS

| | MINIMAL SEDATION | MODERATE SEDATION | DEEP SEDATION | GENERAL ANESTHESIA |
|---|---|---|---|---|
| Responsiveness and consciousness | Normal response to verbal stimulation; impaired cognition and coordination | Purposeful[a] response to verbal or tactile stimulation; depression of consciousness | Purposeful[a] response following repeated painful stimulation; depression of consciousness | Unarousable, even with painful stimulus |
| Airway | No intervention required | No intervention required | Intervention may be required | Intervention often required |
| Spontaneous ventilation | Adequate | Adequate | May be inadequate | Frequently inadequate |
| Cardiovascular function | Maintained | Usually maintained | Usually maintained | May be impaired |

[a]Reflex withdrawal from a painful stimulus is not considered a purposeful response.

Reprinted with permission from Practice Guidelines for Moderate Procedural Sedation and Analgesia 2018: A Report by the American Society of Anesthesiologists Task Force on Moderate Procedural Sedation and Analgesia, the American Association of Oral and Maxillofacial Surgeons, American College of Radiology, American Dental Association, American Society of Dentist Anesthesiologists, and Society of Interventional Radiology. Anesthesiology. 2018; 128(3): 463.[1]

drugs used to establish a level of deep sedation and in the rescue of patients who exhibit adverse physiologic consequences of a deeper-than-intended level of sedation. This training includes the didactic and performance concepts below and may be a formally recognized part of a recently completed Accreditation Council for Graduate Medical Education residency or fellowship training (e.g., within two years), or may be a separate deep sedation educational program that is accredited by Accreditation Council for Continuing Medical Education or equivalent providers recognized for dental, oral surgical and podiatric continuing education.[4] (p. 1)

## INDICATIONS AND CONTRAINDICATIONS

Monitored anesthesia care is indicated for any procedure that requires sedation, regardless of depth. Minimal sedation can be done by MAC because the provider performing the case is not certified to perform sedation. As well, it is done when the non–anesthesia proceduralist feels uncomfortable providing moderate sedation during the case. MAC must be performed by a provider who is qualified to rescue an airway or convert to general anesthesia as needed.[1,3,4]

The main contraindication to MAC is a need to protect the airway with some form of instrumentation. This would include patients with high aspiration risk, such as emergent cases where the patient recently ate, has severe gastric reflux, is obese, or is a pregnant women. Using a qualified anesthesia person during a procedure provides a higher level of care, comfort, and safety to the patient than without one. The risks of not using MAC greatly outweigh the costs of an added provider during the procedure.

## RISKS AND COMPLICATIONS

A common misconception is that the risks increase as the level of sedation increases; however, this does not truly describe the relationship between sedation and hemodynamic instability. At all levels of sedation, there is always concern for a quick and drastic change in the hemodynamic stability of the patient. The anesthesiologist should be able to "rescue" the patient from a deeper level of sedation and bring them back to the intended level of sedation without adverse physiologic consequences.[4,5]

The greatest concern during MAC is the loss of airway at any point. When this happens, the airway can be managed with oral or nasal airway adjuncts or by conversion to a general anesthetic with insertion of a laryngeal mask airway or endotracheal tube.

## ANESTHETIC CONSIDERATIONS

### PREOPERATIVE

Prior to the beginning of a procedure, a preanesthesia evaluation should be completed for any patient receiving MAC.[5]

### INTRAOPERATIVE

All ASA-mandated basic monitoring standards apply intraoperatively. Intravenous access should be maintained throughout the case. Vital functions, hemodynamic stability, airway, and respiration will be monitored by the anesthesia provider. Depth of sedation and its appropriateness for the procedure will be monitored and managed accordingly.

## POSTOPERATIVE

A postoperative anesthesia examination must be completed following completion of the procedure and anesthetic in the postanesthesia care unit and may be performed by a different anesthesiologist than the one who completed the preoperative anesthetic evaluation.

## REFERENCES

1. Practice Guidelines for Moderate Procedural Sedation and Analgesia 2018. A report by the American Society of Anesthesiologists Task Force on Moderate Procedural Sedation and Analgesia, the American Association of Oral and Maxillofacial Surgeons, American College of Radiology, American Dental Association, American Society of Dentist Anesthesiologists, and Society of Interventional Radiology. *Anesthesiology.* 2018;128(3):437–463.

2. American Society of Anesthesiologists. Position on monitored anesthesia care. 2018. https://www.asahq.org/standards-and-guidelines/position-on-monitored-anesthesia-care

3. American Society of Anesthesiologists. Continuum of depth of sedation. 2019. https://www.asahq.org/standards-and-guidelines/continuum-of-depth-of-sedation-definition-of-general-anesthesia-and-levels-of-sedationanalgesia

4. American Society of Anesthesiologists. Distinguishing monitored anesthesia care from moderate sedation/analgesia. 2018. https://www.asahq.org/standards-and-guidelines/distinguishing-monitored-anesthesia-care-mac-from-moderate-sedationanalgesia-conscious-sedation

5. Das S, Ghosh S. Monitored anesthesia care: An overview. *J Anaesthesiol Clin Pharmacol.* 2015;31(1):27–29.

# Part 8

# RESPIRATORY SYSTEM ANATOMY

# DIVISIONS OF BRONCHOSCOPIC ANATOMY

*Matthew Gunst and Christopher Giordano*

## ANATOMY

The initial feature of the airway below the level of the vocal cords is the trachea. The trachea comprises 16 to 20 cartilaginous, C-shaped rings on the anterior portion, with the posterior trachealis smooth muscle completing the cylindrical shape. The trachea ends at the carina in adults, approximately 10 to 12 cm inferior to the vocal cords, and splits into the right and left main bronchi, the primary airways to both lungs.[1] The main conducting airways are divided into secondary bronchi going to each lobe of the lungs, which further divide into tertiary bronchial segments going into the roughly 18 segments of the lungs.[2] The structure of the main bronchi and segmental bronchi is reinforced by cartilage similarly to the trachea, but the cartilaginous rings form complete circles past the carina, as opposed to the C-shaped rings of the trachea. These large, conductive airways do not participate in gas exchange; thus, they function as physiologic dead space. Despite not contributing to gas exchange, these structures play a vital role in transmitting air from the atmosphere or ventilator to the lower portion of the lungs where gas exchange occurs. Altered anatomy secondary to trauma, mucous plugging, infection, tumor, or any number of obstacles can limit airflow to and from the lower portion of the lungs.

The splitting of the trachea into two main bronchi occurs at the carina (Figure 79.1). The carina is a ridge of cartilage marking the point between the left and right main bronchi. Anatomically, the carina most often aligns externally with the sternal angle. At each bifurcation of the lung into further divisions, there are secondary and tertiary "carina" that mark the different lobes and segments of the lungs.

The left main bronchus breaks off at the carina slightly more laterally than the right bronchus and extends for an average of 5 cm in adults. Typically, there is no further division of the left main bronchus that can be seen by bronchoscopy from the carina. With the aid of a bronchoscope, the left main bronchus on average appears smaller in diameter than the opening to the right main bronchus due to its lateral takeoff angle. The left main bronchus bifurcates into the left upper and left lower lobes. The upper lobe of the left lung contains four segments: apical, anterior, inferior, and superior. The lower lobe of the left lung also contains four segments: superior, lateral, posterior, and anteromedial.

The right main bronchus typically breaks from the carina inferiorly. With a bronchoscope, its diameter appears larger. The takeoff for the right upper lobe is often visible from the level of the carina. This takeoff is close to the carina, and approximately 5% of patients have a right upper lobe takeoff at the level of the carina or even higher. This leads to a right mainstem bronchus that is much shorter on average than the left main bronchus, usually 2 to 3 cm long in adults. The membranous posterior portion of the trachea continues into the right main bronchus. The right upper lobe of the lung contains three segments: apical, anterior, and posterior. Following the takeoff of the right upper lobe, the right main bronchus becomes the bronchus intermedius, which continues until bifurcating into the right middle and right lower lobes. The right middle lobe contains two segments: medial and lateral. The right lower lobe contains five segments: superior, medial, anterior, lateral, and posterior.

The average pair of lungs contains 18 segments: 10 on the right and 8 on the left. A helpful pneumonic is ASIA ALPS for the left superior and inferior lobes, respectively. The comparative pneumonic for the right is A PALM Seed Makes Another Little Palm, with the capital letters representing the segments in descending order.

Basic anatomic landmarks help identify the left- and right-sided bronchus: the anterior cartilage rings in the trachea, the posterior smooth muscle descending into the main bronchi, and the early right upper lobe takeoff.

## ANESTHETIC CONSIDERATIONS

Lung isolation is commonly used in numerous procedures, either with double-lumen endotracheal tubes (ETTs) or some form of bronchial blocker.[3] Left double-lumen tubes are primarily used due to the longer left main bronchus and

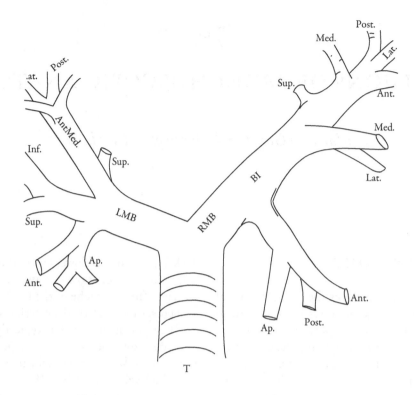

**Figure 79.1** The anatomy and all subsequent divisions of the bronchial tree. Ap., anterior-posterior; Ant., anterior; Ant. Med., anteromedial; BI, bronchus intermedius; Inf., inferior; Lat., lateral; LMB, left main bronchus; Med., medial; Post., posterior; RMB, right main bronchus; Sup., superior; T, trachea.

variable anatomy of the right upper lobe takeoff. The longer distance prior to the first division of the left main bronchus provides a more reliable landing spot for a left-sided, double-lumen ETT under bronchoscopic guidance. Right double-lumen tubes can be used for surgeries that occur near the left main bronchus. These right-sided, double-lumen tubes have an orifice to permit gas exchange for the early right upper lobe takeoff; however, given the variability in right upper lobe origination, it is important to recognize when a patient's anatomy is not conducive to these right-sided tubes.

Knowledge of bronchoscopic anatomy is also vital for placement of bronchial blockers, which are available in several different varieties.

Flexible bronchoscopy is often used in critically ill patients with known lung processes, such as pneumonia or abnormal radiographic findings or in patients who are struggling to liberate from a ventilator.

## REFERENCES

1. Atchabahian A, Gupta R, eds. *The Anesthesia Guide*. McGraw-Hill; 2013:836–840.
2. Barash PG. et al., eds. *Clinical Anesthesia*. 7th ed. Philadelphia, PA: Lippincott Williams & Wilkins; 2013:264–266.
3. Ryan B, et al. Anatomical considerations in bronchoscopy. *J Thorac Dis*. 2017;9(suppl 10):S1123–S1127.

# 80.

# BRONCHIAL AND PULMONARY CIRCULATIONS

*Jordan Brewer and Christopher Giordano*

## ANATOMY

The lung and its supportive components receive blood from two sources: pulmonary and bronchial vasculature (Figure 80.1). The pulmonary vascular system delivers the entirety of deoxygenated cardiac output (approximately 3.5 L/min/m$^2$) to the lungs to participate in gas exchange and return to systemic circulation. Blood from the right ventricle flows from the right ventricle outflow tract to the main pulmonary artery (PA), which splits into right and left PAs. These large-caliber vessels split and travel along connective tissue planes and culminate in a system of 280 million capillaries that bathe alveolar bodies. A single capillary microvasculature (5–10 μm in diameter) allows the passage of one red blood cell at a time and wraps around multiple alveoli, thereby maximizing surface area for gas exchange. Notably, the alveoli receive metabolic substrates from this blood supply. Capillaries coalesce into the pulmonary venules, which ultimately return oxygenated blood to the left atrium (LA) from four pulmonary veins.

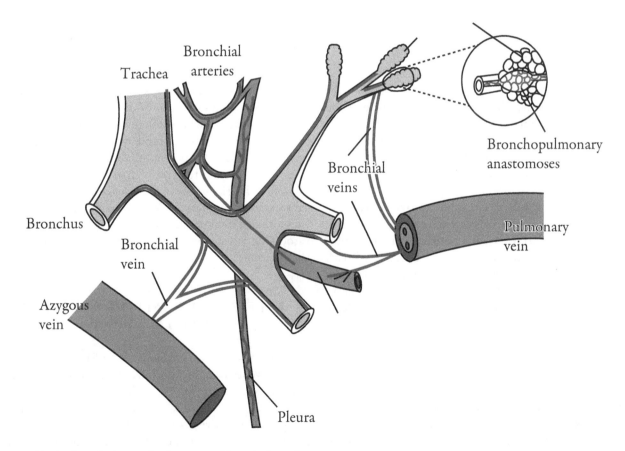

**Figure 80.1** Tracheobronchial tree and pulmonary and bronchial circulations.

Modified from Deffebach ME, Charan NB, Lakshminarayan S, Butler J. The bronchial circulation: small but a vital attribute of the lung. *Am Rev Respir Dis.* 1987; 135:463.

The volume of blood contained in the pulmonary system at any point in time, including the main PA to the LA, is nearly 500 mL or 10% of the estimated blood volume.

The remainder of the lung parenchyma receives blood supply from the bronchial vascular system. It typically arises from branches off the descending thoracic aorta, but it can also originate from intercostal, subclavian, or innominate arteries. This blood supply is a small volume and comprises between 1% and 4% of cardiac output. Left and right bronchial arteries extend to their respective lungs and split into smaller arteries and arterioles as they travel from the trachea to the main bronchi, lobar bronchi, and terminal bronchioles. Bronchial arterioles wrap circumferentially around the terminal bronchioles, providing metabolic substrates to the conductive airways, and they also provide blood supply to the visceral pleural surfaces. Capillary beds return the bronchial blood to prelung circulation (via azygos, hemiazygos, and mediastinal veins) and postlung circulation (via bronchial veins). The mixing of this deoxygenated blood with the pulmonary venous (oxygenated) blood flow provides for an absolute right-to-left shunt between 2% and 5%, which is an expected norm in healthy individuals. Other connections, such as anastomoses between bronchial and pulmonary capillaries, may provide for collateral blood flow in states of occluded flow, such as a pulmonary embolus.

## INNERVATION

Adrenergic receptors ($\alpha$ and $\beta$) are present throughout the pulmonary vasculature, allowing for manipulation of blood flow. Vasoconstriction is achieved through activation of $\alpha_1$-receptors. Vasodilation is achieved through activation of $\beta_2$-receptors. Notably, pulmonary vessels lack V1 receptors, making vasopressin an attractive choice for systemic blood pressure control in patients with pulmonary hypertension or right heart failure. Large pulmonary vessels (>50 $\mu$m) receive sympathetic innervation to the adventitia, which can respond to stretch and chemical stimuli, in turn augmenting smooth muscle contraction. Small vessels lack smooth muscle and receive no sympathetic innervation. Parasympathetic nerves are derived from the vagus nerve (cranial nerve X) and mediate vasodilation via the release of nitric oxide.

## VENTILATION-PERFUSION ZONES

Perfusion to lung segments is driven by gravity and pressure differentials. The typical model description for lung perfusion is broken into three zones (Figure 80.2). In zone 1, alveolar pressure in the lung apex is equal to atmospheric pressure, which is greater than both pulmonary arterial and venous pressures. This results in no blood flow through

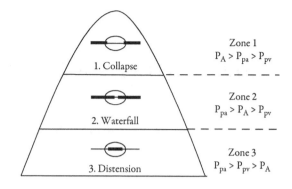

**Figure 80.2** Ventilation-perfusion zones. Relationship of alveolar pressure (PA), PA pressure ($P_{pa}$), and pulmonary venous pressure ($P_{pv}$).

Modified from Barash P. *Clinical Anesthesia*. 2013. 274.

collapsed capillaries, thus establishing an area of dead space ventilation. Zone 2 contains the majority of alveoli surface area, and perfusion and ventilation are well matched due to favorable pressure gradients from the PA and alveoli. Zone 3 is marked by excess blood flow, or shunt, as capillaries become distended due to low alveolar pressures. Flow in this zone depends on the pulmonary arterial and venous pressure gradient.

## HYPOXIC PULMONARY VASOCONSTRICTION

Pulmonary perfusion pressures can be augmented by the arterial response to oxygen tension. In areas of low alveolar oxygenation, blood flow can be diverted to more favorably ventilated lung segments through vasoconstriction. Certain agents and conditions can inhibit hypoxic pulmonary vasoconstriction (HPV): potent inhaled agents, hypothermia, vasodilators (e.g., nitroglycerin), hypocarbia, and metabolic alkalemia. Nitric oxide, an endothelial-derived factor that causes smooth muscle relaxation, is an important consideration. Inhaled nitric oxide can selectively induce pulmonary vasodilation and reverse HPV without causing systemic vasodilation.

## EFFECTS OF POSITIVE PRESSURE VENTILATION

Positive end-expiratory pressure (PEEP) assists with mechanical ventilation by minimizing atelectasis at the distal small alveoli. PEEP also carries the risk of further elevating intrathoracic pressure, which can impede venous return and preload to the right-sided cardiac chambers. It may also impede blood flow at the compressible microvasculature and impair gas exchange. Research on canine pulmonary physiology has demonstrated that low levels of PEEP (3–10 cm $H_2O$) do not hinder pulmonary blood flow; however, at

15 cm $H_2O$ of PEEP, bronchial blood flow exceeded systemic to pulmonary blood flow, indicating decreased anastomotic drainage.

## REFERENCES

1. Tamul PC, et al. Respiratory function in anesthesia. In: Barash P, et al., eds. *Clinical Anesthesia*. 7th ed. Lippincott Williams & Wilkins; 2013:266–275.

2. Butterworth JF, et al. Respiratory physiology & anesthesia. In: Butterworth JF, et al., eds. *Morgan & Mikhail's Clinical Anesthesiology*. 6th ed. New York, NY: McGraw-Hill Education; 2018:487–525.

3. Deffebach ME, et al. The bronchial circulation. *Am Rev Respir Dis*. 1987;135:463–481.

4. Navalesi P, et al. Positive end-expiratory pressure. In: Tobin MJ, ed. *Principles and Practice of Mechanical Ventilation*. 3rd ed. New York, NY: McGraw-Hill; 2013: Chap. 10.

5. The pulmonary circulation. *Thoracic Key* blog. October 11, 2019. https://thoracickey.com/the-pulmonary-circulation-3/

# 81.

# LUNG MECHANICS

*Evan Davidson and Ettore Crimi*

## INTRODUCTION

Oxygen enters the lungs, diffuses into the bloodstream, and reaches the cells, where aerobic respiration can occur. Conversely, the carbon dioxide produced from cellular respiration dissolves into the blood and diffuses out in the lungs to be exhaled into the atmosphere.

## MECHANICS OF INSPIRATION AND EXPIRATION

The respiratory system relies on pressure differences for air to enter and leave the lungs.[1] Air flows from the areas of highest pressure to lowest pressure. Differences in pressure, or pressure gradients, create the force that drives air from the atmosphere into the lungs during spontaneous breathing. Mouth pressure $P_m$ is the air pressure at the level of the mouth and is equal to atmospheric pressure. Interpleural pressure, or $P_{pl}$, is the pressure in the space between the parietal and visceral pleura; it is normally negative with respect to atmospheric pressure (approximately −5 cm $H_2O$) at the end of expiration. During inspiration, $P_{pl}$ normally decreases to approximately −10 cm $H_2O$. Alveolar pressure $P_{alv}$ is the air pressure within the alveoli and directly changes with interpleural pressure.

The transairway pressure $P_{TA}$ is defined as the pressure difference between the mouth pressure (at atmospheric pressure) and the alveolus:

$$P_{TA} = P_m - P_{alv}$$

$P_{TA}$ drives air into the lungs and is affected by airway resistance.

The transthoracic pressure $P_{TT}$ is the difference between the alveolar and body surface (atmospheric pressure):

$$P_{TT} = P_{alv} - P_{bs}$$

$P_{TT}$ is the pressure needed to expand the alveoli against the lung and chest wall forces.

The transpulmonary pressure $P_{TP}$ is the difference between the alveolar and pleural pressure:

$$P_{TP} = P_{alv} - P_{pl}.$$

**Table 81.1** PRESSURE CHANGES DURING SPONTANEOUS BREATHING AND MECHANICAL VENTILATION

|  | SPONTANEOUS BREATHING | MECHANICAL VENTILATION |
|---|---|---|
| Inspiration | $P_{pl} < P_{alv} < P_m$ | $P_m > P_{alv}$ |
| Expiration | $P_{pl} > P_{alv} > P_m$ | $P_m < P_{alv}$ |

$P_{TP}$ is the pressure needed to maintain alveolar inflation.

These pressures change in concert during spontaneous breathing.[2] As the diaphragm contracts and the volume of the thoracic space increases, $P_{pl}$ decreases from −5 to −10 cm $H_2O$ relative to the atmosphere at end inspiration. The decrease in $P_{pl}$ causes a decreased $P_{alv}$ relative to the mouth, which remains at atmospheric pressure. The negative pressure gradient allows air to enter the lungs. The opposite effect occurs during expiration: The diaphragm relaxes, the thoracic cavity decreases in diameter, the pleural and alveolar pressures increase to approximately +5 cm $H_2O$ relative to the atmospheric pressure, and expiration occurs.

In contrast, mechanical ventilation uses positive pressure to deliver a breath (Table 81.1). For a positive pressure breath to occur, the ventilator must increase transrespiratory pressure, the pressure between the mouth and the body surface at atmospheric pressure:

$$P_{TR} = P_m - P_{bs}$$

When delivering a breath, the ventilator increases the $P_m$. This higher pressure is transmitted to the distal airways. Eventually, this positive pressure is delivered to the alveoli, increasing $P_{alv}$ and $P_{TP}$. Airflow stops when these two pressures equal the positive pressure delivered by the ventilator. Then, $P_m$ decreases to less than the higher positive pressure within the alveoli, allowing air to move out of the alveoli into the airways and expiration to occur.

## COMPLIANCE AND RESISTANCE

Elastance and resistance of the respiratory system oppose lung inflation. Elastance, the inverse of compliance, describes the tendency of a lung to return to its resting form following the application of a force changing its shape. Compliance can be defined as the change in volume for any defined pressure:

$$Compliance = \Delta Volume / \Delta Pressure$$

The compliance of the lung is the pressure needed to change the volume of the lung. The compliance of the chest wall is the pressure needed to change the volume of the chest wall.

The more compliant the lung is, the less pressure required to expand it; the less compliant the lung, the more pressure required.

Resistance is the impedance of airflow entering the lung and is represented by the equation

$$Resistance = Pressure / Airflow$$

Respiratory system resistance consists of airway resistance, the impedance of air flowing into airways, and tissue resistance, the viscous impedance of the lung and adjacent tissues on airflow.

Resistance can be calculated from Poiseuille's law as

$$Resistance = 8 \text{ (Viscosity of gas)(Length of tubing)} \text{ (Gas flow rate)} / \pi \text{ (radius of the tube)}^4$$

Resistance is decreased the most with a larger radial tube and increased the most with a smaller radial tube. Airway resistance can be increased by an artificial airway (e.g., endotracheal tube) or airway disease (e.g., asthma, bronchospasm, foreign object, or chronic obstructive pulmonary disease).[3]

## TIME CONSTANT

The time constant, the length of time needed to inflate or deflate the lung to a certain percentage of its volume, is the product of compliance and resistance:

$$TC = C \times R$$

One time constant will allow 63% of the lung to fill or empty, two time constants will allow 86% to empty or fill, and three time constants will allow 98% of the lung to empty or fill. The lung will be completely filled or empty after five time constants.

Various diseases will affect the time constant as they affect the compliance of the lung or airway resistance. For example, a patient with emphysema has a highly compliant lung that fills with a high volume of air in a short time, whereas a patient with pulmonary fibrosis has low-compliant lungs that fill quickly with a small volume of air. A lung with high airway resistance (e.g., bronchospasm) has a low time constant, whereas the time constant will increase once a bronchodilator is administered.[4]

## WORK OF BREATHING

Work is the force necessary to change the volume of a structure and is defined by the equation

$$Work = Pressure \times Change in Volume$$

The work of breathing has two components: elastic work, which consists of work to overcome the elastic recoil of both the chest and lungs, and resistive work, which is work done to overcome the tissue resistance of the lung, chest wall, and airways. Increased work of breathing, such as in the case of high airway resistance during bronchospasm, restrictive disease as in the case of pleural effusions, or high surface tension at the alveolar level as seen in a premature infant, can lead to fatigue and eventual respiratory failure.[4]

## REFERENCES

1. Lumb AB, Thomas C. Elastic forces and lung volumes In: *Nunn's Applied Respiratory Physiology*. 9th ed. Elsevier; 2021:14–26.
2. West JB, Luks AM. Mechanics of breathing In: *West's Respiratory Physiology: The Essentials*. 10th ed. Lippincott Williams & Wilkins; 2016:108–141.
3. Bigatello L, Pesenti A. Respiratory physiology for the anesthesiologist. *Anesthesiology*. 2019;130:1064–1077.
4. Cloutier M. Mechanical properties of lung and chest wall. In: *Respiratory Physiology*. 2nd ed. Elsevier; 2019:15–28.

# 82.

# NORMAL ACID-BASE REGULATION

*Erica Alcibiade and Maggie W. Mechlin*

## INTRODUCTION

Maintaining a normal pH (7.35–7.45) is necessary for normal physiologic function. Beyond a normal range, widespread organ dysfunction ensues. Table 82.1 outlines basic acid-base derangements and compensation; however, in-depth blood gas interpretation is discussed in a separate chapter. Optimal pH is important for enzyme activity, chemical reactions, and transport of oxygen throughout the body. Numerous situations in the operating room (OR) can rapidly alter acid-base balance, such as changes in ventilation, tissue hypoperfusion, intravenous fluids (based on their composition), and electrolyte abnormalities. Controlling derangements is crucial and may be complicated by the fact that general anesthesia hinders the body's homeostatic compensation mechanisms.

The relationship between physiologic factors affecting pH is described by the Henderson Hasselbach equation, $pH = 6.1 + \log [HCO_3^-/(0.03 \times PaCO_2)]$. It demonstrates that pH and $H^+$ have an inverse relationship. Furthermore, as pH decreases, $PaCO_2$ and bicarbonate are expected to increase. There is a second classification system, known as the Fencl-Stewart approach. This method emphasizes the many other cations/anions that play a role in metabolic

*Table 82.1* ACID-BASE, INTERPRETATION, AND NORMAL VALUES

| PRIMARY DISORDER | PH | PACO$_2$ | HCO$_3^-$ | PRIMARY CHANGE | COMPENSATORY RESPONSE |
|---|---|---|---|---|---|
| Normal | 7.35–7.45 | 35–45 | 22–26 | — | — |
| Respiratory acidosis | ↓ | ↑ | Normal (initially) | ↑ PaCO$_2$ | ↑ HCO$_3^-$ |
| Respiratory alkalosis | ↑ | ↓ | Normal (initially) | ↓ PaCO$_2$ | ↓ HCO$_3^-$ |
| Metabolic acidosis | ↓ | Normal (initially) | ↓ | ↓ HCO$_3^-$ | ↓ PaCO$_2$ |
| Metabolic alkalosis | ↑ | Normal (initially) | ↑ | ↑ HCO$_3^-$ | ↑ PaCO$_2$ |

acid-base physiology. This is discussed further in another chapter.

## COMPENSATING FOR CHRONIC ACID-BASE DISORDERS

Under normal conditions, the body has multiple compensatory mechanisms that work to maintain homeostasis within the normal pH range. These can be subdivided into three main categories: weak acid buffers, renal regulation via bicarbonate and $H^+$ absorption and secretion, and respiratory compensation through $CO_2$ retention or excretion. In general, respiratory disorders are compensated through renal mechanisms—with complete compensation taking approximately 2–5 days.[1] Metabolic disorders are compensated through respiratory mechanisms and occur more quickly, with initial response happening instantly and full compensation at approximately 12–36 hours.[1] If compensation takes longer than this to occur, the presence of a second or mixed disorder is possible.

Buffering systems and respiratory compensation begin to occur quickly (within minutes to hours) as the balance begins to shift. There are two major metabolic buffer systems within the human body, bicarbonate and hemoglobin. The bicarbonate system utilizes carbonic anhydrase (present in endothelium, kidney, and red blood cells). The hemoglobin system works via histidine side chains with multiple proton-binding sites that allow uptake of $H^+$ when pH decreases and releasing $H^+$ as pH increases.

Under normal conditions, respiratory compensation is managed by changes in alveolar ventilation. Arterial $CO_2$ is measured and regulated by central chemoreceptors located in the brainstem and peripheral chemoreceptors located in the aortic arch and carotid bodies. Carbon dioxide diffuses across the blood-brain barrier, increasing the $[H^+]$ of the cerebrospinal fluid, which activates central chemoreceptors in the medulla and increases ventilation. Minute ventilation increases 1–4 L/min for each acute 1 mmHg increase in $PaCO_2$.[2] While central chemoreceptors are primarily responsive to $H^+$, peripheral chemoreceptors are more sensitive to $PaO_2$. Patients who have had bilateral carotid endarterectomies lose the peripheral chemoreceptor response and will have little to no hypoxic ventilatory drive.[3] Furthermore, the magnitude of the pulmonary response is greater with metabolic acidosis than metabolic alkalosis. This is because increasing hypoventilation (in response to metabolic alkalosis) often leads to hypoxemia, which triggers $O_2$-sensitive chemoreceptors and limits the compensatory response. These mechanisms are all hindered under general anesthesia, especially in those patients who are mechanically ventilated, thereby relying on the anesthesiologist to manage the patient's minute ventilation.

The final compensatory mechanism occurs through the kidneys. Although renal compensation starts immediately, it does not typically achieve the target effect until 12–24 hours, and maximal effects may not be seen for up to 5 days.[2] Thus, while renal compensation may start in the OR, the result is not usually apparent until the postoperative period. The kidneys have two major roles in acid-base regulation: reabsorption of bicarbonate and excretion of $H^+$. Eighty to ninety percent of bicarbonate is reabsorbed in the proximal convoluted tubule, which allows for highly effective correction of alkalosis through rapid excretion. The hydrogen cation can also be excreted as ammonium. Ammonia passively enters the tubular fluid, where it can combine with hydrogen to form $NH_4^+$. Once this reaction occurs, $NH_4^+$ is trapped within the tubule and is excreted within the urine, effectively eliminating $H^+$ from the body.

## ANESTHETIC MANAGEMENT

### PREOPERATIVE

Preoperatively, it is important to consider the patient's current (and baseline) acid-base status. Common conditions that alter acid-base status and may exist on presentation to the operating room include shock states, vomiting or diarrhea, pain, anxiety, long-standing chronic obstructive pulmonary disease with $CO_2$ retention, metabolic acidosis related to renal failure, and so on. It is also important to recognize whether any existing abnormality is acute or chronic, metabolic or respiratory, and if appropriate compensation is occurring. If the presence of an acid-base disorder or the potential for large swings in acid-base status during the case exists, the anesthesia team may consider placing an arterial line to facilitate easy and frequent blood draws for analysis and management decisions.

### INTRAOPERATIVE

Intraoperative management focuses on keeping a patient's acid-base status near baseline by compensating for the ways in which preexisting comorbidities, general anesthesia, sedation, and surgery will alter this complicated homeostasis. It is important to recognize patients with chronic acid-base abnormalities. For example, patients with a history of obstructive lung disease often retain $CO_2$. Over time, they begin to retain bicarbonate so that they may achieve a normal pH with their elevated $PaCO_2$. It is imperative not to correct the $PaCO_2$ to "normal" as this patient will have a limited respiratory drive at a lower $CO_2$ than usual.

## POSTOPERATIVE

Postoperative management of acid-base status relies on correcting any ongoing major abnormalities. While most patients will not require major ongoing postoperative resuscitation, consideration for transfer to the intensive care unit may be necessary to facilitate closer monitoring and management if large disturbances exist.

## REFERENCES

1. Faust RJ, Trentman TL. *Faust's Anesthesiology Review*. 5th ed. Amsterdam, Netherlands: Elsevier; 2020.
2. Butterworth JF, et al. *Morgan & Mikhail's Clinical Anesthesiology*. 6th ed. New York, NY: McGraw-Hill Education; 2018.
3. Pardo MC, Miller RD. *Basics of Anesthesia*. 7th ed. Philadelphia, PA: Elsevier; 2018.

# 83.

# EFFECTS OF IMBALANCE ON ELECTROLYTES AND ORGAN PERFUSION

*Sarah Maben*

## POTASSIUM

The high intracellular concentration of potassium relative to serum level is necessary to maintain the cell's resting membrane potential. The distal segments of the kidney are the primary route for $K^+$ excretion. Changes in systemic pH affect $K^+$ excretion (Table 83.1). Chronicity of acid-base abnormality plays a role; in chronic acidosis, $K^+$ excretion is promoted secondary to increased filtration at the cortical collecting duct. Acute acidosis reduces $K^+$ excretion. Metabolic and respiratory alkalosis enhances $K^+$ excretion. Acute respiratory acidosis decreases $K^+$ excretion.

## SODIUM

Details regarding body sodium balance are discussed elsewhere. When changes in sodium and chloride are proportional (i.e., an increase or decrease synchronously), excessive hydration or dehydration is often the culprit. Conversely, a change in chloride without a change in sodium indicates an acid-base disorder. A metabolic alkalosis or respiratory acidosis decreases chloride concentration relative to sodium concentration. A respiratory alkalosis or hyperchloremic metabolic acidosis shows an increase in chloride greater than sodium.[1,2]

## H⁺ SECRETION BY THE KIDNEY

Under normal circumstances, the net acid excretion is equivalent to the bicarbonate production in the kidney. Sodium enters the proximal tubule cell in exchange for a hydrogen ion excreted into the urine. The hydrogen ion then reacts with bicarbonate to form $CO_2$ and $H_2O$. The $H^+$ is generated

*Table 83.1* RELATIONSHIP OF K⁺ EXCRETION AND ACID-BASE DISORDER

| ACID-BASE DISORDER | EFFECT ON K⁺ EXCRETION |
| --- | --- |
| Acute metabolic acidosis | Decreased |
| Acute respiratory acidosis | Decreased |
| Acute metabolic alkalosis | Increased |
| Acute respiratory alkalosis | Increased |
| Chronic metabolic alkalosis | Increased |
| Chronic respiratory acidosis | Increased |

Hyperkalemia is often seen in oliguric acute kidney injury due to a reduced glomerular filtration rate. In patients with rhabdomyolysis or tumor lysis syndrome, hyperkalemia is seen due to release of intracellular $K^+$ stores from lysed cells.[1,3]

in the cell via the same biochemical reaction between carbon dioxide and water. Intracellularly, this is catalyzed by carbonic anhydrase. In the distal tubule, the intercalated cells play the most important role in hydrogen ion homeostasis. Type A intercalated cells secrete $H^+$, and type B intercalated cells secrete $HCO_3^-$. Metabolic acidosis with a high anion gap is often seen in patients with acute kidney injury; this is due to decreased excretion of $H^+$ in the kidney.[1]

## ORGAN PERFUSION

Metabolic autoregulation matches tissue oxygen needs with available oxygen, and this process is severely deranged in acidosis via a number of different mechanisms. The cellular environment operates at high efficiency within a narrow physiologic pH. Prolonged exposure to nonphysiologic pH causes cellular deformity and ultimately cell death, including the red blood cells that are required to transport the majority of oxygen in the blood. Cell death leads to a pro-inflammatory state, which causes further cellular damage and impairs organ perfusion. The combination of acidosis, cellular death, and hypoxemia leads to tissue ischemia and production of lactate acid via the reduction of pyruvate to lactate when aerobic metabolism is impaired. This causes a positive-feedback loop of increasing cell death, worsening hypoxemia, and worsening acidosis, leading to cell death.

Severe acidosis also affects cardiac myocytes, leading to arrhythmias, hemodynamic instability, and decreased response to catecholamines. Impaired ventricular contractility and arrhythmias further decrease organ perfusion and contribute to cardiovascular collapse.

## ROLE OF ADMINISTERING EXOGENOUS BICARBONATE IN ACIDEMIA

The role of administering bicarbonate in metabolic acidosis is unclear. In general, most clinicians will administer exogenous bicarbonate therapy when the pH is below 7.2 and the patient has coexisting acute kidney injury. Remember that giving bicarbonate will cause increased production of carbon dioxide, and if the patient cannot compensate with increased alveolar ventilation, there is a risk of inducing iatrogenic respiratory acidosis. Exogenous bicarbonate does not confer a mortality benefit but may prevent initiation of hemodialysis and allow reversal of underlying acidosis in critically ill patients.[3]

## REFERENCES

1. Lee H, et al. Acid-base homeostasis. *Clin J Am Soc Nephrol.* 2015;10:2232–2242.
2. Reddi Alluru S. *Fluid, Electrolyte, and Acid-Base Disorders: Clinical Evaluation and Management.* 2nd ed. SpringerLink; 2018:321–337.
3. Jaber S, et al. BICAR-ICU Study Group. Sodium bicarbonate therapy for patients with severe metabolic acidaemia in the intensive care unit (BICAR-ICU): a multicentre, open-label, randomised controlled, phase 3 trial. *Lancet.* 2018;392(10141):31.

# 84.

# STRONG IONIC DIFFERENCE

*Christopher Giordano and Ravi Patel*

## INTRODUCTION

To appreciate the impact and application of Stewart's strong ion difference (SID) approach to acid-base disturbances, it is helpful to first review other preexisting tools used to decipher acid-base imbalances. The Henderson-Hasselbach equation, created by Lawrence Joseph Henderson in 1908 and modified by Karl Albert Hasselbach in 1917,[1] posits that the pH of a solution can be determined using the concentration of the acid [HA] and conjugate base [A−] in a solution along with the acid dissociation constant [Ka]: pH = pKa + $\log_{10}$ ([A–]/[HA]) = 6.1 + $\log_{10}$ ([HCO$_3^-$]/(0.03 × pCO$_2$)).[1] By studying the changes in [HCO$_3^-$] and pCO$_2$, this traditional approach allows differentiation between acute and chronic respiratory and metabolic derangements and their impact on pH.

$$pH = pKa + \log_{10}([A-/[HA])$$
$$= 6.1 + \log_{10}([HCO_3^-]/(0.03 \times pCO_2))$$

$$AG = \left[Na^+\right] + \left[K^+\right] - [Cl^-] - [HCO_3^-]$$

$$SID = [Na^+] + [K^+] + [Ca^{2+}] + [Mg^{2+}] - [Cl^-] - [Lactate]$$

## ANION GAP

Despite its ability to elucidate many pH disturbances, the Henderson-Hasselbalch approach fails to explain the specific mechanisms leading to the metabolic perturbations. The anion gap (AG), the difference between unmeasured plasma cations and anions, was designed to help classify metabolic disturbances such as normal AG acidosis or increased AG acidosis: AG = [Na$^+$] + [K$^+$] − [Cl$^-$] − [HCO$_3^-$]. The AG is susceptible to changes in albumin concentration because it is the major unmeasured anion in plasma, as well as changes in pH that alter albumin's charge and affect its hydrogen-binding capacity. Thus, the albumin-corrected AG was created to compensate for abnormal albumin concentrations.

## STRONG ION THEORY

In 1981, Peter Stewart introduced a novel approach to the acid-base assessment that redefined independent and dependent variables.[2] Whereas [H$^+$] had previously been assumed to be an independent variable, Stewart's new approach suggested that it was a dependent variable, along with [OH$^-$], [HCO$_3^-$], [HA], and [A–]. The three independent variables that determine the pH in Stewart's approach are PaCO$_2$, total weak acids (ATot), and SID.

## PACO$_2$

Similar to the previous traditional acid-base approaches, Stewart's theory includes respiratory acidosis and alkalosis as potential causes of acid-base disturbances because PaCO$_2$ is an independent variable. However, unlike those approaches, [HCO$_3^-$] is a dependent variable; therefore, it is not a determinant of blood pH. Instead, any metabolic derangements that occur are a result of changes in the SID or total weak acids (Figure 84.1).

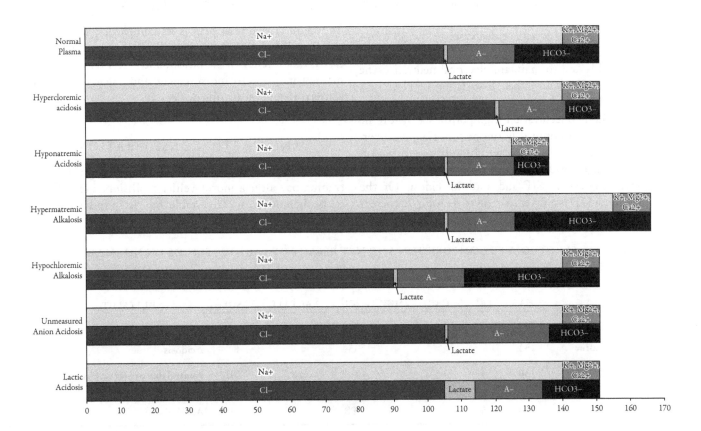

**Figure 84.1** Gamblegrams demonstrating various metabolic abnormalities explained by the Stewart approach.

## ATOT

The total weak acids ATot is the total plasma concentration of nonvolatile weak acids, including albumin, inorganic phosphate, and serum proteins. Disease states with high ATot (e.g., hyperphosphatemia) result in mild acidification because the relative concentration of weak acids increases. Conversely, a low ATot (e.g., hypoalbuminemia) will lead to mild alkalization because the relative concentration of the weak acid decreases.

## STRONG ION DIFFERENCE

The SID is the difference between the strong ions in plasma. A strong ion is defined as a cation or anion that remains completely dissociated at physiologic pH; thus, their ionization state is independent of pH. The strong cations included in this formula are sodium, potassium, calcium, and magnesium. The strong anions include chloride and lactate: $SID = [Na^+] + [K^+] + [Ca^{2+}] + [Mg^{2+}] - [Cl^-] - [Lactate]$. At normal physiologic conditions, SID typically ranges between 38 and 44 mEq/L. The law of electroneutrality requires that the sum of the positive charges must equal the sum of the negative charges; therefore, the SID must be equal to the sum of negative charges composed of weak anions such as bicarbonate, albumin, and phosphate in the body. Thus, under normal conditions, SID plus the sum of negative charges equals zero. With an accumulation of unmeasured anions, SID does not equal the sum of the negative charges.

When the SID of a patient decreases below 38 to 44 mEq/L, there is an excess of anions relative to cations. In response to this and to maintain electrical neutrality, the body generates $H^+$ from either dissociation of $H_2O$ or a donating buffer, which leads to acidosis.[3] Conditions that decrease sodium concentration (e.g., polydipsia, syndrome of inappropriate antidiuretic hormone secretion, glucocorticoid deficiency, etc.) or increase chloride concentration (e.g., iatrogenic chloride administration, renal tubular acidosis, etc.) can decrease SID and result in acidosis. On the contrary, if the SID is greater than 38 to 44 mEq/L, there is a relative cation excess, and the body's response is to trap $H^+$ ions by generating $HCO_3^-$, reassociation of $H_2O$, or weak acids converting to their conjugate base, leading to alkalosis.[4] Conditions that increase sodium concentration (e.g., dehydration, iatrogenic sodium administration, mineralocorticoid or glucocorticoid excess, etc.) or decrease chloride concentration (e.g., excessive vomiting, gastric fluid drainage, diuretic use, etc.) can increase SID and result in alkalosis. This explains why administering intravenous fluids, such as normal saline (NS), that decrease SID can cause acidosis, while administering intravenous fluids, such as Plasma-Lyte, that increase SID will result in alkalosis in the patient (Table 84.1).

## ADVANTAGES

One of the main reasons that the Stewart approach has gained popularity over previous traditional approaches is that it accounts for some clinical events that previous models were unable to explain (e.g., acid-base disturbances in hypoalbuminemic patients and clinical cases discussed below). Another advantage of the Stewart approach is that it accounts for the role of plasma proteins and phosphate in pH, making it more reliable to evaluate critically ill patients who can suffer from hypoproteinemia and hypophosphatemia.

## DISADVANTAGES

The main criticism of SID is its complexity, which does not simplify acid-base disorders. Furthermore, a disadvantage is that it relies on the measurement of several variables, making it prone to measurement and calculation errors across different measuring devices.

## ANESTHETIC CONSIDERATIONS

A previously healthy 22-year-old man is brought into the trauma bay after a motor vehicle collision. He is found to be hemodynamically stable but is found to have a

*Table 84.1* ELECTROLYTE COMPOSITION AND NET EFFECT OF VARIOUS FLUIDS ON NORMAL PHYSIOLOGIC PH

| | NA+ | K+ | CA2+ | MG2+ | CL- | LACTATE | SID | NET EFFECT |
|---|---|---|---|---|---|---|---|---|
| Plasma | 140 | 4 | 2.5 | 1 | 102 | | 38–44 | |
| Normal saline | 154 | | | | 154 | | 0 | Acidosis |
| Lactated Ringer | 130 | 4 | 1.5 | | 109 | 28 | 28 | Neutral due to SID acidosis but dilutional alkalosis |
| Plasma-Lyte | 140 | 5 | | 1.5 | 98 | | 50 | Alkalosis |

positive focused assessment with sonography for trauma. In the trauma bay, he is administered 3 L of NS and no other medications. He is taken to the operating room for emergent exploratory laparotomy. In the operating room, initial arterial blood gas shows a metabolic acidosis with a pH of 7.24 and normal lactate. Appreciating Stewart's SID, one recognizes that the patient received 3 L of a fluid (NS) with a SID of zero, and this lowered the patient's SID, resulting in excess hydrogen ion generation to maintain electrical neutrality but creating a metabolic acidosis in the process. Specifically, the patient experienced a hyperchloremic metabolic acidosis secondary to the 3 L of NS.

A septic patient in the operating room has an ischemic bowel secondary to a small bowel obstruction. The patient's pH is 7.12, and lactate is 8. The surgeon suggests sodium, administering sodium bicarbonate (NaHCO$_3$) to address the metabolic acidosis. Applying the Stewart approach better elucidates the mechanism of action of sodium bicarbonate to correct an acidosis. Administering sodium bicarbonate will increase the patient's plasma sodium.

The bicarbonate will rapidly combine with hydrogen and be metabolized into water and CO$_2$ that is expired. Subsequently, the [HCO$_3^-$] will have minimal impact on the patient's pH, whereas the excess sodium will significantly increase the SID, leading to a cation excess that shifts [H$^+$] out of solution, resulting in a metabolic alkalosis. NaHCO$_3$ should be seen as a fluid that is chloride-free sodium as opposed to a bicarbonate-rich fluid.[5]

## REFERENCES

1. Constable PD. Acid-base assessment: when and how to apply the Henderson-Hasselbalch equation and strong ion difference theory. *Vet Clin North Am Food Anim Pract.* 2014;30(2):295–316, v.
2. Stewart P. *How to Understand Acid-Base.* Elsevier, New York 1981.
3. Schiraldi F, Guiotto G. Base excess, strong ion difference, and expected compensations: as simple as it is. *Eur J Emerg Med.* 2014;21(6):403–408.
4. Morgan TJ. The Stewart approach—one clinician's perspective. *Clin Biochem Rev.* 2009;30(2):41–54.
5. Story DA. Stewart acid-base: a simplified bedside approach. *Anesth Analg.* 2016;123(2):511–515.

# 85.

# ARTERIAL BLOOD GAS INTERPRETATION

*Sarah Maben*

## STEPWISE ALGORITHM FOR ABG INTERPRETATION

1. Identify the primary acid-base disorder using Figure 85.1.
2. Calculate the anion gap (AG). If applicable, calculate the delta gap ($\Delta$AG/$\Delta$HCO$_3^-$).
3. Formulate a differential diagnosis for the primary disorder.
4. Calculate the expected physiologic compensation and compare with patient laboratory values.
5. Identify any additional acid-base disorders, if any.

## PH CONSIDERATIONS

The *Henderson equation* (Equation 85.1) relates the hydrogen ion concentration [H$^+$] to pH.

$$H^+ (nmol/L) = 24 \times (pCO_2 / [HCO_3^-]) \qquad (85.1)$$

A [H$^+$] of 40 nmol/L corresponds to a pH of 7.40. This equation is used to calculate HCO$_3^-$ from an ABG.[1-3] (Figure 85.1).

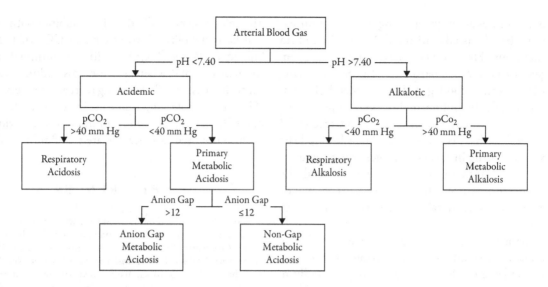

**Figure 85.1** Stepwise algorithm for evaluating an ABG.

## ACIDEMIA

If the pH is less than 7.40, the patient is *acidemic*. Acidemia is the state of having excess [H⁺] in the blood. *Acidosis* is the physiologic cause for the acidemia. When considering the etiology of acidemia, use the following formula (Equation 85.2):

$$CO_2 + H_2O \leftrightarrow H_2CO_3 \leftrightarrow HCO_3^- + H^+ \qquad (85.2)$$

If the $pCO_2$ is greater than 40 mm Hg, then the primary disorder is respiratory acidosis. As seen by Equation 85.2, increasing $CO_2$ drives the equilibrium to the right, increasing [H⁺] and causing acidemia. If the $HCO_3^-$ is decreased (as in metabolic acidosis), this will also drive the equation to the right, causing acidemia.[1,3]

Respiratory acidosis is driven by excessive $pCO_2$, or inability to adequately ventilate the lungs. Carbon dioxide retention can be acute, chronic, or acute-on-chronic. Respiratory acidosis is caused by chronic obstruction pulmonary disease; respiratory depression (from narcotics or after traumatic brain injury); neuromuscular weakness (Guillain-Barré syndrome, myasthenia gravis); or an obstructed airway.[3]

If the pH is less than 7.40 and $pCO_2$ less than 40 mm Hg, the primary disorder is metabolic acidosis. The anion gap (AG) is used to help categorize the pathogenesis of a metabolic acidosis into diagnoses with a high concentration of unmeasured anions (high AG or positive AG metabolic acidosis) or a relative high chloride ion level (normal AG acidosis). The AG is calculated as

$$AG(mEq/L) = \left[ (Na^+) - (Cl^- + HCO_3^-) \right] \qquad (85.3)$$

For a differential diagnosis of metabolic acidosis, see Table 85.1.

## DELTA GAP

If an elevated AG metabolic acidosis is present, the next step is to calculate the delta gap, or the ratio of the change in AG to the change in $HCO_3^-$ ($\Delta AG/\Delta HCO_3^-$). In simple terms, it compares the AG with the change in bicarbonate, and if the ratio is not 1:1, there must be another acid-base disorder present. For example, if a patient has an increased AG metabolic acidosis and the AG = 8, we expect the $HCO_3^-$ to decrease by 8 mEq/L. If the $HCO_3^-$ has decreased by only 5 mEq/L, then there must be a coexisting metabolic alkalosis driving $HCO_3^-$ higher than expected for a pure metabolic acidosis.[1,3]

## ALKALEMIA

When the pH is greater than 7.40, the patient is *alkalemic*. If the $pCO_2$ is low, Equation 85.2 will be driven to the left, causing a decrease in [H⁺]. This is a primary respiratory alkalosis. Respiratory alkalosis frequently results from tachypnea,

*Table 85.1* DIFFERENTIAL DIAGNOSIS OF METABOLIC ACIDOSIS

| INCREASED ANION GAP (AG > 12) | NORMAL ANION GAP (AG ≤ 12) |
|---|---|
| Methanol ingestion | GI loss of $HCO_3^-$ (diarrhea, ileostomy) |
| Uremia | |
| Diabetic ketoacidosis | Renal tubular acidosis (RTA) |
| Isoniazid toxicity | Hyperchloremia (e.g., NaCl administration) |
| Acetaminophen toxicity | |
| Lactic acidosis | Carbonic anhydrase inhibitors |
| Ethylene glycol toxicity | |
| Salicylate toxicity | |

Table created by the author.

such as from pain, anxiety, sepsis, trauma, heat exposure, or high altitude. Pneumonia, pulmonary embolism, pulmonary edema, and severe anemia are other common etiologies. Correlating the patient's clinical history with the ABG will help determine the most likely diagnosis.[3]

Metabolic alkalosis is caused by excessive body bicarbonate content. Diuretics, renal salt wasting and secondary hyperaldosteronism, and refeeding syndrome all causing excess $HCO_3^-$. Gastrointestinal loss of hydrochloric acid (HCl) from vomiting or nasogastric suction also leads to a disproportionate bicarbonate load.[3]

## DETERMINING THE COMPENSATORY RESPONSE

Initially the acid-base abnormality is addressed by buffering immediately using buffers in the body fluid compartment. Over the next hours compensation occurs via the renal system for respiratory acid-base abnormalities and through the respiratory system for metabolic abnormalities. The last phase is correction of the abnormality by eliminating the acid-base disturbance.

Once you have determined the primary acid-base disorder, calculate the expected physiologic compensatory response and compare it to the patient's laboratory values. This will uncover any additional acid-base disorders that may be present.

Respiratory compensation for a primary metabolic acidosis is known as Winter's formula:

$$pCO_2 = HCO_3^- \times 1.5 + (8 \pm 2) \qquad (85.4)$$

Use the patient's $HCO_3^-$ to calculate the expected $pCO_2$. If the actual $pCO_2$ is different, there must be a coexisting respiratory acid-base disorder. If the $pCO_2$ is lower than expected, there is a secondary respiratory alkalosis. If the $pCO_2$ is higher than expected, there is a secondary respiratory acidosis.[3]

Respiratory compensation for a primary metabolic alkalosis is an increase of 0.7 mm Hg $pCO_2$ per mEq/L increase in $HCO_3^-$.

## METABOLIC COMPENSATION OF A PRIMARY RESPIRATORY ACID-BASE DISORDER

For each 10 mm Hg increase in $pCO_2$, the expected $HCO_3^-$ is

|  | Respiratory Acidosis | Respiratory Alkalosis |
|---|---|---|
| Acute | Increased 1 | Decreased 2 |
| Chronic | Increased 3 | Decreased 4–5 |

For every 10 torr change in $PaCO_2$, the PH will change 0.08 unit in the opposite direction. If the bicarbonate is less than expected, there is a secondary metabolic acidosis. If the bicarbonate is greater than expected, there is a secondary metabolic alkalosis.[1,3]

## REFERENCES

1. Gennari FJ, RG Narins, eds. *Maxwell and Kleeman's Clinical Disorders of Fluid and Electrolyte Metabolism*. 5th ed. New York, NY: McGraw-Hill; 1994.
2. Lee H, et al. Acid-base homeostasis. *Clin J Am Soc Nephrol*. 2015;10:2232–2242.
3. Reddi Alluru S. *Fluid, Electrolyte, and Acid-Base Disorders: Clinical Evaluation and Management*. 2nd ed. SpringerLink; 2018.

# 86.

# THE ANION GAP AND METABOLIC ACIDOSIS

*Scott Stayner and Kris Ferguson*

## ANION GAP

To maintain electrochemical neutrality, the concentration of anions (negatively charge ions) and cations (positively charged ions) must remain equal. The commonly measured ions include the cation sodium ($Na^+$) and the anions chloride ($Cl^-$) and bicarbonate ($HCO_3^-$). However, there are also unmeasured cations and unmeasured anions. The anion gap (AG) is a measure of the difference between the unmeasured cations and unmeasured anions, as illustrated by the following equations:

$$[Na^+] + [\text{Unmeasured Cations}]$$
$$= [Cl^-] + [HCO_3^-] + [\text{Unmeasured Anions}]$$

Rearrangement of the equation:

$$\text{Anion Gap} = [\text{Unmeasured Anions}] - [\text{Unmeasured Cations}]$$
$$= [Na^+] - ([Cl^-] + [HCO_3^-])$$

The AG increases with any process that *decreases* [Unmeasured Cations]. Unmeasured cations include $K^+$, $Ca^{2+}$, and $Mg^{2+}$. The AG also increases with an *increase* in [Unmeasured Anions]. Common unmeasured anions include phosphates, sulfates, and plasma proteins. The accepted range for a normal AG is 8–16 mEq/L.[1]

Albumin is an especially prominent anion. The AG is reduced 2.5 mEq/L for every 1 g/dL drop in albumin concentration. The Figge equation can be used to calculate the corrected AG (cAG) to account for the difference in normal albumin versus measured albumin.[2]

$$cAG = AG + 025 \times (\text{normal albumin-measured albumin})$$

## CLINICAL RELEVANCE

### INCREASED ANION GAP METABOLIC ACIDOSIS

Elevated AG acidosis suggests an increase of unmeasured anions, such as lactic acid or keto acids as $HCO_3^-$ is consumed to maintain physiologic pHa. There are several reasons that an increased AG metabolic acidosis occurs (Box 86.1).

Organic acids are typically excreted by the renal system. Patients in renal failure will progress to metabolic acidosis due to the inability to eliminate endogenous organic acids. Also, as the renal function decreases, the ability of the kidneys to excrete $NH_4^+$ decreases, resulting in an excess [$H^+$] and acidotic state. Liver failure and/or cirrhosis results in excess lactic acid accumulation due to decreased conversion of lactate to glucose.

Lactic acid produced in excess (i.e., lactic acidosis) is a common cause of increased AG metabolic acidosis. Hypoxemia and subsequent tissue ischemia can occur when there is a mismatch between tissue oxygen supply and

---

**Box 86.1 COMMON CAUSES OF INCREASED ANION GAP METABOLIC ACIDOSIS**

**Causes of High Anion Gap Metabolic Acidosis**
Lactic acidosis
 Tissue underperfusion—hypoxia, shock, anemia, heart failure
 Excessive oxygen demand—shivering, fever, strenuous exercise
 Drugs—methanol, ethanol, salicylate
Renal failure—accumulation of organic acids
Liver failure—decreased conversion of lactate to glucose
Ketoacidosis—diabetes mellitus, alcohol, starvation

*From Reference 3.*

---

demand. Decreased oxygen supply is a frequent etiology and can occur in severe hypoxia, shock, severe anemia, or in cardiac failure. However, excessive oxygen demand can also cause increased lactic acid production due to shivering, high fever, strenuous exercise, and seizures.

Inability of tissue to utilize oxygen resulting from abnormal pyruvate metabolism can also result in lactic acidosis. This can be due to congenital errors of metabolism such as glucose-6-phosphate dehydrogenase deficiency, fructose 1,6-diphosphonate deficiency, or type 1 glycogen storage disease. Substances such as methanol, ethanol, acetaminophen, and salicylates can also disrupt normal pyruvate metabolism to increase lactic acid production. Hyperglycemia from inadequate insulin can result in the accumulation of β-hydroxybutyric and acetoacetic acids as well as interrupt pyruvate dehydrogenase activity, which leads to excess lactic acid production in addition to keto acid (acetoacetate and β-hydroxyutyrate). Excess keto acid production is also observed in starvation states.

## NORMAL ANION GAP METABOLIC ACIDOSIS

Metabolic acidosis with a normal AG is the result of $HCO_3^-$ loss rather than consumption of $HCO_3^-$ as occurs in metabolic acidosis when $HCO_3^-$ buffers nonvolatile acids. The $[Cl^-]$ in plasma is increased to compensate for the $[HCO_3^-]$ loss and is therefore termed *hyperchloremic metabolic acidosis*. Common causes of normal AG metabolic acidosis are outlined in Box 86.2.

Gastrointestinal loss of $HCO_3^-$ in the form of diarrhea is a common cause of hyperchloremic metabolic acidosis. The fluids in diarrhea are derived from the small bowel, biliary tract, and pancreas, which all have high $[HCO_3^-]$.

Renal dysfunction can also result in normal AG hyperchloremic metabolic acidosis. Kidney dysfunction affects plasma $[K^+]$; therefore, the plasma $[K^+]$ can help elucidate the underlying cause. In renal tubular acidosis, loss of $HCO_3^-$ occurs due to inadequate reabsorption of $HCO_3^-$ (proximal renal tubular acidosis) or impaired $H^+$ secretion (distal renal tubular acidosis). Both proximal and distal renal tubular acidosis are associated with hypokalemia. Type 4 renal tubular acidosis, aldosterone deficiency, and aldosterone resistance also result in a net loss of $HCO_3^-$ but induce hyperkalemia. Multiple drugs can induce a type 4 renal tubular acidosis such as angiotensin-converting enzyme inhibitors, spironolactone trimethoprim, nonsteroidal anti-inflammatory drugs (NSAIDs), and cyclosporine. When the glomerular filtration rate drops to 30–59 mL/min (stage 3), a normokalemia metabolic acidosis occurs.

When the extracellular volume is rapidly expanded with a bicarbonate free fluid, hyperchloremic normal ion gap metabolic acidosis can occur. This is common with rapid volume expansion using normal saline. However, parenteral hyperalimentation as occurs in total parenteral nutrition and administration of ammonium chloride or arginine hydrochloride can also cause a normal AG metabolic acidosis.

## ANESTHETIC CONSIDERATIONS

There are multiple serious consequences of severe acidemia, as outlined in Box 86.3.

---

**Box 86.2** COMMON CAUSES OF NORMAL ANION GAP (HYPERCHLOREMIC) METABOLIC ACIDOSIS

**Causes of Normal Anion Gap (Hyperchloremic) Metabolic Acidosis**
Gastrointestinal bicarbonate loss
　Diarrhea
　Ileostomy
Renal acidosis
　Hypokalemia (proximal and distal renal tubular acidosis
　Hyperkalemia (type 4 renal tubular acidosis, aldosterone deficiency/resistance)
　Normokalemia (chronic kidney disease)
Drug-induced hyperkalemia resulting in renal insufficiency
　K⁺-sparing diuretics (spironolactone triamterene, amiloride)
　NSAIDs
　Cyclosporine
Rapid administration of 0.9% normal saline, hyperalimentation, or other chloride-containing fluid

*From Reference 4.*

---

**Box 86.3** ADVERSE EFFECTS OF SEVERE ACIDEMIA

**Adverse Effects of Severe Acidemia**
Cardiovascular
　Decreased cardiac output
　Cardiac arrhythmia
　Hypotension
　Increased pulmonary vascular resistance
　Insensitivity to catecholamines
Central nervous system
　Decreased level of consciousness
Metabolic
　Increased $O_2$ affinity to hemoglobin, reduced oxygen delivery
　Insulin resistance
　Hypercalcemia

*From Reference 4.*

Assess for volume status and renal function in the preoperative setting. An arterial line should be considered to enable real-time observation of blood pressure and easy access to arterial blood for intraoperative arterial blood gas sample collection. In the case of shock, preload monitoring via pulmonary artery catheterization or echocardiography should be considered.

Although treating the underlying cause of acidosis is the most definitive treatment, it is reasonable to replace lost $HCO_3^-$. This is not without some controversy as controlled studies in humans and animals have not shown any reduction in morbidity and mortality.[5] However, alternative treatments such as Carbicarb and THAM (tris-hydroxymethylamino-methane) have not been widely adopted due to limited clinical control trials and potential side effects. The initial dose of $HCO_3^-$ can be estimated using the following equation, assuming the space distribution of bicarbonate is approximately 50%[4]:

$$HCO_3^- \text{ deficit} = (\text{desired serum } [HCO_3^-]$$
$$- \text{measured } [HCO_3^-]) \times 0.5 \times \text{body weight (kg)}$$

## INTRAOPERATIVE

Intraoperatively, an exaggerated hypotensive response to drugs and positive pressure ventilation should be expected.

Although hyperventilation should be utilized to help elevate pHa, efficacy should be monitored via capnography and serial arterial blood gases. Normal saline should be avoided for fluid resuscitation, and balanced salt solutions such as lactated Ringer should be used to avoid further reduction in pHa.

## POSTOPERATIVE

The patient should be monitored for ongoing metabolic acidosis and potential complications. The severity of the acidosis will dictate disposition to the surgical intensive care unit for further intense monitoring versus extubation and less stringent monitoring in the normal hospital ward.

## REFERENCES

1. Kraut JA, Nagami GT. The serum anion gap in the evaluation of acid-base disorders: what are its limitations and can its effectiveness be improved? *Clin J Am Soc Nephrol.* 2013;8(11):2018–2024.
2. Figge J, et al. Anion gap and hypoalbuminemia. *Crit Care Med.* 1998;26(11):1807–1810.
3. Maloney DG, et al. Anions and the anaesthetist. Published online 2002;15.
4. Lim S. Metabolic acidosis. *Acta Medica Indones.* 2007;39(3):145–150.
5. Mathieu D, et al. Effects of bicarbonate therapy on hemodynamics and tissue oxygenation in patients with lactic acidosis: a prospective, controlled clinical study. *Crit Care Med.* 1991;19(11):1352–1356.

# 87.

# TEMPERATURE EFFECT ON BLOOD GASES
## ALPHA-STAT VERSUS PH-STAT

*Sohail K. Mahboobi and Faraz Mahmood*

## INTRODUCTION

When a blood gas sample is collected and analyzed, it is heated to a temperature of 37°C prior to measurements. In certain clinical situations, the patients are hypothermic or

hyperthermic due to pathologies, illnesses, or treatments. The hyperthermic conditions occurring in clinical practice are fever, sepsis, endocrine problems (thyrotoxicosis), and cerebral injuries. The hypothermic conditions usually encountered are severe sepsis, hypothyroidism, drug overdoses, winter cold exposure, and cardiopulmonary bypass. Therapeutic hypothermia to slow cellular metabolism is being used after resuscitation of cardiac arrest and hypoxic cerebral insults. These temperature shifts result in changes in the properties of gases, which invariably result in differences in $PaCO_2$, $PaO_2$, and pH. There are two blood gas management strategies that are commonly used to manage these changes: alpha-stat and pH-stat.

## EFFECT OF TEMPERATURE ON GAS SOLUBILITY

According to Henry's law, the concentration of a gas in a solution is directly proportional to the partial pressure of the gas and the solubility of $O_2$, and $CO_2$ varies with temperature (Figure 87.1). As temperature decreases, the gases become more soluble with a decrease in partial pressure.[1] This results in a decrease in the protonated form of gasses ($HA \rightleftharpoons H^+ + A^-$), which pushes equilibrium to the left with formation of more HA than $H^+$. In practice, $PaCO_2$ decreases by approximately 2 mm Hg per degree centigrade below 37°C.

Blood gas analyzers are designed to measure gas partial pressures at 37°C.[1] As a blood sample is warmed to 37°C by the analyzer, the partial pressures of $CO_2$ and $O_2$ increase, leading to reported $PaO_2$ and $PaCO_2$ (uncorrected for a patient's temperature) results that are greater than actual values in a hypothermic patient. The obtained value is then corrected to the patient's current temperature.

The two strategies reflect different approaches in management of pH addressing the increased solubility of $CO_2$ at lower temperatures. In the pH-stat method, $CO_2$ is added to maintain a "normal" $PaCO_2$ (40 mm Hg) at the patient's actual hypothermic temperature. On the other hand, alpha-stat is a strategy that prioritizes the body's ability to maintain its own homeostasis and no additional $CO_2$ is added. Instead, the goal is to keep the pH and $PaCO_2$ within a normal range when the measurements are performed at 37°C. To summarize, in the alpha-stat method no temperature correction is applied, and in the pH-stat method a temperature correction is applied to maintain normal blood gas values.

## PH-STAT METHOD

In the pH-stat method, the ideal pH and $PaCO_2$ are attempted to be maintained at 7.40 and 40 mm Hg, respectively, regardless of the patient's actual temperature (Figure 87.2). The alkaline shift is corrected by adding $CO_2$ to keep the arterial carbon dioxide partial pressure at 40 mm Hg and the pH at 7.4 when measured at the patient's actual temperature (corrected to the patient's temperature).[2] This results in relative hypercarbia and acidemia at an uncorrected temperature of 37°C. The eventual result is a higher $PaCO_2$ level, which has several physiological effects. High $CO_2$ levels result in uncoupling of cerebral autoregulation, which can lead to increases in cerebral blood flow independent of metabolic demands. There is also systemic vasodilation, which can result in quicker and even cooling in cardiac bypass patients. The pH-stat method also counteracts the leftward shift of the $O_2$-hemoglobin dissociation curve that results from hypothermia and alkalemia, which theoretically helps increase oxygen unloading and delivery to the tissues.

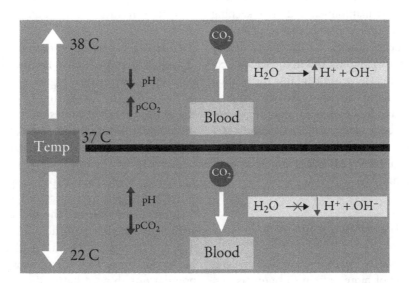

**Figure 87.1** Effect of temperature on solubility of gases in blood. A decrease in temperature causes gases to be more soluble, with a resultant increase in pH and a decrease in $PaCO_2$. A rise in temperature results in less solubility and a lower pH with higher $PaCO_2$.

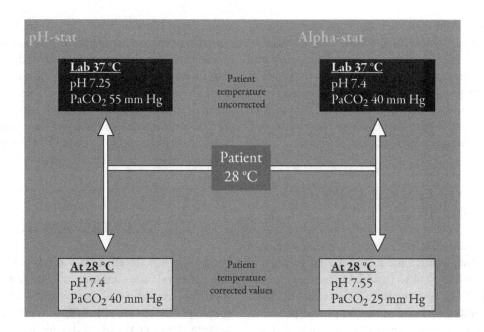

**Figure 87.2** Comparison of pH-stat and alpha-stat methods for a patient at 28°C. Note the difference in temperature-uncorrected and temperature-corrected values of blood gasses in both methods.

## ALPHA-STAT METHOD

The goal of the alpha-stat strategy is to maintain the intracellular acid-base homeostasis by keeping pH of neutrality (pN) in the normal range. pN is considered the pH at which the concentration of hydrogen ions equals hydroxide ions ([H⁺] = [OH⁻]). The pN of 0.55 is optimal for the cellular function. The hypothesis is that pN is a temperature-dependent parameter and not correcting the pH at different temperatures preserves its ability to maintain an optimal pN on both sides of the cell membrane. The name derives from the description of the dissociation of the imidazole groups of the amino acid, histidine, that is present in proteins. With the goal to keep pH uncorrected, the pN is maintained and thus keeping alpha (the degree of dissociation) constant, that is, alpha-stat. The temperature-dependent intracellular protein buffering by imidazole residues on histidine changes in the same direction as the systemic pH changes and maintains the normal pH gradient required for normal functioning of the proteins. Therefore, the pH of 7.4 and pCO$_2$ of 40 mm Hg are appropriate only with a normal body temperature. In the alpha-stat method, when the sample is anaerobically warmed to 37°C, ideally the (temperature uncorrected) values should be a pH of 7.4 and a pCO$_2$ of 40 mm Hg.

## CLINICAL IMPLICATIONS

The pH-stat strategy causes cerebral vasodilation and blood flow with a supply of more oxygen to brain tissues. This strategy is also considered to cause faster recovery of intracellular pH along with recovery of cerebral high-energy metabolites after deep hypothermic circulatory arrest cases.[3] The resultant systemic vasodilation is helpful in quicker and generalized cooling of patients on cardiopulmonary bypass.

The alpha-stat strategy has been shown to preserve cerebral autoregulation, which prevents excessive cerebral blood flow and a rise in intracranial pressure. The resultant alkalemia in alpha-stat is cerebral protective. This method maintains the pN and cellular proteins and enzyme functions. It also avoids the chance of any error in measuring body temperature, which can be catastrophic in pH-stat management, particularly if temperature-corrected results are mistakenly assumed temperature uncorrected.

There are certain potential disadvantages with the alpha-stat strategy, such as less metabolic suppression in hypothermia, requiring a higher hematocrit, and distributed cerebral oxygenation during fast rewarming. In contrast, the pH-stat method causes increased blood flow, increased intracranial pressure, and a loss of cerebral autoregulation and its coupling to cerebral metabolism. This has the potential risk of microembolism to the brain in high-risk procedures like cardiac bypass surgery.[4]

Currently, it is unresolved whether it is necessary to temperature correct the blood gas results in patients with hypothermia. Another view is that the best strategy depends on age, with the pediatric population having better outcomes with the pH-stat method, whereas adult populations showed better outcomes with the alpha-stat strategy.[5]

## REFERENCES

1. Ashwood ER, et al. Temperature correction of blood-gas and pH measurements. *Clin Chem.* 1983;29:1877–1885.
2. Pokela M, et al. Ph-stat versus α-stat perfusion strategy during experimental hypothermic circulatory arrest: a microdialysis study. *Ann Thorac Surg.* 2003;76:1215–1226.
3. Duebener LF, et al. Effects of pH management during deep hypothermic bypass on cerebral microcirculation: α-stat versus pH-stat. *Circulation.* 2002;106(12):1103–1108.
4. Henriksen L. Brain luxury perfusion during cardiopulmonary bypass in humans. A study of the cerebral blood flow response to changes in $CO_2$, $O_2$, and blood pressure. *J Cereb Blood Flow Metab.* 1986;6: 366–378.
5. Aziz KA, Meduoye A. Is pH-stat or alpha-stat the best technique to follow in patients undergoing deep hypothermic circulatory arrest? *Interact Cardiovasc Thorac Surg.* 2010;10:271–282.

# 88.

# LUNG FUNCTION AND CELL PROCESSES

*Amit Prabhakar and Matt Warth*

## INTRODUCTION

The lungs act as the primary conduit for gas exchange and can be categorized by both anatomic and physiologic functionality. Specialized cells in the pulmonary system help to facilitate gas exchange, maintain the structural integrity of the pulmonary architecture, provide immunologic support, and also help to function in enzymatic physiology.

## LUNG ANATOMY AND PHYSIOLOGY

The pulmonary system comprises an intricate network of tissues that form a unique architecture allowing for a multitude of physiologic functions. Diaphragmatic contraction is controlled by the phrenic nerve and results in downward displacement of thoracic contents. This downward displacement promotes inhalation via pulmonary expansion. Air from the environment travels through the non–gas-exchanging upper respiratory system and eventually reaches the lower respiratory system, where gas exchange occurs. The upper respiratory system comprises the mouth, nasal cavity, nasopharynx, oropharynx, pharynx, and larynx.[1] Air movement through the upper respiratory system is called *conduction*. Conduction constitutes the warming,

humidification, and filtration of particulate matter as air travels into the lower respiratory system.

The trachea is the first component of the lower respiratory system and is an approximately 2-cm wide by 12-cm long tubular conduit supported by 16–20 cartilaginous rings. Air travels through the trachea and eventually hits the tracheal bifurcation at the level of the carina. The carina then divides the pulmonary system into the left and right lungs via the primary bronchi. The right bronchus is characterized as having a larger caliber and more vertical orientation, which makes it more susceptible to aspiration compared to the left bronchus. The left lung is divided into two lobes (upper and lower) while the right lung is divided into three lobes (superior, middle, inferior). These mainstem bronchi are then further divided into smaller and smaller segments called secondary and tertiary bronchi, respectively. Tertiary bronchi transition to smaller segments called bronchioles. Bronchioles extend deep into the lungs and further progress into terminal bronchioles, respiratory bronchioles, and then finally to the alveoli, the primary site of gas exchange.[1,2]

## SPECIFIC CELLULAR PROCESSES

The pulmonary architecture discussed comprises of a unique set of cells that help with conduction, facilitate gas exchange, and offer immunologic protection, among other things. Cells of the upper respiratory system allow for conduction of the air prior to entering the lower respiratory system. The interior of the trachea is lined with the respiratory epithelium, composed of specialized epithelial cells called goblet cells and pseudostratified ciliated columnar cells. Respiratory epithelial cells are coated in mucus-containing lysozymes and antimicrobial proteins known as defensins. This mucus is produced by goblet cells and serves as a defense against microbial infection. When foreign particles become trapped in the mucus of the trachea, pseudostratified ciliated columnar cells guide the particles toward the upper respiratory tract through the rhythmic beating of their cilia in a process known as the mucociliary escalator, where the contents are removed into the environment through the upper airway.[3]

Gas exchange occurs in the alveolar sacs. The alveoli are composed of a thin layer of epithelial cells called pneumocytes. The two lineages of pneumocytes are type 1 and type 2, and both are highly permeable to facilitate gas exchange. Type 2 pneumocytes account for only 3%–5% of respiratory epithelial cells, with type 1 cells accounting for the remaining 95%–97%. In addition to facilitating gas exchange, type 1 pneumocytes maintain alveolar ion and fluid balance. Type 2 pneumocytes are responsible for producing a phospholipid- and protein-based layer called surfactant.[4] Surfactant reduces the surface tension in the pulmonary tissue and maintains pulmonary integrity by preventing alveolar collapse. Type 2 pneumocytes can also regenerate into type 1 cells in response to injury or inflammation. Alveolar macrophages also reside in the alveoli and play a significant role in destroying pathogens and clearing inhaled particulates from the pulmonary system.[5]

In addition to the aforementioned cellular processes, regulation of systemic vasomotor activity within the body relies on cooperation with the hormonal and enzymatic metabolic function of lung tissue. In response to systemic vasodilation, the sympathetic nervous system activates the renin-angiotensin system (RAS) with the release of angiotensinogen. After proteolytic cleavage, angiotensinogen is converted to angiotensin 1. The pulmonary endothelium contains angiotensin-converting enzyme (ACE), which cleaves angiotensin 1 to angiotensin 2. Angiotensin 2 then goes on to act on several other sites throughout the body to promote vasoconstriction. ACE activity can be affected by pharmaceutical intervention via ACE inhibitors, preventing the conversion of angiotensin I into angiotensin II, slowing the RS and inducing vasodilation. Other pharmaceuticals targeting lung tissue include anticholinergics, adrenoreceptor agonists, leukotriene inhibitors, and corticosteroid inhalants. The majority of metabolites and byproducts following use are transported to the kidneys through the bloodstream; they are processed in the kidneys and excreted through the urine from the body.

## REFERENCES

1. Ball M, et al. Anatomy, airway. In: *StatPearls*. Treasure Island, FL: StatPearls Publishing; January 2020; updated August 2020. https://www.ncbi.nlm.nih.gov/books/NBK459258/
2. Saran M, et al. Anatomy, head and neck, larynx vocal cords. In: *StatPearls*. Treasure Island, FL: StatPearls Publishing; July 14, 2019.
3. De Rose V, et al. Airway epithelium dysfunction in cystic fibrosis and COPD. *Mediators Inflamm*. 2018;2018:1309746.
4. Basil MC, et al. The cellular and physiological basis for lung repair and regeneration: past, present, and future. *Cell Stem Cell*. 2020;26:482–502.
5. Ochs M, et al. The number of alveoli in the human lung. *Am J Respir Crit Care Med*. 2004;169(1):120–124.

# 89.

# VENTILATION-PERFUSION

*Jarrod Bang and Archit Sharma*

## INTRODUCTION

Gas exchange in the alveoli occurs via diffusion, in the respiratory zone of the lung, where alveoli are present. Hence, the alveolar basement membrane needs to be both ventilated and perfused for efficient gas exchange to occur.

**Perfusion:** The lungs have a dual blood supply that is derived from both the right and left heart. The pulmonary arteries receive blood from the right ventricle and receive the entire cardiac output. The pulmonary vasculature operates at approximately four-fold lower vascular resistance with the same cardiac output as the systemic circulation, resulting in lower pressures than the systemic vasculature under normal conditions. The other blood supply to the lungs is the bronchial arteries, which drain into the pulmonary vasculature and are derived from the systemic circulation. Transplanted lungs have a singular blood supply, from the pulmonary arteries.

**Ventilation:** An understanding of the west zones of the lung is essential to comprehend both lung perfusion and ventilation. West zones describe areas of the lung based on variations in pulmonary arterial pressure (PAP), pulmonary venous pressure (PVP), and alveolar pressure (AP).

The west lung zones are classically defined as three zones, but a fourth zone can be added.[1]

West lung zone 1 is defined by an alveolar pressure that is higher than both arterial and venous pulmonary pressures, resulting in no blood flow.

West lung zone 2 has an alveolar pressure that is less than the arterial pressure but higher than venous pressure, creating a pulsatile blood flow.

Areas with west lung zone 3 physiology have continuous blood flow due to an alveolar pressure that is lower than arterial and venous pressures.

West lung zone 4 introduces effects from increased interstitial pressures, commonly due to pulmonary edema or atelectasis.

The apical region, considered as zone 1, is where $P_A$ (alveolar pressure) can be higher than pulmonary arterial pressure ($P_a$) and pulmonary venous pressure ($P_{xww2}$). Since $P_A > P_a > P_v$ in zone I, no arterial blood flow occurs, and this zone is considered as physiological dead space. In middle zone or zone 2, the difference of $P_a$ to $P_A$ decides the perfusion ($P_a > P_A > P_v$), while in the lower zone or zone 3, the difference of $P_a$ to $P_v$ ($P_a > P_v > P_A$) decides the perfusion.

Figure 89.1 describes the different west zones in a lung and the relevant relationships between various pressures.

**Ventilation-Perfusion Ratio (V/Q Ratio):** The V/Q ratio evaluates the relationship and differences in matching of ventilation (V) to perfusion (Q). There is regional variation in both ventilation and perfusion within the lung. Ventilation is 50% greater at the base than at the apex. The weight of fluid in the pleural cavity increases the intrapleural pressure at the base to a less negative value, causing alveoli to be less expanded and have higher compliance at the base. This leads to a bigger increase in volume on inspiration and increased ventilation. Perfusion is also greater at the base of the lung due to gravity pulling the blood toward the base. Overall, perfusion increases more than the ventilation does at the base of the lung, resulting in lower V/Q ratios in the base of the lung compared to the apex.[2] In a healthy individual, the V/Q ratio is 1 at the middle of the lung, with a minimal spread of V/Q ratios from 0.3 to 2.1 from base to apex.[3] In cases of high V/Q ratios, $PO_2$ increases and $PCO_2$ decreases as alveolar air more closely matches the larger volume of inspired air than perfused blood.[4] On the other hand, low V/Q ratios result in decreased $PO_2$ and an increased $PCO_2$.

## PATHOPHYSIOLOGY

Dead space ventilation is defined as a portion of the respiratory tract that participates in ventilation but does not have perfusion to allow gas exchange to occur. There are two separate types of dead space: anatomic and alveolar. Anatomic dead space includes the respiratory tract from the pharynx to terminal bronchioles, which do not have a blood supply designed to participate in gas exchange. This dead space is unalterable. Alveolar dead space is ventilation to alveoli that could potentially participate in gas exchange but are not perfused (west lung zone 1). Dead

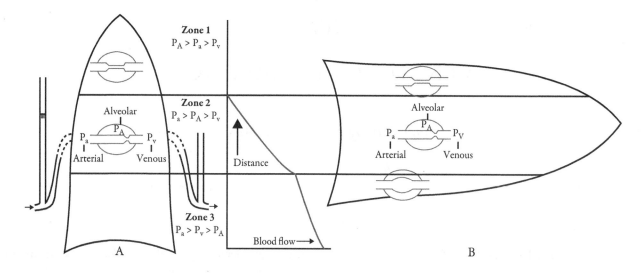

**Figure 89.1** West zones in the lung in the (A) upright position and (B) supine position and the relevant relationships between alveolar pressure ($P_A$), pulmonary arterial pressure ($P_a$), and pulmonary venous pressure ($P_v$).

space ventilation has a V/Q ratio equal to infinity. A pulmonary embolus can restrict blood flow in the pulmonary circulation, resulting in alveoli that are ventilated but not perfused; this results in an increased V/Q ratio and decreased gas exchange.[5]

A shunt refers to blood that flows from the right side of the heart to the left side of the heart without oxygenation. Intrapulmonary shunting occurs when blood flow is present to nonventilated portions of the lung. Hence, in the case of a shunt even though alveoli are perfused, they are not ventilated, causing a complete shunt to have a V/Q ratio of zero.

Hypoxic pulmonary vasoconstriction occurs due to the body's compensatory mechanism to shunt blood away from poorly oxygenated alveoli to well-oxygenated alveoli. Different anesthetics have varying effects on this important mechanism. Volatile anesthetics reduce the degree of hypoxic pulmonary vasoconstriction, while total intravenous anesthesia, including propofol and narcotics, has minimal affects.

## ANESTHETIC CONSIDERATIONS

### PREOPERATIVE

Preoperative assessment involves a review of pulmonary diagnoses, pulmonary medications, history of dyspnea, available tests such as pulmonary function tests, and coexisting heart failure. An important preoperative consideration in patients undergoing thoracoabdominal procedures, especially in a patient with preexisting lung disease, is to maximize their V/Q matching using regional anesthetic techniques that allow for early mobilization and better pulmonary rehabilitation.

### INTRAOPERATIVE

Increased $FiO_2$ (fraction of inspired air) has been shown to increase the shunt fraction up to 10% of the cardiac output, possibly from absorption atelectasis or attenuation of hypoxic pulmonary vasoconstriction.

The functional residual capacity is significantly reduced when a patient moves from an upright position to a supine position. It is also decreased under general anesthesia, and this decrease can be partially prevented with the application of positive end-expiratory pressure.

One-lung ventilation is generally tolerated better by taking advantage of the nonoperative lung being the dependent lung that largely participates in west lung zone 3 physiology and receives a larger portion of the blood supply.

### POSTOPERATIVE

Use of an inspiratory spirometer or similar breathing device can decrease postoperative atelectasis and pneumonia. Application of continuous positive airway pressure can also be useful in decreasing the development of atelectasis.

### REFERENCES

1. Hughes JMB, et al. Effect of lung volume on the distribution of pulmonary blood flow in man. *Respir Physiol.* 1968;4(1):58–72.
2. Hedenstierna G, et al. Ventilation and perfusion of each lung during differential ventilation with selective PEEP. *Anesthesiology.* 1984;61(4):369–376.
3. Wagner PD, et al. Continuous distributions of ventilation-perfusion ratios in normal subjects breathing air and 100% $O_2$. *J Clin Investig.* 1974;54(1):54–68.
4. Petersson J, Glenny RW. Gas exchange and ventilation–perfusion relationships in the lung. 2014;1023–1041.
5. Huet Y, et al. Hypoxemia in acute pulmonary embolism. *Chest.* 1985;88(6):829–836.

# 90.

# LUNG VOLUME

*Sarah Helwege and Archit Sharma*

## INTRODUCTION

Lung volumes, also known as respiratory volumes, refer to the volume of gas in the lungs at a given time during the respiratory cycle. Lung capacities are derived from a summation of different lung volumes. These volumes tend to vary and depend on the depth of respiration, ethnicity, gender, age, body composition, and certain respiratory diseases.[1] Measurement of these volumes and capacities can be done using various methods, such as spirometry, body plethysmography, nitrogen washout, and helium dilution.[2]

**Volumes:** Lung volumes measure the amount of air for a specific function.

**Tidal Volume (TV):** Tidal volume is the volume of gas passively inspired and expired with resting normal breathing (~500 mL). This depicts the functions of the respiratory centers, respiratory muscles, and the mechanics of the lung and chest wall.[3]

**Residual Volume (RV):** This is the volume of gas remaining in the lung after maximum exhalation (~1200 mL). It is indirectly measured from summation of functional residual capacity (FRC) and expiratory reserve volume (ERV) and cannot be measured by spirometry. The residual volume (RV) is high in obstructive lung diseases with features of incomplete emptying of the lungs and air trapping.[4]

**Expiratory Reserve Volume (ERV):** The ERV is the maximum volume that can be exhaled beyond the TV (~1100 mL).

**Inspiratory Reserve Volume (IRV):** The IRV is the maximum volume that can be inhaled beyond the TV (~3000 mL).

**Capacities:** These are calculated values obtained by adding two or more volumes. The different volumes and capacities are described in Figure 90.1.

**Total Lung Capacity (TLC):** This is the IRV + TV + ERV + RV (~5800 mL).

**Vital Capacity (VC):** This is the IRV + TV + ERV.

**Inspiratory Capacity (IC):** This is the IRV + TV.

**Functional Residual Capacity (FRC):** This is the ERV + RV (~2300 mL).

Functional residual capacity is the amount of gas in the lungs at the end of a normal TV breath and is affected by the balance of elastic recoil of the lungs and the passive recoil of the chest wall. The FRC increases with height, age, and obstructive lung diseases. The FRC decreases with obesity, diaphragmatic dysfunction, supine posture, restrictive lung disease, increased abdominal pressure, and in females. A low FRC results in larger portions of collapsed alveoli in between breaths. These alveoli still receive perfusion and therefore have lower $SO_2$, and when mixing with the rest of pulmonary blood cause an overall decrease in $O_2$ saturation.

**Closing Capacity (CC):** The CC is the volume at which small airways begin to close with expiration; it is about on half of FRC when upright and two-thirds of FRC when supine. The CC increases with age, intra-abdominal pressure, decreased pulmonary blood flow, and decreased compliance

**Forced Expiratory Volume (FEV):** The FEV is the volume of gas expired over a given amount of time. Measuring volumes at specific intervals of time allows the severity of obstructive lung disease to be assessed in relation to the FVC. The most commonly used value is $FEV_1$,

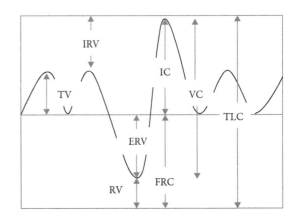

**Figure 90.1** A graphic representation of the different lung volumes and capacities.

which is the expired volume over the first second of expiration. A normal $FEV_1$ is greater than 75% of the FVC. If this ratio is reduced, it is a good indicator of obstructive pathology (chronic obstructive pulmonary disease, asthma).[5] However, since this ratio is often normal in restrictive lung disease, it is a poor index for these diseases.

## ANESTHETIC CONSIDERATIONS

### PREOPERATIVE

The values most frequently evaluated preoperatively are THE $FEV_1$, FVC, RV, FRC, and the diffusing capacity of the lungs for carbon monoxide. Another indication for preoperative pulmonary function tests is patients having thoracic surgery, in which the aim is to identify individuals who would have increased risk of perioperative morbidity and mortality and to help surgeons identify who is better suited for lung resection versus a pneumonectomy.

### INTRAOPERATIVE

Continue assessment of pulmonary function intraoperatively. The patient's capnometry tracing and flow volume loops can tell a lot about lung function. In addition, if a patient's respiratory function is poor enough on preoperative assessment, one might consider alternative means of anesthesia, including regional and monitored anesthesia care in order to avoid airway instrumentation and positive pressure ventilation.

### POSTOPERATIVE

Respiratory complications in the postanesthesia care unit (PACU) can be anticipated and avoided by optimizing the patient intraoperatively for safe extubation via practices such as judicious use of opioids, use of regional anesthesia to prevent shallow breathing secondary to pain, decreasing atelectasis with positive end-expiratory pressure and recruitment maneuvers, ensuring adequate ventilation prior to extubation, and use of a patient's noninvasive respiratory devices such as continuous positive airway pressure or bilevel positive airway pressure machines in the PACU. Patients with an obstructive pattern on preoperative testing might benefit from bronchodilator administration in the recovery area.

## REFERENCES

1. Maiolo C., et al. Body composition and respiratory function. *Acta Diabetol.* 2003;40(1):s32–s38.
2. Ranu H, et al. Pulmonary function tests. *Ulster Med J.* 2011; 80(2):84–90.
3. Hough, A. *Physiotherapy In Respiratory Care: An Evidence-Based Approach to Respiratory and Cardiac Management.* Nelson Thornes; 2001.
4. Arabalibeik H, et al. Classification of restrictive and obstructive pulmonary diseases using spirometry data. *Stud Health Technol Inform.* 2009;142:25–27.
5. Sue DY. Measurement of lung volumes in patients with obstructive lung disease. A matter of time (constants). *Ann Am Thorac Soc.* 2013;10(5):525–530.

# 91.

# PULMONARY FUNCTION TESTS

*Sarah Helwege and Archit Sharma*

Ventilation is the movement of gas into and out of the lungs with inspiration and expiration. Minute ventilation $V_E$ is the sum of all exhaled gas volumes in the span of a minute, determined by respiratory rate (RR), and on average $V_E$ is about 5 L/min. However, not all inspired gas reaches the alveoli to participate in gas exchange; this is referred to as *dead space $V_D$*. The *alveolar ventilation $V_A$* is $V_E - V_D$ and is about 4 L/min; therefore, $V_E = V_A + (RR \times V_D)$

Pulmonary perfusion $Q$ operates at a far lower pressure than the systemic circulation due to short and wide vessels. Since ventilation is about 4 L/min and perfusion is about 5 L/min, the average ventilation to perfusion ratio V/Q is about 0.8.[1] When there is a mismatch in this ratio, hypoxia and/or hypercapnia can result due to creation of a shunt or dead space.

A shunt is a condition whereby blood from the right side of the heart enters the left side without taking part in any gas exchange. Examples of low V/Q are atelectasis, lobe collapse, intracardiac shunts, pneumonia, acute respiratory distress syndrome (ARDS), and the like. In contrast to dead space, a *physiologic shunt* refers to areas of the lung that are perfused but poorly ventilated, resulting in a V/Q less than 1. An estimated 2%–5% of cardiac output is normally shunted via the Thebesian, bronchial, mediastinal, and pleural veins.

A shunt fraction $Q_s/Q_T$ uses the Fick relationship to determine the calculation of a physiologic shunt. The variables include shunt flow per minute $Q_s$, total cardiac output per minute $Q_T$, ideal arterial $O_2$ content $Cc'O_2$, measured arterial $O_2$ content $CaO_2$, and mixed venous $O_2$ content $CvO_2$.[2]

$$Q_s/Q_T = (Cc'O2 - CaO2)/(Cc'O2 - CvO2)$$
$$\text{Arterial } CaO2 = (1.34 \times Hb \times SpO2) + (PaO2 \times 0.003)$$

where 1.34 is the $O_2$ content per gram hemoglobin, and 0.003 is the $O_2$ content dissolved in plasma.

$Q_s/Q_T$ is obtained by acquiring mixed venous and arterial blood gas measurements and calculating ideal $CaO_2$ with an $SpO_2$ of 100%. The oxygen contents in the shunt are approximate by the saturation values for each term; therefore, a simplified equation is as follows:

$$Q_s/Q_T = (1 - S_aO2)/(1 - S_vO2)$$

Dead space $V_D$, as noted above, refers to areas of the lung that are ventilated with poor perfusion or a V/Q ratio greater than 1. Dead space comprises the sum of anatomic dead space and alveolar dead space.[3] *Anatomic dead space* is the fraction of tidal volume that remains in the airways (nose, mouth, trachea, bronchi) and does not participate in gas exchange. Usually, it is about 100–150 mL or 2 mL/kg. *Alveolar dead space* is the gas within the alveoli that does not participate in gas exchange and is typically a negligible volume in a healthy individual. Pathologic causes of increased dead space include mechanisms that increase the size of conducting airways (e.g., bronchiectasis) or interrupt perfusion to alveoli (e.g., pulmonary embolus). Table 91.1 discusses how to differentiate between different reasons for hypoxia. Table 91. 2 discusses multiple pathophysiologic conditions and the mechanisms by which they cause hypoxia.

The ratio of dead space to tidal volume $V_D/V_T$ estimates the fraction of each tidal volume breath that is not participating in gas exchange or in other words physiologic dead space. Normal values are between 0.2 and 0.4 in spontaneously breathing individuals and increase to 0.5 in individuals undergoing positive pressure ventilation.[4] $P_aCO_2$ is determined using the alveolar gas equation, $P_ECO_2$ is measured as the average $CO_2$ in expired gas over several minutes. An increase in the ratio can be due to both an increase in dead space and a decrease in tidal volume.

$$V_D/V_T = (P_aCO2 - P_ECO2) / P_aCO2$$

**Table 91.1** DIFFERENT CAUSES OF HYPOXEMIA AND ITS EFFECT ON OXYGENATION AND VENTILATION PARAMETERS

| | CAUSES OF HYPOXEMIA | | | |
|---|---|---|---|---|
| DISTURBANCE | $PAO_2$ ON ROOM AIR | $PAO_2$ ON OXYGEN | $PAO_2$ WITH EXERCISE | $PACO_2$ |
| Hypoventilation | Low | Normal | No change | High |
| V/Q mismatch | Low | Normal | No change | Normal |
| Shunt | Low | Low | No change | Normal |
| Diffusion impairment | Low | Normal | Low | Normal |

## ASSESSMENT OF OXYGENATION

The alveolar-arterial $O_2$ gradient *A-a gradient* is the difference between calculated alveolar partial pressure of $O_2$ $P_AO_2$) and measured arterial partial pressure of $O_2$ $P_aO_2$ on room air.[5] The normal pressure gradient is usually less than 15 mm Hg but does increase with age. Expected $PaO_2$ can be estimated with the equation

$$Expected\ P_aO2 = 120 - Age/3$$

In order to determine the partial pressure of $O_2$ at the alveoli, the following equation is used:

$$Alveolar\ O_2\ Tension = F_iO2\left(P_{ATM} - P_{H2O}\right)$$

$$= 0.21\left(760\ mmHg - 47\ mmHg\right)$$
$$= 149.7\ mmHg\ (on\ room\ air).$$

The alveolar gas equation calculates expected $P_AO_2$. It is a useful predictor of arterial oxygenation, and clinically it allows recognition of alveolar hypoventilation. Following Dalton's law that each gas in a mixture will contribute to the sum of total pressure, the equation considers that inspired gases are mixed with residual alveolar gas from previous breaths; therefore, measured arterial $CO_2$ needs to be accounted for.

$$P_AO2 = Alveolar\ O2\ Tension - \left(P_aCO2/R\right)$$
$$= 149.7\ mmHg - \left(40\ mmHg/0.8\right) \sim 100\ mmHg$$

The respiratory quotient R is the ratio of oxygen consumed to the amount of carbon dioxide produced. It is dependent on metabolic activity and diet, but on average is about 0.8.

The most common cause of hypoxemia is an increase in the A-a gradient. V/Q mismatch, shunt, dead space ventilation, and diffusion abnormalities can all cause an elevated A-a gradient. Cardiac output also affects the A-a gradient due to its influence on shunting as well as mixed venous oxygen tension.

The arterial-alveolar $CO_2$ gradient *a-ET $PCO_2$* is the difference between measured $PaCO_2$ in the blood and end-tidal $CO_2$ measured with capnography. It is a predictor of dead space and is about 2–5 mm Hg in the average healthy person. The a-ET $PCO_2$ is decreased in children and in pregnant patients due to higher cardiac output states and increased in states of low pulmonary perfusion, such as low cardiac output,

**Table 91.2** DIFFERENT PATHOPHYSIOLOGIC CONDITIONS LEADING TO HYPOXIA THROUGH DIFFERENT MECHANISMS

| | MECHANISMS OF HYPOXIA | | | |
|---|---|---|---|---|
| DISORDER | HYPOVENTILATION | DIFFUSION IMPAIRMENT | V/Q MISMATCH | SHUNT |
| Chronic bronchitis | Yes | No | Yes | No |
| Emphysema | Yes | Yes | Yes | No |
| Asthma | No | No | Yes | No |
| Fibrosis | No | Yes | Yes | Yes |
| Pneumonia | No | No | Yes | Yes |
| Atelectasis | No | No | No | Yes |
| Pulmonary edema | No | Yes | Yes | Yes |
| Pulmonary embolism | No | No | Yes | Yes |
| ARDS | No | No | Yes | Yes |

hypovolemia, excessive positive end expiratory pressure (PEEP), atelectasis, emphysema, or pulmonary embolism.

FEV$_1$ and FVC Relationship: The forced expiratory volume FEV measures how much air a person can exhale during a forced expiration. A spirometer can measure the amount of air exhaled during the first (FEV$_1$), second (FEV$_2$), and/or third (FEV$_3$) seconds of the forced breath. Forced vital capacity (FVC) is the total amount of air exhaled during the FEV test. This helps a clinician calculate a FEV$_1$/FVC ratio, which helps to distinguish between restrictive and obstructive pathology. When the FEV$_1$/FVC ratio is less than 80%, an obstructive lung disease is likely present. However, in restrictive lung diseases, both the FEV$_1$ and FVC measurements decrease proportionally; hence, the FEV$_1$/FVC ratio is preserved. Patients suffering from asthma can be assessed for bronchodilator reversibility by checking postbronchodilator values. An increase in FEV$_1$ and/or FVC of 12% or more over baseline and 200 mL or more is generally considered a positive response.

**Bronchoprovocation Challenge:** A patient with mild or no airflow limitation may not show reversal after bronchodilator administration. In such cases, a bronchial challenge with inhaled methacholine or other modalities would be indicated to demonstrate reversible airflow obstruction.

An increased residual volume (RV ≥ 120% predicted or greater than the upper 95th percentile) is the most common abnormality of all the lung volumes in asthmatic patients, and it is the last to return to normal following treatment. A functional residual capacity (FRC) value of 120% or greater predicted suggests air trapping. A total lung capacity of 120% or greater predicted suggests hyperinflation.

## ANESTHETIC CONSIDERATIONS

### PREOPERATIVE

Many patient factors can affect respiratory mechanics under anesthesia. Age, body mass index, comorbidities, preexisting lung pathology, type of surgery, and patient positioning, and preoperative PFTs, if available, should be accounted for when planning an anesthetic. In addition, discussion with high-risk patients regarding postoperative care, including the possible need for mechanical ventilation and intensive care unit admission, is an important preoperative task.

### INTRAOPERATIVE

Volatile anesthetics can inhibit hypoxic pulmonary vasoconstriction and lead to an increase in physiologic shunting. The use of positive pressure ventilation, which causes an increase in alveolar pressure and results in a higher ratio of dead space to alveolar ventilation. Atelectasis is a common result of the decreased muscle tone caused by anesthetics, resulting in redistribution of inspired gases from the dependent lower portions of the lung to the upper lung regions. This can be overcome to an extent with recruitment maneuvers and PEEP.

### POSTOPERATIVE

It is common for most patients to have periods of hypoventilation and decreased oxygenation immediately postoperatively due to sedation and atelectasis, which can lead to a shunt. Use of an incentive spirometry device will improve oxygenation.

## REFERENCES

1. West JB. Ventilation-perfusion relationships. *Am Rev Respir Dis.* 1977;116(5):919–943.
2. Sandoval J, et al. Independent influence of blood flow rate and mixed venous PO$_2$ on shunt fraction. *J Appl Physiol* 1983;55(4):1128–1133.
3. Fowler WS. Lung function studies. II. The respiratory dead space. *Am J Physiol.* 1948;154(3):405–416.
4. Kline JA, et al. Use of the alveolar dead space fraction (Vd/Vt) and plasma D-dimers to exclude acute pulmonary embolism in ambulatory patients. *Acad Emerg Med.* 1997;4(9):856–863.
5. Stein PD, et al. Alveolar-arterial oxygen gradient in the assessment of acute pulmonary embolism. *Chest.* 1995;107(1):139–143.

# Part 9

# CLINICAL SCIENCE

# 92.

# OBSTRUCTIVE LUNG DISEASE

*Bryan J. Hierlmeier and Anesh Rugnath*

## INTRODUCTION

Obstructive diseases are separated into upper airway (congenital, infectious, neoplastic, traumatic, foreign body, obstructive sleep apnea [OSA]); tracheobronchial (congenital, infectious, neoplastic, traumatic, foreign body); and parenchymal (asthma, bronchitis, emphysema, chronic obstructive pulmonary disease, lung abscess, bronchiectasis, cystic fibrosis, mediastinal masses) disorders.

## OBSTRUCTIVE SLEEP APNEA

Obstructive sleep apnea is a common sleep disorder characterized by episodic, partial, or complete obstruction of the upper airway during sleep associated with snoring and periods of apnea. In adults, OSA is associated with obesity, while in children it is associated with tonsillar hypertrophy. The STOP BANG questionnaire (Table 92.1) was developed as a screening tool for OSA, while the

*Table 92.1* STOP BANG QUESTIONNAIRE

| S (snore) | Do you snore? |
|---|---|
| T (tired) | Do you often feel tired or sleepy during the daytime? |
| O (observed) | Has anyone observed you stop breathing during sleep? |
| P (pressure) | Do you have high blood pressure? |
| B (BMI) | BMI > 35 kg/m$^2$? |
| A (age) | Age > 50 years? |
| N (neck) | Neck circumference > 40cm? |
| G (gender) | Gender male? |

BMI, body mass index.

HIGH risk of OSA= answering "yes" to 3 or more questions.

LOW risk of OSA = answering "yes" to less than 3 questions,

Apnea-Hypopnea Index (Table 92.2) is used to classify the severity. Patients with OSA typically have daytime somnolence, increased incidence of hypoxia, dysrhythmias, hypertension, myocardial ischemia, and pulmonary hypertension. OSA patients have an increased sensitivity to narcotics with respect to respiratory depression, so nonnarcotic analgesics along with regional anesthesia techniques play an important role in caring for these patients. There is an association with redundant airway tissues, making ventilation and intubation a challenge. Desaturation may occur rapidly after induction. Utilization of oral and nasal airways should occur early on, and backup strategies should always be readily available prior to induction. Current practice guidelines recommend that a patient on home continuous positive airway pressure should bring their machine and be allowed to use their own device in the immediate postoperative period and while sleeping unless contraindicated.[1]

## FOREIGN BODY ASPIRATION

Aspiration of a foreign body is a common cause of acute respiratory distress in a child, but it can also occur in adults. Foreign body aspiration can lead to obstruction and may be supraglottic, glottic, or subglottic. Onset is typically acute, stridor and wheezing may be present, but history of aspiration may not be present. Immediate removal is required even if there are no signs of distress. Inhalational induction

*Table 92.2* APNEA SEVERITY: APNEA EVENTS/HOUR OF SLEEP[a]

| Normal | <5 |
|---|---|
| Mild | 5–15 |
| Moderate | 15–30 |
| Severe | >30 |

[a]The Apnea-Hypopnea Index will allow for severity classification of OSA.

is recommended for small children without an intravenous line as attempting one could cause additional distress and could dislodge the foreign body leading to complete airway obstruction. After successful inhalational induction, an intravenous line can be placed and paralytics given prior to insertion of a ridged bronchoscope. Ventilation can be achieved from the side port on the ridged bronchoscope. Once the object is removed, an laryngeal mask airway or endotracheal tube may be used until the patient begins spontaneous breathing.

## CHRONIC OBSTRUCTIVE PULMONARY DISEASE

Obstructive disorders such as chronic obstructive pulmonary disease have resistance to airflow, and as the disease progresses, both forced expiratory volume in 1 second ($FEV_1$) and the $FEV_1/FVC$ (forced vital capacity) ratio are less than 70% predicted.[2] Table 92.3 shows a comparison of lung volumes for obstructive versus restrictive lung disease. The resistance to airflow leads to air trapping, which in turn increases the residual lung volume and total lung capacity.[2] Progressive obstruction typically results first in expiratory wheezing only and then in both inspiratory and expiatory wheezing. Severe obstruction may lead to absent airflow and no breath sounds being appreciated. Extensive history should be completed prior to any anesthetics and should include recent changes in dyspnea, cough, sputum production, wheezing, and hospitalizations. Acute smoking cessation is associated with decreased carboxyhemoglobin levels and an increase in airway reactivity and mucus production. Smoking cessation at least 6–8 weeks prior to surgery is suggested to decrease mucus production and carbon monoxide and reduce pulmonary complications.

*Table 92.3* LUNG VOLUMES FOR OBSTRUCTIVE VERSUS RESTRICTIVE PULMONARY DISEASE

|  | OBSTRUCTIVE | RESTRICTIVE |
| --- | --- | --- |
| TLC | Normal or Increased | Decreased |
| VC | Normal or Decreased | Decreased |
| RV | Increased | Decreased |
| FVC | Normal to Increased | Decreased |
| FRC | Increased | Decreased |
| $FEV_1$ | Decreased(marked) | Normal or Decrease(slight) |
| $FEV_1/FVC$ | Decrease | Normal or Increase |
| $FEF_{25\%-75\%}$ | Decreased | Normal |

$FEF_{25\%-75\%}$, forced expiratory flow, midexpiratory phase; FRC, functional residual capacity; RV, residual volume; TLC, total lung capacity, VC, vital capacity.

## EMPHYSEMA

Emphysema is characterized by destruction of lung parenchyma with loss of elastic recoil and closure of small airways during expiration, which leads to air trapping and dyspnea. Regional anesthesia with avoidance of intubation carries a lower risk or pulmonary complications. Interscalene (phrenic nerve blocked) and high neuroaxial block may worsen pulmonary function. If intubation and general anesthesia are required, then setting lower respiratory rates and increasing the I:E ratio will allow for longer expiration time to avoid air trapping. The use of nitrous oxide has the potential to rupture pulmonary bullae and cause a pneumothorax.

## ASTHMA

Asthmatics have bronchiolar inflammation and a hyperreactive airway in response to a variety of stimuli, which are generally reversible. During an asthma attack, bronchoconstriction, airway edema, and secretion increase resistance to gas flow in the lower airways. A normal or high $PaCO_2$ suggests that the patient can no longer maintain the work of breathing and is an ominous sign. Treatment options for acute attacks include a β-agonist, glucocorticoids, and anticholinergics. Chronic treatment options can include the addition of mast cell–stabilizing agents and leukotriene blockers. Patients with active bronchospasm presenting for emergency surgery should undergo a period of intense treatment if time allows. The most critical time for an asthmatic undergoing anesthesia is typically during intubation and extubation. Intraoperative bronchospasm is treated by deepening the anesthetic and β₂-agonists given as an aerosol through the inspiratory limb. If bronchospasm is so severe that airflow is completely restricted, then intravenous epinephrine (10–20 μcg) should be given for its bronchodilation effect. Drugs associated with histamine release (atracurium, meperidine, morphine) should be avoided if possible.

## MEDIASTINAL MASSES

The most common mediastinal masses in order of frequency in adults are lymphoma (Hodgkin or non-Hodgkin), thymoma, germ cell tumor, granuloma, bronchogenic carcinoma, thyroid tumors, bronchogenic cyst, and cystic hygroma.[3] Mediastinal masses are an anesthetic dilemma and present multiple challenges to the anesthesiologist as induction of anesthesia and loss of airway muscle tone can lead to airway compromise and cardiovascular collapse. A through preoperative assessment of the patient along with a discussion with the surgeon must occur. Postural worsening of respiratory symptoms (dyspnea, cough, syncope) when supine instead of upright are concerning and predictive of airway collapse with induction of anesthesia. Preoperatively, the patient should be asked which position relieves respiratory symptoms. Preoperative echocardiography along with chest computed tomography (CT) should be reviewed for airway and vascular compression (superior vena cava syndrome) prior to anesthetic decision-making. Patients with CT or magnetic resonance imaging scans showing greater than 50% compression of the tracheal cross-sectional area preoperatively are poor candidates for general anesthesia and intubation. Anesthetic agents should be carefully titrated in order to preserve respiratory drive and allow spontaneous ventilation. Induction and maintenance of anesthesia can be accomplished by either inhalational induction or small amounts of intravenous anesthetics along with inhalational agents with the avoidance of paralytics unless absolutely necessary. Insertion of a preoperative arterial line will help with hemodynamic monitoring during induction of anesthesia. If complete airway obstruction occurs, the patient should be repositioned in an attempt to relieve the obstruction. A ridged bronchoscope may be used to bypass the obstruction. If this fails, then extracorporeal membrane oxygenation should be initiated.

## REFERENCES

1. Practice guidelines for the perioperative management of patients with obstructive sleep apnea: an updated report by the American Society of Anesthesiologists Task Force on Perioperative Management of Patients With Obstructive Sleep Apnea. *Anesthesiology.* 2014;120(2):268–286.
2. Butterworth JF, IV, Mackey DC, Wasnick JD, eds. *Morgan & Mikhail's Clinical Anesthesiology, 5e.* McGraw Hill; 2013.
3. Ferguson MK, et al. Selective operative approach for diagnosis and treatment of anterior mediastinal masses. *Ann Thorac Surg.* 1987; 44:583–586.

# 93.

# RESTRICTIVE LUNG DISEASE

*Binoy Samuel and Justin Merkow*

## INTRODUCTION

Restrictive lung disease is characterized by a group of diseases that prevent the lungs from fully expanding, resulting in inadequate ventilation. Compared to obstructive disease, there is no airway resistance, and airflow measures are within normal limits. Pulmonary function tests (PFTs) will reveal a decrease in total lung capacity (TLC), decreased forced expiratory volume in 1 second (FEV$_1$), and decreased forced vital capacity (FVC).[1] The FEV$_1$/FVC ratio remains normal because both values are decreased. The flow volume loop is normal but shows reduced volumes. Functional residual capacity (FRC) and total lung compliance are also reduced. The respiratory rate is often increased to compensate for increased oxygen demand.

Restrictive lung disease can be classified as intrinsic and extrinsic. Intrinsic disorders cause an internal defect, leading to inflammation, stiffening, and/or scarring of the lung tissue. Extrinsic disorders are caused by problems with structures or tissues outside of the lungs and also includes neurological disorders (Table 93.1).

A good mnemonic to help remember anatomical sites of pathology that can cause restrictive lung disease is PAINT. This stands for the following: P, pleural (scarring, empyema, hemothorax, effusions, asbestosis); A, alveolar (edema, hemorrhage); I, interstitial (pulmonary fibrosis, interstitial pneumonia, cryptogenic organizing pneumonia [COP; formerly known as bronchiolitis obliterans]); N, neuromuscular (amyotrophic lateral sclerosis [ALS], myasthenia gravis, myopathy); T, thoracic/extrathoracic (obesity, fractured ribs, kyphoscoliosis, ascites).

*Table 93.1* CAUSES OF RESTRICTIVE LUNG DISEASE

| INTRINSIC | EXTRINSIC |
|---|---|
| • Pneumonia | • Pleural effusions |
| • Tuberculosis | • Scoliosis |
| • Sarcoidosis | • Neuromuscular disease such |
| • Idiopathic pulmonary | as Lou Gehrig disease (ALS), |
| fibrosis | multiple sclerosis, muscular |
| • Interstitial lung disease | dystrophy, myasthenia gravis |
| • Lung cancers | • Malignant tumors |
| • Fibrosis caused by radiation | • Fractured ribs |
| • Rheumatoid arthritis | • Diaphragm paralysis |
| • ARDS | • Kyphosis |
| • Inflammatory bowel disease | • Diaphragmatic hernia |
| (IBD) | • Congestive heart failure |
| • Systemic lupus | • Abdominal distension (SBO, |
| | ascites, obesity) |
| | • Pain related |

## INTRINSIC CAUSES

Diseases with sudden onset and pathophysiology that primarily affects the alveoli are classified as acute intrinsic respiratory disease. Examples include cardiogenic and noncardiogenic pulmonary edema, acute respiratory distress syndrome, hemorrhage, and infectious pneumonia. These pathologies cause an increase in capillary permeability as well as an increase in extravascular lung water, which decreases pulmonary compliance. This results in the classic restrictive pattern seen on PFTs.

Chronic intrinsic restrictive disease is characterized by an insidious onset and chronic inflammation of the lung parenchyma, causing pulmonary fibrosis. Interstitial lung diseases have various etiologies and include nonspecific interstitial pneumonia; COP; pulmonary fibrosis; adverse drug side effects (bleomycin and nitrofurantoin); hypersensitivity pneumonitis from occupational exposure to toxins (asbestosis, silicosis, etc.); radiation pneumonitis; autoimmune diseases; chronic pulmonary aspiration; oxygen toxicity; severe acute respiratory distress syndrome (ARDS); and sarcoidosis.

As the pulmonary fibrosis progresses, gas exchange will be diminished. Patients can present with a nonproductive cough and shortness of breath. Severe disease results in hypoxia and/or hypercapnic respiratory failure. In advanced disease, crackles on lung auscultation and other evidence of cor pulmonale may be present. A characteristic "ground glass opacity" will be seen on chest imaging that will progress to more prominent reticulonodular markings. A "honeycomb" appearance seen on imaging is also consistent with advanced disease. Additionally, PFTs will demonstrate a restrictive pattern, and the carbon dioxide diffusing capacity of the lungs will be diminished.

## EXTRINSIC CAUSES

Musculoskeletal, neuromuscular, or other extrapulmonary disorders affecting the normal expansion of the lungs can be classified as extrinsic restrictive diseases. As with diseases in the other categories, PFTs will show a restrictive pattern. Conditions include myasthenia gravis, ALS, myopathies, pleural effusions, pneumothorax, mediastinal masses, kyphoscoliosis, pectus excavatum, abdominal distension, obesity, ascites, pain related, pregnancy, or intra-abdominal bleeding. We use abdominal causes and pain as examples of how extrinsic factors affect respiratory physiology. TLC is the total volume the lung is able to accommodate, and FRC is the volume that remains in the lung at the end of a normal expiration. Furthermore, closing capacity (CC) is the volume in the lungs during expiration at which point the small airways (bronchioles) collapse. In a young healthy adult, the FRC is greater than the CC, meaning there is enough volume in the lungs with normal passive breathing to prevent small airways from collapsing. However, if the FRC decreases to less than the CC, which can occur with extrinsic disorders, the small airways will collapse to a greater degree during expiration and lead to lower lung volumes and restrictive physiology.

There are various abdominal causes leading to restrictive lung physiology, primarily related to increases in intra-abdominal pressure and distension. Examples include obesity, ascites, and small bowel obstruction. The increasing intra-abdominal pressure results in upward force on the lung parenchyma and thereby reduces its ability to fully expand. This lowers FRC and increases small airway collapse. Obese patient may have a decrease in chest wall expansion as well with similar affect. These patients often require higher inspired fractional concentration of oxygen ($FiO_2$) to maintain their saturation, and this can further increase atelectasis and lower FRC.

Pain-related causes also can induce restrictive physiology. This is especially true of thoracic and abdominal pain as these conditions significantly decrease one's ability to take full breaths. Patients in severe pain often have an increased respiratory rate and lower tidal volume (rapid, shallow breathing). These factors will translate to atelectasis, decreasing FRC and causing a more restrictive respiratory pattern.

## ANESTHESIA CONSIDERATIONS

### PREOPERATIVE

Elective surgery is not indicated in patients with acute intrinsic restrictive disease. If a patient requires an emergent procedure, the underlying cause of the acute disease should be treated perioperatively (antibiotics for infectious pneumonia, diuretics for inotropes in cardiogenic pulmonary edema).[2] ARDS may require ventilation with high positive end expiratory pressures, low tidal volumes (4–6 mL/kg), and permissive hypercapnia to achieve adequate oxygenation.[3] For those with chronic disease, the severity and its effect on pulmonary function should be assessed preoperatively. The systemic effect of the underlying disease should also be evaluated. Patients presenting with a history of dyspnea should be evaluated with PFTs, and an arterial blood gas sample should be drawn. A vital capacity lower than 15 mL/kg (normal is > 70 mL/kg) is indicative of advanced disease. It may be necessary to obtain imaging such as a chest x-ray or computed tomographic scan. A cardiac evaluation may also be indicated. For intra-abdominal causes, actions to decompress the intra-abdominal cavity such as draining ascites or placing an nasogastric tube if indicated will be helpful. Also, adequately addressing pain is imperative and will encourage better lung expansion and FRC.

## INTRAOPERATIVE

Patients with severe restrictive diseases tolerate apnea poorly because of reduced FRC, so rapid hypoxemia following induction of anesthesia should be anticipated intraoperatively. Oxygenation prior to induction should be prolonged to get the highest expired $O_2$ for maximum denitrogenating of the alveoli. The $FiO_2$ should be decreased to the minimum value needed to maintain an appropriate $SpO_2$ (88%–92%) during maintenance of anesthesia since these patients may be at higher risk of oxygen toxicity. High $FiO_2$ can also lead to absorption atelectasis. Peak inspiratory pressures should be kept within an appropriate range as these patients are more susceptible to pneumothorax during positive pressure ventilation. In order to maintain low peak and plateau inspiratory pressures, the I:E ratio can be lowered to 1:1. Finally, limiting abdominal distension will help improve lung mechanics.

## POSTOPERATIVE

Similar principles apply postoperatively for patients with restriction lung disease.

## REFERENCES

1. Kavanagh BP, Hedenstierna G. Respiratory physiology and pathophysiology. In: Gropper M, et al. *Miller's Anesthesia*. 9th ed. Philadelphia, PA: Elsevier; 2020:354–383.
2. Butterworth JF IV, et al. Anesthesia for patients with respiratory disease. *Morgan & Mikhail's Clinical Anesthesiology*. 6th ed. New York, NY: McGraw-Hill; 2020.
3. Tamul PC, Peruzzi WT. Assessment and management of patients with pulmonary disease. *Crit Care Med*. 2004;32:S137–S145.
4. Craig DB. Postoperative recovery of pulmonary function. *Anesth Analg*. 1981;60(1):46–52.

# 94.

# MANAGEMENT OF PATIENTS WITH RESPIRATORY DISEASE
## INTRAOPERATIVE MANAGEMENT

*Dmitry Roberman and Felipe F. Suero*

## INTRODUCTION

Respiratory complications after surgery represent the greatest cost to healthcare.[1] The choice of anesthetic technique should be guided primarily by the requirement of the procedure and by surgeon and patient preferences (Table 94.1). Avoiding general anesthesia with laryngoscopy and tracheal intubation may decrease the risk of bronchospasm, pneumonia, and the potential for prolonged intubation.

Standard American Society of Anesthesiologists (ASA) monitoring is required. All noninvasive and invasive monitors are secured to avoid displacement during repositioning, surgical prepping, and draping. After positioning, access to these may be limited. All patients will have standard noninvasive monitors, including electrocardiography, pulse oximetry, and noninvasive blood pressure cuff measurements.[2] After the airway has been secured, end-tidal $CO_2$ and intermittent airway pressures and volumes are monitored.

Invasive monitors are needed in patients undergoing major pulmonary resection procedures (e.g., lobectomy or pneumonectomy) include an intra-arterial catheter and a bladder catheter. The intra-arterial catheter may be inserted before or after induction of anesthesia, while the bladder catheter is typically inserted after induction but before repositioning the patient for surgery. Healthy patients undergoing a short procedure (e.g., simple wedge resection of a localized lesion in the pulmonary periphery) generally do not require either of these invasive monitors.[3] Intra-arterial catheters provide a wealth of information, including continuous monitoring of arterial blood pressure to immediately recognize problems such as hemodynamic instability due to compression of the heart or major vessels. Blood samples can be drawn frequently to detect hemorrhage, hypoxia, and hypercarbia.

Intermittent arterial blood gas analysis, which allows direct measurement of $PaO_2$ and $PaCO_2$ is important in patients at risk for desaturation. Measurements may be obtained during two-lung ventilation (baseline) following induction of general anesthesia and every 15 to 60 minutes during One Lung Ventilation (OLV), as needed. Final measurements may be obtained after completion of lung resection and reexpansion of the nonventilated lung in order to assess respiratory reserve before extubation.

*Table 94.1* SUMMARY OF IMPORTANT RISK FACTORS FOR PERIOPERATIVE PULMONARY COMPLICATIONS

|  | PATIENT-RELATED FACTORS | PROCEDURE-RELATED FACTORS |
|---|---|---|
| Supported by good evidence | Advanced age | Aortic aneurysm repair |
|  | ASA class > 2 | Thoracic surgery |
|  | Congestive heart failure | Abdominal surgery |
|  | Functional dependency | Neurosurgery |
|  | COPD | Head and neck surgery |
| Supported by fair evidence | Weight loss | Perioperative transfusion |
|  | Impaired sensorium |  |
|  | Cigarette use |  |
|  | Alcohol use |  |
|  | Abnormal chest examination |  |
| Insufficient data | Obstructive sleep apnea | Esophageal surgery |
|  | Poor exercise capacity |  |

From Reference 5.

Other infrequently used invasive monitors include the following[4]:

1. Central venous catheter: Central venous access may be useful for transfusion of blood products and maintenance of intravascular volume and hemodynamic stability if adequate vascular access is not otherwise available.
2. Transesophageal echocardiography (TEE): TEE is not used routinely. However, patients with moderate-to-severe pulmonary hypertension, severe right ventricular (RV) dysfunction, significant valvular heart disease, or intracardiac shunting may benefit from TEE monitoring, particularly during pulmonary artery clamping, which may cause RV dysfunction. TEE may be urgently employed to rapidly diagnose unanticipated causes of severe hemodynamic instability (e.g., hypovolemia or hypervolemia, myocardial ischemia, severe left ventricular or RV dysfunction, or tumor compression or embolization to the heart).
3. Pulmonary artery catheter (PAC): Use of a PAC is rare but may be helpful in the setting of severe RV dysfunction or severe pulmonary hypertension.

Pain control is a major challenge in these patients, and intravenously administered opioid analgesia compromises respiratory drive. Regarding neuraxial anesthesia, epidural anesthesia is a good adjunctive technique for patients with respiratory disease who are undergoing appropriate surgical procedures, particularly if a large thoracic or abdominal surgical incision is planned.[4] Compared with general anesthesia with postoperative systematic opioid analgesia, postoperative neuraxial analgesia provides superior pain control, which may facilitate deep breathing and better ambulation. Neuraxial techniques used as the primary anesthetic for appropriate surgeries also avoid laryngoscopy and tracheal intubation thereby reducing a potential cause of bronchospasm.[3] Theoretical concerns regarding neuroaxial anesthesia for patients with respiratory disease includes muscle weakness and potential increase in bronchomotor tone via a mechanism of sympathectomy.

Peripheral nerve blocks can be used. A regional nerve block is appropriate in some surgical patients with respiratory disease if a surgical site is peripheral and the surgical procedure is of short-to-moderate duration. As with neuroaxial anesthesia, laryngoscopy and tracheal intubation are avoided. Some regional blocks are not appropriate for patients with respiratory disease; for example, the interscalene block has a 100% incidence of phrenic nerve blockade because this nerve courses anterior to the brachial plexus nerve roots.[2] The supraclavicular block also has a high incidence of phrenic nerve blockade. Blockade of the phrenic nerve results in paralysis of the ipsilateral diaphragm, causing a 25% reduction of forced vital capacity, which may not be well tolerated in patients with severe or symptomatic chronic obstructive pulmonary disease (COPD).

General anesthesia is preferred for patients with baseline severe dyspnea, anxiety, inability to lie supine, or persistent coughing. The risk of bronchospasm is lower with mask ventilation or insertion of a laryngeal mask airway (LMA) compared with endotracheal intubation. Endotracheal intubation may be necessary depending on individual patient factors and the surgical procedure. During controlled ventilation via a mask, LMA, or endotracheal tube in patients with COPD, a phenomenon known as breath stacking may occur, causing a sudden decrease in systemic blood pressure. This improves immediately when the anesthesia mask is transiently lifted from the face or the breathing circuit is transiently disconnected.

Lung-protective ventilation for the patient with respiratory disease during anesthesia should include the procedures discussed in this paragraph.[5] Controlled ventilation with reduced tidal volume (5 to 8 mL/kg predicted body weight) is lung protective. Reducing tidal volume helps prevent air trapping and avoids high plateau airway pressure (e.g., > 35 cm $H_2O$), thereby minimizing risk of barotrauma. Reducing tidal volume may decrease minute ventilation, potentially causing hypercapnia and hypoxemia. This can be partially offset by an increase in respiratory rate, as long as expiratory time remains adequate for complete exhalation. Some degree of hypercapnia is acceptable in patients without any specific contraindication for hypercapnia (e.g., elevated intracranial pressure), but adequate oxygenation and a pH of 7.25 or greater should be maintained. Plateau pressures should be maintained at less than 15 to 20 cm $H_2O$. Adjust the fraction of inspired oxygen to the lowest level required to maintain the oxygen saturation greater than 90%. The benefits and risks of positive end-expiratory pressure are unpredictable in an individual patient. COPD patients have an increased risk for development of tension pneumothorax with hypotension due to rupture of bullae during mechanical ventilation.[1]

## REFERENCES

1. Ishikawa S, et al. Acute kidney injury after lung resection surgery: incidence and perioperative risk factors. *Anesth Analg.* 2012;114:1256.
2. Smetana GW, et al. American College of Physicians. Preoperative pulmonary risk stratification for noncardiothoracic surgery: systematic review for the American College of Physicians. *Ann Intern Med.* 2006;144:581.
3. Raphael J, et al. Hemodynamic monitoring in thoracic surgical patients. *Curr Opin Anaesthesiol.* 2017;30:7.
4. Lohser J, Slinger P. Lung injury after one-lung ventilation: a review of the pathophysiologic mechanisms affecting the ventilated and the collapsed lung. *Anesth Analg.* 2015;121:302.
5. Licker M, et al. Risk factors for acute lung injury after thoracic surgery for lung cancer. *Anesth Analg.* 2003;97:1558.

# 95.

# RESPIRATORY ADJUNCTS
## HELIOX, NITRIC OXIDE, EPOPROSTENOL,
## AND INTRAOPERATIVE STEROIDS

## *Michelle McMaster*

## INTRODUCTION

Respiratory adjuvants include heliox, nitric oxide (NO), epoprostenol, and the perioperative use of steroids for respiration pathology.

## HELIOX

Heliox is a mixture of helium and oxygen. Helium is an odorless, nontoxic, inert gas. When mixed with oxygen, the combination has a lower density but similar viscosity when compared to oxygen and nitrogen (the primary components of air). If inhaled, the decreased density of heliox when compared to air increases the proportion of laminar flow versus turbulent flow through the airways. This physical phenomenon is described using the Reynolds number, which is a dimensionless quantity defined as $Re = Density \times Flow\ Speed \times Diameter/Viscosity$. When the Reynolds number is high, turbulent flow predominates. When the Reynolds number is low, laminar flow predominates. Heliox has a lower Reynolds number when compared to air.

Therapeutic utilization of heliox exploits this physical phenomenon to improve ventilation. Unlike other therapeutic modalities that focus on decreasing resistance to airflow by increasing airway caliber, this modality aims to improve airflow by altering gas composition, which makes heliox an attractive treatment option for pathologies that are not amenable to immediate bronchodilation (i.e., a fixed lesion or acute airway edema). Often, heliox is utilized in clinical practice as a temporizing measure to decrease the workload of breathing until more definitive treatments (i.e., tracheostomy or bronchodilators) can be implemented or have time to take effect. Clinical scenarios in which heliox may be reasonable include postextubation edema or stridor, laryngotracheal stenosis, vocal cord paralysis, croup,

angioedema, and airway obstruction related to tumors. While heliox has been used to treat acute asthma, a systematic review found little clinical benefits.[1] Heliox can also be used as the driving gas for nebulizer treatments.

Clinically, heliox is delivered as a 70%–80% helium/ 30%–20% oxygen mix via an open circuit or facemask. For this reason, clinical scenarios that require a high inspired oxygen concentration may not be amenable to heliox therapy. Mechanical ventilators may need recalibration if used with heliox, and most anesthesia machines are not usually fitted for heliox use. If entrained into the anesthesia circuit via an air inlet, airflow meters will be unreliable and may provide inaccurate tidal volume and fraction of inspired oxygen estimations. Some research suggests that helium may reduce the risk for airway fires when compared to air.[2]

## NITRIC OXIDE

Nitric oxide is a colorless, odorless gas and a potent vasodilator. In clinical anesthesia practice, inhaled NO has been used to treat acute hypoxemic respiratory failure in patients with pulmonary hypertension and as a rescue therapy for hypoxic patients with acute right heart failure, although the evidence to support the latter indication is limited. Inhalation of NO is often the preferred route as the vasodilatory effects should theoretically occur preferentially in ventilated alveoli, improving ventilation/perfusion matching. This is in contrast to systemically administered vasodilatory agents, which increase blood flow to ventilated and unventilated alveoli alike. NO is rapidly metabolized when administered via the inhalational route, and therefore inhaled NO has minimal systemic effects. NO toxicity can occur by the spontaneous oxidation of NO into $NO_2$ in the lungs, which can cause pulmonary edema in high concentrations. High doses of NO can also lead to methemoglobinemia. Toxicity is rare with dosing ranges of 20–40 ppm.

## EPOPROSTENOL

Epoprostenol is a naturally occurring prostaglandin. In clinical anesthesia practice, epoprostenol has been used to treat pulmonary hypertension during cardiopulmonary bypass. As a medication, it can be administered via intravenous or inhalational routes, although its use as an inhaled agent is considered off-label. Like NO, inhaled epoprostenol has a short half-life, and its vasodilatory effects are restricted to well-ventilated areas. Standard dosing has not been established; however, patients should be weaned from this drug slowly to prevent rebound hypertension.

## STEROIDS

Intraoperative uses of steroids related to respiratory pathology include prevention of adrenal insufficiency in patients on chronic steroids for chronic obstructive pulmonary disease (COPD), treatment or prevention of bronchospasm associated with anaphylaxis, and treatment or prevention of airway edema after traumatic intubation.

## ADRENAL INSUFFICIENCY

Many patients with COPD (and many other conditions) require chronic oral steroids. In these patients, it is common to administer a stress dose of steroids in the perioperative period to prevent adrenal insufficiency and associated cardiovascular compromise. While chronic steroid therapy is known to impair wound healing and cause hyperglycemia and psychological disturbances, it is not clear if stress-dose steroids worsen these risks. Therefore, the risk of cardiovascular compromise associated with adrenal insufficiency often outweighs the anesthesiologist's assessment of the risks of administering perioperative stress-dose steroids. While there is little evidence to guide this practice, a practical approach is discussed next.

One approach is to divide patients into high, intermediate, or low risk for adrenal crisis[3] (Table 95.1). High-risk patients who would benefit from stress-dose steroids include patients with diagnosed secondary adrenal insufficiency or patients taking more than 20 mg of prednisone per day. Patients at low risk who do not require

*Table 95.1* INTRAOPERATIVE STEROID DOSING

| SURGERY TYPE | ENDOGENOUS CORTISOL SECRETION RATE | EXAMPLE | RECOMMENDED STEROID DOSING |
|---|---|---|---|
| **Superficial** | 8–10 mg per day (baseline) | Dental surgery biopsy | Usual daily dose |
| **Minor** | 50 mg per day | Inguinal hernia repair<br>Colonoscopy<br>Uterine curettage<br>Hand surgery | Usual daily dose<br>*Plus*<br>Hydrocortisone 50 mg IV before incision<br>Hydrocortisone 25 mg IV every 8 h × 24 h<br>Then usual daily dose |
| **Moderate** | 75–150 mg per day | Lower extremity revascularization<br>Total joint replacement<br>Cholecystectomy<br>Colon resection<br>Abdominal hysterectomy | Usual daily dose<br>*Plus*<br>Hydrocortisone 50 mg IV before incision<br>Hydrocortisone 25 mg IV every 8 h × 24 h<br>Then usual daily dose |
| **Major** | 75–150 mg per day | Esophagectomy<br>Total proctocolectomy<br>Major cardiac/vascular<br>Hepaticojejunostomy<br>Delivery<br>Trauma | Usual daily dose<br>*Plus*<br>Hydrocortisone 100 mg IV before incision<br>Followed by continuous IV infusion of 200 mg of hydrocortisone more than 24 h<br>*or*<br>Hydrocortisone 50 mg IV every 8 h × 24 h<br>Taper dose by half per day until usual daily dose reached<br>*plus*<br>Continuous intravenous fluids with 5% dextrose and 0.2%–0.45%NaCl (based on degree of hypoglycemia) |

Reprinted with permission from Liu MM, Reidy AB, Saatee S, Collard CD. Perioperative Steroid Management Approaches Based on Current Evidence. *Anesthesiology.* 2017;127(1):166–172.

stress-dose steroids include patients taking less than 5 mg of prednisone per day AND do not have clinical features of Cushing syndrome. Patients at intermediate risk include patients who do not fall into the high- or low-risk group categories. Intermediate-risk patients may benefit from preoperative short-acting corticotropin testing to determine hypothalamus-pituitary-adrenal axis integrity. Dosing regimens for stress-dose steroids are largely empiric. Factors to consider when choosing a regimen include type of surgery (major or minor), relative glucocorticoid and mineralocorticoid activity, and length of action of the drug chosen. A common strategy involves the continuation of the patient's normal dose of steroids the morning of surgery, a preincision bolus of hydrocortisone (a short-acting steroid with 1:1 glucocorticoid-to-mineralocorticoid activity), and continuation of intravenous supplementation of 25–50 mg intravenous every 8 hours for a minimum of 24 hours.

## BRONCHOSPASM

Intraoperatively, steroids can be utilized to treat or prevent bronchospasm. Bronchospasm can be the result of anaphylaxis and mechanical or pharmacological factors (i.e., as a reaction to intravenous contrast). Regardless of the etiology, systemic steroids are a mainstay of treatment regimens[4] and prophylactic measures (in the case of contrast allergies).

While steroids are recommended in these scenarios, there is no consensus regarding treatment regimens.

## TRAUMATIC INTUBATION

Steroids are also utilized intraoperatively to prevent postoperative stridor and reintubation. Although the optimal dose and administration time remain to be established, at least one meta-analysis[5] suggested that steroids should be administered at least 4 hours prior to extubation in patients at high risk (i.e., after a traumatic intubation with a positive cuff-leak test) to decrease the risk of reintubation.

## REFERENCES

1. Ho AMH, et al. Heliox vs air-oxygen mixtures for the treatment of patients with acute asthma—a systematic overview. *Chest.* 2003;123(3):882–890.
2. Pashayan AG, Gravenstein JS. Helium retards endotracheal-tube fires from carbon-dioxide lasers. *Anesthesiology.* 1985;62(3):274–277.
3. Liu MM, et al. Perioperative steroid management approaches based on current evidence. *Anesthesiology.* 2017;127(1):166–172.
4. Dewachter P, et al. Case scenario: bronchospasm during anesthetic induction. *Anesthesiology.* 2011;114(5):1200–1210.
5. Jaber S, et al. Effects of steroids on reintubation and post-extubation stridor in adults: meta-analysis of randomised controlled trials. *Crit Care.* 2009;13(2):R49.

# 96.

# PREOPERATIVE EVALUATION AND PREPARATION OF THE PATIENT WITH PULMONARY DISEASE

*Anna-Kaye Brown and Ellen Hauck*

## INTRODUCTION

Thorough evaluation and preparation of patients with pulmonary disease are essential before any surgical procedure. The preoperative assessment incorporates the following information: medical records, patient interview, physical examination, consultations with other providers, and findings from medical tests and procedures. This information estimates the patient's preoperative pulmonary reserve, severity of pulmonary disease, and risk for postoperative pulmonary complications (PPCs). History taking should minimally include signs and symptoms of pulmonary and cardiac disease, exercise capacity, tobacco and alcohol use, recent respiratory infections, hospitalizations, exacerbations of cardiopulmonary conditions, steroid dependence or recent use, and chronic pain and its management. Medication reconciliation must be completed. A thorough review of systems follows and may identify cardiovascular risk factors, indications for preoperative testing, and undiagnosed obstructive sleep apnea (OSA). There are screening tools for OSA, including the STOP-BANG questionnaire.[1] Performing a full physical examination is best, but examination of the heart, lungs, and airway are essential. Pulmonary consultation is warranted in patients with unexplained dyspnea on exertion, hypoxemia, hemoptysis, pulmonary hypertension (PH), poorly controlled chronic obstructive pulmonary disease (COPD), abnormal chest imaging, or recent medical attention for acute pulmonary processes.[2] Patients managed by a pulmonologist should consult this specialist preoperatively.[2]

## RISK ASSESSMENT

Findings from the history and physical may provide indications for medical testing and address the perioperative risk for thoracic and nonthoracic surgery. The American Society of Anesthesiologists (ASA) does not recommend routine preoperative testing but indicated testing based on patient findings and/or surgical procedure.[3] Cardiac risk should be determined. Several cardiac risk calculators are in use, including the Lee Revised Cardiac Risk Index (RCRI), Gupta Index, and the American College of Surgeons Surgical Risk Calculator (ACS-SRC). The RCRI has six questions and is easy to use. The Gupta Index assesses risk for perioperative myocardial infarction and cardiac arrest and consists of five questions. The ACS-SRC requires knowledge of a patient's specific surgery and 19 specific patient factors. While more cumbersome, the ACS-SRC is useful because it evaluates risk for 12 complications.[2] Patients with cardiovascular risk factors, cardiocirculatory disease, respiratory disease, or having major surgery may warrant an electrocardiogram (ECG). Patients with risk factors for coronary artery disease need functional status assessment. Unknown functional status or less than 4 metabolic equivalents means pharmacological stress testing if results will impact perioperative care.[2,3] Chest imaging may be indicated for patients with pulmonary symptoms, prior abnormal radiograph, known cardiopulmonary disease, or severe obesity (body mass index > 40).[2] However, such chest imaging changed management in 0.5%–17% of cases.[3] Medical tests can be useful for assessing surgical risk. Elevated serum blood nitrogen (>30 mg/dL), low serum albumin (3.5 mg/dL), and low hemoglobin are associated with increased risk for PPCs.[1] Arterial blood gas

(ABG) concentrations may help plan surgery for high-risk patients; they do not predict PPCs.[1]

Pulmonary risk should be assessed in all preoperative patients, especially those with pulmonary pathology. Patients at high risk for PPCs include those with patient and/or surgical factors as follows: age over 60 years, preexisting lung disease, smoking, previous spirometry changes (forced expiratory volume in the first second of expiration < 1 L), surgical or anesthesia time greater than 3 hours, head and neck surgeries, chest and upper abdomen surgeries, and use of nasogastric tube preoperatively.[4] Several pulmonary risk calculators exist that can be used to estimate the risk of PPCs. The ACS-SRC calculates the risk of pneumonia. Two Gupta pulmonary risk calculators predict respiratory failure and pneumonia.[2] The Assess Respiratory Risk in Surgical Patients in Catalonia calculator predicts risk of many PPCs.[2] The American College of Physicians adopted indices for calculating the risk of several respiratory complications (Table 96.1).[4] Finally, the ASA created a scoring system to determine PPC risk for those with OSA (Table 96.2).[5]

## RECOMMENDED TESTING AND INTERVENTIONS

The preoperative evaluation can guide disease-specific preoperative preparation for patients with PH, obstructive airway disease, restrictive lung disease, and OSA. Patients with PH undergoing noncardiothoracic surgery should have a resting ECG, a 6-minute walk test (6MWT) and an echocardiogram less than 6 months old to assess the severity of PH. Cardiopulmonary exercise testing measures respiratory oxygen uptake, carbon dioxide production, and ventilation and is used in patients with PH to establish prognosis and assess therapeutic response.[4] Preoperatively, medications that decrease blood pressure should be avoided.[1] Perioperatively, avoid pulmonary vasoconstrictors such as hypoxia, inspiratory pressure of greater than 30 mm Hg, high positive end-expiratory pressure (>15 mm Hg), hypercarbia, and acidosis. Promote pulmonary vasodilation by improving oxygenation.[1] Patients with obstructive pulmonary disease may need spirometry to evaluate current status relative to baseline, chest radiography, and ABGs if symptomatic. An ECG is recommended for most patients with COPD. Current medications should be continued prior to and on the day of surgery.[4] Glucocorticosteroid use within the past 6 months means systemic coverage is recommended during the surgical period to avoid the development of adrenal insufficiency, then rapidly tapered during the 24 hours after surgery.[1] Patients with recent exacerbation or poorly controlled COPD should not undergo elective surgery until optimized[42]; preoperative pulmonary rehabilitation reduces postoperative morbidity and

*Table 96.1* RISK ASSESSMENT FOR POSTOPERATIVE (A) ACUTE RESPIRATORY FAILURE AND (B) PNEUMONIA IN GENERAL NONCARDIAC SURGERY

| (A) RISK FACTOR | SCORE |
|---|---|
| Abdominal aortic aneurysm repair | 27 |
| Thoracic | 14 |
| Upper abdominal, peripheral, or vascular neurosurgery | 21 |
| Neck | 11 |
| Emergency surgery | 11 |
| Albumin < 3.0 mg dL$^{-1}$ | 9 |
| Plasma urea > 30 mg dL$^{-1}$ | 8 |
| Totally or partly dependent functional status | 7 |
| COPD | 6 |
| Age ≥ 70 years | 6 |
| Age 60–69 years | 4 |

| CLASS | SCORE | %RISK |
|---|---|---|
| 1 | ≤10 | 0.5 |
| 2 | 11–19 | 1.8 |
| 3 | 20–27 | 4.2 |
| 4 | 28–40 | 10.1 |
| 5 | ≥40 | 26.6 |

| (B) RISK FACTOR | SCORE |
|---|---|
| Type of surgery | |
| Abdominal aortic aneurysm repair | 15 |
| High thoracic | 14 |
| High abdominal | 10 |
| Neck or neurosurgery | 08 |
| Vascular | 03 |
| Age (years) | |
| ≥80 | 17 |
| 70–79 | 13 |
| 60–69 | 09 |
| 50–59 | 04 |
| Functional status | |
| Totally dependent | 10 |
| Partially dependent | 6 |
| Weight loss over 10% in the last 6 months | 7 |
| COPD | 5 |
| General anesthesia | 4 |
| Altered sensorium | 4 |
| Prior stroke | 4 |
| Urea (mg dL$^{-1}$) | |
| <8 | 4 |
| 22–30 | 2 |
| ≥30 | 3 |
| Blood transfusion greater than 4 units | 3 |
| Emergency surgery | 3 |
| Chronic use of corticosteroids | 3 |
| Smoking in the last year | 3 |
| Alcohol intake > 2 doses in the previous 2 weeks | 2 |

| CLASS | SCORE | %RISK |
|---|---|---|
| 1 | 0–15 | 0.24 |
| 2 | 16–25 | 1.2 |
| 3 | 26–40 | 4.0 |
| 4 | 41–55 | 9.4 |
| 5 | >55 | 15.8 |

From Reference 2.

mortality.[2] Adequate hydration decreases the viscosity of secretions.[1] The underlying cause of restrictive lung disease determines perioperative evaluation and management. Pulmonary function tests and exercise testing (6MWT) are recommended. Preoperative ABG analysis determines baseline oxygenation and ventilation.[1] Patients with long-standing hypoxemia should have a recent ECG along with echocardiography if the ECG is abnormal.[2] Patients with OSA should be adherent to continuous positive airway pressure (CPAP) during the preoperative period; this reduces postoperative complications.[1] A preoperative echocardiogram may be warranted for patients with signs and symptoms of OSA.[2]

In the postoperative period, smokers have increased 30-day mortality and major morbidity risk, including PPCs.[2] Smoking cessation 6 to 8 weeks prior to surgery may reduce PPCs.[2,5] Therapies including nicotine replacement therapy, cognitive behavioral therapy, bupropion, and varenicline are recommended.

## ANESTHETIC CONSIDERATIONS

Patients with lung disease undergoing elective surgery require a thorough preoperative evaluation, including indicated medical testing and perioperative risk assessment. Those having thoracic surgery warrant more extensive testing, including prediction of postoperative pulmonary reserve and function. Elective surgery should be postponed until there has been optimization of pulmonary conditions. Preoperative pulmonary rehabilitation has been shown to reduce PPCs. Tobacco smoking cessation is an essential component of preoperative preparation whenever possible.

*Table 96.2* THE ASA SCORING SYSTEM FOR PERIOPERATIVE RISK OF COMPLICATIONS IN PATIENTS WITH OBSTRUCTIVE SLEEP APNEA

A. Severity of sleep apnea based on sleep study (or clinical indicators if sleep study is not available)
   Point score: (0–3) +,*

| Severity of OSA | Points |
|---|---|
| None | 0 |
| Mild | 1 |
| Moderate | 2 |
| Severe | 3 |

B. Invasiveness of surgery and anesthesia
   Point score: (0–3)

| Type of surgery and anesthesia | Points |
|---|---|
| Superficial surgery under local or peripheral nerve block anesthesia without sedation | 0 |
| Superficial surgery with moderate sedation or general anesthesia | 1 |
| Peripheral surgery with spinal or epidural anesthesia (with no more than moderate sedation) | 1 |
| Peripheral surgery with general anesthesia | 2 |
| Airway surgery with moderate sedation | 2 |
| Major surgery, general anesthesia | 3 |
| Airway surgery, general anesthesia | 3 |

C. Requirement for postoperative opioids
   Point score: (0–3)

| Opioid requirement | Points |
|---|---|
| None | 0 |
| Low-dose oral opioids | 1 |
| High-dose oral opioids, parenteral or neuraxial opioids | 3 |

D. Estimation of perioperative risk:
   Overall point score: the score for A plus the greater of the score for either B or C: (0–6)
     Patients with a score of 4 may be at increased perioperative risk from OSA.
     Patients with a score of 5 or 6 may be at significantly increased perioperative risk from OSA.

CPAP, continuous positive airway pressure; NIPPV, noninvasive positive pressure ventilation; OSA, obstructive sleep apnea.

A scoring system similar to the above may be used to estimate whether a patient is at increased perioperative risk of complications from OSA. This example, which has not been clinically validated, is meant only as a guide, and clinical judgment should be used to assess the risk of an individual patient. + One point may be subtracted if a patient has been on CPAP or NIPPV before surgery and will be using his or her appliance consistently during the postoperative period. * One point should be added if a patient with mild or moderate OSA also has a resting $PaCO_2 > 50$ mm Hg. Ω Patients with a score of 4 may be at increased perioperative risk from OSA; patients with a score of 5 or 6 may be at significantly increased perioperative risk from OSA.

From Reference 5.

# REFERENCES

1. Diaz-Fuentes G, et al. Perioperative evaluation of patients with pulmonary conditions undergoing non-cardiothoracic surgery. *Health Serv Insights.* 2016:9(S1):9–23.
2. Selzer A, Sarkiss M. Preoperative pulmonary evaluation. *Med Clin North Am.* 2019;103(3):585–599.
3. Committee on Standards and Practice Parameters; et al. Practice advisory for preanesthesia evaluation: an updated report by the American Society of Anesthesiologists Task Force on Preanesthesia Evaluation. *Anesthesiology.* 2012;116(3):522–538.
4. Degani-Costa LH, et al. Preoperative evaluation of the patient with pulmonary disease. *Braz J Anesthesiol.* 2014;64(1):22–34.
5. American Society of Anesthesiologists Task Force on Perioperative Management of Patients With Obstructive Sleep Apnea. Practice guidelines for the perioperative management of patients with obstructive sleep apnea: an updated report by the American Society of Anesthesiologists Task Force on Perioperative Management of Patients With Obstructive Sleep Apnea. *Anesthesiology.* 2014; 120(2):268–286.

# 97.

# CHOICE OF ANESTHESIA/ANESTHETIC TECHNIQUES IN THORACIC SURGERY

*Callan Bialorucki*

## INTRODUCTION

Common indications for thoracic surgery include thoracic malignancies, lung reduction surgeries, tracheal stenoses, esophageal disease, and chest trauma. With the exception of chest trauma, an overwhelming majority of patients undergoing thoracic surgery have concomitant pulmonary disease with a higher likelihood of having reactive airway disease, thus influencing the anesthetic plan from the preoperative phase through induction, maintenance, and postoperative phases of care. Furthermore, anesthetic management is influenced by physiologic derangements unique to thoracic surgery that arise secondary to the need for lateral decubitus positioning, thoracotomy resulting in open pneumothorax, and one-lung ventilation (OLV).

## PREMEDICATION

The thoracic surgery patient population is more likely to have reactive airway disease and thus have a higher propensity to develop bronchospasm with induction, airway management, and surgical manipulation of the airway.[1,2] Premedication prior to induction of anesthesia can be utilized to mitigate this risk. Lidocaine administered topically or intravenously may be helpful in preventing bronchoconstriction. Short-acting inhaled $\beta_2$-agonists such as albuterol given 5–10 minutes prior to induction may be useful, particularly in patients on chronic $\beta$-agonist therapy. Anticholinergics can be administered prior to induction to block muscarinic effects of acetylcholine to decrease oral and respiratory secretions as well as protect against cholinergic-mediated bronchoconstriction.[1]

## INDUCTION

In most patients, induction of anesthesia can be safely accomplished with propofol or etomidate. However, in patients with reactive airway disease, ketamine can be considered as an adjunct or as the sole agent as it has bronchodilatory properties. It is important to consider that patients undergoing thoracic surgery likely have underlying lung disease, and smoking is a risk factor for not only chronic obstructive pulmonary disease and reactive airway pathology but also coronary artery disease.[2] Appropriate preoperative cardiopulmonary evaluation should guide hemodynamic goals of induction and thus medication selection and dosing. If indicated, such as in patients presenting for tracheal resection secondary to severe upper airway obstruction, an inhalational induction with sevoflurane provides an optimal induction profile.[1] All potent inhaled anesthetics act directly on pulmonary smooth muscle to induce bronchodilation, and sevoflurane is the least irritating to the airway. Intravenous opioids can be given to supplement induction and blunt the sympathetic response to laryngoscopy. Fentanyl would be preferable to morphine given the propensity of morphine to induce the release of histamine. Neuromuscular blockade selection should also take into consideration histamine release.

## AIRWAY MANAGEMENT

Size and type of endotracheal tube (ETT) will be dependent on the patient's body habitus and the surgical procedure. However, regardless of choice of chosen ETT, the anesthetic should be of adequate depth to mitigate risk of bronchospasm with airway manipulation. For surgical procedures requiring OLV, a single-lumen endotracheal tube (SLT) with an inserted bronchial blocker or a double-lumen endotracheal tube (DLT) can be utilized to isolate the operative lung.[3] There are benefits and drawbacks to each available option that should be considered on a case-by-case basis. A DLT can provide better isolation of each lung when hemorrhage or infection of the operative lung are involved. The DLT also provides ease of pulmonary suctioning intraoperatively, whereas an SLT with an endobronchial blocker would require deflation in order to accomplish the same task. However, as compared to the SLT, DLTs take longer to place and require more skill. Furthermore, after using a DLT, patients requiring post-operative mechanical ventilation necessitate an airway exchange for an SLT, which may be difficult as the large DLT increases the risk for laryngeal edema.

## MAINTENANCE

All current anesthetic techniques have been used for thoracic surgery; however, the most commonly utilized remains the combination of an inhaled anesthetic augmented with an opioid.[2] Inhaled agents are advantageous in the setting of thoracic surgery for several reasons. Isoflurane, sevoflurane, and desflurane have a dose-dependent bronchodilatory effect, have a dose-dependent airway reflex depression, can be used in conjunction with concentrations of inspired oxygen, and are rapidly titratable. However, when utilizing OLV with inhaled anesthetics, one must take into consideration the effects on hypoxic pulmonary vasoconstriction (HPV). When initiating OLV in the lateral decubitus position, HPV favorably influences the V/Q (ventilation-perfusion) inherent in this position by causing a time-dependent decrease in blood flow to the nonventilated lung, thus improving V/Q matching.[4] Numerous clinical studies have investigated the effect of inhaled anesthetics on HPV, suggesting a dose-dependent inhibition. Halothane has been demonstrated to inhibit HPV at 0.5 MAC (minimum alveolar concentration); however, modern inhaled anesthetics require higher doses to demonstrate the same effect.[4] Furthermore, studies have demonstrated there does not appear to be any difference in HPV inhibition at MAC equivalent doses of modern inhaled anesthetic agents. Of the modern inhaled anesthetic agents, immunomodulatory effects of sevoflurane on the deflated lung have been demonstrated in comparison to propofol. Decreases in inflammatory mediators and significantly improved clinical outcomes were demonstrated in patients receiving sevoflurane as compared to propofol.[1] However, propofol has been demonstrated to have no dose-dependent inhibition on HPV despite its intrinsic vasodilatory properties.[4] Therefore, maintenance of anesthesia should always be dictated by the needs of the particular patient, and when clinical instability secondary to HPV inhibition is a possibility, consideration should be given to a balanced technique.

One of the most severe pulmonary complications in thoracic surgery is acute lung injury, which is the leading case of mortality in patients undergoing lung resection.[3,5] Anesthetic management plays a role in the prevention of this complication with lung-protective mechanical ventilation and optimal fluid management. Much of the evidence of lung-protective strategies in OLV have been extrapolated from ARDS Network critical care literature suggesting benefit to low tidal volume ventilation with relatively higher positive end-expiratory pressure to maintain oxygenation with the goals of minimizing barotrauma, volutrauma, and atelectrauma while maintaining appropriate oxygenation and ventilation. Fluid management in the thoracic surgery population is a controversial subject, with disadvantages to both liberal and restrictive regimens.[5] Studies have demonstrated that fluid administration of more than 2 L in a pneumonectomy is associated with poorer outcomes; however, restrictive fluid management can also be associated with end-organ malperfusion and acute kidney injury, complicating a patient's postoperative course.[5]

The importance of postoperative pain control in the thoracic surgical patient population cannot be overstated. A balance must be attained between adequate pain control to avoid poor respiratory effort and avoidance of respiratory depression. In addition to multimodal analgesia with nonopioid analgesic medications such as acetaminophen, gabapentinoids, and nonsteroidal anti-inflammatory drugs, an optimal means of alleviating acute postoperative pain is epidural analgesia. While there is debate about type of medication and timing of administration, common practice involves preoperative placement at the thoracic level and administration of a combination local anesthetic and opioid.[1,2]

## REFERENCES

1. Barash P, et al. Anesthesia for thoracic surgery. In: Eisenkraft JB, Cohen E, Neustein SM, eds. Clinical *Anesthesia*. Philadelphia, PA: Lippincott Williams & Wilkins; 2006:1029–1076.
2. Butterworth J, et al. Anesthesia for thoracic surgery. In: *Morgan & Mikhail's Clinical Anesthesiology*. New York, NY: McGraw-Hill; 2013:545–573.
3. Lederman D, et al. Anesthetic considerations for lung resection: preoperative assessment, intraoperative challenges and postoperative analgesia. *Ann Transl Med*. 2019;7(15):356.
4. Lumb AB, Slinger P. Hypoxic pulmonary vasoconstriction: physiology and anesthetic implications. *Anesthesiology* 2015;122(4):932–946.
5. Dinic VD, et al. Enhanced recovery in thoracic surgery: a review. *Front Med*. 2018;5:14.

# 98.

# NONPULMONARY SURGERY, INCLUDING MEDIASTINOSCOPY AND BRONCHOSCOPY

*Christopher O. Fadumiye*

## INTRODUCTION

The provision of anesthesia for surgeries in the thoracic cavity, particularly the mediastinum and bronchoscopy, has changed progressively over the years, from the advent of double-lumen endotracheal tubes, bronchial blockers, TIVA (total intravenous anesthesia), and the use of more refined laryngeal mask airways (LMAs).[1] Surgical procedures have improved in terms of their efficiency and the ability to provide anesthesia for more challenging procedures of the mediastinum. This chapter is divided into two sections. The first part discusses surgical procedures of the mediastinum. The second part of the chapter discusses bronchoscopy, endobronchial ultrasound use in bronchoscopy, perioperative management and considerations, the use of TIVA with bronchoscopy, and ultimate surgical considerations and adverse complications.

## SURGICAL PROCEDURES OF THE MEDIASTINUM

### MEDIASTINAL TUMORS

Mediastinal tumors are described based on their location (anterior, middle, or posterior) and their size. Common tumors include thymoma, lymphoma, and germ cell tumor (anterior). Anterior tumors are usually removed via a median sternotomy, while middle and posterior tumors are resected via a lateral thoracotomy or video-assisted thoracoscopy.[2] Preoperative consideration includes the presence of intrathoracic airway obstruction on induction of anesthesia and baseline comorbidities these patients present with. Notwithstanding, most mediastinal masses do not cause obstruction of the trachea or bronchial tree at rest, but with induction of anesthesia coupled with muscle relaxation, complete airway obstruction is possible.[2]

Most mediastinal resections are performed under general anesthesia with a single-lumen endotracheal tube; large masses can preempt the use of awake fiber-optic endotracheal intubation. Positioning is mostly supine or lateral decubitus depending on the size and location of the mass. Essential monitoring includes basic standard monitors and a good bore intravenous arterial access is indicated depending on the length of surgery and comorbidities of the patient. Morbidity is also usually aligned to excessive bleeding. Some other associated complications or conditions are injury to the recurrent laryngeal nerve, superior vena cava (SVC) syndrome, and injury to a great vessel. A multimodal approach to pain control (opioids, antineuropathic medications, regional anesthesia) are preferred.

It is crucial to evaluate the mass before surgery and establish a plan to deal with any airway obstruction that may occur on induction. A rigid bronchoscope should be available in the operating room in case the mass obstructs the airway on induction; a rigid bronchoscope can be placed through the airway to alleviate this obstruction. If the risk is very high, away fiber-optic intubation can be utilized. In severe cases where obstruction cannot be managed at induction, cardiopulmonary bypass will be the preferred option. Location of the mass in relation to the bronchial tree can significantly impact the plan as well. In conclusion, the anesthesiologist should have plans A, D, and C and choose the safest option to avoid emergency/life-threatening situations.

### MEDIASTINASCOPY

Mediastinascopy is mostly performed to establish a diagnosis or to determine the resectability of a mass. Cervical mediastinoscopy provides access to the pretracheal, paratracheal, and anterior subcarinal nodes.[1] Relative contraindications to this procedure include a previous mediastinoscopy and radiation because scarring obscures the dissection plane. Absolute contraindications include the presence of a thoracic aneurysm or an obstructed SVC; this is because of the high risk of puncturing the vessels with the mediastinal scope. General anesthesia is obtained similar to mediastinal mass resections, with care given to

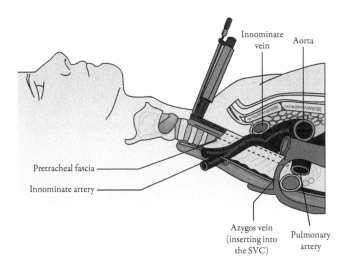

Figure 98.1 Insertion of mediastinoscope.

used for the diagnosis and evaluation of myriad pulmonary conditions, such as pulmonary alveolar proteinosis, bullous emphysema, and cancer.[2] Anesthesia can be attained via general anesthesia or MAC. The use of a rigid bronchoscope is more appropriate for the evaluation of intrabronchial procedures such as mechanical dilation of bronchial or tracheal strictures, removal of foreign bodies, mechanical tumor debridement, and hemoptysis drainage. General anesthesia is the mainstay here with ventilation usually attained from the side port of the rigid bronchoscope. TIVA can also be utilized; the avoidance of volatile anesthetics with the multiple intermittent ventilation attempts allows for reduced inhalation of pungent anesthetic gases by the surgeon and anesthesia provider. Intermittent ventilation or the use of jet ventilation or a venturi ventilator can also be utilized to maintain optimal ventilation. The anesthetic consideration here mostly pertains to reducing hypoxemia and hypercapnia in these patients. Of note also is the baseline presentation of these patients, which can range from asymptomatic to severe respiratory distress presentation. The plan of care with anesthesia should be tailored based on the patient's presentation, their preexisting comorbidities, length of procedure, and overall comfort of the anesthesia provider.

Endobronchial ultrasound with fine-needle aspiration is a less invasive option to mediastinoscopy for staging and diagnosis of a mediastinal mass.[2] The ultrasound device is attached to the distal end of the bronchoscope and thus provides continuous ultrasound waves for the purpose of clinical visualization, identification of vascular structures, and overall improved image visibility. These procedures can be performed under general anesthesia or MAC. LMA use has also been noted, as the use of an LMA allows the visualization and evaluation of upper paratracheal lymph nodes, which will otherwise be difficult to see with an endotracheal tube.[2]

airway obstruction and patients presenting comorbidities (i.e., obesity, myasthenia gravis, obstructive sleep apnea). It is important to state that with the advent of improved computed tomographic scans and magnetic resonance imaging, the need for mediastinoscopy for diagnostic purposes has diminished, notwithstanding its use for biopsies of masses is still in place. Local anesthetic and monitored care anesthesia (MAC) may be considered for patients with active cerebrovascular disease to enable monitoring of cardiovascular function in the awake state. Primary focus from the anesthesia provider is on the right upper extremity blood pressures, as compression of the innominate vein and right subclavian and carotid arteries can occur (Figure 98.1). Reflex bradycardia as a result of aortic compression, arrhythmias, hypovolemia, tension pneumothorax, and compression of the trachea are also notable complications anesthesia requiring provider vigilance.

## BRONCHOSCOPY AND ENDOBRONCHIAL ULTRASOUND

Bronchoscopy is usually performed with either a rigid or flexible bronchoscope. Flexible fiber-optic bronchoscopy is

## REFERENCES

1. Benumof JL, et al. Anesthesia for thoracic surgery. In: *Miller's Anesthesia*. Philadelphia, PA: 1727, 1732–1736.
2. Kulkarni V, et al. Thoracic surgery. In: *Anesthesiologist's Manual of Surgical Procedures*. Philadelphia, PA: 308–311, 315–317.

# 99.

# THORACIC AND PULMONARY SURGERY

*Al-Awwab Mohammad Dabaliz and Christina Stachur*

## INTRODUCTION

Operations involving the trachea, lungs, and chest wall pose unique anesthetic considerations that can provide difficult yet engaging challenges to the anesthesia provider. Special considerations throughout the perioperative period are particularly necessary for pulmonary surgeries. These generally include the following operations: wedge resections, blebectomies, lobectomies, pneumonectomies, and lung volume reduction surgeries. The primary indication for these operations is early stage cancer. Other indications include infections, hemorrhage, and air leak.[1–2]

## ANESTHETIC CONSIDERATIONS

### PREOPERATIVE CONSIDERATIONS

The preoperative evaluation of patients undergoing lung resection should include a complete history, physical examination, and laboratory tests, with the intention of identifying the risk for postoperative complications and optimizing the functional status. The majority of these patients have an extensive smoking history and multiple comorbidities requiring optimization. Patients have to meet minimum requirements during the preoperative respiratory assessment in order to qualify for pulmonary resection. The most valid tests for predicting postoperative complications in this patient population are the forced expiratory volume in 1 second ($FEV_1$), the diffusing lung capacity for carbon monoxide (DLCO), and the maximal oxygen uptake ($VO_2$ max). These reflect respiratory mechanics, parenchymal function, and cardiopulmonary reserve, respectively. Predicted postoperative values of less than 40% for both $FEV_1$ and $D_LCO$ and baseline $VO_2$ max less than 15 mL/kg/min are associated with increased risk of postoperative pulmonary complications (Table 99.1).[1,3]

Other important considerations include performing transthoracic echocardiography to evaluate for the presence of right ventricular dysfunction with concomitant pulmonary hypertension, which may be a contraindication to lung resection, and the association between thoracic neoplasms and myasthenic syndromes.

Tracheal resections generally involve performing a primary anastomosis, which is a contraindication to

*Table 99.1* THREE PARAMETERS OF PRETHORACOTOMY RESPIRATORY ASSESSMENT

| | RESPIRATORY MECHANICS | CARDIOPULMONARY RESERVE | LUNG PARENCHYMAL FUNCTION |
|---|---|---|---|
| Low risk | $ppoFEV_1 > 40\%$ | $VO_2$ max > 15 mL/kg/min | ppoDLCO > 40% |
| Unacceptably high risk | $ppoFEV_1 < 20\%$ | $VO_2$ max < 10 mL/kg/min | ppoDLCO < 20% |
| Other tests and values indicating high risk | MVV < 50% RV/TLC > 50% FVC < 50% | Stair climb < 2 flights 6MWT < 2000 feet Exercise $SpO_2$ > 4% drop | $PaO_2 < 50$ mm Hg $PaCO_2 > 45$ mm Hg |

V/Q scan can be utilized to assess the preoperative contribution of the lung to be resected when the preoperative $FEV_1$ or DLCO are < 80% or when the $ppoFEV_1$ is < 40%.

Calculating predicted postoperative PFT: $ppo = \text{preoperative PFT} \times \left(1 - \dfrac{\textit{percent of functional lung removed}}{100}\right)$.

FVC, forced vital capacity; MVV, maximal voluntary ventilation; 6MWT, 6-minute walk test; $PaCO_2$, partial pressure of carbon dioxide; $PaO_2$, partial pressure of oxygen; ppo, predicted postoperative; RV, residual volume; TLC, total lung capacity.

postoperative mechanical ventilation. Therefore, preoperative pulmonary function tests (PFTs) are also required in these patients.

## INTRAOPERATIVE CONSIDERATIONS

Standard induction and monitoring should be performed. In the majority of these surgeries, the placement of an arterial line, a urinary catheter, and, less frequently, a central venous catheter may be warranted. In many instances, the surgeon will perform bronchoscopic evaluation prior to lung resection. A large, single-lumen endotracheal tube (8.0 mm) should be used initially in such cases and then replaced with an appropriately size double-lumen endotracheal tube (DLT) following bronchoscopy. One-lung ventilation is utilized.[2]

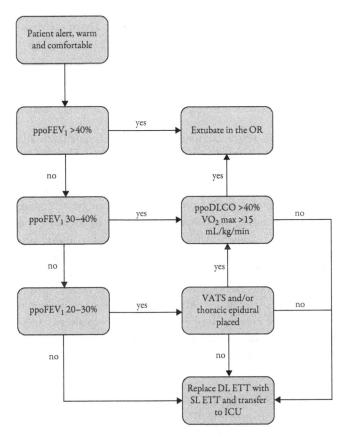

**Figure 99.1** Extubation algorithm. DL, double lumen; ETT, endotracheal tube; ICU, intensive care unit; OR, operating room; SL, single lumen.

If required, it is important to ensure appropriate patient positioning in the lateral decubitus position, including padding the pressure points, along with proper placement of an axillary roll. A common complication associated with turning the patient includes displacement of the endotracheal tube, particularly when a DLT is utilized. This may be associated with a sudden increase in peak airway pressures along with a precipitous drop in expired tidal volumes and oxygen saturation. Bronchoscopic reconfirmation of endotracheal tube positioning after turning the patient is warranted.

Fluid volume restrictive strategies (10–15 mL/kg) are preferred in thoracic surgeries due to increased risk of right ventricular failure and pulmonary edema in overhydrated patients. Consider replacing blood loss with colloids 1:1 to minimize administered volume.[1]

## POSTOPERATIVE CONSIDERATIONS

Life-threatening complications in the immediate postoperative period include cardiac herniation or arrhythmias (most commonly supraventricular, i.e., atrial fibrillation), acute right heart failure, massive hemorrhage, bronchopleural fistulas from disruption of the bronchial stump, tension pneumothorax, torsion and pulmonary infarction, postpneumonectomy pulmonary edema, and acute respiratory failure. Additional complications include renal dysfunction and injuries related to lateral positioning.[1,4]

Interventions that are vital in decreasing postoperative pulmonary complications include providing adequate pain control, early but appropriate extubation (see Figure 99.1), and early ambulation. Pain control may be achieved through neuraxial blockade, intercostal or paravertebral nerve blocks, intrapleural analgesia, cryoneurolysis, nonsteroidal anti-inflammatory drugs, and patient-controlled analgesia.

## REFERENCES

1. Gropper MA, et al., eds. *Miller's Anesthesia.* 2 Vol. Elsevier Health Sciences; October 7, 2019.
2. Jaffe RA, et al., eds. *Anesthesiologist's Manual of Surgical Procedures.* Lippincott Williams & Wilkins; 2014.
3. Yao FS, et al., eds. *Yao & Artusio's Anesthesiology: Problem-Oriented Patient Management.* Lippincott Williams & Wilkins; 2008.
4. Slinger PD, Johnston MR. Preoperative assessment: an anesthesiologist's perspective. *Thorac Surg Clin.* 2005;15(1):11–25.

# 100.

# BRONCHOPLEURAL FISTULA

*Adam Lepkowsky and Dane Coyne*

## INTRODUCTION

A bronchopleural fistula is an abnormal communication between the bronchial tree and the pleural space.[1,2] While rare, bronchopleural fistulas are a dangerous, life-threatening condition, with overall mortality ranging from 5% to 70%.[1,3] A number of surgical and nonsurgical etiologies have been associated with the formation of a bronchopleural fistula, including lung resection, rupture of bronchus or bulla, necrotic lung infection, erosion caused by a carcinoma, and traumatic or iatrogenic penetrating chest wounds.[1–3] Bronchopleural fistulas most commonly occur after lung resection, with higher rates following a pneumonectomy than other surgical lung resections, with an incidence ranging from 2% to 11%.[1–4]

## CLINICAL FEATURES

Bronchopleural fistulas most often occur in the postoperative period between days 8 and 12.[1] Presentation within the first 72 hours postpneumonectomy is usually due to failed bronchial stump closure and can lead to life-threatening tension pneumothorax or asphyxiation from pulmonary flood.[3,4] When bronchopleural fistulas form acutely, they present with an air leak in the chest tube, along with sudden-onset dyspnea, hypotension, subcutaneous emphysema, increasing pneumothorax with shifting of the mediastinum, or increase of air-fluid levels on chest radiograph.[1,3,4] Following a pneumonectomy, both air and fluid are present in the pleural space. Both are usually reabsorbed within the first 24 to 48 hours, with air being gradually reabsorbed first, followed by fluid reabsorption. If empyema is present, rapid filling of fluid in the pleural space will be seen with associated fever, leukocytosis, and cough with expectoration of purulent material due to the connection between the pleural space and the airway. If the patient is coughing up fluid, rapid clearance of fluid levels from the pleural space will be seen on chest radiograph.[1]

Delayed presentations are commonly due to necrotic suture lines associated with infection or insufficient blood flow to the healing stump.[4] These present more gradually and are characterized by wasting malaise, fever, and minimally productive cough. Fibrosis of the pleural space and mediastinum can be present, which prevents shifting of the mediastinum seen in the acute form. These are managed with drainage of the pleural space or with a Clagett procedure.[3]

## DIAGNOSIS

The diagnosis of a bronchopleural fistula is made clinically and is then confirmed with further imaging. Bronchoscopy can be both diagnostic and therapeutic; the fistula can be localized and evaluated for the possible introduction of a sealant, and an infectious etiology can be excluded. Computed tomography scan can be used to identify and localize the fistula, which can then be used to guide further surgical intervention.[1] Other diagnostic tests include administration and detection of certain dyes and inhalants. Methylene blue can be administered in the pleural space; if a fistula is present, it will be detected in the sputum.[1,3] Detection of radionuclide in the pleural space after inhalation of xenon or a mixture of $N_2O$ and $O_2$ also indicates a fistula's presence.[3]

## ANESTHETIC CONSIDERATIONS

### PREOPERATIVE

The challenge an anesthesiologist faces when treating a patient with a bronchopleural fistula is protecting the healthy lung via lung isolation and providing adequate ventilation while avoiding complications and contamination.[2,3] Complications include ineffectively ventilating the patient with positive pressure ventilation due to a large air leak and the potential of forming a tension pneumothorax.[4] Preoperatively, there should be a discussion with the surgeon regarding whether a chest tube should be placed before induction or to be prepared for rapid placement after induction. To avoid lung contamination from an empyema, drainage is performed under local anesthesia preoperatively with the patient positioned sitting upright and leaning toward the affected side.[2,4]

The larger the air leak caused by the bronchopleural fistula, the greater the need for one-lung ventilation, so it is important to estimate the loss of tidal volume preoperatively. A larger fistula will have continuous air bubbles flowing through the chest tube water seal chamber, while smaller fistulas will have an intermittent bubble flow. Reduction in tidal volume can be quantified by the difference between inhaled and exhaled tidal volumes.[3]

## INTRAOPERATIVE

During induction, spontaneous ventilation and discontinuation of chest tube suctioning can reduce the loss of tidal volumes during positive pressure ventilation. The healthy lung needs to be rapidly isolated from the fistula to reduce the likelihood of a tension pneumothorax and possible contamination. This is accomplished using a double-lumen tube or a bronchial blocker.[3,4] This also eliminates the risk of contaminating the healthy lung when the patient is placed in the lateral decubitus position. One-lung ventilation is used to provide adequate positive pressure ventilation to the healthy lung without loss of minute ventilation. Ventilation can be provided using a double-lumen tube, selective single-lung intubation of the healthy lung, high-frequency ventilation to provide lower peak airway pressures, one-way endobronchial valves (close during inspiration and open during expiration) placed in the affected segment, or with differential lung ventilation. (The nondiseased lung can be ventilated normally while the diseased lung is ventilated with a reduced tidal volume, continuous positive airway pressure, or high-frequency ventilation).[3]

The safest and preferred intubation approach is an awake fiber-optic intubation with the patient is breathing spontaneously on supplemental oxygen. Insertion of the double-lumen tube can also be accomplished under general anesthesia, while the patient is breathing spontaneously. Spontaneous breathing will help avoid inadequate positive pressure ventilation from an air leak and the formation of a pneumothorax.[2,3] Rapid sequence induction should be avoided because of its association with tension pneumothorax and contamination. Be aware that there may be an outpouring of pus from the affected lung if an empyema is present, and it should be suctioned appropriately to minimize cross-contamination of the healthy lung.[2] Confirmation of lung isolation is necessary before positive pressure ventilation is applied or the patient is repositioned.[3] The chest tube must be left unclamped intraoperatively to avoid the possibility of developing a tension pneumothorax.[2,3] In the case of multiple fistulas, the use of high-frequency oscillatory ventilation may be considered due to its ability to use lower peak airway pressures and high minimum airway pressures to avoid barotrauma.[3]

## POSTOPERATIVE

Postoperatively, extubation should be attempted as early as possible after the fistula is repaired.[4] This is necessary to avoid barotrauma to the surgical stump caused by positive pressure ventilation.[3]

## REFERENCES

1. Lois M, Noppen M. Bronchopleural fistulas. *Chest.* 2005;128(6): 3955–3965.
2. Eisenkraft JB, Cohen E, Pasternak JJ. Chapter 38: Anesthesia for Thoracic Surgery, In: *Clinical Anesthesia.* 8th ed. Philadelphia, PA: Wolters Kluwer; 2017:1062–1063.
3. Slinger P, Campos JH. Chapter 53: Anesthesia for Thoracic Surgery, In: *Miller's Anesthesia.* 9th ed. Philadelphia, PA: Elsevier; 2020:1698–1699.
4. Butterworth JF, Mackey DC, Wasnick JD. Chapter 25: Anesthesia for Thoracic Surgery. In: *Morgan and Mikhail's Clinical Anesthesiology.* 6th ed. New York, NY: McGraw-Hill Education; 2018:553–582.

# 101.

# ADVANCED ANESTHESIA REVIEW
## ONE-LUNG VENTILATION

*Sohail K. Mahboobi and Dillon B. Coplai*

## INTRODUCTION

One lung ventilation (OLV) is the technique of ventilating one lung while letting the other collapse. Traditionally, it was used for thoracic lung procedures; but with the advancement of surgical techniques, it is being used for esophageal, cardiac, aortic, mediastinal surgeries as well as in critical care units in certain conditions (Box 101.1). There is no absolute contraindication to OLV. Certain conditions may prevent using a specific technique, e.g. intrabronchial tumor. A substitute technique, like contralateral endobronchial single or double lumen tube, can be adapted in these situations.

---

**Box 101.1 INDICATIONS FOR ONE-LUNG VENTILATION**

- Thoracic lung procedure
  - Lobectomies
  - Wedge resection
  - Pneumonectomy
  - Surgeries for bronchopleural fistula
  - Video or robotic assisted thoracic surgeries
- Cardiac Procedures
  - Minimally invasive mitral valve surgeries
  - Minimally invasive coronary artery bypass grafts
  - Thoracic aortic aneurysm surgeries
- Esophageal surgeries
  - Open, video or robotic assisted esophagectomy
  - Surgeries for tracheoesophageal fistula
- Miscellaneous
  - Pulmonary artery rupture
  - Differential ventilation of one lung e.g. in single lung lavage procedures

---

## TECHNIQUES FOR ONE-LUNG VENTILATION

The commonly used technique is using a right or left double lumen tube (DLT). Others are bronchial blockers and single lumen endotracheal tubes advanced endobronchially.

Double Lumen Tubes (DLT) consist of a bronchial and tracheal lumen, each can be ventilated independently by application of an external clamp or using the in-build flow blocker. The tracheal opening stays above carina while the angulated bronchial lumen fits into the respective main stem bronchus. DLT is available in 26 to 41 Fr (number indicates the tube's external diameter in centimeters) sizes. Size 41, 39, 37, 35 and 28 Fr are equal to diameter of 6.5, 6, 5.5, 5 and 4.5 mm respectively. The DLT cuffs and connectors are color-coded, to ensure proper assembly and selective ventilation. The bronchial cuff is blue colored to help identification with the fiberoptic bronchoscope. Due to the close proximity of the right upper lobe bronchus to the carina, the right DLT has a modified bronchial cuff with an opening (Murphy's eye) embedded in the cuff to align with the right upper lobe. Bronchopleural fistula, protecting one lung from contamination of other lung's contents as in abscess and hemorrhage, and to perform one lung lavage as in alveolar proteinosis are absolute indications for double lumen tube placement (Box 101.2). The left sided DLT can be used for most thoracic procedures requiring one lung ventilation regardless of the operative side. In left sided surgery the endobronchial portion of the left sided tube can be withdrawn into the trachea at the time of clamping the left main stem.

Left sided placement is contraindicated in carinal or proximal left mainstem lesions that could be traumatized by a left-sided tube. Whenever easible, a left sided tube is always preferred.

Bronchial blockers are used to occlude the operative side mainstem bronchus and can be placed through a single

Double-lumen tube (DLT):
- Advantages:
  - Easy placement even without visualization with fiberoptic bronchoscope
  - Available in various sizes to be used according to patient's tracheal diameter
  - CPAP application and suctioning of the operative lung is possible
  - Lung isolation can be performed on both sides alternatively using the same DLT
- Disadvantages:
  - Placement can cause airway trauma
  - Challenging to place in patients with difficult airway
  - Need replacement with a single lumen endotracheal tube if postoperative ventilation is required

Bronchial blocker
- Advantages
  - Easy placement with already in place single lumen endotracheal tube
  - Technique of choice in difficult airway or when DLT placement is not possible
  - Postoperative ventilation is possible with single lumen tube after removing the blocker
  - Selective lobar occlusion is possible
- Disadvantages
  - Requires training and practice and has a learning curve
  - Cannot be placed without fiberoptic bronchoscope
  - Application of CPAP, bronchoscopy and suctioning of the operative lung is not possible
  - Operative lung collapse is not faster as it requires absorption of the trapped air
  - Alternate lung isolation cannot be performed if required during procedure
  - Difficult placement in right mainstem bronchus due to shorter anatomical landing zone

Single-lumen endobronchial tube
- Advantages:
  - Easy placement without requirement of extra training and equipment, particularly in difficult airway and emergency situations
- Disadvantages
  - Tendency to go to right mainstem bronchus and difficulty in forwarding to left mainstem bronchus
  - Application of CPAP, bronchoscopy and suctioning of the operative lung is not possible
  - Cuff is not designed for lung isolation

lumen tube (easier) or adjacent to it (difficult). The most commonly used is Arndt wire guided bronchial blocker and is available in sizes 5, 7, and 9 Fr. The 9 Fr blocker is recommended for endotracheal tubes of 7.5 mm and above, 7 Fr for 6.0 to 7.0 mm, and 5 Fr for 4.5 to 5.5 mm. It requires a special adapter for placement that has four ports: a standard 15-mm adaptor for the circuit, a connector to the endotracheal tube, port for the bronchial blocker that can be tightened around, and port for the fiberoptic bronchoscope. These blockers can be used with tracheostomies or in nasal intubations. Blockers should be considered in patients already intubated to avoid complications of reintubation and unexpected airway loss.

Another OLV technique is to advance a single lumen endotracheal tube further into the nonoperative mainstem bronchus. This technique was previously performed in difficult DLT placement but with advancement in blockers, it is now rarely used.

## ANESTHETIC CONSIDERATIONS

### PREOPERATIVE CONSIDERATIONS

Patients should be assessed for any history of or signs of difficult airway. Majority of the cases, regardless of the side of the lung procedure, can be done with the left sided tube due to easy placement. Right sided DLT is required in procedures involving left mainstem bronchus, left pneumonectomy, left lung transplant, large descending thoracic aortic aneurysm and anatomical disruption of left tracheobronchial tree. The ventilation of the right lung with the left DLT in flexed right lateral decubitus position can result in narrowing and partial obstruction of the right mainstem bronchus, requiring higher insufflation ventilatory pressures with chances of air trapping and development of auto PEEP. Traditionally, a size 39 Fr has been used for males and 37 Fr for females. Ideal technique is measuring the left mainstem bronchus on chest x-ray or

CT scan and using a table to select appropriate size DLT.[1] Additionally, review any imaging for findings that may foreshadow perioperative complications such as bullae on the ventilated lung (risk of pneumothorax) or atelectasis, effusions, consolidations (risk of hypoxemia). The ACCP recommends using forced expiratory volume-one second (FEV1) and diffusing capacity of the lungs for carbon monoxide (DLCO) to determine predicted post-operative (PPO) values.[2] No further testing required if both are > 60%, exercise test to measure maximum oxygen consumption if < 30% and stair climbing test if between 30-60%.

## INTRAOPERATIVE CONSIDERATIONS

A balanced anesthetic technique using opioids, muscle relaxants and inhalational agent is most commonly used. Total intravenous anesthesia can also be used. In patients with reassuring airway, conventional laryngoscopy is used for DLT placement. Once the bronchial cuff passes vocal cords, the stylet should be removed and the tube should be turned 90 degrees counterclockwise for the left DLT and clockwise for the right sided DLT. Fiberoptic bronchoscope is inserted through the tracheal lumen to confirm placement of the bronchial lumen. For right sided DLT, the fiberoptic scope should be placed through the bronchial lumen to visualize proper alignment of the Murphy's eye with the right upper lobe bronchus.

In case of difficult airway, video laryngoscopy and video stylets to place DLT, bronchial blocker via single lumen tube (placed with either video laryngoscopy or fiberoptic bronchoscope), tube exchanger (e.g. Cook exchanger, Cook Medical, USA) to replace single lumen tube with DLT or endobronchial single lumen tube, can be considered.[3] For patients with tracheostomy, the bronchial blocker assembly can be used by attaching it to the tracheostomy tube.

One lung ventilation is not physiological and can cause acute lung injury to the ventilated lung due to barotrauma, volutrauma and biotrauma. A protective lung ventilation strategy (tidal volume of 6 ml/kg and peak pressure < 35 cm H2O with PEEP) should be used to ventilate the nonoperative lung.

During OLV, the deflated lung is perfused but not ventilated, causing a shunt and ventilation/perfusion (V/Q) mismatch and decreased oxygenation. Hypoxic pulmonary vasoconstriction (HPV) is the body's physiological response to divert pulmonary blood from hypoxic to ventilated alveoli. Some of the anesthetic agents decrease HPV like use of inhalational agents and vasodilators. Intraoperative hypoxia during one lung ventilation can be treated with several interventions that can improve oxygenation:

- Ensure proper placement of the DLT/blocker with fiberoptic bronchoscope
- If it isn't already, increase FiO2 to 1.0
- Maintain sufficient perfusion and hemodynamics
- Recruitment maneuvers of the ventilated lung
- Adjust PEEP to avoid atelectasis, use cautiously as increasing PEEP can divert more blood to non-ventilated lung[4]
- Apply external continuous positive airway pressure (CPAP) 5-15 cm H2O to the non-ventilated lung
- Clamp the pulmonary artery of the deflated lung
- Resume bilateral lung ventilation in severe and refractory hypoxemia

## POSTOPERATIVE CONSIDERATIONS

At the end of the procedure, the patient should be evaluated according to extubation criteria. If postoperative ventilation is required, DLT can be replaced with a single lumen tube for postoperative ventilation either with conventional laryngoscopy or by using a tube exchange catheter.[5]

## REFERENCES

1. Brodsky JB, Lemmens JMH. Left double lumen tubes: clinical experience with 1,170 patients. *J Cardiothorac Vasc Anesth.* 2003;*17*:289–298.
2. Liptay, MJ et al. Diffusion lung capacity for carbon monoxide (DLCO) is an independent prognostic factor for long-term survival after curative lung resection for cancer. *Journal of Surgical Oncology.* 2009;*100*(8),703–707.
3. Hagihara S et al. One-lung ventilation in patients with difficult airways. *J Cardiothorac Vasc Anesth.* 1998;*12*:186–188.
4. Fugiwara M et al. The effects of positive end-expiratory pressure and continuous positive airway pressure on the oxygenation and shunt fraction during one-lung ventilation with propofol anesthesia. *J Clin Anesth* 2001;*13*:473–477.
5. Şentürk M et al. Intraoperative mechanical ventilation strategies for one-lung ventilation. *Best Pract Res Clin Anaesthesiol.* 2015;*29*: 357–369.

# 102.

# THORACOSCOPY

*Al-Awwab Mohammad Dabaliz and Christina Stachur*

## INTRODUCTION

Video-assisted thoracoscopic surgery (VATS) techniques are used for both diagnostic and therapeutic purposes across a variety of pleural diseases (e.g., pleurodesis, drainage of effusions, decortication of early empyema); pulmonary resections (e.g., wedge resections, lobectomies); and peripheral biopsies. Other nonpulmonary indications for VATS include esophageal surgeries (e.g., myotomies, esophagectomy); upper dorsal sympathectomies; and minimally invasive cardiac surgeries.

Simple diagnostic and therapeutic procedures may be performed under local (chest wall infiltration) or regional (intercostal blocks, epidural) anesthesia with light sedation. The main limitation with these anesthetic modalities is that the patient is required to breathe spontaneously. This is not well tolerated for longer and more extensive procedures, in which general anesthesia is necessary. Frequently, general anesthesia is preferred as it provides better surgical exposure along with a secure airway.[1–3]

## ANESTHETIC CONSIDERATIONS

### PREOPERATIVE

Given the wide range of indications, patients undergoing VATS have diverse underlying conditions. Preoperative evaluation should focus on the patient's comorbidities and planned intervention. Optimization through pretreatment with bronchodilators and treating respiratory infections as indicated, in addition to smoking cessation for several weeks, may improve preoperative pulmonary function. One should examine available chest imaging (radiograph and computed tomographic scan) and pulmonary function tests to assess feasibility of lung isolation and risk of hypoxemia during one-lung ventilation (OLV).[4]

### INTRAOPERATIVE

Video-assisted thoracoscopic surgery is performed with the patient in the lateral decubitus position, with the operative lung up and collapsed, while the dependent lung is ventilated. The operative field is visualized by inserting a camera and trocars into three to five ports along the chest wall.

If local or regional anesthesia is chosen, care must be taken to properly explain to the patient what the plan is and have their cooperation. A combination of techniques can be used, which include, but are not limited to, infiltration of the skin with local anesthetic, intercostal nerve blocks (at the level of the incision as well as two levels above and below), and thoracic epidurals. To aid in patient comfort and cooperation, an ipsilateral stellate ganglion block can be performed to inhibit the cough reflex, as well as the administration of intravenous sedation. If the patient cannot tolerate regional anesthesia, if intraoperative extension of the surgery is needed, or if the anesthesiologist needs to secure the airway, conversion to general anesthesia is appropriate. Note, to secure the airway with a double-lumen tube (DLT), the patient may need to be repositioned supine.[1]

For general anesthesia, standard induction and monitoring should be performed. Arterial catheters may be required based on the patient's comorbidities and surgical proximity to great vessels. As per most thoracic surgeries, lung isolation (preferably with a double-lumen endotracheal tube or alternatively bronchial blockers), lateral positioning, and OLV are necessary for appropriate surgical exposure. If a bronchopleural fistula is suspected, lung isolation should be achieved prior to initiation of positive pressure mechanical ventilation.[3]

Compared to open thoracotomy, lung collapse in VATS is slower due to incomplete exposure to atmospheric pressure. If managed incorrectly, this may lead to suboptimal surgical exposure and worse outcomes, including the need to convert to an open thoracotomy. Early initiation of OLV, applying gentle suction to the unventilated lung (-20 cm $H_2O$), denitrogenating the operative lung using a fraction of inspired oxygen ($FiO_2$) of 1 prior to initiating OLV, ensuring trocars are open to atmosphere for 30–60 seconds prior to inserting instruments, and $CO_2$ insufflation can all be used to accelerate lung collapse. Sudden $CO_2$ insufflation may cause hemodynamic collapse due to increased intrathoracic pressure. Furthermore, there is an increased risk of venous gas embolism and hypercarbia.[1,5]

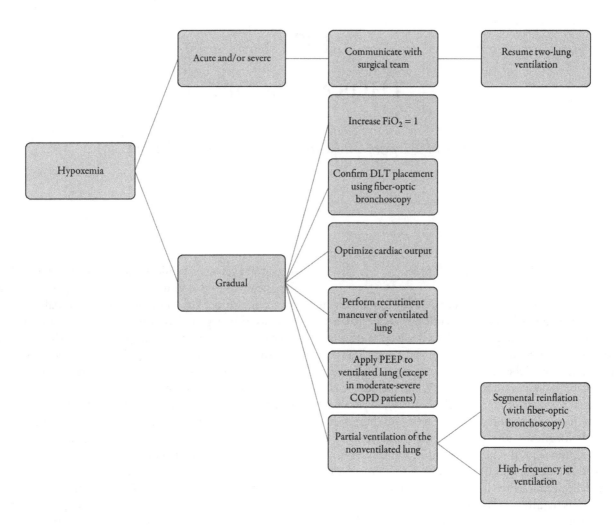

**Figure 102.1** Management of hypoxemia during thoracoscopic surgery under OLV. Adapted from Cohen E. Anesthesia for Video-Assisted Thoracoscopic Surgery. Springer; 2011.

Notably, initiating OLV prior to surgical incision may lead to passive paradoxical ventilation in the nonventilated lung if the lumen of the DLT is open to atmosphere (closed-chest OLV; approximately 130 mL/breath), which further delays desired collapse. The passive air movement should halt once the chest is open to atmospheric pressure.[1]

Managing intraoperative hypoxemia during OLV depends on its acuity and severity. Severe or acute hypoxemia may necessitate the immediate resumption of two-lung ventilation. Conversely, the management of gradual desaturation can be achieved in a stepwise approach (see Figure 102.1). In both instances, communication with the surgical team is essential.

Injury to intrathoracic structures or excessive hemorrhage may dictate conversion to open thoracotomy.

## POSTOPERATIVE CONSIDERATIONS

Patients are typically extubated in the operating room. The greatest concern in the postoperative period is from an unidentified air leak leading to tension pneumothorax. In instances where there is a concern for air leak, a chest tube will be placed, and postoperative serial chest radiographs are obtained. Pain scores are generally less than for open thoracotomies but are not insignificant. Local (i.e., intrapleural infiltration), regional, and systemic modalities may all be used to treat postoperative pain. In general, patients with underlying pulmonary disease have a decreased risk of postoperative respiratory complications with VATS compared with open thoracotomies.[2]

## REFERENCES

1. Cohen E. Anesthesia for video-assisted thoracoscopic surgery. In: Slinger P, ed. *Principles and Practice of Anesthesia for Thoracic Surgery*. New York, NY: Springer; 2011:331–340.
2. Gropper MA, et al. *Miller's Anesthesia*. 2 Vol. Elsevier Health Sciences; October 7, 2019.
3. Jaffe RA, et al., eds. *Anesthesiologist's Manual of Surgical Procedures*. Lippincott Williams & Wilkins; 2014.
4. Slinger PD, Johnston MR. Preoperative assessment: an anesthesiologist's perspective. *Thorac Surg Clin*. 2005;15(1):11–25.
5. Yao FS, et al., eds. *Yao & Artusio's Anesthesiology: Problem-Oriented Patient Management*. Lippincott Williams & Wilkins; 2008.

# 103.

# POSTOPERATIVE PAIN

*Nasir Hussain and Tristan E. Weaver*

## INTRODUCTION

The International Association for the Study of Pain defines chronic postsurgical or posttraumatic pain as pain that develops or increases in intensity after a surgical procedure or a tissue injury and persists beyond the healing process (i.e., at least 3 months after the surgery or tissue trauma).[1] Prompt treatment of acute postoperative pain is essential as findings have shown that this reduces the acute neuroplastic responses, such central sensitization and windup, that can present after tissue injury.[2] Chronic postsurgical pain (CPSP) can have detrimental effects on a patient's quality of life and may lead to sleep and mood disturbances. CPSP is more than anecdotal in frequency, with 2%–10% of all surgical patients experiencing significant pain symptoms well into a chronic phase.[3] Multimodal analgesia is considered to be the most optimal approach.

Multimodal analgesia deploys pharmacological interventions with synergistic and additive properties that affect different receptors and sites throughout the peripheral and central nervous systems. The ultimate goal of using a multimodal approach is to provide optimal pain control while decreasing side effects and limiting the use of opioids after a surgical procedure.[3] Furthermore, adequate postoperative analgesia, whether through a parenteral or neuraxial route of administration, can also have significant impact on reducing postoperative complications and ventilatory dysfunction. We highlight both pharmacological and adjunctive treatments that may be used in a multimodal, postoperative analgesia regimen and special considerations for their use (Table 103.1, Table 103.2). Each is discussed in detail through other chapters in this review book.

## ADJUNCTIVE TECHNIQUES

### TRANSCUTANEOUS ELECTRICAL NERVE STIMULATION

Transcutaneous electrical nerve stimulation (TENS) stimulation is an easily applied and relatively cheap adjunct in the treatment of chronic pain. One proposed mechanism by which

TENS reduces postoperative pain by is by electrical fields though direct modulation of the gating mechanisms at the dorsal horn system to decrease pain transmission to the brain and spinal cord.[4] It has been found to reduce mild-to-moderate postsurgical pain without any significant risk to the patient.[3]

### CRYOTHERAPY

Cold is often used to decrease inflammation, edema, and pain during the first 48 hours after an acute injury, such as a surgical event. Other indications for cryotherapy include edema, muscle spasm, and hemorrhage. Use of cryotherapy leads to vasoconstriction, followed by vasodilation and decreased metabolic and enzymatic activity. This leads to decreased oxygen demand in local tissues. Treatment is usually applied by means of ice packs at -12°C with layered towels in order to protect the skin. Application times over superficial nerves should not exceed 30 minutes to prevent neuropraxia.[4]

### ACUPUNCTURE

Acupuncture is an essential component of traditional Chinese medicine and consists of mechanical stimulation via needle insertion and thermal input by either moxa (a chinse herb) or a heat lamp applied over the needles (moxibustion). It is thought to modulate pain by activating a mixture of bioactive chemicals, including opioids, serotonin, and norepinephrine, through peripheral, spinal, and supraspinal mechanisms. At this time, clinical data are not definitive but is certainly promising in its use for acute postoperative pain control.[4]

### HYPNOSIS

A growing body of evidence exists for the use of hypnosis as a first-line or adjunctive measure in the treatment of postoperative pain. Several proposed mechanisms of actions exist, with psychological dissociation a common theme among mechanistic proposals. Little to no contraindications exist for its use, and the treatment is relatively cost-effective. It also may help decrease the incidence of side effects that are associated with the more common medicinal approaches to pain relief.[5]

*Table 103.1* ANALGESIC MEDICATION CLASSES WITH HIGH-YIELD COMMENTS

| MEDICATION CLASS TO REDUCE POSTOPERATIVE PAIN | HIGH-YIELD COMMENTS |
| --- | --- |
| Opioids | • Can be given through IM, IV, oral or transdermal routes<br>• Common side effects include respiratory depression, nausea and vomiting, impaired gastrointestinal motility, urinary retention, pruritus, delirium and cognitive dysfunction<br>• No analgesic ceiling |
| Local anesthetics (i.e., intravenous lidocaine infusion) | • Opioid sparing<br>• Reduced pain scores, nausea, vomiting and duration of ileus up to 72h after abdominal surgery<br>• May be useful agent to treat acute neuropathic pain<br>• Reduced length of stay for open procedures |
| $\alpha_2$-Agonist | • Improves perioperative opioid analgesia and leads to decreased opioid requirements and opioid side effects<br>• Common side effects include sedation, hypotension, bradycardia |
| Nonsteroidal anti-inflammatory drugs (NSAIDs) | • Reduces opioid consumption and incidence of nausea, vomiting, and sedation<br>• Incidence of perioperative renal impairment is low<br>• Risk of gastropathy increased when ketorolac use exceeds five days and patients should be well hydrated and without significant kidney disease<br>• Leads to platelet dysfunction<br>• Ketorolac and ibuprofen are available through IV route of administration |
| *N*-Methyl-D-aspartate (NMDA) receptor blockers (i.e., ketamine) | • Effective adjuvant for pain associated with central sensitization (i.e. severe acute pain, neuropathic pain, opioid-resistant pain)<br>• May reduce CPSP and opioid-induced tolerance/hyperalgesia<br>• Opioid sparing and reduces incidence of nausea and vomiting<br>• Safe and effective analgesic for painful procedures in pediatrics<br>• Uncertain optimal dosing regimen |
| Mixed agonist-antagonists | • Poor choice for patients with severe pain<br>• Analgesic ceiling<br>• If combined with a pure opioid agonist, may precipitate acute pain and opioid withdrawal |
| Antidepressants: tricyclic antidepressants (TCAs) and selective serotonin and norepinephrine reuptake inhibitors (SSRIs and SNRIs) | • Useful for acute neuropathic pain<br>• Side effects: excessive sedation and cardiac arrhythmias (TCAs) and changes in appetite, insomnia, and sexual dysfunction (SNRIs) |

IM, intramuscular; IV, intravenous; SNRI, serotonin norepinephrine reuptake inhibitor; SSRI, selective serotonin reuptake inhibitor; TCA, tricyclic antidepressants.

From References 3 and 4.

*Table 103.2* ANALGESIC MEDICATION CLASSES WITH HIGH-YIELD COMMENTS

| ROUTE OF ADMINISTRATION | HIGH-YIELD COMMENTS |
| --- | --- |
| Oral | • Simple, inexpensive<br>• May not be suitable in many surgical considerations<br>• Subject to first-pass effect<br>• Slow onset of action relative to intravenous route |
| Subcutaneous (SC) | • Avoid first-pass effect<br>• Faster onset of analgesia compared with most oral preparations, though slower than intravenous administration<br>• Uncomplicated access in patients with poor venous access |
| Transcutaneous | • Improved patient compliance<br>• Avoidance of first-pass metabolism<br>• Control of absorption<br>• May cause local allergic cutaneous reactions |

*Table 103.2* CONTINUED

| ROUTE OF ADMINISTRATION | HIGH-YIELD COMMENTS |
|---|---|
| Intramuscular (IM) | • Intramuscular ketamine often used in difficult patient populations (pediatric or those with behavioral issues) as a sedative |
| Intravenous (IV) | • Avoid first-pass effect<br>• Patient-controlled analgesia (PCA):<br>  ○ Better pain control, satisfaction, and fewer opioid side effects when compared to on-demand opioids<br>  ○ Children less than 4 years old not good candidates for PCA use |
| Neuraxial | • Less pain seen in comparison to systemic opioids and reduced opioid requirements<br>• Reduced cardiac/pulmonary morbidity<br>• Earlier return of gastrointestinal tract function<br>• Side effects/risks<br>  ○ Epidural local anesthetic: hypotension; sensory deficits; motor weakness; urinary retention<br>  ○ Epidural opioids: nausea; vomiting; pruritus; respiratory depression<br>  ○ Technique related: backache; postdural puncture headache; neurologic injury; epidural hematoma; epidural abscess |
| Interpleural | • No difference in opioid consumption or pain scores when compared to epidural analgesia in patients undergoing thoracotomy with fewer side effects and complications<br>• Side effects: hypotension; urinary retention; nausea/vomiting |

From References 3 and 4.

## REFERENCES

1. Schug SA, et al. The IASP classification of chronic pain for ICD-11: chronic postsurgical or posttraumatic pain. *Pain.* 2019;160:45–52.
2. Kehlet H, et al. Persistent postsurgical pain: risk factors and prevention. *Lancet.* 2006;367:1618–1625.
3. Lovich-Sapola J, et al. Postoperative pain control. *Surg Clin North Am.* 2015;95:301–318.
4. Benzon HT, et al. *Essentials of Pain Medicine.* 3rd ed. Philadelphia, PA: Elsevier/Saunders; 2011
5. Jensen MP, et al. Mechanisms of hypnosis: toward the development of a biopsychosocial model. *Int J Clin Exp Hypn.* 2015;63:34–75.

# 104.

# VENTILATOR SUPPORT AND EXTUBATION CRITERIA

*Benjamin B. G. Mori and Abayomi Akintorin*

## ANATOMY AND PHYSIOLOGY

During physiologic negative pressure ventilation (NPV), the work of breathing (WOB) refers to contraction of the diaphragm and accessory respiratory muscles, leading to an increased intrathoracic volume and mounting of negative intrapleural pressure from -5 cm $H_2O$, at the end of expiration, to -10 cm$H_2O$, at the end of inspiration. This negative pressure is transmitted to the alveolar space, where air flows from the pharynx (at atmospheric pressure) driven by the transpulmonary pressure gradient. As inspiratory volume increases, alveolar pressure approaches zero, and inspiration ends. Exhalation is a passive process occurring with respiratory muscle relaxation, intrathoracic volume decrease, and air forced out of the alveoli. When pressure in the alveoli equals atmospheric pressure, expiration ends.

Compliance refers to the ability of the lung and chest wall tissue to stretch with inspiration; it is reduced in restrictive disease. Static compliance is measured at a fixed lung volume and allows for compliance monitoring in ventilated patients. Resistance to airflow is the result of conductive airway anatomy and tissue viscous resistance within. It is increased with restrictive disease, but often remains constant during mechanical ventilation (MV). The ability of air to flow through the airways depends on the gas density, viscosity, flow rate, and length and diameter of the anatomic/artificial airways. Typically, airway length, gas density, and viscosity remain constant, where resistance is increased with a reduction in airway diameter (e.g., bronchospasm, kinked endotracheal tube [ETT]) and increasing flow rates. As resistance increases, pressure is disproportionally transmitted to the conductive airways compared to the alveoli, resulting in less fractional gas exchange. Moreover, higher pressures are required to deliver gas through narrowed airways, leading to an increased WOB with spontaneous breathing and an elevated risk of barotrauma with MV.

During positive pressure ventilation (PPV), air is driven into the airways via an artificial conduit (e.g., ETT). During inspiration, inflating pressure at the upper airway equals the sum of pressures required to overcome pulmonary compliance and airway resistance. The pressure in the alveoli progressively becomes more positive, which is transmitted across the visceral pleura, resulting in increased intrapleural pressure at the end of inspiration, and the ventilator stops inflation. The upper airway pressure then returns to ambient pressure while the alveolar pressure remains positive, resulting in passive exhalation.[1] Table 104.1 summarizes the important pressures involved in PPV.

## MODES AND TECHNIQUES OF MECHANICAL VENTILATION

There are three control variables: volume, pressure, and flow. One control variable is set (independent), and the two others will be dependent. If the volume is set (i.e., volume controlled), pressure varies inversely with airway compliance. If pressure is set (i.e., pressure controlled), the volume delivered is proportional to compliance.

The phase variable trigger determines what prompts the ventilator to initiate a breath. There are four main triggers: (1) time or mandatory respiratory rate (RR); (2) flow, where a breath is initiated when an inhalational effort results in a set threshold flow rate; (3) pressure, where a threshold negative inspiratory pressure is reached; and (4) volume trigger breathing when a breath is initiated when the patient inhales a set volume.

*Table 104.1* SUMMARY OF THE IMPORTANT PRESSURES MONITORED DURING PPV

| PRESSURES IN PPV | DEFINITIONS AND IMPORTANT NOTES |
| --- | --- |
| Baseline pressure | Normally zero (i.e., atmospheric), indicating no pressure is applied into the airway during expiration and before inspiration. The baseline pressure is higher than zero if positive end-expiratory pressure (PEEP) is applied. Pressures are compared to a baseline pressure. |
| Positive end-expiratory pressure (PEEP) | PEEP prevents the patient exhaling to zero pressure and increases the volume of gas in the lungs at the end of expiration (↑ functional residual capacity). *Extrinsic PEEP*: PEEP applied by the ventilator, which prevents alveolar derecruitment (i.e., collapse). The PEEP to prevent derecruitment is less than the PEEP needed to recruit (i.e., open) alveoli. *Intrinsic PEEP (Auto-PEEP)*: A complication of PPV resulting in air trapping in the lungs. This occurs when the patient does not have enough time to exhale before the ventilator delivers another breath. |
| Peak inspiratory pressure (PIP) | The highest pressure recorded at the end of inspiration. The pressure rises progressively to a peak pressure during PPV. The pressures measured during inspiration are the sum of the pressures required to force gas through the resistance of the airways and the pressure of the gas volume as it fills the alveoli. |
| Plateau pressure | Measured after a breath has been delivered and before exhalation. This is achieved with an end-inspiratory pause (0.5–1.5 seconds), where exhalation is prevented. The plateau pressure reflects the elastic recoil on the volume inside the alveoli and breathing circuit (i.e., compliance/elastance). |
| End exhalation pressure | At the end of exhalation, airway pressure should return to baseline if the patient has enough time to exhale. End exhalation pressure will be greater than baseline pressure with intrinsic PEEP. |

From Reference 1.

A phase variable cycle is what triggers the ventilator to switch between inhalation and exhalation phases. Breathing effort is stopped and exhalation begins when a set volume, pressure, and flow rate have been achieved or the elapsed time has passed, depending on which variable has been selected. A phase variable limit is what stops a breath—the set limit value cannot be exceeded during inspiration. There can be limits to volume, pressure, flow, and minute ventilation.[1]

There are four conventionally used MV modes, which are summarized in Table 104.2. Advancements in ventilator technology have allowed for numerous specialized modes of MV, but these are less commonly used.

| MODES OF MECHANICAL VENTILATION | DESCRIPTION |
|---|---|
| Pressure support ventilation (PSV) | PSV is a form of augmented spontaneous breathing. The patient determines their RR (flow triggered) and inspiratory/expiratory flow rates. $V_T$ is dependent on the combined efforts of the patient and the inspiratory pressure prescribed to each breath. Time cycling can be used as a backup mode (i.e., intermittent mandatory ventilation).<br>*Advantages*: Most comfortable mode, ↓ WOB, excellent mode for weaning.<br>*Disadvantages*: Risk of hypoventilation with ↓ patient effort and ↓ compliance conditions, poorly tolerated in chronic obstructive pulmonary disease. |
| Assist-controlled ventilation (ACV) | A lower limit RR and $V_T$ are set. The patient can trigger a breath (variable trigger). The set $V_T$ is delivered at a constant flow rate regardless if it is a Ventilator (time-triggered) or a patient-initiated breath.<br>*Advantages*: ↓ WOB, provides adequate VE.<br>*Disadvantages*: ↑ Risk of barotrauma, auto-PEEP, discomfort due to constant flow through inhalational cycle, prolonged use can result in respiratory muscle deconditioning, ↑ risk of respiratory alkalosis with overbreathing (i.e., patient-initiated RR > prescribed RR). |
| Synchronized intermittent ventilation (SIMV) | A lower limit RR and $V_T$ are set; similar to ACV (time triggered). In contrast to ACV, the patient-initiated breaths (variable trigger) are pressure supported, rather than simply acting as a trigger to deliver a predetermined $V_T$. As such, TV can vary with spontaneous breathing depending on patient effort. The ventilator attempts to synchronize the delivery of mandatory breaths with the spontaneous efforts of the patient. In contrast to ACV, SIMV can deliver spontaneous volumes that are 100% driven by patient effort.<br>*Advantages*: ↑ Patient comfort, provides adequate VE, ↓ risk of respiratory alkalosis and respiratory muscle deconditioning.<br>*Disadvantages*: ↑ WOB if inadequate pressure support is applied to spontaneous breaths. |
| Pressure-controlled ventilation (PCV) | RR and inspiratory pressure are set. Does not allow for patient-initiated breaths (time triggered). $V_T$ will vary with each breath, with higher $V_T$ achieved with increased prescribed pressure.<br>*Advantages*: ↓ Risk of barotrauma in low-compliance conditions, ↑ oxygenation due to ↑ lung distension during inspiration.<br>*Disadvantages*: ↓ Control of $V_T$ and VE. |

Respiratory rate (RR), tidal volume ($V_T$), minute ventilation (VE), work of breathing (WOB).

From Reference 1.

Ventilation ($PaCO_2$) and oxygenation ($PaO_2$) can be altered and improved with changes in ventilator settings as shown in Table 104.3.

On initiation of MV, select the ventilation mode, $FiO_2$, and controlled variables, which are mode dependent. As a rough starting point in healthy adults, the following variables can be set: TV 6–8 mL/Kg; RR 10–12 breaths/min; flow rate 40–100 L/min; inspiratory/expiratory ratio 1:2; fraction of inspired oxygen ($FiO_2$) 100%; and positive end-expiratory pressure (PEEP) may be applied.[1,2] Variables should be titrated to patient physiology.[2] An example MV protocol is shown in Table 104.4.

## COMPLICATIONS OF MECHANICAL VENTILATION

There are complications associated with MV. High $V_T$ can lead to alveolar shear stress (i.e., volutrauma). Conversely, low $V_T$ is associated with atelectasis (i.e., atelectrauma).[3] Hyperoxia is associated with lung injury and increased mortality.[1,3] The $FiO_2$ should be titrated to the lowest possible level to maintain an $SpO_2$ (oxygen saturation as measured by pulse oximetry) greater than 90%.[1] MV can induce diaphragm dysfunction and can be prevented with modes that encourage patient effort. Barotrauma can occur with elevated pressures (plateau pressure > 35 mm Hg). Aspiration injury can be prevented with oral hygiene, head

*Table 104.3* EFFECT OF VENTILATOR SETTINGS ON
$PACO_2$ AND $PAO_2$

| VENTILATOR VARIABLE | EFFECT ON $PACO_2$ | EFFECT ON $PAO_2$ |
|---|---|---|
| ↑ Inspiration/expiration ratio | — | ↑ |
| ↑ $FiO_2$ | — | ↑ |
| ↑ PEEP | ↑ | ↑ |
| ↑ PIP | ↓ | ↑ |
| ↑ RR | ↓ | ↑ |
| ↑ $V_T$ | ↓ | ↑ |

From Reference 1.

*Table 104.4* EXAMPLE OF AN EVIDENCE-BASED PROTOCOL FOR INITIATING MECHANICAL VENTILATION IN AN ADULT

| | |
|---|---|
| Set TV | • $V_T$ 6–8 mL/kg predicted body weight |
| Airway pressures (volutrauma) | • Limit plateau pressure < 30 cm $H_2O$ (check every 4 hours)<br>• Higher pressures are acceptable with stiff chest walls<br>• Plateau pressure > 30 cm $H_2O \rightarrow \downarrow V_T$ in 1-mL/kg increments<br>• Plateau pressure < 25 cm $H_2O$ and $V_T$ M 6 mL/kg $\rightarrow \uparrow V_T$ in 1-mL/kg increments until > 25 cm $H_2O$ of $V_T$ = 6 mL/kg<br>• Plateau pressure < 30 cm $H_2O$ and auto-PEEP/dyssynchrony $\rightarrow \uparrow$ VT in 1-mL/kg increments to 7–8 mL/kg or plateau pressure > 30 cm $H_2O$ |
| PEEP (atelectrauma) | • Set PEEP ≥ 5 cm $H_2O$<br>• ↑ PEEP in obesity (8 cm $H_2O$ for body mass index (BMI) 30–40 kg/m², 10 cm $H_2O$ for BMI > 40 kg/m²) |
| Oxygenation | • Initiate $FiO_2$ at 100% (i.e., 1.0) and immediately $\downarrow FiO_2$ to 30%–40% after intubation<br>• Titrate $FiO_2$ to an $SpO_2$ of 90%–95% or $PaO_2$ of 55–60 mm Hg<br>• $FiO_2$-PEEP combination can be used to optimize both oxygenation and airway pressures |
| Ventilation | • Set RR at 10–12 breaths/min and set I:E ratio at 1:1<br>• Monitor end-expiratory pressure and $\downarrow$ RR with auto-PEEP |
| pH goal | • pH > 7.45 $\rightarrow \downarrow$ RR<br>• pH < 7.30 $\rightarrow \uparrow$ RR to 35 breaths/min maximum and until pH > 7.30 or $PaCO_2$ < 25 mm Hg<br>• pH < 7.15 $\rightarrow \uparrow$ RR to 37 breaths/min maximum and $\uparrow$ TV 1 mL/kg until pH > 7.15 |
| Aspiration prevention | • Elevate head of bed ≥ 30°<br>• Place nasogastric/orogastric tube to decompress stomach |

From Reference 1.

elevation, and intubation. PPV, especially with high $V_T$ and PEEP, can reduce preload and worsen hemodynamics in some circumstances (e.g., hypovolemic shock). In these cases, spontaneous breathing (i.e., NPV) may be more appropriate.[1] The risk of ventilator-associated pneumonia increases with prolonged MV (>72 hours) and carries a high rate of morbidity/mortality.[1,3]

## LIBERATION (WEANING) FROM MECHANICAL VENTILATION

A patient should be continually assessed for their ability to be weaned from MV, and the degree of respiratory support should be titrated to progress toward ventilator liberation, which should be done as early as possible.[1,4] Patients can be considered for weaning when three criteria are met. First, resolution of the cause of intubation/MV must have occurred.[4] Second, the patient must be in stable condition (i.e., systolic blood pressure > 90 mm Hg without significant vasopressor/ionotropic support). There should be minimal ventilator support (i.e., $FiO_2$ < 40%, pressure support and PEEP ≤ 5 mm Hg, and normal WOB).[1,4] the patient should be afebrile and have a normal acid-base status, phosphorus, and potassium level.[1] The patient should be conscious and have intact airway reflexes on minimal sedation. Last, normal lung mechanics are required with spontaneous breathing (i.e., vital capacity [VC] ≥ 10 mL/min,

rapid shallow breathing index < 105, negative inspiratory force ≤ 30 mm Hg, measured WOB < 0.8 J/L).[1,4] Also to be considered is the absence (or reduction) of excessive airway secretions.

After the above criteria are met, a spontaneous breathing trial (SBT) can be performed using a T-piece trial, PSV 5 cm $H_2O$ or less, with PEEP 5 or less, or automatic tube compensation ventilator mode. The patient can be extubated 30 minutes after SBT initiation if the following criteria are met: no signs of respiratory distress, no tachycardia, $PaO_2$ greater than 60 mm Hg ($SpO_2$ > 90%), pH 7.30 or greater, and TV greater than 4 mL/kg.[1,4] High-risk airways can be extubated over exchange catheter, and high-risk patients can be extubated to noninvasive ventilation or high-flow nasal cannula to reduce the risk of reintubation.[1]

## REFERENCES

1. Abou Leila AM, et al. Ventilator management. In: Reichman EF, ed. *Reichman's Emergency Medicine Procedures*. 3rd ed. New York, NY: McGraw-Hill Education; 2019:288–299.
2. Guo L, et al. Mechanical ventilation strategies for intensive care unit patients without acute lung injury or acute respiratory distress syndrome: a systematic review and network meta-analysis. *Crit Care.* 2016;20(1):226.
3. Pierson DJ. Complications associated with mechanical ventilation. *Crit Care Clin.* 1990;6(3):711–724.
4. Epstein SK. Weaning from mechanical ventilation. *Respir Care.* 2002;47(4):454–466; discussion 466–468.

# 105.

# MANAGEMENT OF RESPIRATORY FAILURE

*Phil Boysen and Patrick Newman*

## INTRODUCTION

Respiratory failure is the loss of the body's ability to maintain appropriate oxygen delivery to the blood and removal of carbon dioxide from the blood.[1] Respiratory failure can be classified as hypoxemic, defined as $PaO_2$ less than 60 mm Hg; hypercarbic, defined as $PaCO_2$ greater than 45 mm Hg; or mixed. The timeline is also used to describe it: acute, chronic, and acute on chronic. Significant morbidity and mortality occur due to respiratory failure, which is a common reason for hospital and intensive care unit (ICU) admission.

## NONVENTILATORY SUPPORT

Nonventilatory oxygen support is useful for patients with mild-to-moderate hypoxic respiratory failure. This can be accomplished with something as simple as a nasal cannula (NC) or may require more support, which can be delivered by a nonrebreather mask or high-flow nasal cannula (HFNC). The HFNC allows titration of flow and fraction of inspired oxygen ($FiO_2$). Flow rates can be titrated up to 60 L/min on some machines.[1] At these flow rates, the HFNC offers some positive end-expiratory pressure (PEEP) to the patient.

## NONINVASIVE MECHANICAL VENTILATION

While the NC or HFNC may be sufficient for some, patients who require ventilatory support for hypercarbia or have more severe hypoxic respiratory failure will require mechanical ventilation. Noninvasive ventilation with continuous positive airway pressure or bilevel positive airway pressure (BiPAP) will provide appropriate support for many patients. These modes are beneficial for patients with chronic obstructive pulmonary disease or congestive heart failure (CHF) exacerbations.[1] BiPAP allows for titration of inspiratory and expiratory pressures, respiratory rate,

and $FiO_2$. BiPAP has not been shown to be beneficial for patients with acute respiratory distress syndrome (ARDS).

## INVASIVE MECHANICAL VENTILATION

If the above therapies fail or the patient presents with severe hypoxic or hypercarbic respiratory failure, invasive mechanical ventilation will be necessary. Careful selection and management of the ventilator settings are required to provide the support the patient needs without causing damage to the patient's lungs. While it has long been established that lung-protective settings are vital in patients with ARDS, more evidence is showing that these settings are beneficial to the vast majority of patients in the ICU and operating room (OR). Lung-protective settings include a tidal volume of 6–8 mL/kg predicted body weight, higher levels of PEEP, and keeping plateau pressure less than 30 cm $H_2O$.[1–3] While there are many ways to select the ideal PEEP for each patient, one common way is use of a pressure-volume loop and the lower inflection point. The pressure at this point is selected as the PEEP. Figure 105.1 shows a pressure-volume loop with the lower inflection point identified.

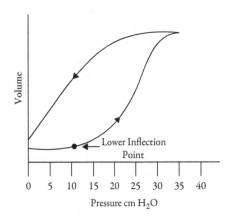

Figure 105.1 Pressure-volume loop.

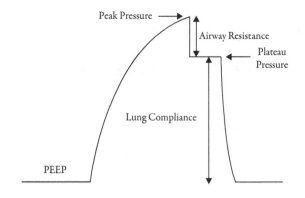

**Figure 105.2** Peak versus plateau pressure.

Limiting plateau pressure to less than 30 cm $H_2O$ helps prevent barotrauma. Figure 105.2 shows a pressure curve with peak and plateau pressures identified. This curve is helpful to select lung-protective ventilator settings and troubleshoot compliance issues as increased peak and plateau pressures have different causes. Peak pressure elevations with normal plateau pressures are indicative of increased airway resistance as would be seen in endotracheal tube kinking, bronchospasm, or mucous plugging. Increases in plateau pressures are indicative of decreases in lung compliance, as would be seen in ARDS, pulmonary edema, or atelectasis.

## MEDICATIONS AND THERAPIES

In patients with severe hypoxic respiratory failure, mechanical ventilation alone may not be enough, especially if their p/f ratios ($PaO_2/FiO_2$) are less than 150 mm Hg.[1] In these patients, proning, paralytics, and inhaled vasodilators may be beneficial. Paralytics increase oxygenation in patients who have ventilator dyssynchrony. Improving ventilator synchrony allows for more precise volume delivery at lower pressures and better PEEP control. Inhaled vasodilators such as nitric oxide or epoprostenol increase oxygenation by improving ventilation-perfusion (V/Q) matching. As these medications are inhaled, they are delivered to lung segments that are actively participating in ventilation. The vasodilators will then diffuse across to the blood vessels that are perfusing these lung segments, selectively dilating the blood vessels that are perfusing well-ventilated lung segments without producing systemic vasodilation.[1,4] Proning improves oxygenation by optimizing V/Q matching throughout the lung and improving compliance by removing the chest wall mechanics.

Bronchoscopy can be beneficial in the OR and ICU as it is both diagnostic and therapeutic. Bronchoscopy allows for airway inspection, collection of cultures, and clearing of secretions or mucous plugs in the airway that could limit oxygenation or ventilation.

## ANESTHETIC CONSIDERATIONS

### PREOPERATIVE

One very important preoperative consideration for a patient in respiratory failure scheduled for surgery is the reproducibility of the ventilator settings in the OR. The majority of ICU ventilators have advanced modes and settings that cannot be reproduced on anesthesia machines. If patients are on one of the advanced modes or are requiring high ventilator settings, the anesthesia, surgery, and ICU teams need to make a decision on the necessity of surgery and plan for the respiratory management in the perioperative period.

Disconnecting the ventilator from the endotracheal tube can happen multiple times during a transport from the ICU to the OR. While this act may be harmless in some patients, it derecruits the lungs, which can be extremely detrimental to patients who are PEEP dependent. One technique to limit the derecruitment is to clamp the endotracheal tube prior to disconnection in an effort to maintain the airway pressure.

### INTRAOPERATIVE

Hypoxic pulmonary vasoconstriction (HPV) is the body's attempt to improve oxygenation by limiting perfusion to poorly ventilated lung segments. Intraoperatively, volatile anesthetics can inhibit HPV, worsening a patient's oxygenation. Intravenous anesthetics have no effect on HPV.[3] Inhibition of HPV should be considered for any patient in respiratory failure with acute worsening hypoxia in the OR.

### POSTOPERATIVE

While fluid management is important postoperatively for all patients, critically ill patients in respiratory failure are at high risk of worsening respiratory failure with inappropriate fluid use. Fluids should only be administered to patients who are fluid responsive with the goal of improving organ perfusion. Excess fluids can lead to pulmonary edema, which can worsen oxygenation and pulmonary compliance.[2]

## REFERENCES

1. Vincent JL, et al. *Textbook of Critical Care*. 7th ed. Elsevier; 2017:30–37.
2. Marino P. *The ICU Book*. 3rd ed. Lippincott, Williams & Wilkins; 2007:426–431.
3. Barash PG. *Clinical Anesthesia*. 7th ed. Wolters Kluwer; 2013:469, 1595–1596.
4. Miller R, et al. *Basics of Anesthesia*. 4th ed. Churchill Livingstone/Elsevier; 2000:440–441.

# 106.

# MODE OF VENTILATION

*Katarina Kapisoda and Ettore Crimi*

## INTRODUCTION

The principle of mechanical ventilation is regulated by the equation of motion[1]:

Pvent + Pmus = Volume/Compliance + (Inspiratory Flow × Resistance)

The amount of pressure that can be generated by the ventilator (Pvent) and by the respiratory muscles (Pmus) to deliver a volume of gas into the lung depends on the elastic properties of the respiratory system (determined by compliance and tidal volume) and resistive properties of the respiratory system (determined by airways resistance and inspiratory flow). In apneic patients, all of the pressure is generated by the ventilator. The four variables controlled by the ventilator to deliver a breath are pressure, volume, flow, and time. Ventilators can control one variable at a time. When breath delivery is pressure controlled, airway pressure will be constant regardless of changes in compliance and resistance and determine flow and volume. When breath delivery is volume controlled, flow and volume delivery will not change and determine airway pressure.

The so-called phase variables (trigger, limit, and cycle) regulate the beginning, duration, and end of an inspiration. The trigger variable, responsible for initiation of inspiration (either time or patient initiated) includes pressure, flow, or volume triggering. The limit variable represents the maximum preset pressure, volume, or flow during inspiration. The cycle variable causes the end of inspiration: it is volume or time during volume-controlled ventilation, time during pressure-controlled ventilation (PCV), and flow during pressure support ventilation (PSV). Breath type can be spontaneous when a patient triggers and cycles the breath or mandatory when ventilator triggers and cycles.

## CONTINUOUS MANDATORY VENTILATION

Continuous mandatory ventilation (CMV), also known as assist-control (A/C) ventilation, combines assisted and/or controlled ventilation. Mechanical breaths are either volume or pressure controlled, ventilator or patient triggered, limited by volume and/or flow, and cycled by volume or time. The physician presets a minimum rate and tidal volume or pressure; the patient can trigger additional breaths at the same parameters as the controlled breaths (Figure 106.1). This mode provides full ventilator support, reduces the work of breathing by unloading the inspiratory muscles and improves gas exchange.[2]

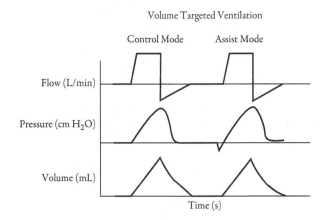

**Figure 106.1** Assist/control mode: flow, pressure, and volume waveforms. Note that in assist mode the negative change of the pressure waveform suggests a spontaneous inspiratory effort.

## SYNCHRONIZED INTERMITTENT MANDATORY VENTILATION

Synchronized intermittent mandatory ventilation (SIMV) guarantees a set number of controlled breaths that are synchronized with the patient's inspiratory effort. Mandatory breaths are volume, pressure, or adaptive pressure controlled. In between the mandatory breaths, the patient can breathe spontaneously, and each breath is supported with pressure support. Synchronization of spontaneous and controlled breaths may reduce patient-ventilator dyssynchrony.[2]

## PRESSURE CONTROLLED VENTILATION AND INVERSE RATIO VENTILATION

Pressure-controlled ventilation is a pressure-controlled, time-cycled mode that requires three parameters to be set: inspiratory pressure, mandatory frequency, and inspiratory time. The inspiratory flow is determined by airway resistance and respiratory compliance. PCV maintains airway pressure constant while tidal volumes change depending on the compliance and resistance of the respiratory system (Figure 106.2). Compared to volume-controlled ventilation, PCV delivers volume early, improving gas distribution and usually resulting in lower peak pressure and higher mean pressure. Pressure-controlled inverse ratio ventilation is an alternative modality of PCV where the inspiratory time is longer than the expiratory time. The longer inspiratory time increases mean airway pressure, prolongs lung recruitment, and improves oxygenation. The shorter expiratory time can promote air trapping and auto-PEEP (positive end-expiratory pressure), which can lead to barotrauma and hemodynamic instability.[2,3]

## PRESSURE SUPPORT VENTILATION

Pressure support ventilation is an assisted spontaneous breathing mode that supports all of the patient's respiratory efforts. It is patient triggered and flow cycled. The clinician sets a level of inspiratory pressure to assist patient-triggered breaths. The patient controls the rate, tidal volume, inspiratory flow, and time. The inspiratory phase ends when the flow rate is less than a set minimum (usually 5 L/min) or decreases to less than 25% of the patient's peak flow. It augments a patient's spontaneous tidal volume and decreases the respiratory rate and work of breathing. PSV requires an intact respiratory drive and does not guarantee a constant tidal volume that changes depending on the set pressure, patient's effort, and respiratory mechanics.[2]

## AIRWAY PRESSURE RELEASE VENTILATION

Airway pressure release ventilation (APRV) is an advanced ventilator mode that provides two-level continuous positive airway pressure (CPAP; P high and P low) and allows spontaneous breathing during either the low or high pressure level. The clinician sets level of P high (25–30 cm $H_2O$) and P low (0–5 cm $H_2O$) and the duration of P high (Time high: 4–6 seconds) and P low (Time low: 0.6–1.5 seconds). Tidal volume is determined by the difference between P high and P low. Switching from P high to P low allows exhalation and ventilation. Pressure support can be added to the spontaneous breaths. Careful monitoring of the minute ventilation ensures adequacy of ventilation and prevention of hypercapnia. APRV limits peak airway pressures, increases mean airway pressure, and improves alveolar recruitment, and oxygenation through optimization of ventilation/perfusion match. It is used in patients with refractory hypoxemia secondary to acute lung injury and acute respiratory distress syndrome.[4]

## HIGH-FREQUENCY VENTILATION

High-frequency ventilation (HFV) defines a group of modes of mechanical ventilation that utilize high respiratory rates (above 150 breaths/min) or frequencies (cycles/s). HFV delivers small tidal with higher mean airway pressures. The primary mechanisms of gas exchange are molecular diffusion and convection. HFV includes the following modalities: high-frequency jet ventilation (HFJV), high-frequency oscillatory ventilation (HFOV), and high-frequency percussive ventilation (HFPV). HFJV delivers gas at rates of 150 cycles/s while allowing passive expiration. It can be used during tracheal/bronchial and cardiac ablation procedures and to provide percutaneous transtracheal ventilation when an airway cannot be established (Table 106.1). HFOV uses small pressure oscillations at rates of 180–900 cycles/s where both inspiration and expiration are actively caused by the oscillator. Peak pressures and tidal

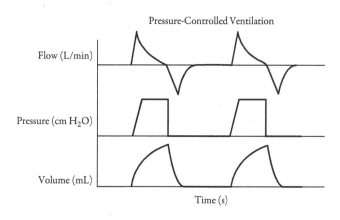

Figure 106.2 Pressure mode: flow, pressure, and volume waveforms.

**Table 106.1 HIGH-FLOW JET VENTILATION VERSUS HIGH-FLOW OSCILLATORY VENTILATION**

|  | HFJV | HFOV |
| --- | --- | --- |
| Frequency (cycles per minute) | 12–150 | 180–900 |
| Allows ETCO$_2$ sampling | No | No |
| Allows passive exhalation | Yes | No |
| Set driving pressure | Yes | No |
| Continuous lung distending pressure | No | Yes |

volume cannot be monitored. Both HFJV and HFOV require paralysis or heavy sedation and active humidification. They do not allow sampling end-tidal CO$_2$ (ETCO$_2$); thus, frequent arterial blood gas tests are required to measure arterial CO$_2$ (PaCO$_2$) to monitor adequacy of CO$_2$ exchange.

HFPV uses rates of 200–900 (cycles/s) and has been used in burn centers in patients with inhalational injuries due to its ability to aid in clearance of respiratory secretions.[5]

## REFERENCES

1. Hess DR. Respiratory mechanics in mechanically ventilated patients. *Respir Care.* 2014;59:1773–1794.
2. Hess DR, Kacmarek RM. Traditional modes of mechanical ventilation. In: Hess, Kacmarek, ed. *Essentials of Mechanical Ventilation.* 4th ed. New York, NY: McGraw-Hill; 2019:50–60.
3. Amato MP, Marini JJ. Pressure-controlled and inverse-ratio ventilation. In: Tobin MJ, ed. *Principles and Practice of Mechanical Ventilation.* 3rd ed. New York, NY: McGraw-Hill; 2013:227–251.
4. Lim J, Litton E. Airway pressure release ventilation in adult patients with acute hypoxemic respiratory failure: a systematic review and meta-analysis. *Crit Care Med.* 2019;47:1794–1799.
5. Hess DR, Kacmarek RM. High-frequency ventilation. In: Hess, Kacmarek, ed. *Essentials of Mechanical Ventilation.* 4th ed. New York, NY: McGraw-Hill; 2019:100–107.

# 107.

# BIPAP, AIRWAY PRESSURE RELEASE VENTILATION, AND PRONE VENTILATION

*Neisaliz Marrero-Figueroa and Ettore Crimi*

## INTRODUCTION

The mainstay of the management of patients with acute lung injury/acute respiratory distress syndrome (ALI/ARDS) requiring mechanical ventilation is a lung-protective strategy using lower tidal volumes (4–8 mL/kg predicted body weight) and lower inspiratory pressures (plateau pressure ≤ 30 cm H$_2$O). Biphasic positive airway pressure (BiPAP), airway pressure release ventilation (APRV), and prone ventilation are used as rescue therapies for refractory hypoxemia in patients with ALI/ARDS. Both BiPAP and APRV use a high level of continuous positive pressure while allowing spontaneous breathing to recruit collapsed alveoli, decrease ventilation-perfusion mismatch, and ultimately improve oxygenation. Ventilation in prone position determines a rapid

and sustained improvement in oxygenation secondary to more uniform lung inflation, improved lung recruitment, increase in functional residual capacity, redistribution of regional lung perfusion, variations in diaphragm movement, and better clearance of secretions. Prone position can reduce mortality in patients with ALI/ARDS.[1]

## AIRWAY PRESSURE RELEASE VENTILATION AND BIPHASIC POSITIVE AIRWAY PRESSURE

Biphasic positive airway pressure and APRV are two similar invasive mode of ventilation that provide two levels of continuous positive airway pressure (CPAP) and allow the patient to breathe spontaneously throughout the ventilatory cycle.

Airway pressure release ventilation, also referred to as Bilevel Airway Pressure depending on the manufacturer, is a form of pressure-controlled, time-cycled mode of ventilation that provides two different levels of CPAP (P high and P low) with an inverse I:E ratio and allows spontaneous breathing at both levels of CPAP. In the absence of spontaneous effort, APRV is similar to pressure-controlled inverse ratio ventilation.[2]

The mandatory breaths are machine triggered, pressure targeted, and time cycled. APRV settings include (1) P high, the highest preset level of CPAP (15–30 cm $H_2O$); (2) T high, inspiratory time (4–6 seconds); (3) P low, the lowest preset level of CPAP (0–5 cm $H_2O$); (4) T low, expiratory/release time (0.6–1.5 seconds). The mechanical breath results from the brief and intermittent interruption of P high and its quick restoration (Figure 107.1). Spontaneous breaths can occur throughout and between the mandatory breaths and are assisted by pressure support. Minute ventilation depends on lung compliance, airway resistance, the degree of the pressure gradient, and the patient's spontaneous effort.

Oxygenation depends on the level of P high and the ventilation ($CO_2$ removal) on the frequency and duration (T low) of the airway pressure release. The duration of T low should guarantee complete lung deflation to prevent the development of significant auto-PEEP (positive end-expiratory pressure). APRV recruits collapsed alveoli at lower airway pressure than traditional modes of ventilation, preserves spontaneous breathing, and improves ventilation-perfusion (V/Q) mismatch and oxygenation.

Although commonly the names of BiPAP and APRV are utilized interchangeably, differences exist between these two modes. BiPAP does not uses extreme inverse I:E ratios greater than 1:1, and there are no restrictions with the duration of the T low. Compared to APRV, BiPAP typically uses shorter T high, longer T low, and higher P low.[3]

Spontaneous ventilation and improved alveolar recruitment and oxygenation are allowed by APRV/BiPAP; tidal volume is variable and requires close monitoring. Auto-PEEP is usually present and can be deleterious in hemodynamically unstable patients.

## PRONE VENTILATION

Prone position is used to improve oxygenation in patients with acute respiratory distress syndrome (ARDS) and severe hypoxemia.[4] Mechanisms that can explain its beneficial effects include a reduced pleural pressure gradient with more uniform lung inflation and improved lung recruitment, an increase in functional residual capacity, redistribution of regional lung perfusion, variations in diaphragm movement, and better clearance of secretions.[5] Prone position causes a more uniform distribution of transpulmonary pressure secondary to the change of the gravitational center. In prone position, the heart, the diaphragm, and the abdominal viscera no longer affect the size of the intrathoracic cavity secondary to weight transmission. As a result, the posterior nondependent lung regions with greater alveolar density are recruited more homogeneously and become available for ventilation. Thus, there will be an improvement in V/Q matching and a reduction in the intrapulmonary shunt. Increased lung volume and more homogeneous distribution of ventilation also reduce pulmonary vascular resistance and right heart strain. Altogether, prone ventilation

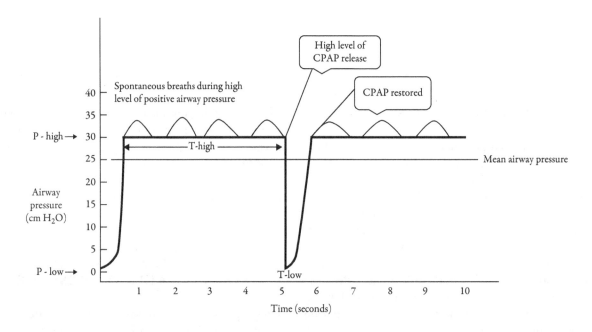

**Figure 107.1** APRV: airway pressure waveform.

contributes to a steady oxygenation improvement over time in over 70% of patients with severe ARDS and a decrease in mortality as well.

The most significant benefits from prone position are obtained when it is instituted earlier in the course of ARDS or within 7 to 10 days after mechanical ventilation was initiated. This time window usually coincides with the early exudative phase of ARDS, characterized by diffuse alveolar damage. Prone position is not effective during the late phase of ARDS with pulmonary fibrosis. Clinical improvement time can vary from 1 hour (rapid responders) up to 6 hours (slow responders).[4] Prone ventilation can be associated with several complications, such as transient hemodynamic instability, transient desaturation, accidental extubation and loss of intravascular lines, pressure ulcerations, facial edema, endotracheal tube obstruction with copious secretions, need for excessive sedation, neuropraxia or permanent loss of nerve function due to prolonged nerve compression, and ischemic optic neuropathy. Experienced personnel, use of a checklist and specialized equipment (rotating bed), and close monitoring can prevent most of these complications.

## REFERENCES

1. Hess D, Kacmarek R. Advanced modes of mechanical ventilation In: Hess, Kamareck ed. *Essentials of Mechanical Ventilation*. 4th ed. McGraw-Hill; 2019:73–86.
2. Putensen C. Airway pressure release ventilation. In: Tobin M, ed. *Principles and Practice of Mechanical Ventilation*. 3rd ed. McGraw-Hill; 2013:305–313.
3. Lim J, Litton E. Airway pressure release ventilation in adult patients with acute hypoxemic respiratory failure: a systematic review and meta-analysis. *Crit Care Med*. 2019;47:1794–1799.
4. Guérin C, et al. Prone positioning in severe acute respiratory distress syndrome. *N Engl J Med*. 2013;368:2159–2168.
5. Kallet RH. A comprehensive review of prone position in ARDS. *Respir Care*. 2015;60:1660–1687.

# 108.

## SLEEP APNEA

*Sohail K. Mahboobi*

## INTRODUCTION

Obstructive sleep apnea (OSA) is the most common type of sleep apnea encountered by anesthesiologists and characterized by upper airway obstruction during sleep that results in hypoxemia, arterial oxygen desaturation, and disturbed sleep. These obstructive episodes usually occur due to anatomic features like narrowing of the upper airway, relaxed muscular tone, or excessive airway soft tissues. OSA usually occurs in obese patients, but certain anatomic conditions, like tonsillar hypertrophy, can result in this condition in nonobese population. Recurrent hypoxia leads to secondary pulmonary hypertension, cardiac rhythm disturbances, and eventually right ventricular failure. Identifying patients at high risk for OSA before surgery may help reduce perioperative patient complications.

## ANESTHETIC CONSIDERATIONS

### PREOPERATIVE

An OSA patient should be assessed preoperatively with a review of available previous medical records, questioning the patient and family for the presence of symptoms and signs of OSA, and physical examination. OSA does occur in both sexes, thin individuals, and all age groups, although majority of patients are middle-aged male. Review of previous records includes a history of airway difficulty, hypertension, and other cardiovascular problems. The patient and family should be asked questions related to snoring, episodes of apnea, frequent arousals during sleep, and daytime somnolence. There are preoperative screening questionnaires available that help in identifying patients at risk of OSA. Some of these are Berlin Questionnaire, the American Society of Anesthesiologists checklist, and the STOP-BANG questionnaire. The STOP-BANG questionnaire is most commonly used.[1] Physical examination of high-risk OSA patients includes an examination of the airway along with neck circumference and mouth opening, tongue, and tonsils. Obese patients with fat distribution predominantly to the upper part of the body are at higher risk of having OSA. Examination should include assessment of signs of systemic or pulmonary hypertension and heart failure as chronic hypoxemia can lead to right heart failure.[2] Additional tests such as an echocardiogram or pulmonary function tests can be ordered if physical examination findings require further evaluation. If after assessment the patient is suspected of having OSA, then detailed planning with the surgical team is required about further investigations (e.g., sleep studies vs. proceeding with the planned surgery). Discussion should also include optimization of the patient's condition; perioperative management, including postoperative monitoring; analgesia; and whether the procedure should be performed in an inpatient or outpatient setting. The patient and the family should be informed of the potential outcomes of the perioperative course.

If there is no urgency in performing the surgical procedure, the patient should be optimized before surgery. Optimization includes regular use of a continuous positive airway pressure (CPAP) or mandibular advancement devices and weight loss. CPAP therapy should start early, particularly in high-risk or symptomatic patients.

## INTRAOPERATIVE

The mainstay of intraoperative care of these patients includes safe anesthetic technique, airway management, and adequate monitoring. These patients are sensitive to the respiratory depressant effects of sedatives, opioids, and inhaled anesthetics, especially if untreated. For this reason, choice of anesthetic agents should be done cautiously. Consider using local anesthesia or nerve blocks with minimal sedation in superficial procedures and neuraxial anesthesia (spinal/epidural) for lower extremity procedures. Capnography should be continuously performed in all cases, including sedation to detect early airway obstruction. General anesthesia is preferable for procedures that require a deep level of anesthesia. A combination of regional and general anesthesia is helpful in reducing the use of opioids and other respiratory depressants. These patients are at increased risk for aspiration at the time of induction, and rapid sequence induction should be considered. Obtaining reliable intravenous access can also be challenging. Due to obesity, the functional residual capacity is reduced, which makes them prone to

develop hypoxia faster than other patients. This fact, particularly in the presence of possible difficult airway, requires careful planning and availability of a surgical airway.[3] In some cases, an awake fiber-optic intubation may be required. At the end of the procedure, muscle relaxants should be completely reversed, and the patient should be completely awake before extubation except in conditions requiring smooth deep extubation (e.g., after intracranial procedures). Extubation and recovery should be carried out in the upright position for better respiratory function.

## POSTOPERATIVE

Postoperatively, these patients require monitoring, with particular attention to analgesia, oxygenation, positioning, and respiration. Patients with severe OSA undergoing a major surgical procedure and receiving opioids are at higher risk of developing postoperative respiratory depression. Additionally, the airway can be narrowed from swelling and inflammation after prolonged perioperative intubation, making the patient more susceptible to airway obstruction.[4]

Multimodal analgesia should be considered for pain management. Continuous basal infusions should not be used with patient-controlled analgesia. Nonsteroidal anti-inflammatory agents and acetaminophen should be considered to reduce opioid requirements. Other simultaneous use of sedatives should be avoided. The patient should be receiving oxygen therapy continuously until baseline oxygen saturation on room air is achieved. CPAP should be used after surgery to help oxygenation if the surgical procedure did not involve the head and neck area.[5] Patients should be advised to bring their own equipment as it improves compliance. Patients should be placed in a semiupright position throughout the recovery process to improve breathing efforts. These patients should be continuously monitored with pulse oximetry during the hospital stay and should not be placed in an unmonitored area. These patients should be assessed before discharge from the hospital and be breathing room air, particularly during sleep.

## REFERENCES

1. Chung F, et al. STOP-Bang questionnaire: a practical approach to screen for obstructive sleep apnea. Chest. 2016;149(3):631–638.
2. Shahar E, et al. Sleep disordered breathing and cardiovascular disease: cross sectional results of the Sleep Heart Health Study. Am J Respir Crit Care Med. 2001;163:19–25.
3. Kaw R, et al. Postoperative complications in patients with obstructive sleep apnea. Chest. 2012;141:436–441.
4. Gentil B, et al. Difficult intubation and obstructive sleep apnoea syndrome. Br J Anaesth. 1994;72:368.
5. Practice guidelines for the perioperative management of patients with obstructive sleep apnea: an updated report by the American Society of Anesthesiologists Task Force on Perioperative Management of Patients With Obstructive Sleep Apnea. American Society of Anesthesiologists Task Force on Perioperative Management of Patients With Obstructive Sleep Apnea. Anesthesiology. 2014;120:268–286.

# 109.

# COMPLICATIONS AND SIDE EFFECTS OF MECHANICAL VENTILATION

*Sohail K. Mahboobi and Mahad Sohail*

## INTRODUCTION

Initially, mechanical ventilation was limited to critical care units, and over time, patients have been mechanically ventilated in postanesthesia care units, step downs, and even regular floors. Mechanical ventilation, though life-saving, is not free of complications.

## PULMONARY COMPLICATIONS

### AUTO–POSITIVE END-EXPIRATORY PRESSURE

Auto-PEEP (positive end-expiratory pressure) occurs due to incomplete exhalation and trapping of air in the lungs at the end of expiration.[1] It occurs when mechanical inspiration is initiated before the expiratory flow from the previous breath has completed. A larger tidal volume, increased rate, and decreased expiratory time will result in auto-PEEP. Auto-PEEP increases the risk of pulmonary barotrauma and can cause hemodynamic instability by decreasing venous return. It can be diagnosed by applying an expiratory pause and measuring the airway pressure. Once diagnosed, various ventilator strategies (e.g., increasing the inspiratory flow rate, decreasing the respiratory rate and tidal volume to allow exhalation) can be used.

### VENTILATION-PERFUSION MISMATCH

Ventilation in the alveoli that do not have perfusion can increase dead space with mechanical ventilation resulting in V/Q mismatch. Similarly, it can reduce shunting if these alveoli have adequate perfusion, particularly if PEEP is added.

## BAROTRAUMA, VOLUTRAUMA, AND BIOTRAUMA

Excessive tidal volume can result in barotrauma, which can cause pneumothorax. Pneumothorax should be suspected in sudden desaturation, tachypnea, tachycardia, hypotension, elevated peak airway pressures, and reduced breath sounds on one side. Chest x-ray or ultrasound can help confirm the diagnosis. Another complication of large tidal volume is volutrauma; large tidal volumes can result in alveolar edema and increased permeability irrespective of airway pressures. Biotrauma is the result of mechanical stress from high inspiratory pressures; this stretches alveolar epithelial cells and triggers an inflammatory process.

## REDUCED IMMUNITY AND PULMONARY INFECTIONS

Mechanical ventilation can induce inflammation in the patients who received large tidal volumes and low PEEP. Ventilator-associated pneumonia (VAP) is defined as the pneumonia that occurs after 48 hours of mechanical ventilation. The risk of developing VAP increases with duration of intubation and mechanical ventilation. Oropharyngeal and gastric secretions can leak around the endotracheal tube cuff folds and serve as the primary reason for infection. Certain steps can be helpful in decreasing the incidence of aspiration, such as elevating the head of the bed to 30° and suctioning the subglottic secretions, along with checking and maintaining the endotracheal cuff pressure at least 20 cm $H_2O$. Chlorhexidine can be used to clean the oral cavity and reduce pneumonia. Prophylactic use of antibiotics is not recommended. Presence of an infiltrate on chest x-ray consistent with a consolidation in the presence of fever, leukocytosis, and purulent sputum (two of the last three) is diagnostic of VAP. Mechanically ventilated patients usually have nasogastric tubes placed, which can cause sinusitis.

This should be suspected in patients with fever and purulent nasal discharge. Diagnosis can be confirmed by x-ray or computed tomographic scan of the sinuses.

## MYOPATHY AND RESPIRATORY MUSCLE DYSFUNCTION

Mechanical ventilation, particularly if controlled, can cause a type of disuse atrophy involving the diaphragm and respiratory muscles. Long-term mechanical ventilation and difficulty weaning are associated with diaphragmatic muscle injury, atrophy, and proteolysis.[2] The mechanism of myopathy and respiratory muscle weakness is probably prolonged use of sedatives; use of neuromuscular blocking agents, particularly steroid muscle relaxants; and critical illness. Early mobilization and exercise (i.e., physical and occupational therapy) may help in recovery. Mechanical ventilation also impairs mucociliary motility in the airways associated with retention of secretions and possible pneumonia.

## CARDIOVASCULAR COMPLICATIONS

Intrathoracic pressure increases during mechanical ventilation, causing reduced venous return. The reduced venous return is further aggravated by PEEP, auto-PEEP, or hypovolemia.[3] Exaggerated respiratory variation on the arterial pressure waveform is a sign that mechanical ventilation is significantly affecting venous return and cardiac output. A reduction in right ventricular output can shift the interventricular septum to the left and cause impaired diastolic filling of the left ventricle. Keeping the patient euvolemic or slightly hypervolemic can overcome this decrease in ventricular output. In patients with impaired left ventricular function, increased intrathoracic pressure can improve left ventricular performance by decreasing both venous return and left afterload.

## GASTROINTESTINAL AND HEPATIC COMPLICATIONS

The gastric mucosa does not have autoregulatory capability, and mechanical ventilation (greater than 48 hours) can cause stress-induced gastric ulceration due to decreased cardiac output, decreased splanchnic perfusion, and increased gastric venous pressure.[4] Similarly, it can adversely affect hepatic function by decreased cardiac output, increased hepatic vascular resistance, and elevated bile duct pressure.

Other complications include erosive esophagitis, diarrhea, acalculous cholecystitis, and hypomotility.

## RENAL COMPLICATIONS

Mechanical ventilation can cause acute renal failure due to the release of inflammatory mediators (e.g., interleukin 6) and impaired renal blood flow, increased sympathetic tone, or activation of humoral pathways.

## CENTRAL NERVOUS SYSTEM COMPLICATIONS

Mechanical ventilation increases intracranial pressure (ICP) as a result of elevated intrathoracic pressure impairing cerebral venous outflow, which may lead to hippocampal neuronal apoptosis, resulting in delirium.

## SLEEP DISORDERS

Sleep is not normal among mechanically ventilated patients. Environmental, disease, and treatment-related factors are possible causes of the disordered sleep. These patients have atypical sleep with sleep fragmentation and the absence of rapid eye movement. The mode of mechanical ventilation may also influence sleep quality, and it is recommended to use assist-controlled ventilation rather than pressure support ventilation during nights.[5]

## ENDOTRACHEAL TUBE COMPLICATIONS

Placement of an endotracheal tube can result in laryngeal injury due to traumatic intubation. Prolonged intubation may result in laryngeal edema, mucosal ulcers, granulomas, and vocal cord paralysis. Usually laryngeal injuries recover spontaneously without intervention. Steroid therapy is recommended to treat laryngeal edema.

## MISCELLANEOUS COMPLICATIONS

Mechanical ventilation with prolonged bed rest has also been associated with insulin resistance, venous thromboembolic disease, and joint contractures. During mechanical ventilation, the head of the bed is frequently raised to prevent aspiration and ventilator-acquired pneumonia, which may increase the risk of sacral pressure ulcers by increasing the pressure on the skin in the sacral region.

## REFERENCES

1. Pepe PE, Marini JJ. Occult positive end-expiratory pressure in mechanically ventilated patients with airflow obstruction: the auto-PEEP effect. *Am Rev Respir Dis.* 1982;126:166–170.
2. Jaber S, et al. Rapidly progressing diaphragmatic weakness and injury during mechanical ventilation in humans. *Am J Crit Care Med.* 2011;183:364–371.
3. Qvist J, et al. Hemodynamic responses to mechanical ventilation with PEEP: the effect of hypovolemia. *Anesthesiology.* 1975;42:45–55.
4. Backer DD. The effects of positive end-expiratory pressure on the splanchnic circulation. *Intensive Care Med.* 2000;26:361–363.
5. Rittayamai N, et al. Positive and negative effects of mechanical ventilation on sleep in the ICU: a review with clinical recommendations. *Intensive Care Med.* 2016;42:531–541.

# 110.

# VOLUTRAUMA, BAROTRAUMA, AND BIOTRAUMA

*Sohail K. Mahboobi and Joshua F. Bolanos*

## INTRODUCTION

Mechanical ventilation may pose harmful effects on lungs, collectively known as ventilator-induced lung injury (VILI). All mechanically ventilated patients are at risk for developing VILI. Risk factors include intrinsic lung disease, acute lung injury, acute respiratory distress syndrome (ARDS), or any condition resulting in reduced lung compliance. There are three types of VILI: barotrauma, volutrauma, and biotrauma.[1] Some signs of VILI can be nonspecific, including hypoxemia, tachypnea, and tachycardia.

## BAROTRAUMA

Barotrauma is the lung injury caused by high inflation pressure that results in high transpulmonary pressures (the pressure difference between airway and pleura) and subsequent rupture of alveoli. Therefore, high tidal volumes in addition to pressure play a role in increasing the risk of developing barotrauma. The rise in volume and pressure within an alveolus leads to the development of a pressure gradient between the alveolus and the perivascular sheath. If the pressure increases beyond a certain threshold, the alveoli can rupture, causing air to infiltrate into the extra-alveolar tissues and move toward the mediastinum and can lead to perivascular interstitial edema. Air traveling through tissue can cause subcutaneous emphysema, pneumopericardium, pneumoperitoneum, or a bronchopleural fistula. The most serious consequence is the development of a pneumothorax or tension pneumothorax. Fortunately, most of the barotrauma complications require just supportive treatment, except for pneumothorax or tension pneumothorax. In clinical practice, the plateau pressure can be used as a representative of transpulmonary pressure in assessing the probability of barotrauma.

An effective way to minimize the risk of developing barotrauma is to maintain the plateau pressures less than 30 cm $H_2O$, keeping peak inspiratory pressures less than 40 cm $H_2O$, and employing low tidal volumes of 6–8 mL/kg of ideal body weight.[2] Another consideration is sedating or paralyzing the patient if they become dyssynchronous with the ventilator. However, in patients with a chronically rigid chest wall, the plateau pressure may be high. This does not necessarily mean the presence of barotrauma or alveolar damage. In this case, the high plateau pressure is the result of the pressure required by the ventilator to expand the chest wall versus the lungs. During mechanical ventilation, there may be an unequal distribution of ventilation, particularly in diseased and atelectatic lung parenchyma, which can expose certain alveoli to higher tidal volumes and pressures than others. High levels of positive end-expiratory pressure (PEEP) may or may not increase the risk of barotrauma. Adopting a high PEEP may distend atelectatic alveoli and improve ventilation. If the applied PEEP does not lead to recruitment of the collapsed alveoli and further dilate patent alveoli, it can lead to an increased risk of barotrauma.

## VOLUTRAUMA

Volutrauma is caused by overdistension of the lung alveoli due to excessive ventilatory volume. In normal respiration, alveolar walls reduce elastic strain due to tidal volume by unfolding and stretching to their maximum capacity. The strain caused by the distension results in lipid trafficking to the cell membrane to help repair the damage and to provide more surface area.[3] When the maximum stretch capacity is achieved, any further increase in volume results in increased strain, which ultimately causes cellular detachment, disruption of the basement membrane and intracellular junctions, and eventually increased capillary permeability and alveolar edema.[4] As described, lower tidal volumes can also cause damage when the lung alveoli receive an unequal distribution of ventilation, with more compliant alveoli receiving higher volumes, leading to their overdistension (e.g., in lungs with lower compliance). Adjusting tidal volumes to 6–8 mL/kg of ideal body weight can reduce the risk of developing volutrauma.

The overdistension of some alveoli and collapse of others lead to a condition known as atelectrauma. Atelectrauma is damage done to alveoli from "cyclical atelectasis" or repetitive opening and closing during inspiration and expiration. This repetitive motion leads to a shearing force on the alveoli. Even alveoli that remain patent and are not atelectatic but are nearby to atelectatic alveoli may become susceptible to damage. Using adequate amounts of at PEEP 3–5 cm $H_2O$ to maintain alveolar patency and provide recruitment maneuvers may reduce the risk of developing atelectrauma. While in the operating room, providing a recruitment breath or placing the patient in the prone position may recruit alveoli and prevent atelectrauma. Administering a lower fraction of inspired air ($FiO_2$) may decrease absorption atelectasis and atelectatic injury during mechanical ventilation.

## BIOTRAUMA

Biotrauma is the lung and multiorgan injury due to release of inflammatory products in response to mechanical ventilation. The ventilatory mechanical stress creates an inflammatory reaction in the lungs as high inspiratory pressures stretch alveolar epithelial cells, resulting in cell injury and triggering of cytokine and inflammatory products like interleukin 6 and tumor necrosis factor $\alpha$.[5] Volutrauma and barotrauma can lead to the release of inflammatory mediators from neutrophils. The inflammatory mediator levels can rise quickly, even within 1 hour if ventilation settings are not lung protective. Biotrauma can increase the risk of pulmonary fibrosis and in severe cases cause multiorgan failure. Because the lungs are well perfused, cytokines, chemokines, and other inflammatory mediators can spread hematogenously throughout the body, which can lead to a systemic inflammatory response and organ dysfunction. Particularly, it affects renal and gastrointestinal systems as well as bacterial translocation into the bloodstream from the lungs. Reducing mechanical stress on alveolar walls by using ventilator strategies to avoid end-expiratory collapse reduces levels of inflammatory markers.

## REFERENCES

1. Slutsky AS. History of mechanical ventilation. From Vesalius to ventilator-induced lung injury. *Am J Respir Crit Care Med.* 2015;191(10):1106–1115.
2. Acute Respiratory Distress Syndrome Network. Ventilation with lower tidal volumes as compared with traditional tidal volumes for acute lung injury and the acute respiratory distress syndrome. *N Engl J Med.* 2000;342(18):1301–1308.
3. Vlahakis NE, et al. Role of deformation-induced lipid trafficking in the prevention of plasma membrane stress failure. *Am J Respir Crit Care Med.* 2002;166(9):1282–1289.
4. Fu Z, et al. High lung volume increases stress failure in pulmonary capillaries. *J Appl Physiol.* 1992;73(1):123–133.
5. Curley GF, et al. Biotrauma and ventilator-induced lung injury: clinical implications. *Chest.* 2016;150:1109–1117.

# 111.

# MANAGEMENT OF BRONCHOSPASM

*Jeffery James Eapen and Jason Bang*

## INTRODUCTION

Bronchospasm is a respiratory condition in which the smooth muscle surrounding the bronchioles constricts, resulting in airflow obstruction, primarily in the expiratory phase of the respiratory cycle. Reactive airway disease such as asthma, chronic obstructive pulmonary disease, anaphylaxis, or intervention by an anesthesiologist increases the risk of bronchospasm. Bronchospasm occurs 0.2% of the time during general anesthesia, but the incidence increases to 6% in patients who have reactive airway disease.[1]

Risk factors for bronchospasm include asthma, upper respiratory tract infection, smoking history, and carcinoid syndrome. Noxious stimuli such as allergens, dust, cold air, endotracheal intubation, secretions, desflurane, β-blockers, nonsteroidal anti-inflammatory drugs, cholinesterase inhibitors, and histamine-releasing drugs such as morphine can result in stimulation of afferent sensory fibers that eventually stimulate the nucleus tractus solitarius, which in turn stimulates efferent fibers of the vagus nerve to result in bronchial smooth muscle contraction.[1]

Release of inflammatory mediators is another cause of bronchospasm. These inflammatory mediators can be a result of allergic reactions or anaphylactic shock in which bronchospasm is either mediated by anaphylactoid or immunoglobulin E–mediated anaphylaxis. Bronchospasm is also a complication seen in carcinoid syndrome, occurring in 15%–19% of patients.[2]

## CLINICAL FEATURES

Perioperative bronchospasm can occur following a noxious stimulus, such as endotracheal intubation. Observed signs and symptoms during bronchospasm are dependent on whether the patient is being mechanically ventilated. If the patient is not being mechanically ventilated, respiratory distress is noted with physical examination findings of decreased breath sounds and expiratory wheezing. While mechanically ventilated, a rapid rise in peak airway pressures from baseline are observed. Capnography will show delayed rise in end-tidal carbon dioxide, and decreased exhaled tidal volumes are noted.[3] If bronchospasm persists, the patient will begin to desaturate, and hypotension is often experienced due to decreased preload from air trapping, resulting in increased intrathoracic pressure.

## MANAGEMENT

If bronchospasm is suspected, quick action should be taken to prevent further complications. Management should aim to increase delivered oxygen content to the patient, improve ventilation, relax bronchial smooth muscle, and stop stimulation such as surgery.[3] Increasing the inspired oxygen concentration to 100%, increasing the inspired concentration of nonnoxious volatile anesthetics for their bronchodilating properties. Intravenous agents such as propofol and ketamine are often employed in scenarios of continued bronchospasm. Ketamine in particular is a known bronchodilator. Initiate manual ventilation as it can serve as a diagnostic tool for ruling out mechanical complications and assessment of pulmonary compliance during the bronchospasm. The $\beta_2$-agonists such as albuterol are often used to manage bronchospasm via metered dose inhalator or nebulized forms introduced into the endotracheal tube. If the bronchospasm is refractory to various techniques employed to terminate the bronchospasm, epinephrine should be used, usually starting with 10 μg IV per dose.[3]

## ANESTHETIC CONSIDERATIONS

### PREOPERATIVE

Preoperatively, identification of and appropriate planning for the management in patients who are at increased risk of bronchospasm can impact the incidence and outcomes of bronchospasm. Physical examination by auscultation and taking a history from the patient are vital on the day of the surgery to assess if further action is necessary to optimize the patient's respiratory status prior to proceeding with the anesthetic plan. Patients should be counseled about smoking cessation 6–8 weeks prior to surgery as this reduces the risk of respiratory complications, including bronchospasm.[4] Respiratory infections should have resolved, with the absence of symptoms for 2 weeks to decrease the chance of bronchospasm.[5] In patients with reactive airways such as asthma, pretreatment with β-agonist nebulized agents 30 minutes prior to the procedure has been associated with decreased incidence of bronchospasm.[3]

## INTRAOPERATIVE

On induction, appropriate depth of anesthesia should be a goal prior to proceeding with laryngoscopy and intubation as this can promote the development of bronchospasm intraoperatively. Emergency medications such as epinephrine should be prepared in anticipation of refractory bronchospasm. During the maintenance of general anesthesia, avoid histamine-releasing drugs and maintain an adequate depth of anesthesia. At the end of the procedure, consider a deep extubation as this can decrease the stimulatory effects of extubation on the smooth muscle of the bronchioles.

## POSTOPERATIVE

During recovery, the patient should be assessed for continued airway reactivity; this can necessitate continued use of bronchodilator therapy, corticosteroids, and chest physiotherapy postoperatively.

A chest radiograph should be obtained to evaluate for pulmonary edema or pneumothorax. If anaphylaxis was a suspected cause, ordering a tryptase level is warranted.[3]

## REFERENCES

1. Freeman B. *Anesthesiology Core Review*. McGraw-Hill; 2014: 390–392.
2. Ferrari AC, et al. Carcinoid syndrome: update on the pathophysiology and treatment. *Clinics (Sao Paulo)*. 2018;73(suppl 1):e490s.
3. Looseley A. Update in anaesthesia. Accessed August 30, 2020. https://www.wfsahq.org/components/com_virtual_library/media/3fe4887e14541ff43fc8b0d7c6c477f8-Bronchospasm-During-Anaesthesia--Update-27-2011-.pdf
4. Dudzińska K, Mayzner-Zawadzka E. Tobacco smoking and the perioperative period. *Anestezjol Intens Ter*. 2008;40:108–113.
5. Nandwani N, et al. Effects of an upper respiratory tract infection on upper airway reactivity. *Br J Anaesth*. 1997;78:352.

# 112.

# LUNG TRANSPLANTATION

*Yamah Amiri and Dinesh J. Kurian*

## INTRODUCTION

Important to consider multiple factors including disease specific and surgical factors. Furthermore, patients with transplanted lungs provide unique anesthetic challenges for non-transplant surgeries.

## END-STAGE LUNG DISEASE FALL INTO FOUR CATEGORIES

The following are some examples of end-stage lung disease[1]:

1. Obstructive lung disease
   - Emphysema
   - Chronic bronchitis
   - Bronchiolitis obliterans
2. Suppurative lung disease
   - Cystic fibrosis
   - Ciliary dyskinesia
   - Bronchiectasis
3. Interstitial lung disease
   - Idiopathic pulmonary fibrosis
   - Hypersensitivity pneumonia
   - Nonspecific pneumonia
4. Pulmonary artery hypertension (PAH)

# ANESTHETIC CONSIDERATIONS

## PREOPERATIVE

Preoperative tests utilize disease-specific factors to evaluate patient's candidacy for transplant, which are used to calculate their lung allocation score (LAS) to help determine priority and survival.[2] Factors that go into the LAS are listed in Table 112.1.[2]

Patients may not be candidates if they have contraindications like active malignancy, significant dysfunction of another major organ, heart disease, unstable medical condition or infection, uncorrectable bleeding disorder, or psychosocial barriers.

Patients with a history of cystic fibrosis can have drug-resistant bacterial colonization, pancreatic exocrine deficiency, and malnutrition (including insufficiency of vitamin K–dependent factors). Patients with chronic obstructive pulmonary disease or interstitial pulmonary fibrosis may present with chronic steroid use and often at an older age, which could come with a history of cardiovascular disease.[1]

Review heart catheterization and echocardiography to evaluate left ventricular and right ventricular (RV) function, chest computed tomography to assess tracheal and bronchial anatomy, and ventilation/perfusion (VQ) scans to assess which lung should be transplanted first. Many of these patients have high pulmonary vascular resistance, requiring contingency planning to manage acute RV failure. Overpreparation for potential difficult airway is advised as many patients are at risk of becoming hypoxemic quickly, and placement of a double-lumen tube can be challenging

*Table 112.1* LUNG ALLOCATION SCORE

| FACTORS USED TO PREDICT WAIT-LIST SURVIVAL | FACTORS USED TO PREDICT POSTTRANSPLANT SURVIVAL |
|---|---|
| Predicted FVC % | Predicted FVC |
| PA systolic pressure | PCW mean pressure > 20 mm Hg |
| O₂ at rest, L/min | Mechanical ventilation |
| Age at offer | Age at transplant |
| BMI | Serum creatinine |
| NYHA functional status | NYHA functional status |
| Diagnosis | Diagnosis |
| Six-minute walk distance < 150 | |
| Mechanical ventilation | |
| Diabetes | |

BMI, body mass index; FVC, forced vital capacity; NYHA, New York Heart Association; PA, pulmonary artery; PCW, pulmonary capillary wedge (pressure).

in any patient with pulmonary fibrosis causing traction on the trachea.

## INTRAOPERATIVE

Understanding common surgical techniques is helpful for preparing the ideal anesthetic plan. Prior to incision, it is important to consider whether cardiopulmonary bypass (CPB) will be required. CPB indications include concomitant intracardiac procedure (atrial septal defect/ventricular septal defect closure or valve repair), RV failure due to severe PAH, or inability to position a double-lumen endotracheal tube. The primary argument against CPB is that it is associated with a higher risk of primary graft dysfunction (PGD).[3]

Positioning and surgical access will differ for single- versus double-lung transplant. Single-lung transplants may be performed via thoracotomy, often in the lateral position. Double-lung transplants typically involve a clamshell bilateral thoracotomy in the supine position. When CPB is planned, the surgical approach is via a median sternotomy. Patients with adhesions from prior surgery, a history of cystic fibrosis, or previous pleurodesis may be at high bleeding risk.

The first native lung to be isolated should be determined by V/Q tests. The poorly perfused lung is more likely to hemodynamically tolerate pulmonary clamping and reduces risk of refractory hypoxemia. A clamp is placed across the pulmonary artery of the first lung, and anticoagulation with systemic heparin may be required (typically a goal activated clotting time of 200–300 seconds). The recipient native pneumonectomy involves access to the hilar pericardium, stapling the pulmonary vessels, dividing the mainstem bronchus, and ligating the recipient bronchial arteries.

Transplantation of the donor lung commonly begins with the anastomosis of the most posterior membranous area of the bronchus, moving anteriorly. After completion of the bronchial anastomosis, the integrity of the connection is tested with an air leak test or bronchoscopy. The bronchial arteries are typically not reconnected. Next, the vascular anastomosis begins with the main pulmonary arteries, then the pulmonary veins. During this step, hemodynamic instability can occur due to obstructive shock physiology from traction or obstruction on the left atrium. Prior to completion of the pulmonary venous anastomosis, the PA clamp is partially released to flush the air from the donor lung, potentially resulting in 500–1000 mL acute blood loss, which can result in hemodynamic instability from hypovolemia and postreperfusion syndrome. Cell salvage techniques may effectively preserve red cells, though dilutional coagulopathy may still occur though loss of plasma proteins and mechanical degradation of platelets. For double-lung transplantation, this process is repeated for the second lung.[4,5]

Airway equipment should include an appropriate size double-lumen endotracheal tube (with a backup single-lumen tube), suction catheters, and airway exchange catheters. Vascular access includes an arterial line for hemodynamic monitoring and laboratory sampling. A central line will be required for nearly all cases, and the site of placement should be discussed with the surgical team, as the right internal jugular vein may be needed for the extracorporeal membrane oxygenation (ECMO) cannula. For blood loss during the operation, large-bore peripheral access may also be required. Gas exchange during the lung transplant may be difficult to ascertain, so a bispectral index (BIS) monitor is useful to ensure adequate anesthesia. Additionally, coagulation status should be monitored given the high risk of developing coagulopathy independent of any heparin effect from dilutional thrombocytopenia or hypofibrinogenemia. Transesophageal echocardiography may be valuable for differentiation of the causes of hemodynamic instability and useful to assess the quality of the pulmonary venous anastomosis. Finally, because the donor and native lungs require different ventilation strategies, a second ventilator may be required intraoperatively.

To minimize pulmonary edema from excess volume administration, vasoactive support to temporize hypotension or RV dysfunction is appropriate. Common choices include epinephrine, norepinephrine, vasopressin, and inhaled nitric oxide. Immunosuppression should be coordinated with the pulmonary transplant team and may include mycophenolate, basiliximab, and steroids. If renal function is normal, calcineurin inhibitors may be used. Some patients may require rabbit antithymoglobulin or intravenous immunoglobulin. Antimicrobial prophylaxis should cover gram-positive organisms, including methicillin-resistant staphylococcus, gram-negative organisms, antifungal prophylaxis, and possible cytomegalovirus coverage. Patients with a history of drug-resistant organisms may require additional prophylaxis.

Ventilator management in the native lungs can be determined as needed, including liberal use of the fraction of inspired oxygen ($FiO_2$). Hypercapnia may be well tolerated in patients with chronic respiratory insufficiency, and vent settings should be adjusted to correct pH. Ventilation of the first donor lung may require a separate ventilator with low tidal volumes and the lowest $FiO_2$ tolerated to minimize risk of graft dysfunction due to ischemia/reperfusion injury from hyperoxia.[3] The lowest mean airway pressure tolerated should be used to avoid breakdown of the bronchial anastomosis. If the second ventilator cannot deliver volatile anesthetic, it may be essential to transition to an intravenous anesthetic with BIS monitoring.

## POSTOPERATIVE

Patient's arrive to the intensive care unit (ICU) intubated with early postoperative goals of lung-protective ventilation

*Table 112.2* PGD SCORES

| GRADE | PULMONARY EDEMA ON X-RAY | PAO₂/FIO₂ RATIO |
|-------|--------------------------|------------------|
| 0 | No | Normal |
| 1 | Yes | >300 |
| 2 | Yes | 200–300 |
| 3 | Yes | <200 |

with early extubation as tolerated, hemodynamic stability, restrictive fluid management, arrhythmia management, continuing immunosuppression, and prophylactic antibiotics. In order to maintain anastomosis and avoid barotrauma, tidal volumes are set to 6 mL/kg–8 mL/kg of ideal body weight, conservative PEEP, and plateau pressures less than 35 mm Hg. Furthermore, chest x-rays are monitored with $PaO_2$ to $FiO_2$ ratio to evaluate for hypoxia in the first 72 hours after transplantation, which could represent PGD. PGD scores are assigned as 0 to 3 depending on pulmonary edema on x-ray and worsening ratio scores, and a high score could indicate poor prognosis, such as chronic lung allograft dysfunction, retransplantation, longer ventilator application, long ICU stay, and increased need for dialysis (Table 112.2).

Treatment includes reducing pulmonary edema with diuresis, protective lung ventilation, and inhaled nitric oxide, and the last line would be initiating venovenous ECMO.[6] Once inotropes and vasopressors are weaned off, patients are at high risk for atrial fibrillation after transplant, and prevention can include utilizing calcium channel blockers, β-blockers, or amiodarone pending institutional guidelines. Appropriate pain management that includes thoracic epidural is encouraged to avoid splinting, atelectasis, and infection development. Speech therapists should evaluate the patient prior to advancing diets to avoid aspiration of new lungs. Last, it will be critical to continue working with the lung transplant medicine team and infectious disease team to ensure the patient is on appropriate immunosuppression and prophylactic antibiotics.

## CONSIDERATIONS FOR LUNG TRANSPLANT RECIPIENTS UNDERGOING NONTRANSPLANT SURGERY

Patients with a history of lung transplantation may require nontransplant surgery. It is important to address any number of complications following their transplant: infection due to immunosuppressed status, rejection causing bronchiolitis obliterans, or breakdown of the bronchial anastomosis. These changes may affect the strategy used for mechanical ventilation. It is essential to consider all comorbid conditions associated with the underlying pathology that required transplantation as these may not have resolved. Also, preoperative optimization can be challenging with ensuring all the appropriate medication and antimicrobial prophylaxis have been given the day of surgery.

Patients should be considered as having aspiration precautions as the immunosuppression medications can lower esophageal sphincter tone. Calcineurin inhibitors increase the risk of acute kidney injury, which should be considered for any patient undergoing procedures associated with renal injury. Many of these medications may also result in anemia, and CMV-negative patients should receive leukoreduced blood products if required. Patients are at higher risk of developing pulmonary edema or pleural effusion as the lymphatic connections are not restored, so use caution fluid with management.

Due to immunosuppression, minimize infection risk and perform all procedures with strict attention to aseptic technique.[6]

## REFERENCES

1. Nicoara A, Anderson-Dam J. Anesthesia for lung transplantation. *Anesthesiology Clin.* 2017;35(3):473–489.
2. Egan TM, et al. Development of a new lung allocation system in the United States. *Am J Transplant.* 2006;2:1212–1227.
3. Diamond JM, et al. Clinical risk factors for primary graft dysfunction after lung transplantation. *Am J Respir Crit Care Med.* 2013;187(5):527–534.
4. Gust L, D'Journo X-B, et al. Single-lung and double-lung transplantation: technique and tips. *J Thorac Dis.* 2018;10(4):2508–2518.
5. Hayanga JWA, D'Cunha J. The surgical technique of bilateral sequential lung transplantation. *J Thorac Dis.* 2014;6(8):1063–1069.
6. Kim SY, et al. Critical care after lung transplantation. *Acute Crit Care.* 2018;33(4):206–215.

# Part 10

# CARDIOVASCULAR SYSTEM ANATOMY

# 113.

# NORMAL ANATOMY OF HEART AND MAJOR VESSELS

*Marc Rodrigue and Subramanya Bandi*

## INTRODUCTION

Cardiac anatomy plays a vital role in cardiac function. An in-depth knowledge of cardiac anatomy, and resulting clinical implications, cannot be undervalued in the practice of anesthesiology.

## GROSS ANATOMY

The heart in its simplest form is a muscular and cartilaginous organ that comprises four chambers (left and right atria/ventricles) and the corresponding avascular fibrous valves (tricuspid, pulmonic, mitral, and aortic) separating the chambers within the heart, as well as the pulmonic and aortic roots. Coronary artery vessels (left and right, with divisions) arise from the aortic root to supply the myocardium with oxygen and nutrient-rich blood.

## MYOCARDIUM

Of the muscular layers within the heart, it is the myocardium that makes up the bulk of the tissue of the heart, rather than the endocardial or epicardial layers. The muscular walls of the two atria are thinner in comparison to the thickened left ventricle (LV), whose fibers are arranged in a multiplane orientation. This allows the LV to contract in a twisting motion, creating maximum ejection of its volume and, conversely, creates optimal filling conditions when relaxing. The right ventricle (RV) however, is thinner walled, more compliant, crescent shaped, and located anterior and to the right of the LV. Its peristalsis-like systolic motion is only able to produce about 20% of the total stroke work of the LV, but it is able to eject similar stroke volume with assistance from the contracting LV and shared septal wall.[1]

## VALVES

The valves within the heart are both bileaflet (mitral) and trileaflet (tricuspid, pulmonic, and aortic). These cartilaginous, avascular structures open and close with the pressure changes of the cardiac cycle, ensuring blood flow in a single direction.

The mitral valve is composed of anterior (oval shaped) and posterior (crescent shaped) leaflets. In a three-dimensional reconstruction, it resembles a saddle-like shape when closed.[2] It allows blood to flow from the left atrium (LA) to the LV during diastole. The leaflets are supported during systole by chordae tendinae, rope-like structures that restrict the leaflets' superior motion when closing, allowing proper coaptation and eliminating regurgitation.[1] The chordae tendinae are attached inferiorly by two papillary muscles within the LV and are named according to their anatomic location, anterolateral and posteromedial. Rupture of the posteriomedial papillary muscle due to inferior wall ischemia (i.e., non–ST-segment elevation myocardial infarction) is a common cause of acute mitral regurgitation in certain populations.[3]

The tricuspid valve and its positional named leaflets (anterior, posterior, and septal), ensure blood flows from the right atrium (RA) to the RV without regurgitation back into the central venous system. The tricuspid leaflets are rooted in the atrioventricular (AV) septum that separates the RA and RV, which is different from the annulus of the mitral valve.[1]

The aortic and pulmonic valves are both trileaflet structures, separating the LV and RV from the aorta and the main pulmonary artery, respectively. The pulmonic valve lies anterior to the aortic valve within the mediastinum. Its three valves are named for their anatomic orientation: anterior, left, and right. The aortic valve also has a left and right cusps and are oriented as such. However, the third leaflet, the noncoronary cusp, is located posterior to the other two cusps and is adjacent to the fibrous interventricular septum.[4]

## CORONARY VESSELS

The two major epicardial vessels that supply the myocardium have their root in the aortic sinus of Valsalva. The left coronary artery (LCA) and right coronary artery (RCA) each have their own supply distribution, and dominance of circulation is determined by which major coronary artery supplies the posterior descending artery (PDA). Approximately 80% of the population has a right-dominant circulation, meaning the RCA supplies the PDA.[1] Clinically, this is significant because occlusion of the dominant circulatory route, left or right, can result in complete heart blockade of the AV node, which the PDA supplies.

During the cardiac cycle, changes in pressure within the LV exceed the aortosystolic pressure within the coronary system. This means the LV myocardium is only supplied with blood flow during diastole, when the intraventricular pressure is lowest. In contrast, the pressures within the RA, RV, and LA rarely exceed systemic pressure and are therefore perfused throughout the cardiac cycle.[1]

Drainage of the cardiac vascular beds occurs via three major coronary veins: the great cardiac vein, which runs alongside of the left anterior descending coronary artery, the anterior cardiac vein (RCA), and middle cardiac vein (PDA). About 85% of the LV coronary venous blood returns to the coronary sinus via the great cardiac vein. The remaining the 15% of venous drainage empties directly into the ventricular chamber through Thebesian veins. This is in contrast to the RV coronary venous return, which empties into the RA via the anterior cardiac vein.[1]

## ELECTRICAL CONDUCTION SYSTEM

The sinoatrial node is the primary conducting pacemaker of the heart. Situated in the superior portion of the RA, there are three internodal pathways that conduct from the sinotrial node to the AV node: the anterior, middle (Wenkebach), and posterior (Thorel) pathways. These pathways penetrate the cartilage layers that divide the atrium from the ventricles, allowing conduction to reach the AV node. The Bachmann bundle, a division of the anterior pathway, carries conduction signals through the interatrial septum to supply the LA. Abnormal, aberrant, or excessive conduction within these conduction bundles results in a multitude of atrial dysrhythmias. From the AV node, the depolarization continues through the bundle of His, which then divides into the left and right bundle branches, terminating in the Purkinje fibers within the endocardium of each ventricle.[1]

## REFERENCES

1. Barash PG, et al. Clinical Anesthesia. 8th ed. Philadelphia, PA: Wolters Kluwer; 2017:278–282.
2. Sidebotham DA, et al. Intraoperative transesophageal echocardiography for surgical repair of mitral regurgitation. *J Am Soc Echocardiogr.* 2014;27:345–366.
3. Fradley MG, Picard MH. Rupture of the posteromedial papillary muscle leading to partial flail of the anterior mitral leaflet. *Circulation.* 2011;123:1044–1045.
4. Netter FHI. *Atlas of Human Anatomy.* 5th ed. Philadelphia, PA: Saunders/Elsevier; 2010:216.

# 114.

# ECHO HEART ANATOMY

*Christina Gibson and Matthew McConnell*

## INTRODUCTION

Perioperative transesophageal echocardiography (TEE) is a relatively safe diagnostic method with a mortality rate of less than 0.01% and a morbidity rate of 0.2%–1.2%.[1]

## MIDESOPHAGEAL FOUR-CHAMBER VIEW

The midesophageal (ME) four-chamber view is obtained at approximately at a depth of 30–35 cm, posterior to the left atrium. Ensure the mitral valve is centered while adjusting the image depth to optimize the left ventricular (LV) apex. The multiplane can be rotated 10°–20°. Structures seen include the right atrium, interatrial septum, left atrium, mitral valve, tricuspid valve, LV, right ventricle (RV), and interventricular septum. Diagnoses that can be obtained from this view include LV (anterior lateral and inferior septal) and RV function, chamber volume and function, mitral valve, and tricuspid valve (Figure 114.1).[2,3]

## MIDESOPHAGEAL TWO-CHAMBER VIEW

The ME two-chamber view is obtained by rotating the multiplane from the ME four-chamber view to 80°–100° when the RV disappears from view. Structures seen include the left atrium, mitral valve, LV, and left atrial appendage. Diagnoses include LV function (anterior and inferior walls), mitral valve, and atrial appendage (Figure 114.2).[2,3]

## MIDESOPHAGEAL LONG-AXIS VIEW

The ME long-axis (LAX) view is obtained by rotating the multiplane from the ME two-chamber view to 120°–160° as the left ventricular outflow tract (LVOT) and aortic valve are seen. Structures seen include the left atrium, mitral valve, LV, LVOT, aortic valve, and proximal ascending aorta. Diagnoses include chamber volume and function (anterior septal and inferior lateral walls of the LV), LVOT pathology, and aortic and mitral valves (Figure 114.3).[2,3]

## MIDESOPHAGEAL ASCENDING AORTIC LONG-AXIS VIEW

The ME ascending aortic LAX view is obtained by withdrawing the probe from the ME LAX view. Visualized structures include the ascending aorta, main pulmonary artery (PA), and pulmonic valve with counterclockwise rotation. Diagnoses include proximal pulmonary emboli, aortic dissection, and Doppler of the RVOT (Figure 114.4).[2,3]

## MIDESOPHAGEAL ASCENDING AORTIC SHORT-AXIS VIEW

The ME ascending aortic short-axis (SAX) view is obtained by rotating the multiplane back to 20°–40° from the image of the main PA. Structures include the PA (right PA is usually seen), ascending aorta, and superior vena cava. Diagnoses include pulmonary emboli, confirmation of PA catheter placement, and Doppler measurements of the PA (Figure 114.5).[2,3]

## MIDESOPHAGEAL AORTIC VALVE SHORT-AXIS VIEW

The ME aortic valve SAX view is obtained by advancing the probe from the ME ascending aortic SAX view. Structures include the aortic valve cusps as described in the image. Diagnoses include aortic valve pathology, including aortic regurgitation and stenosis; bicuspid valves, patent foramen ovale (PFO), RV function, tricuspid valve, and pulmonic valve (Figure 114.6).[2,3]

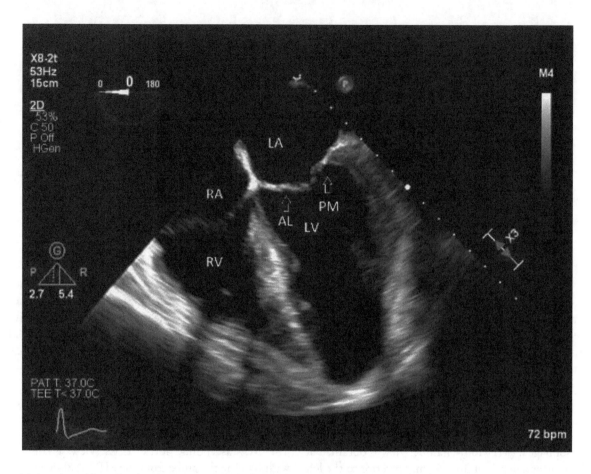

**Figure 114.1** Midesophageal four-chamber view. AL, anterior leaflet MV; PL, posterior leaflet MV; LA, left atrium; LV, left ventricle; RA, right atrium; RV, right ventricle.

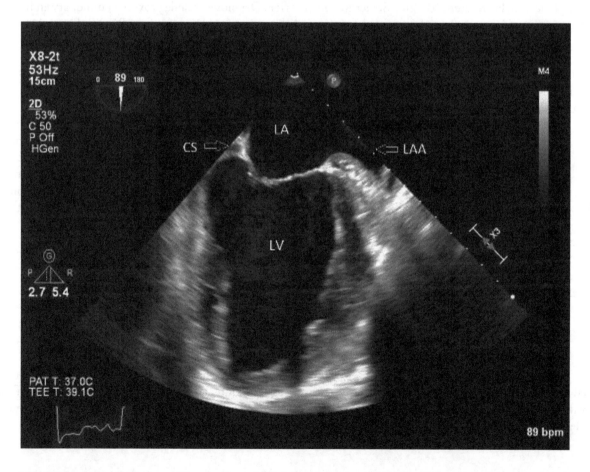

**Figure 114.2** Midesophageal two-chamber view. CS, coronary sinus; LA, left atrium; LAA, left atrial appendage; LV, left ventricle.

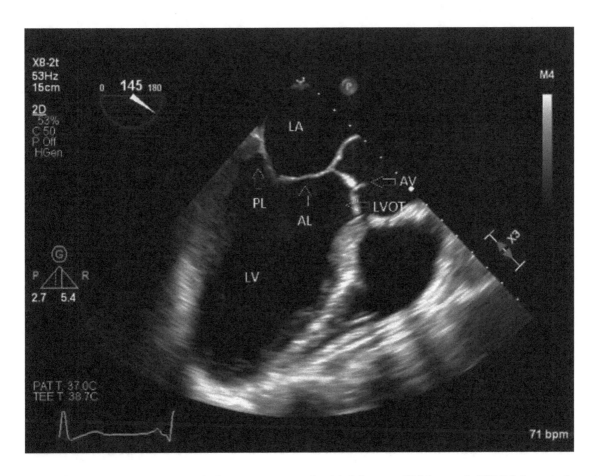

**Figure 114.3** Midesophageal LAX view. AL, anterior leaflet MV; AV, aortic valve; LA, left atrium; LV, left ventricle; LVOT, left ventricular outflow tract; PL, posterior leaflet MV; RV, right ventricle.

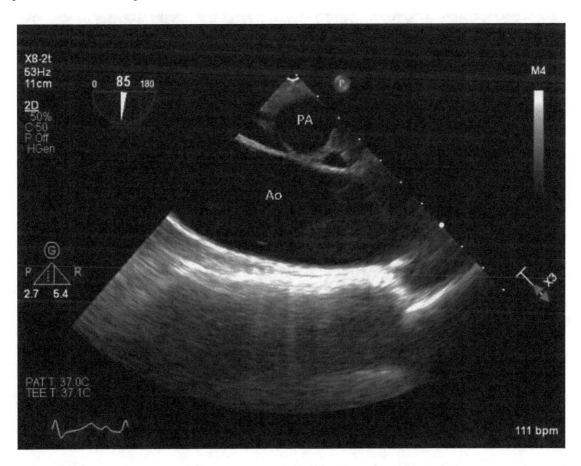

**Figure 114.4** Midesophageal ascending aortic LAX view. Ao, aorta; PA, pulmonary artery.

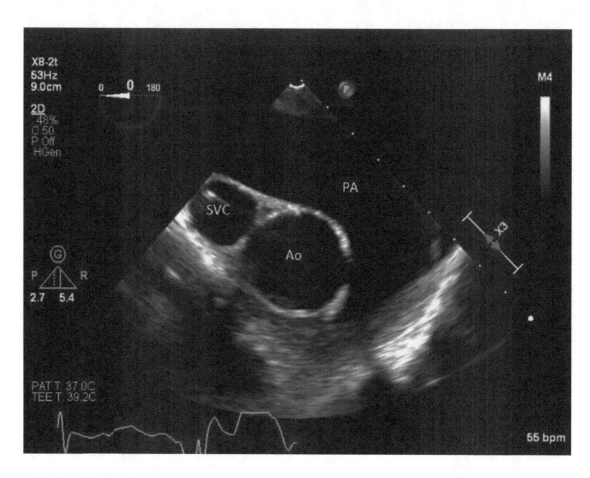

**Figure 114.5** Midesophageal ascending aortic SAX view. Ao, aorta; PA, pulmonary artery; SVC, superior vena cava.

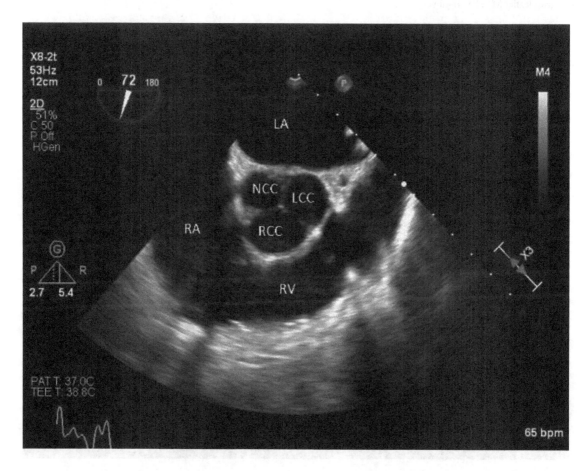

**Figure 114.6** Midesophageal aortic valve SAX view. LA, left atrium; LCC, left coronary cusp; NCC, noncoronary cusp; RA, right atrium; RCC, right coronary cusp.

## MIDESOPHAGEAL RIGHT VENTRICLE INFLOW-OUTFLOW VIEW

The ME RV inflow-outflow view is obtained from the ME ascending aortic SAX view by rotating the multiplane to 60°–90°. Structures include the left atrium, right atrium, tricuspid valve, RV, pulmonic valve, main PA, RV free wall, and RVOT. Diagnoses include RV function, tricuspid and pulmonic valve function, and RV systolic pressure (Figure 114.7).[2,3]

## MIDESOPHAGEAL BICAVAL VIEW

The ME bicaval view is obtained from the ME RV inflow-outflow view by rotating the multiplane 90°–100° with the probe turned clockwise. Structures include superior vena cava, inferior vena cava, left atrium, right atrium, right atrial appendage, and interatrial septum. Diagnoses include interatrial shunt, PFO, ostium secundum, line placement, and tricuspid valve (Figure 114.8).[2,3]

## TRANSGASTRIC MIDPAPILLARY SHORT-AXIS VIEW

The transgastric midpapillary SAX view is obtained from the ME four-chamber view by advancing the probe into the stomach until the posteromedial papillary muscle (PMP) comes into view, then anteflexion will allow visualization of the anterolateral papillary muscle (ALP). Structures viewed are the ALP; PMP; anterior, inferior, septal, and lateral walls of the LV; interventricular septum; and RV (if the probe is turned to the right). Diagnoses include LV volume status, systolic function, and regional wall motion (Figure 114.9).[2,3]

## DESCENDING AORTIC SHORT-AXIS VIEW

The descending aortic SAX view is obtained by turning the probe to the left from the ME four-chamber view until the descending thoracic aorta comes into display at an angle of 0°. Structures visualized include the descending aorta. While keeping the aorta in the center, the probe can be advanced and withdrawn to image the entire aorta. Diagnoses

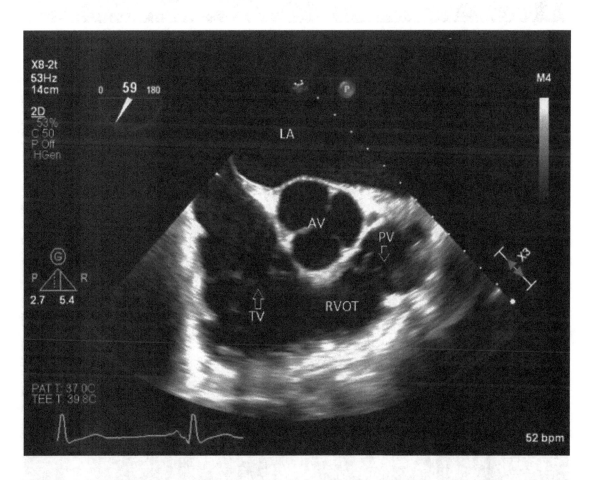

**Figure 114.7** Midesophageal RV inflow-outflow view. AV, aortic valve; LA, left atrium; PV, pulmonic valve; RVOT, right ventricular outflow tract; TV, tricuspid valve.

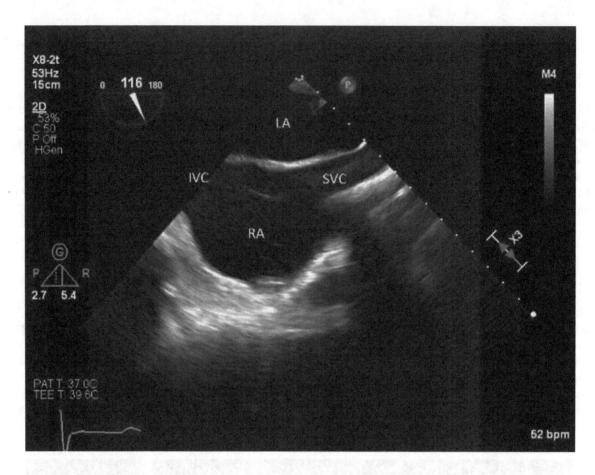

**Figure 114.8** Midesophageal bicaval view. IVC, inferior vena cava; LA, left atrium; RA, right atrium; SVC, superior vena cava.

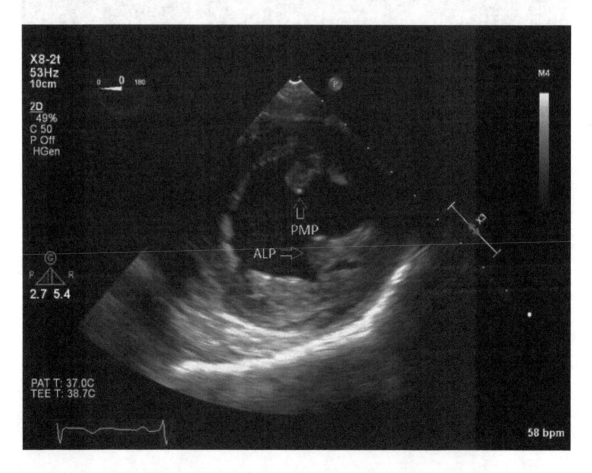

**Figure 114.9** Transgastric midpapillary SAX view. ALP, anterior lateral papillary muscle; PMP, posterior medial papillary muscle.

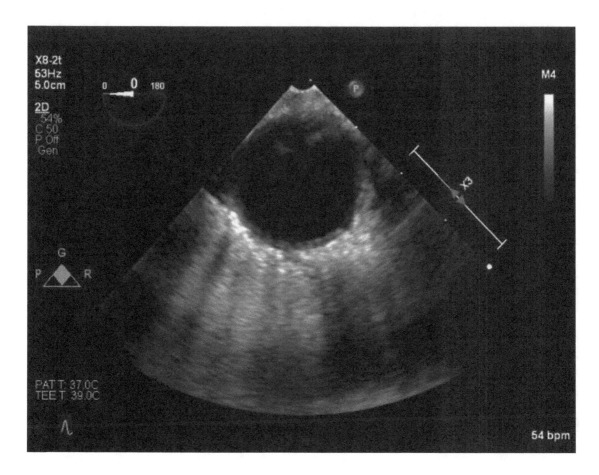

**Figure 114.10** Descending aortic SAX view.

include aortic pathology, aortic diameter, atherosclerosis, and aortic dissection (Figure 114.10).[2,3]

## DESCENDING AORTIC LONG-AXIS VIEW

The descending aortic LAX view is obtained by turning the probe to the left from the ME four-chamber view until the descending thoracic aorta comes into display at an angle of 90°. Structures visualized include the descending aorta. While keeping the aorta in the center, the probe can be advanced and withdrawn to image the entire descending aorta. Diagnoses include aortic pathology, aortic diameter, atherosclerosis, and aortic dissection. Additionally, left pleural effusions can be seen in the far field, and right pleural effusions can be seen if the probe is turned further clockwise (Figure 114.11).[2,3]

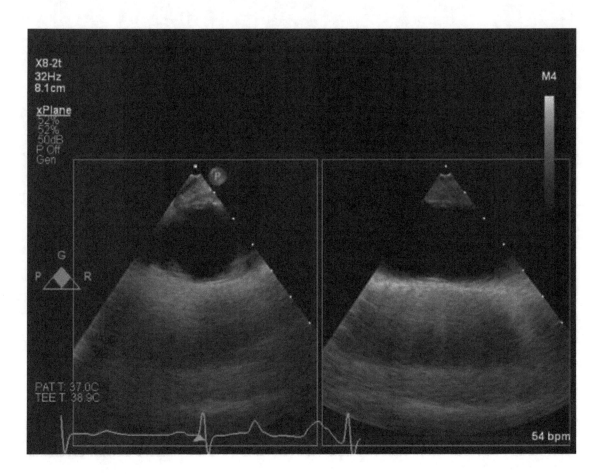

**Figure 114.11** Descending aortic LAX view.

## REFERENCES

1. Hilberath J, et al. Safety of transesophageal echocardiography. *J Am Soc Echocardiogr.* 2010;23(11):1115–1127.
2. Perrino A, et al. *A Practical Approach to Transesophageal Echocardiography.* 4th ed. Lippincott, Williams & Wilkins; 2019.
3. Reeves S, et al. Basic perioperative transesophageal echocardiography examination: a consensus statement of the American Society of Echocardiography and the Society of Cardiovascular Anesthesiologists. *J Am Soc Echocardiogr.* 2013;26(5):443–456.

# 115.

# CARDIAC CATHETERIZATION

*Virgilio de Gala and Iwan Soffan*

## INTRODUCTION

Cardiac catheterization procedures include left and right heart catheterization, coronary angiography, electrophysiological studies, implantation of pacemakers and defibrillators, percutaneous closure of septal defects, and transcatheter cardiac valve implantations.[1] Structural heart procedures (Watchman, MitraClip, etc.) and cardiac assist device placements (intra-aortic balloon pump, Impella, etc.) are also becoming more common.

Often located outside of the main operating room, cardiac catheterization laboratory procedures present unique anesthetic challenges. These include an unfamiliar environment, limited workspaces, exposure to radiation, and limited access to backup equipment and personnel.[1]

## CARDIAC CATHETERIZATION

Cardiac catheterizations are typically done under fluoroscopy to assess either the left or the right heart anatomies and functions. The ALARA principle, "as low as reasonably achievable," is usually employed to reduce radiation exposure. Access is obtained at the femoral, radial, or brachial sites. Using the Seldinger technique, a sheath is placed for arterial or venous access for the duration of the procedure.[1]

### RIGHT HEART CATHETERIZATION

Right heart catheterization remains the gold standard in the assessment of pulmonary artery (PA) hemodynamics, and pulmonary hypertension (PH).[1,2] Cardiac output/index are traditionally measured using the direct Fick method[2]; however, a Swan-Ganz catheter can calculate cardiac output using the thermodilution method (normal CO 5 L/min, CI 2.5–4.0 L/min/m²).[2] These catheters are also indicated in cardiogenic shock and in the diagnosis and follow-up of PH.[2]

The catheter is inserted into a central vein, directed into the right atrium (RA), and advanced through the right heart. Measurements and information obtained include RA pressure (normal 2–6 mm Hg); right ventricular (RV) systolic (15–25 mm Hg)/diastolic pressures (0–8 mm Hg); PA systolic (15–25 mm Hg)/diastolic (8–15 mm Hg); mean pressures (<25 mm Hg); and PA wedge pressure (6–12 mm Hg).[2,3] Oxygen saturations in the superior vena cava, inferior vena cava, RA, RV, PA, left atrium, and pulmonary veins (when possible) can also be measured.[2] Pulmonary vascular resistance (normal 30–180 dynes/s/cm⁻⁵) and response to acute vasodilators, such as nitric oxide or milrinone, can also be observed.[2,3]

## LEFT HEART CATHETERIZATION

Left heart catheterization can measure left ventricular end-diastolic pressure, LV size, ejection fraction, regional wall motion abnormalities, aneurysms, filling defects/clots, and mitral regurgitation. Withdrawing the catheter through the aortic valve (AV) allows the measurement of the transvalvular aortic gradient, correlating with the degree of aortic stenosis. The size of the ascending aorta, number of AV cusps, any possible vein grafts, and severity of aortic insufficiency can also be assessed.[4]

## CORONARY ANGIOGRAPHY

Coronary angiography is performed to diagnose, and sometimes treat, coronary artery disease (CAD). Some indications include patients with acute coronary syndromes, symptoms of heart failure, and refractory angina undergoing high-risk surgery.[4] Treatments during angiography include balloon angioplasty, stent placement, or occasionally an intra-aortic balloon pump for acute support.

The two main coronary arteries originate from their respective aortic cusps. The left main bifurcates into the left anterior descending artery (LAD) and left circumflex artery (LCx). The LAD descends toward the apex in the interventricular groove. It can be divided into thirds, termed the proximal, mid, and distal segments. The LAD branches include the diagonal and septal arteries. The LAD supplies the anteroseptal, anterior, and anterolateral

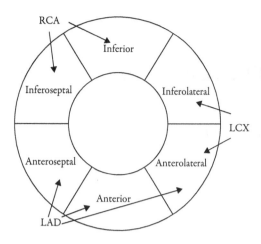

**Figure 115.1** Left ventricular segments and coronary distributions.

walls of the LV. The LCx travels along the left atrioventricular groove, moving inferiorly and posteriorly while giving off branches to the obtuse marginal arteries to supply the inferolateral wall and a portion of the anterolateral wall.[4] The right coronary artery (RCA), like the LAD, can be divided into proximal, mid, and distal segments. The RCA continues as the posterior descending artery to supply the inferior and inferoseptal segments of the LV wall.[4]

The LV can be divided longitudinally into three sections: the base, mid, and apex. These can then be subdivided into six basal segments, six midcavity segments (Figure 115.1), four apical segments, and the true apex as the 17th segment.[5] While there are significant anatomic variants among patients, in general, the coronary distribution of the LV correlates well.[4,5]

## ANESTHETIC CONSIDERATIONS

### PREOPERATIVE

The majority of patients in the catheterization laboratories will have significant heart disease. Some of the pertinent cardiac histories include obstructive CAD, arrhythmias, valvular abnormalities, poor left or right heart functions, and anticoagulation medications. Each procedure will have its own unique considerations, but most will involve large catheters in major vessels and the heart itself. There is always a risk of significant cardiovascular events, such malignant arrhythmia, cardiac tamponade, and cardiac arrest. Preoperative case preparation should include ensuring the ability to induce general endotracheal anesthesia, administer vasopressor boluses, and start drips and transfusions.

### INTRAOPERATIVE

Intraoperatively, catheterization laboratory rooms are usually smaller and have various cardiology devices that can limit access to the patient. There might also be variations in anesthesia equipment, gas outlets, and standard or emergency drug availability. The patient may also be located further away, while the procedure table itself may be mobile to facilitate the fluoroscopy. Extended breathing circuits and long monitoring lines may be required. The fluoroscope will likely need to be moved during induction and intubation so the airway can be secured.[1]

While most procedures may be performed under sedation, general anesthesia may be preferred for longer procedures, especially in those patients who are unable to tolerate light-to-moderate sedation.[1] Other anesthetic techniques that have been used include epidural anesthesia for patients with lower extremity stents to promote vascular patency and high-frequency jet ventilation to reduce respiratory variations and diaphragmatic movement.[1]

### POSTOPERATIVE

Cardiac catheterization and coronary angiography are usually regarded as low-risk procedures. Major complications may occur in less than 1% of patients and include myocardial infarction, heart failure, major bleeding, tamponade, arrhythmias, stroke, renal failure, vascular damage, anaphylactic reactions, and death.[4] Stable hemodynamics should remain one of the primary concerns and typical extubation criteria may be used.

### REFERENCES

1. Hamid M. Anesthesia for cardiac catheterization procedures. *Heart, Lung, Vessels*. 2014;6(4):225–231.
2. D'Alto M, et al. Right heart catheterization for the diagnosis of pulmonary hypertension. Controversies and practical issues. *Heart Fail Clin*. 2018;14(3):467–477.
3. Naderi N. Hemodynamic study. *Pract Cardiol*. 2014;183–191.
4. Zahedmehr A. Catheterization and angiography. *Pract Cardiol*. 2014;173–181.
5. Cerqueira M, et al. Standardized myocardial segmentation and nomenclature for tomographic imaging of the heart. *Circulation*. 2002;105:539–542.

# Part 11

# CLINICAL SCIENCES

# 116.

# ISCHEMIC HEART DISEASE

*Daniel Ramirez Parga and Tatiana Jamroz*

## INTRODUCTION

Ischemic heart disease (ISHD) is a group of clinical syndromes resulting from myocardial ischemia or an imbalance between myocardial blood supply and demand. Atherosclerosis of the coronary arteries is the leading cause of the decreased blood flow to the myocardium. Imbalance between myocardial blood supply and demand can also occur in the absence of coronary blood flow obstruction. An example would be increased oxygen demand in situations that lead to increases in preload, afterload, myocardial tension, and tachyarrhythmias—as is seen in myocardial hypertrophy, aortic stenosis, aortic regurgitation, anemia, or hyperthyroidism. Variant angina is the form of ISHD caused by coronary vasospasm, while syndrome X is caused by microvascular dysfunction of the coronary circulation.[1]

Ischemic heart disease is the most common cause of death in both developed and developing countries.

Coronary artery disease (CAD)—as ISHD is often referred to—is also highly prevalent, and thus around 30% of patients presenting for surgery will also have ISHD.[1]

Patients suffering from ISHD may present with symptoms of chronic stable angina or acutely with symptoms of one of the acute coronary syndromes (ACSs). Sudden cardiac death, where no testing is available, frequently is due to cardiac dysrhythmias as a result of ISHD.[1]

## RISK FACTORS

Atherosclerosis and smoking are the principal contributors to coronary artery disease. Other risk factors are male gender, advanced age, diabetes, family history of heart disease, hypertension, obesity, physical inactivity, and high cholesterol.[1]

## CLINICAL FEATURES

Ischemic heart disease may manifest by symptoms of myocardial ischemia, infarction, arrhythmias, heart failure, or sudden cardiac death. Classically, it presents in the chronic form as chronic stable angina or as an ACS[1] (Figure 116.1).

Acute coronary syndrome due to acute or worsening imbalance of myocardial oxygen supply and demand may present as an unstable angina, characterized by new intensity or frequency in the setting of previously stable angina. There are usually nonspecific electrocardiographic (ECG) changes present, but no elevations of cardiac-specific biomarkers are detected.

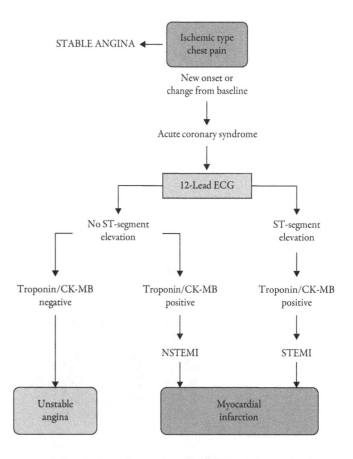

**Figure 116.1** Terminology of acute coronary syndrome. Reprinted with permission from Akhtar S. Ischemic Heart Disease. In: Hines RL, Marschall KE. *Stoelting's Anesthesia and Co-Existing Disease.* 7th ed. Philadelphia: Elsevier; 2018: 79–106.

Myocardial infarction (MI) is another form of ACS. It involves symptoms of angina with cardiac-specific biomarkers either elevated or changed in their value within a certain time frame. ECG changes will further specify the MI as non–ST segment elevation myocardial infarction (NSTEMI) or ST segment elevation MI (STEMI).

The fourth Universal Definition of Myocardial Infarction (UDMI) categorizes MI into five different types based on the reasons that led to elevations of cardiac troponin (cTn) values. According to the fourth UDMI, the *myocardial injury* is a detection of an elevated cTn value, while *MI* is the presence of acute myocardial injury *AND* clinical evidence of acute myocardial ischemia.[2]

Type 1 MI is a myocardial injury related to acute coronary atherosclerotic plaque rupture or erosion, often with thrombosis (most STEMIs), while type 2 classifies myocardial injury as related to acute myocardial ischemia from oxygen supply-and-demand imbalance from other causes than atherosclerosis with thrombosis (most NSTEMIs)[2] (Figure 116.2).

## DIAGNOSIS

- Clinically: Chest pain, shortness of breath, sweating, tachycardia, pain irradiated to jaw or arm
- ECG: ST elevation or depression, T-wave inversion, Q waves; exercise ECG is useful for detecting ischemia and for evaluation of exercise capacity
- Echocardiography

- Nuclear cardiology techniques: Electron beam computed tomography (CT), CT angiography, positron emission tomography
- Coronary angiography
- Biomarkers:
  - Cardiac troponin: Released to bloodstream from ischemia-damaged cardiomyocytes, and change in its values can be used to define acute events.
  - High-sensitivity cTn assays: Can detect a significantly lower concentration of cTn, but also may detect chronically elevated cTn in other noncardiac conditions, such as end-stage renal disease.[3]
  - Natriuretic peptides: Brain natriuretic peptides (BNPs) and the inactive N-terminal pro-BNP (NTpro-BNP) are released into the bloodstream in response to not only left atrial stretching but also ischemia and inflammation.[4]

## TREATMENT

There are several goals in the treatment of ISHD: decrease in myocardial oxygen requirement, improvement in coronary blood flow, plaque stabilization, thrombosis prevention, and remodeling of the injured myocardium. Treating physicians must also identify the cause of the disease while aiming for risk reduction and lifestyle modification.

In addition to percutaneous coronary intervention (PCI) and revascularization by coronary artery bypass grafting, there are several pharmacological options used

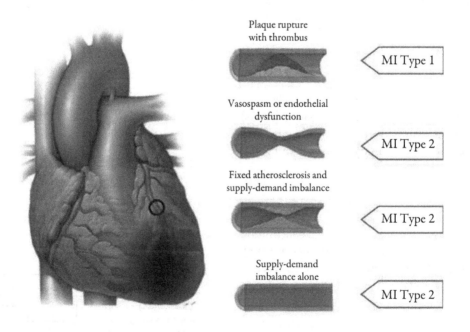

**Figure 116.2** Differentiation between myocardial infarction (MI) types 1 and 2 according to the condition of the coronary arteries. Reprinted with permission from Thygesen K, Alpert JS, Jaffe AS, et al. Writing Group on behalf of the Joint European Society of Cardiology (ESC)/ACC/AHA/WHF Task Force for the Universal Definition of Myocardial Infarction. Third Universal Definition of MI (2012). *Circulation.* 2012; 126:2020–2035.

for reduction of symptoms and progression of the disease. They include antiplatelet drugs (e.g., aspirin), nitrates, β-blockers, calcium channel blockers, angiotensin-converting enzyme inhibitors, and angiotensin receptor blockers. The β-blockers are the only drugs that have shown a decrease in mortality and myocardial reinfarction.[1]

## ANESTHETIC CONSIDERATIONS

### PREOPERATIVE

#### Risk Assessment

Preoperatively, patients should have their perioperative risks assessed, and if time permits, these should be optimized. Multiple scoring systems are available to predict major adverse cardiac events (MACEs). Lee's Revised Cardiac Risk Index (RCRI) is a simple and widely used scoring system that predicts risks of MACE based on the presence of six independent factors (Box 116.1).

Other important risk factors include recent MI, recent revascularization with coronary stents, elevated preoperative cTn, valvular disease, decompensated heart failure, and arrthythmias.[3]

The RCRI was incorporated into the 2014 American Heart Association/American College of Cardiology (ACC/AHA) guidelines for perioperative cardiovascular evaluations for noncardiac surgery, where patients are categorized into two groups: low risk and elevated risk. It is important to note that patients with two or more RCRI risk factors are considered to be at elevated risk (i.e., having more than a 1% chance of MACE during the perioperative period of noncardiac surgery).[1,3]

### Optimization

The main goal of the preoperative stratification according to the ACC/AHA algorithm is to identify patients at increased risk and manage them pharmacologically or through interventions that lessen the risk or severity of perioperative cardiac events. These could include surgical revascularization, revascularization by PCI, and optimal medical management.[1]

- Noninvasive cardiac stress testing: According to the 2014 AHA/ACC guidelines, preoperative stress testing is indicated if[3]
  - Surgery is elective.
  - The patient has poor functional capacity.
  - The patient has elevated perioperative risk of MACEs.
  - Testing will impact the decision for perioperative care.
- Coronary revascularization: Indications for revascularization in the perioperative setting are the same as outside the perioperative setting. There is no benefit from prophylactic revascularization in patients with stable coronary artery disease.[3] If patients undergo revascularization/reperfusion, they are in significantly higher risk of perioperative MACEs, and their surgery should be delayed[1,3] (Table 116.1).

---

**Box 116.1** CARDIAC RISK FACTORS IN PATIENTS UNDERGOING ELECTIVE MAJOR NONCARDIAC SURGERY

1. High-risk surgery
   Abdominal aortic aneurysm
   Peripheral vascular operation
   Thoracotomy
   Major abdominal operation
2. Ischemic heart disease
   History of myocardial infarction
   History of a positive finding on exercise testing
   Current complaints of angina pectoris
   Use of nitrate therapy
   Presence of Q waves on ECG
3. Congestive heart failure
   History of congestive heart failure
   History of pulmonary edema
   History of paroxysmal nocturnal dyspnea
   Physical examination showing rales or $S_3$ gallop
   Chest radiograph showing pulmonary vascular redistribution
4. Cerebrovascular disease
   History of stroke
   History of transient ischemic attack
5. Insulin-dependent diabetes mellitus
6. Preoperative serum creatinine concentration > 2 mg/dL

*Reprinted with permission from Akhtar S. Ischemic Heart Disease. In: Hines RL, Marschall KE. Stoelting's Anesthesia and Co-Existing Disease. 7th ed. Philadelphia: Elsevier; 2018: 79–106.*

---

*Table 116.1* RECOMMENDED TIME INTERVALS TO WAIT FOR ELECTIVE NONCARDIAC SURGERY AFTER CORONARY REVASCULARIZATION

| PROCEDURE | TIME TO WAIT FOR ELECTIVE SURGERY |
|---|---|
| Angioplasty without stenting | 2–4 weeks |
| Bare-metal stent placement | At least 30 days; 12 weeks preferable |
| Coronary artery bypass grafting | At least 6 weeks; 12 weeks preferable |
| Drug-eluting stent placement | At least 12 months |

Reprinted with permission from Akhtar S. Ischemic Heart Disease. In: Hines RL, Marschall KE. *Stoelting's Anesthesia and Co-Existing Disease.* 7th ed. Philadelphia: Elsevier; 2018: 79–106.

- Medication considerations:
  - β-Blockers should be continued by those patients already taking them.
  - Aspirin: For patients who are on aspirin, the decision to continue aspirin should be based on individual risk of perioperative bleeding.
  - Statins: These may reduce the incidence of perioperative MI and should be continued if patients are already on them and could be initiated at least 2 weeks preoperatively in patients undergoing vascular surgery.[3]

## INTRAOPERATIVE

Intraoperative management consists of appropriate monitoring and prevention of the myocardial oxygen supply-demand imbalance. Special attention should be given to identifying and treating intraoperative myocardial ischemia.

### Anesthetic Technique

The majority of evidence suggests there is no difference between general, neuraxial, or regional anesthetic technique.[3]

- Intraoperative monitoring
  - Electrocardiography: The addition of precordial leads to the standard three-lead monitoring increases the sensitivity for detection of ischemia. The ST baseline should be recorded, and any depression or elevation should be treated promptly.
  - Blood pressure (BP) monitoring: Intraoperative hypotension is associated with adverse cardiac events. Severity and duration of hypotension are key determinants of myocardial injury, recognizing that patients with preexisting cardiovascular disease are especially vulnerable. Accurate BP measurement and timely treatment of hypotension (and hypertension) are important in this group of patients, and invasive BP monitoring should be considered.[3,5]
  - Transesophageal echocardiography (TEE): Intraoperative echocardiography detects regional wall motion abnormalities. It requires an experienced operator and is used mostly in response to persistent intraoperative hemodynamic instability.[3]
- Diagnosis of intraoperative ischemia and infarction[3]

Myocardial ischemia is identified by a patient's symptoms and signs or from ECG abnormalities. Symptoms of ischemia may be absent in the perioperative setting where anesthesia and analgesic modalities were administered. Other signs of ischemia include tachycardia, bradycardia, hemodynamic instability, and pulmonary congestion.

ECG criteria to diagnose acute myocardial ischemia require at least two anatomically contiguous leads with the following:

- ST elevation at the J point of at least 1 mm, or
- ST depression of at least 0.5 mm and/or T-wave inversion

Myocardial infarction is defined as myocardial cell death and is diagnosed by a rise of cardiac biomarkers and at least one of the following:

- Symptoms of ischemia.
- New ST segment changes or new left bundle-branch block.
- New pathological Q waves.
- Imaging evidence of new loss of viable myocardium or new regional wall motion abnormality.
- Identification of an intracoronary thrombus by angiography or autopsy.
- OR: Cardiac death with symptoms suggestive of myocardial ischemia.
  - Management of myocardial ischemia[3]
- Confirm diagnosis: Obtain a 12-lead ECG, consider TEE, obtain baseline and 4-hour cTn level.
- Optimize myocardial oxygen supply-and-demand balance: Pause surgery if appropriate while the situation is stabilized and maintain physiologic goals of low/normal heart rate, normal blood pressure, and normal oxygen saturation with the least fraction of inspired oxygen possible and avoid hypothermia and excessive fluid. Administer β-blockers to achieve a low/normal heart rate if BP permits; consider giving aspirin via nasogastric tube and nitroglycerin infusion.
- Obtain cardiology consultation.
- Consider use of intra-aortic balloon pump, abandoning surgery and urgent need for PCI.

## POSTOPERATIVE

Postoperative considerations will depend on intraoperative events and the risk category of the patients. If appropriate, patients should be monitored continuously with telemetry or in an intensive care unit.[3] Avoid postoperative hypotension. Most postoperative MI and myocardial injury after noncardiac surgery occur within 48 hours after surgery. An elevated cTn value within 2 days postoperatively increases perioperative 30-day mortality and 1-year cardiovascular morbidity.[5] Consider serial ECG and cTn.

Maintain good postoperative analgesia, euvolemia, and the addition of β-blockers to minimize tachycardia. Ensure normal oxygen saturation.

Cardiology consultation should guide further therapy.[3]

## REFERENCES

1. Akhtar S. Ischemic heart disease. In: Hines RL, Marschall KE. *Stoelting's Anesthesia and Co-Existing Disease.* 7th ed. Philadelphia, PA: Elsevier; 2018:79–106.
2. Thygesen K, et al. Executive Group on behalf of the Joint European Society of Cardiology (ESC)/ACC/AHA/WHF Task Force for the Universal Definition of Myocardial Infarction. Fourth Universal Definition of MI (2018). *Circulation.* 2018;138:e618–e651.
3. De Hert S, Lurati Buse GA. Cardiac biomarkers for the prediction and detection of adverse cardiac events after noncardiac surgery: a narrative review. *Anesth Analg.* 2020;131:187–195.
4. Short H. Perioperative myocardial ischaemia in non-cardiac surgery. Anaesthesia Tutorial Of The Week by World Federation of Societies of Anaesthesiologists, General anaesthesia, Tutorial 375. March 20, 2018.
5. Ruetzler K, et al. Myocardial injury after noncardiac surgery: preoperative, intraoperative, and postoperative aspects, implications, and directions. *Anesth Analg.* 2020;131:173–186.

# 117.

# CORONARY ARTERY BYPASS PROCEDURES

*Andaleeb A. Ahmed*

## INTRODUCTION

Primary indications for myocardial revascularization, with either coronary artery bypass grafting (CABG) or percutaneous coronary intervention (PCI), are to relieve anginal symptoms and/or improve patient survival. Despite expanding indications for PCI and technical improvement in stent design, CABG remains the mainstay for many patients with multivessel disease. Anatomical complexity of coronary artery disease (CAD) (SYNTAX [synergy between percutaneous coronary intervention with TAXUS and cardiac surgery] score),[1,2] predicted surgical mortality (risk stratification), and anticipated completion of revascularization are some of the crucial factors in deciding revascularization strategy (Figure 117.1).[3]

### ACC/AHA CLASS 1 INDICATIONS FOR CABG

The following are the ACC/AHA class 2 indications for CABG[3]:

- Left main disease greater than 50%
- Three-vessel CAD of greater than 70% with or without proximal left anterior descending coronary artery (LAD) involvement

- Two-vessel disease: LAD plus one other major artery
- One or more significant stenosis greater than 70% in a patient with significant anginal symptoms despite maximal medical therapy
- One-vessel disease greater than 70% in a survivor of sudden cardiac death with ischemia-related ventricular tachycardia

## SURGICAL TECHNIQUE

Standard CABG is performed through a median sternotomy incision and involves the institution of cardiopulmonary bypass (CPB). In addition to on-pump (with CPB) CABG, off-pump CABG, minimally invasive direct CABG, robotic, and hybrid revascularization strategies are increasingly being used. In standard on-pump CABG, vascular conduits (saphenous vein, internal thoracic artery, radial artery, etc.) are grafted between the ascending aorta and coronary artery distal to its obstruction. Once the vascular conduits are chosen and prepared, the patient undergoes CPB. CPB redirects blood to an extracorporeal circuit, allowing the surgeon to operate on a motionless heart with a relatively "bloodless" surgical field. During the period of asystolic arrest, myocardial protection is achieved with hypothermia and intermittent reperfusion of cardioplegia.

| Factors favoring PCI | Factors favoring CABG | Assessment of anatomical complexity of CAD using SYNTAX score. |
|---|---|---|
| • Multivessel disease (SYNTAX < 22)<br>• Severe comorbidities not reflected in EuroSCORE II and STS model<br>• Reduced life expectency, fraility, and advanced age.<br>• History of radiation to the chest<br>• Porcelain aorta<br>• Severe scoliosis or thoracic deformity<br>• Lack of conduits limiting complete myocardial revascularization | • Left main disease or complex multivessel disease (SYNTAX < 22)<br>• Diabetes<br>• Reduced left ventricular function (<35%)<br>• Contraindications to dual antiplatelet therapy<br>• Recurrent diffuse stent restenosis<br>• Severe coronary artery calcification<br>• Indication for concomitant heart surgery<br>• Predicted inability to achieve complete revascularization | 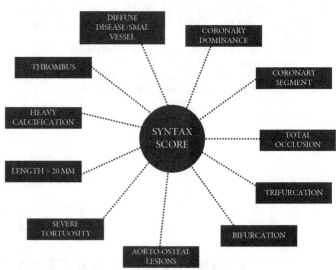 |

Important factors for assessing revascularization strategy

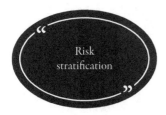 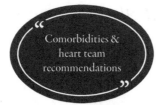 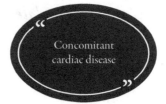 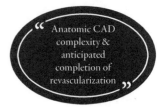

**Figure 117.1** Top left: List of clinical factors favoring PCI and CABG. Top right: Anatomical assessment of CAD using SYNTAX scoring[1]. Bottom panel: The important factors for assessing revascularization strategy (PCI vs. CABG). CABG, coronary artery bypass grafting; PCI, percutaneous coronary intervention; SYNTAX, synergy between percutaneous coronary intervention with TAXUS and cardiac surgery.

The period of CABG is divided into three stages: (1) pre-CPB; (2) CPB; and (3) post-CPB.

## ANESTHETIC CONSIDERATIONS

### PRE–CARDIOPULMONARY BYPASS PERIOD

The pre-CPB period consists of skin incision, median sternotomy, harvesting of the left internal thoracic/internal mammary artery and saphenous vein grafts, and cannulation. For standard on-pump CABG, the most common sites of cannulation are the ascending aorta and right atrium. The primary anesthetic goal during the pre-CPB period is to maintain coronary perfusion pressure and avoid of tachycardia (Figure 117.2). Tight glycemic control and prevention, recognition, and treatment of myocardial ischemia are of paramount importance. High-risk preoperative characteristics include the following:

• Advanced age
• Active ischemia/infarction

• Severe left ventricular dysfunction (ejection fraction < 30%)
• Left main/proximal LAD lesion
• Reoperative cardiac surgery
• Emergent CABG
• Cardiogenic shock
• Significant valvular heart disease
• Aortic calcification
• Stroke with neurological deficits

Monitoring for the CABG procedure includes standard American Society of Anesthesiologists monitors, continuous electrocardiography, arterial blood pressure monitoring, central venous pressure and transesophageal echocardiography (TEE). Routine pulmonary artery catheter (PAC) placement is unnecessary, and the decision to place a PAC should be individualized. General anesthesia can be induced using a variety of agents, provided tachycardia, hypotension, and hypertension can be avoided. Small doses of short-acting narcotics (like fentanyl) with induction agents like propofol and etomidate are typically used for induction. Vasopressors like phenylephrine and

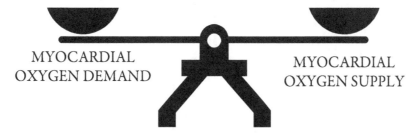

WALL STRESS: $\dfrac{\text{PRESSURE X RADIUS}}{2 \text{ X WALL THICKNESS}}$

- CORONARY BLOOD FLOW
  - DIASTOLIC PRESSURE
  - LV END-DIASTOLIC PRESSURE
  - DIASTOLIC TIME
  - COLLATERALS, CAPILLARY DENSITY
- OXYGEN (O2) CONTENT
  - HEMOGLOBIN (HB)
  - ARTERIAL O2 SATURATION
- O2 EXTRACTION/HB-O2 DISSOCIATION CURVE

- PRELOAD
- AFTERLOAD

- HEART RATE
- CONTRACTILITY

MYOCARDIAL OXYGEN DEMAND

MYOCARDIAL OXYGEN SUPPLY

DETERMINANTS OF MYOCARDIAL OXYGEN BALANCE

**Figure 117.2** Determinants of myocardial oxygen balance. LV, left ventricle.

ephedrine should be readily available to counteract hypotension. After securing the airway, central venous access is obtained, typically through the right internal jugular vein. Prior to cannulation, the patient is anticoagulated with intravenous unfractionated heparin (usual initial dose 300 units/kg). The heparin dose is titrated to achieve an activated clotting time (ACT) goal of more than 400 seconds. Important events in the pre-CPB and post-CPB periods are summarized in Table 117.1.

## CARDIOPULMONARY BYPASS PERIOD

The CPB period simulates the heart and lung by draining deoxygenated caval blood from the patient, oxygenating and eliminating carbon dioxide, and returning blood to the patient's arterial circulation. The elements of a CPB circuit are shown in Figure 117.3. Once CPB is initiated, aortic cross-clamping is applied, and the cardioplegia solution is

*Table 117.1* IMPORTANT EVENTS IN THE PRE-CPB AND POST-CPB PERIODS

| EVENT | IMPLICATION | ACTION |
|---|---|---|
| - Sternotomy | - Risk of lung/right ventricular injury with sternal saw<br>- Higher risk of injury during redo cardiac surgery | - Pause mechanical ventilation<br>- Banked blood readily available |
| - Sternal retraction and harvesting of left internal thoracic artery (ITA) | - Period of low stimulation<br>- May impair functioning of ipsilateral catheters | - Avoid hypotension and myocardial ischemia<br>- Check arterial/venous catheters |
| - Saphenous vein harvest | - Risk of venous gas embolism (if $CO_2$ is used) | - Monitor with TEE |
| - Papaverine use with ITA<br>- Clamping of ITA | - Hypotension<br>- Thrombosis of harvested ITA | - Watch<br>- Intravenous heparin |
| - Arterial and venous cannulation | - Risk of aortic dissection<br>- Risk of arrhythmias | - Avoid hypertension during aortic cannulation<br>- Defibrillation/cardioversion with internal paddles<br>- Ensure full heparinization and adequate ACT |
| - "Retrograde prime" (if used) | - Risk of severe hypotension | - Support blood pressure with vasopressors |

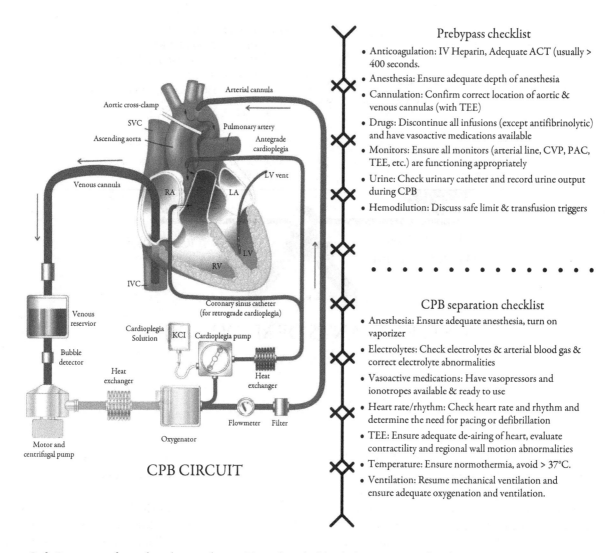

**Prebypass checklist**

- Anticoagulation: IV Heparin, Adequate ACT (usually > 400 seconds.
- Anesthesia: Ensure adequate depth of anesthesia
- Cannulation: Confirm correct location of aortic & venous cannulas (with TEE)
- Drugs: Discontinue all infusions (except antifibrinolytic) and have vasoactive medications available
- Monitors: Ensure all monitors (arterial line, CVP, PAC, TEE, etc.) are functioning appropriately
- Urine: Check urinary catheter and record urine output during CPB
- Hemodilution: Discuss safe limit & transfusion triggers

**CPB separation checklist**

- Anesthesia: Ensure adequate anesthesia, turn on vaporizer
- Electrolytes: Check electrolytes & arterial blood gas & correct electrolyte abnormalities
- Vasoactive medications: Have vasopressors and ionotropes available & ready to use
- Heart rate/rhythm: Check heart rate and rhythm and determine the need for pacing or defibrillation
- TEE: Ensure adequate de-airing of heart, evaluate contractility and regional wall motion abnormalities
- Temperature: Ensure normothermia, avoid > 37°C.
- Ventilation: Resume mechanical ventilation and ensure adequate oxygenation and ventilation.

**CPB CIRCUIT**

**Figure 117.3** Left: Basic circuit for cardiopulmonary bypass. Top right: Checklist before initiation of cardiopulmonary bypass (CPB). Bottom right: Checklist before weaning CPB. ACT, activated clotting time; CVP, central venous pressure; IVC, inferior vena cava; LA, left atrium; LV, left ventricle; PAC, pulmonary artery catheter; RA, right atrium; RV, right ventricle; SVC, superior vena cava; TEE, transesophageal echocardiography.

administered through catheters in the aortic root (antegrade) or coronary sinus (retrograde). Cardioplegia provides myocardial protection by reducing myocardial metabolic demand and ensures a motionless heart by inducing diastolic arrest. Proximal and distal anastomoses are performed during CPB.

## POST-CARDIOPULMONARY BYPASS PERIOD

After anastomoses of vascular conduits, the grafts are checked, and the patient is prepared for separation from CPB. The heart is filled with blood, air is evacuated, and the aortic cross-clamp is removed. Epicardial pacing leads are placed, and CBP is then gradually weaned off. The heart is decannulated, and protamine is administered for heparin reversal. After the placement of mediastinal drains, the sternum is approximated with sternal wires, the

incision is closed, and the patient is transferred to the intensive care unit.

## REFERENCES

1. Morice MC, et al. Outcomes in patients with de novo left main disease treated with either percutaneous coronary intervention using paclitaxel-eluting stents or coronary artery bypass graft treatment in the Synergy Between Percutaneous Coronary Intervention with TAXUS and Cardiac Surgery (SYNTAX) trial. *Circulation.* 2010;121(24):2645–2653.
2. Nashef SA, et al. EuroSCORE II. *Eur J Cardiothorac Surg.* 2012;41(4):734–745.
3. Hillis LD, et al. 2011 ACCF/AHA guideline for coronary artery bypass graft surgery: executive summary: a report of the American College of Cardiology Foundation/American Heart Association Task Force on Practice Guidelines. *Circulation.* 2011;124(23):2610–2642.
4. Shahian DM, et al. The Society of Thoracic Surgeons 2008 cardiac surgery risk models: part 3—valve plus coronary artery bypass grafting surgery. *Ann Thorac Surg.* 2009;88(1 suppl):S43–S62.

# 118.

# VALVULAR HEART DISEASE

*Michael Morkos and Matthew McConnell*

## INTRODUCTION

The heart can largely be thought of as two separate circuits arranged in parallel. The central venous system supplies the right side of the heart, which feeds into the pulmonary vasculature. The blood then returns to the left side of the heart, which functions to provide continuous blood flow to the systemic vasculature. Four valves are involved throughout this process, functioning to preserve pressure gradients and allow for continual forward flow.

## AORTIC STENOSIS

Aortic stenosis (AS) is the most common valvular lesion in the United States.[1] It can be subvalvular, valvular, or supravalvular, with valvular being the most common. Two primary etiologic factors are associated with higher risk for AS: aging, which results in leaflet calcification, and a bicuspid aortic valve, which promotes early-onset fibrosis and aortic root dilation (Figure 118.1). Rheumatic AS is usually associated with mitral valve involvement.

The stenotic lesion decreases the aortic valve area (normally 3–4 cm$^2$) necessary to eject an adequate stroke volume, leading to systemic signs, including dyspnea, angina, and syncopal episodes. Severe aortic stenosis is characterized by a valve area less than 0.8 cm$^2$, transvalvular pressure gradients greater than 40 mm Hg, and jet velocity greater than 4.0 m/s.[1,2] The diagnosis carries a significant risk of sudden death as a result of cardiac arrhythmias.

The majority of patients with AS are asymptomatic. Auscultation reveals a systolic murmur over the right sternal border with radiation to the carotid artery. Diagnosis is confirmed by echocardiography, which is also used to evaluate severity of disease and the need for an aortic valve replacement.

Asymptomatic patients are medically managed, although periodic physical examinations are needed to monitor severity. Once symptoms develop (dyspnea, syncope, angina), aortic valve replacement is recommended to provide a drastic improvement in symptoms and quality of life. The last decade has seen an emergence of transcatheter aortic valve replacement (TAVR) in patients considered "high risk" for surgery. Candidates

## Valvular heart disease

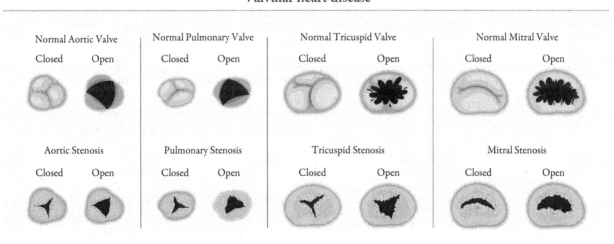

**Figure 118.1** Demonstration of the valvular orifice seen in a normal valves in comparison to a stenotic lesion of the aortic, mitral, tricuspid, and pulmonary valves.

for TAVR must have a tricuspid aortic valve, New York Heart Association 2 or greater and have severe/symptomatic AS creating unsafe conditions to initiate and maintain general anesthesia.

## ANESTHETIC MANAGEMENT

Elucidating symptom severity is crucial due to the increased risk of perioperative complications.[2] A recent electrocardiogram (ECG) and echo reading should be reviewed. Induction may be accomplished with an opioid in cases with diminished left ventricular function.[2] Maintenance of anesthesia may be provided by a combination of inhalation agents, opioids, and nitrous oxide in an attempt to maintain systemic vascular resistance (SVR).[2] In particular, patients with severe AS may benefit from an opioid-centered anesthetic approach to maintain SVR, which they heavily rely on for adequate systemic perfusion. Intraoperative monitoring of AS requires standard American Society of Anesthesiologists monitoring. Additional modalities are typically used, including an arterial line, central venous catheter, pulmonary artery catheter, and transesophageal echo. Hemodynamic goals are listed in Box 118.1. Many comorbidities exist in association with AS, which need close intraoperative monitoring.

## AORTIC INSUFFICIENCY

Aortic insufficiency (AI) causes regurgitation of a portion of the stroke volume during diastole due to improper leaflet coaptation. The most common causes include rheumatic heart disease, infective endocarditis, bicuspid aortic valve, and aortic root pathology.[1]

A diastolic murmur may be heard along the right sternal border along with widened pulse pressure, bounding pulses, and a decreased diastolic pressure. Symptoms may be absent until severe pathology is present. The most common etiology is left ventricular failure, which may be observed on echocardiography.[2]

Treatment is centered on surgical valve replacement before left ventricular failure becomes permanent. A useful indicator of declining ventricular function is an ejection fraction decrease below 55%.[2] Surgery is urgent in symptomatic patients in particular as these patients have a 10% annual mortality rate due to heart failure complications.

---

Box 118.1 HEMODYNAMIC GOALS FOR
AORTIC STENOSIS

- Avoid hypotension
- Avoid abrupt increases in systemic vascular resistance
- Optimize intravascular volume
- Avoid bradycardia and tachycardia

---

Box 118.2 HEMODYNAMIC GOALS FOR AORTIC
INSUFFICIENCY

- Avoid bradycardia
- Avoid drastic increases in systemic vascular resistance
- Avoid myocardial depression

---

## ANESTHETIC MANAGEMENT

The anesthetic plan is devised to ensure forward flow of stroke volume. This is best designed by decreasing time spent in diastole and decreasing the pressure gradient across the valve.[2] Maintaining an elevated heart rate aids in preventing left ventricular overload leading to ischemic changes. Induction may be achieved using a combination of volatile agents, opioids, and nitrous oxide. Volatile agents provide a layer of cardioprotection by decreasing the afterload experienced by the contracting left ventricle, thereby reducing oxygen requirements of the heart.[2] In cases with significant left ventricular dysfunction, an anesthetic heavily dependent on opioids may be preferred. Hemodynamic goals are described in Box 118.2.

## MITRAL STENOSIS

Mitral stenosis (MS) is infrequently encountered in the United States due to the decreased incidence of rheumatic fever, a primary etiology of MS. The lesion progresses slowly, with patients often remaining asymptomatic for the initial 20–30 years, until calcification of the leaflets and annulus diminish the valve area from 4–6 cm$^2$ to 1.5 cm$^2$ or less, as seen in Figure 118.1.[1] The left atrium is initially able to compensate for the increase in volume with a likewise increase in pressure to maintain left ventricular stroke volume. Atrial fibrillation is a concern in this patient population as a result of left atrial dilation. As the leaflets continue to fuse, pressure begins to accumulate in the pulmonary vasculature, resulting in pleural edema, shortness of breath, and dyspnea on exertion.[2]

Proper diagnosis requires echocardiography to evaluate the extent of leaflet mobility, transvalvular pressure gradient, and valve area. It is routine to assess chamber dimensions and pulmonary pressures and evaluate for possible thrombus formation in the left atrium.

## ANESTHETIC MANAGEMENT

Providing anesthesia requires vigilance in preventing pulmonary edema and tachycardia, which results in a decrease in cardiac output. Nearly all anesthetics may be used, with the exception of ketamine due to its tendency to increase heart rate. If atrial fibrillation develops acutely, attempts to revert to normal sinus rhythm using amiodarone, β-blockers, calcium channel blockers, or cardioversion if the patient is hemodynamically unstable should be attempted.[3] In cases with preexisting atrial fibrillation, it is often difficult to convert to normal sinus rhythm. Due to elevated pulmonary pressures, it is prudent to avoid hypoxia and hypercarbia, which may exacerbate preexisting pulmonary hypertension. Postoperatively, hemodynamic status should continue to be evaluated due to the continued risk of pulmonary edema resulting in right heart failure.

## MITRAL REGURGITATION

Mitral regurgitation is one of the most common valvular pathologies in the United States. It usually occurs secondary to ischemic heart disease, annular dilation, and disease of the chordae tendineae/papillary muscle.

Similar to aortic regurgitation, a portion of the volume ejected into the left ventricle is returned to the left atrium, causing volume and pressure overload. The following contraction ejects a larger volume of blood, eventually causing remodeling of the left ventricle into a larger and more compliant chamber. The left atrium also expands due to the larger volume experienced during diastole. Determinants of severity include area of the mitral valve orifice, transvalvular pressure gradient, and the heart rate.[2,3]

Mitral regurgitation is often heard as a holosystolic murmur radiating to the axilla. ECG and chest x-ray may show signs consistent with enlargement of the left atrium and left ventricle. Echocardiography is used to confirm the cause and severity of the lesion, as well as to assess chamber volume, pressure, and ventricular function. Color flow, pulsed wave Doppler, and three-dimensional imaging may prove to be useful in determining regurgitant volume and area of the regurgitant jet.

### ANESTHETIC MANAGEMENT

For anesthetic management, focus on sustaining forward flow by elevating heart rate to reduce time spent in diastole. Induction may be done with intravenous anesthetics while avoiding bradycardia.[3] Volatile agents are ideal for maintenance of anesthesia due to the reduction in SVR with an increase in heart rate.

## TRICUSPID REGURGITATION

The tricuspid valve is the largest valve of the heart and contains three leaflets (septal, anterior, and posterior). The pathology of the leaflets or annulus may contribute to tricuspid regurgitation, with annular dilation being the most common culprit.[1] Many other causes must be considered, including rheumatic heart disease, endocarditis, carcinoid syndrome, infarction, and tumors preventing coaptation of the leaflets. On evaluation, patients will typically have symptoms of fatigue, peripheral edema, and possibly atrial fibrillation due to enlargement of the right atrium.[1]

Diagnosis is made with echocardiography, using color Doppler to determine regurgitant jet size, orifice diameter, and area of the valve annulus to define mild, moderate, or severe pathology. In the setting of severe regurgitation, there is a high likelihood of associated liver damage as a result of hepatic venous congestion.[2,3] The valve may be replaced with a prosthetic valve or repaired with ring annuloplasty under cardiopulmonary bypass.

## TRICUSPID STENOSIS

In general, tricuspid stenosis is less frequently encountered than regurgitation. The majority of cases are attributed to rheumatic fever, although radiation, systemic lupus erythematosus, and carcinoid syndrome are also causes.

Echocardiographic diagnosis is definitive. Color flow Doppler shows a high-velocity jet and turbulent flow into the right ventricle (Figure 118.1). Anesthesiologists may determine hemodyncamically severe TR by measuring a pressure gradient of 5 mm Hg or greater, valve area of 1 cm$^2$ or less, and an inflow time-velocity integral greater than 60 cm.[2,3]

Replacement of the valve in this patient population is performed only in symptomatic cases (fatigue, hepatomegaly, ascites) or severely stenotic valves.

## PULMONIC REGURGITATION

The pulmonic valve is a semilunar valve of the heart composed of three leaflets (anterior, right, and left) that serve as a bridge between the right ventricular outflow tract and the pulmonary vasculature. Transthoracic echocardiography provides the best imaging as it is the most anterior of the four valves. The most common etiology of pulmonic regurgitation is pulmonary hypertension resulting in right ventricular enlargement.[3] The vast majority of patients remain asymptomatic, but if the regurgitation is severe, it may present with signs of right heart failure.

## PULMONIC STENOSIS

Stenotic lesions of the pulmonary valve are most frequently encountered as congenital malformations in tetralogy of Fallot.[1] Adult pathology is rarely encountered (Figure 118.1) but is often seen in association with 5-hydroxyindoleacetic acid release from carcinoid tumors. Surgical correction is reserved for symptomatic patients exhibiting signs of syncopal episodes, dyspnea, or right-sided heart failure.

## SUBACUTE BACTERIAL ENDOCARDITIS PROPHYLAXIS

Antibiotic prophylaxis is recommended in patients with certain structural heart disease (Box 118.3) to prevent infective endocarditis. The most common antibiotic used is 2 g oral amoxicillin 30–60 minutes before the start of the procedure involving manipulation of gingival or respiratory tract tissue.[3] Prophylaxis is not required for gastrointestinal or genitourinary procedures.

---

**Box 118.3 PATIENTS REQUIRING INFECTIVE ENDOCARDITIS PROPHYLAXIS**

- Prosthetic heart valve (including transcatheter prosthetic valves and annuloplasty rings)
- History of infective endocarditis
- Unrepaired cyanotic congenital heart disease
- Congenital heart disease repaired within the last 6 months
- Congenital heart disease with adjacent structural defect
- Heart transplant with resultant valvular pathology

---

## REFERENCES

1. Frogel J, Dragos G. Anesthetic considerations for patients with advanced valvular heart disease undergoing noncardiac surgery. *Anesthesiol Clin.* 2010;28:67–85.
2. Mittnacht AJ, et al. Anesthetic considerations in the patient with valvular heart disease undergoing noncardiac surgery. *Semin Chardiothorac Vasc Anesth.* 2008;12:33–59.
3. Shipton B, Wahba H. Valvular heart disease: review and update. *Am Fam Physician.* 2001;63:2201–2209.
4. Nishimura RA, et al. 2017AHA/ACC focused update of the 2014 AHA/ACC guideline for the management of patients with valvular heart disease: a report of the American College of Cardiology/American Heart Association Task Force on Clinical Practice Guidelines. Circulation. 2017;135:e1159–e1195.

# 119.

## SUBACUTE BACTERIAL ENDOCARDITIS PROPHYLAXIS

*Melissa Anne Burger and Todd Everett Jones*

### INTRODUCTION

Subacute bacterial endocarditis (SBE) occurs when bacteria adhere to the surface of damaged endothelium of cardiac valves, leading to an indolent but progressive infection that may become fulminant, with high morbidity and mortality.[1] Bacteria cannot easily adhere to normal valvular endothelium. However, in the setting of endothelial damage or "jet lesions" due to turbulent blood flow, chronic inflammation due to degenerative or rheumatic valvular disease, or artificial heart valves, circulating bacteria may adhere to fibrinous deposits or thrombi on the valves and proliferate to form vegetations.[2,3]

In theory, antibiotic prophylaxis during procedures that cause transient bacteremia could prevent the development of SBE and thereby reduce the need for treatment of a potentially lethal disease with prolonged courses of antibiotic therapy or curative surgery. Animal models have demonstrated that antibiotic administration can reduce the development of endocarditis following injection of pathogenic bacteria after traumatization of heart valves.[2] Thus, by extension, it had been assumed that humans, particularly those with prosthetic valves or valvular disease, would benefit from antibiotic prophylaxis during gastrointestinal, genitourinary, or dental procedures, which are most likely to generate bacteremia with pathogens more commonly responsible for SBE.[3] However, most human studies evaluating the efficacy of antibiotic prophylaxis showed a reduction of bacteremia as the endpoint but did not evaluate if this reduced development of infective endocarditis.

In reality, daily activities such as eating or brushing teeth are more likely to be the source of SBE as they produce more transient bacteremia than dental work or more invasive gastrointestinal or genitourinary procedures. Guidelines now emphasize the importance of good daily oral hygiene and routine professional cleaning and care.[1–3] Antibiotic prophylaxis likely prevents a vanishingly small percentage of cases of SBE, and this benefit is outweighed by antibiotic-related adverse events when considered over a large population. For these reasons, the American College of Cardiology and American Heart Association (ACC/AHA) guidelines for SBE prophylaxis underwent significant revisions in 2007, and these changes were reiterated in the most recent 2017 guidelines.[1,2] Antibiotic prophylaxis is no longer recommended for low- and moderate-risk patients.

## ANESTHETIC CONSIDERATIONS: PREOPERATIVE ASSESSMENT OF RISK

The need for SBE prophylaxis is determined based on the patient's risk stratification and the type of procedure being performed. Antibiotics are now reserved for only high-risk patients. This includes patients with the following[1]:

1. Prosthetic cardiac valves, including transcatheter-implanted prostheses and homografts
2. Prosthetic material used for cardiac valve repair, such as annuloplasty rings and chords
3. Previous infective endocarditis
4. Unrepaired cyanotic congenital heart disease or repaired congenital heart disease, with residual shunts or valvular regurgitation at the site of, or adjacent to the site of, a prosthetic patch or prosthetic device
5. Cardiac transplant with valve regurgitation attributed to a structurally abnormal valve

The highest risk of bacteremia that may lead to SBE is associated with invasive dental procedures.[1,2] Prophylaxis should be given for routine dental cleanings as well as any dental work involving manipulation of gingival tissues or the periapical region of teeth or perforation of the oral mucosa, including tooth extractions or drainage of dental abscesses in high-risk patients. A significant change in the 2007 AHA/ACC guidelines was the elimination of the recommendation for dental prophylaxis in low- or moderate-risk patients. Prophylaxis is not recommended in cases of trauma to the lips or oral mucosa.[2]

High-risk patients should receive prophylaxis for procedures involving the incision or biopsy of the respiratory tract mucosa, such as tonsillectomy and adenoidectomy or bronchoscopy with a biopsy but not bronchoscopy alone. Prophylaxis should be given for procedures involving infected skin, skin structures, or musculoskeletal tissue.[1,2]

Subacute bacterial endocarditis prophylaxis is *not* recommended for procedures of the gastrointestinal or genitourinary tract, such as esophagogastroduodenoscopy, colonoscopy, cystoscopy, or transesophageal echocardiography, in the absence of active infection.[1,2]

The AHA does not recommend that high-risk patients receive SBE prophylaxis during labor and vaginal delivery.[2] However, based on level B evidence, the American College of Obstetricians and Gynecologists (ACOG) recommends SBE prophylaxis 30 minutes prior to delivery for patients at the highest risk of infective endocarditis, specifically those with cyanotic cardiac disease, prosthetic valves, or both. ACOG does not recommend SBE prophylaxis prior to vaginal delivery for women with acquired or congenital structural heart disease unless infection is present. Patients undergoing a cesarean delivery or an obstetric anal sphincter repair should receive the same antimicrobial prophylaxis as those not at risk for SBE as the standard antibiotic dose will simultaneously protect against SBE.[4]

## ANESTHETIC CONSIDERATIONS: ANTIBIOTIC SELECTION

*Streptococcus viridans* is the most likely pathogen to cause SBE following invasive dental or respiratory procedures and thus is the primary target of antibiotic prophylaxis.[5] If active infection is present, antibiotic selection should also cover *Staphylococcus aureus,* with consideration for the patient's risk of methicillin-resistant *S. aureus* (MRSA).

Antibiotic selection is based on the patient's ability to take oral medication and any allergy to penicillin (Figure 119.1).[2] For most adult patients, a single oral dose of amoxicillin 2 g can be given 30 to 60 minutes prior to incision. For penicillin-allergic adults, a single oral dose of cephalexin 2 g, oral clindamycin 600 mg, or oral clarithromycin 500 mg may be substituted. For adult patients unable to tolerate oral medication, ampicillin 2 g IV or IM, cefazolin 1 g IV or IM, or ceftriaxone 1 g IV or IM may be given. If the patient is allergic to penicillin and unable to tolerate oral medication, an intravenous or intramuscular dose of cefazolin 1 g, ceftriaxone 1 g, or clindamycin 600 mg may be used. Cephalosporins should not be given if there is a history of anaphylaxis, angioedema, or urticarial reaction following any type of penicillin.

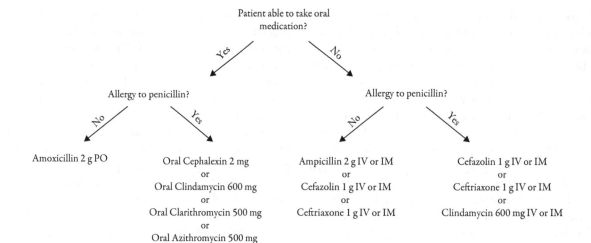

**Figure 119.1**

# REFERENCES

1. Nishimura RA, et al. 2017 AHA/ACC focused update of the 2014 AHA/ACC guideline for the management of patients with valvular heart disease: a report of the American College of Cardiology/ American Heart Association Task Force on Clinical Practice Guidelines. *Circulation*. 2017;135(25):e1159–e1195.
2. Wilson W, et al. Prevention of infective endocarditis: guidelines from the American Heart Association: a guideline from the American Heart Association Rheumatic Fever, Endocarditis, and Kawasaki Disease Committee, Council on Cardiovascular Disease in the Young, and the Council on Clinical Cardiology, Council on Cardiovascular Surgery and Anesthesia, and the Quality of Care and Outcomes Research Interdisciplinary Working Group. *Circulation*. 2007;116(15):1736–1754.
3. Habib G, et al. Guidelines on the prevention, diagnosis, and treatment of infective endocarditis (new version 2009): the Task Force on the Prevention, Diagnosis, and Treatment of Infective Endocarditis of the European Society of Cardiology (ESC). *Eur Heart J*. 2009;30(19):2369–2413.
4. Committee on Practice Bulletins-Obstetrics. ACOG Practice Bulletin No. 199: use of prophylactic antibiotics in labor and delivery. *Obstet Gynecol*. 2018;132(3):e103–e119.
5. Baddour LM, et al. Infective endocarditis in adults: diagnosis, antimicrobial therapy, and management of complications: a scientific statement for healthcare professionals from the American Heart Association. *Circulation*. 2015;132(15):1435–1486.

# 120.

# CONDUCTION ABNORMALITIES AND RHYTHM DEFECTS

*Ellyn Gray and Archit Sharma*

## PERIOPERATIVE ARRHYTHMIAS

*Etiology*: The causes of these conduction abnormalities can be reversible, with etiologies including the following:

- Underlying structural myocardial disease
- Neurohormonal factors and catecholamine imbalance
- Electrolyte abnormalities: hypokalemia and hypomagnesemia
- Drug toxicities: sympathomimetic drugs, QT-prolonging medications, diuretics
- Hypothermia
- Myocardial hypoperfusion.
- Valve abnormalities or surgical interventions

*Diagnosis* of all of these arrhythmias involves obtaining a 12-lead electrocardiogram (ECG) at minimum and evaluation by a clinician. Further abnormalities might trigger further evaluation in the form of echocardiography and coronary angiography.

*Bradyarrhythmias* are the result of inadequate firing of the sinoatrial (SA) node or impaired conduction of electrical signals traveling from the atrium to the ventricles.[1]

1. *Sinus bradycardia* refers to a very slow heart rate of less than 60 beats per minute and can be secondary to age, ischemia, sinus node dysfunction, and certain medications, such as parasympathetic agents and β-blockers. Symptoms include lightheadedness, presyncope, worsening angina, and exercise intolerance.
2. *Sick sinus syndrome* is a group of abnormal rhythms caused by the SA node firing too slowly, having periods of asystole, and occasionally periods of atrial tachycardia. The etiology is the same as sinus bradycardia, and symptoms include lightheadedness, presyncope, worsening angina, and exercise intolerance.
3. *Atrioventricular (AV) blocks* involve slowed, incomplete, or failure of conduction through the AV conduction system. These can be caused by to ischemic heart disease, myocarditis, congenital heart disease, hereditary or familial AV blocks (Lenegre disease), electrolyte imbalance, and endocrine abnormalities such as hypothyroidism. The presentation consists of the patient complaining of lightheadedness, presyncope, worsening angina, and exercise intolerance.
   *First-degree AV block* is diagnosed by a prolonged PR interval (greater than 200 ms).
   *Second-degree AV block*: There are two types of second-degree AV block.
   *Mobitz I*, also known as *Wenckebach*, is marked by a PR interval that progressively lengthens with each subsequent beat until there is a QRS interval that does not follow the P wave.
   *Mobitz II* has a constant PR interval with intermittent dropped QRS complexes (nonconducting beats).
   *Third-degree AV block*, also known as complete heart block, involves failure of conduction through the AV junction with complete atrial and ventricular dissociation. Figure 120.1 depicts the ECG representation of these conduction abnormalities.
4. *Bundle-branch blocks (BBB)* are another AV conduction abnormality that cause abnormal ventricular depolarization and a prolonged QRS complex.
   *Right BBBs* present with a QRS duration greater than or equal to 120 ms in adults an rSR′ in V1 (M shape) and S wave of greater duration than R wave or greater than 40 ms in leads I and V6. They can represent a congenital abnormality or underlying heart disease, primarily right heart disease, such as pulmonary embolism and cor pulmonale.
   *Left BBBs* present with a QRS duration greater than or equal to 120 ms in adults; broad notched or slurred R wave in leads I, aVL, V5, and V6; and delayed upstroke in V5 and almost always indicate

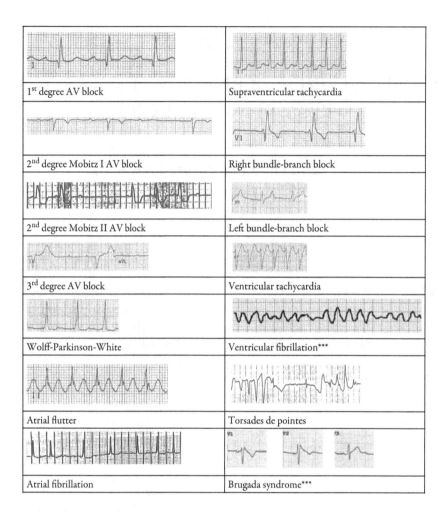

| | |
|---|---|
| 1st degree AV block | Supraventricular tachycardia |
| 2nd degree Mobitz I AV block | Right bundle-branch block |
| 2nd degree Mobitz II AV block | Left bundle-branch block |
| 3rd degree AV block | Ventricular tachycardia |
| Wolff-Parkinson-White | Ventricular fibrillation*** |
| Atrial flutter | Torsades de pointes |
| Atrial fibrillation | Brugada syndrome*** |

**Figure 120.1** Electrocardiographic representation of the conduction abnormalities.

underlying heart disease. They are more common in patients who have had a myocardial infarction, endocarditis, myocarditis, hypertension, and cardiomyopathy. Figure 120.1 depicts the ECG representation of these conduction abnormalities.

Treatment of all these blocks is dependent on the etiology. Based on the etiology, the treatment options include revascularization of the coronaries to counteract ischemia, medical management and decreasing nodal-blocking agents such as β-blockers and calcium channel blockers, and use of temporary and permanent pacemakers for pacing these patients to generate a normal cardiac output or in cases of hemodynamic instability.

## TYPES OF ARRHYTHMIAS

### SUPRAVENTRICULAR ARRHYTHMIAS

Supraventricular tachycardia (SVT) is a broad term for tachyarrhythmias originating above the ventricles (atrial or junctional).[2]

1. *Paroxysmal supraventricular tachycardia (PSVT)* is an abrupt-onset, abrupt-offset, narrow-complex tachycardia. PSVT is part of the narrow QRS complex tachycardias with a regular ventricular response, in contrast to multifocal atrial tachycardia, atrial fibrillation, and atrial flutter. It can occur due to an array of reasons such as hyperthyroidism; increased caffeine consumption; medications (amphetamines, albuterol, cocaine); myocardial infarction; pulmonary embolism; and pericarditis. Treatment includes vagal maneuvers initially and then using adenosine to treat the arrhythmia.

2. *AV node reentrant tachycardia* involves a reentrant conduction circuit within or near the AV node with a slow and fast pathway, with a QRS duration of less than 120 ms. It most commonly causes palpitations and is treated with vagal maneuvers, carotid massage, adenosine, cardioversion, and radio-frequency ablation.

3. *Wolff-Parkinson-White (WPW) syndrome* is a conduction pattern in which there is an accessory pathway through which antegrade signals can propagate, resulting in preexcitation of part of

the ventricles. This results in a slurred upstroke of the QRS complex (delta wave) with a narrow PR interval. The most common form of tachycardia associated with WPW is an AV reentrant tachycardia. Because conduction through the accessory pathway is more rapid than through the AV node, drugs traditionally used to slow conduction through the AV node can have deleterious effects for patients with WPW.

4. *Atrial flutter* is a narrow, complex tachyarrhythmia, characterized by rapid, regular atrial depolarizations at a characteristic rate of approximately 300 beats/min and a regular ventricular rate of about 150 beats/min. It can lead to symptoms of palpitations, shortness of breath, fatigue, or lightheadedness and presents as the characteristic sawtoothed pattern on an ECG. Treatment includes rate control with β-blockers and calcium channel blockers or chemical/electrical cardioversion if unstable.

5. *Atrial fibrillation* presents as an irregularly irregular rhythm, with an irregular R-R interval, with an absence of P waves. Treatment includes rate control with β-blockers and calcium channel blockers or chemical/electrical cardioversion if unstable. In addition to treatment of cardiac arrhythmias with medications, ablation therapy can be used for atrial flutter, atrial fibrillation, paroxysmal supraventricular tachycardia, WPW syndrome, and ventricular tachycardia.[3]

## PREMATURE BEATS

Premature conduction beats can be atrial, junctional, or ventricular in nature. Atrial and junctional premature beats can be secondary to sympathetic stimulation; exogenous stimulants (amphetamines, caffeine); toxins; hyperthyroidism; digoxin toxicity; and atrial stretch. Premature ventricular contractions, particularly when complex (i.e., multifocal or couplets, which are two premature ventricular contractions in a row) may be predictors of more malignant arrhythmias and sudden cardiac death. Treatment includes treating the etiology and ablation in advanced cases.

## VENTRICULAR ARRHYTHMIAS

Ventricular tachyarrhythmias are more life-threatening arrhythmias that can rapidly progress to cardiac arrest.

1. *Ventricular tachycardia* is a regular wide-complex arrhythmia that does not have a discernable P wave before each QRS. They can be caused by ischemic cardiomyopathy, heart failure, dyselectrolytemia, and medications. They can usually lead to palpitations and dizziness and can lead to syncope.

2. *Ventricular fibrillation* features irregularly irregular wide QRS complexes. Treatment includes defibrillation, cardiopulmonary resuscitation, epinephrine, and amiodarone. They can usually lead to palpitations and dizziness and can lead to syncope or cardiac arrest since the fibrillation is a nonperfusing rhythm.

3. *Torsade de pointes* is a ventricular tachyarrhythmia in which polymorphic QRS complexes appear to be twisting around an isoelectric baseline. Treatment includes magnesium and electrical cardioversion.

4. *Brugada syndrome* is an autosomal dominant disorder, more common in men, that presents with ventricular arrhythmias, syncope, and sudden death.[4] The ECG will demonstrate a pseudo–right BBB and ST elevation in V1 to V3, without a wide S wave in the lateral leads. Patients with Brugada syndrome should be evaluated for automated implanted cardioverter-defibrillator (AICD) implantation.

*Treatment*: Most ventricular arrhythmias are managed with the use of medications such as β-blockers, antiarrhythmic agents (amiodarone, sotalol), and in cases of unstable hemodynamics electrical cardioversion. AICDs are placed for primary and secondary prevention of death secondary to cardiac arrest from recurring ventricular arrhythmias. Primary prevention indications include an ejection fraction less than 35%, sustained or unstable ventricular tachyarrhythmias, hypertrophic cardiomyopathy, and a strong family history of sudden cardiac death.[5]

## REFERENCES

1. Vogler J, et al. Bradyarrhythmias and conduction blocks. *Rev Esp Cardiol (Engl Ed)*. 2012;65(7):656–667.
2. DiMarco JP, et al. Diagnostic and therapeutic use of adenosine in patients with supraventricular tachyarrhythmias. *J Am Coll Cardiol*. 1985;6(2):417–425.
3. Calkins H, et al. A new system for catheter ablation of atrial fibrillation. *Am J Cardiol*. 1999;83(5):227–236.
4. Gropper MA, et al. *Miller's Anesthesia*. 2 Vol.. Elsevier Health Sciences; 2019.
5. Madhavan M, et al. Outcomes after implantable cardioverter-defibrillator generator replacement for primary prevention of sudden cardiac death. *Circ Arrhythm Electrophysiol*. 2016;9(3): e003283.

# 121.

# PACEMAKERS AND AUTOMATED IMPLANTABLE CARDIOVERTER/DEFIBRILLATOR (AICD) IMPLANTATION

*Jayakar Guruswamy and Snigdha Parikh*

## INTRODUCTION

Cardiac implantable electronic devices (CIEDs) refer to a permanently implanted cardiac pacemaker, an implantable cardioverter-defibrillator (ICD), or a cardiac resynchronization therapy (CRT) device.[1] Approximately 3 million people in the United States have a pacemaker, and close to 300,000 people have an ICD, making patients with CIEDs a growing population in the perioperative arena. An aging population with increased prevalence of cardiac disease is an important driver for the increased utilization of CIEDs.

## PACEMAKERS

Pacemakers are devices placed for bradyarrhythmias and are the only effective treatment for symptomatic bradycardia. Standard pacemakers have either one or two (atrial and ventricular) leads. Pacing systems consist of an impulse generator and lead(s). Leads can have one (unipolar), two (bipolar), or multiple (multipolar) electrodes. Most pacemaker systems use bipolar, which require less energy and are more resistant to interference.

A patient is pacemaker dependent if they suffer significant symptoms or even experience cardiac arrest on the cessation of pacing. Some of the common indications for permanent pacemaker placement include symptomatic bradyarrhythmias, asymptomatic Mobitz II or greater, sinus node disease, atrioventricular node disease, long QT syndrome, some types of supraventricular tachycardia or ventricular tachycardia (VT), orthotopic heart transplantation, hypertrophic obstructive cardiomyopathy, and dilated cardiomyopathy.[2]

Indications for temporary pacemakers include following cardiac surgery, treatment of drug toxicity resulting in arrhythmias, certain arrhythmias associated with myocardial infarction, permanent generator failure, and cardiac arrest.

Most pacemakers have the capability of varying the pacing rate. In the rate-adaptive mode, the pacemakers sense the patient's level of activity and accordingly adjust the pacing rate using sensors that detect body motion transmitted from underlying muscles or detection of the respiratory rate and/or volume using bioimpedance sensors.

All pacemakers generate a pulse of current to depolarize a small region of the myocardium; the wave then spontaneously spreads to the rest of the myocardium. The pacing capture *threshold* is the minimum current required to pace the atrium/ventricle. *Sensitivity* is the voltage level that must be exceeded to detect a P or R wave; lowering the sensitivity makes the device more sensitive to native P/R waves. *Capture* denotes to the pacing current causing ventricular contraction.

The North American Society of Pacing and Electrophysiology (NASPE) and the British Pacing and Electrophysiology Group (BPEG) initially published a generic pacemaker code (NBG code) in 1987 that was revised in 2002 (see Table 121.1.)[3]

Dual-chamber, adaptive-rate pacing (DDDR), dual-chamber pacing without atrium synchronous ventricular pacing (DDIR), and dual-chamber asynchronous pacing are common perioperative settings. DDDR defines a pacemaker programmed to pace the atrium and/or ventricle, sense the atrium and/or ventricle, inhibit or trigger pacing output in response to a sensed event, and have a rate-responsive sensor that is able to alter paced rates due to changes in perceived metabolic demand; it is commonly used for patients with sick sinus syndrome and/or heart block. DDIR is a common pacing mode for patients with supraventricular tachyarrhythmias (SVTs).

An asynchronous mode or nontracking mode will pace the atrium and ventricle at a set rate, regardless of the

*Table 121.1* NASPE/BPEG GENERIC PACEMAKER CODE (NBG)

| POSITION I | POSITION II | POSITION III | POSITION IV | POSITION V |
|---|---|---|---|---|
| Chambers paced | Chambers sensed | Response to sensing | Programmability | Multisite pacing |
| O = None | O = None | O = None | O = None | O = None |
| A = Atrium | A = Atrium | I = Inhibited | R = Rate modulation | A = Atrium |
| V = Ventricle | V = Ventricle | T = Triggered | | V = Ventricle |
| D = Dual (A + V) | D = Dual (A + V) | D = Dual (T+I) | | D = Dual (A + V) |

underlying rate and rhythm. This is advantageous in order to avoid the pacemaker oversensing the monopolar electrocautery as intrinsic cardiac conduction and inhibit pacing, especially in pacemaker-dependent patients. The point of pacemaker sensing is to avoid R on T. Asynchronous pacing can lead to R on T, which may cause VT or VF. As such, the asynchronous mode should be used only in a monitored setting.

A leadless, intracardiac, ventricular-only pacemaker called the Micra Transcatheter Pacemaker System (Medtronic) is available now that has no magnet response.

## IMPLANTABLE CARDIOVERTER-DEFIBRILLATORS

Implantable cardioverter-defibrillators are implanted in patients for primary or secondary prevention of cardiac arrest. Primary prevention refers to ICD placement for patients who have not had any episodes of ventricular arrhythmias but who are at risk of future events. Secondary prevention refers to ICD placement for patients who have had prior ventricular arrhythmias.[2] There is strong evidence that ICDs implanted for primary prevention improve mortality in high-risk patients compared to optimal medical therapy. ICDs reduce mortality by approximately 30% in patients with ischemic and nonischemic cardiomyopathy compared to antiarrhythmic medical therapy.

The ICDs sense atrial or ventricular electrical activity, classify these signals to various programmed "heart rate zones," deliver tiered therapies to terminate VT or VF, and pace for bradycardia. All modern ICDs are pacemakers, and this has important perioperative applications.

The ICDs measure the R-R interval and categorize these as normal, too fast (short R-R intervals), or too slow (long R-R intervals). When the device detects a sufficient number of short R-R intervals, an antitachycardia event will begin. The device will choose between overdrive pacing and shock. In addition, the ICD will have the capability for antibradycardia pacing when the R-R interval is prolonged.

Inappropriate shocks are common (30% to 50% of all shocks) and are most commonly the result of inappropriate treatment of SVT. Inappropriate shocks are proarrhythmic, can lead to anxiety and depression, and decrease patient quality of life. Discrimination between VT and SVT is critical for ICDs to avoid inappropriate therapy. There are several methods by which ICDs discriminate between SVT and VT, such as *onset criteria* (usually, VT onset is abrupt, whereas SVT onset has sequentially shortening R-R intervals); *stability criteria* (R-R intervals of VT are relatively constant, whereas R-R intervals of AF with rapid ventricular response are quite variable); and *QRS width criteria* (usually, QRS width in SVT is narrow [<110 ms], whereas QRS width in VT is wide [>120 ms]). The sensitivity and specificity for VT detection by QRS morphology is more than 90%.

*Table 121.2* NASPE/BPEG DEFIBRILLATOR CODE

| POSITION I | POSITION II | POSITION III | POSITION IV |
|---|---|---|---|
| Shock chambers | Antitachycardia pacing chambers | Tachycardia detection | Antibradycardia pacing chambers |
| O = None | O = None | E = Electrogram | O = None |
| A = Atrium[1] | A = Atrium | H = Hemodynamic | A = Atrium |
| V = Ventricle | V = Ventricle | | V = Ventricle |
| D = Dual (A + V) | D = Dual (A + V) | | D = Dual (A + V) |

Implantable cardioverter-defibrillators terminate ventricular arrhythmias by either antitachycardia pacing (ATP) or defibrillation. ATP is desirable because it reduces inappropriate shocks, is better tolerated by the patient, utilizes less energy, and prolongs battery life. For VT that is not terminated by ATP or for VF, defibrillation is the treatment of choice.

The NASPE and the BPEG initially published a generic ICD code (NBG code) in 1987 that was revised in 2002 (Table 121.2).[3]

The subcutaneous ICD introduced by Boston Scientific in 2012 is different from the transvenous ICDs in that it cannot provide pacemaker or resynchronization therapy.

## REFERENCES

1. Practice advisory for the perioperative management of patients with cardiac implantable electronic devices: pacemakers and implantable cardioverter–defibrillators 2020: an updated report by the American Society of Anesthesiologists Task Force on Perioperative Management of Patients With Cardiac Implantable Electronic Devices. *Anesthesiology*. 2020;132(2):225–252.
2. Rourke RA, et al. Hurst's *The Heart Manual of Cardiology*, 11th ed.; Epstein AE, et al. ACC/AHA/HRS 2008 *Guidelines for Device-Based Therapy of Cardiac Rhythm Abnormalities*. *Heart Rhythm*. 2008;5(6):e1–e62.
3. Bernstein AD, et al. The revised NASPE/BPEG generic code for antibradycardia, adaptive-rate, and multisite pacing. *J Pacing Clin Electrophysiol*. 2002;25(2):260–264.

# 122.

# PERIOPERATIVE IMPLICATIONS OF PACEMAKERS AND AICDS

*Jayakar Guruswamy and Snigdha Parikh*

## INTRODUCTION

The goal of the perioperative evaluation of a patient with a cardiac implantable electronic device (CIED) consists of determining type of CIED (whether it is a pacemaker [PM] or automated implanted cardioverter-defibrillator [AICD]), manufacturer, primary indication for device placement, current setting of the device, if the patient is device dependent, and the possibility of electromagnetic interference (EMI).

## PREOPERATIVE EVALUATION

Conducting a focused history and physical is an important aspect of anesthesia management for determining whether a patient has a cardiac implantable device.

Obtaining a detailed history of the cardiac implantable device include determining the type of CIED, manufacturer, and primary indication for the placement of the device. This information can be obtained by reviewing the most recent device interrogation report.[1] If this report is not available, obtaining the manufacturer's identification card from the patient can also play a vital role in providing the information. If no other data are available, especially in emergency settings, obtain a chest x-ray as most implantable devices have an x-ray inscribed code on the generator of the device that helps in identification of the device.[2] Also, the presence of a shocking coil in the x-ray helps differentiate a PM from an AICD, as shown in Figure 122.1.

In emergency situations, application of a magnet can help identify devices given the unique consistent magnet response of the devices. For example, a Medtronic device will switch to 85 beats/min and Boston scientific to 100 beats/min.

Determining whether a patient is PM dependent or not is also essential. Reviewing electrocardiographic (ECG)

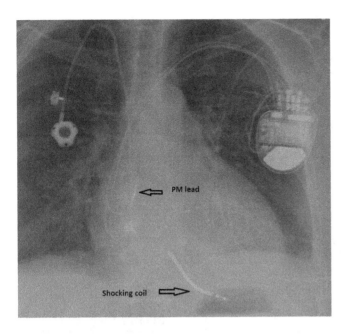

PM lead

Shocking coil

Figure 122.1 Presence of shocking coil differentiates an ICD from a pacemaker.

and interrogation reports can be used to obtain this information. The ECG will show "pacing spikes" before every ORS if the patient is PM dependent. A CIED interrogation that shows no evidence of spontaneous ventricular activity when the PM function of the CIED is programmed to the lowest programmable rate is the most reliable method to determine dependency.[1]

Reviewing the most recent interrogation report or reinterrogating the device will help determine the current setting of the device and ensure that the device is functioning as prescribed. *Early failure* of a CIED is usually due to displaced or broken electrodes, while *late failure* is usually due to premature battery failure.

Preoperative preparation for patient safety includes determining potential sources of **EMI**. The main concern regarding EMI is device malfunction, which might lead to inappropriate antitachycardia therapy in the case of an AICD and loss of pacing with PMs. While electrocautery is one of the most common causes of EMI, other potential EMI sources include external defibrillation, electroconvulsive therapy , transcutaneous electrical nerve stimulation, and radio-frequency waves used in ablation procedures. More interference is expected if the EMI is near the pulse generator and the path of EMI crosses over the CIED generator.

Some of the methods to reduce the possibility or effect of EMI is by increasing the distance between the EMI source and the CIED to more than 15 cm, utilization of bipolar as opposed to monopolar electrocautery, using short bursts of electrocautery (less than 10 seconds), using

lower electrocautery power settings, and ensuring proper positioning of the electrocautery return pad to minimize the flow of current across the CIED.

Hyperkalemia, hypokalemia, arterial hypoxemia, myocardial infarction, catecholamines, and abnormal antiarrhythmic drug level are some of the perioperative factors that may alter the threshold of cardiac PMs.

Magnet response varies depending on whether the device is a PM or an ICD. While a PM will pace asynchronously after magnet application, in general a magnet applied to an ICD will disable tachycardia therapy and will not have any effect on the PM. The Heart Rhythm Society recommends magnet placement when needed where the magnet behavior is known, appropriate for the patient, the patient is supine, the magnet can be observed, and access to the magnet is possible. The Anesthesia Patient Safety Foundation has published an algorithm for perioperative management of CIEDs (Figure 122.2).[3]

## INTRAOPERATIVE MANAGEMENT

The patient's underlying disease processes and the nature of the surgery should be taken into while managing these patients intraoperatively. As for any other anesthetics, it is essential to have standard American Society of Anesthesiologists monitors. The presence of a CIED should not affect the choice of anesthetic agents used, as they do not alter the current or the voltage threshold of the PM. However, skeletal myopotential due to a depolarizing neuromuscular blocker can potentially inappropriately inhibit or trigger PM stimulation.

Potential sources of EMI include use of monopolar electrocautery above the umbilicus, radio-frequency ablation, lithotripsy, magnetic resonance imaging, radio-frequency identification devices, and electroconvulsive therapy. Whenever possible, it is essential to use bipolar cautery because it causes less EMI.

It is essential not to use electrocautery within 15 cm of a PM. When unipolar cautery is used, the grounding pad should be placed as close to the operative site as possible and as far from the CIED as possible. It is important to limit the use of electrocautery to a few-second bursts to avoid asystole.[1] Atropine and isoproterenol should be readily available. It is also important to ensure that there is temporary pacing and defibrillation equipment available.

External defibrillation can be used in a patient with an implanted ICD. Paddles should be oriented away from the implanted electrodes, and the lowest effective energy should be used.

In certain instances, the AICD may be disabled, and external defibrillator paddles will be placed on the patient

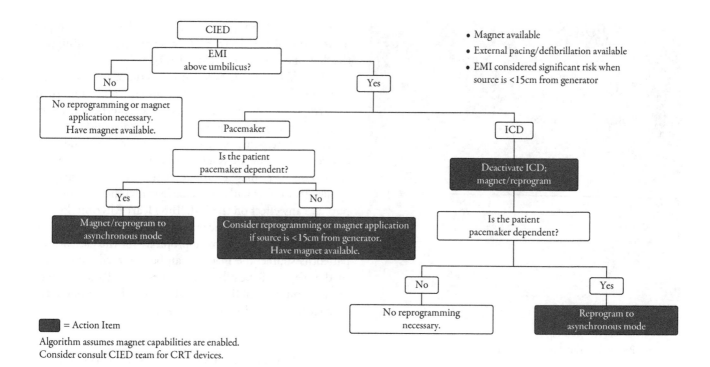

**Figure 122.2** Algorithm for perioperative management of CIEDs.

(perpendicular to the implanted leads and away from the implanted generator).

## POSTOPERATIVE MANAGEMENT

Postoperative management of CIEDs includes restoring devices to their prescribed function and ensuring that the devices are interrogated postoperatively as needed. It is also important that the patient remains in a monitored environment until the device is restored to its permanent setting.

## REFERENCES

1. Practice advisory for the perioperative management of patients with cardiac implantable electronic devices: pacemakers and implantable cardioverter defibrillators: an updated report by the American Society of Anesthesiologists Task Force on Perioperative Management of Patients With Cardiac Implantable Electronic Devices. *Anesthesiology.* 2020;132:225–252.
2. Jacob S, et al. Cardiac rhythm device identification algorithm using x-rays: CaRDIA-X. *Heart Rhythm.* 2011;8(6):915–922. doi:10.1016/j.hrthm.2011.01.012
3. Neelankavil J, et al. Managing cardiovascular implantable electronic devices (CIEDs) during perioperative care. *APSF Newsletter.* 2013;28(2):29–48.

# 123.

# VENTRICULAR SYNCHRONIZATION

*Jayakar Guruswamy and Snigdha Parikh*

## VENTRICULAR SYNCHRONIZATION

Cardiac resynchronization therapy (CRT) devices, also called biventricular pacing, play an important role in the management of heart failure. These devices are commonly encountered by anesthesiologists because of the large prevalence of heart failure in the United States. These devices are indicated in select patients with heart failure, systolic dysfunction, and a prolonged QRS. Patients with systolic heart failure often have conduction abnormalities. Of these patients, 25% to 40% have a prolonged QRS complex (>120

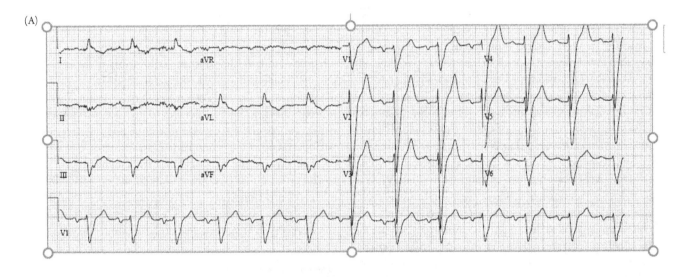

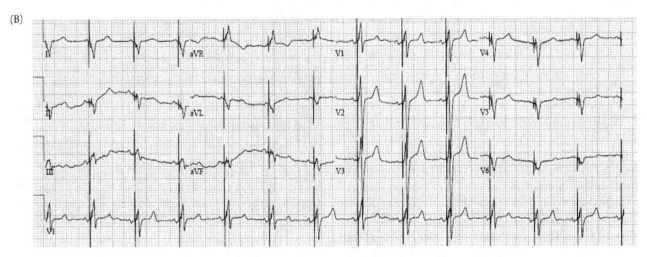

**Figure 123.1** Electrocardiogram before (A) and after (B) initiation of cardiac resynchronization therapy.

**Table 123.1** INDICATIONS FOR CARDIAC RESYNCHRONIZATION THERAPY

| | LVEF (%) | QRS DURATION (MS) | NYHA CLASS | BRADYCARDIA, PACER DEPENDENCE |
|---|---|---|---|---|
| CRT-D | <35 | >120 | III, IV (I, II) | +/− |
| CRT-P | <35 (no ICD preferred) | >120 | III, IV (I, II) | +/− |

CRT, cardiac resynchronization therapy; CRT-D, cardiac resynchronization therapy with automatic implantable cardioverter-defibrillator; CRT-P, biventricular pacing; ICD, implantable cardioverter-defibrillator; LVEF, left ventricular ejection fraction; NYHA, New York Heart Association.

ms), in whom cardiac depolarization spreads slowly through the myocardium, leading to intraventricular dyssynchrony[1] During intraventricular dyssynchrony, the left ventricular (LV) septal wall contracts earlier than the lateral wall, which leads to less efficient ejection from the LV and decreased diastolic filling. The goal of CRT is to maintain sequential atrioventricular (AV) contraction and to restore synchronous contraction of the LV and to optimize timing of LV and right ventricular (RV) ejection. While a dual-chamber pacemaker successfully maintains sequential AV contraction between the right atrium (RA) and the RV, RV pacing often results in delayed depolarization of the LV inferior or inferolateral wall because of a conduction delay. This is overcome through biventricular pacing using a standard RV lead and an LV lead placed adjacent to the inferolateral wall via the coronary sinus (CS). Figure 123.1 shows an electrocardiogram before and after successful CRT showing the narrowing of QRS. The "CS lead" is another passive fixation lead that is frequently maintained in place by removing a guide, which allows the lead to take a bent shape in the vessel lumen. In contrast to the RA or RV leads, which are endocardial, a lead placed in the CS results in epicardial pacing. Biventricular pacing in the RV and the LV leads to improved hemodynamic variables, including systolic blood pressure, stroke volume, and cardiac output. CRT improves cardiac performance with reductions in myocardial metabolic demand, in contrast to pharmacological means of improving systolic function. CRT has also been shown to reverse ventricular remodeling over time and thereby improve mitral regurgitation (MR) and New York Heart Association (NYHA) function class.

Indications for CRT have expanded in recent years. Standard indications for CRT are left ventricle ejection fraction (LVEF) less than 35% with QRS greater than 120 ms, sinus rhythm, and NYHA class III or IV after optimal medical therapy, as shown in Table 123.1. Left bundle branch block is the most common conduction abnormality in patients undergoing CRT.

The fifth position of the standard pacemaker codes, the NBG coding system conveys unique and valuable information to the practitioner regarding either multiple leads in a single chamber or leads in multiple chambers. The presence of a CRT device can often be picked up on x-ray, where the CS lead can be seen as shown in Figure 123.2. Because most patients who qualify for CRT also meet indications for implantable cardioverter-defibrillator (AICD) therapy, most CRT patients will have CRT-D (cardiac resynchronization therapy with automatic implantable cardioverter-defibrillator) devices. The CRT-D devices pose a unique problem for perioperative management because a magnet application will only deactivate the implantable cardioverter-defibrillator (ICD) portion of the device. Given that the goal of CRT is the synchronization of ventricular contraction and the associated increase in cardiac output, these patients might be considered "*functionally*" *pacemaker dependent*, though they often have an adequate underlying rhythm. Inhibition of biventricular pacing by electromagnetic interference (EMI) may result in a reduction in cardiac output and hypotension. Therefore, reprogramming CRT-D devices to an asynchronous mode would be required to guarantee continued pacing in the perioperative period when EMI is anticipated.

The ultimate location of the CS lead has been generalized to the posterior or basal inferolateral location, but in fact, optimization does vary. However, despite optimal placement, approximately 30% of patients meeting selection criteria for CRT do not respond to biventricular pacing.

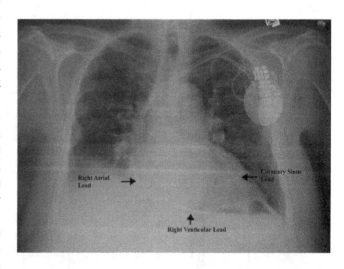

**Figure 123.2** Chest x-ray showing coronary sinus lead suggestive of biventricular pacing.

Risk factors for failure to respond to CRT include ischemic cardiomyopathy, sustained ventricular tachycardia, severe MR, and dilated LV cavity.

Cardiac resynchronization therapy has been shown to reduce mortality, heart failure symptoms, and also heart failure hospitalizations. Patients with CRT should be considered pacemaker dependent because of the constant pacing they undergo to synchronize the ventricle.

## REFERENCES

1. Owen JS, et al. Cardiac resynchronization therapy. *Ochsner J.* 2009;9(4):248–256.
2. US Department of Health and Human Services. Heart failure fact sheet. https://www.cdc.gov/heartdisease/heart_failure.htm
3. Jeon DS, Park JS. Rapid and potent antiarrhythmic effect of cardiac resynchronization therapy in a patient with advanced dilated cardiomyopathy and a large ventricular arrhythmia burden. *Korean Circ J.* 2017;42(4):523–527. doi.org/10.4070/kcj.2016.0361

# 124.

# ABLATIONS, CRYOTHERAPY, AND MAZE PROCEDURE

*Anna Moskal*

## INTRODUCTION

Cardiac arrhythmias are common and an important source of mortality and morbidity. Current management options include surgical and catheter ablative techniques using surgical incisions, cryotherapy, or radio-frequency (RF) energy. General indications include drug-resistant arrhythmias, drug intolerance, severe symptoms, or a desire to avoid lifelong symptoms. Ablative procedures can abolish the origins of arrhythmias by interposition of scar tissue along a reentry pathway or by isolating an ectopic area. Diagnosis of the underlying mechanisms of arrhythmia requires invasive electrophysiologic testing. A mapping catheter is passed through a femoral venous sheath into the heart. Intracardiac electrograms are recorded to understand the arrhythmia and guide the ablation catheter to the correct position (Figure 124.1). Various catheter navigation systems have been developed to facilitate mapping and improve catheter position and stability. During a stereotaxis-guided procedure, a catheter with an internal permanent magnet is steered into position via a magnetic navigational device. The catheter has two distal electrodes for endocardial pacing, recording, and RF ablation.[1]

## RADIO-FREQUENCY ABLATION

Radio-frequency energy consists of alternating current with a frequency range of 100 to 2000 kHz, which causes resistive heating of a narrow rim (<1 mm) of tissue that is in direct contact with the ablation electrode.[2] Lesion size is proportional to the temperature at the electrode-tissue interface, the size of the ablation electrode, optimal electrode-tissue contact, and duration of RF delivery. Single-point RF catheters are associated with char formation on the ablation electrode, which results in a rapid rise in electrical impedance with loss of effective tissue heating and less effective ablation. In addition, heat generated by RF energy can cause thrombus formation, which can lead to cerebral embolism. Open-loop irrigated tip catheters were introduced to overcome these limitations. Infusion of saline over the catheter tip reduces temperatures at the electrode-tissue interface and thus allows continued delivery of RF current into the surrounding tissue, as shown in Figure 124.2B. This ablation system creates larger and deeper ablation lesions and minimizes thrombus formation, but excessive intramyocardial heating still may occur. When tissue temperature reaches 100°C, an

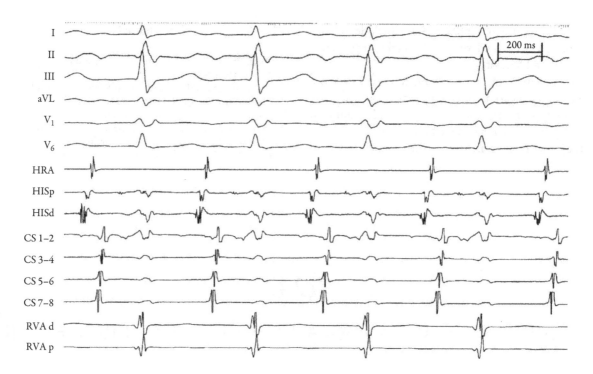

**Figure 124.1** Intracardiac e-grams. From MC Ashley Elizabeth. Anesthesia for electrophysiology procedure in the cardiac catheter laboratory. Cont Ed Anaesth Crit Care Pain. 2012; 12 (5):230-6. Copyright © 2020. Elsevier. Reprinted with permission.

intramyocardial explosion leads to the production of gas and an audible sound called a steam pop. It is a potentially severe complication, which has been associated with cardiac perforation and ventricular septal defect. The new "contact force sensing" RF catheters are able to apply just the right amount of pressure to create transmural lesions while avoiding steam pops.

## CRYOTHERAPY

During pulmonary vein isolation (PVI) cryoablation procedures, the guide wire is passed into the pulmonary vein, and then a balloon is inflated in the pulmonary vein ostia, causing vein occlusion. The refrigerant nitrous oxide is delivered into the balloon, where it undergoes a liquid-to-gas phase change, resulting in cooling the temperature to approximately -80°C. The entire pulmonary vein is isolated by cryoablation in one-balloon inflation, as shown in Figure 124.2A. The first-generation cryoballoon only distributes refrigerant to an equatorial belt on the balloon's surface, while the second generation of the balloon has a larger surface area of coolant distribution, which encompasses the distal hemisphere of the balloon. The design allows for more uniform and distal cooling and decreased standard freezing time. The cryoablation procedures are less complex, shorter, and less painful to the patient. The mechanism of ablation using cryotherapy results in distinct lesion qualities advantageous to RF

with preservation of tissue ultrastructure and less extensive endothelial damage and thrombus formation.

## MAZE PROCEDURE

Surgical therapy for atrial fibrillation (AF) was introduced by James Cox with the principal goals of interrupting possible routes of macro reentrant circuits leading to the arrhythmia, restoring sinus rhythm, and preserving nodal conduction, atrioventricular synchrony, and atrial mechanical function. The maze I procedure consisted of the cut-and-sew technique, with multiple atrial incisions created in a maze-like pattern around the sinoatrial node and atrial–superior vena cava junction. This technique was complicated by a blunted chronotropic response to exercise and high rate of pacemaker implantation.[3] For these reasons, the procedure was further modified into the Cox–maze III, which is considered the gold standard of lesion sets. The procedure includes seven distinct left atrial lesions, including PVI and left atrial appendage closure. The right atrial lesion set decreases the risk of atrial flutter and is important for patients with persistent AF. Unfortunately, the Cox–maze III procedure was seldom performed due to technical complexity and prolonged cardiopulmonary bypass time. Later, it was modified to the Cox–maze IV by replacing most of the original incision lines with a combination of bipolar RF and cryothermy ablation. In select patients, this procedure can be performed through a right minithoracotomy.

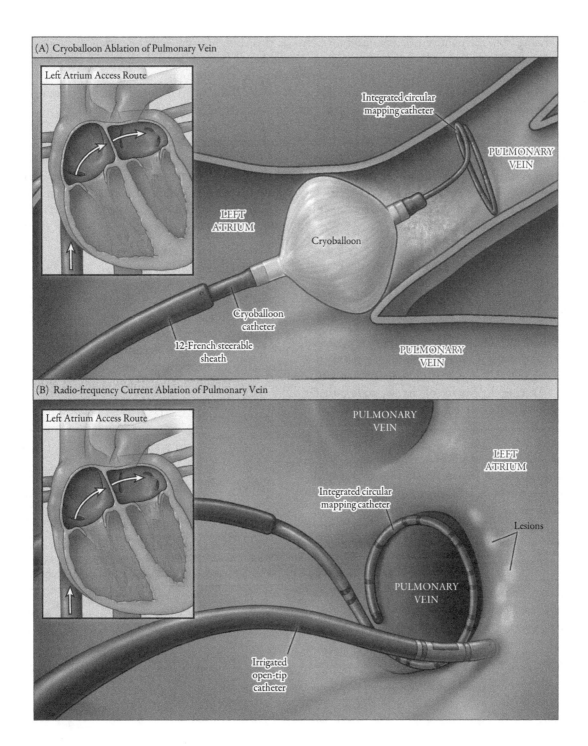

**Figure 124.2** Catheter ablation methods. From Kuck K.H., Brugada J., Furnkranz A., Metzner A., Ouyang F., Chun K.R.J., Elvan A., Arentz T., Bestehorn K., Pocock S.J., Albenque J.P., Tondo C. Cryoablation or Radiofrequency Ablation for Paroxysmal Atrial Fibrillation. N Engl J Med 2016; 374: 2235-45. Copyright © 2020. Massachusetts Medical Society. Reprinted with permission.

## ANESTHETIC CONSIDERATIONS

### PREOPERATIVE

Advantages of proceeding with monitored anesthesia care (MAC) include the ability to avoid volatile and other intravenous anesthetics, which may have adverse effects on the patient's hemodynamic stability. Protracted procedures such as those concerning persistent AF may require general anesthesia. The patient's discomfort and movement from lying on a table for a long period of time may result in the need for remapping of the arrhythmia and decrease the procedure's efficacy. Shorter procedures such as paroxysmal atrial fibrillation, which involves only PVI or right-sided lesions, such as atrial flutter, AVNRT, or ventricular tachycardia arising from the right ventricular outflow track can be ablated under MAC.[2]

In case of AF ablation, several factors should be considered to determine the risk of thrombotic events. These factors include duration of arrhythmia (paroxysmal vs. chronic), presence of systemic anticoagulation, the patient's CHADS2 score, and left atrium size. The CHADS2 score is a composite number that takes into account the presence of congestive heart failure, hypertension, increased age, diabetes mellitus, and previous stroke. The higher the risk for stroke, the lower the threshold should be to perform preoperative transesophageal echocardiography.[1]

## INTRAOPERATIVE

Intraoperatively, placement of the arterial line depends on the patient's comorbidities and duration of arrhythmia induced for mapping. If general anesthesia is needed, reduced tidal volumes with an increased respiratory rate are preferred to decrease chest excursion while maintaining minute ventilation. Anticoagulation is necessary if transseptal puncture is performed. During the passage of the electrode catheter into the left atrium, thrombi may form and cause systemic embolization. Activated clotting time is maintained between 250 and 300 seconds. Placement of the esophageal temperature probe reduces the risk of esophageal injury, which is a serious complication occurring due to close proximity to the posterior wall of the left atrium. The mechanism is thought to be direct thermal injury from RF current. An atrial-esophageal fistula may lead to air emboli and sepsis, with high mortality. A more common esophageal complication is an esophageal ulcer, which can be managed conservatively. Phrenic nerve injury can occur during cryoablation of the right upper pulmonary vein. During this portion of the procedure, cardiologists may pace the diaphragm and request the patient not be paralyzed. A low dose of opioid at this time may prevent the patient from coughing. Any sudden increased hemodynamic instability should warrant concern about pericardial effusion and cardiac tamponade. Treatment includes reversal of anticoagulation, administration of fluids and vasopressors, and placement of a pericardial drain if the effusion is large. Definitive surgical treatment may be needed if bleeding continues. The use of open irrigated RF catheters for ablation can lead to fluid overload. It is important to monitor fluid balance and administer furosemide if pulmonary edema is diagnosed. Smooth reversal and extubation are important to control groin hematoma.

## POSTOPERATIVE

Typically, anticoagulation should be resumed 4 to 6 hours after femoral sheaths from the procedure have been removed, but in the face of postoperative bleeding, it should not be resumed until bleeding has subsided. If a patient appears to be hypovolemic despite a negative echocardiogram, retroperitoneal bleeding should be suspected as a result of trauma to the femoral or iliac artery.

## REFERENCES

1. Malladi V, et al. Endovascular ablation of atrial fibrillation. *Anesthesiology.* 2014;120:1513–1519.
2. Ashley EMC. Anaesthesia for electrophysiology procedures in the cardiac catheter laboratory. *Cont Ed Anaesth Crit Care Pain.* 2012;12(5):230–236.
3. Kik Ch, Bogers Ad JJC. Maze procedures for atrial fibrillation, from history to practice. *Cardiol Res.* 2011;2(5):201–207.
4. Kuck KH, et al. Cryoablation or radiofrequency ablation for paroxysmal atrial fibrillation. *N Engl J Med.* 2016;374: 2235–2245.
5. Badhwar V, et al. The Society of Thoracic Surgeons 2017 clinical practice guidelines for the surgical treatment of atrial fibrillation. *Ann Thorac Surg.* 2017;103:329–341.

# HEART FAILURE AND CARDIOMYOPATHY

*Lovkesh L. Arora and Surangama Sharma*

## INTRODUCTION

Heart failure (HF) is defined as a clinical condition arising from impaired ventricular relaxation or systolic ejection of the cardiac ventricles. Its major clinical manifestations are dyspnea, fatigue, and fluid retention. It is the result of variable underlying pathology, including ischemic heart disease (i.e., ischemic cardiomyopathy); hypertension; valvular heart disease; myocarditis; infiltrative disorder (e.g., sarcoidosis, amyloidosis); and peripartum cardiomyopathy.

## CLASSIFICATION

The New York Heart Association (NYHA) classification system is most commonly used to quantify the degree of functional limitation, and it assigns patients to one of four functional classes[1]:

- Class I—Patients with heart disease without resulting limitation of physical activity. Ordinary physical activity does not cause HF symptoms such as fatigue or dyspnea.
- Class II—Patients with heart disease resulting in slight limitation of physical activity. Symptoms of HF develop with ordinary activity, but there are no symptoms at rest.
- Class III—Patients with heart disease resulting in marked limitation of physical activity. Symptoms of HF develop with less-than-ordinary physical activity, but there are no symptoms at rest.
- Class IV—Patients with heart disease resulting in inability to carry on any physical activity without discomfort. Symptoms of HF may occur even at rest.

### STAGES IN THE DEVELOPMENT OF HF

As outlined by the American College of Cardiology (ACC) Foundation/American Heart Association (AHA) guidelines[2]:

- Stage A—At high risk for HF but without structural heart disease or symptoms of HF.

- Stage B—Structural heart disease but without signs or symptoms of HF. This stage includes patients in NYHA functional class I with no prior or current symptoms or signs of HF.
- Stage C—Structural heart disease with prior or current symptoms of HF. This stage includes patients in any NYHA functional class (including class I with prior symptoms).
- Stage D—Refractory HF requiring specialized interventions. This stage includes patients in NYHA functional class IV with refractory HF.

Heart failure can also be classified based on the severity of ventricular systolic dysfunction, namely, HF with reduced ejection fraction (HFrEF) versus HF with preserved ejection fraction (HFpEF). Most medical therapy for improving morbidity and mortality in HF (i.e., angiotensin-converting enzyme inhibitor [ACEI], angiotensin receptor blocker [ARB], aldosterone antagonist, β-adrenergic blocker, ivabradine) have only demonstrated efficacy in HFrEF. In contrast, medical therapy for HFpEF is largely aimed at symptoms and underlying conditions (e.g., hypertension).[3]

## ANESTHETIC CONSIDERATIONS

### PREOPERATIVE

Symptomatic HF has been consistently identified as a risk factor for adverse perioperative outcomes and a component of the Revised Cardiac Index. *Among patients with HF, perioperative risk may be higher in patients with HFrEF versus HFpEF.* The prognostic importance of asymptomatic systolic dysfunction is less clear, and that is why the current ACC/AHA guidelines discourage routine preoperative assessment of ventricular function but recommends it reasonable to perform in patients with dyspnea of unknown origin.[4]

*The clinical stability of HF symptoms prior to surgery is another important determinant of perioperative risk,* and the European Society of Cardiology (ESC) and the European Society of Anaesthesiology (ESA) guidelines recommend that elective intermediate-risk and high-risk noncardiac procedures be deferred for at least 3 months after initiation of medical therapy in patients with newly diagnosed HF.[5]

The *preoperative history pertaining to HF* should clarify its type, etiology, severity, stability, recent investigations, and current therapy. Inquire about recent weight gain, fatigue, shortness of breath, orthopnea, paroxysmal nocturnal dyspnea, nocturnal cough, peripheral edema, hospitalizations, and recent changes in medical management. *The patient's functional status should be classified according to the NYHA categories.*

A chest radiograph may provide further diagnostic guidance, especially in dyspneic patients, with pulmonary vascular redistribution and interstitial edema useful findings for supporting the presence of HF. Natriuretic peptide measurement can further clarify whether a patient has HF. *Both brain natriuretic peptide and N-terminal pro-BNP have excellent diagnostic performance, and their concentrations are markers of perioperative cardiac risk.* While routine preoperative echocardiography is not useful, such specialized testing is helpful for assessment of dyspnea of unknown origin or recent altered clinical status in an individual with known HF. Other tests for patients with HF include electrocardiograms and blood sampling to measure electrolyte and creatinine concentration.

## PHARMACOTHERAPY AND OPTIMIZATION

Consideration should be given for collaborative perioperative management with a cardiologist or HF specialist of severely affected HF patients (i.e., NYHA III or IV; decompensated HF) who will undergo intermediate-risk or high-risk procedures. Most medical therapy, including β-adrenergic blockers, hydralazine, nitrates, and digoxin, should be continued preoperatively. Loop diuretics (e.g., furosemide) can be continued on the day of surgery for most procedures since this strategy does not increase risks of intraoperative hypotension or adverse cardiac events. The exception is lengthy high-risk procedures with projected significant blood loss or fluid requirements, in which potent diuretics should be held on the morning of surgery. Since ACEI and ARB administration within 24 hours before surgery is associated with increased risks of intraoperative hypotension and postoperative myocardial injury, it is reasonable to withhold these medications for 24 hours before surgery, provided that they are restarted postoperatively once patients are hemodynamically stable. Patients on anticoagulant therapy will likely need these medications temporarily discontinued before surgery.

## INTRAOPERATIVE

In addition to standard monitoring tools, monitoring the volume status in these patients is important because they are very sensitive to volume changes due to surgical bleeding and sympathetic tone changes due to anesthesia in the perioperative period. Thus, invasive arterial monitoring for indirect assessments of preload by stroke volume variance and frequent blood sampling are advisable. In major or vascular surgery, central venous catheterization, pulmonary artery catheterization, and/or transesophageal echocardiography may be needed, which can contribute to intraoperative evaluation of intravascular volume during anesthesia.

## POSTOPERATIVE

In the postoperative period, hypoxemia and/or atrial fibrillation are the most common complications because restored vascular sympathetic tone due to emergence and resolution from general or regional anesthesia causes a volume shift to central blood volume. The subsequent volume overload can result in pulmonary edema and/or atrial fibrillation due to decompensation.

Deterioration can happen acutely in a patient with an initially stable appearance; therefore, continuous and careful postoperative monitoring is essential. It is reasonable to transfer patients to intensive care in longer duration procedures or intermediate- and high-risk surgeries.

## REFERENCES

1. The Criteria Committee of the New York Heart Association. *Nomenclature and Criteria for Diagnosis of Diseases of the Heart and Great Vessels* (9th ed.). Boston: Little, Brown & Co. 1994:253–256.
2. Yancy CW, et al. 2013 ACCF/AHA guideline for the management of heart failure: a report of the American College of Cardiology Foundation/American Heart Association Task Force on Practice Guidelines. *J Am Coll Cardiol.* 2013;62(16):e147–e239.
3. Iwano H, Little WC. Heart failure: what does ejection fraction have to do with it? *J Cardiol.* 2013;62(1):1–3.
4. Fleisher LA, et al. 2014 ACC/AHA guideline on perioperative cardiovascular evaluation and management of patients undergoing noncardiac surgery: a report of the American College of Cardiology/American Heart Association Task Force on Practice Guidelines. *Circulation.* 2014;130(24):e278–e333.
5. Kristensen SD, et al. 2014 ESC/ESA guidelines on non-cardiac surgery: cardiovascular assessment and management: the Joint Task Force on Non-cardiac Surgery: cardiovascular assessment and management of the European Society of Cardiology (ESC) and the European Society of Anaesthesiology (ESA). *Eur J Anaesthesiol.* 2014;31(10):517–573.

# 126.

# SYSTOLIC VERSUS DIASTOLIC DYSFUNCTION

*Andaleeb A. Ahmed and Sohail K. Mahboobi*

## INTRODUCTION

An intricate interplay between diastolic and systolic function is required to maintain adequate cardiac output (Figure 126.1). Ventricular dysfunction can be categorized into systolic and diastolic dysfunction. Systolic dysfunction occurs when the ventricle fails to eject blood normally, leading to reduced stroke volume. Diastolic dysfunction is the inability to fill the left ventricle (LV) to an adequate end-diastolic volume while maintaining a normal left atrial pressure. Both systolic and diastolic dysfunction can lead to heart failure (HF). The clinical syndrome of heart failure secondary to systolic dysfunction is termed *heart failure with reduced ejection fraction* (HFrEF), and heart failure in the presence of diastolic dysfunction with normal or near-normal ejection fraction (EF) (>50%) is termed *heart failure with preserved ejection fraction* (HFpEF).[1] HFpEF and HFrEF have distinct etiologies with considerable overlap. Important adaptive and maladaptive compensatory mechanisms in patients with HF include increased preload, fluid retention, activation of sympathetic nervous system, and activation of renin-angiotensin-aldosterone.

The HFpEF syndrome is more common in female and elderly patients with hypertension, obesity, and diabetes. Anesthetic management of patients with HFpEF and

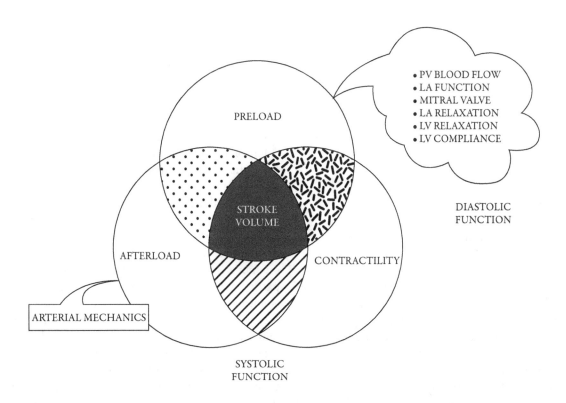

**Figure 126.1** The determinants of systolic and diastolic function. LA, left atrium; LV, left ventricle; PV, Pulmonary vein.

HFrEF requires careful assessment and optimization of preload, afterload, and contractility.

## SYSTOLIC DYSFUNCTION

Systolic contraction of the heart utilizes three movements: (1) base-to-apex longitudinal contraction, (2) radial thickening, and (3) circumferential torsion. Normal LV function is dependent on myocardial contractility and loading conditions. The gold standard for assessing LV systolic function is cardiac magnetic resonance imaging. However, the most common modality for assessing LV function is echocardiography. The hallmark of systolic dysfunction is reduced EF. The EF represents the fraction of blood ejected with each heartbeat.

$$\text{Ejection fraction} = \frac{LVEDV - LVESV}{LVEDV} \times 100\%$$

where LVEDV is LV end-diastolic volume, and LVESV is LV end-systolic volume.

Using echocardiography, EF is calculated by Simpson's method of disks. Other echocardiographic methods of assessing systolic function include fractional shortening, fractional area change, Quinones method, dP/dT, myocardial performance index, and three-dimensional echocardiography.

Three primary mechanisms of systolic dysfunction are (1) impaired myocardial contractility, (2) pressure overload, and (3) volume overload. Systolic dysfunction is categorized as mild (EF < 50%), moderate (EF 30%–40%), and severe (EF < 30%) categories.

The etiology of systolic dysfunction is as follows:

- Coronary artery disease
- Hypertension
- Valvular heart disease
- Chronic lung disease
- Nonischemic dilated cardiomyopathy
- Toxic/metabolic/viral cardiomyopathy
- Chronic tachyarrhythmias and bradyarrhythmias

There is considerable overlap between LV systolic dysfunction and the clinical syndrome of HF. Symptoms of LV systolic dysfunction can range from asymptotic systolic dysfunction to symptoms of overt congestive HF (HFrEF). It is often associated with secondary involvement of the right ventricle, dilated LV, regional wall motion abnormality (with coronary artery disease), impaired contractility, and LV hypertrophy. Diuretics, vasodilators, β-blockers, angiotensin-converting enzyme inhibitor, and angiotensin II receptor blocker are established therapies for treatment of HF.[2]

## DIASTOLIC DYSFUNCTION

The diastolic phase of the heart is the period between aortic valve closure and mitral valve closure. The LV diastolic phase can be further divided into four phases:

- *Isovolumic relaxation time (IVRT)*: Period when aortic and mitral valve are closed; normal IVRT is 70–90 milliseconds
- *Rapid early LV filling*: Responsible for 70%–80% LV diastolic filling
- *Diastasis*: Equalization of left atrial (LA) and LV diastolic pressures
- *LA systole ("atrial kick")*: Responsible for 20%–25% of LV filling

Diastolic dysfunction is characterized by impaired relaxation and/or increased chamber stiffness. The LA serves as a reservoir during ventricular systole, as a conduit during early diastole, and as a pump during late diastole.[3] Progressive diastolic dysfunction leads to increased LA pressure at rest or with exercise, LA remodeling, and increased LA volume. A LAVI (LA volume index) that is indexed to body surface area greater than 34 mL/m$^2$ is an important feature of diastolic dysfunction. Patients with significant diastolic dysfunction can remain asymptomatic for long periods. Signs and symptoms of HF diastolic dysfunction arise from elevated LA pressure.

Common causes of diastolic dysfunction are the following:

- Age
- Hypertension
- Diabetes
- Coronary artery disease
- Chronic kidney disease
- Cardiomyopathy (hypertrophic, restrictive, and dilated)
- Valvular heart disease
- Pericardial disease

Nearly one-half of patients with HF have a normal or near-normal EF.[4] Diastolic dysfunction and HFpEF are not synonymous, but diastolic dysfunction is the fundamental pathophysiology behind HFpEF. Other pathophysiologic abnormalities associated with HFpEF include impaired LA function, abnormal right ventricular–pulmonary artery coupling, chronotropic incompetence, impaired microvascular function, reduced systemic vascular compliance, and pulmonary vascular impairment.[4] Patients with restrictive diastolic dysfunction poorly tolerate fluid challenges and tachyarrhythmias and can readily develop pulmonary congestion.[4]

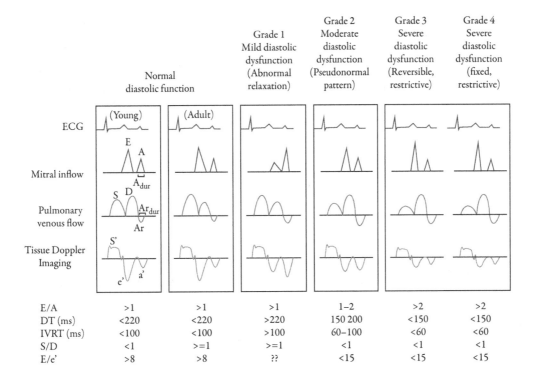

| | Normal diastolic function | Grade 1 Mild diastolic dysfunction (Abnormal relaxation) | Grade 2 Moderate diastolic dysfunction (Pseudonormal pattern) | Grade 3 Severe diastolic dysfunction (Reversible, restrictive) | Grade 4 Severe diastolic dysfunction (fixed, restrictive) |
|---|---|---|---|---|---|
| E/A | >1 | >1 | >1 | 1–2 | >2 | >2 |
| DT (ms) | <220 | <220 | >220 | 150 200 | <150 | <150 |
| IVRT (ms) | <100 | <100 | >100 | 60–100 | <60 | <60 |
| S/D | <1 | >=1 | >=1 | <1 | <1 | <1 |
| E/e' | >8 | >8 | ?? | <15 | <15 | <15 |

**Figure 126.2** Grades of diastolic dysfunction. *A*, Mitral filling waveform at atrial contraction; *a'*, tissue Doppler mitral annular late diastolic velocity; *Adur*, mitral filling wave at atrial contraction duration; *Ar*, pulmonary venous reverse flow velocity at atrial contraction; *D*, pulmonary venous diastolic flow; DT, deceleration time of E wave; *E*, mitral early filling wave; *e'*, tissue Doppler mitral annular early diastolic tissue velocity; IVRT, isovolumic relaxation time; *S*, pulmonary venous systolic flow; *s'*, tissue Doppler mitral annular systolic velocity.

Left ventricular diastolic dysfunction is detected and quantified by echocardiography. Primary echocardiographic parameters used to grade diastolic dysfunction include (1) transmitral Doppler flow (E and A waves); (2)

**Table 126.1** DIFFERENCES BETWEEN SYSTOLIC AND DIASTOLIC DYSFUNCTION

| | SYSTOLIC DYSFUNCTION | DIASTOLIC DYSFUNCTION |
|---|---|---|
| Ejection fraction | Reduced | Normal or near normal |
| Stroke volume | Reduced | Normal or ↓ |
| Primary mechanism | Impaired contractility | Impaired LV filling/relaxation |
| LV cavity size | Normal or decreased | Increased |
| LV wall thickness | Decreased | Increased |
| End-diastolic volume | Increased | Normal |
| End-systolic volume | Increased | Normal or decreased |
| LV geometry | Spherical | Usually unchanged |
| *LVmass/Cavity* | Normal or decreased | Increased |

pulmonary venous Doppler flow (S, D waves); (3) tissue Doppler mitral annular motion (e' and a' wave); (4) LAVI; and (5) tricuspid regurgitation jet velocity.[3] Figure 126.2 outlines the grades of diastolic dysfunction based on Doppler echocardiographic parameters.

Grades of diastolic dysfunction are as follows:

- Grade 1: Impaired LV relaxation; lower E/A ratio, prolonged IVRT and deceleration time
- Grade 2: Pseudonormal pattern; normal E/A ratio, S/D less than 1
- Grade 3: Restrictive diastolic dysfunction (reversible): tall narrow E wave, E/A greater than 2, short IVRT and deceleration time (DT)
- Grade 4: Restrictive diastolic dysfunction (fixed): Similar to above but dysfunction is permanent

Main differences between systolic and diastolic dysfunction are summarized in Table 126.1.

## REFERENCES

1. van der Meer P, et al. ACC/AHA versus ESC guidelines on heart failure: JACC guideline comparison. *J Am Coll Cardiol.* 2019;73(21):2756–2768.
2. Yancy CW, et al. 2017 ACC/AHA/HFSA focused update of the 2013 ACCF/AHA guideline for the management of heart failure:

a report of the American College of Cardiology/American Heart Association Task Force on Clinical Practice Guidelines and the Heart Failure Society of America. *J Card Fail.* 2017;23(8): 628–651.

3. Sharkey A, et al. Diastolic dysfunction—what an anesthesiologist needs to know? *Best Pract Res Clin Anaesthesiol.* 2019;33(2): 221–228.

4. Pagel PS, et al. Heart failure with preserved ejection fraction: a comprehensive review and update of diagnosis, pathophysiology, treatment, and perioperative implications. *J Cardiothorac Vasc Anesth.* 2021;35(6):1839–1859.

5. Obokata M, et al. Diastolic dysfunction and heart failure with preserved ejection fraction: understanding mechanisms by using noninvasive methods. *JACC Cardiovasc Imaging.* 2020;13(1 pt 2):245–257.

# 127.

# POSTOBSTRUCTIVE PULMONARY EDEMA

*Benjamin Kloesel and Balazs Horvath*

## INTRODUCTION

Postobstructive pulmonary edema (POPE) describes a unique form of gas exchange impairment that can be encountered in the perioperative period. It is triggered by vigorous respiratory efforts against an obstructed airway, which leads to a chain of events that facilitate transvascular fluid filtration. The resulting pulmonary edema causes impairment of gas exchange, which manifests as hypoxemia, dyspnea, tachypnea, and expectoration of pink, frothy sputum. Airway obstruction can have many different etiologies, but in anesthetic practice, the most frequent situations that lead to POPE include laryngospasm and occlusion of the endotracheal tube caused by the patient biting down when no protective bite block is in place.

## PATHOPHYSIOLOGY

The main pathophysiological factor for the development of POPE remains the generation of negative pleural pressures significantly below the physiological level during the attempt to spontaneously inhale against an obstructed airway (modified Mueller maneuver).[1] During physiologic breathing via an unobstructed upper airway, the diaphragm generates negative inspiratory pressures of -2 to -8 cm $H_2O$, while forceful inspiration against an obstructed airway can

result in negative inspiratory pressures of up to -140 cm $H_2O$ (Figure 126.1).[2] Some sources categorize POPE into two different types: Type I occurs after relief of an acute upper airway obstruction, while type II is characterized by occurrence after relief of a chronic upper airway obstruction, for example, after tonsillectomy or airway tumor removal.[3]

During type I POPE, inhalation against an obstructed airway generates an increase in right ventricular preload along with negative intrapleural pressures that are transmitted to the alveoli. Negative pleural pressure facilitates an increase in venous return and creates a large gradient between alveoli and pulmonary capillaries, resulting in fluid movement into the interstitial space. Furthermore, high pressure gradients can disrupt pulmonary epithelium and blood vessel membranes, resulting in microhemorrhage and further fluid translocation.[3] In type II POPE, patients experience long-standing, intermittent episodes of airway obstruction resulting in wide swings in intrathoracic pressure, generation of intrinsic positive end-expiratory pressure (PEEP), hypoventilation, and hypercarbia. Sudden relief of the obstruction removes intrinsic PEEP and causes an increase in venous return and right ventricular preload. Chronic changes from the long-standing obstructive episodes, such as systemic vasoconstriction, hypoxic pulmonary vasoconstriction, increased pulmonary artery pressures, and myocardial dysfunction, impair the body's ability to handle the sudden fluid load

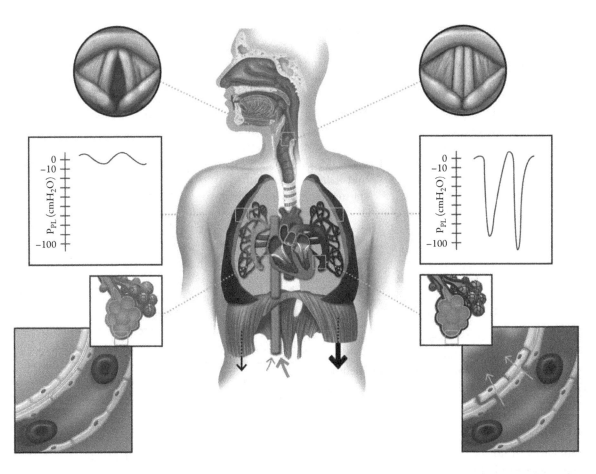

**Figure 127.1** As shown in the *left* of the illustration, breathing through the normally open upper airway requires minimal diaphragmatic efforts (thin black arrow) that generate small levels (-2 to -8 cm $H_2O$) of negative pleural pressure ($P_{PL}$) during inspiration. In normal conditions, the alveolar–capillary pressure gradient is small, and when hydrostatic pressures slightly increase in the pulmonary capillary bed, the fluid overload may be offset by increased lymphatic drainage. Conversely, inspiration against an obstructed upper airway—as represented by closed vocal cords in the *right* of the illustration—requires forceful diaphragmatic efforts (large black arrow) generating high levels (-50 to -140 cm $H_2O$) of negative $P_{PL}$ that increase venous return to the right side of the heart (large arrow next to the inferior vena cava). This may result in higher hydrostatic pressures in the pulmonary capillaries and a sudden drop of pressures in the alveolar spaces, creating a huge pressure gradient across the pulmonary capillary wall and disruption of the alveolar–capillary membrane, leading to alveolar flooding and pulmonary edema (thin arrows at bottom right picture). Adapted under the creative commons license from Lemyze et al.[2]

imposed on the pulmonary circulation and result in development of pulmonary edema.[3]

due to their ability to generate large negative intrathoracic pressures.[1,4]

## ETIOLOGY AND RISK FACTORS

The most common triggering factors of POPE differ within the pediatric and adult population. In children, the majority of upper airway obstruction resulting in POPE is caused by infectious croup or epiglottitis. In adults, postextubation laryngospasm, upper airway infection, and tumors are the predominant etiologic factors. Other risk factors include difficult intubation, hanging, strangulation, goiter, expanding hematoma, obstructive sleep apnea, airway foreign body, and bilateral vocal cord paralysis. Young, healthy adults are at higher risk for development of POPE

## DIAGNOSIS

The first and probably most important clue for the diagnosis should be drawn from the situation in which POPE occurs and the time frame to symptom onset. Events such as laryngospasm in the perioperative phase, the patient biting down on the endotracheal tube, or airway obstructions after medication administration should raise the index of suspicion for POPE if the patient develops otherwise unexplained hypoxemia and dyspnea. POPE is furthermore characterized by a rapid onset of symptoms (seconds to minutes after the precipitating event), although delayed presentations (30–60 minutes and even 24 hours after a precipitating event) have been reported.[5] The patient may exhibit tachycardia, tachypnea, dyspnea, agitation, and cough. Expectoration of pink frothy sputum or even frank hemoptysis may occur. Auscultation of the lungs may reveal rales and rhonchi. A chest x-ray can show alveolar and/or interstitial edema, typically in a bilateral distribution. Bronchoscopy is often unnecessary for diagnosis but may show bloody return consistent with alveolar hemorrhage. The differential diagnosis for POPE should include cardiogenic pulmonary edema, neurogenic pulmonary edema, aspiration pneumonia, anaphylaxis, and iatrogenic fluid overload.[4]

## ANESTHETIC CONSIDERATIONS

### PREOPERATIVE

Typically, POPE occurs in the postoperative period. Risk factors such as potential difficult intubation, obesity, and obstructive sleep apnea that may predispose a patient to develop POPE should be elicited preoperatively.

### INTRAOPERATIVE/POSTOPERATIVE

Most frequently, POPE occurs after extubation or in the postanesthesia care unit, but cases occurring during induction of anesthesia have also been reported.[2] The most important step to address POPE is relieving the precipitating airway obstruction, either by simple basic life support maneuvers (head extension, jaw thrust) or more advanced techniques (oropharyngeal/nasopharyngeal airway, supraglottic airway device, endotracheal intubation). Further treatment of POPE is supportive. A majority of cases can be managed with supplemental oxygen and patient observation.[2] If hypoxemia is refractory, noninvasive positive pressure ventilation may be trialed. This allows application of oxygen to address hypoxemia along with continuous positive airway pressure, which supports fluid resorption from the alveoli back into the vascular space.[2,4] If noninvasive positive pressure ventilation is unsuccessful or not possible, the patient may require endotracheal intubation and mechanical ventilation. A lung-protective ventilation strategy should be targeted (e.g., tidal volume of 4–8 mL/kg predicted body weight with target plateau pressures less than 30 cm $H_2O$), and PEEP should be utilized to facilitate fluid resorption. Diuretics have been used but are often unnecessary; they may hasten the resolution of pulmonary edema, although care must be taken to avoid the administration in a hypovolemic patient.[2,3] Some sources recommend the use of inhaled $\beta_2$-agonists, although it is important to point out that both interventions (diuretics and inhaled $\beta_2$-agonists) have not been studied in POPE and are therefore use is not evidence based.[3,5] Rescue therapies for severe refractory hypoxemia despite mechanical ventilation include neuromuscular blockade, prone positioning, and extracorporeal membrane oxygenation. The majority of cases resolve within 12 to 48 hours. Sequelae are uncommon, and patients usually experience a full recovery.[1]

## REFERENCES

1. Bhattacharya M, et al. Negative-pressure pulmonary edema. *Chest*. 2016;150(4):927–933.
2. Lemyze M, Mallat J. Understanding negative pressure pulmonary edema. *Intensive Care Med*. 2014;40(8):1140–1143.
3. Udeshi A, et al. Postobstructive pulmonary edema. *J Crit Care*. 2010;25(3):508.e1–5.
4. Krodel DJ, et al. Case scenario: acute postoperative negative pressure pulmonary edema. *Anesthesiology*. 2010;113(1):200–207.
5. Liu R, et al. Negative pressure pulmonary edema after general anesthesia: a case report and literature review. *Medicine (Baltimore)*. 2019;98(17):e15389.

# 128.

# PULMONARY HYPERTENSION

*Frank Barrack and Bryan Noorda*

## INTRODUCTION

Until recently, pulmonary hypertension was defined as a mean pulmonary artery pressure (PAP) greater than 25 mm Hg.[1,2] After the Sixth World Symposium on Pulmonary Hypertension, the definition was revised to a mean pulmonary artery pressure (mPAP) greater than 20 mm Hg, or more than two standard deviations above the average mPAP of 14 mm Hg in healthy individuals.[3] Patients with pulmonary hypertension can experience a range of symptoms, from shortness of breath, chest pains, fatigue, to syncope. Hypoxemia, jugular venous distension, edema, and ascites are also seen in patients with pulmonary hypertension. These effects on the body stem from increased right heart strain and eventually right heart failure in advanced disease.[1] Echocardiography offers a noninvasive way to evaluate elevated right heart pressures via measurement of the right ventricular systolic pressure. Magnetic resonance imaging also provides a way to evaluate right heart strain. Right heart catheterization is the gold standard for diagnosis of pulmonary hypertension.[2]

The causes of pulmonary hypertension are many, but can be categorized into five different groups. Group 1 pulmonary hypertension is due to primary pulmonary vascular disease. This category is also termed pulmonary arterial hypertension (PAH). PAH is defined as mPAP greater than 20 mm Hg, pulmonary capillary wedge pressure below 15 mm Hg, and pulmonary vascular resistance (PVR) greater than 3 Woods units (WU) in the absence of chronic lung disease, left heart disease, or chronic thromboembolic disease.[2,3] PAH affects about four times as many women as men, although men have a higher mortality rate. PAH results from several different mechanisms, including endothelial dysfunction of the pulmonary vasculature, impaired vasodilator release, inflammatory processes, and fibrosis.[1,2] These changes result in right ventricle remodeling and eventually right ventricular failure. Treatment generally focuses on pulmonary vasodilation through medical therapy, including phosphodiesterase-5 inhibitors, guanylate cyclase stimulators, endothelin receptor antagonists, epoprostenol, prostacyclin analogues, and prostacyclin receptor agonists.[4]

Group 2 pulmonary hypertension is due to left heart disease causing increased PAPs. Poor left heart function causes increased back pressure in the pulmonary circulation and increases pulmonary vascular pressures. The PVR is normal. Treatment focuses on improving left heart function, and in most cases pulmonary vasodilators actually worsen symptoms.[1]

Group 3 pulmonary hypertension results from chronic lung disease or hypoxia. Chronic lung diseases such as chronic obstructive pulmonary disease, interstitial lung disease, and persistent damage from smoking cause inflammation, mechanical stress from hyperinflated lungs, and remodeling of the pulmonary vasculature, leading to increased pulmonary pressures. Chronic hypoxia from conditions such as obstructive sleep apnea or chronic hypoventilation similarly induces pulmonary hypertension from chronic hypoxic vasoconstriction. Treatment focuses on management of the underlying lung disease.[1]

Pulmonary hypertension due to thromboembolic disease makes up group 4. Repeated emboli to the lungs cause arterial obstruction in the pulmonary vasculature and can lead to fibrosis. Pulmonary vasodilators may improve symptoms. Pulmonary thromboendarterectomy in patients appropriate for surgical intervention may be curative. Group 5 consists of pulmonary hypertension due to unknown or multifactorial causes, and treatment focuses on management of the underlying disease states and use of pulmonary vasodilation as necessary.[1]

## ANESTHETIC CONSIDERATIONS

### PREOPERATIVE

Pulmonary hypertension is an independent predictor of perioperative mortality (4%–24%). Poor functional capacity as indicated by New York Heart Association designation greater than class II, a 6-minute walk less than 300 m, duration of anesthesia less than 3 hours, and use of vasopressors increase mortality and morbidity. Evaluation of pertinent symptoms, including dyspnea, syncope, fatigue, and chest pain, is necessary. Review of pertinent preoperative workup, including routine blood tests, chest imaging, electrocardiography, echocardiography, pulmonary function testing, blood gases, and right heart catheterization results. Echocardiography can underestimate mPAPs. Right heart catheterization gives the most accurate assessment of mPAP, helps differentiate pre- and post–capillary pulmonary hypertension, and demonstrates whether the pulmonary vasculature will be reactive to vasodilators. Pulmonary hypertension medications should be continued through the day of surgery.[1]

## INTRAOPERATIVE

Patients with pulmonary hypertension undergoing surgical procedures are more likely to require close hemodynamic monitoring via arterial blood pressure and pulmonary artery catheters. Temperature monitoring is important as hyperthermia can worsen pulmonary hypertension. Transesophageal echocardiography is invaluable for evaluating right heart strain, directing fluid management, and early detection of ischemia. Intraoperatively, general anesthesia and positive pressure ventilation can increase pulmonary arterial pressure. Vasodilators such as milrinone may ease the afterload for the right ventricle but should be used cautiously in patients with borderline or low blood pressure.[1] Maintain left ventricular afterload. Regional techniques avoid anesthetic-related increases in PAP. However, care must be taken to avoid hypoventilation, as hypercarbia and hypoxia increase PVR and can increase right heart strain and decrease right coronary perfusion. Avoid spinal anesthesia because of rapid onset of sympathetic blockade.

## POSTOPERATIVE

Postoperative monitoring and a comprehensive pain management plan are important for patients with pulmonary hypertension. Respiratory failure and right heart failure are major risks postoperatively. Regional blocks and nonopioid analgesics will minimize hypoventilation and potentially prevent worsening PVR.[1] Atrial tachyarrhythmias may also occur in the postoperative period. β-Blockers are poorly tolerated in these patients; therefore, amiodarone to restore rhythm or digoxin for rate control is recommended. Vasodilators that may have been initiated intraoperatively should be slowly weaned and/or transitioned to the preoperative oral regimen.[1]

## PRIMARY PULMONARY HYPERTENSION IN PREGNANCY

Primary pulmonary hypertension (PPH) mainly affects young women and is associated with high mortality (between 30% and 55%) from right heart failure during pregnancy. Vaginal delivery results in less dramatic hemodynamic shifts for pregnant patients with PPH but is associated with a chance for unplanned emergency cesarean delivery. Labor pain may also affect PVR, and neuraxial analgesia with dilute local anesthetic with opioids can provide analgesia with minimal changes in systemic vascular resistance (SVR). Scheduled cesarean delivery, if possible, offers the opportunity to deliver in a more controlled manner with optimized conditions. Spinal anesthesia may abruptly decrease SVR in patients presenting for cesarean delivery; however, gradual induction of epidural anesthesia may be able to mitigate this change. General anesthesia presents risks for increased PAPs during intubation, decreased venous return from positive pressure ventilation, and negative inotropy from volatile anesthetics.[5]

## REFERENCES

1. Sarkar MS, Desai PM. Pulmonary hypertension and cardiac anesthesia: anesthesiologist's perspective. *Ann Card Anaesth.* 2018;21(2):116–122.
2. Thenappan T, et al. Pulmonary arterial hypertension: pathogenesis and clinical management. *BMJ.* 2018;360:j5492.
3. Galiè N, et al. An overview of the 6th World Symposium on Pulmonary Hypertension. *Eur Respir J.* 2019;53(1):1802148.
4. Hansmann G. Pulmonary hypertension in infants, children, and young adults. *J Am Coll Cardiol.* 2017;69(20):2551–2569.
5. Barash P, et al. *Clinical Anesthesia.* 8th ed. Philadelphia, PA: Wolters Kluwer; 2017:1162.

# 129.

# HEART TRANSPLANTATION

*James Leonardi and Daniel Cormican*

## INTRODUCTION

Heart failure (HF) encompasses structural or functional cardiac disorders that impair the ability of either ventricle to produce cardiac output. Cardiac transplant is indicated for intractable HF that is classified as a New York Heart Association class III or IV. Worldwide, the most common indication for heart transplantation is nonischemic cardiomyopathy, followed by ischemic cardiomyopathy. Patient "transplant status" reflects a potential recipient's degree of cardiac dysfunction, amount of required cardiac support, and urgency for receiving a transplant, as per the Organ Procurement and Transplantation Network (OPTN) as shown in Table 129.1.

## ANESTHETIC MANAGEMENT OF THE HEART TRANSPLANT RECIPIENT

### PREOPERATIVE

Patients scheduled for cardiac transplantation are functionally compromised; it is important to consider many patients will present preoperatively with inotropic infusions, a ventricular assist device (VAD), or extracorporeal membrane oxygenation (ECMO) support. Multiple concomitant organ systems may also be impaired by end-stage HF: Acute or chronic renal failure can be associated with hypoperfusion; renal failure brings electrolyte derangements and metabolic disturbances. Hepatic dysfunction and transaminitis may be noted due to liver engorgement. Pulmonary compromise may be seen—pulmonary edema and pleural effusions are not uncommon due to the "back pressure" created when left ventricular and left atrial pressures increase due to HF. Importantly, changes to the pulmonary vasculature due to HF can result in significant pulmonary hypertension; this pulmonary hypertension can impair the function of newly transplanted heart if severe. Many patients present with a pacemaker or defibrillator and are risk for life-threatening ventricular arrhythmias.[1] Those on a left VAD or ECMO support require anticoagulation. Total body volume overload may manifest as peripheral edema, which may complicate placement of invasive monitors.

### INTRAOPERATIVE

The orthotopic heart transplantation (OHT) recipient requires standard monitors intraoperatively. Consideration should be given for a preinduction arterial catheter if one is not already present. Patients undergoing OHT should be considered "full stomach" as the timing is dictated by donor availability, and rapid sequence intubation should be considered to reduce to risk of aspiration. External defibrillation pads are indicated if the recipient has an implantable-cardioverter defibrillator that may need to inactivated intraoperatively.[1] Anesthetic induction should maintain cardiac output and systemic vascular resistance; inotropic infusions should be maintained to ensure the hemodynamic stability. Anesthesia maintenance with volatile agents is used with relatively low concentrations to maintain hemodynamic stability and end-organ perfusion. Lung-protective ventilator strategies are aimed at preventing an increase in pulmonary vascular resistance by overdistension of alveolar vessels and minimizing right ventricular (RV) afterload.

Regarding vascular access, large-bore central venous access is required. Many centers place a pulmonary artery catheter for perioperative monitoring. Some centers avoid catheterization of the right internal jugular vein to preserve a conduit for future endomyocardial biopsies. The transplant recipient may be placed on cardiopulmonary bypass (CPB) via cannulation of the femoral vessels with repeat sternotomy. Blood should be immediately available in the room if the case is a repeat sternotomy due to an increased risk of injury to intrathoracic vessels.

Implantation of the donor graft immediately follows explantation of the native heart. Native atrial appendages are removed due to a risk of postoperative thrombus formation. If a patent foramen ovale has been identified in the donor graft, it is surgically repaired; in most contemporary transplant practices, the "bicaval technique" is used for graft

**Table 129.1** 2018 ORGAN PROCUREMENT AND TRANSPLANTATION NETWORK CRITERIA FOR MEDICAL URGENCY STATUS: ORTHOTROPIC HEART TRANSPLANTATION

| 2018 STATUS | INDICATIONS |
| --- | --- |
| 1 | ECMO[1] <br> Non-dischargeable VAD[2] <br> MVS with life threatening arrhythmia[2] |
| 2 | Non-dischargeable LVAD[2] <br> Percutaneous endovascular LVAD[2] <br> IABP[2] <br> VT/VF without MCS[2] <br> MCS with mechanical failure[2] <br> Dischargeable BiVAD/RVAD/TAH[2] |
| 3 | Dischargeable LVAD[3] <br> High dose inotrope/multiple inotropes requiring monitoring[2] <br> MCS with: <br> Hemolysis[2] <br> Pump thrombosis[2] <br> RV failure[2] <br> Infection[6] <br> Mucosal bleeding[7] <br> Aortic insufficiency[8] <br> ECMO[4] <br> Non-Dischargeable LVAD[5] <br> Percutaneous Endovascular LVAD[5] <br> IABP[5] |
| 4 | Congenital heart disease[8] <br> Hypertrophic cardiomyopathy[8] <br> Restrictive cardiomyopathy[8] <br> Dischargeable LVAD[8] <br> Inotropes without monitoring[8] <br> Intractable angina[8] <br> Re-transplant[8] |
| 5 | Multi–organ transplant[9] |
| 6 | All others[9] |

1: Renewable every 7 days. 2: Renewable every 14 days. 3: Discretionary 30-day period. 4: If Status 1 is not renewed. 5: If Status 2 is not renewed. 6: 14 days if clinical evidence of driveline infection, 42 days if bacteremia requiring antibiotic, 90 days if device pocket infection or recurrent bacteremia. 7: 14 days if two hospitalizations in 6 months, 90 days if 3 times in past 6 months. 8: Renewable every 90 days. 9: 180 days.

Reproduced with permission from Stein LH, Choudhary M, Silvestry SC. ©2018. http://dx.doi.org/10.5772/intechopen.74819

anastomosis, although some centers may use the "biatrial technique." Two surgical techniques for OHT are briefly reviewed:

- Biatrial implantation refers to the anastomosis of the donor heart to the recipient's left (LA) and right atria (RA). This approach places the sinoatrial node at risk of injury, atrial dysrhythmias, and tricuspid insufficiency secondary to distortion of the RA.[2]

- Bicaval implantation refers to the anastomosis of the recipient's LA cuff containing the PVs to the donor heart with lower risk of dysrhythmias, lower RA pressures, and lower incidence of tricuspid insufficiency.[2]

Immunosuppression (often in the form of high-dose steroids) may be given prior to removal of the aortic cross clamp. Once the donor and recipient aorta are united, the aortic cross clamp is removed, and the patient is placed in Trendelenburg position to decrease the risk of an air embolism. Transesophageal echocardiographic guidance is utilized to swiftly identify global contractility, evidence of profound valvulopathy, or signs of anastomotic stenosis, among other considerations. Acute RV failure is of particular concern. Treatment goals for post-CPB RV failure include adequate coronary perfusion by maintaining aortic pressure, optimizing preload, and maintaining adequate filling pressures, which can be obtained with inhaled Flolan or nitric oxide as an adjunct to lower pulmonary vascular resistance prior to CPB wean and help prevent right HF.[3] The heart rate post-CPB wean is normally kept 100–120 beats per minute, thus preventing excessive diastolic filling time in the RV. Refractory RV failure requires a right VAD or ECMO placement.

## POSTOPERATIVE

Important considerations postoperatively include autonomic denervation as the transplanted heart lacks the cardiac autonomic plexus, resulting in loss of vagal neurons and postganglionic sympathetic nerves from the stellate ganglion to the myocardium.[4] This manifests as an elevated resting heart rate, commonly seen from 90 to 100 beats per minute. The transplanted heart responds to direct acting β-adrenergic agonists, such as isoproterenol or dobutamine. RV failure may arise postoperatively as well; management options are similar to those discussed previously.

## PROGNOSIS

The OPTN data from 2011 through 2013 reveal the overall survival after OHT at 1 year, 3 years, and 5 years was 90.3%, 84.7%, and 79.6%, respectively.[5] Risk factors for increased mortality after undergoing heart transplantation include prior transplantation due to acute graft failure, poor human leukocyte antigen matching, preoperative ventilator dependence, advanced as well as younger recipients and older donors.[6] After immunosuppression, there is risk for infection; chronic immunosuppression increases the risk of malignancies.

## REFERENCES

1. Chia PL, Foo D. Overview of implantable cardioverter defibrillator and cardiac resynchronisation therapy in heart failure management. *Singapore Med J.* 2016;57(7):354–359.
2. el Gamel A et al. Orthotopic cardiac transplantation: a comparison of standard and bicaval Wythenshawe techniques. *J Thorac Cardiovasc Surg.* 1995;109(4):721–729.
3. Cheng A, Slaughter MS. Heart transplantation. *J Thorac Dis.* 2014;6(8):1105–1109.
4. Awad M, et al. Early denervation and later reinnervation of the heart following cardiac transplantation: a review. *J Am Heart Assoc.* 2016;5(11):e004070.
5. Adult Heart Transplant. Scientific Registry of Transplant Recipients. OPTN/SRTR 2018 annual data report: heart. Accessed August 12, 2020. https://srtr.transplant.hrsa.gov/annual_reports/2018/Heart.aspx
6. Stehlik J, et al. The Registry of the International Society for Heart and Lung Transplantation: twenty-seventh official adult heart transplant report–2010. J Heart Lung Transplant. 2010;29:1089–1103.

# 130.

# CARDIAC TAMPONADE

*Ravi K. Grandhi and Alaa Abd-Elsayed*

## INTRODUCTION

Etiologies of pericardial tamponade vary based on whether they are inflammatory or noninflammatory.[1] The pericardium is composed of two layers of tissue, the serous visceral and fibrous parietal layers, which have less than 50 mL of serous fluid. By definition, a pericardial effusion is when the amount of fluid exceeds this amount.

## ETIOLOGY

A number of disease processes can cause pericardial effusions, but few etiologies progress to cardiac tamponade. The most likely causes include malignancy, end-stage renal disease, bacterial or fungal infections, and effusions 3–7 days after cardiac surgery.[2] Pericardial effusions caused by bacterial or fungal etiologies are often exudative in nature. In the developing world, the most common cause is tuberculosis. Idiopathic reasons may also cause it.

Cardiac tamponade can be

- Acute, which occurs within minutes due to trauma or rupture of the heart. This type will have a presentation similar to cardiogenic shock.

- Subacute, which occurs within days to weeks due to neoplastic, uremic, or idiopathic pericarditis.
- Low pressure (occult), which is a subset of subacute cardiac tamponade and usually occurs in patients who are severely hypovolemic.
- Regional, which occurs when the tamponade is loculated. It can be caused by a localized hematoma, and it will exert pressure/compression on the related chamber.

## DIAGNOSIS

Diagnosis is based on history, physical, and imaging modalities. Critical findings include tachycardia, dyspnea, diminished arterial and cardiac pulsations, muffled heart sounds, chest discomfort, increased jugular venous pressures, diaphoresis, and pulsus paradoxus (also known as paradoxic pulse), which is an abnormally large decrease in stroke volume, systolic blood pressure, and pulse wave amplitude during inspiration. The normal decrease in systolic blood pressure is less than 10 mm Hg. So, a drop a higher will be seen with pulsus paradoxus. The hemodynamics are related to decreased pericardial compliance, ventricular interdependence, and inspiratory decrease in pressure gradient for left ventricular filling.[1] An electrocardiogram (ECG) shows diffuse low voltage and electrical alternans (alternating QRS amplitude that is seen in one or all leads on an ECG with no changes to conduction pathways of the heart), which occurs due to swinging of the heart in the fluid-filled pericardial sac. Chest x-ray is also used and may indicate a normal size heart until the effusion is more than 200 mL.

As the volume of the pericardium increases, there is increased central venous and pulmonary artery occlusion pressures. A ECG shows increased intrapericardial and intracardiac filling pressure, and diastolic volumes decrease, dramatically impairing cardiac filling and reducing cardiac output.[2] These changes are more dramatic for the thin-walled right atrium and ventricle, which have lower pressures and are less muscular than the left ventricle.[2] Left atrium collapse, which occurs rarely, is highly specific. There may also be paradoxical motion of the intraventricular septum. If a pulmonary artery catheter (PAC) is placed, it may show equilibration of central venous, pulmonary artery, and pulmonary artery occlusion pressures.

## ANESTHETIC CONSIDERATIONS

Cardiac tamponade is a medical emergency.

### PREOPERATIVE

Preoperatively, assess for hemodynamic stability. For patients who are hemodynamically unstable, pericardial drainage may be performed with local anesthetic infiltration and low-dose sedatives. In those patients who are hemodynamically stable or acquired stability after partial drainage with local anesthetic, general anesthesia may be employed. Consider placing an arterial line and a PAC.

### INTRAOPERATIVE

Induction agents that minimally depress cardiac function are preferred intraoperatively. There is no difference in outcome between those that receive local anesthesia and those receiving general anesthesia.[2] However, with general anesthesia it is possible to completely evacuate the pericardial contents. Hemodynamic goals are fast, full, and tight by using fluids and inotropes to maintain heart rate, preload, and afterload.

Mechanical ventilation, especially positive pressure ventilation, may increase pulmonary vascular resistance and decrease right ventricular outflow, further exacerbating septal shift, impairing left ventricular filling, and potentially worsening systemic hypotension. The key is to avoid large tidal volumes and high peak airway pressures or to use spontaneous ventilation if possible.

### POSTOPERATIVE

Continue monitoring during the postoperative period.

### REFERENCES

1. Vakamudi S, et al. Pericardial effusions: causes, diagnosis, and management. *Prog Cardiovasc Dis.* 2017;59(4):380–388.
2. O'Connor CJ, Tuman KJ. The intraoperative management of patients with pericardial tamponade. *Anesthesiol Clin.* 2010;28(1):87–96.

# 131.

# CONSTRICTIVE PERICARDITIS

*Ravi K. Grandhi and Alaa Abd-Elsayed*

## INTRODUCTION

Constrictive pericarditis (CP) is caused by a fibrotic pericardium. CP can be symmetric or asymmetric, affecting the right or left side predominantly, and affecting ventricular interdependence.

## ETIOLOGY

Constrictive pericarditis most commonly occurs after pericardial disease or cardiac surgery or for idiopathic reasons.[1] In the developing world and immunocompromised patients, tuberculosis has to be considered. Other rarer causes include connective tissue disorders, malignancy, trauma, medications, asbestos, or sarcoidosis.

## DIAGNOSIS

Diagnosis of CP is based on history, physical, and diagnostic modalities. On physical examination, there is elevated jugular venous pressure associated with a deep y descent with right heart catheterization.[2] There may also be evidence of a Kussmaul sign (a paradoxical rise in jugular venous pressure [JVP] on inspiration or a failure in the appropriate fall of the JVP with inspiration) and pericardial knock (a high-pitched, early diastolic sound that occurs when unyielding pericardium results in sudden arrest of ventricular filling). An electrocardiogram (ECG) may show nonspecific ST-segment and T-wave changes associated with low-voltage QRS. The ECG shows reduced diastolic filling and thus diastolic heart failure, with preserved systolic function. There is also diastolic equalization of the pressures in the right atrium, right ventricle, and pulmonary wedge pressures. The diastolic filling is reduced by an inelastic pericardium, which may present as an increased pericardial thickness on imaging. There may

also be exaggerated ventricular interdependence. Chest x-ray may show pericardial calcifications, along with pleural effusions.[3]

## TREATMENT

Mild cases can be treated with anti-inflammatory medications. Severe cases will require pericardiectomy.

## ANESTHETIC CONSIDERATIONS

### PREOPERATIVE

In the preoperative period, it is important to assess for severity.

### INTRAOPERATIVE

Primary anesthetic considerations intraoperatively include preserving myocardial function, avoiding bradycardia, and avoiding excessive volume administration. Titrating to urine output can be important in avoiding major fluid shifts. Diuretics can also be used to maintain euvolemia.

### POSTOPERATIVE

Continue monitoring during the postoperative period.

## REFERENCES

1. Khandaker MH, et al. Pericardial disease: diagnosis and management. *Mayo Clin Proc.* 2010;85(6):572–593.
2. Yusuf SW, et al. Pericardial disease: a clinical review. *Expert Rev Cardiovasc Ther.* 2016;14(4):525–539.
3. Schwefer M, et al. Constrictive pericarditis, still a diagnostic challenge: comprehensive review of clinical management. *Eur J Cardiothorac Surg.* 2009;36(3):502–510.

# 132.

# MECHANICAL CIRCULATORY ASSIST DEVICES

*James Leonardi and Daniel Cormican*

## INTRODUCTION

Mechanical circulatory support refers to a broad list of devices used to aid or replace cardiac output in patients with heart failure (HF). These devices can be used when shock is either attributable to cardiogenic insult or the indirect result of systemic pathologic process (i.e., septic shock). Important anesthetic considerations consistent across all circulatory support devices include indications for device placement (i.e., acute myocardial infarction, myocarditis, post–cardiotomy shock, etc.); anticoagulation requirements; changes to/absence of pulsatility; and technical aspects of the device.

## VENTRICULAR ASSIST DEVICES

The ventricular assist devices (VADs) are surgically implanted pumps intended to provide significant or complete unloading of the ventricle in which it is implanted, such as a left VAD (LVAD) for left ventricular support. Contemporary LVADs are small pumps of either axial impellers or centrifugal rotational devices; the HeartMate II LVAD (Abbott, Abbott Park, IL, USA) is the most commonly encountered axial device. HeartMate 3 LVAD and Heartware HVAD (Medtronic, Minneapolis, MN, USA) are the available centrifugal devices. Both devices provide continuous flow, which creates minimal to no pulsatility in the arterial system. LVADs have an inflow cannula placed into the apex of the left ventricle (LV), a pump, an outflow cannula placed into the aorta, and a driveline that connects to an extracorporeal controller. The pump's speed is programed into the controller after optimal speed settings have been determined by a physician. Batteries connected to the controller power the device, and patients are discharged from the hospital with the LVAD after clinical stability is obtained. Failure to care for the LVAD may lead to catastrophic consequences, like driveline infection or battery failure.

Implantation of the LVAD is indicated for patients with New York Heart Association class IV HF symptoms that are not improved despite maximal guideline-directed medical therapies and who have a severely depressed ejection fraction. The LVAD is intended to provide patients sufficient cardiac output to improve comorbidities associated with HF, relieve symptoms of severe HF, and improve quality of life. LVADs may be implanted as definitive care ("destination therapy"), to support a patient until cardiac transplantation ("bridge to transplant"), or to allow for reversal of severe HF ("bridge to recovery"). Contraindications to LVAD placement include severe right ventricular (RV) dysfunction, known terminal medical comorbidity, or lack of stable resources to meticulously care for the LVAD and its requisite components.

Device-related complications include driveline infection; pump thrombosis; RV failure; arrhythmias; life-threatening gastrointestinal bleeding; cerebrovascular accidents; and hemolysis. These are well-described adverse events.

Right ventricular assist devices have been granted Food and Drug Administration approval for RV failure following LVAD implantation, acute myocardial infarction, or cardiac transplant. These devices are rarely used in isolation.

Temporary VADs include smaller devices, which are often percutaneously placed, that provide the same theoretical benefit as the durable VAD; the temporary devices are intended for a much shorter duration of use, require hospitalization in an intensive care unit, and are almost always placed in emergency situations where overwhelming cardiogenic shock has suddenly presented. Common contemporary temporary VADs include the Impella (Abiomed, Danvers, MA, USA) and TandemHeart (CardiacAssist Inc., Pittsburgh, PA, USA).

## ANESTHETIC CONSIDERATIONS

### PREOPERATIVE

The anesthetic provider should be aware preoperatively of the device type, implantation date, pump speed, pump flow, and pulsatility flow index as well as indication for LVAD implantation and any prior VAD-related complications. Cardiac function might also be impaired, with RV failure commonly following LVAD implantation.[1] In patients undergoing noncardiac procedures, anticoagulation is rarely discontinued in the perioperative period; notable exceptions are with intracranial and ophthalmic procedures in which compression of vascular structures to control hemorrhage is not feasible. The provider should consult with both the VAD team and surgeon regarding bridging anticoagulation with heparin.

## INTRAOPERATIVE

Standard monitors should be applied intraoperatively prior to induction of anesthesia with one caveat: Continuous flow VADs typically do not produce a palpable pulse and minimal to no arterial pulse pressure. In such scenarios, blood pressure monitoring is performed by either Doppler ultrasound or arterial catheterization, which remains the gold standard. Doppler pressure has been shown to closely approximate mean arterial pressure (MAP) via arterial catheterization in patients with HeartMate II and HVAD.[2]

The VADs are dependent on preload to maintain pump flow; changes in position (i.e., Trendenlenburg or reverse Trendelenburg), excessively large respiratory tidal volumes, or high intra-abdominal pressures can decrease venous return to the heart: Anticipating such hemodynamic changes is vital to maintenance of cardiac output.

When intravascular volume is not adequate to maintain LVAD flow, a "suction event" may precipitate in which the walls of the LV adjacent to the inflow conduit collapse and may lead to ventricular arrhythmias and hemodynamic compromise.

In the event of severe hypotension or cardiac arrest, it is paramount to initially determine if the device is functioning: A VAD produces a "hum" that signals a functional device. In the setting of end-tidal carbon dioxide less than 20 mm Hg in the setting of shock with MAP less than 50 mm Hg, relatively gentle chest compressions should be initiated; if time allows, the decision to begin compressions should be made in consultation with a cardiac surgeon or cardiologist intimately familiar with VADs.[3] Fatal dislodgement of the intraventricular or aortic cannulae can occur with aggressive chest compressions.[4] If no hum is audibly appreciated, the power source must be thoroughly investigated to rule out power failure. Patients who experience loss of VAD function for greater than 30 minutes are at increased risk of developing a thrombus and may require VAD exchange.

## POSTOPERATIVE

Disposition of the patient postoperatively must include a fully monitored setting in addition to ensuring the VAD is connected to an external power outlet and ensuring emergency batteries are charged if needed for further transport. If anticoagulation was withheld, resumption should be considered at this point for prophylaxis of thrombus formation. Any changes to the VAD settings should be promptly communicated with the VAD team to ensure safe and appropriate discharge.

## REFERENCES

1. Stone ME, et al. Implantable left ventricular assist device therapy—recent advances and outcomes. *J Cardiothorac Vasc Anesth.* 2018;32:2019.
2. Li S, et al. Accuracy of Doppler blood pressure measurement in continuous-flow left ventricular assist device patients. *ESC Heart Fail.* 2019;6(4):793–798.
3. Peberdy MA, et al. Cardiopulmonary resuscitation in adults and children with mechanical circulatory support: a scientific statement from the American Heart Association. *Circulation.* 2017;135(24):e1115–e1134.
4. Mabvuure NT, Rodrigues JN. External cardiac compression during cardiopulmonary resuscitation of patients with left ventricular assist devices. *Interact Cardiovasc Thorac Surg.* 2014;19(2):286.

# 133.

# CARDIOPULMONARY BYPASS

*Kim Sung and Lovkesh L. Arora*

## INTRODUCTION

Cardiopulmonary bypass (CPB) is an essential method to provide a bloodless field for cardiac surgeries. CPB is a type of extracorporeal circuit that drains venous blood and returns it to the arterial side. Additionally, the CPB machine allows for oxygenation, temperature regulation, electrolyte balance, and pH balance.

## CARDIOPULMONARY BYPASS COMPONENTS AND PRIMING

Cardiopulmonary bypass is made up of six important components: arterial circulation, venous circulation, reservoir, pump, heat exchanger, and oxygenator. Arterial and venous cannulae are currently made of polyvinylchloride and wire reinforcement. A right atrial cannula is the source of drainage into the venous reservoir. Blood exits the reservoir to a pump and then to an oxygenator, which mostly has a heat exchanger. Then blood passes through an arterial line filter before entering the aortic cannula.

Different types of cannulae and cannulation can occur at different sites to meet the needs of the type of surgery. The venous and arterial cannulae and connected tubing are primed with a mixture of crystalloid and colloid solutions with heparin. Priming volume can be anywhere from 750 to 2000 mL depending on the circuit length in adults. This volume can cause a significant drop in hematocrit. To circumvent and minimize hemodilution during CPB, tubing can be filled with blood in a retrograde manner, and part of the priming solution can be discarded. However, it is important that the patient continues to have enough blood volume to support the total circulating volume. Autologous priming is a class I recommendation. There are many studies to find an optimal target hematocrit during CPB, and lower hematocrit is associated with a higher risk of mortality and morbidity, such as renal failure. The current class I recommendation states that packed red blood cells (pRBCs) should be transfused if the hematocrit is less than 18%, class IIb recommendation to transfuse pRBCs if

the hematocrit is between 18% and 24%, and class III recommendation to withhold transfusion if the hematocrit is greater than 24%.[1,2]

## TYPES OF CPB

There are two main types of pumps: roller and centrifugal. Although more roller pumps are used in the United States, centrifugal pumps have significant usage in CPB. One benefit of the roller pump is that it costs less than the centrifugal pumps. There is a concern that due to the occlusive nature of the roller pump to the tubing, it may generate hemolysis and spallation inside the tubing. Centrifugal pumps avoid this problem. The disadvantage of a centrifugal pump is that a sudden change in afterload or preload can dramatically affect its function. It is a class IIa recommendation to use a centrifugal pump for surgeries that require longer CPB times.[1,3]

## APPROACH TO ANTICOAGULATION DURING CPB

Proper management of anticoagulation during CPB is critical for the safety of patients in cardiac surgery. Unfractionated heparin is most widely used as it binds to antithrombin and potentiates inactivation of thrombin and factor Xa. Anticoagulation status is monitored with activated clotting time (ACT). ACT can be influenced by temperature, low hematocrit, and platelet counts. The most common starting dose of heparin for CPB is between 300 to 500 U/kg, and the target ACT to initiate CPB is greater than 480 seconds (class IIa). If the patient fails to reach the target ACT, the patient most likely has a type of heparin resistance. There are different management approaches, including an additional 5,000–10,000 units of heparin, transfusion of fresh frozen plasma, or injection of antithrombin III. Antithrombin III is made from human plasma; therefore, it has a theoretical risk of Creutzfeldt-Jakob disease.[1,3]

After weaning from CPB, anticoagulation from heparin must be reversed. Protamine is a medication of choice to reverse the effect of heparin. Protamine works by binding to heparin to form a heparin-protamine complex, and once the complex is formed, heparin is detached from antithrombin. There are three important side effects of protamine: anaphylactic reaction, systemic hypotension, and pulmonary hypertension. A "test" dose is frequently given for early detection of these reactions, and slow infusion of protamine is recommended to reduce systemic hypotension and pulmonary hypertension.[1,3]

## CARDIOPLEGIA AND HEART PROTECTION

Cardioplegia is a potassium-rich solution delivered to the myocardium during CPB to provide surgeons with a bloodless and motionless field while operating. Cardioplegia also provides protection from ischemic damage to the myocardium. The concentration of potassium varies from 8 to 20 mEq/L and causes depolarized arrest of the myocardium. Cardioplegia can be delivered either antegrade or retrograde. Antegrade cardioplegia is delivered through either the root or direct ostial methods to the left main coronary and the right coronary artery. Retrograde cardioplegia is delivered through the coronary sinus via a coronary sinus catheter. Antegrade cardioplegia has far better cardioprotection compare to retrograde cardioplegia; however, retrograde cardioplegia is indicated in patients with aortic valve insufficiency or left main disease.[1,3]

## ANESTHETIC AND HEMODYNAMIC MONITORING ON CPB

The anesthetic plan must be carefully planned and discussed with the perfusionist while the patient is on CPB. Volatile anesthetic or total intravenous anesthesia can be used during CPB. Volatile anesthetic brings a unique challenge due to mild induced hypothermia. Hypothermia increases the blood/gas partition coefficient, decreases minimum alveolar concentration requirements, reduces systemic vascular resistance (which offsets increased systemic vascular resistance associated with hemodilution), and decreases oxygen requirement. However, during the initiation of the CPB, hemodilution is common due to the priming solution in the circuit leading to a decrease in the blood/gas partition coefficient. Decreased blood viscosity associated with hemodilution reduces systemic vascular resistance. During the rewarming phase of CPB, the reverse is true in that increases in blood temperature lower the blood/gas partition coefficient. Proper depth of anesthesia can be difficult to assess and manage due to significant and sudden changes in physiology. Electroencephalography-based bispectral index monitors have been suggested for use during CPB for guidance of the depth of anesthesia.[1,4] During CPB, the patient's blood pressure is monitored via an invasive arterial cannula. Since there is no pulsatility while on CPB, mean arterial pressure (MAP) is monitored throughout CPB. Maintaining and monitoring appropriate perfusion pressure is important to protect all end organs, such as the brain, kidneys, and the gastrointestinal tract. Vasoplegia during CPB occurs mainly due to the surge of pro-inflammatory cytokines. There is no current consensus on optimal mean arterial pressure during CPB as large randomized control studies comparing MAP goals of 70–80 versus 40–50 mm Hg showed no difference in cerebral injury. Current class I recommendation is to maintain a MAP between 50 and 80 mm Hg, and the use of $\alpha_1$-adrenergic agonist vasopressor is recommended for vasoplegia.[1,2]

## REFERENCES

1. Wahba A, et al. 2019 EACTS/EACTA/EBCP guidelines on cardiopulmonary bypass in adult cardiac surgery. *Eur J Cardiothorac Surg.* 2020;57:210.
2. Ranucci M, et al. Lowest hematocrit on cardiopulmonary bypass impairs the outcome in coronary surgery: an Italian multicenter study from the National Cardioanesthesia Database. *Tex Heart Inst J.* 2006;33(3):300–305.
3. Barry AE, et al. Anesthetic management during cardiopulmonary bypass: a systematic review. *Anesth Analg.* 2015;120:749.
4. Campbell JA, et al. Influence of intraoperative fluid volume on cardiopulmonary bypass hematocrit and blood transfusions in coronary artery bypass surgery. *J Extra Corpor Technol.* 2008;40(2):99–108.

# 134.

# MYOCARDIAL PRESERVATION DURING CARDIAC SURGERY

*Jay Trusheim and Marisa Pappas*

## INTRODUCTION

Myocardial preservation is an important aspect of cardiac surgery involving cardiopulmonary bypass. When a cross clamp is applied to the aorta, the heart will no longer receive perfusion. Therefore, mechanisms must be put in place to protect the myocardium during this time of ischemia. The three main ways the myocardium is protected are with cardioplegia solution, hypothermia, and venous drainage. There are different ways to achieve each of these, with the ultimate goal being (I think you need being or something similar here for a complete thought) a protected myocardium that is capable of separation from bypass.

## CARDIOPLEGIA

Cardioplegia is induced heart arrest (e.g., for cardiopulmonary bypass). The cardioplegia is induced by a potassium-rich solution cardioplegia solution that achieves electromechanical arrest of the heart, silencing cellular activity, and thereby decreasing cellular oxygen demand. The cardioplegia solution composition can vary by institution, but the main components include crystalloid solution or blood solution, potassium, bicarbonate, mannitol, glutamate, magnesium, and calcium.[1] These solutions are most often delivered at cold temperatures and can be given intermittently, typically every 20 minutes, or as a continuous bolus. The delivery location of cardioplegia is an important consideration.

The myocardial blood supply is delivered via coronary arteries, which originate from coronary ostia at the aortic root. The right coronary artery can be found at the right coronary cusp of the aortic valve, and the left main coronary artery originates at the left coronary cusp of the aortic valve. The left main coronary artery then bifurcates into the left anterior descending artery and left circumflex artery. Venous drainage of the myocardium occurs via multiple cardiac veins, most of which ultimately empty into the coronary sinus (Figure 134.1).

The delivery of cardioplegia can be accomplished either anterograde or retrograde. Anterograde cardioplegia is accomplished when an aortic root vent is inserted proximal to the aortic cross clamp. The cardioplegia solution is blocked from entering systemic circulation via the cross clamp and is delivered to the myocardium via the right and left coronary arteries. This results in electromechanical arrest of the heart. Another option for delivery of antegrade cardioplegia is with handheld cannulae under direct visualization. Once the aorta is open, the surgeon can directly deliver a set amount of cardioplegia solution to the coronary arteries.

Retrograde cardioplegia is necessary in two main circumstances. The first is aortic insufficiency. Anterograde cardioplegia will result in inadequate arrest of the heart since the solution will not pool in the coronary ostia and traverse down the coronary arteries, but instead reflux into the left ventricle. This process not only does not arrest the heart, but also results in left ventricular distention. The second instance in which retrograde cardioplegia may be necessary is advanced coronary artery disease or complete occlusion of coronary arteries. In these situations, a cannula is advanced into the coronary sinus, and cardioplegia solution is delivered. This solution reaches the myocardium in the opposite direction of traditional blood flow, achieving mechanical arrest.

The placement of a retrograde coronary sinus catheter can be accomplished with intraoperative transesophageal echocardiography. Additionally, one can transduce the pressure at which the solution is delivered as an added precaution. Pressures exceeding 40 mm Hg can result in damage to the coronary sinus. It is important to note, however, that the use of retrograde cardioplegia alone carries a risk of inadequate right ventricular protection while on cardiopulmonary bypass as right ventricular venous drainage is primarily via anterior cardiac veins and Thebesian veins, neither of which traditionally share a connection to the

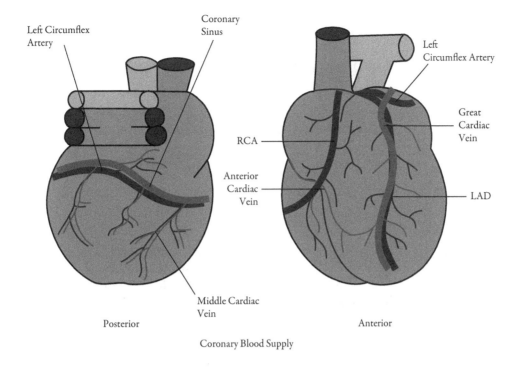

Left Circumflex Artery

Coronary Sinus

RCA

Anterior Cardiac Vein

Middle Cardiac Vein

Posterior

Left Circumflex Artery

Great Cardiac Vein

LAD

Anterior

Coronary Blood Supply

**Figure 134.1** Coronary arteries. LAD, left anterior descending coronary artery; RCA, right coronary artery.

coronary sinus.[2] This could manifest as right ventricular dysfunction or failure when attempting to wean from cardiopulmonary bypass.

## HYPOTHERMIA

Hypothermia is an additional mechanism of myocardial preservation and can be accomplished by several routes. Application of ice slush to the heart directly in the surgical field is a frequently employed method, as is the use of cold cardioplegia. Additionally, the patient can be actively cooled via the cardioplulmonary bypass circuit and through the use of underbody cooling blankets. Cooling reduces the metabolic rate at the cellular level, decreasing oxygen demand and consumption. Thus, the myocardium is further protected.

## DECOMPRESSION

During cardiopulmonary bypass, an arterial cannula is typically placed in the ascending aorta, and venous cannulae are placed in either the vena cava or right atrium to provide adequate venous drainage. Venous drainage is often accomplished passively and relies on gravity. Optimal positioning of the cannula is required to ensure adequate flow, and ideal placement may require transesophageal echocardiography. Additionally, a left ventricular vent can be placed to allow

for drainage from blood return to the heart via Thebesian and bronchial veins. This decompression of the myocardium offers additional myocardial protection due to the lack of pressure and wall tension.

## MYOCARDIAL PRESERVATION: ANESTHETIC CONSIDERATIONS

Myocardial preservation is accomplished during cardiac surgery via three main mechanisms and is frequently a task that involves anesthesia providers, perfusionists, and surgeons. Cardioplegia, especially when retrograde cannulae are required, may require transesophageal echocardiography to confirm placement and the addition of a pressure transducing line to monitor delivery. Additionally, hypothermia can be aided by the use of cooling blankets, and temperature should be monitored through the procedure to ensure optimal temperature is achieved. Finally, decompression of the heart ensures decreased wall tension, and localization of venous cannulae via transesophageal echocardiography may be necessary if inadequate drainage is encountered.

## REFERENCES

1. Ota T, et al. Short-term outcomes in adult cardiac surgery in the use of Del Nido cardioplegia solution. *Perfusion*. 2016;31(1):27–33.
2. Sutter F, et al. Right ventricular protection with coronary sinus retrograde cardioplegia. *Clin Anat*. 1994;7(5):257–262.

# 135.

# PRECONDITIONING

*Mada Helou and Ryan Nazemian*

## INTRODUCTION

The concept that brief manipulation(s) could protect an organ or tissue from subsequent ischemic injury was first put forth by Bob Jennings of Duke University. In their landmark 1986 paper,[1] Jennings's group reported results from dogs that underwent four bouts of brief occlusion of the circumflex artery (5 minutes) prior to a sustained period of ischemia (40 minutes); the control group just underwent the 40 minutes of occlusion. Subsequent histologic assessments conducted[2] days later determined that occlusive preconditioning produced a 75% decline in coronary infarct size (Figure 135.1).

In the ensuing 35 years, ischemic preconditioning has been shown in preclinical studies to protect all commonly transplanted organs from myriad pathophysiologic insults; however the translation of this phenomenon into clinical practice has not been smooth. Nonetheless, under controlled scenarios where there is a high probability of an ischemic event, various human preconditioning trials have demonstrated benefit with respect to improved organ function and reduced morbidity and mortality.[2] Practical

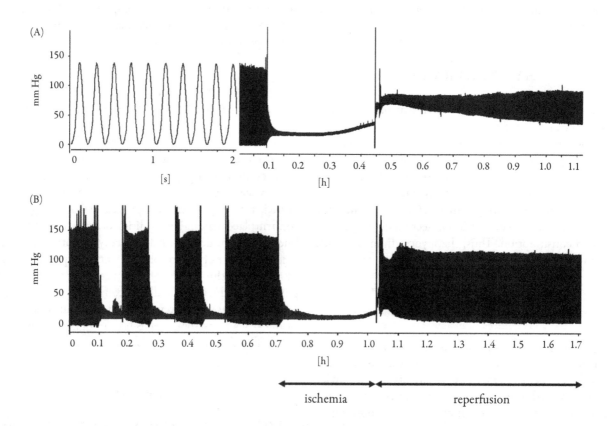

**Figure 135.1** Native records of contractile activity of the left ventricle of isolated rat heart perfused under Langendorff technique. Curve A, contractile function of the heart is greatly depressed after ischemia-reperfusion. Curve B, a set of short ischemic episodes (ischemic preconditioning) before prolonged ischemia provided functional recovery of contractile activity of the heart at reperfusion. By Goshovska—Own work, CC BY-SA 4.0, https://commons.wikimedia.org/w/index.php?curid=44044521.

constraints on physically reducing blood flow (e.g., access, duration of occlusion, etc.) have led to the search for pharmacological alternatives, and one of the first recognized drug categories to provide cell protection was the volatile anesthetics (VAs). VAs, specifically defined as halogenated compounds such as isoflurane and sevoflurane, have been shown to directly precondition or indirectly enhance ischemic preconditioning of a variety of different organs.[3] In a key example that modeled Jennings's study, Kersten and colleagues used a canine protocol to demonstrate that isoflurane (1 MAC for 65 minutes) prior to 60 minutes of coronary artery occlusion produced an equivalent reduction in infarct size as ischemic preconditioning[4]; additional positive preclinical reports soon followed. Anesthetic preconditioning has now been well documented to also occur in humans.[5] Importantly, the cellular and metabolic changes that are integral to ischemic preconditioning occur within minutes of exposure and can persist for hours.

## MECHANISM

Mechanisms of preconditioning are not well established, but there is a preponderance of evidence from animal studies that it can reduce both necrosis and apoptosis through receptor-mediated pathways involving activation of a number of protein kinases (specifically protein kinase C and mitochondrial $K_{ATP}$ channels). Future studies to elucidate the underlying mechanisms in preconditioning would facilitate development of suitable and targeted pharmacological agents that would mimic preconditioning.

## IMPLICATIONS FOR GENERAL ANESTHESIA

The importance of preconditioning and its implications during general anesthesia and specifically during surgery is still controversial. In recent years, many studies investigated the clinical importance of anesthetic preconditioning by using surrogate markers such as troponin (correlated strongly with worse clinical outcome) or inflammatory markers (e.g., interleukin [IL] 1, IL-6, and tumor necrosis factor $\alpha$).

There is substantial evidence from clinical proof-of-concept trials that all major volatile anesthetics (isoflurane, desflurane, and sevoflurane) are potentially cardioprotective, potentially depending on the pattern of administration (e.g., during the whole surgical procedure and intermittently before cardiopulmonary bypass). Also, there is evidence that a combination of volatile anesthetics and a high dose of propofol during bypass and reperfusion might increase myocardial protection as well.

## REFERENCES

1. Murry CE, et al. *Circulation*. 1986;74:1124.
2. Tomai F, et al. *Circulation*. 1999;100:559.
3. McMullan V, et al. *Perfusion*. 2015;30:6.
4. Kersten JR, et al. *Anesthesiology*. 1997;87:361.
5. Conzen PF, et al. *Anesthesiology*. 2003;99:826.

# 136.

# OFF-PUMP CORONARY ARTERY BYPASS (OPCAB)

*Ryan Krebs and Joseph Sanders*

## INTRODUCTION

The first off-pump coronary artery bypass graft surgery (OPCAB) was performed in 1967.[1] This procedure is performed similarly to coronary artery bypass grafting (CABG) and involves one or more coronary arteries bypassed via a midline sternotomy approach. However, OPCAB is performed without use of cardiopulmonary bypass (CPB). Avoiding CPB has many advantages, such as decreased risks of coagulopathy and the inflammatory response and avoidance of cross clamping the aorta. However, compared to the use of CPB, the lack of optimal surgical conditions and increased hemodynamic instability with OPCAB are challenges the surgeon and anesthesiologist will face.[1]

## ANESTHETIC CONSIDERATIONS

### PREOPERATIVE

A preoperative patient selection procedure is important to properly identify patients for whom OPCAB is appropriate.[2] Some of the many considerations include surgeon expertise, degree of atheromatous plaque, and the health of the patient regarding pulmonary and renal function. Also, special considerations should be given to determining the primary targets for bypass. The location and severity of the lesions play an important role in anticipating hemodynamic stability during the procedure.[2] For example, compared to the left anterior descending artery, the left circumflex artery requires more significant repositioning of the heart, leading to increased hemodynamic instability.[3]

### INTRAOPERATIVE

Induction of anesthesia during OPCAB should be performed as for any patient with coronary artery disease. Quality intraoperative patient care requires a thorough understanding of the procedure and the causes of hemodynamic changes. Good communication with the surgical team is essential. With OPCAB, surgeons use special equipment to stabilize the beating heart, which may alter hemodynamics. In addition, snaring the vessel to be bypassed could potentially lead to ischemia, which can be observed by ST changes on the electrocardiogram (ECG).[4] During stabilization and shunting of the vessel to be bypassed, hemodynamic compromise can occur; therefore, the anesthesiologist must determine if this compromise is from myocardial ischemia, hypovolemia, or cardiac chamber compression and then treat the patient appropriately (Table 136.1). Transesophageal echocardiography (TEE), pulmonary artery catheter, and ECG are helpful in diagnosing the cause of hemodynamic changes, and anticipation of these hemodynamic changes is common practice. Deep Trendelenburg position, fluid boluses, and vasopressors are used to maintain collateral flow to the vessel to be bypassed.[4] At our institution, we titrate norepinephrine. Manipulation of the heart during OPCAB surgery also may lead to lethal arrhythmias. Lidocaine infusion is sometimes used as a preventive measure, although there is no clear evidence for the effectiveness of this practice. If a patient is persistently acidotic and if hemodynamics are difficult to maintain despite the aforementioned maneuvers, then cardiac bypass should be readily available. Heparin dosing is institution dependent,

*Table 136.1* HEMODYNAMIC COMPROMISE AND TREATMENT DURING OFF-PUMP CARDIOPULMONARY BYPASS

| HEMODYNAMICS | TREATMENT |
| --- | --- |
| Hypovolemia | Fluids, Trendelenburg position |
| Cardiac chamber compression | Fluids, Trendelenburg position |
| Ischemia | Pressor, inotropes, fluids |
| Arrhythmia | Lidocaine |
| Continuous acidosis and hemodynamic compromise | Consider cardiopulmonary bypass |

but much lower doses are typically needed with OPCAB compared to CABG. TEE to differentiate regional wall abnormalities is more difficult with OPCAB since the surgeon uses special equipment to stabilize the heart, which could lead to a false-positive regional wall motion abnormality. Data suggest that approximately 3% of these cases will emergently convert to on-pump CABG.[4]

## POSTOPERATIVE

Similar to CABG, early extubation in the operating room has been described for OPCAB and can be done successfully in appropriate patients. Postoperative care is similar to the care for CABG patients.

## OUTCOMES

An outstanding question is whether OPCAB is better than CABG. Several large trials have compared these two surgical methods. The Randomized On/Off Bypass (ROOBY) trial in 2009 showed that patients in the off-pump group had a more unfavorable rate in the 1-year composite outcome and graft patency than did patients in the on-pump group.[4] Surgeons only had to previously perform 20 OPCAB procedures to be considered "expert" and enroll

in the study. In contrast, the CABG Off or On Pump Revascularization Study (CORONARY) required the surgeon to complete at least 100 OPCAB procedures and have 2 years of OPCAB surgical experience. The CORONARY study found no significant difference between the two procedures for primary outcomes such as death, nonfatal stroke, nonfatal myocardial infarction, or nonfatal new onset renal failure at 30 days.[5] The differences between the two procedures appear insignificant and may be more related to surgical expertise and experience.

## REFERENCES

1. Couture P, et al. Mechanisms of hemodynamic changes during off-pump coronary artery bypass surgery. *Can J Anaesth.* 2002 Oct;49(8):835–849.
2. Shanewise JS, et al. Off-pump coronary surgery: how do the anesthetic considerations differ? *Anesthesiol Clin North Am.* 2003 Sep;21(3):613–623.
3. Gründeman PF, et al. Exposure of circumflex branches in the tilted, beating porcine heart: echocardiographic evidence of right ventricular deformation and the effect of right or left heart bypass. *J Thorac Cardiovasc Surg.* 1999 Aug;118(2):316–323.
4. Gropper MA, et al, eds. *Miller's Anesthesia.* 9th ed. Elsevier; 2020.
5. Lamy A, et al. CORONARY Investigators. Effects of off-pump and on-pump coronary-artery bypass grafting at 1 year. *N Engl J Med.* 2013 Mar 28;368(13):1179–1188.

# 137.

# MINIMALLY INVASIVE DIRECT CORONARY ARTERY BYPASS GRAFTING (MIDCAB)

*John K. Kim and Iwan Sofjan*

## INTRODUCTION

Minimally invasive direct coronary artery bypass grafting (MIDCAB) is an increasingly popular alternative to the standard coronary artery bypass grafting (CABG). Some advantages of the MIDCAB approach are smaller incision, decreased bleeding, less postoperative pain, shorter hospital

stay, and faster overall recovery.[1,2] It is most commonly used to treat either a single-vessel disease, typically the left anterior descending coronary artery (LAD), or as part of a hybrid revascularization therapy with coronary stents. The main surgical steps include a small left anterior thoracotomy, left internal mammary artery (LIMA) harvesting, and anastomosis to the target coronary artery.[2]

## PROCEDURAL DETAILS

The patient is positioned supine with a pressure bag under the left scapula in order to elevate the left hemithorax. Defibrillation pads should always be placed since the nature of the surgery prevents use of open heart paddles. One-lung ventilation is typically utilized and can be achieved with either a double-lumen endotracheal tube or a bronchial blocker. Occasionally, two-lung ventilation may be sufficient if smaller tidal volumes are used. After sternal and intercostal landmarks are identified, an oblique 5- to 7-cm thoracotomy incision is made lateral to the left sternal border. Through this incision, the fourth intercostal space is identified and opened. Once the LIMA is identified, the pericardium is opened, exposing the LAD. The LIMA graft is then harvested and the adequate length established. The distal end is then anastomosed to the LAD on a beating heart, assisted by a suction or pressure stabilizer and $CO_2$ blower. During the creation of the anastomosis, coronary artery blood flow is diverted by proximal occlusion or intracoronary shunt. A test occlusion of 3–8 minutes of the target coronary artery is often performed prior to creation of the anastomosis to assess the patient's ability to tolerate off-pump revascularization. A reduced dose (100–200 U/kg) of heparin is given in between distal transection of the LIMA and coronary artery occlusion. Once the anastomosis is completed, the left lung is reinflated carefully to minimize excessive tension on the graft; protamine is administered, and surgical closure can begin.[1,3]

Off-pump coronary artery bypass is performed through a median sternotomy and can be used for grafting multiple vessels. MIDCAB avoids the median sternotomy and the associated risk of infection, but it can cause more trauma to costal cartilage and provides limited exposure.

## ANESTHETIC CONSIDERATIONS

### PREOPERATIVE

Typically, MIDCAB is reserved for patients with single-vessel disease requiring LIMA-LAD grafting that is not amenable to angioplasty. Several factors can make the MIDCAB approach difficult. A completely intramyocardial LAD course is a contraindication because the LAD is more difficult to locate, and the LIMA graft is often too short to reach the apical LAD segment.[1] Morbid obesity can make surgical landmark identification difficult and complicates airway management and one-lung ventilation. Atrial fibrillation may make inducing bradycardia difficult if required (as discussed below) and may lead to significant hemodynamic instability in patients relying on an atrial kick for

diastolic filling. The degree of coronary obstruction may correlate with the amount of hemodynamic instability and arrhythmias that may present in the operating room during vessel occlusion; the lesser the degree of obstruction, the more likely these complications will be encountered, as sufficient collateralization may not have developed. Other factors to be considered preoperatively and that can negatively affect MIDCAB include prior cardiac surgery, peripheral vascular disease, aortic atheroma, congestive heart failure, chronic lung disease, chest irradiation, and pulmonary hypertension.[1,4,5]

Patients requiring coronary revascularization also often have a number of comorbidities regardless of the surgical technique utilized, such as diabetes, chronic kidney disease, and cerebrovascular disease, all of which can increase surgical mortality and morbidity. Ultimately, determining which patients are appropriate candidates for MIDCAB takes several considerations into account.

### INTRAOPERATIVE

While avoidance of cardiopulmonary bypass (CPB) can offer several benefits for the patient, operating on a beating heart presents a number of intraoperative challenges for both the surgeon and anesthesiologist. Manipulation of the heart and myocardial ischemia caused by coronary artery occlusion during creation of the graft anastomosis can lead to significant hemodynamic instability, and communication during this time period is critical. Occasionally, suction/pressure stabilizers may be insufficient to provide stability of the surgical site, and the anesthesiologist may need to administer β-blockers or adenosine to further decrease motion caused by a beating heart. Diltiazem and neostigmine have also been used successfully to induce bradycardia.[5]

In addition to hemodynamic concerns, one-lung ventilation can lead to oxygenation and ventilation issues due to shunting of the nondependent lung and atelectasis of the dependent lung. Patients presenting for coronary revascularization frequently have concurrent smoking history and other pulmonary comorbidities, which can affect the ability to tolerate one-lung ventilation.[5]

Occasionally, CPB may be used in conjunction with a minimally invasive surgical technique. In these situations, the arterial inflow cannula is normally placed in the femoral artery, while the venous drainage cannula is placed in the femoral or internal jugular vein. If necessary, the anesthesiologist may be required to place a retrograde cardioplegia cannula through an internal jugular catheter assisted by transesophageal echocardiogram. Last, if revascularization is unsuccessful with MIDCAB or if an emergency occurs intraoperatively, conversion to sternotomy and CPB remain a possibility.[5]

## POSTOPERATIVE

Despite being smaller than a traditional sternotomy, the thoracotomy incision used in MIDCAB may cause significant pain. Intravenous opioid and nonopioid analgesic techniques have traditionally been used for pain management postoperatively. Thoracic epidural catheters and single-shot intrathecal opioids have also been used successfully, but carry the risk of epidural hematoma in systemically anticoagulated patients and can lead to further hemodynamic instability via sympathetic blockade. Intercostal nerve blocks can be performed under direct visualization by the surgeon.[5] In addition, paravertebral and erector spinae blocks have been used to decrease postoperative narcotic requirements while avoiding the risks associated with neuraxial analgesia.

## REFERENCES

1. Tekin Aİ, Arslan Ü. Perioperative outcomes in minimally invasive direct coronary artery bypass versus off-pump coronary artery bypass with sternotomy. *Wideochir Inne Tech Maloinwazyjne.* 2017;12(3):285–290.
2. Kotowicz V, et al. How to perform a MIDCAB procedure step-by-step in single-vessel disease. *CTSNet.* July 2018. doi:10.25373/ctsnet.6713054.v1. https://www.ctsnet.org/article/how-perform-midcab-procedure-step-step-single-vessel-disease
3. Repossini A, et al. MIDCAB: tips and tricks for a successful procedure. *Multi-media Manual of Cardo-Thoracic Surgery.* May 22, 2020. https://mmcts.org/tutorial/1470
4. Malik V, et al. Anesthetic challenges in minimally invasive cardiac surgery: Are we moving in a right direction? *Ann Card Anaesth.* 2016;19(3):489–497.
5. Schell RM. Anesthesia for minimally invasive cardiac surgery. In: Estafanous FG, ed. *Cardiac Anesthesia: Principles and Clinical Practice.* Philadelphia, PA: Lippincott, Williams & Wilkins; 2001: Chap 25.

# 138.

# PERCUTANEOUS VALVE REPAIR/REPLACEMENT

*Asif Neil Mohammed and Iordan Potchileev*

## INTRODUCTION

Valvular heart disease and resultant heart failure are a leading cause of morbidity and mortality in the United States. As a result, the need for cardiac surgery or percutaneous structural heart repair continues to increase, with percutaneous valve repair or replacement becoming one of the most rapidly developing areas in cardiology.

In developed countries, the most common valvular lesions are aortic stenosis (AS), due to calcific deposits, and mitral regurgitation (MR), due to either degenerative disease or secondary causes, such as ischemic heart disease or nonischemic cardiomyopathy. Several procedures have been developed over the past several decades to facilitate less invasive methods of repairing or replacing valves. These procedures include balloon valvuloplasty (BAV), annuloplasty, edge-to-edge repair, and complete replacement of the valve.

## AORTIC VALVE

Aortic valve replacement is the definitive therapy for those with severe AS or severe aortic regurgitation, characterized by symptoms according to the New York Heart Association classification system. However, surgical aortic valve replacement exposes patients to the risks associated with the invasiveness of a sternotomy, cardiopulmonary bypass, and cardiac arrest. Thus, transcatheter aortic valve implantation (TAVI), is being performed for high-risk patients with promising outcomes.

The transfemoral arterial approach is the most common method of implantation, although subclavian, axillary, transaortic, or transapical approaches can also be performed based on the patient's condition. When the technique was first developed, general anesthesia (GA) was preferred as it allowed intraoperative transesophageal echocardiography (TEE) monitoring to provide technical guidance and to identify perivalvular leaks.[1] However, an increasing amount of these procedures are being performed under moderate sedation, without the use of TEE monitoring. Studies demonstrated that moderate sedation is associated with lower mortality risk, lower inotrope use, and shorter hospital stays.[2] Current systems include the balloon-delivered Edwards SAPIEN, SAPIEN XT, and SAPIEN 3 valves (Edwards Lifesciences, Irvine, CA) versus self-expanding valves (CoreValve, Medtronic Inc., Minneapolis, MN).

## MITRAL VALVE

Mitral valve pathology is stratified by Carpentier classification (I, II, IIIa, IIIb). Currently available transcatheter repairs include the widely used edge-to-edge repair (Figure 138.1). The MitraClip (Abbott Vascular, Santa Clara, CA) is currently the only percutaneous therapy for MR approved by the Food and Drug Administration, but several other transcatheter platforms, including transcatheter mitral valve replacement systems, are either in development or being clinically evaluated.

On the contrary, patients with severe mitral stenosis (MS) can benefit from percutaneous mitral balloon valvotomy under mild or moderate sedation and often do not require GA or intraoperative TEE monitoring.

## PULMONIC VALVE

In select patients with severe pulmonary regurgitation or severe right ventricular outflow obstruction, percutaneous pulmonic valve implantation is the preferred treatment. The two most common commercially available valves are the Melody™ Transcatheter Pulmonary Valve (TPV) or Edwards valve. The procedure can be performed both under GA or moderate sedation, and the valve is most commonly implanted through a femoral vein approach, although entrance through the jugular vein is also accepted.

Complications include left main coronary artery compression, conduit rupture, stent fracture, and endocarditis.[5]

## TRICUSPID VALVE

Current tricuspid valve devices are investigational in the United States and have not been commercially approved. However, the Abbott Triclip™ and Edwards PASCAL™ valves have been approved for use in Europe.

## ANESTHETIC CONSIDERATIONS

### PREOPERATIVE

The goal of the preanesthetic preoperative evaluation is to develop an anesthetic plan that minimizes risk to the patient while taking into account the patient's comorbidities. A physical examination should be performed and must take into consideration ease of venous or arterial access, ability to lay supine with positive pressure, any existing infections that pose a risk to a newly implanted prosthetic valve, esophageal disease that precludes the use of TEE if required, and the possibility of a difficult airway. Multiple scoring systems have been developed to assess the preoperative risk for patients undergoing cardiac surgery, such as the EuroSCORE, which takes into account factors such as patient's age, sex, insulin-dependent diabetes mellitus, chronic pulmonary disease, impaired mobility, and renal disease, in addition to, the CARE score, which factors in whether or not a patient has stable cardiac disease and whether or not the surgery is considered complex.

The anesthesiologist should review any existing laboratory or imaging data. Medication lists should be reviewed, and special attention should be paid to cardiovascular medications, such as β-blockers, platelet inhibitors, or oral anticoagulants.

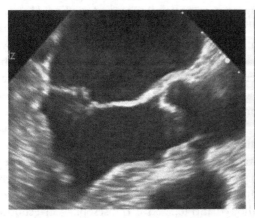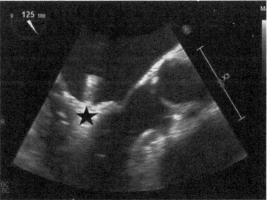

**Figure 138.1** (Left) TEE of mitral valve with P2 prolapse. (Right) Mitral valve with edge-to-edge clip in place, black star on clip.

## INTRAOPERATIVE

The overall intraoperative hemodynamic goals for an anesthesiologist are to maintain sinus rhythm, preload, and afterload and to maintain contractility through inotropic support. However, there are a few key differences according to the valvular lesion being treated. In patients with AS, hemodynamic instability must be anticipated and treated when the TAVI valve is advanced across the native atrioventricular (AV) annulus. To correctly position the percutaneous aortic valve, many centers will perform a BAV to increase the stenotic valve opening to accommodate the new AV apparatus. After BAV and before deployment, the patient is usually rapidly paced to 120–180 beats per minute to allow for proper positioning.

For mitral valve lesions, it is important to maintain right ventricular contractility by avoiding drugs that cause myocardial depression. If inotropic support is needed, milrinone or dobutamine are the preferred agents. Peripheral vascular resistance should be minimized by avoiding hypoxemia or hypercarbia. All percutaneous interventions for the mitral valve require a transseptal puncture, which may lead to embolic sequelae. Prior to crossing the interatrial septum, intravenous heparin is administered to obtain an activated clotting time of more than 250 seconds.

## POSTOPERATIVE

Patients undergoing percutaneous valve replacements or repairs currently require postoperative intensive care unit care. Common complications include hematoma at the venous/arterial access points, intra-atrial puncture, aortic valve annulus injury, and embolic events.

Currently, TAVI patients are monitored for heart block, arrhythmias, stroke, heart failure, and postoperative respiratory failure. Post–mitral valve edge-to-edge repair patients are monitored for arrhythmia, signs of clip embolization, and signs of MS or MR. Echocardiographic follow-up is imperative to assess the function of the new valve. Post-TAVI, some centers may start antiplatelet therapy per American Heart Association recommendations.

## REFERENCES

1. Teeter EG, et al. Assessment of paravalvular leak after transcatheter aortic valve replacement: transesophageal echocardiography compared with transthoracic echocardiography. *J Cardiothorac Vasc Anesth*. 2017;31(4):1278–1284.
2. Hyman MC, et al. Conscious sedation versus general anesthesia for transcatheter aortic valve replacement. *Circulation*. 2017;136(22):2132–2140.
3. Hilberath JN, et al. Intraoperative evaluation of transmitral pressure gradients after edge-to-edge mitral valve repair. *PLoS One*. 2013;8(9):e73617.
4. Estévez-Loureiro R, et al. Percutaneous mitral valve repair for acute mitral regurgitation after an acute myocardial infarction. *J Am Coll Cardiol*. 2015;66(1):91–92.
5. Eicken A, et al. Percutaneous pulmonary valve implantation: two-centre experience with more than 100 patients. *Eur Heart J*. 2011;32(10):1260–1265.

# 139.

# INTRA-AORTIC BALLOON PUMPS

*Frank Barrack and Bryan Noorda*

## INTRODUCTION

Several mechanical supports for the failing heart exist. One frequently utilized left ventricular assist device is the intra-aortic balloon pump (IABP). The IABP is designed to improve the oxygen supply/demand ratio in failing hearts.[1]

The IABP is the most common and readily available form of mechanical support for a failing heart.[1,2] An IABP is a long balloon measuring around 25 cm mounted on a 90-cm catheter, which is usually inserted via the femoral artery or, less often, via the ascending aorta. The balloon is advanced so that the distal tip rests distal to the left subclavian artery and the proximal tip above the renal arteries. The device connects to an external console, which contains a cylinder of gas, usually helium, for balloon inflation, a valve unit monitor to track the patient's electrocardiogram and arterial line tracings, and a control unit to coordinate the measurements with balloon function.[2]

The IABPs decrease myocardial oxygen consumption while also increasing the oxygen supply to the myocardium, improving the oxygen supply/demand balance.[1] The mechanism by which this is achieved is called counterpulsation. The IABP synchronizes with the heartbeat to inflate during diastole and deflate during systole, effectively moving blood in a direction counter to normal flow.[2] Coronary artery perfusion occurs during diastole. Inflation of the IABP during diastole increases diastolic pressure, augmenting coronary perfusion and improving oxygen supply to potentially ischemic areas. Subsequent deflation during systole decreases the afterload faced by the left ventricle, decreasing myocardial oxygen consumption. Effective synchronization with the heartbeat is necessary to maximize these beneficial effects. Controlling heart rate and preventing dysrhythmias promotes synchronicity. Myocardial function often improves with improved oxygen supply and systolic unloading, improving systemic perfusion to end organs.[1]

General indications for IABP placement are based on the beneficial physiological effects of the device. One is temporary support or bridging for the left ventricle following myocardial infarction (MI), intraoperative injury, or heart failure. The other is preservation of myocardium and limiting continued ischemic damage by improving the oxygen supply/demand balance. Specific examples reflect one or both of these ideas. Placement of an IABP for unstable angina refractory to medical therapy may provide relief of chest pain, improvement in ST segment changes, and prevent associated ventricular tachyarrhythmias.[1,2]

In MI, IABPs minimize extension of the ischemic zone and provide a bridge to revascularization therapy. Another complication of MI is papillary muscle rupture, usually after right coronary artery territory infarction, resulting in mitral valve regurgitation.[2]. IABPs minimize regurgitant volume by promoting anterograde flow with systolic unloading. Similarly, IABPs benefit patients who undergo rupture of the interventricular septum following MI. In the event of medically intractable tachyarrhythmias due to MI, IABP placement can also assist in the acute period prior to cardiac catheterization or coronary artery bypass grafting. During high-risk cardiac catheterizations with percutaneous coronary intervention, IABPs are either kept on standby or placed prophylactically in the event of complications such as MI.[2]

Other less common indications include using IABPs as a bridge for cardiac transplantation, for high-risk patients undergoing noncardiac procedures, for inability to wean from cardiopulmonary bypass, and for use in pediatric patients with severe valvular disease or congestive heart failure. Use of IABPs in pediatrics is complicated due to the size of the device relative to the aorta, the elasticity of the aorta, and the small stroke volume in this population.[2] Contraindications to IABPs include severe aortic regurgitation, irreversible brain damage, irreversible cardiac disease, or inability to insert the device.[1]

Complications of IABP arise from the process of placing the device or vascular injury associated with the prolonged use of IABPs. Malposition of the device is fairly common and can cause problems, such as kidney injury in the case of juxtarenal malposition.[1,2] Clinically silent complications such as aortoiliac dissection or arterial emboli may occur. Occasionally, these result in ischemia to extremities requiring balloon removal or other intervention. Mild thrombocytopenia is common, occurring in around half of patients with IABPs. Extended duration of IABP use predisposes to higher rates of infection and thrombosis. Very rarely, the balloon can rupture causing the helium to react with blood and form a hard clot, trapping the balloon in the aorta.[2]

## ANESTHETIC CONSIDERATIONS

### PREOPERATIVE

Only emergent procedures should be performed on patients reliant on an IABP. Proper IABP placement should be confirmed prior to the procedure. Providers must undertake careful transport for patients with these devices to ensure the position remains the same. Unless required for the procedure, preoperative heparin anticoagulation is not usually necessary. A current type and screen should be available in case of complications.[3]

### INTRAOPERATIVE

It is reasonable intraoperatively to have a goal mean arterial pressure over 65 mm Hg for patients with IABPs. The arterial line waveform on the operating room monitors will have a pronounced diastolic wave reflecting inflation of the balloon during diastole. Electrocautery during a procedure can cause changes in the detected electrocardiogram and potentially precipitate asynchronous balloon inflation and deflation. In this event, the monitoring unit can be switched to reading the native arterial waveform.[3]

### POSTOPERATIVE

Postoperative considerations mirror the preoperative considerations.

## REFERENCES

1. Barash P, et al. *Clinical Anesthesia*. 8th ed. Philadelphia, PA: Wolters Kluwer; 2017:1162.

2. Parissis H, et al. IABP: history-evolution-pathophysiology-indications: what we need to know. *J Cardiothorac Surg.* 2016;11(1):122.

3. Tickoo M, Bardia A. Anesthesia at the edge of life: mechanical circulatory support. *Anesthesiol Clin.* 2020;38(1):19–33.

# 140.

# EXTRACORPOREAL MEMBRANE OXYGENATION (ECMO)

*Michael Morkos and Daniel Cormican*

## INTRODUCTION

The use of extracorporeal membrane oxygenation (ECMO) has increased dramatically over the past 30 years due to drastic improvements in equipment and technique. ECMO can reliably perform the physiological functions of oxygenation, carbon dioxide removal, and perfusion of vital organs. The device has proven to be invaluable in the temporary bypass of the heart and/or lungs in critically ill patients unresponsive to standard therapy.

## BASIC PRINCIPLES

The standard ECMO circuit drains deoxygenated blood into a pump (centrifugal or roller), with the blood then sent to an oxygenator. The oxygenator contains a semipermeable membrane separating blood from fresh gas (a combination of air and oxygen, also termed "sweep gas"). Following equilibration of gases, oxygenated blood is pumped back to the patient via return cannulas. Blood oxygenation is primarily determined by the fraction of oxygen delivered through the sweep gas, blood flow through circuit, and the ability of the patient's lungs to participate in gas exchange. Similarly, removal of carbon dioxide is determined by the rate of blood flow and sweep gas flow.[1]

## MODES

Two modes of ECMO are currently available and dependent on patient requirements: venous-arterial (VA) and venous-venous (VV). Of the two, VA ECMO is most analogous to conventional cardiopulmonary bypass as it provides both cardiovascular and pulmonary support. Arterial cannulation is often done peripherally via the femoral artery (the subclavian and axillary arteries may also be used; Figure 140.1) or centrally through the aorta, which requires a thoracotomy.[2] VA ECMO is reserved for patients in cardiogenic failure displaying a cardiac index below 2 L/min/m², systolic pressure below 90 mm Hg, and lactic acidosis despite adequate volume resuscitation, inotropic support, and use of an intra-aortic balloon pump.[1,3]

Venous-venous ECMO is used in cases of respiratory failure that require selective pulmonary support. This configuration drains deoxygenated blood from the central venous circulation (typically from the common femoral vein), which is then returned to the left side of the heart. VV ECMO is used in respiratory failure to facilitate recovery of damaged lungs or as a bridge to transplant.[1,3] Specific indications for VA and VV ECMO are listed in Table 140.1.

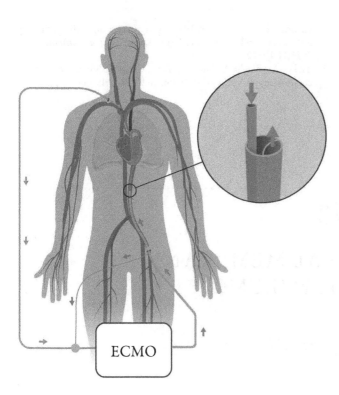

**Figure 140.1** VA ECMO is shown, with the blue arrow indicating the draining cannula from the internal jugular. After passing through the oxygenator, blood returns to the patient through the femoral artery in retrograde fashion, indicated by the red arrow.

## CONTRAINDICATIONS

Absolute contraindications to all ECMO include multiorgan failure (cirrhosis, end-stage renal disease), malignant dissemination, and existing intracranial hemorrhage.[1,3,4] Specific contraindications to each mode are listed in Table 140.2. Relative contraindications include obesity, advanced age, pregnancy, and severe peripheral vessel disease.[3,4]

*Table 140.1* INDICATIONS FOR VA AND VV ECMO

| INDICATIONS FOR VA ECMO | INDICATIONS FOR VV ECMO |
|---|---|
| • Inability to wean from bypass<br>• Cardiogenic shock<br>• Drug toxicity<br>• Pulmonary embolism<br>• Trauma to the heart or major vessels<br>• Refractory dysrhythmias<br>• High risk percutaneous interventions (percutaneous coronary intervention, poorly controlled comorbidities)<br>• Bridge to heart transplant | • Acute respiratory distress syndrome<br>• Bridge to lung transplant<br>• Graft failure following lung transplant<br>• $PaO_2{:}FiO_2 < 150$<br>• Severe pulmonary contusion<br>• Complete, irreversible airway obstruction<br>• Status asthmaticus<br>• Severe pulmonary hemorrhage |

*Table 140.2* ABSOLUTE CONTRAINDICATIONS FOR VA AND VV ECMO

| CONTRAINDICATIONS TO VA ECMO | CONTRAINDICATIONS TO VV ECMO |
|---|---|
| • Irreversible heart damage not amenable to transplant or assist device<br>• Aortic dissection<br>• Severe aortic regurgitation | • Irreversible pulmonary pathology<br>• Significant brain injury<br>• Immunosuppression (neutrophil count < 400) |

## COMPLICATIONS

Extracorporeal membrane oxygenation is associated with morbidity and mortality due to the patient's underlying comorbidities as well as complications due to the ECMO circuit itself (cannulation, anticoagulation, thrombosis).[1,4] As a general rule, VA ECMO has more complications than VV ECMO. In particular, blood return may overwhelm a failing left ventricle, resulting in left ventricular distension and possibly ventricular fibrillation. VV ECMO may result in "recirculation," wherein the draining and return cannulas are too close in proximity, resulting in the newly returned oxygenated blood being immediately removed by the draining cannula.[4]

Hemorrhage is the most common complication in ECMO patients, with an incidence between 10% and 30%.[1] Bleeding is largely attributed to hemodilution of coagulation factors, platelet dysfunction, and systemic heparinization. Bleeding often occurs at cannulation sites and into the retroperitoneal and abdominal cavities. Therapy is focused on reversing anticoagulation by decreasing heparin dosage and infusion of fresh frozen plasma and platelets as needed.

Due to the continuous heparin infusion, heparin-induced thrombocytopenia (HIT) must be considered when platelets decrease. When HIT is diagnosed, heparin should immediately be discontinued and transition to a novel anticoagulant, such as argatroban (ideal due to its short half-life) or bivalirudin, initiated.[1,4]

## ANESTHETIC CONSIDERATIONS

Surgical procedures for patients on ECMO are only performed in emergent situations due to the high risk of complications. When a procedure is required, appropriate blood products should be available. Activated clotting time levels should be checked preoperatively with titration of systemic anticoagulation as needed. Intraoperatively, monitoring should include an arterial line for frequent blood gas analysis and to ensure appropriate mean arterial pressure. It must be noted that standard monitors, specifically capnography, may not be reliable as the sweep gas removes $CO_2$ much more efficiently than the ventilator. Pulse oximetry and non-invasive blood pressure will also be unreliable with VA ECMO as loss of pulsatility prevents either modality from detecting a signal. Following the procedure, full anticoagulation may be resumed.

## REFERENCES

1. Makdisi G, Wang I. Extracorporeal membrane oxygenation (ECMO): review of a lifesaving technology. *J Thorac Dis.* 2015;7:166–176.
2. Pavlushkov E, et al. Cannulation techniques for extracorporeal life support. *Ann Trans Med.* 2017;5:70.
3. Zangrillo A. The criteria of eligibility to the extracorporeal treatment. *HSR Proc Intensive Care Cardiovasc Anesth.* 2012;4:271–273.
4. Pillai AK, et al. Management of vascular complications of extracorporeal membrane oxygenation. *Cardiovasc Diagn Ther.* 2018;8: 372–377.

# 141.

# VENTRICULAR ASSIST DEVICES

*Priyanka H. Patel and Matthew McConnell*

## INTRODUCTION

Ventricular assist devices (VADs) have been utilized for over two decades for patients with progressive heart failure in whom medical therapy is no longer effective. The utilization of VADs in management of heart failure has been shown superior to medical treatment alone.[1] VAD is a broad term encompassing any device that can be utilized to help ventricular function. Such devices include Impella (right and left) and ventricular assist devices (right and left). Here we focus predominantly on left ventricular assist devices (LVADs).

## INDICATIONS AND UTILITY

Traditional medical treatment for heart failure, such as β-blockers, diuretics, angiotensin-converting enzyme inhibitors, and inotropic agents, have not been shown to improve mortality in patients with end-stage heart failure.[2] The Randomized Evaluation of Mechanical Assistance for the Treatment of Congestive Heart Failure (REMATCH) trial, a landmark study, evaluated the efficacy of VADs as a destination therapy in 2001 and showed that LVADs,

specifically, can improve the survival and quality of life for patients when compared to medical therapy.

The use of VADs can be long or short term. The clinical applications of VADs are bridge to transplant (BTT), bridge to recovery, and destination therapy. BTT is limited due to lack of available donor hearts.

## CONTRAINDICATIONS

Absolute contraindications for the placement of VADs include irreversible hepatic or renal failure unrelated to cardiac failure, metastatic cancer, and cerebrovascular accident with deficits. Relative contraindications include active coagulopathy, active infection, mechanical cardiac valves, arrhythmias, and severe aortic regurgitation.

### FIRST GENERATION

First-generation LVADs have been widely replaced by second- and third-generation devices in clinical practice. First-generation LVADs can give up to 1 year of support due to limited durability.[3]

## SECOND GENERATION

Second-generation LVADs (HeartMate II) provide nonpulsatile flow and use axial flow pumps. Second-generation LVADs are more durable and consist of smaller drivelines, decreasing the risk of infections.[3]

## THIRD GENERATION

Third-generation LVADs (HeartWare and HeartMate 3) are continuous flow centrifugal pumps, lowering the risk of thrombosis and hemolysis.[1] These are overall smaller in size compared to the previous generation of VADs. Third-generation LVADs do not have mechanical bearings within, increasing their durability.[3]

## MECHANISM

The LVAD, specifically second-generation LVADs, consists of an inflow conduit, inlet, rotor, motor, outlet, and outflow graft.[2] The inlet, rotor, motor, and outlet components make up the main pump of the LVAD (Figure 141.1A). The external power source and controller are connected to the device via a percutaneous lead. The inflow conduit is placed at the apex of the left ventricle, wherein the blood in the ventricle is drained into the device with the use of the rotor. The outflow graft is attached at the ascending aorta into which the blood is propelled.[2] The third-generation LVAD is a continuous flow pump, circular in shape with a short inlet placed at the apex of the left ventricle (Figure 141.1B). Similar to the second generation, the third-generation LVAD has an outflow graft at the ascending aorta.[1]

## MANAGEMENT OF CARDIOPULMONARY ARREST IN PATIENTS WITH VADS

During a cardiac arrest, standard advanced cardiac life support should be carried out. Previously, chest compressions were not recommended due to concern for dislodging the machinery. The 2017 guidelines by the American Heart Association indicated that in a low-flow state, the end-tidal $CO_2$ should be used to evaluate systemic perfusion. In a pulseless, unresponsive, and intubated LVAD patient, an end-tidal $CO_2$ of 20 mm Hg or less indicates a low-flow state, and cardiopulmonary resuscitation should be performed.[4]

## COMPLICATIONS

1. *Immediately postimplantation*: Postoperatively, right heart failure (RHF) can occur. Patients with biventricular cardiovascular disease are more prone to RHF and may require ionotropic support or a right VAD.[3]
2. *Thrombosis*: Patients with VADs require systemic anticoagulation. Thromboembolic events are not uncommon with VADs; these events include stroke, pulmonary embolus, mesenteric ischemia, and device thrombosis.[2] Pump thrombosis can be treated with tissue plasminogen activator but is associated with increased mortality. Device replacement may be necessary.[3]
3. *Infection*: Infections may include superficial infections involving the transcutaneous drive

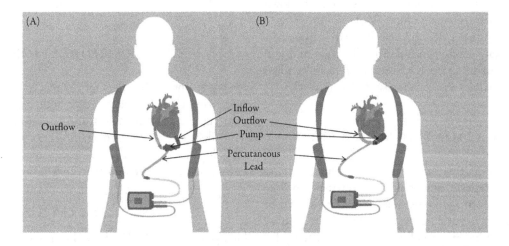

**Figure 141.1** (A) HeartMate II, Second-Generation LVAD is depicted in this image. (B) HeartMate 3, Third-Generation LVAD is illustrated in this image. HeartMate II and HeartMate 3 are trademarks of Abbott or its related companies. Reproduced with permission of Abbott, © 2020. All rights reserved.

catheters or endocarditis involving native and/or prosthetic valves.[2] Many patients are on broad-spectrum antibiotics for prolonged durations due to recurrent VAD infections.

## ANESTHETIC CONSIDERATIONS

### PREOPERATIVE

There are no contraindications of types of anesthesia or positioning of patients with VADs.[3] A thorough history and physical examination should be performed in the preoperative setting. It is important to note the type of VAD the patient has and the basic settings of the device. The type of therapy the patient is on should be addressed with the patient and the VAD multidisciplinary team.[1,5]

Baseline coagulation and hematocrit levels should be obtained prior to the surgery. Patients with VADs are likely to have an extensive transfusion history, resulting in the development of antibodies; thus, a blood type and screen is indicated. Assessing change in the patient's cardiovascular function after the VAD placement is critical. Reviewing a recent echocardiogram is important to establish baseline function. In preparation for intrathoracic and abdominal cases, the review of medical imaging may aid in avoiding iatrogenic injury to machinery and drivelines. VADs can also have an automated implanted cardioverter-defibrillator (AICD function) and thus may have to be reprogrammed prior to the procedure.

A preinduction arterial line should be considered in patients with known right ventricular (RV) dysfunction, recent hospitalization, or inotrope requirement. A pulse may not be palpable in continuous-flow devices, and an ultrasound may be required for placement of the arterial line.[1]

### INTRAOPERATIVE

During a noncardiac procedure, the mean arterial pressure should be maintained at 70–90 mm Hg, adequate preload should be provided, and caution must be taken to avoid RV strain. As always, standard American Society of Anesthesiologists monitors are required intraoperatively. However, a pulse oximeter may be unreliable given the nonpulsatile blood flow compounded by hypotension induced by anesthetic agents. In situations like these, cerebral oximetry can be utilized to better assess perfusion.[3] For the above reasons, noninvasive blood pressure (BP) monitoring may also be imprecise. While manual BP monitoring with the use of Doppler ultrasound is often more useful than automated noninvasive BP monitors, arterial line BP monitoring remains the gold standard for patients with VADs.

Certain patients requiring higher inotropic support may require central venous access for monitoring of central venous pressure and delivery of medications. Intraoperative echocardiography may also be useful in assessing volume status and overall cardiac function.[1]

### POSTOPERATIVE

Patients should be monitored closely postoperatively for hypoxia and hypercarbia, as they may lead to RV dysfunction. The care team should be informed if the AICD was reprogrammed so proper steps are taken to reset the device to the appropriate settings. Anticoagulation should be coordinated with the cardiology and surgical teams.[1]

## REFERENCES

1. Tickoo M, Bardia A. Anesthesia at the edge of life. *Anesthesiol Clin.* 2020;38(1):19–33.
2. Thunberg CA, et al. Ventricular assist devices today and tomorrow. *J Cardiothorac Vasc Anesth.* 2010;24(4):656–680.
3. Freeman R. *Anesthesiology Core Review: Advanced Exam.* New York, NY: McGraw-Hill Education; 2016.
4. Peberdy MA, et al. Cardiopulmonary resuscitation in adults and children with mechanical circulatory support: a scientific statement from the American Heart Association. *Circulation.* 2017;135(24).
5. Jorde UP, et al. Continuous-flow left ventricular assist device survival improves with multidisciplinary approach. *Ann Thorac Surg.* 2019;108(2):508–516.

# 142.

# PULMONARY EMBOLISM

*Lovkesh L. Arora and Surangama Sharma*

## INTRODUCTION

Acute pulmonary embolism (PE) is a life-threatening condition that can lead to both acute and long-term morbidity and mortality. It occurs when a blood clot from a peripheral vein, most commonly in the legs, dislodges, embolizes, and travels to the pulmonary vasculature, leading to vascular obstruction. The incidence of PE is approximately 100 per 100,000 person-years and increases with age. The severity of PE ranges from asymptomatic, with no hemodynamic effects, to life threatening with circulatory collapse. Despite advances in treatment, the mortality rate in patients with shock approaches 50%.[1]

## CLASSIFICATION OF PE

The American Heart Association classifies PE into three categories: massive, submassive, and low risk. Massive PE is defined as a PE that has caused hemodynamic instability. Submassive PE represents a group without hemodynamic instability but with evidence of cardiac dysfunction, seen on blood testing, electrocardiography, or transthoracic echocardiography (TTE). Low-risk PE refers to patients without hemodynamic instability and without evidence of cardiac dysfunction.[2]

## RISK STRATIFICATION

The current treatment approach for PE is based on rapid assessment of severity risk to determine therapy. Severity of PE is classified as low risk, intermediate risk, or high risk based on the presence of shock, right ventricle (RV) dysfunction, and biomarker elevation, with the PE severity correlating with mortality risk.[3] High-risk PE is defined by the presence of shock or hypotension. Patients with intermediate-risk PE have evidence of RV dysfunction based on abnormalities in TTE or computed tomography (CT) or have elevations in cardiac biomarkers, specifically troponin and brain natriuretic peptide. Even

if TTE is not available, the CT angiogram of the chest may provide useful information, as a RV to left ventricle ratio greater than 0.9 is associated with increased mortality risk. Finally, those with low-risk PE have no evidence of shock, hypotension, RV dysfunction, or biomarker elevation.

## ANESTHETIC CONSIDERATIONS

### PERIOPERATIVE DIAGNOSIS

Accurate detection of PE remains difficult, and the differential diagnosis is extensive. Manifestation under anesthesia can be acute severe hypoxia and hypotension. *Tachypnea, tachycardia, arterial hypoxemia, and hypercapnia are the most common signs* of PE but are nonspecific. Electrocardiographic findings in the majority of patients with acute PE include ST-T wave changes and right axis deviation. Peaked P waves, atrial fibrillation, and right bundle-branch block may be present if the PE is sufficiently large to cause acute cor pulmonale. *Capnography will demonstrate a decrease in end-tidal carbon dioxide tension, representing an increase in dead-space ventilation.* Laboratory testing like a D-dimer test can aid in diagnosis as the negative predictive value of the D-dimer test is above 99%. Troponin levels may be elevated and may represent RV myocyte damage caused by acute RV strain. *TTE may be particularly useful in critically ill patients suspected of having PE* and can help identify RV pressure overload as well as myocardial infarction, aortic dissection, and pericardial tamponade, which can mimic PE. The European Society of Cardiology recommends TTE only in hemodynamically unstable patients, where an echocardiogram may facilitate the diagnosis of PE, and in stable patients with diagnosed PE, it may further classify intermediate-risk patients. The American Society of Echocardiography guidelines for the evaluation of a cardiac source of emboli state that "echocardiography is not a diagnostic modality of choice for the diagnosis of PE per se but is used for patient risk stratification."[4]

*Echocardiographic features consistent with the submassive classification include RV dilation, RV dysfunction, septal bulging, increased RV systolic pressure, and visualization of right heart thrombi.*[5] Ventilation-perfusion lung scanning and ultrasonography of leg veins are other noninvasive tests that can aid in the diagnosis of deep venous thrombosis and/or PE. In patients who are candidates for percutaneous embolectomy, conventional pulmonary angiography can be performed to confirm the diagnosis of PE immediately before the embolectomy procedure.

## PERIOPERATIVE MANAGEMENT

Treatment options for acute PE include noninvasive management with anticoagulation or thrombolytic therapy depending on risk classification and invasive management with inferior vena cava filter placement, catheter-induced thrombolytic lysis, and surgical embolectomy. *Heparin remains the cornerstone of treatment for acute PE. An intravenous bolus of unfractionated heparin (5000 to 10,000 U) followed by a continuous intravenous infusion should be administered immediately to any patient considered to have a high clinical likelihood of PE.* An alternative is low-molecular-weight heparin given subcutaneously. *Thrombolytic therapy* may be considered to hasten dissolution of pulmonary emboli, especially if there is hemodynamic instability or severe hypoxemia. Hemorrhage is the principal adverse effect of thrombolytic therapy, so this treatment is contraindicated in patients at high risk of bleeding. The extended period of anticoagulation is usually accomplished with warfarin in a dosage that maintains an international normalized ratio of 2.0 to 3.0. Patients who cannot undergo anticoagulation, experience significant bleeding while being treated with anticoagulants, or have recurrent pulmonary emboli despite receiving anticoagulant therapy may require insertion of a vena cava filter to prevent lower extremity thrombi from becoming pulmonary emboli. The use of vena cava filters should be reserved for patients with contraindications to anticoagulant treatment. *Supportive management* includes use of inotropes such as dopamine and dobutamine or a vasoconstrictor such as norepinephrine. A pulmonary vasodilator may be needed to help control pulmonary hypertension. Tracheal intubation and mechanical ventilation may be necessary in patients who do not have a definitive airway in place. Analgesics to treat the pain associated with PE are important but must be administered very carefully because of the underlying cardiovascular instability. Pulmonary artery embolectomy is reserved for patients who have a massive PE that is unresponsive to medical therapy and who cannot receive thrombolytic therapy.

Patients with shock may also require additional hemodynamic support with extracorporeal membrane oxygenation.[6]

## REFERENCES

1. Witkin AS. Acute and chronic pulmonary embolism: the role of the pulmonary embolism response team. *Curr Opin Cardiol.* 2017;32:672–678.
2. Jaff MR, et al. Management of massive and submassive pulmonary embolism, iliofemoral deep vein thrombosis, and chronic thromboembolic pulmonary hypertension: a scientific statement from the American Heart Association. *Circulation.* 2011;123:1788–1830.
3. Becattini C, Agnelli G. Risk stratification and management of acute pulmonary embolism. *Hematol Am Soc Hematol Educ Program.* 2016:404–412.
4. Saric M, Armour AC, Arnaout MS, Chaudhry FA, Grimm RA, Kronzon I, Landeck BF, Maganti K, Michelena HI, Tolstrup K. Guidelines for the use of echocardiography in the evaluation of a cardiac source of embolism. *J Am Soc Echocardiogr.* 2016 Jan;29(1):1–42.
5. Dutta T, et al. Echocardiography in the evaluation of pulmonary embolism. *Cardiol Rev.* 2017;25:309–314.
6. Cormican D, et al. Acute perioperative pulmonary embolism-management strategies and outcomes. *J Cardiothorac Vasc Anesth.* 2020;34:1972–1984.

# 143.

# PULMONARY EDEMA

*Sangini Punia and Lovkesh L. Arora*

## INTRODUCTION

Pulmonary edema refers broadly to the abnormal accumulation of fluid within the extravascular lung tissue, adversely affecting gas exchange across the capillary membrane. Perioperative pulmonary edema may be due to cardiogenic or noncardiogenic causes, which are described further in this chapter. It can occur acutely in the intraoperative or immediate postoperative period. The overall incidence of postoperative pulmonary complications, including pulmonary edema, following noncardiac surgery is about 5%–10%.[1] Of these, pulmonary edema is relatively uncommon, comprising less than 1% of pulmonary complications.[2] However, despite this, it is an important cause of perioperative morbidity and should be evaluated to ascertain the cause and initiate the appropriate management.

## PATHOPHYSIOLOGY AND CLASSIFICATION

Most cases of pulmonary edema are caused due to an imbalance of Starling forces across the alveolar membrane. The Starling relationship can predict the net flow of fluid across a membrane. It is calculated with the following equation:

$$\text{Net filtration} = Kf \times (\Delta \text{Hydrostatic pressure} - \Delta \text{Oncotic pressure})$$

where *Kf* is the filtration coefficient.

For pulmonary edema to occur, there must be a change in hydrostatic or oncotic pressure across the membrane that results in fluid moving into the extravascular tissue. This results in a transudative collection of extravascular fluid.

A change in membrane permeability may also result in pulmonary edema, as seen in case of sepsis or acute respiratory distress syndrome (ARDS). In this case, due to leakage of plasma proteins, the collection of fluid is exudative.

Broadly, the cause of pulmonary edema may be classified as cardiogenic and noncardiogenic.

## CARDIOGENIC PULMONARY EDEMA

Cardiogenic pulmonary edema is a result of acute decompensated heart failure from left ventricular impairment, valve abnormalities, or coronary artery disease. The decompensated heart failure itself may be a result of primary cardiac disease, extreme fluid overload, or severe hypertension. A rapid increase in left ventricular filling pressures leads to fluid transudation into the extravascular pulmonary tissue, leading to hypoxia and impaired gas exchange.

## NONCARDIOGENIC PULMONARY EDEMA

In the noncardiogenic case, pulmonary edema occurs without evidence of cardiac dysfunction, as evidenced by normal left ventricular filling pressures and pulmonary artery wedge pressure. Patients undergoing anesthesia may have noncardiogenic causes of pulmonary edema more commonly. The causes are varied and include post–airway obstruction (e.g., negative pressure pulmonary edema), anaphylaxis, ARDS, neurogenic pulmonary edema from acute sympathetic surge, aspiration, and transfusion-related lung injury. Negative pressure pulmonary edema is uncommon (<0.1% incidence in some studies), but quite unique to the practice of anesthesia. The main risk factors are male gender, younger age, and head and neck surgery. It occurs as a result of sudden, deep inhalation against a closed glottis, for example during laryngospasm or when a patient bites down on the endotracheal tube during emergence. The massive negative intrathoracic pressure that is generated leads to an increase in left ventricular preload and an increase in transmural pressure, leading to pulmonary edema. One quick method to prevent negative pressure pulmonary edema in an intubated patient is to deflate the cuff of the endotracheal tube immediately to prevent the sudden increase in intrathoracic negative pressure. Other causes of noncardiogenic pulmonary edema worth noting include acute spinal cord injuries or severe head trauma. These can lead to a catecholamine surge, leading to left ventricular dysfunction and acute pulmonary edema. Sudden cate-cholamine surge can also be caused with naloxone admin-istration. Even a small dose (80–500 μg) can cause severe pulmonary hypertension and pulmonary edema, which is potentially fatal in healthy young adults. Hypothermia can lead to increased vasoconstriction, causing increased afterload, which can result in pulmonary edema. Warm patients are unlikely to develop pulmonary edema due to excess capacitance secondary to vasodilation; hence, normothermia is critical to optimal volume management. Preeclampsia can also result in pulmonary edema as a re-sult of circulatory overload, aspiration during convulsions, or heart failure.

## DIAGNOSIS

Pulmonary edema is usually a clinical diagnosis, as the signs, symptoms, and pertinent history will readily identify the pathology as cardiogenic or noncardiogenic. However, sometimes it may be difficult to differentiate, and in such cases it may be necessary to obtain specific investigations.

*Symptoms*: The awake patient may complain of dyspnea and air hunger and may appear to be in respiratory dis-tress. There may be associated chest discomfort if there is a cardiogenic cause.

*Signs*: Tachypnea, tachycardia, hypoxia, and crepitations on auscultation are signs. In intubated patients, the pres-ence of pink frothy sputum within the endotracheal tube is pathognomonic for pulmonary edema. Acute pulmo-nary edema is a clinical diagnosis, and treatment should be initiated empirically while definitive imaging or laboratory work is pursued.

*Laboratory Tests*: Consider obtaining a plasma brain natriuretic peptide value, which is usually normal in noncardiogenic pulmonary edema, and cardiac enzymes if cardiac ischemia is suspected. Other laboratory tests can be obtained based on clinical suspicion to rule out sepsis and anaphylaxis.

*Imaging*: Chest x-ray will demonstrate signs of fluid overload, including cephalization of pulmonary vessels, Kerly B lines, peribronchial cuffing, "batwing" pattern, and patchy ground glass appearance.

*Cardiac*: Echocardiography can be used to assess left ventricular function and valve dysfunction. Electro-cardiography to rule out acute ST segment elevation my-ocardial infarction, arrhythmia, or new bundle-branch blocks may be useful. Pulmonary artery catheterization to measure cardiac filling pressures can differentiate between cardiogenic and noncardiogenic pulmonary edema.

## MANAGEMENT

The initial supportive management of pulmonary edema should take place as soon as a clinical diagnosis is made. More targeted management can then be implemented based on whether it is cardiogenic or noncardiogenic in origin.

Initial supportive management includes

- Increased inspired oxygen concentration to treat hypoxia
- Head-up position if possible
- Application of noninvasive positive pressure if patient is extubated
- Consideration of early intubation if the patient seems to be acutely decompensating or coughing up pink frothy sputum.
- Cardiovascular support with inotropic infusions as necessary to maintain hemodynamic stability
- Consider transfer of patient to the intensive care unit for monitoring.

After the initial supportive therapy is initiated, the goal is to identify and treat the inciting cause of pulmonary edema.

In cardiogenic pulmonary edema, treatment of fluid overload with diuretics (furosemide) is indicated. If hy-potensive, inotropic support should be provided with epi-nephrine infusion titrated to the patient's hemodynamics. Further management is directed based on the findings of echocardiography and pulmonary artery catheterization.

In case of noncardiogenic pulmonary edema, contin-uous positive airway pressure is the most beneficial therapy. If the suspected cause is ARDS or transfusion-related acute lung injury (TRALI), lung-protective ventilation strategies should be initiated as described by ARDSnet.[3] The use of intravenous steroids is not recommended for TRALI and ARDS.[4]

## REFERENCES

1. Fischer SP, et al. Preoperative evaluation. In: Miller RD, et al., eds. *Miller's Anaesthesia*. 7th ed. New York, NY: Churchill, Livingstone; 2010:1019–1022.
2. Chapman MJ, et al. Crisis management during anaesthesia: pulmo-nary oedema. *QualSaf Health Care*. 2005;14:e8.
3. ARDSnet. NIH NHLBI ARDS clinical network mechanical venti-lation protocol summary. http://www.ardsnet.org/files/ventilator_protocol_2008-07.pdf
4. Steinberg KP, et al. National Heart, Lung, and Blood Institute Acute Respiratory Distress Syndrome (ARDS) Clinical Trials Network. Efficacy and safety of corticosteroids for persistent acute respiratory distress syndrome. *N Engl J Med*. 2006;354(16):1671–1684.

# 144.

# HYPERTENSION

*Kim Sung and Lovkesh L. Arora*

## INTRODUCTION

According to the American College of Cardiology/ American Heart Association 2017 guidelines, hypertension is defined by two stages. Stage 1 hypertension has a systolic pressure of 130 to 139 mm Hg or diastolic pressure of 80 to 89 mm Hg, and stage 2 hypertension has a systolic pressure of at least 140 mm Hg or diastolic pressure of at least 90 mm Hg. There are two types of hypertension: primary hypertension and secondary hypertension. The etiology of the disease can be complex, and causes of primary hypertension are not yet fully understood; however, genetic and environmental risk factors (age, obesity, race, high-sodium diet, and inactivity) are thought to contribute. Secondary hypertension is due to either a medical condition or medication. Some of the medical conditions include primary aldosteronism, obstructive sleep apnea, pheochromocytoma, and coarctation of the aorta. Medications that can lead to hypertension include oral contraceptives, decongestants, stimulants, chronic nonsteroidal anti-inflammatory drug use, cyclosporine, tacrolimus, tyrosine kinase inhibitors, tricyclic antidepressants, monoamine oxidase inhibitors, corticosteroids, and angiogenesis inhibitors.[1,2]

## CONSEQUENCES OF CHRONIC HYPERTENSION

Hypertension has numerous downstream effects on cardiovascular, renal, and neurophysiology. Hypertension can lead to left ventricular hypertrophy and ischemic heart disease. Left ventricular hypertrophy can develop due to pressure or volume overload accompanying hypertension. This remodeling process can lead to acute myocardial infarction and heart failure with preserved and reduced ejection fractions. Hypertension can also cause ischemic stroke and intracerebral hemorrhage. It has a detrimental effect on the renal system, leading to chronic kidney disease and end-stage renal disease.[1,2]

The American College of Cardiology/American Heart Association and International Society of Hypertension Global Hypertension practice guidelines both recommend that management of primary hypertension should focus on the amount of blood pressure reduction rather than the choice of medication class for initial monotherapy. This recommendation was based on numerous, trials including Captopril Prevention Project (CAPPP), Swedish Trial in Old Patients with Hypertension (STOP-Hypertension-2), Nordic diltiazem (NORDIL), United Kingdom Prospective Diabetes Study (UKPDS), and Intervention as a Goal in Hypertension Treatment (INSIGHT).

## ANESTHETIC CONSIDERATIONS

### PREOPERATIVE

Current evidence indicates elective surgery in a hypertensive patient does not need to be delayed if diastolic blood pressure is less than 110 mm Hg and systolic blood pressure is less than 180 mm Hg. When patients have higher blood pressure in the preoperative setting, there is no evidence to suggest that initiating a new therapy to achieve normal blood pressure is beneficial, and it may even be harmful if it results in low diastolic blood pressure. Therefore, maintaining blood pressure within 10%–20% of the patient's baseline and keeping mean arterial blood pressure more than 65 mm Hg is the most widely accepted approach to management. For patients with chronic hypertension, the duration and degree of hypotension (mean arterial blood pressure less than 65 mm Hg) are well correlated with adverse postoperative outcomes, including acute kidney injury, myocardial infarction, and stroke. Although invasive blood pressure monitoring systems such as intra-arterial catheters are not currently recommended for every patient with hypertension, frequent and vigilant blood pressure monitoring is recommended with a noninvasive blood pressure method.[3]

Medications such as β-blockers and centrally acting sympatholytics should be continued as they can cause withdrawal symptoms if they are held. On the other hand, angiotensin-converting enzyme inhibitors or angiotensin II receptor blockers are associated with an increased risk of intraoperative hypotension, and it is reasonable to hold them 12–24 hours prior to surgery. Angiotensin-converting enzyme inhibitors or angiotensin II receptor blockers work at angiotensin II receptors for a more complete renin-angiotensin system blockade. The combined antagonistic effect of this receptor from the medication with anesthesia-induced reduction of systemic vascular resistance and pre-load may cause significant hypotension. Chronic use of these medications can also reduce the α-agonistic response leading to a blunted response to phenylephrine and ephedrine. Treatment of choice for intraoperative hypotension secondary to angiotensin-converting enzyme inhibitors or angiotensin II receptor blockers is a bit controversial, but currently norepinephrine is suggested, followed by vasopressin.[3,4]

## INTRAOPERATIVE

Acute hypertension during intraoperative periods often can occur. During induction of anesthesia, laryngoscopy and endotracheal intubation are crucial procedures to secure an airway. Sympathetic response to these procedures typically increases blood pressures by 20–25 mm Hg in normotensive patients and even more in hypertensive patients. Use of intravenous anesthetics (propofol), short-acting opioids (fentanyl, alfentanil, and remifentanil), and/or volatile anesthetics can effectively blunt this systemic response. β-Blockers such as esmolol and topical lidocaine on the pharynx and larynx may also be considered. Similar treatment with short-acting intravenous agents or increasing volatile anesthetics can be used during the surgical stimulus, which also leads to a surge in sympathetic activity.[5]

Hypoxemia and/or hypercarbia during the intraoperative period may cause hypertension and tachycardia due to sympathetic stimulation. It is important to have adequate minute ventilation and a higher fraction of inspired oxygen to avoid such a response. It is also important to recognize some of the less common causes of intraoperative hypertension, such as chronic antihypertensive medication withdrawal (β-blockers and clonidine), bladder distension, increase in intracranial pressure, and history of acute amphetamine or cocaine usage. In a severely hypertensive pregnant or postpartum patient, the recommended first-line agent of treatment is labetalol or hydralazine, and the second line is an initiation of nicardipine, esmolol, or nitroglycerin infusion.[1,2]

## POSTOPERATIVE

Postoperative hypertension is more common in patients with chronic hypertension. In the postanesthesia care unit, blood pressure should be less than 160 mm Hg. Medications including labetalol, hydralazine, or nicardipine may be used to treat the blood pressure. However, it is important to recognize the underlying causes of hypertension. The most common causes are due to noxious stimuli such as pain, nausea, shivering, and bladder distension. Assuming the patient is not in a hypertensive crisis, treating the underlying conditions should be a priority before using hemodynamic-altering medications. Undiagnosed obstructive sleep apnea can cause hypertension during the recovery period. General anesthesia may exacerbate symptoms of obstructive sleep apnea in the postoperative period, leading to hypoxemia and hypercarbia. If the patient has risk factors such as body mass index greater than 35 $km/m^2$, advanced lung disease, elevated serum bicarbonate, neuromuscular disease, higher opioid requirements, and major invasive surgeries, it is reasonable to initiate positive airway pressure.[5]

## REFERENCES

1. Fleisher LA, et al. 2014 ACC/AHA guideline on perioperative cardiovascular evaluation and management of patients undergoing noncardiac surgery: a report of the American College of Cardiology/American Heart Association Task Force on Practice Guidelines. *J Am Coll Cardiol.* 2014;64:e77.
2. Kristensen SD, et al. 2014 ESC/ESA guidelines on non-cardiac surgery: cardiovascular assessment and management: the Joint Task Force on Non-cardiac Surgery: cardiovascular assessment and management of the European Society of Cardiology (ESC) and the European Society of Anaesthesiology (ESA). *Eur Heart J.* 2014;35:2383.
3. Hartle A, et al. The measurement of adult blood pressure and management of hypertension before elective surgery: joint guidelines from the Association of Anaesthetists of Great Britain and Ireland and the British Hypertension Society. *Anaesthesia.* 2016;71:326.
4. Hollmann C, et al. A systematic review of outcomes associated with withholding or continuing angiotensin-converting enzyme inhibitors and angiotensin receptor blockers before noncardiac surgery. *Anesth Analg.* 2018;127:678.
5. Travieso-Gonzalez A, et al. Management of arterial hypertension: 2018 ACC/AHA versus ESC guidelines and perioperative implications. *J Cardiothorac Vasc Anesth.* 2019;33(12):3496–3503.

# 145.

# EFFECT OF INTRACARDIAC SHUNTS ON INHALATION INDUCTION

*Elie Geara and Caroline Alhaddadin*

## INTRODUCTION

Congenital heart disease (CHD) encompasses a variety of abnormalities that are mostly detected in infancy, early childhood, or less commonly adulthood. With the current surgical and medical treatment, an increasing number of patients with CHD may survive to adulthood and be encountered during non cardiac procedures.[1] Stable inhalational anesthetic induction in patients with CHD has its special challenges. The anesthesiologist needs an in-depth understanding of the effect of intracardiac shunts on the uptake, delivery, and balance of anesthetic drugs. Intracardiac shunts can alter the speed and time of induction, so careful titration is warranted to avoid any undesirable myocardial depression. Most patients present with cyanosis or congestive heart failure or are generally asymptomatic. Cyanosis in particular is a result of an abnormal intracardiac communication that allows unoxygenated blood to reach the systemic arterial circulation; another term is right-to-left shunting. Congestive heart failure is prominent, with obstructions to the left ventricular outflow or any markedly increased pulmonary blood flow, which is caused by left-to-right shunting returning the oxygenated blood to the right side.

## INHALATIONAL INDUCTION

Inhalational induction is not a common practice for adults. On the other hands, many pediatric patients arrive to the operating room without intravenous access, and nearly all would be traumatized from an intravenous line, especially when they have been without oral intake, making inhalational induction one of the preferable methods of induction.[2]

Typically, the child is coaxed into breathing an odorless mixture of nitrous oxide (70%) and oxygen (30%). Sevoflurane is added to the gas mixture in 0.5% increments every one to two breaths. Alternatively, single-breath induction could be used with sevoflurane at 7%–8% in 60% nitrous oxide to speed induction. Once an adequate level of anesthesia is achieved, an intravenous line can be started, and intravenous induction with appropriate drugs can facilitate intubation.[2]

Normally, pulmonary blood flow Qp and systemic blood flow Qs do not mix. All the systemic venous return goes to the systemic arterial circulation. But, when an abnormal communication or a defect between two separate structures exists, part of the venous return is redirected back to the arterial outflow of the same circulation. The relative pressures of the communicating structures dictate the direction of the shunt flow, and shunting is limited by the size of the defect. Small defects tend to be restrictive with limited flow versus large defects, which tend to be nonrestrictive with unimpaired flow.

Three factors determine inhalational anesthetic uptake: Anesthetic gas solubility [$\lambda$, cardiac output Q, and alveolar-to-venous anesthetic partial pressure difference (PA $\mp$ PV). The anesthetic balance between the alveoli, arterial blood, and brain determines the speed of induction. Patients with right-to-left shunts have a delayed speed of inhalational induction compared to patients with left-to-right shunts.[3]

## QP TO QS RATIO IN MIXING LESIONS

In a balanced blood circulation, the ratio of Qp to Qs is 1. Any preferential flow toward the aorta will increase the systemic blood flow Qs at the expense of greater desaturation and therefore less oxygen delivery, and any preferential flow to the pulmonary artery will increase pulmonary blood flow Qp, resulting in greater oxygen saturation of the mixed blood but at the expense of a systemic cardiac output. The flow resistance of the two circulations, composed of pulmonary vascular resistance and systemic vascular resistance determine the Qp to Qs ratio.[4]

A ratio greater than 1 usually indicates a left-to-right shunt, whereas a ratio less than 1 indicates a right-to-left shunt. A ratio of 1 indicates either no shunting or a bidirectional shunt of opposing magnitudes.

## RIGHT-TO-LEFT SHUNTS

Shunts in the right-to-left shunt group (sometimes also called mixing lesions) occur when the systemic venous return is redirected to the systemic arterial outflow bypassing the lungs. The hallmark of these lesions is hypoxemia because the pulmonary venous return mixes with recirculated systemic venous blood; the resulting arterial oxygen saturation will decrease. The degree of desaturation is proportionate to the magnitude of the right-to-left shunt. A right-to-left intracardiac shunt slows the rate of induction.[1] The decrease in pulmonary blood flow secondary to a right-to-left shunt will directly decrease the rate of rise of partial pressure of the soluble inhalational anesthetic in the arterial blood. The last physiology is described as dilution of inhalational anesthetics due to mixing of blood in the left ventricle that increases the time to raise the partial pressures in the brain, resulting in a delayed induction.

## LEFT-TO-RIGHT SHUNTS

A left-to-right shunt happens when a part of the pulmonary venous return is redirected toward the arterial system. Left-to-right shunts are mostly intracardiac, either ventricular or atrial septal defects, but can take place at the great vessels like a patent ductus arteriosus. They usually are associated with increased pulmonary blood flow, which does not have a real effect on the rate of induction of anesthesia. Due to the high pressure of the left side of the heart, the blood flows across from left to right, which increases blood flow to the right heart and lungs. The large increase in pulmonary blood flow produces pulmonary vascular congestion. Recirculation through the lungs decreases uptake from the alveoli, which increases the alveolar partial pressure of the anesthetic; this is compensated by the increase in the pulmonary blood flow, which in turns enhances the anesthetic uptake.[4]

The inhalational induction of anesthesia is delayed in patients with a right-to-left shunt compared to patients with a left-to-right shunt. The anesthesiologist needs to have an in-depth understanding of the physiology and effect of shunt lesions on the uptake, delivery, and equilibration of anesthetic drugs.

## REFERENCES

1. Tanner GE, et al. Effect of left-to-right, mixed left-to-right, and right-to-left shunts on inhalational anesthetic induction in children: a computer model. *Anesth Analg.* 1985;64(2):101–107.
2. Morgan, GE, et al. *Clinical Anesthesiology.* New York, NY: Lange Medical Books/McGraw Hill Medical Publications Division; 2006.
3. Hasija S, et al. Comparison of speed of inhalational induction in children with and without congenital heart disease. *Ann Card Anaesth.* 2016;19(3):468–474.
4. Miller, RD, et al. *Basics of Anesthesia.* Philadelphia, PA: Elsevier/Saunders; 2011.

# Part 12

# VASCULAR DISEASES

# 146.

# CAROTID ENDARTERECTOMY

*Ravi K. Grandhi and Claire Joseph*

## INTRODUCTION

Carotid endarterectomy (CEA) and carotid artery stunting (CAS) are both options to assist in the revascularization of the carotid artery due to atherosclerotic disease. A number of studies have shown that CAS has a higher risk of heart attack, stroke, and death.[1] As a result, CEA is the more common procedure.

Carotid endarterectomy is a procedure during which atherosclerotic plaque is removed from inside the vessels to help reduce the risk of ischemic stroke. Plaque is most commonly removed from the location of maximum turbulence where the common carotid artery divides into the internal and external carotid artery. The National Institute for Health and Clinical Excellence recommends that people with moderate-to-severe (50%–99% blockage) stenosis and symptoms have urgent endarterectomy within 2 weeks.[2] Even if the plaque is asymptomatic, there is an increased risk of symptoms compared to the general population. In these settings, surgery can be done if the patient is expected to live at least 5 years with a carotid artery stenosis of greater than 70% and the anticipated that the risk of complication is less than 3%.[3]

## ANESTHETIC CONSIDERATIONS

### PREOPERATIVE

Preoperatively, identify and optimize the cardiovascular status of the patient. Initial therapy on diagnosis includes aggressive blood pressure control with β-blockers, antiplatelet agents, statins, and smoking cessation. Cardiology consultation maybe warranted. At a minimum, a 12-lead electrocardiogram is required for all patients. The majority of patients are moderate- to high-risk surgical candidates according to the Revised Cardiac Risk Index. High-risk criteria for CEA includes elderly (greater than 80 years), class 3 or 4 congestive heart failure, class 3 or 4 angina pectoris, left main or multivessel coronary artery disease, need for open heart surgery within 30 days, left ventricular ejection fraction less than 30%, recent (less than 30 days) heart attack, severe lung disease or chronic obstructive lung disease, severe renal disease, high cervical or intrathoracic lesion, prior radical neck surgery or radiation therapy, contralateral carotid artery occlusion, prior ipsilateral CEA, contralateral laryngeal nerve injury, or tracheostomy.[4]

## INTRAOPERATIVE

Regional or general anesthesia is used intraoperatively to provide optimal conditions for the surgical procedure. Arterial lines are placed for close hemodynamic monitoring. Due to the significant past medical history and to minimize induction-associated hemodynamic changes, the arterial lines are placed preinduction. If regional techniques are chosen, a deep cervical plexus block can be performed, which will block C2, C3, and C4 nerve roots. The advantages of regional techniques are that the patient can assist with the neurologic examination, and there is less postoperative hypertension. However, the patient has to be cooperative. If there are any complications associated with the surgery such as hemiplegia and the patient has to be emergently intubated, it can be challenging with a sterile field. Further, anxious patients have increased sympathetic drive, increasing the risk for myocardial ischemia in a subset of patients already prone to cardiac events. If general anesthetic techniques are used, as is the case more often, somatosensory evoked potentials (SSEPs) and electroencephalograms (EEGs) are monitored. Both anesthetic techniques have similar overall rates of morbidity and mortality.

During a CEA, there is temporary clamping of the carotid artery, which places the ipsilateral side dependent on the collateral blood flow from the vertebral arteries and contralateral carotid artery through the circle of Willis. On occasion, systolic pressure beyond the carotid clamp is measured by placing a needle into the distal carotid artery. Stump pressure should be greater than 40 mm Hg. If there is any ischemia noted or there are reduced stump pressures, a shunt can be placed to provide temporary revascularization.

Shunts are placed more often with regional anesthesia. In addition, depth of anesthesia and use of vasopressors such as phenylephrine can be titrated to the EEG. Anesthetic agents reduce the cerebral metabolic rate, which may offer some degree of cerebral protection. Often, blood pressure is kept about 20% above baseline to maintain appropriate collateral circulation. However, anesthesiologists must balance the competing needs for increased blood pressure with reducing myocardial workload. General anesthesia is associated with labile blood pressures. When the surgeon is dissecting close to the carotid artery, there may be stimulation of the carotid baroreceptor, which may cause bradycardia. The effects of bradycardia can be limited with local anesthetic infiltration, anticholinergic agents such as glycopyrolate, and halting the surgical procedure briefly.

Electroencephalographic records spontaneous electrical activity of cortical surfaces, which is the area more susceptible to decreased perfusion. EEG changes occur in about 20% of patients during carotid occlusion and may indicate serious ischemia. Changes lasting greater than 10 minutes correlate with postoperative neurological deficits. Regional blood flow is around 50–55 mL/min/100 g brain tissue; however, ischemia occurs around 18–20 mL/min/100 g and tissue death at around 8–10 mL/min/100 g. EEG deterioration begins around 20 mL/min/100 g, with suppressed $\alpha$- or $\beta$-activity. EEG does not monitor the deep structures, and preexisting defects reduce predictive value. EEG is also affected by changes in temperature, blood pressure, $PaCO_2$, and anesthetic depth. SSEPs are based on detection of cortical potentials after electrical stimuli are presented to a peripheral nerve. SSEPs are better predictors in patients with previous stroke or EEG changes. However, EEG is not as sensitive or specific for ischemia during CEA, and it monitors only certain areas of the brain. Ischemia manifests as decreased amplitude and prolonged latency. Together with EEGs, SSEPs can provide a more comprehensive picture. Because of the use of neuromonitoring, volatile anesthetics are avoided in favor of a total intravenous anesthetic technique using propofol and remifentanyl. Less than 1 minimum alveolar concentration (MAC) of volatile anesthetic should be used if necessary. Avoid long-acting narcotics to assess postoperative cognitive changes.

## POSTOPERATIVE

Most important postoperative complications include embolic stroke secondary to dislodgment of carotid plaque and myocardial ischemia or infarction. Other potential postoperative complications include neck hematoma and airway compromise. The patient should be monitored for changes in blood pressure during extubation and awakening and should avoid coughing or straining to the extent possible. Hypertension should be avoided to reduce the risk of hyperperfusion syndrome.[5] Blood pressure should be controlled so that it is within normal limits. Monitoring neurologic status postoperatively as frequently as every 15 minutes allows the care team to monitor for any new neurologic deficits and provide early reintervention if necessary. Postoperative hypertension might be related to impaired carotid baroreceptor function. Denervation of the carotid sinus can cause sympathomimetic symptoms. Dissection at the bifurcation may improve previously impaired baroreceptor function if carotid sinus afferent fibers are left intact, possibly causing postoperative hypotension. Impairment of carotid body function may occur after bilateral CEA, which in turn abolishes the cardiorespiratory responses to hypoxemia and makes respiratory regulation totally dependent on changes in $PaCO_2$.

## REFERENCES

1. Sidawy AN, et al. Risk-adjusted 30-day outcomes of carotid stenting and endarterectomy: results from the SVS Vascular Registry. *J Vasc Surg.* 2009;49(1):71–79.
2. Swain S et al. Diagnosis and initial management of acute stroke and transient ischaemic attack: summary of NICE guidance, BMJ 2008;337:a786.
3. American Academy of Neurology. Five things physicians and patients should question. Choosing Wisely: an initiative of the ABIM Foundation, American Academy of Neurology. February 2013. Accessed August 1, 2013.
4. Fairman RM. Carotid endarterectomy. In: Eidt JF, et al., eds. *UpToDate.* Waltham, MA: UpToDate; February 2020. Accessed September 6, 2020.
5. Fairman RM. Complications of carotid endarterectomy. In: Eidt JF, eds. *UpToDate.* Waltham, MA: UpToDate; June 2019. Accessed September 6, 2020.

# 147.

# PERIPHERAL ARTERIOSCLEROTIC DISEASE

*Racha Tadros and Nasir Hussain*

## INTRODUCTION

Peripheral arteriosclerotic disease (PAD) is highly prevalent in the United States, affecting more than 8.5 million people over the age of 40, and it is associated with substantial morbidity, mortality, and impairment of quality of life. The disease causes luminal narrowing of the medium and large arteries through deposition of lipid and fibrous material between the intimal and medial layers of the vessel. Atherosclerosis is by far the most common cause of arterial luminal narrowing and insufficiency, although there are many other disease processes that can cause this, including fibrosis, inflammation, and thrombosis. PAD affects the lower extremities more often than the upper extremities. It typically localizes within a particular vascular segment, such as the aortoiliac, femoropopliteal, or infrapopliteal segments in the proximal to mid portions of the vascular bed but can also occur more distally. The clinical features of the disease depend on the severity and location of occlusion/stenosis and can vary (discussed further in the chapter). Furthermore, it is associated with a higher risk of adverse cardiovascular events, including heart attacks and stroke.[1,2]

## CLINICAL FEATURES

According to the American College of Cardiology/American Heart Association guidelines on PAD, the following are risk factors for its development:

- Age more than 65 years
- Age 50 to 64 years with risk factors for atherosclerosis (e.g., diabetes mellitus, history of smoking, hypertension, hyperlipidemia)
- Age less than 50 years with one additional risk factor for atherosclerosis
- Individuals with known atherosclerotic disease in another vascular bed (e.g., coronary, carotid, subclavian, mesenteric artery stenosis)[1]

Symptoms of PAD can vary significantly and depend mainly on the location and degree of the occlusion/stenosis, number of arteries affected, and the activity level of the patient. Multiple studies have found that most patients with PAD are either asymptomatic or have atypical leg symptoms (i.e., non–joint-related limb symptoms). Other patients may experience the classic symptom of PAD, claudication, which is a reproducible muscle pain that is brought on by exertion, relieved by rest, and occurs due to an imbalance between supply and demand of blood flow. Unfortunately, 1%–2% of patients with PAD present with advanced chronic limb-threatening ischemia, where they exhibit pain at rest and have gangrene or the presence of a lower extremity ulcer for more than 2 weeks.[3]

## DIAGNOSIS

To properly evaluate a patient with increased risk for PAD, a thorough history, review of systems, and physical examination need to be performed. A vascular examination for PAD includes checking lower extremity pulses, listening for femoral bruits, and inspecting the legs and feet. For most patients, the presence of risk factors, symptoms, and physical examination findings are enough to make the diagnosis.[1] For those who are asymptomatic or have an equivocal pulse examination, an ankle-brachial index (ABI) less than 0.9 is diagnostic for PAD. An ABI can be obtained by measuring the systolic blood pressure of the arms (brachial) and legs (dorsalis pedis or posterior tibial) and dividing the highest upper extremity value with the highest lower extremity value. Other physiologic tests may also be necessary for diagnosis and include an exercise treadmill ABI, toe-brachial index, and perfusion studies (e.g., transcutaneous oxygen pressure or skin perfusion pressure) (Figure 147.1). Patients who are symptomatic and are candidates for revascularization may need further imaging studies, such as duplex ultrasound, computed topography angiography, or invasive angiography.[1]

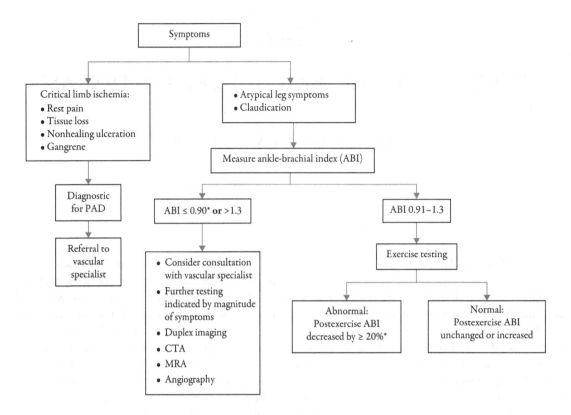

**Figure 147.1** Algorithm for testing patients with suspected PAD. From Reference 5.

## TREATMENT

The gold standard for managing PAD is goal-directed medical therapy (GDMT), which is aimed at treating risk factors to prevent adverse cardiovascular events. GDMT primarily includes structured exercise and lifestyle modification. Smoking cessation is also critical for a patient with PAD. Exercise therapy through a rehabilitation program or supervised exercise has also been shown to improve walking parameters for those who exhibit symptoms of claudication.[1] A customized pharmacotherapy plan should be incorporated into the initial management of the patient based on their individual risk factors. Pharmacotherapy for patients with PAD typically involves antiplatelet therapy and a statin, as well as medication for hypertension or diabetes if they have those comorbidities. For patients with lifestyle limitation due to claudication, cilastazol, a phosphodiesterase inhibitor, may be trialed, although it is associated with many undesirable side effects, such as headaches, diarrhea, dizziness, and palpitations. Patient education regarding foot care is paramount to preventing tissue loss. Finally, the last resort is surgical revascularization, which is typically reserved for patients on GDMT who continue to have poor quality of life from claudication, rather than for the purpose of limb salvage. Endovascular techniques include balloon dilation (angioplasty), stents, and atherectomy.[4,5]

## REFERENCES

1. Gerhard-Herman M, et al. 2016 AHA/ACC guideline on the management of patients with lower extremity peripheral artery disease: executive summary: a report of the American College of Cardiology/American Heart Association Task Force on Clinical Practice Guidelines. *Circulation.* 2017;135(12):e686–e725.
2. Creager MA, Loscalzo J. Arterial diseases of the extremities. In: Jameson JL, et al., eds. *Harrison's Principles of Internal Medicine.* New York, NY: McGraw-Hill Medical Publishing Division; 2015: Chap. 275.
3. Schorr E, Treat-Jacobson D. Methods of symptom evaluation and their impact on peripheral artery disease (PAD) symptom prevalence: a review. *Vasc Med.* 2013;18(2):95–111.
4. Hirsch A, et al. ACC/AHA 2005 practice guidelines for the management of patients with peripheral arterial disease (lower extremity, renal, mesenteric, and abdominal aortic). Circulation. 2006;113(11):e463–e654.
5. Layden J, et al. Diagnosis and management of lower limb peripheral arterial disease: summary of NICE guidance. *BMJ.* 2012;345: e4947–e4947.

# 148.

# AORTIC ANEURYSMS

*Jarrod Bang and Lovkesh L. Arora*

## INTRODUCTION

Aortic aneurysms can be broadly differentiated according to the segment involved as thoracic aneurysms and thoracoabdominal or abdominal aortic aneurysms, as per the Crawford classification system (Figure 148.1). The location and extent of the aortic aneurysm, and associated disease, greatly affect surgical intervention and therefore anesthetic management. Open repairs are highly invasive procedures resulting in wide swings in hemodynamics, fluid shifts, neuroendocrine changes, acute metabolic derangements, and end-organ perfusion mismatch. Open repair carries a relatively higher perioperative mortality rate. Endovascular repairs incur significantly fewer physiologic derangements; however, each component must still be monitored, and conversion to open repair may be necessary sometimes. Endovascular repair compared to open repair decreases perioperative and early mortality, but it has statistically insignificant mortality benefit at 3 years and requires more frequent reinterventions.[1]

## DIAGNOSIS

Abdominal aortic aneurysms (AAAs) occur in approximately 8% of the population. The underlying mechanism can be variable and is incompletely understood; however, the loss of aortic connective tissue due to chronic inflammation is an important portion of the pathophysiology. Risk factors include male gender, increasing age, family history of AAA, smoking, hypertension, obesity, and other atherosclerotic disease. The natural progression of aortic aneurysms, defined by a size greater than 4 cm in diameter, is progressive enlargement and eventual rupture. Indication for intervention includes a diameter greater than 5 cm and interval size increase of greater than 0.5 cm in 6 months.

Thoracic aortic aneurysms (TAAs) are result primarily from degenerative atherosclerosis (80%) but also occur secondary to chronic aortic dissection (17%). Indication for intervention is based on aneurysm enlargement or diameter greater than 5 cm. Diagnosis and surveillance of both types of aneurysms is mainly by computed tomogaphic angiography; however, AAAs may be diagnosed and monitored via ultrasound. All iodinated contrast studies should be performed well in advance of the planned procedure to avoid contrast-related acute kidney injury.[2]

## ANESTHETIC CONSIDERATIONS

### PREOPERATIVE

The preoperative goal is to diagnose comorbidities, assess the risk of adverse outcome, optimize medical status, and plan an anesthetic technique that reduces the risk of complications. Accurate assessment of baseline cardiac function is essential in determining need for further testing. Preoperative kidney function should be assessed with a basic metabolic panel. Chronic kidney disease (serum creatinine > 1.5 mg/dL) is one of the strongest predictors of renal failure, carrying a high perioperative mortality, following aortic surgery. Special emphasis on evaluation of cardiac function and, if warranted, coronary perfusion is extremely important. Pulmonary function tests may be indicated if preexisting disease is present, especially if the patient is undergoing repair of a TAA.

### INTRAOPERATIVE

Intraoperatively, open repairs are almost exclusively conducted under general anesthesia. Depending on planned duration and method of arterial access for endovascular repair, local or regional anesthesia techniques may be utilized. Arterial access for continuous blood pressure monitoring and close laboratory value monitoring is required and usually employed via right radial artery cannulation. If bypass techniques are planned, an arterial monitor distal to the aneurysm should be employed. Large-bore intravenous access is necessary for all procedures due to the possibility of rapid, large-volume blood loss. Central access is necessary for more extensive aneurysm repairs for both central venous pressure monitoring and

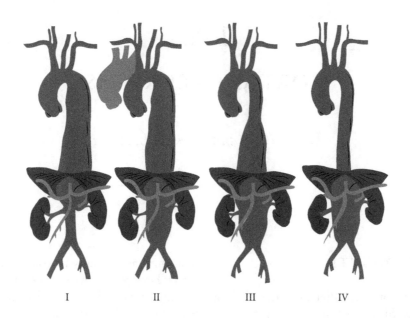

**Figure 148.1** The Crawford classification of thoracoabdominal aortic aneurysms is defined by anatomic location and the extent of involvement. Type I aneurysms involve all or most of the descending thoracic aorta and the upper abdominal aorta; type II aneurysms involve all or most of the descending thoracic aorta and all or most of the abdominal aorta; type III aneurysms involve the lower portion of the descending thoracic aorta and most of the abdominal aorta; and type IV aneurysms involve all or most of the abdominal aorta, including the visceral segment. From Anesthesia for Vascular surgery. Miller's Anesthesia.

*Table 148.1* IMPACT OF CROSS-CLAMP APPLICATION AND RELEASE

| CROSS-CLAMP APPLICATION | CROSS-CLAMP RELEASE |
|---|---|
| Increased blood pressure | Decreased blood pressure |
| Increased systemic vascular resistance | Decreased systemic vascular resistence |
| Increased left ventricular wall tension | Decreased myocardial contractility |
| Decreased ejection fraction | Decreased ejection fraction |
| Decreased cardiac output | Decreased cardiac output |
| Increased central venous pressure | Decreased central venous pressure |
| Increased wall motion abnormalities | Increased pulmonary vascular resisteance |
| Decreased oxygen consumption | Increased oxygen consumption |
| Decreased $CO_2$ production | Increased circulating myocardial depressing factors |
| Increased epinephrine and norepinephrine release | Hypothermia |
| Decreased renal blood flow | Increased lactic acid |
| Metabolic acidosis | Metabolic acidosis |
| Respiratory alkalosis | |

vasoactive medication administration. Pulmonary artery catheters should be used selectively based mainly on patient comorbidities. Transesophageal echocardiography may be useful in directing surgical intervention in thoracic aneurysm repair and can be utilized for cardiac optimization, especially immediately following cross-clamp application and release. Temperature monitoring of core temperature should be employed at two locations, above and below the level of anticipated cross-clamp application. Importantly, bair huggers should not be utilized on hypoperfused tissues as this will increase metabolic demand. Lung isolation may be necessary for thoracic aortic repairs. Cell-saver techniques should be routine. Acute normovolemic hemodilution may be considered.[1]

Cross-clamp application and release result in a variety of physiologic changes that become more pronounced with more proximal clamp location (Table 148.1). The tolerance of aortic clamping and unclamping is highly dependent on volume status, ventricular function, coronary patency, duration of clamping, and diverting circulatory support. Due to the changes described following cross-clamp application, treatment with rapid-acting afterload-reducing agents (e.g., nitroprusside or increased anesthetic depth) and/or preload-reducing agents (e.g., nitroglycerin) is a necessity to avoid left ventricular dilation and failure. Prior to cross clamp, mannitol is often administered to increase cortical blood flow and provide kidney protection, although its benefits have not been proven. Prior to cross-clamp release, fluid resuscitation should be optimized, vasodilators and venodilators decreased, and anesthetic level decreased. Once the cross clamp is removed, further fluid resuscitation may be necessary along with the use of vasocontricting medications and buffering of acidemia with bicarbonate and increased minute ventilation. If refractory hypotension ensues, re-application of the cross clamp for further optimization prior to release may be indicated. Hyperkalemia should be monitored for both by laboratory value and signs on electrocardiogram and treated aggressively.[3]

Coagulopathy may be encountered due to coagulation factor dilution, large-volume transfusion, hypothermia, heparin administration, and liver ischemia. Monitoring with prothrombin time, partial thromboplastin time, fibrinogen level, platelet count, and thromboelastography can all help guide treatment of coagulopathy. In addition to blood products, aminocaproic acid may be beneficial in a bleeding patient.

The spinal cord is perfused via two posterior spinal arteries and one anterior spinal artery. The anterior spinal artery supplies 75% of the spinal cord and arises from the vertebral arteries cranially and the radicular arteries caudally. The largest of these radicular arteries is the great radicular artery, or artery of Adamkiewicz. This artery may arise anywhere from T5 and L5, but 75% of the time it arises from between T9 and T12. Patients are at high risk for spinal cord ischemia during extensive repairs or involving the T9 to T12 levels. Intraoperative motor evoked potentials may be useful in identifying acute spinal cord ischemia. Lumbar drain for cerebrospinal fluid (CSF) pressure monitoring and CSF drainage allow improved control of spinal cord perfusion and mean arterial pressure minus central venous pressure or CSF pressure and may improve neurological outcomes.

## POSTOPERATIVE

With the possible exception of uncomplicated endovascular infrarenal aneurysm repairs, aneurysm repairs require postoperative care in the intensive care unit (ICU) due to hemodynamic monitoring; respiratory care, including possible mechanical ventilation; and close neurological monitoring. Extubation in the operating room, extubation on arrival to the ICU, or continued mechanical ventilation depends on the extent of the repair, required volume resuscitation, normothermia, hemodynamic stability, and preoperative pulmonary status, in addition to standard extubation criteria. Continued fluid shifts may require ongoing fluid resuscitation. Vasoactive medications are commonly continued postoperatively for tight blood pressure parameters in order to avoid hypertension while maintaining perfusing pressures. Frequent neurological assessment is a necessity as over one-third of initial onset of neurological deficit occurs in the postoperative period, and restoring adequate spinal cord perfusion pressure may reverse these deficits.

## REFERENCES

1. Miller RD, Cohen NH. *Miller's Anesthesia*. 8th ed. Philadelphia, PA: Elsevier, Saunders; 2015).
2. Moxon JV. Diagnosis and monitoring of abdominal aortic aneurysm: current status and future prospects. *Curr Probl Cardiol*. 2010;35(10):512–548.
3. Biebuyck JF. The pathophysiology of aortic cross-clamping and unclamping (976470370 757123353 D. Phil, Ed.). *Anesthesiology*. 1995;82:1026–1057.

# 149.

# ADVANCED CARDIOPULMONARY RESUSCITATION
## ADULTS AND CHILDREN

*Donnie Laborde*

## ADVANCED CARDIAC LIFE SUPPORT

After completing the initial basic life support assessment with high-quality cardiopulmonary resuscitation (CPR), healthcare providers should follow the American Heart Association's cardiac arrest algorithms. Simultaneously, all healthcare providers involved in the code should be diagnosing the underlying cause of the patient's condition. Recommended goals to increase survival rates include (1) minimizing intervals between stopping chest compressions and delivering defibrillator shocks; (2) defibrillate as soon as possible, preferably within 3–5 minutes of collapse; (3) high-quality chest compressions with advanced life support strategies, including defibrillation, medications, and advanced airways; and (4) minimize interruption in compressions to less than 10 seconds.[1,2]

## SHOCKABLE RHYTHMS

Shockable rhythms, such as ventricular tachycardia and ventricular fibrillation, are caused by an alteration of the electrical activity of the heart. Ventricular tachycardia, a visually wide and rapid rhythm, may or may not have a pulse. Most are unresponsive and pulseless, and defibrillation will allow the sinoatrial node to restart. The cardiac arrest algorithm allows treatment to begin with the following steps:

1. Begin high-quality CPR, attach defibrillator pads, and provide oxygen.
2. Determine if the rhythm is shockable by viewing the defibrillator.
3. If shockable rhythm is present, provide shock (biphasic dose = 120–220 J; monophasic dose = 360 J).
4. Begin 2 minutes of CPR and obtain intravenous/intraosseous (IV/IO) access.
5. After 2 minutes of CPR, determine the rhythm via defibrillator and provide a shock if a shockable rhythm is present.

6. Continue CPR for 2 minutes, administer epinephrine (1 mg) every 3–5 minutes. Consider an advanced airway with use of capnography.
7. Determine the rhythm via defibrillator and provide a shock if shockable rhythm is present.
8. Continue 2 minutes of CPR, administer amiodarone (300 mg), and treat any reversable causes (see material that follows).

After completion of step 8, revert back to step 5 to determine rhythm via defibrillator and continue cycling steps 5–8 until return of spontaneous circulation (ROSC) is achieved. When cycling, the epinephrine dose remains 1 mg every 3–5 minutes. However, the amiodarone dose should only be administered as an initial bolus dose of 300 mg followed by a second 150-mg dose. Step 6 advanced airway possibilities include endotracheal intubation or supraglottic advanced airway. Waveform capnography will confirm endotracheal tube placement. When the advanced airway is in place, administer 1 breath every 6 seconds. When searching for reversable causes, remember "H's and T's:" hypovolemia, hypoxia, hydrogen ion (acidosis), hypokalemia, hyperkalemia, hypothermia, tension pneumothorax, tamponade (cardiac), toxins, thrombosis (pulmonary or coronary).

## NONSHOCKABLE RHYTHMS

The cardiac arrest algorithm allows treatment to begin with the following steps:

1. Begin high-quality CPR, attach defibrillator pads, and provide oxygen.
2. Determine if the rhythm is shockable by viewing the defibrillator. If nonshockable rhythm is present, continue.
3. Provide CPR for 2 minutes; administer epinephrine (1 mg) every 3–5 minutes. Consider an advanced airway with use of capnography.
4. Determine the rhythm via defibrillator.

5. If nonshockable rhythm is present, continue CPR for 2 minutes and treat reversible causes.
6. Determine the rhythm via defibrillator. If a nonshockable rhythm is present and there no signs of ROSC, continue repeating. If rhythm becomes shockable, revert to shockable rhythm algorithm beginning at step 2. If ROSC is achieved, post–cardiac arrest care will need to be provided.

## IMMEDIATE POST–CARDIAC ARREST CARE

Post–cardiac arrest care begins with ROSC. The steps involved include ensuring ventilation and oxygenation and maintaining oxygen at 94%. If the patient is unconscious or unresponsive, an advanced airway with continuous waveform capnography is needed. Give one ventilation every 5–6 seconds. Avoid overventilation. If systolic pressure is less than 90 mm Hg, treat with appropriate intravenous fluid and/or pharmacotherapies. Look for causes and remember the H's and T's. Conduct an electrocardiogram (ECG) to determine if a ST segment elevation myocardial infarction (STEMI) occurred or if there is need for percutaneous coronary intervention. If a STEMI occurred or if there is high suspicion of an acute myocardial infarction (MI), attempt coronary reperfusion. Continue ECG monitoring until deemed clinically unnecessary. Consider implementing targeted temperature management protocols, especially if patient is nonverbal. After coronary reperfusion interventions, or in cases where the ECG reveals no suspicion of an acute MI, transfer the patient to intensive care.[3])

## Bradycardia

Treatment for bradycardia consists of maintaining or assisting the airway and providing oxygen when necessary, obtaining intravenous access, and performing a 12-lead ECG. If bradycardia is causing hypotension, altered mental status, signs of shock, chest discomfort, or acute heart failure, administer atropine. If atropine is ineffective, consider transcutaneous pacing or a dopamine infusion. If the patient does not respond to any of these interventions, consider expert consultation. If the patient goes into cardiac arrest, seek the cardiac arrest algorithm.[2]

## Tachycardia

Tachycardia can occur with both a present and an absent pulse. If a pulse is present, determine whether the patient is stable or unstable, then provide treatment based on the rhythm. Tachycardia treatment consists of (1) maintaining the airway and assisting with oxygen if needed and (2) placing the patient on a cardiac monitor while simultaneously monitoring blood pressure and oxygen levels. If the patient is symptomatic with hypotension, altered mental status, shock, chest discomfort, or acute heart failure, immediate synchronized cardioversion is needed. If a patient is stable and the QRS complex is wide (≥0.12 seconds), seek expert consultation. If a patient has a narrow QRS with a regular rhythm, attempt vagal maneuvers. If this is unsuccessful, administer adenosine. Treat recurrence with adenosine or longer-acting arteriovenous nodal blocking agents (e.g., nondihydropyridine calcium channel blockers or β-blockers). Obtain expert consultation if tachycardia reoccurs. Do not administer adenosine for unstable, irregular, or polymorphic wide-complex tachycardia.[2]

## PEDIATRIC ADVANCED LIFE SUPPORT

Recommended goals for pediatric advanced life support (PALS) are similar, but not identical, to advanced cardiac life support (ACLS) and include the following:

1. Push hard (infants 1½ inches, children 2 inches).
2. Push fast (100–120 compressions per minute).
3. Allow complete chest recoil.
4. Minimize interruptions to less than 10 seconds.
5. Continuous compressions once advanced airway is in place.
6. Avoid excess ventilation.
7. Use an automated external defibrillator (AED) as soon as possible. If available, use child pads for children under 8 years old. Adult pads may also be used as long as the provider ensures the pads do not overlap.[4]

Determine if the infant or child requires interventions by examining their appearance, work of breathing, circulation, and level of consciousness. If a child is unresponsive and not breathing, activate emergency response and begin CPR immediately. If there is no effective breathing with a pulse, perform rescue breathing (1 breath every 3–5 seconds) and provide oxygen as soon as possible. If the victim's pulse is less than 60 beats per minute with signs of poor perfusion, provide chest compressions and ventilation. Attach a heart monitor and pulse oximeter to the victim. When interpreting pulse oximetry readings, understand that lights of different wavelengths capture saturation levels of hemoglobin. Carbon monoxide will reveal a false high oxygen saturation level. Increased respiratory rates during distress may reveal normal oxygen saturation due to increased rate and supplemental oxygen being administered. If a pulse oximeter heart rate is not matching the ECG monitor, then consider the oxygen saturation unreliable.

## CARDIAC ARREST

The pediatric cardiac arrest algorithm allows treatment to begin with the following steps:

1. Activate emergency medical services, send for an AED, check pulse.
2. Begin high-quality CPR, attach defibrillator pads, and provide oxygen.
3. Determine if the rhythm is shockable by viewing the defibrillator (VF/pVT). If shockable rhythm is present, continue with the following steps:
4. Deliver shock (2 J/kg) if manual AED, CPR for 2 minutes, and obtain IO/IV access.
5. Deliver shock if shockable rhythm is present (second shock is 4 J/kg; subsequent shocks ≥ 4 J/kg; maximum is 10 J/kg or adult dose).
6. Administer CPR for 2 minutes.
7. Administer epinephrine 0.01 mg/kg (0.1 mL/kg of 1:10,000 concentration). Repeat epinephrine dosage every 3–5 minutes.
8. Deliver shock if shockable rhythm is present.
9. Administer either amiodarone (5 mg/kg bolus; may repeat up to two times for refractory VF/pulseless VT) OR lidocaine (1 mg/kg loading dose; maintenance 20–50 µg/kg via infusion) and treat reversable causes.

If initial rhythm is initially not shockable or becomes nonshockable during the above steps:

1. Administer CPR for 2 minutes and obtain IO/IV access; give epinephrine every 3–5 minutes (see dosage above); consider advanced airway.
2. Check rhythm with AED. If still nonshockable, conduct 2 minutes of CPR and treat reversible causes.
3. If an organized rhythm occurs and a pulse is present (ROSC), administer post–cardiac arrest care.

## BRADYCARDIA

Pediatric bradycardia is most commonly the result of progressive hypoxemia, respiratory failure, or shock. The priority should be to ensure an adequate airway to support oxygenation and ventilation. With a slow heart rate and subsequent decreased cardiac output, infants' and children's ability to compensate by increasing stroke volume (SV) is limited.

If the heart rate is less than 60 beats/min with poor perfusion despite oxygenation and ventilation and persistent bradycardia, follow these steps: Administer epinephrine (0.01 mg/kg; repeat every 3–5 minutes); administer atropine (0.02 mg/kg; may repeat once; minimum is 0.1 mg; maximum is 0.5 mg); consider transthoracic pacing/

transvenous pacing, treat underlying causes, and if pulseless arrest, follow the pediatric cardiac arrest algorithm given previously.

## TACHYCARDIA

Pediatric tachycardia is defined as a heart rate that is rapid in comparison to the normal heart rate in relation to the child's age. An increased heart rate can shorten diastole, decreasing SV and increasing myocardial oxygen demand. Signs of this include hypotension, altered mental status, shock, sudden collapse with rapid/weak pulse, and/or respiratory distress/failure. Tachycardia is classified by the QRS complex. Narrow tachycardia is ≤ 0.09 seconds versus wide tachycardia ≥ 0.09 seconds.

### Narrow Tachycardia Treatment

1. Sinus tachycardia
   a. P wave present/normal
   b. Variable R-R, constant P-R
   c. Search for and treat causes
2. Probable supraventricular tachycardia
   a. P waves absent/abnormal
   b. Heart rate not variable
   c. Consider vagal maneuvers (no delays)
   d. IV/IO adenosine (first dose 0.1 mg/kg rapid bolus, second dose 0.2 mg/kg rapid bolus/maximum 12 mg) OR procainamide (15 mg over 30–60 minutes)
      i. If ineffective, synchronize cardioversion.

### Wide Tachycardia Treatment

1. Possible ventricular tachycardia with symptoms including hypotension, acutely altered mental status, and signs of shock.
   a. Synchronized cardioversion
   b. If not revealing cardiopulmonary compromise signs:
      i. Administer adenosine if regular rhythm and monomorphic QRS are present, with expert consultation advised.
      ii. Amiodarone (5 mg/kg over 20–60 minutes).
      iii. Procainamide IV/IO (15 mg/kg over 30–560 minutes).

**Do not routinely administer amiodarone and procainamide together.**

## SHOCK MANAGEMENT

Shock is a result of tissues not receiving adequate oxygen to sustain metabolic demands, impairing the organ's functions. There will be poor outcomes if shock leads to cardiac arrest. There are four basic types of shock: hypovolemic, cardiogenic, distributive, and obstructive.

Diagnosing and treating the underlying cause of shock should be prompt and are critical to the patient's survival. Consider the following steps: (1) improve oxygen content and delivery; (2) improve blood volume (bolus fluid); and (3) reduce oxygen demand (support breathing and treat pain, anxiety, and fever) and address metabolic issues.

For further assistance or a more in-depth/high-quality summary on PALS or ACLS, please reference the American Heart Association website and texts.

## REFERENCES

1. Andersen LW, et al. The prevalence and significance of abnormal vital signs prior to in-hospital cardiac arrest. *Resuscitation.* 2016;98:112–117.

2. Panchal AR, et al. 2019 American Heart Association focused update on advanced cardiovascular life support: use of advanced airways, vasopressors, and extracorporeal cardiopulmonary resuscitation during cardiac arrest: an update to the American Heart Association guidelines for cardiopulmonary resuscitation and emergency cardiovascular care. *Circulation.* 2019;140:e881–e894.

3. Callaway CW, et al. Part 8: post-cardiac arrest care: 2015 American Heart Association guidelines update for cardiopulmonary resuscitation and emergency cardiovascular care. *Circulation.* 2015;132(18):S465–S482.

4. De Caen AR, et al. Part 12: pediatric advanced life support: 2015 American Heart Association guidelines update for cardiopulmonary resuscitation and emergency cardiovascular care. *Circulation.* 2015;132(18):S526–S542.

5. Panchal AR, et al. 2018 American Heart Association focused update on advanced cardiovascular life support use of antiarrhythmic drugs during and immediately after cardiac arrest: an update to the American Heart Association guidelines for cardiopulmonary resuscitation and emergency cardiovascular care. *Circulation.* 2018;138(23):e740–e749.

# Part 13

# GASTROINTESTINAL AND HEPATIC SYSTEMS

# 150.

# PARENTERAL NUTRITION

*Mohamed Fayed and Arif Valliani*

## INTRODUCTION

Nutritional support with parenteral nutrition (PN) may be indicated for individuals with malnutrition requiring surgical intervention or for healthy individuals undergoing major surgery with an anticipated lengthy recovery time to return of normal gastrointestinal function. It is still unclear when the appropriate time to start parenteral nutritional support is; the decision should be made with involvement of nutritional support services. Daily requirements are presented in Table 150.1.

## DAILY REQUIREMENTS

Absolute indications:

- Short bowel syndrome
- Small bowel obstruction

*Table 150.1* STANDARD DAILY REQUIREMENTS FOR VARIOUS NUTRITIONAL COMPONENTS

| | REQUIREMENTS |
|---|---|
| Energy | Under 65 years old: 25 kcal/kg/d<br>Over 65 years old: 20 kcal/kg/d |
| Carbohydrate | Should provide 70% of nonprotein calories |
| Lipid | Should provide 30% of nonprotein calories |
| Protein | Normally 1–1.5 g/kg/d; increased to 1.5–2 g/kg/d in hypercatabolic states (e.g., burns, major trauma) |
| Water | 30 mL/kg/d |
| Electrolytes | Sodium 1–2 mmol/kg/d<br>Potassium 0.7–1 mmol/kg/d<br>Calcium 0.1 mmol/kg/d<br>Magnesium 0.1 mmol/kg/d<br>Phosphate 0.4 mmol/kg/d |
| Trace elements | Role is unclear; selenium might have mortality benefit |

- Pseudo-obstruction with complete intolerance to food
- High-output enteric-cutaneous fistulas (unless a feeding tube can be passed distal to the fistula)

Relative indications:

- Non-healing moderate-output enteric-cutaneous fistulas
- Requirement for bowel rest, such as during acute radiation enteritis
- Chylothorax unresponsive to a medium-chain triglyceride diet
- Other situations in which the enteral route does not provide adequate nutrition

Complications:

- Access related: central venous line insertion
- Liver related: hepatic steatosis, cholestasis
- Increased risk of sepsis
- Increased risk of hyperglycemia

## ENTERAL VERSUS PARENTERAL

- A large, pragmatic, multicenter trial[1] that compared early PN with enteral nutrition (EN), found no difference in mortality at 30 days; EN was associated with a higher risk of vomiting and hypoglycemia. The authors concluded that "early nutritional support through the parenteral route is neither more harmful nor more beneficial than such support through the enteral route."[1]

## TIMING OF NUTRITION

- Timing of nutritional intervention (either EN or PN) is generally divided into "early" or "late."
- While there is no absolute consensus on the timings these terms represent, early is generally taken to represent less than 48 hours after intensive care unit

(ICU) admission and late greater than 7 days after admission.
- While high-grade evidence is lacking, there is general consensus that, where possible, EN should be initiated early; this may improve mortality.
- If the enteral route is not available, early initiation of PN is slightly more controversial as evidence shows worse outcomes with early PN.
- In patients with preexisting malnutrition, the need for early nutrition is probably greater.

## IMMUNE-ENHANCING NUTRITION

**Glutamine:** This is the preferred energy source for leukocytes and enterocytes. There is evidence that it has a beneficial role in the inflammatory response, oxidative stress, and gut integrity. Outcome benefit has been demonstrated in trauma and burn patients.[2]

**L-Arginine:** Essential during metabolic stress. It upregulates macrophage activity. High-dose supplementation has been demonstrated to enhance wound healing and to reduce infection in the elective surgical population; it may increase mortality in other groups.

**Omega 3:** Exhibits potent immunomodulatory activity via arachadonic acid inhibition Some evidence exists of improved outcomes in acute respiratory distress syndrome.

## CONSEQUENCES OF MALNUTRITION IN CRITICAL ILLNESS

- Poor wound healing.
- Impaired immune function and increased risk of sepsis.
- Muscle wasting due to protein catabolism; this leads to muscle weakness with consequence of weaning from mechanical ventilation, decreased mobility, and associated complications.
- Mucosal atrophy and diminished barrier function of the gut.
- Increased duration of ICU stay.
- Increased in-hospital mortality.

## OVERFEEDING CONSEQUENCES

- Excessive protein intake: risk of azotemia, hypertonic dehydration, and metabolic acidosis.

- Excessive carbohydrate: risk of hyperglycemia, hypertriglyceridemia, and hepatic steatosis.
- Excessive fat: risk of hypertriglyceridemia and fat-overload syndrome
- Hypercapnia and refeeding syndrome have also been caused by aggressive overfeeding.

## REFEEDING SYNDROME

### ETIOLOGY

Refeeding syndrome develops when a carbohydrate load is delivered following a prolonged fast.

### PATHOPHYSIOLOGY

Hypoinsulinemia is common during fasting, and the sudden increase in circulating insulin provokes the intracellular movement of glucose with potassium and magnesium. Glucose will be phosphorylated during the first step in glycolysis; this will lead to decrease serum phosphate. Hypophophatemia will lead to a decrease in available phosphate for adenosine triphosphate and cyclic adenosine monophosphate. This will lead to failure of tissues with high-energy requirements, such as heart, diaphragm, muscles.

The electrolyte disturbance can provoke cardiac failure and circulatory collapse, as well as symptoms of particular electrolyte losses.[3]

### MANAGEMENT

- Prior to start feeding, all patients at risk of refeeding syndrome should have prophylactic thiamine replacement, normalization of electrolytes, and frequent measurement of electrolytes (first 24–72 hours).
- Feeding should be commenced at lower rates (10 kcal/kg/d).

### REFERENCES

1. Harvey SE, et al. Trial of the route of early nutritional support in critically ill adults. *N Engl J Med.* 2014;371(18):1673–1684. doi:10.1056/NEJMoa1409860
2. Grau T, et al. The effect of L-alanyl-L-glutamine dipeptide supplemented total parenteral nutrition on infectious morbidity and insulin sensitivity in critically ill patients. *Crit Care Med.* 2011;39(6):1263–1268.
3. Fuentebella J, Kerner JA. Refeeding syndrome. *Pediatr Clin North Am.* 2009;56(5):1201–1210.

# 151.

# MORBID OBESITY/ANESTHESIA FOR BARIATRIC SURGERY

*Vincent Roth and Christopher Giordano*

## OVERVIEW OF OBESITY PATHOPHYSIOLOGY

Obesity, defined as a body mass index (BMI) of 30–49.9 kg/m$^2$ and superobesity as greater than 50 kg/m$^2$, is an inflammatory state that impacts every organ system. The highly metabolically active nature of visceral fat contributes to a number of comorbid states, including nonalcoholic fatty liver disease, dyslipidemia, and type 2 diabetes. Metabolic syndrome itself, which is directly related to obesity, carries a number of morbidity and mortality risks, including endothelial dysfunction, microalbuminuria, and hypertension.[1] Some of these conditions directly alter how we deliver anesthesia, discussed next.

**Respiratory:** Increased abdominal and thoracic weight lead to decreased chest wall compliance and increased work of breathing. This restrictive pathology leads to a decreased functional residual capacity (FRC) by decreasing the expiratory reserve volume while maintaining the residual volume; atelectasis formation; and subsequent pulmonary shunting in dependent lung regions.[2] Furthermore, adipose tissue is highly vascular and metabolically active, necessitating a higher baseline oxygen demand and subsequently greater oxygen consumption. These forces work together to cause a rapid decline in oxygen levels with cessation of respiration. To put this in context, the safe apnea period (SAP), or time period between apnea and a lethal decrease in oxygen saturation (SpO$_2$), decreases from about 8–10 minutes in a normal weight patient to just 2–3 minutes in obese patients.[3]

**Cardiovascular:** Obesity increases cardiac output, circulating blood volumes, and cardiac workload.[2,4] Interestingly, circulating blood volumes are lower in obese patients when calculated relative to weight (~45 mL/kg in obese patients versus ~70 mL/kg in normal weight patients), despite higher total circulating blood volumes, which may increase the risk of hemodynamic instability when delivering an anesthetic.[4] The highly vascular adipose tissue creates greater circulation demands, which can translate to left ventricular wall stress, dysfunction, and ultimately heart failure that begins as diastolic dysfunction and can result in systolic dysfunction. Fatty infiltration of the conduction system can also lead to sinoatrial node dysfunction and resultant arrhythmias.[2] Obesity commonly enhances sympathetic activity, which may lead to increased hemodynamic instability during surgical stress.[4] Obese patients generally have higher rates of cardiovascular comorbidities, such as coronary artery disease, ischemic cardiomyopathy, hypertension, and cor pulmonale. Cor pulmonale is closely linked to the respiratory pathophysiology of obesity, in which restricted breathing patterns lead to hypoventilation, increasing CO$_2$ retention, and subsequent pulmonary hypertension, which ultimately strains the right heart and causes right ventricular failure.

**Airway Anatomy:** Obese patients often have adipose tissue deposits in the oral and pharyngeal tissue, leading to narrowing of the airway and obstruction with a loss of consciousness that can lead to obstructive sleep apnea (OSA). OSA more than doubles the risk of postoperative desaturation, respiratory failure, postoperative cardiac events, and intensive care unit admisisons.[1,2] As nighttime hypoventilation elevates PaCO$_2$ levels causing a respiratory acidosis, metabolic compensation occurs with the kidney resorbing bicarbonate. This chronic hypercapnia can cause daytime somnolence from repeated nighttime arousal episodes and continue to insidiously elevate resulting in CO$_2$ narcosis, which exacerbates disordered breathing and maintaining consciousness. This phenomenon is known as obesity hypoventilation syndrome, or Pickwickian syndrome, in which an obese patient's daytime somnolence further impairs alveolar hypoventilation, which exacerbates baseline hypoxia and hypercapnia and can lead to a lethal CO$_2$ narcosis.

## ANESTHETIC CONSIDERATIONS

### PREOPERATIVE

Bariatric patients have predictable healthcare risks related to the previously discussed pathophysiological changes that

**Table 151.1** THE STOP-BANG SCREENING QUESTIONNAIRE FOR OBSTRUCTIVE SLEEP APNEA (OSA)

| | |
|---|---|
| **S**noring | Do you snore loudly? (can be heard through a door or louder than talking) |
| **T**ired | Do you often feel tired, fatigued, or fall asleep during the day? |
| **O**bserved | Have you been observed choking, gasping, or not breathing during sleep? |
| Blood **P**ressure | Do you have (or are you being treated for) high blood pressure? |
| **B**MI | BMI > 35 kg/m$^2$ |
| **A**ge | Age > 50 years |
| **N**eck | Circumference > 43 cm for males; > 41 cm for females |
| **G**ender | Male |

One point is scored for each positive feature/response; a score ≥ 5 indicates high risk for OSA.

should be included in screening.[2] In order to prepare for complications related to OSA, the STOP-BANG questionnaire should be administered (Table 151.1), with a score of 5 or more suggesting sleep-disordered breathing, and positive screening should be followed up with overnight oximetry or polysomnography testing.[2] An arterial blood gas can also help detect the severity of OSA as well as the success of continuous positive airway pressure (CPAP) therapy by recognizing the plasma's bicarbonate value. Metabolic compensation can reflect the severity of respiratory acidosis with bicarbonate values greater than 30–31 mEq/L and signify a lack of or inadequate treatment. Premedication with benzodiazepines should be avoided as they may exacerbate chronic hypercapnia, which could result in carbon dioxide narcosis.

The American Heart Association (AHA) recommends a 12-lead electrocardiogram for all surgical patients with at least one risk factor for coronary artery disease—of which obesity is one. The preoperative clinic visit should elicit information about exercise tolerance and other comorbidities that might warrant further cardiac investigation.[2] It is also an appropriate time to discuss smoking cessation, thromboprophylaxis, and the importance of early mobilization. Obesity independently is an indication for pharmacological thromboprophylaxis—ideally dose-adjusted low-molecular-weight heparin.[2] Studies have demonstrated that obesity is not correlated with gastroesophageal reflux disease or increased aspiration risk, so aspiration prophylaxis is not indicated unless there is an identifiable risk factor.[1] Some obese patients have gastric volume greater than 25 mL and a PH below 2.5. However, obese patients frequently have diabetes mellitus, which can result

in gastroparesis and subsequently place the patient at an increased risk of aspiration.

## INTRAOPERATIVE

**Positioning:** As positioning pertains to airway manipulation, the ramped positioning of the thorax and head (Figure 151.1) typically provides the optimal view for intubation as this best aligns the airway axis and creates the traditional "sniffing position." This can be appreciated with the external auditory canal level with the sternal notch. Reverse Trendelenburg positioning minimizes the restrictive effects of abdominal and thoracic adipose tissue compressing the chest wall, reducing compliance, decreasing FRC, and reducing the SAP.[2,5] Delicate patient positioning during the procedure in obesity is exceptionally important as excess weight and pressure in dependent areas may lead to nerve compression, skin and muscle breakdown, and concomitant rhabdomyolysis.[1]

**Intravenous Access and Monitoring:** Establishing intravenous access in obese patients is often challenging and may require use of ultrasound to locate peripheral veins.[2] Obesity alone is not an indication for invasive monitoring; rather, obese patients more often have comorbidities such as obesity-hypoventilation syndrome, which might require invasive monitoring like an artery catheter for frequent blood gas measurements or to avert a poorly fitting noninvasive blood pressure cuff.[1]

**Airway:** Results from studies investigating difficulties associated with establishing an airway in obese patients are complicated primarily because the meaning of "difficult" is uncertain: effort, success, time for setup, and time to complete access. Some of these challenges result from anatomical obstacles that include shorter, thicker necks; larger tongues; redundant pharyngeal soft tissue; heavy heads; as well as the SAP time challenge. The common theme, however, is that with proper ramped head positioning (Figure 151.1) and reverse Trendelenburg positioning, tracheal intubation by direct laryngoscopy should be as successful as with normal habitus patients.[1,5]

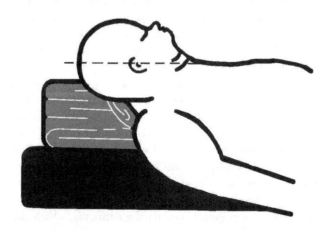

Figure 151.1

**Drugs:** Drugs with high lipophilicity will have a greater volume of distribution in an obese patient and a longer half-life. To account for this variability, drugs may be dosed according to total body weight (TBW) or ideal body weight (IBW), which essentially is lean body weight. Drugs with high lipophilicity (midazolam, succinylcholine, fentanyl, and sufentanil) distribute to peripheral fat compartments and need to be dosed according to the TBW. Alternatively, drugs such as vecuronium, rocuronium, and remifentanil that are hydrophilic do not distribute to the fat compartment and can be dosed according to the IBW.[1] Generally speaking, drugs with less distribution to the peripheral fat compartment tend to have shorter, more predictable clinical effects. Thus, it would be prudent to choose a drug like remifentanil for pain control over fentanyl, as it does not accumulate in adipose tissue and therefore wears off quickly once the infusion is stopped.

## POSTOPERATIVE

In the immediate postoperative period, it is important to consider respiratory support and pain control options for bariatric patients. The use of CPAP, aggressive pulmonary toilet, and early ambulation are vital following surgery. Implementing a multimodal approach to pain control intraoperatively that extends postoperatively by utilizing gabapentin, ketamine, nonsteroidal analgesics, acetaminophen, or regional anesthesia will help avert narcotic-induced respiratory depression and encourage early ambulation.[4]

## REFERENCES

1. Eckmann DM. Anesthesia for bariatric surgery. In: Miller RD, et al. *Miller's Anesthesia E-Book*. Elsevier Health Sciences; 2014:2200–2215.
2. Nightingale CE, et al. Peri-operative management of the obese surgical patient 2015: Association of Anaesthetists of Great Britain and Ireland Society for Obesity and Bariatric Anaesthesia. *Anaesthesia*. 2015;70(7):859–876.
3. Bazurro S, et al. Perioperative management of obese patient. *Curr Opin Crit Care*. 2018;24(6):560–567.
4. Huschak G, et al. Obesity in anesthesia and intensive care. *Best Pract Res Clin Endocrinol Metab*. 2013;27(2):247–260.
5. Boyce JR, et al. A preliminary study of the optimal anesthesia positioning for the morbidly obese patient. Obes Surg. 2003;13(1):4–9.

# 152.

# POSTOPERATIVE HEPATIC DYSFUNCTION

*Peter Nielson and Michael Kaufman*

## INTRODUCTION

The metabolic function of the liver is measured by glucose homeostasis (glucose is transformed to glycogen, which is stored in the liver; insulin stimulates glycogenesis, while glucagon and epinephrine inhibit it); fat metabolism; protein synthesis (all plasma proteins are produced in the liver except γ-globulins and antihemophiliac factor VIII); drug biotransformation; and bilirubin formation and excretion.

Liver function tests and their values are as follows:

- Albumin, normal level 3.5–5.5 g/dL. It is an indirect measurement of the synthetic capacity of the liver.
- Prothrombin time, normal time is 8.4–12.0 seconds. It measures the synthetic ability of the liver. All coagulation factors are synthetized in the liver except factor VIII.
- Bilirubin, normal unconjugated (water-insoluble) level 0.2–0.8 mg/dL. Normal unconjugated (water-soluble) level is 0–0.3 mg/dL.
- Transaminases: Aspartate aminotransferase (AST) normal level is 12–31 U/L and alanine aminotransferase (ALT) normal level is 10–32 U/L.
- Alkaline phosphatase, normal level 90–240 U/dL. It is also present in the skeleton, gastrointestinal tract, pancreas, and placenta (none specific for liver dysfunction).

Postoperative hepatic dysfunction is often diagnosed by development of unexpected jaundice and laboratory confirmation or by incidental laboratory finding alone. The particular liver function test (LFT) that is elevated helps guide the diagnosis and likely insult. Many cases recover with supportive care alone. Drug-induced liver injury should be considered, especially given increasing polypharmacy of patients coming to the operating room. Many LFTs will be elevated transiently after surgery; elevations over two times the normal limit should elicit prompt evaluation for causes of hepatocellular injury, biliary pathology, or both.

## POSTOPERATIVE HYPERBILIRUBINEMIA

Jaundice can be a presenting symptom, but often abnormal LFTs will be noticed before the appearance of skin color changes and scleral icterus; (Table 152.1) provides common differentials. Elevated bilirubin can be either indirect (unconjugated) or, after it is processed by the liver, direct (conjugated). Indirect hyperbilirubinemia is typically caused by an excess of heme breakdown. This can be due to multiple transfusions as up to 10% of red blood cells hemolyze within a day of transfusion. Reabsorption of hematomas is another major contributor to indirect bilirubin. Any causes of shear stress, such as cardiac bypass pumps, may increase release of heme into the blood as well. In short, any process that breaks down red blood cells and releases heme will result in an indirect bilirubinemia if the release is faster than the liver can process the indirect bilirubin.[1]

Blood levels of conjugated bilirubin will increase if excretion of it is hindered. Benign postoperative cholestasis is a poorly understood but somewhat common reason for elevated conjugated bilirubinemia. Opioids may play a role given their capacity to contract the sphincter of Oddi. In these cases, bilirubin is removed from circulation and conjugated but is not excreted. Hepatocellular injury can be a cause of increased bilirubin if the liver is damaged enough that it cannot conjugate bilirubin, but often one will see greater elevations in AST and ALT first, suggesting hepatitis before an increase in other LFTs.[2] Any surgery in the upper abdomen may be a source of a mechanical injury to

### Table 152.1 DIFFERENTIALS OF DIRECT VERSUS INDIRECT POSTOPERATIVE BILIRUBINEMIA

| DIRECT BILIRUBENEMIA | INDIRECT BILIRUBINEMIA |
|---|---|
| • Biliary stone | • Hematoma |
| • Surgical trauma to biliary tree | • Blood transfusions |
| • Postoperative cholestasis | • Genetic hemolytic disease (e.g., G6PD deficiency) |
| • Preexisting liver dysfunction | • Preexisting liver shunt (e.g., patient with TIPS) |

the biliary system, and consultation with the surgical team may be warranted. Of particular concern in cholecystectomy is a retained stone causing obstruction of the biliary system. Congenital disorders of bilirubin excretion may be exacerbated by surgery, and a history of these disorders should raise clinical suspicion of a perioperative exacerbation of the patient's disorder.

## POSTOPERATIVE HEPATITIS

Hepatitis is inflammation of the liver often diagnosed by an elevation in liver enzymes (AST and ALT) greater than two times the normal values. Slight elevations are common and usually transient. Of note, AST is not specific to the liver, while ALT is mainly from the liver.

## DRUG-RELATED CAUSES

Halothane is a drug-related cause of hepatitis of historical significance, but other halogenated anesthetics can also cause hepatitis, although at greatly reduced rates. The mechanism is believed to be due to liver metabolism of the anesthetic releasing byproducts that are immunogenic, leading to immune-modulated inflammation of the liver. Inhaled anesthetic–induced hepatitis is often thought of as a diagnosis of exclusion.[3] Other drug-induced liver injuries are possible, especially if multiple drugs commonly associated with liver toxicity are given in the perioperative period. Concern for continuing rise in LFTs may prompt specialist consult for further workup that may include biopsy.

## ISCHEMIC CAUSES

Another frequently encountered reason for elevations of liver enzymes after surgery is due to a low-flow state to the liver in the perioperative period. Surgical reasons such as upper abdominal surgery or hepatic surgery are obvious risk factors for direct liver injury or damage to vessels supplying the liver. Several drugs used routinely in the course of anesthesia can reduce hepatic blood flow either directly or indirectly. Anesthetics and cardiac depressants decrease flow, while pressors may constrict vessels supplying the liver. "Shock liver" is also possible in situations such as trauma, high blood loss surgery, or excessively deep anesthetic. Avoiding hypotension will aid in prevention of liver dysfunction as well as other morbidities. Decreased blood flow for excessive amounts of time will lead to hepatocellular necrosis and can increase the burden on the remaining hepatocytes. Postoperative dysfunction may also be related to the amount of hepatocytes left after a partial hepatic resection, in addition to any injury or vascular insult during the surgery itself. Patients may also have undiagnosed preexisting liver disease that presents in the postoperative period that may have been precipitated by effects of decreased hepatic blood flow during surgery.[4]

## REFERENCES

1. Tholey D. Postoperative liver dysfunction—hepatic and biliary disorders. *Merck Manuals Professional Edition*. October 2019. Accessed July 25, 2020. https://www.merckmanuals.com/professional/hepatic-and-biliary-disorders/approach-to-the-patient-with-liver-disease/postoperative-liver-dysfunction

2. Barash PG, et al. The liver: surgery and anesthesia. In: *Clinical Anesthesia*. Wolters Kluwer; 2017:1298–1322.

3. Toimil B. Postoperative hepatic dysfunction. *Open Anesthesia*. Accessed July 25, 2020.https://selfstudyplus.openanesthesia.org/kw/entry/-LfpscqH6rYkRvPWa30W

4. Levine W, Allain R. *Handbook of Clinical Anesthesia Procedures of the Massachusetts General Hospital*. 8th ed. Philadelphia: Wolters Kluwer Health/Lippincott, Williams & Wilkins; 2010:57.

# 153.

# LIVER TRANSPLANT SURGERY

*John Mattimore and Michael Kaufman*

## INTRODUCTION

Liver transplantation was pioneered in the 1960s by Thomas Starzl, who completed the first successful liver transplantation in 1967. To date, liver transplantation has become the mainstay treatment for most causes of hepatic failure, with 8250 cases performed in the United States in 2018, and graft 1-year survival rates reaching greater than 91%.[1] Patients with hepatocellular dysfunction with a Model for End-Stage Liver Disease (MELD) score of 15 or higher should be evaluated for a liver transplantation. MELD scores are based on objective measurements, including a patient's total serum bilirubin, creatinine, international normalized ratio, and serum sodium levels (Table 153.1). This validated formula predicts mortality at 90 days after registration. Contraindications to transplantation include active sepsis; AIDS-defining illness (not HIV-positive patients); fewer than 6 months of sobriety/cessation of substance abuse; severe portopulmonary hypertension with mean pulmonary pressures (mPAPs) greater than 45 mm Hg; extremes in size; extrahepatic malignancy; psychosocial issues (the inability to care for the new organ); and severe cardiovascular disease.

## EVALUATION

Potential recipients undergo an extensive preoperative workup to screen for coexisting conditions that will affect surgical outcomes. Transthoracic echocardiography (TTE) is used to assess heart function and screen for the presence of portopulmonary hypertension and hepatopulmonary syndrome. When estimated pulmonary artery systolic pressures are found to be greater than 45 mm Hg by TTE,

*Table 153.1* NINETY-DAY FOR MODEL FOR END-STAGE LIVER DISEASE SODIUM (MELD-NA) SCORE

| MELD-NA SCORE | NINETY-DAY MORTALITY |
|---|---|
| <9 | 1.9% mortality |
| 10–19 | 6.0% mortality |
| 20–29 | 19.6% mortality |
| 30–39 | 52.6% mortality |
| >40 | 71.3% mortality |

From Reference 6.

and additional testing with a right heart catheterization (RHC) is indicated.

If the RHC shows a mPAP greater than 45 mm Hg, with a wedge pressure of less than 15 mm Hg, and pulmonary vascular resistance of greater than 240 dynes/cm$^2$, the patient has severe pulmonary hypertension. Intraoperative liver transplant mortality rates reach 100% when pulmonary artery pressures are severe.[2] However, these patients may still be eligible for transplant if vasodilator therapies are able to lower their mPAPs. If the TTE uncovers wall motion abnormalities, a depressed ejection fraction, or moderate-to-severe valvular dysfunction on an adequate dobutamine stress echocardiogram, a cardiologist should be consulted to optimize the patient before surgery.

Many patients with end-stage liver disease have hepatorenal syndrome (HRS), which can be screened for via basic laboratory work. HRS is caused by portal hypertension decreasing the perfusion pressure of the kidneys. Type 1 HRS may be diagnosed when serum creatinine doubles to a value greater than 2.5 mg/dL in less than 2 weeks. Type 2 HRS requires the same criteria to be met, but takes longer than 2 weeks to develop. Renal failure significantly increases the 1-month mortality risk of these patients.[3] All patients with renal dysfunction should undergo an extensive workup to determine the cause of their renal dysfunction prior to surgery.

Hyponatremia, a consequence of cirrhosis, will place the patient at higher risk for central pontine myolysis and pulmonary edema; adult patients will require liters of fluids for resuscitation through the surgery, and care must be taken not to overcorrect the sodium through the case. Patients may be optimized preoperatively with diuretics and fluid restriction. High serum ammonia levels, in conjunction with confirmatory neuropsychology testing, is indicative of encephalopathy. Particularly important when assessing liver transplant candidates is the identification of patients with acute hepatic failure. Acute increases in serum ammonia levels place patients at risk for cerebral edema and brain herniation. Neuropsychological examination may uncover lethargy or inappropriate behaviors, somnolence, and coma depending on the severity of the encephalopathy. These patients may be evaluated with head computed tomographic scan, and neurosurgery may be consulted for consideration of intracranial pressure monitoring.

## SURGERY

Once removed from the donor, the hepatic allograft has a 10-hour maximum cold ischemia time; thus preparations for a deceased liver donation surgery occur precipitously and preferentially before the harvest has occurred. Living donor surgeries may be scheduled in different operating rooms and occur concurrently at the same institution or nearby institutions. Once underway, the anesthesiologist must be prepared to place multiple invasive monitors and catheters, including central and peripheral arterial lines, central lines, and large-bore intravenous lines (14-gauge) or a rapid infusion catheter, with potential placement of a Swan-Ganz catheter. Swan-Ganz catheters are rarely required for pediatric liver transplants. TEE placement and monitoring are recommended for most patients.[4] A rapid infusion transfusion device, cell-saver device, continuous venovenous hemofiltration device, and a venovenous bypass device should be available.

Liver transplant recipient surgery can be divided into three stages: the preanhepatic (dissection) phase, the anhepatic phase, and the neohepatic phase. Each stage of the transplant surgery presents the anesthesiologist with its own unique set of challenges (Table 153.2).

Increasingly, during the anhepatic phase surgeons are performing a "piggyback technique" instead of a traditional caval reconstruction. A piggyback technique involves preserving part of the donor's inferior vena cava (IVC) and sewing it to the recipient's retrohepatic vena cava in a side-to-side anastomosis. This technique enables the surgeons to only clamp part of the recipient's native IVC, allowing for some of the patient's lower extremity blood supply to return to the patient's heart, thereby eliminating the need for venovenous bypass for complete IVC occlusion.

However, the most critical time of the surgery occurs during the transition from the anhepatic stage to the neohepatic stage: the reperfusion of the donor organ. Once the IVC clamp is released, the liver is now perfused, and it sends cold, acidotic, and potassium-rich blood with microthrombi back to the patient's heart, causing profound hemodynamic instability. This is treated with calcium chloride to stabilize the cardiac myocyte membranes, sodium bicarbonate for hyperkalemia, and vasopressors for vasoplegia. Post–reperfusion syndrome occurs when vasopressors are required for longer than 3 minutes. Cardiac arrhythmias and myocyte dysfunction can occur from electrolyte abnormalities, hypothermia, and preexisting coronary artery disease. Venovenous bypass, decreasing the cold perfusion time of the donor organ, central venovenous hemodialysis, and careful electrolyte management prior to reperfusion will help minimize the reperfusion effects.

## POSTOPERATIVE ALLOGRAFT FUNCTION

Allograft function in the postoperative period is monitored using laboratory measurements and the presence of encephalopathy. Graft nonfunction will require an emergency retransplantation for the patient to survive. Early allograft dysfunction has been defined differently by different authors; however, commonly used determinants include laboratory measurements of hepatic synthetic function,

**Table 153.2 LIVER TRANSPLANTATION SURGERY STAGES, CONCERNS, AND ELECTROLYTE CONSIDERATIONS**

| SURGICAL EVENTS | ANESTHESIOLOGY CONCERNS | ELECTROLYTE DISTURBANCES |
|---|---|---|
| Preanehaptic stage<br><br>- Incision, exposure, and dissection<br>- Hepatic artery cross clamp | - Prepare for bleeding during exposure.<br>- Rapid decreases in preload due to surgical manipulation. | Correct: ↑ or ↓[K], ↓[Mg], ↓[Ca²⁺]<br>Do Not Correct: ↓[Na] |
| Anhepatic stage<br><br>- IVC, portal vein cross clamping, and recipient hepatectomy<br>- Reconstruction of the graft to the patient's IVC | - The patient's preload will drop with the partial or full clamp applied to the patient's IVC and complete portal clamping. Different surgical techniques alter the magnitude of the hemodynamic changes. | Correct: ↑[K] and ↓[Ca²⁺]<br>Do Not Correct: ↓[Na] |
| Neohepatic stage<br><br>- Opening of the portal vein<br>- Flush of the donor liver<br>- Release of the IVC<br>- Anastomoses of the hepatic artery and of the biliary tree<br>- Closure | - Hypovolemia will occur during the flush of the donor liver.<br>- Vasoplegia, hyperkalemia, and acidosis will occur with the reperfusion of the donor liver.<br>- Correcting coagulopathies, acidemia, volume status to prepare for/consider extubation. | Correct:: ↑[K] and ↓[Ca²⁺]<br>Do Not Correct: ↓[Na] |

including bilirubin; prothrombin time, international normalized ratio, and aminotransferase levels.[5] It occurs within the first 7 days following transplantation and is associated with poor outcomes.

## REFERENCES

1. 2018 annual report of the U.S. Organ Procurement and Transplantation Network and the Scientific Registry of Transplant Recipients: transplant data 2007–2018. Department of Health and Human Services, Health Resources and Services Administration, Healthcare Systems Bureau, Division of Transplantation, Rockville, MD; United Network for Organ Sharing, Richmond, VA; University Renal Research and Education Association, Ann Arbor, MI.

2. Swanson KL, et al. Survival in portopulmonary hypertension: Mayo Clinic experience categorized by treatment subgroups. *Am J Transplant*. 2008;8(11):2445–2453.

3. Fede G, et al. Renal failure and cirrhosis: a systematic review of mortality and prognosis. *J Hepatol*. 2012;56(4):810–818.

4. De Marchi L, et al. Safety and benefit of transesophageal echocardiography in liver transplant surgery: a position paper from the Society for the Advancement of Transplant Anesthesia (SATA). *Liver Transplant*. 2020;26(8):1019–1029.

5. Agopian VG, et al. Evaluation of early allograft function using the liver graft assessment following transplantation risk score model. *JAMA Surg*. 2018;153(5):436–444.

6. Kim WR, et al. Hyponatremia and mortality among patients on the liver-transplant waiting list. *N Engl J Med*. 2008;359(10):1018–1026.

# 154.

# ANESTHESIA FOR UPPER AND LOWER GI ENDOSCOPY

*Ethan H. Leer*

## INTRODUCTION

With advances in minimally invasive techniques, an increasing number of gastrointestinal (GI) endoscopic procedures are being performed.[1] GI procedures showed the highest rate of increase among non–operating room anesthesia cases between 2010 and 2013 according to data from the National Anesthesia Clinical Outcomes Registry.[2]

These procedures provide diagnostic and therapeutic interventions for a variety of conditions. Colonoscopy/flexible sigmoidoscopy is typically performed for screening cancer, biopsies, polyp resection, and evaluation of lower GI symptoms such as bleeding. Routine esophagogastroduodenoscopy (EGD) is used for evaluation of nausea/vomiting, heartburn, abdominal pain, dysphagia, unexplained weight loss, and upper GI bleeding. It could also be utilized to remove foreign body or treat esophageal varices. Advanced upper endoscopies such as esophageal dilation/stenting can be used for esophageal/anastomotic strictures or malignant dysphagia. Balloon-assisted deep enteroscopy is useful for evaluation of a surgically altered GI tract. Endoscopic ultrasound can evaluate mural lesions of the upper GI tract and adjacent structures, and it facilitates fine-needle aspiration. Other advanced upper endoscopies include percutaneous endoscopic gastrostomy (PEG) tube placement and endoscopic mucosal resection/submucosal dissection. More recent techniques that combine minimally invasive surgery and endoscopy are natural orifice transluminal endoscopic surgeries; endoscopic cystogastrostomy for symptomatic pancreatic pseudocysts and infected walled-off necrosis, and peroral endoscopic myotomy for treatment of achalasia.[1,2]

Different levels of sedation (Table 154.1) are employed for endoscopic procedures, from minimal sedation to general anesthesia. Simple diagnostic EGD, 15 to 30 minutes in duration, can be performed under sedation/analgesia or monitored anesthesia care (MAC) with propofol sedation. Some advanced upper GI procedures can also be performed under similar levels of sedation as in PEG or esophageal dilation/stenting. However, more complex advanced endoscopic procedures require a deeper level of sedation due to patient discomfort, duration, and complexity of the procedure itself.[1]

For minimal and moderate sedation, benzodiazepine (midazolam) for anxiety and a narcotic (fentanyl) are typically used due to short onset and duration of action.[4] Although other sedatives/hypnotics can be used, propofol, with its rapid onset and offset effect, is more

**Table 154.1** CONTINUUM OF DEPTH OF SEDATION: DEFINITION OF GENERAL ANESTHESIA AND LEVELS OF SEDATION/ANALGESIA[3]

| | MINIMAL SEDATION (ANXIOLYSIS) | MODERATE SEDATION/ ANALGESIA (CONSCIOUS SEDATION) | DEEP SEDATION/ ANALGESIA | GENERAL ANESHTESIA |
|---|---|---|---|---|
| Responsiveness | Normal resoponse to verbal stimulation | Purposeful* response to verbal or tactile stimulation | Purposeful* response after repeated or painful stimulation | Unarousable, even with painful stimulus |
| Airway | Unaffected | No intervention required | Intervention may be required | Intervention often required |
| Spontaneous ventilation | Unaffected | Adequate | May be inadequate | Frequently inadequate |
| Cardiovascular function | Unaffected | Usually maintained | Usually maintained | May be impaired |

effective at achieving moderate sedation, and patient satisfaction is higher compared with the combination of benzodiazepine and a narcotic.[4] Propofol, however, has a narrow therapeutic window, and patient response is not uniform, thus increasing the possibility of the level of sedation transitioning to a deeper level than initially intended.[5] This may require rescue from the deeper sedation level, airway management, and emergent intubation. Because of this danger, the Advisory on Granting Privileges for Deep Sedation to Non-Anesthesiologist Physicians advocated that anesthesiologists should be involved in all deep sedation for patient safety.[6] Despite this, gastroenterologists continue to support the use of propofol sedation by nonanesthesiologists (nonanesthesiologists-administered propofol [NAAP] and nurse-administered propofol sedation [NAPS]), citing the safety and efficacy in the literature. At this time, regulations on propofol administration are determined at the state, regional, and local levels, and state and institutional regulations dictate who can administer MAC.[4]

## ANESTHETIC CONSIDERATIONS

### PREOPERATIVE

During upper endoscopic procedures, the airway reflex is diminished under sedation. The airway is shared with the procedurist's endoscope, and anesthesiologists' access to the airway is further limited due to patient positioning (typically left lateral). Therefore, in addition to standard preanesthetic evaluation for preexisting comorbidities, careful examination of the airway through focused history and physical examination is paramount: prior history of difficulty with anesthesia/sedation, stridor/snoring, sleep apnea (also use the STOP-BANG questionnaire), severe rheumatoid arthritis, cervical spine disease, body mass index, dysmorphic facial features, short neck, large neck circumference, limited neck extension, decreased hyoid-mental distance (<3 cm), small mouth opening (<3 cm), edentulous dentition, protruding incisors, loose or capped teeth, high arched palate, macroglossia, tonsillar hypertrophy, the Mallampati classification, and micrognathia. Also, assessment of risks for pulmonary aspiration is critical; fasting status, elective versus emergent procedure, and impaired gastric emptying.[3] Based on these evaluations, along with procedure variables (duration, complexity, and patient's discomfort level), a decision has to be made whether the adequate level of sedation can be achieved safely and effectively or the airway needs to be secured with endotracheal intubation.

### INTRAOPERATIVE

During the procedure with sedation, standard American Society of Anesthesiologists monitoring must be employed.

Intraoperatively, the ventilation status should be assessed for its adequacy to detect apnea and airway obstruction via capnography. With a pulse oximeter alone there can be significant delay in detecting hypoxemia, especially when supplemental oxygen is being administered, even if oxygen desaturation is detected.[3–5]

### POSTOPERATIVE

Typically after routine endoscopic procedures, patients are expected to recover quickly. Even though the incidence of postoperative complications is low, patients should be monitored to fully recover from anesthesia, and observed for complications specific to the procedure or sedation until they meet discharge criteria.[5]

## ENDOSCOPIC RETROGRADE CHOLANGIOPANCREATOGRAPHY

By combining endoscopic and fluoroscopic imaging techniques, endoscopic retrograde cholangiopancreatography (ERCP) can be diagnostic and therapeutic for biliary and pancreatic pathologies, namely, for choledocholithiasis, biliary obstruction/stricture, or bile leak, by placement of stent and removal of a stone. Along with similar preoperative considerations for other endoscopic procedures, thorough assessment of the airway is utmost important because access to the airway could be more challenging due to the patient in a prone position and fluoroscopic equipment in the room. Therefore, although MAC with propofol can be deployed, general anesthesia with endotracheal intubation should be considered for each patient based on individual risk factors. Patients requiring ERCP may also be post–liver transplant, cholecystectomy, or laparotomy after trauma with abdominal incision. For such patients, the procedure should be performed in supine position and the airway secured with an endotracheal tube. Gastroenterologists may request an antispasmodic such as glucagon or intravenous hyoscyamine to facilitate the procedure. Transient bacteremia is possible, and patients should be monitored closely postoperatively. Complications from ERCP include acute pancreatitis, hemorrhage and perforation with a rate of 5%–10%, and a mortality of 0.1%–1%.[1,2]

## REFERENCES

1. Sharp CD, et al. Anesthesia for routine and advanced upper gastrointestinal endoscopic procedures. *Anesthesiol Clin.* 2017;35(4): 669–677.
2. Souter KJ, et al. Nonoperating room anesthesia. In: Barash P, et al., eds. *Clinical Anesthesia.* 8th ed. Philadelphia, PA: Lippincott, Williams and Wilkins; 2017:880–895.

3. American Society of Anesthesiologists Task Force on Sedation and Analgesia by Non-Anesthesiologists. Practice guidelines for sedation and analgesia by non-anesthesiologists. *Anesthesiology.* 2002;96(4):1004–1017.
4. ASGE Standards of Practice Committee, Early DS, et al. Guidelines for sedation and anesthesia in GI endoscopy. *Gastrointest Endosc.* 2018;87(2):327–337.
5. Bryson EO, Sejpal D. Anesthesia in remote locations: radiology and beyond, international anesthesiology clinics: gastroenterology: endoscopy, colonoscopy, and ERCP. *Int Anesthesiol Clin.* 2009;47(2): 69–80.
6. American Society of Anesthesiologists, Committee on Quality Management and Departmental Administration. Advisory on granting privileges for deep sedation to non-anesthesiologist physicians. 2017. https://www.asahq.org/standards-and-guidelines/advisory-on-granting-privileges-for-deep-sedation-to-non-anesthesiologist-physicians

# Part 14

# RENAL AND URINARY SYSTEMS/
# ELECTROLYTE BALANCE

# 155.

# RENAL ANATOMY

*Erika Taco and Edward Noguera*

## INTRODUCTION

The kidneys are vital organs that can be injured directly during surgery or indirectly as part of postoperative recovery. Left pneumothorax is more common during left nephrectomies due to anatomical reasons.[1]

## MACROSCOPIC ANATOMY

Kidneys are paired organs located in the retroperitoneum and lying on the posterior abdominal wall. Each kidney has a superior and inferior pole, a convex lateral border, and a concave medial border. The medial border has a depression, the hilum, which contains renal vessels and renal pelvis. The right kidney has a mean length of 10 × 5 × 3 cm thick, whereas the left kidney presents a mean length of 11 × 5 × 3 cm thick.[2] Kidney ultrasound showing enlarged kidneys is usually a sign of chronic kidney disease, such as hypertension.

## ANATOMICAL LANDMARKS

The right kidney is situated about 1–2 cm lower than the left kidney because of the position of the liver. Anteriorly, the right kidney is bordered by the liver and the right colonic flexure. The right hilum is in close relation with the head of the pancreas and the descending part of the duodenum. The left kidney is bordered anteriorly by the left colonic flexure. The left renal hilum overlies the body of the pancreas and the splenic vessels. Posteriorly, the diaphragm covers the upper third of the kidneys[1] (Figure 155.1).

## CAPSULE

Gerota's fascia encloses the kidney, adrenal gland, and perinephric fat. Its layers are fused superiorly, laterally, and medially, but not inferiorly. The renal hilum is formed from anterior to posterior by the renal vein, artery, and pelvis.[1,2]

## ARTERIAL SUPPLY

In approximately 75% of cases, the abdominal aorta raises a single renal artery caudal to the origin of the superior mesenteric artery. The renal artery is usually located posterior to the renal vein, but in about 30% is located anteriorly. The right artery passes behind the inferior vena cava (IVC), and it is lower than the left renal artery in relation to the renal pelvis. The renal artery divides into two before entering the hilum, an anterior and posterior division that contribute to 75% and 25%, respectively, of the kidneys' blood supply.

From the arterial divisions, five segmental arteries originate that are end arteries and do not provide adequate collateral circulation. Ligation of a segmental artery could cause a segmental renal infarction. At the level of the fornix, segmental arteries give rise to the interlobar arteries, and these continue in the interlobar septae between the pyramids. Each interlobar artery branches into five to seven arcuate arteries at the corticomedullary junction, which in turn branch into interlobular arteries. Interlobular arteries supply the afferent glomerular arteries.[1]

## VENOUS SYSTEM

The peritubular capillary venous plexus drains to venae rectae into the arcuate veins. Equally to the arterial system, arcuate veins drain into the interlobular vein, forming several trunks that merge as the renal vein anterior to the renal pelvis. In two-thirds of cases, a retropelvic vein is present, which drains some of the posterior part of the kidney. The right renal vein drains directly into the IVC, and rarely, the right gonadal vein may drain into the right renal vein. Duplication is found in 15%–20% of cases. The left renal vein is two to three times longer than the right renal vein, enters the IVC anterior to the aorta, and is infrequently duplicated. The left renal vein drains the gonadal, adrenal, and inferior phrenic; the first or second lumbar; and the paravertebral veins in one-third of cases.[1]

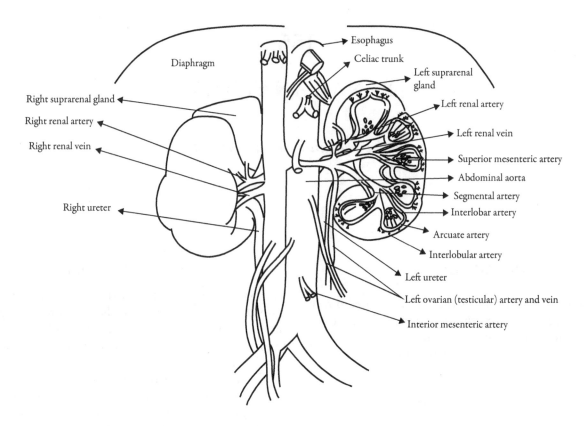

**Figure 155.1** Anatomical landmarks.

## MICROSCOPIC ANATOMY

The kidneys are responsible for regulating volume status, maintaining acid-base equilibrium, eliminating toxins, and producing active hormones, including renin, erythropoietin, and vitamin D.[3] The kidneys have up to 1 million functional nephrons. There are two main components in the nephron: the corpuscle and renal tubules. The kidney is divided into cortex and medulla. Nephrons are classified as cortical and juxtamedullary. All corpuscles are located in the cortex[3] (Figures 155.2A, 155.2B).

### RENAL CORPUSCLE

Each renal corpuscle is composed of a glomerulus, which contains tufts of capillaries, and it is involved by Bowman's capsule. The blood flow comes from an afferent arteriole, divides into capillaries in the glomerulus, and exits as a single efferent arteriole. The glomerular filtration barrier is composed of a fenestrated capillary endothelium (70–100 nm), a basement membrane with type IV collagen, chains and heparan sulfate, and an epithelial layer consisting of podocyte foot processes. These interdigitate tightly between each other and provide an effective and small diaphragm slit (about 25 nm). This barrier has a net negative charge, favoring filtration of cations over anions.[4]

## PROXIMAL CONVOLUTED TUBULE

From the ultrafiltrate about 65%–75% is normally reabsorbed in the proximal renal tubules. During reabsorption, most substances cross the tubular (apical or luminal) side of the cell and then traverse the basolateral cell membrane into the renal interstitium before entering the peritubular capillaries.

The major function of the proximal tubule is reabsorption of 65% to 80% of the filtrated sodium. Sodium is actively transported at the basolateral cell side by Na-K-adenosine triphosphatase (Na–K-ATPase). The low intracellular concentration of sodium allows passive movement of sodium down its gradient from tubular fluid into epithelial cells. Specific carrier proteins use the low concentration of $Na^+$ inside cells to absorb all glucose and amino acids. Sodium reabsorption at the luminal membrane is coupled with hydrogen secretion. Around 60% of isotonic water is reabsorbed at the PCT. The PCT secretes organic cations and anions. Proximal convoluted tubule cells convert 25-OH vitamin $D_3$ to 1,25-$(OH)_2$ vitamin $D_3$ (calcitriol, active form).[4]

## LOOP OF HENLE

The loop of Henle consists of descending and ascending portions. The thin descending segment is a continuation

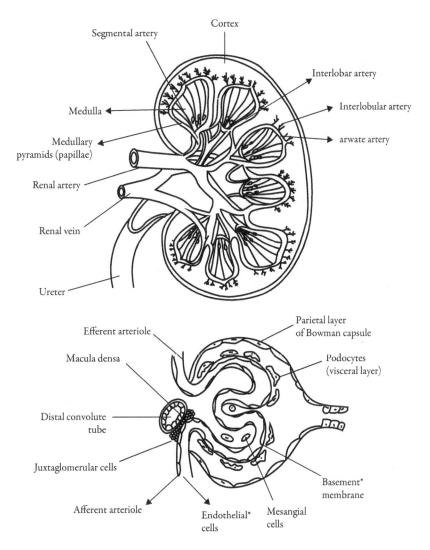

Figure 155.2 (A), (B) Microscopic anatomy.

of the proximal tubule and descends from the renal cortex into the renal medulla. In the medulla, the descending portion acutely turns back on itself and rises back up toward the cortex as the ascending portion. The ascending portion consists of a functionally distinct, thin, ascending limb and medullary and cortical thick ascending limbs.[4]

The thin descending portion is responsible to passively reabsorb water via medullary hypertonicity (impermeable to $Na^+$). Concentrating segment that makes urine hypertonic.[3]

In the ascending thick segment, however, $Na^+$, $Cl^-$, and $K^+$ are reabsorbed in excess of water. $Cl^-$ in tubular fluid appears to be the rate-limiting factor. Active $Na^+$ reabsorption 10%–20% of sodium is absorbed here. It is an important site for calcium and magnesium reabsorption. The thick ascending loop of Henle is impermeable to water; as a result, tubular fluid flowing out of the loop of Henle is hypotonic (100–200 mOsm/L), and the interstitium surrounding the loop of Henle is therefore hypertonic. Urea concentrations also increase within the medulla and contribute to the hypertonicity. The countercurrent mechanism includes the loop of Henle, the cortical and medullary collecting tubules, and their respective capillaries (vasarecta).[4]

## DISTAL TUBULE

The distal tubule receives hypotonic fluid from the loop of Henle and is normally responsible for only minor modifications of tubular fluid. The distal nephron has very tight junctions and is somewhat impermeable to water and sodium. Sodium reabsorption in the distal tubule normally accounts for only about 5% of the filtered sodium load. Sodium reabsorption in this segment is directly proportional to $Na^+$ delivery. The distal tubule is the major site of parathyroid hormone- and vitamin D-mediated calcium reabsorption.[4]

## COLLECTING TUBULE

The collecting tubule has cortical and medullary portions. Both will normally absorb about 5%–7% of the sodium load.[3]

### Cortical Collecting Tubule

The cortical collecting tubule part of the nephron consists of two cell types:

1. The principal cells (P cells), which primarily secrete potassium and participate in aldosterone-stimulated $Na^+$ reabsorption
2. The intercalated cells (I cells) are responsible for acid-base regulation. Since P cells absorb $Na^+$ against the electrical gradient, $Cl^-$ or $K^+$ must be reabsorbed to maintain electroneutrality. Aldosterone activates the H-ATPase at the luminal side.[4]

### Medullary Collecting Tubule

The medullary collecting tubule joins the other nephrons to form the ureter. The collecting tubule is the main site of action for antidiuretic hormone (ADH). ADH acts on the V2 receptors and enhances the expression of the water channel protein, aquaporin 2. ADH secretion is stimulated by dehydration, rendering the luminal side permeable to water. As a result, urine will be more concentrated up to 1400 mOsm/ L. On the other side, hydration suppresses ADH secretion, leading to fluid water loss with hypotonic urine (100–200 mOsm/L).

## JUXTAGLOMERULAR APPARATUS

Mesangial cells are located between the basement membrane and epithelial cells. The juxtaglomerular (JG) cells are modified smooth muscle of the afferent arteriole. Macula densa cells are part of the distal convoluted tube (DCT) and act as a NaCl sensor. All three form the JG apparatus.[3,4] JG cells secrete renin when the RBF decreases or in response to sympathetic $\beta_1$-receptors. Macula densa cells sense low NaCl levels at the DCT, producing renin and producing vasoconstriction of the efferent arteriole, increasing the glomerular filtration rate.[2]

## REFERENCES

1. Klatte T, et al. A literature review of renal surgical anatomy and surgical strategies for partial nephrectomy. *Eur Urol.* 2015;68(6): 980–992.
2. Sampaio FJ. Renal anatomy: endourologic considerations. *Urol Clin.* 2000;27(4):585–607.
3. Hall JE. *Guyton and Hall Textbook of Medical Physiology E-Book.* Elsevier Health Sciences; 2010: Unit V.
4. Butterworth JF, et al. *Morgan and Mikhail's Clinical Anesthesiology.* McGraw-Hill Education; 2018.

# 156.

# PATHOPHYSIOLOGY OF RENAL DISEASE

*Erika Taco and Edward Noguera*

## INTRODUCTION

One of the most common postoperative complications is acute kidney injury (AKI), occurring in 20% to 40% of high-risk patients. Even minor changes in creatinine are associated with increased mortality and hospital length of stay by 2 days. Mortality associated with AKI can be as high as 13% in the hospital and 26% at 1 year.[1]

## ASSESSMENT OF KIDNEY FUNCTION

The blood (serum) urea nitrogen (BUN) is a metabolite from urea that is used as a biomarker to evaluate kidney function. It is not secreted but reabsorbed by renal tubules, and its production can be elevated in gastrointestinal bleeding, corticosteroid therapy, and a high-protein diet. In the noncatabolic state with mildly reduced glomerular filtration rate (GFR), the daily BUN can increase up to 10 to 15 mg/dL and creatinine less than 1.5 mg/dL. On the other hand, in high catabolic states the nitrogen production can increase the BUN to more than 50 mg/dL. During low renal perfusion states, the BUN increases independently from creatinine due to the activation of the renin-angiotensin-aldosterone system and the upregulation of vasopressin and its receptors. It increases the absorption of water and sodium. Thus, urine osmolality increases above 500 mOsm/kg. These findings are highly suggestive of prerenal AKI.

The fractional excretion of sodium (FENa) is a measure of the extraction of sodium and water from the glomerular filtrate. In an euvolemic person, the FENa is 1%. In prerenal azotemia, the proximal tubules reabsorb filtered sodium, resulting in a very low urine concentration (<20 mml/L) and FENa is less than 1%, whereas in intrinsic AKI the urinary sodium concentration is greater than 40 mmol/L and results in a FENa greater than 1%. Fractional excretion of urea (FEUrea) is a calculation based on the same principle as FENa. However, urea reabsorption occurs mainly at the proximal tubule, which in theory makes FEUrea more reliable than FENa during use of diuretic agents, which usually act distally to the proximal tubule. Studies have shown FEUrea can be increased with aging and sepsis.

Creatinine is an end product of skeletal muscle catabolism and is excreted solely by the kidney. Given that its levels are dependent on muscle mass, it can be normal in the elderly despite marked reduction in kidney function.

Creatinine clearance (normal value 110–150 mL/min. This measures glomerular ability to filter creatinine, and it is the most reliable clinical measure of GFR.

Renal blood flow can be experimentally measured by measuring para-aminohippurate clearance.

Urine osmolarity can be a measure of the urine concentrating and diluting ability of the kidney (normal value 300 mOsm/kg).

Regarding the urinary acidification capacity, urine pH is typically below 6.5. This can be tested by giving ammonium chloride orally. If the urine pH is not below 5.5 when the serum pH is below 7.35 and $HCO_3$ is below 20 mEq/L, a renal acidification defect is present.

It is important to note that both BUN and creatinine are late indicators of kidney dysfunction; they increase when the GFR is reduced by about 75%.

Table 156.1 shows the factors that affect urinary excretion of different substances used to assess renal function.

## ACUTE KIDNEY INJURY

Acute kidney injury is broadly defined as an abrupt and sustained decline in the GFR that leads to progressive accumulation of nitrogenous waste products and uremic toxins. Table 156.2 summarizes the criteria for diagnosis of AKI.[1,2,3]

## PATHOPHYSIOLOGY

Normal kidneys can autoregulate themselves to maintain the GFR during constant changes of arterial pressure and volume status. Once autoregulation mechanisms are exhausted, there is an activation of the sympathetic system and a release of the renin-angiotensin aldosterone system, increasing angiotensin II and antidiuretic hormones.[2] AKI

*Table 156.1* FACTORS AFFECTING KIDNEY EXCRETION OF DIFFERENT SUBSTANCES USED TO ASSESS RENAL FUNCTION

| CONSTITUENT | BLOOD LEVEL OR URINE EXCRETION | FACTORS AFFECTING URINARY EXCRETION |
|---|---|---|
| Urea | B = 15–40 mg/dL<br>U = 15–30 g/d | Dietary proteins, protein catabolism, renal blood flow |
| Creatinine | B = 0.7–1.4 mg/dL (M)<br>B = 0.4–1.3 mg/dL (F)<br>U = 1–2 g/d | GFR, tubular secretion, age, sex, muscle mass |
| Uric acid | B = 3–7 mg/dL (M)<br>B = 2–5 mg/dL (F)<br>U = 0.5–0.8 g/d | Purine catabolism, tubular excretion |
| Sodium | B = 135–142 mmol/L | State of hydration, dietary sodium, renal function |
| Potassium | B = 3.5–5 mmol/L | Dietary potassium, acid-base balance, renal function |
| Calcium | B = 9–11 mg/dL | Dietary calcium, PTH, calcitonin, renal function |

*Table 156.2* CRITERIA FOR DIAGNOSIS OF AKI

| RIFLE[a] | AKIN[b] | KDIGO[c] |
|---|---|---|
| **Risk**<br>Increased sCr × 1.5 or GFR decrease > 25%<br>or UOP < 0.5 mL/kg/h for 6 h | **Stage 1**<br>Increased sCr × 1.5–2 or SCr increase > 0.3 mg/dL<br>or UOP < 0.5 mL/kg/h for 6 h | **Stage 1**<br>Increased sCr ×1.5–1.9 within 7 days or SCr increase > 0.3 mg/dL within 48 h<br>or UOP 0.5 mL/kg/h for 6–12 h |
| **Injury**<br>Increased sCr × 2 or GFR decrease > 50%<br>or UOP < 0.5 mL/kg/h for 12 h | **Stage 2**<br>Increased sCr × 2–3<br>or UOP < 0.5 mL/kg/h for > 12 h | **Stage 2**<br>Increased sCr × 2–2.9 or UOP 0.5 mL/kg/h for > 12 h |
| **Failure**<br>Increased sCr × 3 or GFR decrease > 75% or SCr > 4 mg/dL<br>or UOP < 0.3 mL/kg/h for 24 h or anuria for 12 h | **Stage 3**<br>Increased sCr × ≥ 3 or SCr > 4mg/dL with acute rise in sCr ≥ 0.5 mg/dL<br>or UOP < 0.3 mL/kg/h for 24 h or anuria for 12 h | **Stage 3**<br>Increased sCr ≥ 3 or ≥ 4 or initiation of RRT of GFR < 35 in patients < 18 years old<br>or UOP < 0.3 mL/kg/h for > 24 h or anuria > 12 h |
| **Loss**<br>Persistent failure > 4 weeks | | |
| **ESRD**<br>End-stage kidney disease > 3 months | | |

[a]RIFLE, Risk, Injury, Failure, Loss of kidney function, and End-stage kidney disease.

[b]AKIN: Acute Kidney Injury Network.

[c]KDIGO: Kidney Disease: Improving Global Outcomes.

causes are traditionally divided into prerenal, intrinsic, and postrenal (Tables 156.3, 156.4 and 156.5). The most common cause for AKI in hospitalized patients is sepsis, followed by major surgery and acute decompensated heart failure.[1]

## DIAGNOSIS

Serum creatinine (sCr) does not fully assess GFR. sCr starts to increase after the GFR has decreased 50%. Thus, there is a "creatinine blind window" in AKI.[1,3] The tests in Table 156.6 help in the differential diagnosis of AKI.

## PREOPERATIVE ASSESSMENT AND MANAGEMENT

### Prevention

Anesthesiologists can play a big role in assessing the risk of developing perioperative AKI. The most influential factors to prevent AKI are the prevention of hypovolemia and exposure to nephrotoxic agents. The anesthesiologist should plan for ways to effectively manage large-volume shifts, prevent prolonged periods of hypotension intraoperatively, and minimize perioperative exposure to nephrotoxic agents. Sevoflurane was associated with increased production of the haloalkene called "compound A"; nonetheless, it has

*Table 156.3* PRERENAL CAUSES OF AKI

| PREOPERATIVE | INTRA- OR POSTOPERATIVE |
|---|---|
| Hypovolemia | Hypovolemia |
| Sepsis | Hypotension |
| Heart failure | Low cardiac output states |
| Intra-abdominal hypertension | Aortic cross clamp |
| Cirrhosis, hepatorenal syndrome | |
| Nephrotoxic drugs | |

*Table 156.4* INTRINSIC CAUSES OF AKI

| PREOPERATIVE | INTRA- OR POSTOPERATIVE |
|---|---|
| Renal vasculature: thrombosis, emboli | Hypovolemia |
| Interstitial injury: lymphoma | Sepsis |
| Tubular injury: drugs, toxins, ischemia | Heart failure |
| Rhabdomyolysis | Radiocontrast agents |
| TTP/HUS | Fluids (Cl-rich, starches) |

*Table 156.5* POSTRENAL CAUSES OF AKI

| PREOPERATIVE | INTRA- OR POSTOPERATIVE |
|---|---|
| Tumor | Injury: bladder, ureter |
| Prostate enlargement | Dysfunctional Foley catheter |
| Calculi | |
| Blood clots | |
| Neurogenic bladder | |

Adapted from Reference 2.

been extensively proved safe. Sympathetic block by epidural anesthesia does not change renal blood flow in healthy volunteers. A new cohort study did not show any difference between general and neuraxial anesthesia.[1]

If a patient is on chronic renal replacement therapy, the ideal timing for dialysis is the day before surgery. Assessment of baseline dry weight, volume status, and electrolytes status is important. Check the electrolytes and an electro-cardiogram for signs of hyperkalemia or hypercalcemia, ischemia, conduction block, and ventricular hypertrophy. The anesthesiologist should also identify indications for dialysis, such as persistent acidosis; hyperkalemia; intoxication syndromes (methanol, ethylene glycol, metformin, lithium, valproic acid, salicylates, barbiturates, theophylline poisoning); uremic syndrome; and fluid overload.[4]

## Treatment

Of all pharmacological interventions, avoidance of hypovolemia and hypotension is probably the most effective way to prevent postoperative AKI. Close monitoring of volume and oliguria is mandatory to optimize resuscitation.[1,2]

*Table 156.6* DIFFERENTIAL DIAGNOSIS OF AKI

| TEST | PRERENAL | INTRARENAL | POSTRENAL |
|---|---|---|---|
| BUN/sCr ratio | >20 | <20 | <20 |
| Urine osmolality | >500 | <400 | <400 |
| Urine Na$^+$ | <20 | >20 | >20 |
| Urine sediment | Normal | Cellular debris, casts | Cellular debris |
| Urine/sCr ratio | >40 | <20 | <20 |
| FeNa | <1 | >2 | >2 |
| FeUrea | <35% | >50% | N/A |
| FeUric acid | <7% | >15% | N/A |

Fluid administration prevents hypovolemia and improves renal perfusion. Intraoperative hemodialysis should be considered when criteria are met.

## Impact of Intravenous Fluid Composition

### Normal Saline

Normal saline (0.9% sodium chloride) is a common and cost-effective intravenous fluid. However, it increases acid-base imbalances, causes renal vasoconstriction, reduces the GFR, and increases risk of AKI and death. Several randomized clinical trials have assessed the safety of normal saline. A lower incidence of major adverse kidney events in the balanced crystalloid group was present even in the non–critically ill adult patient group. Balanced solutions are preferred for volume resuscitation.[1]

### Starches

Among sepsis and intensive care unit (ICU) patients, hydroxyethyl starch is associated with AKI, need for renal replacement therapy, and death. A black box safety warning for the use of hydroxyethyl starch has been issued.[1]

## Hyperglycemia Avoidance

The KDIGO (Kidney Disease: Improving Global Outcomes) recommends maintaining blood glucose concentrations between 110 and 149 mg/dL in critically ill patients. The European society has increased the range up to 180 mg/dL to minimize perioperative hyperglycemia associated with increased mortality, surgical complications, and AKI risk.[2]

## POSTOPERATIVE

Renal replacement therapy is the only support therapy available for AKI. Neither intermittent hemodialysis nor continuous hemodialysis improves mortality or length of stay in the hospital. Early or late initiation of RRT does not seem to reduce 90-day mortality.[1]

## REFERENCES

1. Gumbert SD, et al. Perioperative acute kidney injury. *Anesthesiology.* 2020;132(1):180–204.
2. Goren O, Matot I. Perioperative acute kidney injury. *Br J Anaesth.* 2015;115(suppl 2):ii3–ii14.
3. Butterworth JF, et al. *Morgan and Mikhail's clinical anesthesiology.* McGraw-Hill Education; 2018.
4. Meersch M, et al. Perioperative acute kidney injury: an under-recognized problem. *Anesth Analg.* 2017;125(4):1223–1232.
5. Vasudevan D, et al. Kidney function tests. In: *Text of biochemistry for medical students.* Jaypee Brother Medical Publishers (P) Ltd.: January 2017:370–383.

# 157.

# MANAGEMENT IN RENAL FAILURE AND ARTERIOVENOUS (AV) SHUNTS

*Lacey Haugen and Jai Jani*

## INTRODUCTION

Anesthetic management of patients with end-stage renal disease (ESRD) and arteriovenous (AV) shunts is complicated due to the physiologic changes of ESRD and the kidney's role in metabolism and excretion of medications (Table 157.1).[1]

## RENAL PHYSIOLOGY AND PATHOPHYSIOLOGY OF ESRD

### RENAL BLOOD FLOW AND GLOMERULAR FILTRATION RATE

Kidneys receive 20% of cardiac output. The renal cortex receives 94% of blood flow and the medulla 6%. Normal glomerular filtration rat (GFR) is 125 mL/min and remains constant despite changes in renal blood flow (RBF) with a mean arterial pressure between 60 and 160 mm Hg due to autoregulation of the renal arterioles.[2] Autoregulation is reset by chronic hypertension and can be abolished in the diabetic kidney.

### INTRAVASCULAR VOLUME

With a GFR less than 15 mL/min, failure of sodium and free water excretion leads to anuria and volume overload, necessitating dialysis. Patients undergoing dialysis have unpredictable intravascular fluid volumes. Surgery too soon after dialysis results in hypovolemia, hypotension, and hypokalemia immediately after dialysis. Problems with not dialyzing soon before surgery include electrolyte abnormalities (hyperkalemia), uremia, acidosis, and hypervolemia.

### HYPERTENSION

Renin is synthesized in response to decreased renal perfusion. Activation of the renin angiotensin aldosterone system (RAAS) increases blood pressure *directly* through Angiotensin II (ATII), causing systemic vasoconstriction and *indirectly* by stimulating secretion of aldosterone, leading to increased sodium and water absorption and increased circulating volume.

## CARDIAC

Hypervolemia and excessive activation of the RAAS system leads to hypertension, left ventricle hypertrophy, heart failure with preserved ejection fraction, and pulmonary edema.[1,2] Activation of Angiotensin I (AT1) receptors on cardiomyocytes leads to cardiac remodeling, increased catecholamine levels, inotropy, chronotropy, and increased systemic vascular resistance due to increased aldosterone and vasopressin secretion. Angiotensin-converting enzyme inhibitors (ACEIs) decrease remodeling of the heart induced by AT1 receptor stimulation. Buildup of uremic toxins and metabolic acidosis lead to poor myocardial contractility and heart failure with reduced ejection fraction. Increased triglycerides, decreased high-density lipoprotein, impaired endothelial function, and low-grade inflammation accelerate atherosclerosis and lead to pericardial disease and cardiac arrhythmias.[1] Many patients have renal disease secondary to diabetes mellitus, which further contributes to cardiac disease.

## ACID-BASE

As the GFR decreases, the kidneys' ability to excrete the daily acid load in the form of ammonia decreases, bicarbonate reabsorption is reduced, and insufficient renal bicarbonate production cause a non–anion gap metabolic acidosis that progresses to anion gap acidosis as the disease advances.[1] Acidosis then causes insulin resistance, thyroid dysfunction, elevated cortisol levels, reduced insulin-like growth factor 1, and increased protein turnover, which leads to decreased serum albumin concentration.[1]

*Table 157.1* IMPACT OF DIFFERENT MEDICATIONS ON THE KIDNEY

| DRUG | METABOLITE | ACTIVE | SIDE EFFECT |
|---|---|---|---|
| Sevoflurane | Compound A | No | Nephrotoxic in animals, although it has never been shown to have clinical effects in humans. |
| Vecuronium | 3-Desacetyl-vecuronium | Yes | 80% as potent as its parent compound. |
| Atricurium and cisatricurium | Laudanosine | No | Metabolized to 80% inactive metabolite laudanosine, which is renally cleared and can cause seizures. More laudanosine is produced with atricurium because it is much less potent than cisatricurium and administered in larger doses. |
| Tramadol | O-Demethyl tramadol | Yes | T½ is increased due to active metabolite with analgesic properties. |
| Morphine | Morphine-3-glucuronide (M3G) | No | Neuroexcitatory effects, including myoclonus, allodynia, and seizure. |
|  | Morphine-6-glucuronide (M6G) | Yes | 100 times more potent than morphine and can build up to cause respiratory depression. |
| Meperidine | Normeperidine | No | Neuroexcitation, including tremors and seizures. |
| Midazolam | 1-Hydrodxymidazolam | Yes | Central nervous system depression. |
| Diazepam | Oxazepam and temazepam | Yes | Metabolites with T½ of 30–100 hours. |
| Nitroprusside | Cyanide | No | Weakness, metabolic acidosis, renal failure, rhabdomyolysis, central nervous system, cardiopulmonary, and gastrointestinal symptoms. |

From References 1, 2, 4, 5.

## ELECTROLYTE

End-stage renal disease leads to decreased ability to excrete electrolytes and free water, resulting in hyperkalemia, hypermagnesemia, hyperphosphatemia, and hyponatremia. Hyperkalemia leads to flaccid paralysis, respiratory distress, and cardiac arrhythmias. Hypermagnesemia causes hypotension and bradycardia and potentiates neuromuscular blockers (NMBs). Hyperphosphatemia results in vascular calcification, cardiac disease, and hypocalcemia in early ESRD. Hypocalcemia increases the risk for laryngospasm, prolonged QT, and cardiac arrhythmias.[1] Low serum calcitriol levels, hypocalcemia, and hyperphosphatemia eventually lead to secondary hyperparathyroidism, which results in mobilization of calcium and phosphate from bone, hypercalcemia, and fragile bones, requiring careful positioning to avoid pathologic fractures.[1]

## HEMATOLOGIC

Uremia leads to abnormal platelet function and increased bleeding times due to decreased platelet factor III activity, interference with von Willebrand factor formation and release, abnormal function of glycoprotein IIb and glycoprotein IIIa, and increased prostacyclin and nitric oxide synthesis. Antithrombin III levels are also reduced, leading to hypercoagulability and potential insensitivity to heparin. ESRD also causes a normochromic, normocytic anemia secondary to decreased renal production of erythropoietin.[2]

Treatments include desmopressin, cryoprecipitate, blood transfusion, conjugated estrogen, iron, and erythropoietin.[1,2]

## EFFECTS ON PHARMACOKINETICS

End-stage renal disease causes decreased expression of cytochrome P450 and suppression of phase II metabolic reactions due to uremic toxins. Most drugs are renally excreted and can build up with ESRD. Proximal renal tubules allow elimination of metabolites from liver and unchanged hydrophilic molecules, whereas high-molecular-weight drugs such as NMBs are excreted in bile.

There are three broad categories of drugs that have increased duration of action or side effects with ESRD:

1. Drugs such as phenobarbital, nadolol, and atenolol that are excreted unchanged in the kidneys.
2. Drugs that undergo metabolism to active compounds or metabolites with side effects that are excreted in the urine (see Table 157.1).
3. Drugs such as barbiturates and most intravenous induction agents (except ketamine) that are highly protein bound. Decreased serum proteins and uremia lead to increased sensitivity due to decreased protein binding of drugs and higher concentrations of free, active molecules.[3,4]

# ANESTHESIA FOR ARTERIOVENOUS SHUNTS

Regional anesthesia (RA) has the benefit of hemodynamic stability, avoiding airway manipulation, improved postoperative analgesia, accelerated recovery, and decreased side effects from accumulation of drugs and their metabolites.[5] RA produces vasodilation and higher blood flow due to sympathectomy, leading to shorter maturation times, lower fistula failure rates, and higher patency rates when compared to local anesthesia (LA) or general anesthesia (GA).[3] Risks of RA include neuropathy, neuronal ischemia and neurotoxicity secondary to intraneuronal injection of LA, hematoma, infection, and LA systemic toxicity.

General anesthesia can be used in patients with difficult anatomy or contraindications to RA, such as an inability to tolerate hemidiaphragm paralysis.[3,5] GA causes potential drug interactions, increased stress response, hemodynamic instability, risk of residual muscle relaxant, respiratory depression, and poor postoperative pain control.

Local anesthesia infiltration is simple and has similar benefits as RA in regard to avoiding GA and its unwanted side effects; however, there is no sympathectomy, resulting in higher fistula failure rates.[3,5] Metabolic acidosis leads to decreased protein binding, resulting in an increased percentage of unbound drug and higher risk of LA toxicity.[3,4]

## PREOPERATIVE

Cardiac risk should be assessed and cardiac consultation considered.[2,3] Hemoglobin, blood pressure, hemoglobin $A_{1c}$, and electrolytes should be optimized prior to surgery.[1] HD should be performed the day prior to surgery[1,5] and elective surgery scheduled at least 6 hours after HD with heparinization.[1]

## INTRAOPERATIVE

Uremic patients should be considered as having a full stomach.[2] Arterial line placement can be useful for hemodynamic monitoring, and stroke volume variation is a useful indicator of intravascular volume and can guide fluid replacement.[1] ESRD patients have high risk of acute kidney injury, so care must be taken to ensure normovolemia and adequate oxygen delivery.[2] The corticomedullary region with the thick ascending loop of Henle is most at risk of hypoxia and acute tubular necrosis with decreased RBF and GFR. Perioperatively, hyperkalemia is precipitated by reduced GFR secondary to medications and hypotension, transcellular shifts, protein catabolism, hemolysis, transfusion of stored red blood cellss,[5] and many drugs, including nonselective β-blockers, potassium-sparing diuretics, mannitol, nonsteroidal anti-inflammatory drugs, ACEIs/angiotensin receptor blockers, digitalis, heparin, and succinylcholine.[2] As such, ACEI and β-blockers (BBs) should be avoided, and calcium channel blockers are the antihypertensives of choice as they increase RBF and GFR. Fenoldopam is also good for a hypertensive crisis with renal impairment. Washing red blood cells will reduce extracellular potassium. Volatile anesthetics reversibly decrease RBF and GFR. Urine output decreases due to increased antidiuretic hormone and sympathetic tone.[2] Decreasing tidal volumes to less than 6 mL/kg can decrease renal injury by decreasing cytokine release. Fentanyl and methadone are the safest opioids with ESRD, and remifentanil is also a good choice. Recurarization with anticholinesterase inhibitors is less likely in ESRD because their action is prolonged more than nondepolarized NMBs.[1]

## POSTOPERATIVE

Postoperative dialysis may be needed to correct fluid imbalances and electrolytes. Certain drugs cannot be dialyzed, including amiodarone, apixaban, and rivaroxaban.

## REFERENCES

1. Kanda H, et al. Perioperative management of patients with end-stage renal disease. *J Cardiothorac Vasc Anesth.* 2017;31(6):2251–2267.
2. Miller RD, ed. *Miller's Anesthesia.* 7th ed. Churchill Livingstone/Elsevier; 2010.
3. Bradley T, et al. Anaesthetic management of patients requiring vascular access surgery for renal dialysis. *BJA Educ.* 2017;17(8):269–274.
4. Pham PC, et al. 2017 update on pain management in patients with chronic kidney disease. *Clin Kidney J.* 2017;10(5):688–697.
5. Nandate K, et al. Anesthetic management of surgical vascular access for hemodialysis. *Austin J Anesth Analg.* 2018;6(2):1071.

# 158.

# ANESTHETIC MANAGEMENT OF KIDNEY TRANSPLANTATION

*Mada Helou and Ryan Nazemian*

## INTRODUCTION

Kidney transplantation is the treatment of choice for end-stage renal disease (ESRD). With recent advancements in the field of transplantation, especially with an expanded donor pool and postoperative care, kidney transplants are now viewed as a relatively straightforward surgery. The majority of transplanted kidneys are procured from deceased donors, either following death by neurological criteria or after cardiac death). Living donation is on the rise but still accounts for less than 20% of the kidneys transplanted annually. Based on the most recent tracking data from the Organ Procurement and Transplantation Network, more than 23,000 kidney transplants were done in the United States in 2019, compared to 2018 a more than 10% increase.[1] Yet there still remains a major unmet need for more organs: As of June 20, 2020, there were more than 93,000 patients on the waiting list to receive a kidney transplant. Thus, optimum anesthetic management is an integral part of patient and graft survival.

## PREOPERATIVE EVALUATION

The preoperative evaluation of a kidney transplant recipient is dependent on the donor source. In most centers, living donors and recipients go through routine preoperative evaluations. But for most deceased donor recipients, due to the unpredictable and emergent nature of the surgery, unique considerations need to be addressed in addition to the routine preoperative evaluation. These include, but are not limited to, the following:

- Fasting status: These patients are usually called from home and they are commonly considered to have a full stomach unless otherwise clarified with the patient. In addition, many ESRD patients are diabetic, and gastroparesis is very common.

- Dialysis: For patients who receive either hemodialysis or peritoneal dialysis, timing of the last dialysis session is of utmost importance. As most patients are familiar with their "dry weight," their volume status can also be assessed by weight. Patients can be hypervolemic or hypovolemic. For those who did not have a recent session, electrolyte imbalance is common, including hyperkalemia, metabolic acidosis, and/or hypocalcemia. For most centers, potassium above 5.5 mEq/L is unacceptable, and the patient might need a dialysis session before surgery.

- Coagulation status: Due to potential uremic platelet dysfunction, coagulation screening with partial thromboplastin time, prothrombin time, international normalized ratio, fibrinogen, and Plt count is necessary. If significant abnormalities are found, urgent correction might be indicated.

- Anemia: The incidence of anemia is due to reduced amounts of erythropoietin secreted from end-stage kidneys. Other contributing factors include blood loss from dialysis and low levels of iron, vitamin $B_{12}$, and folate. Therefore, a complete blood count (CBC) is warranted, and blood products are usually placed on hold for surgery.

- Cardiovascular status: A detailed cardiac history, including history of coronary artery disease, hypertension, arrhythmias, and uremic cardiomyopathy, needs to be detailed. The most recent electrocardiogram and echocardiography (if any) need to be reviewed, and if any particular concerns are present, urgent cardiology clearance might be needed.

## INTRAOPERATIVE MANAGEMENT

- Monitoring: Standard American Society of Anesthesiologists monitors will be used for all patients. With the discretion of the attending anesthesiologist, continuous blood pressure monitoring with an arterial line may be indicated (i.e., if the patient has a prior history of cardiac disease, significant blood loss is expected, cuff measurement is imprecise, etc.). Most centers have opted out of using central venous catheters to assess volume status unless adequate intravenous access (usually two large-bore intravenous lines) cannot be obtained.

- Transplant medications: Appropriate prophylactic antibiotics and immunosuppressive medications (usually methylprednisolone, mycophenolate, and thymoglobulin or basiliximab) should be given in a timely manner based on institutional guidelines.
- Induction: With the exception of rapid sequence induction for a full stomach, standard anesthesia induction can be used for these patients. Of note, succinylcholine is not contraindicated in these patients, but potassium levels should be considered.
- Maintenance: Due to low creatinine clearance, judicious doses of opioids (commonly fentanyl or hydromorphone) and muscle relaxants (cisatracurium as drug of choice or rocuronium) should be used. The maintenance intravenous fluid of choice is 0.9% sodium chloride (normal saline) because it does not contain potassium, but lactated Ringer's is not contraindicated. It is typical for patients to receive 2–3 L of intravenous fluids before and during the vascular anastomoses and before graft reperfusion. If significant blood loss is present, colloids or blood products may be indicated. Desmopressin is the treatment of choice for bleeding due to uremic platelet dysfunction. Surgeons normally ask for bolus administration of diuretics, including mannitol and/or furosemide, before reperfusion of the graft. Adequate renal perfusion during reperfusion is of paramount importance, and hypotension should be avoided. During this period, reduced levels of volatile anesthetic concentration might be required. Vasopressors should be avoided unless life-saving measures are needed, and close communication with the surgical team is required.

Dopamine infusion is commonly used for hypotension or low urine output, but its effects on renal perfusion are controversial.[2]

## POSTOPERATIVE CONSIDERATIONS

After emergence from anesthesia, most patients can be extubated and return to the postanesthesia care unit (PACU) for postoperative care. About 1% of patients might require intensive care unit admission, and most common indications are hypotension, significant blood loss, hypoxic and/or hypercarbic respiratory failure (due to hypervolemia), significant electrolyte imbalance, and sepsis. But the majority have an uneventful recovery in the PACU and go to regular nursing floors after meeting discharge criteria. Many centers have developed their unique enhanced recovery after surgery protocols for their patients,[3] including fluid and proper pain management in the PACU. Multimodal analgesia is highly recommended. Of note, due to reduced renal function and creatinine clearance (glomerular filtration rate), patients usually require smaller and less frequent doses of opioids. Peripheral nerve blocks such as transverse abdominis plane, quadratus lumborum, or erector spinae plane blocks have successfully been used for these patients.[4,5]

## REFERENCES

1. United Network for Organ Sharing. More deceased-donor organ transplants than ever. https://unos.org/data/transplant-trends/
2. Burton CJ, Tomson CRV. Can the use of low-dose dopamine for treatment of acute renal failure be justified? *Postgrad Med J.* 1999;**75**:269–274.
3. Espino KA, et al. Benefits of multimodal enhanced recovery pathway in patients undergoing kidney transplantation. *Clin Transplant.* 2018;32(2):10.1111/ctr.13173.
4. Temirov T, et al. Erector spinae plane block in management of pain after kidney transplantation. *Pain Med.* 2019;20(5):1053–1054.
5. Farag E, et al. Continuous transversus abdominis plane block catheter analgesia for postoperative pain control in renal transplant. *J Anesth.* 2015;29(1):4–8.

# 159.

# ANESTHESIA FOR EXTRACORPOREAL SHOCK WAVE LITHOTRIPSY

*Alain Harb and Elie Geara*

## INTRODUCTION

Extracorporeal shock wave lithotripsy (ESWL) is utilized primarily for 4-mm to 2-cm intrarenal stones, whereas percutaneous and laparoscopic nephrolithotomy are for larger or impacted stones. Medical expulsive therapy (MET) has become the treatment of choice among many clinicians for acute episodes of urolithiasis: For stones up to 10 mm in diameter, administration of β-blockers or the calcium channel blocker lessens the pain of acute urolithiasis and increases the rate of stone expulsion over several days to weeks. Along with MET, the treatment of kidney stones has shifted from primarily open surgical procedures to less invasive techniques: flexible ureteroscopy with stone extraction, stent placement, and intracorporeal lithotripsy (laser or electrohydraulic). Repetitive high-energy shocks (sound waves) are generated and focused on the stone during ESWL, causing its fragmentation into small pieces. A conducting gel is used to couple the device to the patient. Ureteral stents are often placed cystoscopically prior to the procedure. Tissue destruction can occur if the acoustic energy is inadvertently focused at air-tissue interfaces, such as in the lung and intestine. Several shock wave generators are available for clinical use: electrohydraulic, electromagnetic, or piezoelectric. The older electrohydraulic units, currently not in clinical use, needed the patient to be immersed in a heated water bath. Both fluoroscopic and ultrasound localization are currently available with modern electromagnetic or piezoelectric generators.

## PREOPERATIVE CONSIDERATIONS

Patients with a pacemaker can undergo lithotripsy safely if placed pectorally to avoid the field of shock waves and programmed to a nondemand mode in case the shock waves interfere with its function. Synchronization of the shock waves with the electrocardiogram R wave decreases the incidence of arrhythmias during ESWL; the shock waves are usually timed to be 20 ms after the R wave to correspond with the ventricular refractory period. Dual-chamber pacemakers tend to be more sensitive to interference,[1] so treatment should start at a low-energy level and be gradually increased while keeping an eye on the pacemaker function. Automated implanted cardioverter-defibrillator devices should be shut off immediately before lithotripsy and then reactivated immediately after treatment as the manufacturers consider them a contraindication.

## INTRAOPERATIVE CONSIDERATIONS

The amount of pain during lithotripsy is directly related to the energy density of the shock wave at the skin entry site. Older water bath lithotripsy unit requires high-intensity shock waves that are not tolerated by patients without regional or general anesthesia. In contrast, the new lithotripsy unit requires lower intensity shock waves, making sedation a good anesthesia option.

## PHYSIOLOGY OF IMMERSION DURING ESWL

The heated water bath (36°C–37°C) initially results in vasodilation, leading to transient hypotension. But as venous blood is redistributed centrally due to hydrostatic pressure from water on the body, systemic blood pressure rises, systemic vascular resistance increases, and cardiac output decreases, precipitating congestive heart failure in patients with borderline reserves. This increase in intrathoracic blood volume reduces functional residual capacity by 30%–60% and may predispose some patients to hypoxemia. The work of breathing increases with water immersion, and respiration can become fast and shallow. Antidiuretic hormone and prostaglandins decrease, which leads to diuresis, natriuresis, and kaliuresis.

## ANESTHESIA METHODS DURING ESWL

### REGIONAL ANESTHESIA

Regional anesthesia with sedation has a major advantage as it greatly facilitates positioning and monitoring. Continuous epidural anesthesia is commonly employed. Renal innervation is derived from T10 to L2, so a T6 sensory level coverage is needed to ensure adequate anesthesia.[2] During the epidural catheter placement, saline should be used instead of air for the loss-of-resistance technique. Air in the epidural space can dissipate shock waves and promote injury to neural tissue. In animal experiments, it was shown that epidural tissue damage after injection of air and exposure to shock waves can happen.[3] Foam tape also should not be used for the same reason as air in the epidural. Spinal anesthesia has a faster onset compared to an epidural and can be used but has less control over the sensory level, which could be an issue when the duration of the procedure is uncertain. The major disadvantage of using regional anesthesia is the inability to control respiratory movements; excessive diaphragmatic excursion during spontaneous ventilation can distort the stone location compared to the wave focus and may prolong the procedure. Asking the patient to breath rapid, shallow breaths could partially help with this problem.

### GENERAL ANESTHESIA

The major advantage of general endotracheal anesthesia is the control of diaphragmatic movement during lithotripsy, especially when using older water bath lithotripters. But the procedure can be complicated by the logistic of moving an intubated patient from the supine position to a chair, elevating and then lowering the chair into a water bath to shoulder depth, and then reversing the sequence at the end.[3]

### MONITORED ANESTHESIA CARE

Modern low-energy lithotripsy allows intravenous sedation with midazolam and fentanyl or low-dose propofol infusions with or without midazolam and opioid supplementation to be used.[4]

## Complications

Flank pain, nausea, and vomiting and hypertension are immediate postoperative reported side effects. Also common is skin bruising at the entry site of the shock wave, which could last several days. Renal parenchymal injury secondary to shock waves almost universally causes hematuria. Patients with a previous medical history of hypertension, diabetes, or coronary artery atherosclerosis; and the elderly and patients with coagulopathy are at an increased risk of a bleeding complication, but not to the point requiring transfusion. Total obstruction (1%–5%) can happen due to stone fragments accumulating in the ureter instead of being excreted in the urine. Air-filled alveoli in the lungs present a resistance interface, so shock waves hitting the lungs may liberate some of the energy and cause alveolar rupture, leading to hemoptysis; this could be avoided by protecting the lungs using styrofoam padding for children and any short stature adult under 48 inches. Cardiac arrhythmias have been described and were more common in patients who had been treated with the first-generation lithotripters but now are quite rare. Some can be programmed to deliver shock waves using "electrocardiogram gating," which minimizes the risk of an R-on-T phenomenon and subsequent ventricular arrhythmias. Pancreatitis and bowel injury resulting in rectal bleeding have been reported.

## Contraindications

The only two contraindications to lithotripsy are pregnancy and untreated bleeding disorders. Every women of childbearing age should have a negative pregnancy test before the procedure. Standard tests of coagulation—platelet count, prothrombin time, and partial thromboplastin time—should be ordered if indicated by the medical history. Patients with orthopedic prostheses (hip prostheses or Harrington rods) can be treated safely as long as the prostheses are not in the blast path.

## REFERENCES

1. Weber W, et al. Anesthetic considerations in patients with cardiac pacemakers undergoing extracorporeal shock wave lithotripsy. *Anesth Analg.* 1988;67:S251.
2. Lander CJ, et al. Epidural anesthesia and extracorporeal shock wave lithotripsy: pathologic effects on the epidural space. *Anesthesiology.* 1987;67(3A):A227.
3. Coloma M, et al. Fast-tracking after immersion lithotripsy: general anesthesia versus monitored anesthesia care. *Anesth Analg.* 2000;91:92–96.
4. Morgan GE, et al. *Clinical anesthesiology.* New York: Lange Medical Books/McGraw Hill Medical Publishing Division; 2006.

# 160.

# PERIOPERATIVE OLIGURIA AND ANURIA

*Brent Earls and Eellan Sivanesan*

## INTRODUCTION

Oliguria is broadly defined as any urine output value less than 0.5 mL/kg/h, while anuria is the absence of urine production or less than 50 mL/d.[1] Historically, this value has been used in hospitalized patients to gauge intravascular volume status and the risk of developing acute kidney injury (AKI); however, this utility is limited since urine output is not simply a function of intravascular volume. In fact, urine output can decrease through the action of antidiuretic hormone in response to pain, nausea, and surgical intervention. Increases in aldosterone concentration can also decrease urine output. Perioperative factors such as physiological stress, intra-abdominal pressure, interstitial edema, congestive heart failure, and medications can all induce oliguria without volume depletion. Although oliguria includes a continuum of decreasing urine output values, the degree of intraoperative oliguria is not necessarily associated with an increasing risk of postoperative AKI.[2]

## ETIOLOGY

### PRERENAL

- Hypovolemia (dehydration, hemorrhage, diarrhea/vomiting, burns)
- Decreased cardiac output (heart failure, myocardial infarction)
- Decreased peripheral vascular resistance (septic shock, anaphylaxis)
- Decreased renovascular blood flow (bilateral renal vein stenosis)

### RENAL

- Nephrotoxic injury (drugs, contrast dye, crush injury)
- Interstitial nephritis (allergies/antibiotics, infections)
- Acute glomerulonephritis (malignant hypertension)
- Thrombotic disorders

### POSTRENAL

- Benign prostatic hypertrophy
- Bladder cancer
- Calculi formation (kidney stones)
- Spinal cord disorders

## CLASSIFICATION

Several criteria have been proposed to better classify risk of AKI by integrating changes in urine output with changes in serum creatinine and glomerular filtration rate. In 2004, the Acute Dialysis Quality Initiative Group developed a system for the diagnosis and classification of acute impairment of kidney function.[1] The acronym RIFLE stands for the increasing classification severity: Risk, Injury, and Failure, and the two outcome classes, Loss and End-Stage Renal Disease (ESRD). The three severity grades are defined by changes in serum creatinine or urine output, with the worst of each criterion selected. Development of these criteria allowed researchers to make significant progress in the prevention and management of AKI by identifying physiological endpoints to test the efficacy of new interventions.

In 2006, the Acute Kidney Injury Network (AKIN), an international network of AKI researchers, organized a summit of nephrology and critical care societies that endorsed the RIFLE criteria with a small modification to include small changes in serum creatinine (sCr) (>0.3 mg/dL or > 26.5 mmol/L) when they occur within a 48-hour period (Table 160.1). Then in 2012, the Kidney Disease: Improving Global Outcomes (KDIGO) clinical practice guidelines were published and combined the strengths of RIFLE and AKIN.[1] As with AKIN, the KDIGO guidelines stratify AKI into three stages of severity and maintain the minimum creatinine threshold for the diagnosis of AKI as a rise of 0.3 mg/dL or 50% from baseline. However, while an absolute rise is required to occur in less than 48 hours, the 50% rise from baseline may occur over 7 days, as with RIFLE.

*Table 160.1* RIFLE CRITERIA

| RIFLE CATEGORY | SCR AND GFR CRITERIA | URINE OUTPUT CRITERIA |
|---|---|---|
| Risk | sCr increase to 1.5-fold or GFR decrease > 25% from baseline | <0.5 mL/kg/h for ≥ 6 hours |
| Injury | sCr increase to 2-fold or GFR decrease > 50% from baseline | <0.5 mL/kg/h for ≥ 12 hours |
| Failure | sCr increase to 3-fold or GFR decrease > 75% from baseline or sCr ≥ 4 mg/dL (≥354 μmol/L) with an acute increase of at least 0.5 mg/dL (44 μmol/L) | Anuria for ≥ 12 hours |
| Loss | Complete loss of function (RRT) for > 4 weeks | |
| ESKD | RRT > 3 months | |
| AKIN Criteria | sCr Criteria | Urine Output Criteria |
| Stage 1 | sCr increase ≥ 0.3 mg/dL (≥27 μmol/L) or 1.5 to 2-fold from baseline | <0.5 mL/kg/h for ≥ 6 hours |
| Stage 2 | sCr increase > 2- to 3-fold from baseline | <0.5 mL/kg/h for ≥ 12 hours |
| Stage 3 | sCr increase > 3-fold from baseline or sCr ≥ 4 mg/dL (≥354 μmol/L) with an acute increase of at least 0.5 mg/dL (≥44 μmol/L) or need for RRT | <0.3 mL/kg/h for ≥ 24 hours or anuria for ≥ 12 hours |
| KDIGO criteria | sCr Criteria | Urine Output Criteria |
| Stage 1 | sCr increase ≥ 0.3 mg/dL (≥27 μmol/L) or 1.5–1.9 times from baseline | <0.5 mL/kg/h for 6–12 hours |
| Stage 2 | sCr increase 2–2.9 times from baseline | <0.5 mL/kg/h for ≥ 12 hours |
| Stage 3 | sCr increase 3 times from baseline, or sCr ≥ 4 mg/dL (≥354 μmol/L), or need for RRT, or eGFR < 35 mL/min/1.73 m² (<0.34 mL/s/m) in patients < 18 years | Anuria for ≥ 12 hours |

eGFR, estimated GFR; GFR, glomerular filtration rate; RRT, renal replacement therapy; sCr, serum creatinine; ESKD, end-stage kidney disease.

## ANESTHETIC CONSIDERATIONS

The mainstay of prevention is maintenance of hemodynamic stability and adequate renal perfusion. Anesthetic considerations are presented in Table 160.2. Studies show adequate perfusion may be dependent on cardiac output and mean arterial pressure (MAP), not just MAP alone.[1] Anemia is associated with kidney injury (demand vs. delivery mismatch, 1.1–2.0 g/dL = 50% increased risk; > 4.0 g/dL = ~5 times the risk); however, transfusion is also associated with postoperative AKI. Therefore, other non–transfusion-related therapies to improve preoperative hemoglobin have been advocated. For example, the use of erythropoietin has been shown to reduce the risk of AKI by over 20% in coronary artery bypass graft surgery.[3]

Sepsis is a common risk factor associated with perioperative AKI and has been shown to be the causative factor of AKI in almost 50% of critically ill patients.[3] There is limited knowledge of preoperative treatment of infections to reduce postoperative AKI. The routine use of medications such as furosemide, mannitol, fenoldopam, or dopamine is not recommended in the prevention or treatment of perioperative AKI. Studies evaluated in the current KDIGO guidelines found no evidence that these commonly used drugs reduce the incidence or duration of AKI, and there is even mounting evidence that some could worsen kidney injury and increase mortality.[1]

Use of synthetic colloids (e.g., gelatin, dextran) increased the risk of AKI requiring renal replacement therapy (RRT) in patients undergoing surgery on the lung and with sepsis. A recent Cochrane review also revealed that hetastarch products increased the risk of AKI in all patient populations.[1] A number of common medications have been associated with perioperative AKI, including angiotensin-converting enzyme (ACE) inhibitors and angiotensin II receptor (ARB) inhibitors, and nonsteroidal anti-inflammatory drugs (NSAIDs). Aspirin and statins have been noted to have a protective effect in select populations.[4]

*Table 160.2* ANESTHETIC CONSIDERATIONS

| SURGERY PHASE | RECOMMENDATIONS | COMMENTS |
|---|---|---|
| Preoperative | • Assess patient for risk of AKI<br>• Discontinue known medications associated with AKI, such as ACE inhibitors/ARB drugs, NSAIDs; consider giving aspirin and/or statin<br>• Consider delaying surgery after radiocontrast dye exposure (3 hours)<br>• Minimize blood draws<br>• Recommend minimally invasive technique (i.e., laparoscopic vs. open)<br>• Optimize high-risk patient | Evaluate for known variables that convey risk of AKI (age > 59, emergent or high-risk surgery, congestive heart failure, COPD, CKD, PVD, liver disease, sepsis, BMI > 32) |
| Intraoperative | • Maintain MAP > 55 mm Hg<br>• Avoid synthetic colloids during volume resuscitation (HES)<br>• Avoid diuretics to improve urine output<br>• Implement goal-directed hemodynamic therapy in high-risk patients<br>• Implement blood-sparing therapies<br>• Avoid blood transfusion when possible | May require higher MAPs<br>Including natriuretic peptide, fluids and vasopressors, antifibrinolytics, cell salvage |
| Postoperative | • Maintain appropriate renal perfusion<br>• Monitor for severe/refractory hyperkalemia, metabolic acidosis, volume overload, overt uremic manifestations and intoxications<br><br>• Early RRT initiation has been associated with improved survival | Options for bedside assessment include lactate clearance, SVV, abdominal perfusion pressure, esophageal Doppler<br><br>Timing remains controversial, no large trials regarding ideal timing of initiation |

ACE, angiotensin-converting enzyme; AKI, acute kidney injury; ARB, angiotensin receptor blocker; BMI, body mass index; COPD, chronic obstructive pulmonary disease; CKD, chronic kidney disease; HES, hydroxyethyl starch; MAP, mean arterial pressure; NSAID, nonsteroidal anti-inflammatory drug; PVD, peripheral vascular disease; SVV, stroke volume variation.

# REFERENCES

1. KDIGO: Kidney Disease: Improving Global Outcomes (KDIGO) Acute Kidney Injury Work Group. KDIGO clinical practice guideline for acute kidney injury. *Kidney Int Suppl.* 2012;2:1–138.
2. Mira K, et al. Intraoperative oliguria: physiological or beginning acute kidney injury? *Anesth Analg.* 2018;127(5):1109–1110.
3. Charuhas V, et al. *Perioperative Kidney Injury: Principles of Risk Assessment, Diagnosis and Treatment.* New York, NY: Springer; 2014.
4. Xiong B, et al. Preoperative statin treatment for the prevention of acute kidney injury in patients undergoing cardiac surgery: a meta-analysis of randomised controlled trials. *Heart Lung Circ.* 2017;26(11):1200–1207.

# 161.

# DIALYSIS AND HEMOFILTRATION

*Michael J. Gyorfi and Alaa Abd-Elsayed*

## RENAL REPLACEMENT THERAPY OVERVIEW

Renal replacement therapies (RRT) are often broken down into hemodialysis (HD), hemofiltration (HF), and peritoneal dialysis (PD). During HD, blood flows through a filter made of numerous hollow fibers. The dialysate solution (with varying ion concentrations depending on your goal) bathes the fibers while it flows in the opposite direction. The ion differences between the blood and dialysate utilize concentration gradients to diffuse through the pores in the fibrous filter. Diffusion is most apt for correcting small solutes: sodium chloride, potassium, bicarbonate, calcium, urea, and creatinine. Dialysate waste is termed effluent and is subsequently discarded.[1,2]

Hemofiltration, in comparison, does not rely on diffusion. HF utilizes convection through a large-pore, semipermeable hemofilter without a dialysate. HF mimics the Bowman's capsule and the glomerular capillary bed. Pressure is applied across the large hemofilter, pushing the plasma fluid and solutes through the membrane, creating an ultrafiltrate. Due to the large removal of volume with HF, fluid is replaced both pre- and postdilution. Both HD and HF are often used in combination, which is termed hemodiafiltration. Endocrine abnormalities prevalent in renal failure, such as decreased erythropoietin and 1,25-dihydroxyvitamin $D_3$ are not corrected with RRT.[1,2]

Renal replacement therapy often requires anticoagulation with either heparin or regional citrate infusion. The latter is often preferred due to the complications surrounding systemic heparinization. Citrate binds calcium and prevents coagulation. This requires reinfusion of calcium as the blood returns from the machine.[1–3]

Renal replacement therapy can also be broken down into continuous versus intermittent filtration depending on its indication. Continuous filtration is used primarily for acute kidney injuries and hypercatabolic and azotemic states. It is often better tolerated due to the volume being removed at a slower rate.[1] This is done with one of two techniques: continuous arteriovenous hemofiltration (CAVH) and continuous venovenous hemofiltration (CVVH). CAVH uses the arterial pressure from a fistula to force blood through the filter. In comparison, CVVH requires a pump with a double-lumen catheter to return blood into the same vein. CVVH has the advantages of more reliable blood flow with a pump and does not require arterial access.[1,3]

Peritoneal dialysis is another form of RRT. It differs from HD and HF in several ways. PD utilizes the patient's peritoneum as the membrane through which the fluid is filtered. It is also used to remove excess fluid and toxins along with correcting electrolyte abnormalities. Advantages to PD are its ease of use, particularly if the patient lives far from a dialysis center. It also does not require the same vascular access needed in HD and HF. However, there are major limitations to PD that affect its utility. PD is not capable of treating life-threatening abnormalities to the same degree as exterior HD/HF. PD also requires abdominal access, which may not be available with intra-abdominal pathology and surgery.[1–3]

The indications for dialysis can be broken down into acidosis, electrolyte abnormalities, intoxications, fluid overload, and uremia symptoms. These indications have a wide interpretation and should be considered semiobjective. RRT is often initiated due to persistent acute kidney injuries without any of the criteria that follow.[3]

Contraindications vary depending on the type of RRT. PD should not be pursued with acute abdominal pathology, cirrhosis with ascites, or marked hypoalbuminemia. HD traditionally does not have any absolute contraindications. Relative contraindications include recurrent access problems, hemodynamic instability, advanced malignancy, and terminal illnesses.[2,3]

## ANESTHETIC CONSIDERATIONS

### PREOPERATIVE

An accurate dialysis history is important. The type, frequency, last treatment date, route of access, target weight, and electrolyte abnormalities are all important aspects to note before surgery. For elective operations, HD is generally performed 12 to 24 hours preceding surgery.[4] In contrast, PD is often performed daily and can be continued up to just before the surgery; drainage of the peritoneal dialysate should happen preoperatively. Vascular access should be obtained preoperatively without relying on arteriovenous fistula sites unless absolutely necessary.[3,4]

Nonelective surgery may result in gaps between dialysis treatments up to 72 hours or even longer if treatments have been missed. Serum urea, creatinine, and potassium levels must be checked. For elective cases, preoperative dialysis should be performed for a potassium level greater than 5.5 mEq/L. Preoperative hyperkalemia in the setting of an urgent surgery is managed based on electrocardiographic (ECG) changes. A stable patient without hyperkalemic ECG changes may undergo surgery with a continuous ECG intraoperatively with frequent potassium checks. One to 2 hours of dialysis is sufficient to reduce total body potassium and should be performed if pathologic ECG changes from hyperkalemia are present. If surgery cannot wait for dialysis to be performed, the anesthesiologist must manage the hyperkalemia intraoperatively. This can be done with a combination of intravenous calcium, insulin, and bicarbonate. Intraoperative RRT can be performed if the proper personnel are present.[4]

Anticoagulation is an important factor for patients receiving dialysis. Systemic heparinization the day of surgery should be assessed for the need of protamine reversal. Patients who have missed dialysis may have uremia, causing an increased risk of bleeding requiring intravenous desmopressin (DDAVP) with possible need for platelet replacement.[3,4]

## INTRAOPERATIVE

Patients requiring dialysis often have end-stage kidney disease (ESKD), resulting in impaired glomerular filtration, renal tubular reabsorption, and plasma protein concentrations.[1-4] This can result in decreased anesthetic clearance and altered plasma protein binding of metabolites intraoperatively. This can cause fluctuations in drug plasma concentrations throughout the case in addition to severe electrolyte abnormalities. Succinylcholine (SCh), a depolarizing neuromuscular blocking agent (NMBA), is contraindicated for dialysis-dependent patients going to urgent surgery with electrolyte abnormalities due to its potential to exacerbate hyperkalemia. The typical transient increase in potassium after SCh is 0.5 to 1 mEq/L; however, plasma cholinesterase levels are reduced in ESKD, causing the neuromuscular blockade metabolism to fluctuate and be unpredictable. Nondepolarizing agents are preferred in dialysis-dependent patients particularly with a potassium value greater than 5.5 mEq/

L. Atracurium and cisatracurium are the preferred NMBAs due to their lack of active metabolites from Hofmann elimination. Neostigmine is used for reversal of paralysis if required. Sugammadex creates complexes after chelating rocuronium/vecuronium, which may be retained in ESKD.

Maintaining anesthesia is often accomplished with volatile agents. This is regarded as safe in urgent dialysis cases due to elimination occurring predominantly via exhalation independent of renal function. Monitored anesthesia care (MAC) is the preferred method for dialysis-dependent patients undergoing urgent surgery. Medications for sedation and analgesia during MAC cases should be reduced and slowly titrated to effect.[4] Regional anesthesia plays an important role in reducing nephrotoxic anesthetic agents while also providing adequate analgesia. A partial thromboplastin time and international normalized ratio should be checked before performing neuraxial anesthetic procedures due to the potential for increased bleeding risk inherent to dialysis-dependent patients.[4,5]

Fentanyl and sufentanil are not affected by ESKD due to elimination occurring primarily in the liver. Acute alkalinization occurring with intraoperative dialysis may increase the distribution of opioids across the blood-brain barrier and should be slowly titrated to prevent respiratory depression. Remifentanil is broken down by nonspecific plasma esterases and is not adjusted for ESKD.[4,5]

## POSTOPERATIVE

Fluid and electrolyte management are important aspects postoperatively for dialysis-dependent patients. Most patients can be managed in a postanesthesia care unit (PACU). Serum creatinine, electrolytes, and urea levels should be monitored once in the PACU. If postoperative dialysis is indicated, heparinization of the circuit may be reduced in attempts to diminish the risk of postoperative bleeding.[4]

## REFERENCES

1. Tandukar S, Palevsky PM. Continuous renal replacement therapy: who, when, why, and how. *Chest*. 2019;155(3):626–638.
2. Acute Kidney Injury Work Group. KDIGO (Kidney Disease: Improving Global Outcomes) clinical practice guideline for acute kidney injury. *Kidney Int Suppl*. 2012;2(1):89–115.
3. Continuous renal replacement therapies. In: Hanson C III, ed. Procedures in Critical Care. McGraw-Hill; 2009: Chap. 50. https://accessanesthesiology.mhmedical.com/content.aspx?bookid=414&sectionid=41840279
4. Trainor D, et al. Perioperative management of the hemodialysis patient. *Semin Dial*. 2011;24(3):314–326.
5. Dean M. Opioids in renal failure and dialysis patients. *J Pain Symptom Manage*. 2004;28(5):497–504.

# 162.

# PHARMACOLOGIC PREVENTION AND TREATMENT OF RENAL FAILURE

*Anureet Walia and Archit Sharma*

## INTRODUCTION

Acute kidney injury (AKI) affects up to 50% of critically ill patients and is independently associated with both short- and long-term morbidity and mortality; the most frequent causes of AKI in the critically ill are sepsis and hypovolemia, followed by nephrotoxic agents. The RIFLE (Risk, Injury, Failure, Loss of kidney function, and End-stage kidney disease), Acute Kidney Injury Network (AKIN), and Kidney Disease: Improving Global Outcomes (KDIGO) classifications are used in order to define and stratify the severity of AKI. Since the diagnosis of AKI in a patient is in general dependent on the findings of the decline in GFR (glomerular filtration rate; increase in serum creatinine, cystatin C, or other parameters of GFR), many of the preventive measures that are employed are in fact secondary interventions with the aim to either stabilize renal function or improve it toward normal.

## IDENTIFICATION OF AT-RISK INDIVIDUALS

General risk factors for AKI that are consistent across multiple causes include age; hypovolemia; hypotension; sepsis; preexisting renal, hepatic, or cardiac dysfunction; diabetes mellitus; and exposure to nephrotoxins (e.g., aminoglycosides, amphotericin, immunosuppressive agents, nonsteroidal anti-inflammatory drugs [NSAIDs], angiotensin-converting enzyme inhibitors [ACEIs] and/or angiotensin receptor blockers [ARBs], parenteral contrast media [CM]). Preoperative use of ACEIs/ARBs was associated with a 27.6% higher risk for AKI postoperatively.[1] Stopping ACEIs or ARBs before surgery may reduce the incidence of AKI. In patients at increased risk, or in the phase of incipient AKI, emphasis should be put on nonpharmacological interventions, such as ensuring adequate renal perfusion pressure by optimizing volume status and maintaining adequate hemodynamic status by the use

of vasopressors and avoidance of further injury by removing or decreasing the effect of any nephrotoxic substances.

## VOLUME EXPANSION AND FLUID THERAPY

Despite the recognition of volume depletion as an important risk factor for AKI, there are no randomized controlled trials (RCTs) that have directly evaluated the role of fluid hydration versus placebo in the prevention of AKI. However, RCTs have compared different fluids and have combined fluid hydration with other interventions. Solomon et al. demonstrated that in patients with chronic renal insufficiency who are undergoing cardiac angiography, hydration with 0.45% saline provided better protection against acute decreases in renal function induced by radiocontrast agents than hydration with 0.45% saline plus mannitol or furosemide.[2] Results of the Saline versus Albumin Fluid Evaluation (SAFE) study, a randomized comparison of human albumin with crystalloid in the intensive care unit seemed to indicate that albumin is safe, albeit not more effective than saline, for fluid resuscitation.[3] SAFE demonstrated further no difference in renal outcomes (including incidence of AKI, need for renal replacement therapy [RRT] or duration of RRT). At present there is no evidence that the anionic composition of currently available crystalloids increases the risk of AKI in humans. However, it should be remembered that large-volume administration of saline leads to hyperchloremic acidosis, which may be associated with hyperkalemia and blood coagulation disturbances.

## AVOIDANCE OF DRUG-INDUCED AKI

The ACEIs, ARBs, and NSAIDs interfere with the autoregulation of renal blood flow (RBF) and GFR and can provoke acute hemodynamically mediated renal dysfunction. Particularly, ACEIs and ARBs may be associated more commonly with renal dysfunction because any decline in intraglomerular pressure due to blood pressure lowering will be exaggerated by concomitant vasodilation of the efferent arteriole. Acute inhibition of cyclooxygenase (type 1 or 2) by NSAIDs can reduce GFR and RBF in states of renal hypoperfusion, such as sodium depletion, diuretic use, hypotension, and sodium-avid states such as cirrhosis, nephrotic syndrome, and congestive heart failure. Aminoglycoside nephrotoxicity develops in about 10%–15% of patients treated with aminoglycosides. Among the available pharmacological options for prevention or treatment of acute tubular necrosis (ATN), there is a remarkable lack of definitive evidence supporting specific therapy in any setting.

Although loop diuretics, mannitol, and dopamine are frequently used for prevention and/or treatment of ATN, clinical studies have failed to prove value. Other drugs with theoretical value, specifically atrial natriuretic peptide analogues, adenosine blockers, and calcium antagonists, have been insufficiently studied to recommend use. *Low-dose* or "renal" dose dopamine has been advocated in the past to prevent selective renal vasoconstriction in a variety of conditions. This may not be the case in complex clinical conditions, where low-dose dopamine may even worsen renal perfusion. Several meta-analyses have concluded that renal-dose dopamine has no benefit in either preventing or ameliorating AKI in the critically ill.[4]

Ensuring adequate intravascular fluid volume remains the only approach to managing ATN that can be considered relatively effective and safe. Although it seems prudent to correct hypovolemia before contrast administration, prophylactic volume expansion in critically ill patients who are euvolemic cannot be recommended on the basis of current data.

## CONTRAST-INDUCED NEPHROPATHY

Iodinated CM can be categorized according to osmolality, high-osmolal CM (~2000 mOsm/kg), low-osmolal CM (600–800 mOsm/kg), and iso-osmolal CM (290 mOsm/kg). Evidence to date suggests that compared to low- and high-osmolal formulations, the iso-osmolal, nonionic CM are the least nephrotoxic, particularly after intravascular administration.[5] Another approach to prevent contrast-induced nephropathy (CIN) is to use an alternative, less nephrotoxic contrast agent (i.e., gadolinium salts). Results from several case series and isolated case reports suggest improved renal safety in patients with pre-existing CKD.

Mueller et al. found that intravenous hydration using a 0.9% saline solution compared with a 0.45% saline solution in dextrose in 1620 patients undergoing coronary angiography significantly reduced CIN.[6] The sustained administration of isotonic saline before and after radiocontrast injection thus seems to be more protective than equivalent volumes of hypotonic saline and saline. Based on a few prospective studies, administration of bicarbonate does not seem to be more efficient than saline.

N-Acetylcysteine (NAC), a thiol-containing antioxidant, is one of the antioxidants that has been investigated extensively as an agent for CIN prevention. There have been mixed data on whether prophylactic oral and intravenous NAC administration reduces the incidence of CIN in small trials and even in meta-analyses, although its use is generally recommended, given its low cost, easy availability, and favorable side-effect profile.

## REFERENCES

1. Arora P, et al. Preoperative use of angiotensin-converting enzyme inhibitors/angiotensin receptor blockers is associated with increased risk for acute kidney injury after cardiovascular surgery. *Clin J Am Soc Nephrol*. 2008;3(5):1266–1273.
2. Solomon R, et al. Effects of saline, mannitol, and furosemide on acute decreases in renal function induced by radiocontrast agents. *N Engl J Med*. 1994;331(21):1416–1420. doi:10.1056/NEJM199411243312104
3. Finfer S, et al. A comparison of albumin and saline for fluid resuscitation in the intensive care unit. *N Engl J Med*. 2004;350:2247–2256.
4. Friedrich JO et al. Meta-analysis: low-dose dopamine increases urine output but does not prevent renal dysfunction or death. *Ann Intern Med*. 2005;142(7):510–524.
5. Aspelin P, et al. Nephrotoxic effects in high-risk patients undergoing angiography. *N Engl J Med*. 2003;348(6):491–499.
6. Mueller C, et al. Prevention of contrast media–associated nephropathy: randomized comparison of 2 hydration regimens in 1620 patients undergoing coronary angioplasty. *Arch Intern Med*. 2002;162(3), 329–336.

# 163.

# UROLOGIC SURGERY

*Allison K. Dalton*

## INTRODUCTION

Urologic surgery encompasses a wide range of surgical procedures, from simple cystoscopy to laparoscopic and open procedures.

## CYSTOSCOPY

Common indications for cystoscopy are hematuria, malignancy, urinary obstruction, urinary incontinence, recurrent urinary tract infections, renal calculi, and concern for trauma or fistula. Cystoscopy may be performed as a singular procedure or in conjunction with other procedures, including biopsy; transurethral resection of tumors (i.e., bladder, prostate); intravesicular chemotherapy; stone extraction; or placement of urinary stents.

Cystoscopy may be complicated by bladder perforation, transurethral resection of the prostate (TURP) syndrome and sepsis. Fluid extravasation is heralded by poor return of the fluid from the bladder as well as nausea, abdominal pain, hypertension, hypotension, bradycardia, and increased airway pressures in ventilated patients. The use of hypotonic irrigation solutions during cystoscopy for bladder resection may lead to TURP syndrome, a rare complication in which the patient may experience headache, confusion, dyspnea, arrhythmias, hypotension, and seizures as a result of the effects of circulatory overload and hyponatremia from water intoxication.

## RENAL SURGERY

Renal surgery may be performed for benign or oncologic indications. Nephrectomy may be performed as an open, hand-assisted laparoscopic, laparoscopic, or robot-assisted laparoscopic procedure. Patients may be candidates for partial, simple, or radical nephrectomy based on the indication for surgery and the patient's preoperative renal function.

Hematuria, flank pain, and a palpable mass is the classic triad for the diagnosis of renal cancer but is only present in a small percentage of patients. Renal cell carcinoma may be associated with hypertension, hypercalcemia, and erythrocytosis and is strongly associated with tobacco use. A small percentage of renal cell carcinomas have growth into the renal vein and inferior vena cava and may extend as far as the right atrium.

## PROSTATE SURGERY

Prostate cancer is the most common cancer in men. Roughly one in nine men will be diagnosed with prostate cancer in their lifetime. Prostate cancer may be treated with active surveillance, hormonal therapy, external beam radiotherapy, brachytherapy, and radical prostatectomy. Prostatectomy may be performed via open retropubic or laparoscopic approach. Open prostatectomy can be associated with significant blood loss. Currently, robotic-assisted laparoscopic prostatectomy is the most common surgical approach.

## CYSTECTOMY

After prostate cancer, bladder cancer is the most common urologic malignancy. Bladder cancer may be treated surgically via transurethral resection or via radical resection. Urinary diversion may be provided by construction of a conduit (i.e., ileal, jejunal, colonic) or neobladder. Cystectomy is associated with the highest morbidity and mortality rates of all urologic cancer procedures.[1] Robotic-assisted cystectomy can mitigate the risk with lower rates of postoperative complications, lower blood loss, and shorter hospital length of stay.[2]

Anesthetic management goals specific to cystectomy include ensuring adequate hydration to promote urinary flow as sluggish urinary flow through a new jejunal conduit may result in hyponatremia, hypochloremia, hyperkalemia, and metabolic acidosis. Hyperchloremic metabolic acidosis may occur with colonic or ileal conduit.

## TESTICULAR CANCER SURGERY/ RETROPERITONEAL LYMPH NODE DISSECTION

Testicular cancer tumors may be treated with radiation, chemotherapy, or surgery. Retroperitoneal lymph node dissection is utilized for disease management as well as for staging.

Neoadjuvant chemotherapy may predispose the patient to renal insufficiency (cisplatin) and neuropathy (vincristine). Patients with a history of bleomycin therapy may be at risk for pulmonary fibrosis. Anesthesiologists should practice judicious intraoperative fluid administration and use of the lowest inspired oxygen fraction possible.

## ROBOTIC-ASSISTED UROLOGIC SURGERY

Select urologic procedures (i.e., prostatectomy, cystectomy, nephrectomy) may be performed with robotic assistance. Advantages of robotic-assisted surgery include better precision and mobility with the surgical instruments and improved three-dimensional visualization.[3] In order to facilitate robot-assisted pelvic surgery, patients are placed in the steep Trendelenburg position, and the abdomen is insufflated with $CO_2$. Pneumoperitoneum increases the partial pressure of carbon dioxide ($PaCO_2$), and increased minute ventilation is often required intraoperatively. In addition, insufflation results in increased intrathoracic pressures, decreased functional residual capacity (FRC) and expiratory reserve volume (ERV), leading to atelectasis and possible desaturation events intraoperatively or during recovery.

## ANESTHETIC MANAGEMENT

### PREOPERATIVE

Preoperative assessment should focus on the presence of coexisting diseases, laboratory examinations, and imaging studies. Urologic malignancies are associated with tobacco use, leading to increased rates of coexisting coronary artery disease and chronic obstructive pulmonary disease in surgical patients. There is also an increased prevalence of hypertension and diabetes. Due to symptoms of hematuria as well as coexisting disease, patients may be at risk for anemia. Renal function and electrolytes should be evaluated prior to major surgery. For patients at risk for significant intraoperative bleeding (i.e., cystectomy, nephrectomy with venous extension), advanced planning for blood preparation is advised. Preoperative tumor embolization may be considered for patients with extensive vascular tumor burden.

### INTRAOPERATIVE

Minor procedures (i.e., cystoscopy) are performed under neuraxial or general anesthesia. Major urologic surgeries often necessitate general endotracheal anesthesia. Due to risk for blood loss from vascular tumors as well as the potential for vascular tumor spread, adequate intravenous access is paramount intraoperatively. This may include central venous access. Arterial catheter placement is indicated for patients with significant comorbidities or those at risk for hemorrhage. Transesophageal echocardiography may be indicated for patients with significant vascular spread (i.e., right atrial thrombus) or for patients with significant cardiac disease. For patients with tumors extending to the right atrium, intraoperative cardiopulmonary bypass may be required.

Lithotomy position is utilized in many major and minor urologic procedures. Care should be taken to ensure that the legs are appropriately padded (especially on the lateral aspects) to avoid peroneal nerve injury. Prolonged lithotomy positioning has resulted in pressure sores, compartment syndrome, and rhabdomyolysis. Renal surgery is typically performed in the lateral position with flexion of the table. In order to prevent compression injury to the brachial plexus, an "axillary roll" should be placed under the chest on the dependent side. Avoidance of excess dorsal and lateral extension of the neck must be avoided to prevent stretch injuries. Robotic-assisted pelvic surgery is performed in the steep (>30°) Trendelenburg position (Figure 163.1), which is associated with increases in peak and plateau pressures and decreases in FRC and ERV. Steep Trendelenburg positioning also increases risk of facial and airway edema, brachial plexus injuries, and increased intracerebral and intraocular pressures.

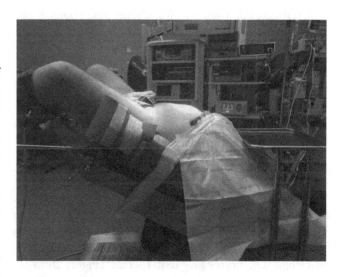

**Figure 163.1** Steep Trendelenburg position utilized for robotic-assisted urologic surgery.

Pain control may be challenging. Epidural analgesia is an effective way to treat postoperative pain associated with large lateral and midline incisions. One may also consider paravertebral or transversus abdominis plane blocks for postoperative pain control. Nonsteroidal anti-inflammatory drugs and drugs that require renal metabolism should be used with caution.

## REFERENCES

1. Patel HD, et al. Morbidity of urological surgical procedures: an analysis of rates, risk factors, and outcomes. *Urology*. 2015;85(3):552–560.
2. Li K, et al. Systematic review and meta-analysis of comparative studies reporting early outcomes after robot-assisted radical cystectomy versus open radical cystectomy. *Cancer Treat Rev*. 2013;39(6): 551–560.
3. Kakar PN, et al. Robotic invasion of operation theatre and associated anaesthetic issues: a review. *Indian J Anaesth*. 2011;55(1):18–25.

# 164.

# PERIOPERATIVE ELECTROLYTE ABNORMALITIES

## Brent Earls and Eellan Sivanesan

## INTRODUCTION

Major electrolytes, such as sodium ($Na^+$), potassium ($K^+$), calcium ($Ca^{2+}$), magnesium ($Mg^{2+}$), and phosphate ($PO_4^{3-}$), are involved in critical and basic physiologic functions and are thus tightly regulated through sophisticated homeostatic mechanisms.[1–5] Disturbances in electrolyte concentration are some of the most frequent disorders in hospitalized and critically ill patients. We discuss the etiology and management of common electrolyte disturbances in the perioperative domain (Table 164.1).

## ANESTHETIC CONSIDERATIONS

*Hyponatremia* can manifest as anorexia, weakness, seizure, nausea/vomiting, altered level of consciousness, coma, and/or cramps. Hyponatremia can be isotonic (plasma osmolality [Posm] 280–295 mOsm/kg), hypotonic (Posm < 280 mOsm/kg), or hypertonic (Posm > 295 mOsm/kg). Treatment can vary greatly depending on the underlying cause, ranging from free water restriction, infusion of 0.9% saline solution, hypertonic (3%) saline boluses, and pharmacological agents for long-term therapy[4] (Figure 164.1).

Sodium deficit (mEq/L) = 0.6 (Weight in kg) × (125-Measured sodium)

*Hypernatremia* can manifest as stupor, renal insufficiency, coma, seizures, and/or decreased urinary concentrating ability. A common condition resulting in excessive renal losses of free water is diabetes insipidus

*Table 164.1* MAJOR ELECTROLYTES AND INTRINSIC REGULATORY MECHANISMS

| ELECTROLYTE | REGULATION |
|---|---|
| Sodium ($Na^+$)[3] | • Aldosterone<br>• Atrial natriuretic peptide<br>• Antidiuretic hormone |
| Potassium ($K^+$)[4] | • Aldosterone<br>• Epinephrine<br>• Insulin<br>• Intrinsic renal mechanisms |
| Calcium ($Ca^{2+}$)[3,4] | • Parathyroid hormone (PTH)<br>• Vitamin D<br>• Calcitonin |
| Magnesium ($Mg^{2+}$)[1,4] | • Intrinsic renal mechanisms in the distal tubule (primary) and thick ascending limb<br>• Parathyroid hormone<br>• Vitamin D |
| Phosphorus ($PO_4^{3-}$)[2,4] | • Parathyroid hormone<br>• Insulin-like growth factor |

Hyponatremia

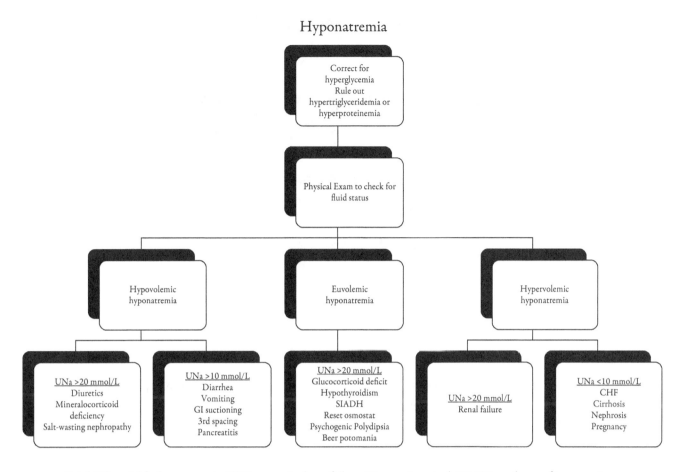

Figure 164.1 Brief differential for hyponatremia. CHF, congestive heart failure; GI, gastrointestinal; SIADH, syndrome of inappropriate antidiuretic hormone secretion.

(DI), both central and nephrogenic. Treatment produced by water loss consists of repleting water and correction of associated deficits in total body Na⁺ (Figure 164.2).[4] Hypernatremia must be corrected slowly due to the risk of neurologic sequelae such as seizures or cerebral edema. The two most suitable agents for correcting central DI (antidiuretic hormone–deficiency syndrome) are desmopressin (DDAVP) and aqueous vasopressin.[3]

*Hypokalemia* can manifest as muscle twitching, weakness, fatigue, and/or cardiac rhythm disturbances. Dysrhythmias are the most dangerous complications of hypokalemia, which include ventricular escape activity,

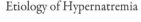

Etiology of Hypernatremia

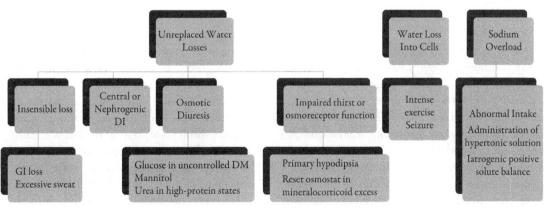

Figure 164.2 Brief differential for hypernatremia. DM, diabetes mellitus.

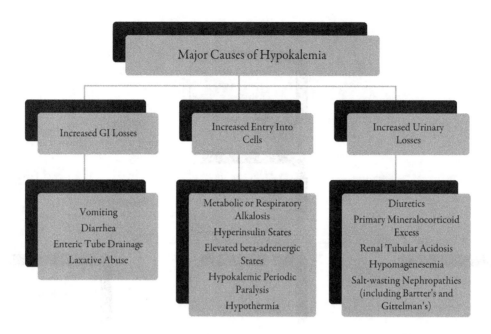

**Figure 164.3** Brief differential for hypokalemia.

reentrant and ectopic tachycardias, and delayed conduction.[4] Electrocardiographic (ECG) changes include PR prolongation, QRS prolongation, and high U wave. Common causes include poor dietary intake, alcoholism (also causes hypomagnesemia), states of insulin excess, and elevated catecholamine states[3] (Figure 164.3). Treatment consists of K+ repletion, correction of alkalemia, and removal of offending drugs.

*Hyperkalemia* can manifest as weakness, flaccid paralysis, and/or cardiac rhythm disturbances. Lethal manifestations of hyperkalemia involve the cardiac conduction system: dysrhythmias, conduction abnormalities, and cardiac arrest. ECG changes include PR prolongation, QRS prolongation, ST elevation, and peaked T wave. Medications, including nonsteroidal anti-inflammatory drugs, angiotensin-converting enzyme inhibitors, cyclosporin, and potassium-sparing diuretics, are now the most common cause of hyperkalemia.[4] Other common causes include acute or chronic kidney dysfunction, acidosis, insulin deficiency or diabetic ketoacidosis, aldosterone deficiency, and tumor lysis syndrome (Figure 164.4).

*Hypocalcemia* can manifest as neuromuscular irritability (tetany), positive Trousseau sign, prolonged QT interval, perioral numbness, positive Chvostek sign, laryngospasm, paresthesias, and/or seizures. Hypocalcemia often results from failure of parathyroid hormone (PTH) and calcitriol action or due to chelation or precipitation, rather than Ca2+ deficiency alone. PTH deficiency can be seen as a result of surgical trauma or following thyroidectomy with subsequent removal of the parathyroid gland. Proper treatment requires identification of the underlying cause and discontinuing offending drugs. In the intensive care unit, the most common causes of hypocalcemia are magnesium

depletion and sepsis. Calcium replacement can help to avoid the severe side effects of hypocalcemia. Calcium chloride contains 13.6 mEq elemental calcium, while calcium gluconate contains 4.5 mEq elemental calcium.

*Hypercalcemia* can manifest as lethargy, constipation, nephrolithiasis, fatigue/muscle weakness, shortened QT interval, polyuria, and/or stupor. Hypercalcemia is most commonly caused by an excess of bone resorption over bone formation. This can be secondary to malignant disease, hyperparathyroidism, hypocalciuric hypercalcemia, thyrotoxicosis, immobilization, or granulomatous diseases.[4] Mainstays of treatment include hydration, correction of associated electrolyte abnormalities, removal of offending drugs, dietary Ca2+ restriction, and increased physical activity. Medications, such as loop diuretics or bisphosphonates, may be introduced to aid in Ca2+ excretion or osteoclast inhibition, respectively.[4]

**Hypomagnesemia** can manifest as tremor, tetany, weakness, and/or widening of the QRS interval and peaking of T waves. Common conditions that precipitate hypomagnesemia include acute or chronic diarrhea, malabsorption or steatorrhea, and small bowel bypass surgery. The most common renal losses of magnesium are medication induced, acute kidney injury, acute tubular necrosis, or other electrolyte abnormalities, most notably hypocalcemia and hypokalemia.[3] Intravenous administration of magnesium can inhibit resorption in the kidney, leading to a large amount of the infused magnesium excreted in the urine.[1] Oral replacement is preferred in patients without severe features who can tolerate oral supplementation.

**Hypermagnesemia** can manifest as nausea, flushing, drowsiness, hypotension, diminished deep tendon reflexes, and/or prolongation of the PR interval, and an increase

# Hyperkalemia Evaluation

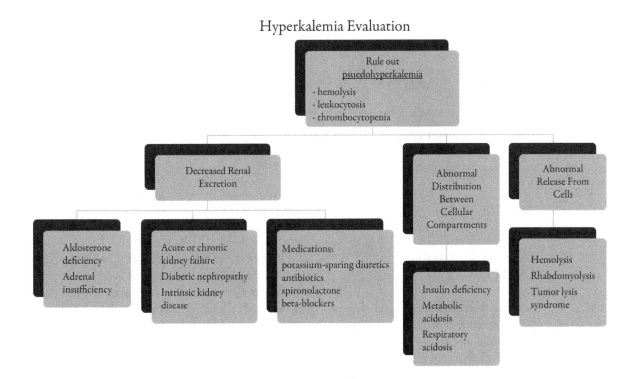

**Figure 164.4** Brief differential for hyperkalemia.

in QRS duration and interval. Hypermagnesemia is an uncommon problem in the absence of exogenous administration or kidney failure.[1] Hypermagnesemia is more commonly seen in the perioperative setting due to administration in antacids, enemas, or total parenteral nutrition. Rarer causes include hypothyroidism and Addison disease. Treatment involves volume expansion and diuresis with a combination of fluid and loop diuretics.[4] Calcium can be administered as a temporary antagonist until more definitive measures are put into place. In the case of renal failure, $Mg^{2+}$ can be removed through dialysis.[5] The earliest manifestations of hypermagnesemia are loss of patellar reflex, double vision, flushing, and somnolence, which occur at a concentration of 8–12 mg/dL. Next, you will see muscle paralysis and respiratory arrest at 15–20 mg/dL, and last, cardiac arrest at levels above 25 mg/dL.[5]

*Hypophosphatemia* can manifest as muscle weakness, hemolytic anemia, rhabdomyolysis, and/or change in mental status. Most commonly seen in patients with alcohol use disorder, burns, or starvation, hypophosphatemia is caused by three primary abnormalities in $P_i$ homeostasis: intracellular shift, increased renal loss, or reduced gastrointestinal absorption. Refeeding syndrome, carbohydrate-induced hypophosphatemia, is the type most commonly encountered in hospitalized patients[4] but it also occurs during medical management of diabetic ketoacidosis. Phosphate should be administered cautiously to hypocalcemic patients because of the risk of precipitating more severe hypocalcemia and

should be given cautiously to patients with renal insufficiency because of impaired excretory ability.

*Hyperphosphatemia* can manifest as phosphate nephropathy, renal tubule damage, and/or metastatic calcification of soft tissue. This can happen as a result of high phosphate load, rapid extracellular shift, or intrinsic kidney disease.[4] High phosphate loads can be seen through exogenous supplementation, tumor lysis syndrome, or rhabdomyolysis. Extracellular shifts are a less common cause but occur with metabolic acidosis and less frequently with respiratory acidosis. In acute and chronic kidney disease, diminished filtration can lead to excess serum phosphate. Proximal tubule phosphate reabsorption can also be affected by circumstances such as hypoparathyroidism or bisphosphonate therapy.[2]

## REFERENCES

1. de Baaij JH, et al. Regulation of magnesium balance: lessons learned from human genetic disease. *Clin Kidney J.* 2012;5(suppl 1):i15–i24.
2. Murer H, et al. Cellular mechanisms in proximal tubular reabsorption of inorganic phosphate. *Am J Physiol.* 1991;260:C885–C899.
3. Charuhas T, et al. *Perioperative Kidney Injury: Principles of Risk Assessment, Diagnosis and Treatment.* New York, NY: Springer; 2014.
4. Svenson C. Electrolytes and diuretics. In: Hemmings HC, Egan TD, eds. *Pharmacology and Physiology for Anesthesia: Foundations and Clinical Application.* Philadelphia, PA: Elsevier; 2019:814–835.
5. Dyer R, Swanevelder J. Hypertensive disorders. In Chestnut DH, ed. *Obstetric Anesthesia: Principles and Practice.* Philadelphia, PA: Mosby/Elsevier; 2009:840–878.

# 165.

# FLUID THERAPY AND HOMEOSTASIS

*Miguel Rovira and Christopher Giordano*

## FLUID MANAGEMENT STRATEGIES

In the operating room, the management of fluid therapy is vital for physiological homeostasis and effective postoperative management. Human physiologic water content changes as we progress from birth to old age: Human water volume peaks in utero or as premature neonates (about 95 mL/kg) and then decreases into adulthood, with men having a slightly greater water volume (75 mL/kg) than women (65 mL/kg).[1,2]

In the 1950s, two pediatricians, Malcolm Holliday and William Segar, investigated the metabolic requirements for fluid resuscitation in fasting states. Graphing the metabolic requirements versus weight, they calculated that children require 4 mL per hour for the first 10 kg of body weight, then 2 mL for the next 10 kg, and 1 mL for every 1 kg thereafter. Since this study came out, clinicians have adopted this strategy for adults as well. For example, a 70-kg person would be estimated to require 40 mL for the first 10 kg, 20 mL for the next 10 kg, and 50 mL for the remaining 50 kg,

totaling a per hour maintenance requirement of 110 mL/h. This fluid requirement calculation is typically employed as an estimate because it does not take into account kidney function and comorbidities such as congestive heart failure, sepsis, and the like.[3]

Types of Intravenous FluidsWhile the types of intravenous fluids that can be administered to patients is limited, their indications and contraindications are nuanced and specific (Table 165.1). The decision on which intravenous fluid to incorporate into the patient's management starts with deciding between crystalloids and colloids. Crystalloids can be further subcategorized into balanced and unbalanced, which describes how close the solution is to physiologic electrolyte concentrations. Furthermore, balanced solutions contain a buffer compound to maintain pH.

Lactated Ringer (LR) solution is perhaps one of the more well-known balanced crystalloids. It contains sodium, chloride, potassium, and calcium at near physiologic concentrations, with the caveat of being slightly hyponatremic at around 130 mEq/L and hyperchloremic at

*Table 165.1* APPROXIMATE VALUES OF ELECTROLYTE CONTENT[a]

| ELECTROLYTE/SOLUTE | LACTATED RINGER | PLASMALYTE | NORMAL SALINE | HUMAN PLASMA |
|---|---|---|---|---|
| Sodium (mEq/L) | 130 | 140 | 154 | 140 |
| Chloride (mEq/L) | 109 | 98 | 154 | 102 |
| Potassium (mEq/L) | 4 | 5 | — | 4.5 |
| Calcium (mg/dL) | 4 | — | — | 3.7 |
| Magnesium (mg/dL) | — | 3 | — | 2.5 |
| Buffer (mmol/L) | Lactate (28) | Acetate (27), gluconate (23) | — | $HCO_3$ (25) |
| pH | 6.5 | 7.4 | 5.7 | 7.4 |
| Osmolarity (mosm/L) | 273 | 295 | 308 | 291 |
| Price | $2.5/L | $5/L | $2/L | — |

[a]Concentrations may vary between distributors.

109 mEq/L. It is also slightly hypo-osmolar at 273 mOsm/ L compared to normal human plasma, which is typically around 291 mEq/L. When choosing LR, it is important to remember that because it contains the buffer lactate there is an increased risk of hyperlactatemia in patients with shock or liver failure, which can further exacerbate acidotic states. Another very important precaution is to avoid using LR to prime your red blood cell or fresh frozen plasma (FFP) transfusion lines. This is because LR contains calcium, which can overwhelm the binding capacity of citrate within banked blood products and result in the precipitation of micro or macro blood clots, occluding intravenous lines or transfusing emboli into the patient.

PlasmaLyte is another commonly used crystalloid that has the closest osmolarity to human plasma at around 295 mOsm/L. Unlike LR, PlasmaLyte contains acetate and gluconate as opposed to lactate, which act as safer buffers for patients in shock burns, liver failure, or other acidotic states. Additionally, it is safer to infuse with blood products because PlasmaLyte does not contain calcium.

The most frequently used unbalanced crystalloid is normal saline (NS), which contains equal contents of sodium and chloride at 154 mEq/L of each. At an osmolarity around 308 mOsm/L, its iso-osmolarity to hyperosmolarity relative to human blood makes it an ideal choice for neurosurgery cases. Because of the elevated chloride content compared to the normal 105 mEq/L, large infusions of NS put the patient at risk of hyperchloremic acidosis (non–anion gap). The larger concentration of chloride contributes to the strong ion difference, which shifts the pH to an acidotic state. Furthermore, this hyperchloremia and acidosis can also lead to immune system dysfunction, vascular permeability, and vasodilation.[4]

Hypotonic solutions include ½ NS, D5 (dextrose 5%) ½ NS, and D10 (dextrose 10%). These solutions are typically reserved for either preventing or managing hypoglycemia (the dextrose-containing solutions) or hypernatremia (the hyponatremic solutions) or slowly attempting to correct hyponatremia in order to avert quick overcorrection and risk central pontine myelinolysis.[5]

Alternatively, the other major category for fluid resuscitation is colloids, which are different from crystalloids in that they are solutions containing large organic compounds or cellular products as opposed to only the cations and anions used in crystalloids. The most commonly used colloid is albumin, which is produced naturally by the liver and works by elevating oncotic pressure and increases the intravascular volume at a near 1:1 volume. This differs from crystalloids, which contribute about a third of the administered volume to the intravascular space. Albumin's main contraindication is use in patients with traumatic brain injury, where the SAFE (Saline versus Albumin Fluid Evaluation) trial demonstrated increased mortality. However, the same study showed an increased benefit of colloids over crystalloids in patients with sepsis.[5] Albumin is heat sterilized to prevent the transmission of infective viruses and bacteria; however, this process cannot eliminate prions from the colloid product. Subsequently, countries with epidemics of bovine spongiform encephalopathy must destroy all albumin collectively in order to avert its spread. Blood products such as red blood cells, platelets, and FFP are also colloids but their indications will not be discussed in this chapter.

## ANESTHETIC CONSIDERATIONS

### PREOPERATIVE

These fluid deficits are typically calculated using the 4–2–1 rule over the time patients are fasting; however, preoperatively more institutions are permitting clear fluids up until 2 hours prior to surgery. This practice has largely changed the approach to the aforementioned fasting resuscitation.

When preparing to administer intravenous solutions, it is ideal to spike the solution bag no more than 1 hour prior to administering the solution in order to prevent bacteria on the outside from entering the solution.

### INTRAOPERATIVE

The type of surgery and medical conditions (e.g., end-stage renal disease, heart failure) determine how much fluids are lost intraoperatively. For example, open abdominal surgeries have much more insensible fluid losses as compared to a laparoscopic surgery, and the manipulation of bowel inadvertently traumatizes it, resulting in cellular swelling that draws from intravascular volume. These losses can be estimated with various formulas or treated according to monitors that can gauge fluid responsiveness. Blood loss, urine output, gastric contents, and other outputs need to be replaced accordingly as well.

Last, the speed at which fluids are administered is determined by the length, diameter, and connectors (e.g., needleless, which slows speed). Being cognizant of these equipment features will be particularly useful in planning before and during a tenuous case.

### POSTOPERATIVE

Detailing an accurate record of total ins and outs during a case is important for postoperative fluid management, whether the patient is sent to the PACU or ICU. Hemodynamic changes will have to be assessed in the setting of recovery from anesthesia as well as the treatment of post-operative pain. Clinical judgment of volume status will depend on combining these findings along with the physical exam as well as the intra-operative course.

## REFERENCES

1. Open Anesthesia. Maximum ABL calculation. https://www.ope nanesthesia.org/maximum_abl_calculation/
2. Holliday M, Segar W. The maintenance need for water in parenteral fluid therapy. *Pediatrics.* 1957;19(5):823–832.
3. Butterworth J, et al. Fluid management and blood component therapy. In: *Morgan & Mikhail's Clinical Anesthesiology* edited by Jason Maley and Christie Naglierei. McGraw-Hill Education; 2018:Chap. 51, 1194–1196.
4. Han JW, et al. Comparison of intraoperative basal fluid requirements in distal pancreatectomy: laparotomy vs. laparoscopy: a retrospective cohort study. *Medicine.* 2017; 6(47):e8763.
5. Marino P, et al. Resuscitation fluids. In: *Marino's the Little ICU Book.* Wolters Kluwer; 2017: Chap. 5.

# 166.

# FLUID BALANCE DURING SURGERY
## THE ROLE OF THE ENDOTHELIAL GLYCOCALYX

*Charlotte Streetzel and Christopher Giordano*

## FLUID BALANCE DURING SURGERY: THE ROLE OF THE ENDOTHELIAL GLYCOCALYX

### STRUCTURE AND FUNCTION OF THE ENDOTHELIAL GLYCOCALYX

The endothelial glycocalyx (EG) is a network of molecules that constitutes the innermost layer of the vasculature. The EG has a backbone of glycoproteins and proteoglycans, which physically anchor the EG to the endothelial wall, and various side chains, the majority of which are heparan sulfates.[1] The soluble components of the EG, including albumin, superoxide dismutase 3, antithrombin III (ATIII), and angiotensin-converting enzyme, are bound to a layer of the EG that is in contact with the vascular contents. Cellular adhesion molecules, as well as the glycoproteins that regulate coagulation, fibrinolysis, and hemostasis, are found within the EG.[1]

The EG also plays a role in body fluid homeostasis, modulation of inflammatory reactions, and the recruitment and adhesion of leukocytes and platelets.[1,2] These functions are mediated via the interaction between the EG and molecules that are delivered by the contents of the circulatory system, which allows for control of the filtration of fluids and molecules, vascular tone, and cellular trafficking. Components of the EG contribute to regulation of the coagulation cascade.[2–5] ATIII, activated factors IX and X, and thrombin undergo enhanced activity after binding to the EG.[2]

### STARLING FORCES REVISED

The revised Starling principle, which takes into account the oncotic pressure of the glycocalyx $\pi_g$,[1] is founded on the idea that the filtration of the capillary is regulated at the initial site where the filtration occurs. Also, forces do not occur across the entire capillary wall, but only across the EG.[2] It is now understood that the oncotic pressure difference is built up within a small protein-free zone just beneath the EG, known as the subglycocalyx, as illustrated in Figure 166.1.[1] The barrier can undergo destruction, such as when atrial natriuretic peptide (ANP) is released into circulation secondary to volume overload. ANP activates enzymes that create pores in the EG, causing fluid extravasation and resultant tissue edema.[5] Additionally, low serum albumin increases leakage of albumin into the interstitial space.[1] Even at low concentrations, infusing albumin is beneficial in maintaining the EG.[2,3]

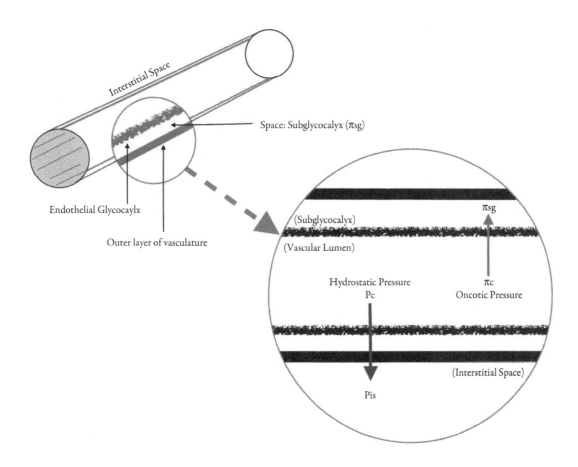

**Figure 166.1** The endothelial glycocalyx. Pc, hydrostatic pressure of capillary; Pis, hydrostatic pressure of interstitium; πc, oncotic pressure of capillary; πsg, oncotic pressure of subglycocalyx.

## INTRAOPERATIVE CONSIDERATIONS

### PATHOLOGIES THAT DIMINISH THE INTEGRITY OF THE EG

Breakdown of the EG in response to inflammation, sheer stress, ischemia, and trauma impairs the function of the barrier.[1] The overwhelming result of this damage manifests as edema, increased platelet aggregation, hypercoagulability, and accelerated inflammation. These conditions should be considered because they will affect management of patients in the perioperative period.[2,3] The clinical pathologies implicated in EG degradation include heart failure, nephrotic syndrome, cirrhosis, acute lung injury, sepsis, trauma, and volume overload. EG breakdown may be detected by measuring EG degradation products.[1]

### ELECTROLYTE DERANGEMENTS

Severe hypernatremia is directly toxic to the EG by causing shedding and reducing its thickness by half.[5] Fluid shifting out of the intracellular spaces results in cellular shrinkage. EG shedding in the setting of hyperglycemia involves induction of enzymes, which creates reactive oxygen species that directly damage the EG.[5] Hyperglycemia causes thinning of the EG and incompetent shedding.[2]

### ACUTE LUNG INJURY AND PULMONARY EDEMA

Regardless of the etiology, noncardiogenic pulmonary edema and acute respiratory distress syndrome have a shared pathophysiology: breakdown of the alveolocapillary barrier, increased fluid extravasation, and a severe inflammatory response.[4,5] In cases in which the cells of the vasculature express syndecan 1, administration of plasma products aids in the reconstitution of the integrity and function of the pulmonary vascular EG.[5]

### HEART FAILURE

Patients with heart failure often have clinical volume overload. The role of the EG in these cases is to buffer increases in total body sodium without retaining excess water.[1] As this ability diminishes due to EG damage, large amounts of sodium are not cleared by the kidneys, resulting in further edema. As such, these patients are sensitive to minor changes in fluid administration and retention.

## NEPHROTIC SYNDROME

The proper function of glomeruli depends on a functional EG. Data have indicated that a disruption in the EG leads to increased permeability throughout the glomerular capillary, leading to an increased permeability to albumin. Uncharged albumin, however, is not altered by damage to the EG, which indicates a disruption to the ability of the EG to select molecules based on charge.[2] A patient will experience edema prior to proteinuria or a decrease in serum albumin; however, increased syndecan 1 is observed in the earliest stages of nephrotic syndromes.[1]

## SEPSIS

The integrity of the vascular endothelium is diminished in sepsis due to direct alterations in charge and structure, as well as increases in adhesion molecule signaling, which directly damages the EG.[1] As the EG becomes destroyed, the ability to regulate fluids between compartments is diminished. The result is increased permeability throughout the vasculature and increased leakage of fluid into the interstitium. In addition to direct damage to the EG, there is a decreased ability to regulate vascular tone. This further intensifies the damage to the EG by causing peripheral pooling of blood, degradation of heparan sulfate, and the resultant deadly procoagulant state. Crystalloid fluids are recommended to correct hypotension in patients with sepsis; however, large volumes should be avoided due to the inevitable extravasation and loss of the ability to retain volume in the intravascular space.[1]

## TRAUMA

The "endotheliopathy of trauma" is a concomitant microvascular disorder, and a trauma patient almost immediately has elevated serum levels of syndical 1.[1] Damage to the EG causes a state of hyperfibrinolysis, which may be implicated in damage to the EG. In trauma patients who have received tranexamic acid, improved survival has been observed.[5] Additionally, patients who received fresh frozen plasma or factor concentrates have an increased ability to rebuild the EG.[5] Other types of damage such as local ischemia and reperfusion also degrade the EG.[2,5] This damage causes cellular swelling and degradation of the EG, followed by recruitment of leukocytes and tissue edema. Hypoalbuminemia increases damage to the EG in trauma patients; early administration of albumin is recommended to maintain the integrity of the EG and physiologic fluid status.[1]

## ANESTHETIC CONSIDERATIONS

- When the EG is damaged, colloids can move throughout the endothelium freely; there is no significant difference in mortality outcomes in patients treated with crystals versus colloids.[3]
- Avoiding fluid overload by using goal-directed management is crucial for proper fluid status and vascular functioning.[3]
- There is evidence that cardiopulmonary bypass causes damage to the EG. Acute fluid loading preoperatively, hyperoxia (defined as $PaO_2 > 185$ mm Hg) with the creation of free radicals, and the formation of gaseous microemboli in the cerebral vasculature during cardiopulmonary bypass contribute to EG degradation and patient morbidity.

## REFERENCES

1. Kundra P, Goswami S. Endothelial glycocalyx: role in body fluid homeostasis and fluid management. *Indian J Anaesth.* 2019;63:6–14.
2. Alphonsus CS, Rodseth RN. The endothelial glycocalyx: a review of the vascular barrier. *Anaesthesia.* 2014;69:777–784.
3. Myers GJ, Wegner J. Endothelial glycocalyx and cardiopulmonary bypass. *J Extra Corpor Technol.* 2017;49:174–181.
4. Collins SR, et al. Special article: the endothelial glycocalyx: emerging concepts in pulmonary edema and acute lung injury. *Anesth Analg.* 2013;117:664–674.
5. Jedlicka J, et al. Endothelial glycocaylx. Crit Care Clin. 2020;36:217–232.

# 167.

# ASSESSMENT OF FLUID RESPONSIVENESS AND GOAL-DIRECTED THERAPIES

*Jacqueline Sohn and Connor McNamara*

## INTRODUCTION

The clinical assessment of a patient's intravascular volume is very challenging and controversial. However, maintenance of euvolemia is critical to electrolyte homeostasis and oxygen delivery to the tissues.[1] Thus, an accurate assessment of intravascular volume status and appropriate reaction to this assessment are essential for managing critically ill patients in both the operating rooms and the intensive care units. Fluid management has been studied and heavily debated through the years. Traditionally, intravenous fluids were given more liberally during and after surgery because it was perceived to replace the amount of fluids lost during the preoperative period from fasting, third spacing, and insensible losses.[1] However, over the years, this liberal approach was found to lead to severe complications, such as pulmonary congestion, decreased tissue oxygenation, decreased wound healing, and delayed recovery.[1,2] Then, the restrictive approach to fluid management gained popularity with the widespread advocacy for enhanced recovery after surgery pathways.[1]

There are many modalities to assess a patient's volume status. The initial assessment though should always include a thorough history taking and a physical examination. Common physiological signs such as oliguria, supine hypotension, and a positive tilt test may suggest dehydration or hypovolemia but are not very sensitive or reliable.[3] Furthermore, the classic way of administering fluid based on the patient's physiological signs or static values such as central venous pressure (CVP) or pulmonary artery occlusion pressure (PAOP) do not accurately predict fluid responsiveness.[3] Fluid responsiveness is conceptually defined as an increase in stroke volume (SV) in response to intravascular volume expansion from a fluid administration.

A quantitative measurement can be used to assess fluid responsiveness, which is defined as a 10% or more increase in SV or in cardiac index after administering 250–500 mL of either colloid or crystalloid fluid.[1,4,5] This is referred to as a fluid challenge test. It is derived from the idea that if the patient's heart function is at the steep portion of the

Frank-Starling curve (Figure 167.1), then a small increase in left ventricular end-diastolic volume (LVEDV) preload will increase the SV.[4] A caveat to using the fluid challenge test as a predictor for fluid responsiveness is that a patient can be fluid responsive regardless of their actual volume status.[3] In other words, "all hypovolemic patients are fluid responsive but not all fluid responsive patients are hypovolemic." Patients can still be fluid responsive when they are euvolemic or hypervolemic if they are in a state of recruitable SV, and nonresponsiveness to fluid also does not indicate hypervolemia.[5] Therefore, the use of static values to measure a volume status such as CVP and PAOP has been slowly decreased through the years.

Since the right ventricular (RV) stroke volume is equivalent to the left ventricular (LV) filling volume, the CVP has been thought of as an indirect measurement of LV preload. However, in critically ill patients, due to the changes in venous tone, intrathoracic pressures, and cardiac compliance, the correlation between the CVP and the actual RV end-diastolic volume may be poor.[2] As a result, many other techniques for assessing volume status and fluid responsiveness, such

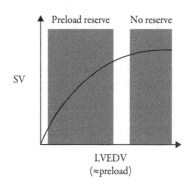

**Figure 167.1** Frank-Starling relationship. When the heart is functioning at the steep part of the curve, there is a reserve to recruit SV, which will increase SV with fluid administration. However, when the heart is functioning at the flat part of the curve, at the maximum capacity, there is no reserve to recruit more SV with fluid administration.

as echocardiography, global end-diastolic volume index measured by transpulmonary thermodilution, esophageal Doppler, pulse pressure variation (PPV), SV variation, pulse contour analysis, and end-expiratory occlusion test, have been gaining more popularity and are being studied more.[2,5] These dynamic monitoring modalities allow better estimation of the patient's position on the Frank-Starling curve and thus provide better prediction of their fluid responsiveness.[2]

## ESOPHAGEAL DOPPLER

Esophageal Doppler is a disposable probe that is about pencil-size thickness that emits continuous-wave ultrasound. It is inserted orally to the depth of the fifth/sixth thoracic vertebrae, and it measures the descending thoracic aortic blood flow. The Doppler provides a velocity versus time waveform, and the area under the curve represents the stroke distance. Then, the device converts the measurement using the patient's age, weight, and height to calculated variables such as SV, cardiac output (CO), and flow time. The esophageal Doppler is a validated method to assess CO, and goal-directed fluid therapies using esophageal Doppler have shown decreased complications and length of stay in high-risk surgical procedures.[1] Limitations of this modality include need of sedation and analgesia, operator dependence, need for probe adjustments, and unreliable results in patients with aortic pathologies.[3]

## PULSE PRESSURE VARIATION AND PULSE CONTOUR ANALYSIS

Pulse pressure (PP) is the difference between the systolic pressure and the diastolic blood pressure in a single cardiac cycle. PPV, systolic pressure variation (SPV), and stroke volume variation (SVV) are dynamic variables to assess fluid status and responsiveness, which are derived from arterial waveforms. The PPV is calculated using the difference between the maximum and the minimum PP as a proportion of the mean over a time period. The SPV is calculated by the difference between the systolic pressure during inspiration and expiration in one mechanical ventilatory cycle.[4] The SVV is calculated using the pulse contour analysis, which includes the area under the systolic pressure waveform and analysis of the shape of the waveform.[3] The principle for these techniques is derived from the simple physiology of heart and lung interaction. In a mechanically ventilated patient, increased intrathoracic pressure during inspiration results in decreased RV preload and increased RV afterload. This results in decreased LV SV, which is clinically seen in two to three beats later on the arterial line due to the pulmonary circulation time[2] (Figure 167.2). This results in decreased PP during expiration and increased PP during inspiration. This difference is exaggerated in a patient who is on the steep portion of the Frank-Starling curve (Figure 167.1), where there is room for SV recruitment. The PPV and SPV are directly measurable

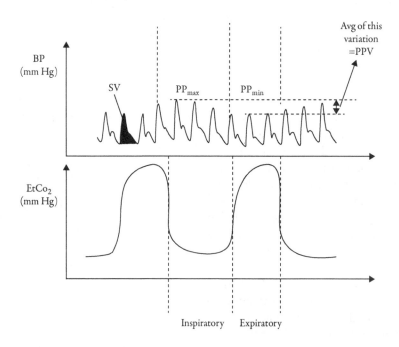

**Figure 167.2** Pulse pressure variation and stroke volume variation. During inspiration, RV preload decreases and RV afterload increases, which results in decreased stroke volume from LV. However, this effect is clinically seen during the expiratory phase due to the delay through pulmonary circulation. Therefore, maximum pulse pressure is seen during inspiration and minimum pulse pressure is seen during expiration. The PPV is calculated by taking the average of the difference between those two values in two to three beats. The SV is the area under the curve in arterial blood pressure monitoring.

using an arterial line waveform. However, the SVV is usually calculated by monitoring devices such as the PiCCO plus system (Pulsion Medical Systems, Munich, Germany); LiDCO plus technique (LiDCO Ltd., London, UK); or the FloTrac/Vigileo system (Edwards Lifesciences, Irvine, CA, USA). Each monitoring system uses a slightly different method to obtain the measurements, but the principle behind is that the area under the curve of systolic pressure corresponds to the SV. A meta-analysis done by Marik et al. showed that these dynamic variables predicted fluid response with high accuracy. The threshold of 11% to 13% of PPV, SVV, or SPV had a very high sensitivity and specificity in predicting fluid responsiveness. Furthermore, it also showed that PPV had more statistically significant diagnostic accuracy than the other variables. However, these variables have limitations. They are only consistently reliable when the tidal volume is about 8–10 mL/kg. Also, there are other conditions that can affect these variables such as open chest, arrhythmia, increased intra-abdominal pressures, elevated positive end-expiratory pressure, use of vasoactive drugs such as norepinephrine, and spontaneous breathing.[2]

## FLUID REPLACEMENT STRATEGIES AND CONTROVERSIES

With the widespread advocacy for enhanced recovery after surgery pathways, a multicenter study called Restrictive versus Liberal Fluid Therapy for Major Abdominal Surgery (RELIEF) trial emerged. This study showed a significantly higher risk of acute kidney injury with the restrictive intravenous fluid group. In conclusion, the authors suggested moderate fluid management with net positive fluid balance of 1 to 2 L at the end of surgery.[1]

Another angle to approach fluid management has been goal-directed therapy (GDT) using dynamic variables derived from advanced monitoring devices. The first large study on GDT was the OPTIMISE (Effect of a Perioperative, Cardiac Output-Guided Hemodynamic Therapy Algorithm on Outcomes Following Major Gastrointestinal Surgery), which was a multicenter trial that utilized CO-guided hemodynamic therapy in patients undergoing major abdominal surgeries. This study did not show any significant reduction in morbidity or mortality, but the study did show a statistically significantly decreased postoperative infection rate and the duration of hospital stay. More recently, the FEDORA trial (Effect of Goal directed haemdynamic therapy on postoperative complications in low-moderate risk surgical patients: a multicentre randomised controlled trial), which was another multicenter trial that utilized an esophageal Doppler monitor to guide hemodynamic therapy, also showed a decrease in hospital length of stay and complications such as acute kidney disease, pulmonary edema, wound infections, and respiratory distress syndrome.[1]

## REFERENCES

1. Miller TE, Myles PS. Perioperative fluid therapy for major surgery. *Anesthesiology*. 2019;130:825–832.
2. Marik PE, et al. Hemodynamic parameters to guide fluid therapy. *Ann Intensive Care*. 2011;1(1):1–9.
3. Van Der Mullen J, et al. Assessment of hypovolemia in the critically ill. Anesthesiol Intensive Therapy. 2018;50(2):150–159.
4. Marik PE, et al. Dynamic changes in arterial waveform derived variables and fluid responsiveness in mechanically ventilated patients: a systematic review of the literature. *Crit Care Med*. 2009;37(9):2642–2647.
5. Martin GS, et al. Perioperative Quality Initiative (POQI) consensus statement on fundamental concepts in perioperative fluid management: fluid responsiveness and venous capacitance. Perioper Med. 2020;9:1–12.

# 168.

## ESOPHAGEAL DOPPLER

*Roy Kim and Alaa Abd-Elsayed*

### INTRODUCTION

Esophageal Doppler monitoring measures blood flow velocity in the descending thoracic aorta using a flexible ultrasound probe that is much smaller than an ordinary transesophageal echocardiographic (TEE) probe; this makes it less invasive with a very good safety record (Figure 168.1). Using information about the patient (age, height, weight), one can estimate cardiac output and stroke volume by using a nomogram-based estimate of aortic cross-sectional area. In addition, intravascular volume status or preload of the left ventricle can be optimized by titrating fluid based on the Frank-Starling principle.[1-3]

With advancing age and increasing comorbidities in patients, the need for monitoring devices in the perioperative period is increasing; tracking variables such as cardiac output (CO), fluid responsiveness, and tissue perfusion is critical for good outcomes. Until recently, either pulmonary artery catheterization or TEE was the only tool available to anesthesiologists to monitor CO. Esophageal Doppler has proven itself to be a reliable, cost-effective, noninvasive tool for monitoring CO and guiding goal-directed therapy.[4]

### INDICATIONS

1. Surgery with large fluid shifts
2. High-risk patients
3. Hemodynamic instability

### CONTRAINDICATIONS

1. Presence of intra-aortic balloon pump
2. Severe coarctation of the aorta
3. Presence of pharyngoesophageal pathology
4. Severe bleeding

### PRINCIPLES

Esophageal Doppler is simply an ultrasound probe that uses the Doppler principle for measuring blood flow. A Doppler shift in frequency occurs when the ultrasound wave is reflected back from moving red blood cells, with the shift in frequency proportional to the velocity of blood flow.

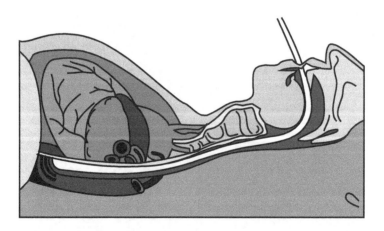

**Figure 168.1** Esophageal Doppler placement.

## INFORMATION OBTAINED

- Cardiac output (Q = SV × HR)
  SV is stroke volume, and HR is heart rate. Q is estimated by minute distance.
- Stroke volume is measured by stroke distance times the aortic root diameter.
  Stroke distance (AUC) × HR, linear cardiac output parameter, distance moved by a column of blood through the aorta in 1 minute (1200cm = high-flow state).
- Corrected (systolic) flow time FTc indicates preload
- Peak velocity (PV) indicates contractility
- Heart rate

## EVIDENCE

There have been no case reports of esophageal perforation during placement of an esophageal Doppler monitoring probe and only minor complications such as soft tissue mucosal trauma and endobronchial placement.[3] A frequent use for an intraoperative esophageal Doppler is to guide fluid replacement. A systematic review analyzing fluid replacement in major abdominal surgery from five studies and 420 patients found reduced hospital stay, fewer complications, fewer intensive care unit admissions, and fewer inotropes required in the intervention group (fluid treatment guided by monitoring ventricular filling via esophageal Doppler vs. conventional parameters).[1] Furthermore, another meta-analysis concluded that using esophageal Doppler monitoring can increase use of colloid fluid and reduce hospital length of stay, time to resume full oral diet or bowel function, and complications after major surgery.[3]

Numerous randomized controlled trials studying fluid optimization using esophageal Doppler have concluded significant positive outcomes in patients undergoing various surgeries, including gynecological cancer surgery, colorectal resection surgery, and laparoscopic surgery to name a few.[3] The Agency for Healthcare Research and Quality,[5] after reviewing over 300 articles, stated that the clinical evidence was strong for esophageal Doppler use in patients undergoing surgical procedures with expected substantial blood loss or fluid compartment shifts requiring fluid replacement. The Centers for Medicare and Medicaid Services (2007) determined it would provide reimbursement for esophageal Doppler use for monitoring CO for ventilated patients in the intensive care unit and operative patients with a need for intraoperative fluid optimization.[5]

## REFERENCES

1. Abbas SM, Hill AG. Systematic review of the literature for the use of esophageal Doppler monitor for fluid replacement in major abdominal surgery. *Anaesthesia*. 2008;63(1):44–51.
2. Marik PE. Pulmonary artery catheterization and esophageal Doppler monitoring in the ICU. *Chest*. 1999;116(4):1085–1091.
3. Phan TD, et al. Improving perioperative outcomes: fluid optimization with the esophageal Doppler monitor, a metaanalysis and review. *J Am Coll Surg*. 2008;207(6):935–941.
4. Funk DJ, et al. Minimally invasive cardiac output monitoring in the perioperative setting. *Anesth Analg*. 2009;108(3):887–897.
5. ECRI Evidence-Based Practice Center. *Esophageal Doppler Ultrasound-Based Cardiac Output Monitoring for Real-Time Therapeutic Management of Hospitalized Patients. A Review*. Prepared by the ECRI Evidence-based Practice Center under contract to the Agency for Healthcare Research and Quality (AHRQ). Contract No. 290-02-0019. Rockville, MD: AHRQ; January 16, 2007.

# 169.

# COMPLICATIONS OF TRANSURETHRAL RESECTION OF THE PROSTATE

*Jacob Justinger and Soozan S. Abouhassan*

## SURGICAL TECHNIQUE

For transurethral resection of the prostate (TURP), the patient is placed in lithotomy position. Small strips of hyperplastic tissue are removed from the periurethral zone of the prostate with a diathermy loop through a resectoscope. Efforts are made to spare the surgical capsule, though there is often not a well-defined surgical plane. Throughout the procedure, the bladder is continuously irrigated to remove surgical debris and allow for surgical visualization. The procedure typically lasts 30 to 90 minutes. At the completion of the procedure, a three-lumen catheter is placed, and irrigation is continued for up to 24 hours postoperatively.[1]

## ANESTHETIC CONSIDERATIONS

### PREOPERATIVE

As incidence of benign prostatic hyperplasia (BPH) increases with age, patients presenting for TURP are elderly, with an average age of 69, and a reported 77% have significant preexisting medical disease. Preoperative preparation should include evaluation and optimization of preexisting medical comorbidities.[1] Long-standing urinary outflow obstruction may result in clinically significant renal impairment. Patients treated with diuretic therapy may present with electrolyte abnormalities or dehydration.[1,2]

### INTRAOPERATIVE

Large volumes of irrigation are used in TURP procedures to dilate the bladder and clear debris. Typically, a hypo-osmolar solution of glycine, sorbitol, or glucose is used. Patients may absorb up to 30 mL of irrigating fluid per minute thru the prostatic venous sinuses. The amount and rate of fluid absorption are affected by the size of the gland, number of open sinuses, hydrostatic pressure of irrigation, duration of the procedure, and vascularity of the prostate.

Collectively, the symptoms that can be seen from absorption of large volumes of irrigation fluid are referred to as TURP syndrome. TURP syndrome occurs in 1% to 8% of cases, with onset from 15 minutes after resection begins up to 24 hours postoperatively.[1]

A variety of irrigation solutions are used each, with its own constellation of disadvantages. Distilled water, while inexpensive and electrically inert, can lead to hyponatremia, hemolysis, hemoglobinemia, and hemoglobinuria. Glycine solutions have a lower incidence of TURP syndrome but may result in hyperammonemia from glycine metabolism, hyperoxaluria, encephalopathy, transient postoperative visual syndrome, central nervous system, cardiac, and renal toxicity. Normal saline and lactated Ringer solutions, while posing a low risk of TURP syndrome, are ionized solutions and pose a risk of electrical conduction when used with electrocautery. Mannitol solutions result in an osmotic diuresis and intravascular expansion. Sorbitol solutions may result in osmotic diuresis, lactic acidosis, and hyperglycemia. Glucose solutions pose a risk of hyperglycemia. Urea solutions pose a risk of increased blood urea.[1,3]

Intravascular volume expansion occurs secondary to absorption of irrigation solution by the prostatic sinuses. This expansion in intravascular volume may result in pulmonary edema, congestive heart failure, and hyponatremia. The resultant hyponatremia may result in severe neurologic consequences, ranging from confusion to ventricular arrhythmia, seizure, and coma.[1,2]

Patients of advanced age are at increased risk of perioperatively hypothermia due to changes in body composition that occur with aging. The large volume of irrigation fluid used in TURP creates an active cooling process. The anesthetic provider must be proactive in monitoring and maintaining normothermia.[2]

Blood loss of approximately 500 mL is typical for a TURP procedure. However, the large volume of irrigation fluid used and the closed nature of the surgery makes intraoperative assessment of blood loss difficult. Visual assessment of the waste irrigation is an unreliable assessment, and advanced measures of quantifying blood loss such as hemoglobin concentration assay may be necessary. Factors increasing intraoperative blood loss include large gland (>60 g) and prolonged surgery time (greater than 1 hour) Additionally, large-volume irrigation can potentially disrupt normal coagulation through hemodilution or metabolic derangement. Further impairment of coagulation may occur secondary to urokinase release from the prostatic tissue, resulting in increased fibrinolysis. Approximately 8% of patients undergoing TURP will require transfusion.[1,2]

If TURP syndrome occurs, termination of the surgery and treatment of the sequelae should occur as quickly as possible. The patient should be intubated for airway protection and oxygenation. Fluid should be restricted with a discontinuation of intravenous fluids. Hypertonic saline may be indicated to correct symptomatic hyponatremia. Loop diuretics may be required to mitigate the effects of circulatory overload.[1,3]

Bladder perforation occurs in approximately 1% of cases due to surgical instrumentation or overdistention with fluid irrigation. Bladder perforation manifests as a sudden decrease in irrigation solution return, pain in the suprapubic region, generalized abdominal pain, shoulder tip pain, and abdominal rigidity.[1]

## POSTOPERATIVE

Postoperative complications can include painful bladder spasm, clot retention, ureteral stricture, erectile dysfunction, retrograde ejaculation, and bacteremia. Bacteremia and septicemia may occur secondary to release of bacteria from prostatic tissue, perioperative indwelling urinary catheter, or preoperative urinary tract infection.[2,4]

## REFERENCES

1. Aidan M. O'Donnell, Irwin T. H. Foo. Anaesthesia for transurethral resection of the prostate. *Continuing Education in Anaesth Crit Care Pain*. 2009;9(3):92–96. https://doi.org/10.1093/bjaceaccp/mkp012
2. Chrouser K, et al. Optimizing outcomes in Urologic Surgery. Retrieved from American Urological Association: https://www.auanet.org/
3. Open Anesthesia. TURP solutions—neuro complications. 2020. https://www.openanesthesia.org/aba_turp_solutions_-_neuro_complications/
4. Rassweiler J, Teber D, Kuntz R, Hofmann R. Complications of transurethral resection of the prostate (TURP)—incidence, management, and prevention. *Eur Urol*. 2006 Nov;50(5):969–79; discussion 980. doi:10.1016/j.eururo.2005.12.042. Epub 2006 Jan 30. PMID: 16469429.

# Part 15

# HEMATOLOGIC SYSTEM

# 170.

# ANEMIA

*Victoria Shapiro and Heather Brosnan*

## INTRODUCTION

Anemia is characterized by a decrease in red cell mass and clinically manifests as a decrease in circulating red blood cells (RBCs). The World Health Organization (WHO) definition is hemoglobin less than 12 g/dL in nonpregnant females and less than 13 g/dL in males and can be classified by morphology and average size of circulating RBCs or mean corpuscular volume (MCV).[1] The most common causes of chronic anemia are iron deficiency, anemia of chronic disease, thalassemia, and ongoing blood loss (Table 170.1). Preoperative anemia is a significant risk factor for blood transfusions, as well as an independent predictor of perioperative morbidity and mortality.[2] It has been associated with increased length of hospital stay and readmissions, infection risk, respiratory complications, kidney injury, and perioperative cardiac events.[1]

At a physiological level, a low RBC count decreases the oxygen-carrying capacity of blood, leading to decreased tissue oxygenation. Acutely, cardiac output increases secondary to enhanced sympathetic outflow, while eventually leading to high-output cardiac failure. There is also a rightward shift of the oxyhemoglobin dissociation curve to release oxygen from hemoglobin to the tissues.[3] Low hematocrit levels also decrease blood viscosity, which increases flow (Poiseille's law) and result in hypotension and contributes to reduced diffusing lung capacity for carbon monoxide on pulmonary function tests.

Clinical symptoms of anemia include fatigue, orthopnea, and dyspnea on exertion; poor exercise tolerance, lightheadedness, and dizziness. Patients can appear pale since blood is redistributed from skin and muscle to vital organs, or may appear jaundiced with scleral icteris in patients with hemolysis. Patients may be tachycardic and hypotensive due to hypovolemia or low blood viscosity, and hepatomegaly and splenomegaly may be palpated. Other signs and symptoms include melena due to gastrointestinal blood losses, pain due to sickle cell crisis, or neurological symptoms associated with $B_{12}$ deficiency.[1]

## DIAGNOSIS

Diagnosis starts with laboratory testing of hemoglobin and hematocrit levels, followed by MCV, ferritin, transferrin, iron levels, total iron-binding capacity, and reticulocyte counts. A peripheral smear can be helpful in determining the etiology of anemia, as is obtaining a menstrual history from female patients (e.g., menorrhagia). Orthostatic vitals can be helpful in estimating volume status in a patient with suspected hypovolemia and anemia due to blood loss.[1,2]

## TREATMENT

Treatment is based on the underlying cause. Oral and intravenous iron supplementation, $B_{12}$, and folate are recommended for deficiencies severe enough to cause anemia. Erythropoiesis stimulating agents can be considered for anemic patients without a nutritional deficiency, and are often administered to patients with chronic kidney disease during dialysis. Blood transfusion should be considered for patients with severe anemia, symptomatic patients, or those undergoing surgery, as per guidelines described below.[1,2]

## PERIOPERATIVE CONSIDERATIONS

### PREOPERATIVE

Routine preoperative hemoglobin and hematocrit levels are not recommended for healthy, asymptomatic patients. Laboratory work is warranted, however, in symptomatic patients; those with a history of anemia, bleeding, or other hematological disorder; liver disease; or based on type and invasiveness of the planned procedure, including anticipated risk of blood loss.[4] The underlying cause of anemia should be treated. In order to minimize intraoperative blood loss, patients should also be screened preoperatively for use of anticoagulants/antiplatelet agents and personal or family history of bleeding disorders. A type and screen should be done for patients undergoing procedures with increased bleeding risk, with a lower threshold for those with preoperative anemia.

## INTRAOPERATIVE

Ensure adequate ventilation and oxygenation and maintain cardiac output and blood pressure. Blood loss should be closely monitored and replaced as needed. The decision to transfuse should be based on the lost circulating blood volume, hemoglobin level, ongoing bleeding, and the risk of end-organ dysfunction due to hypoxemia. Calculating maximum allowable blood loss preoperatively can assist in monitoring blood loss and estimating a transfusion threshold (see the equation that follows). Restrictive transfusion protocols currently recommend transfusing for hemoglobin less than 7 g/dL in most patients and less than 8 g/dL in patients with cardiovascular or other risk factors; however, these guidelines are not absolute, and the physician should take into consideration the patient's hemodynamic status and rate of intraoperative blood loss when deciding the treatment plan. Liberal transfusion guidelines recommend transfusion for hemoglobin levels less than 10 g/dL. Generally, loss of more than 30%–40% of total blood volume requires RBC transfusion to restore oxygen-carrying capacity.[3] Cell salvage, hemodilution, hemostatic agents (e.g., tranexamic acid), and blood-conserving techniques should also be considered.[2] An arterial line may be necessary if multiple blood draws are anticipated to monitor intraoperative hemoglobin levels.

*Equation for maximum allowable blood loss* (MABL): EBV is estimated blood volume (estimates vary by source but can be approximated as 65 mL/kg for an adult female, 75 mL/kg for an adult male, 80 mL/kg for an infant, 85 mL/kg for a full-term neonate, and 95 mL/kg for a premature neonate. $H_{initial}$ is the patient's starting hemoglobin or hematocrit. $H_{final}$ is the lowest acceptable hemoglobin or hematocrit level specific to the patient and their comorbidities (a hemoglobin level of 7-8 g/dL or hematocrit of 20%–30% is commonly used academically).

## POSTOPERATIVE

Acute or chronic anemia should be on the differential diagnosis for hypotension and/or tachycardia in the postanesthesia care unit. Obtain laboratory tests to evaluate hemoglobin and hematocrit levels and coagulation status if there is concern for active bleeding. Ventilation and oxygenation should be optimized with supplemental oxygen if needed. Oxygen consumption should be minimized by ensuring adequate pain control and maintaining normothermia. Treatment for known preoperative anemia should continue in the postoperative period.[2]

## SICKLE CELL DISEASE

Sickle cell disease (SCD) is an inherited disorder of hemoglobin characterized by chronic hemolytic anemia, recurrent episodes of vaso-occlusion, and severe pain. In hemoglobin S (HbS), a valine is substituted for glutamic acid in the sixth amino acid position of the β-globulin chain.[5] Heterozygous mutations (HbS) cause a benign sickle cell trait, while homozygous mutation (HbSS) leads to a variable clinical course ranging from mild to severe, with vascular damage, organ failure, and early death.[5] Patients with SCD are also at risk for acute chest syndrome (vaso-occlusive crisis of the lungs), hypertension, restrictive lung disease, splenic infarct and fibrosis, renal insufficiency, cholelithiasis, stroke, and chronic pain. Patients at increased age, pregnant, or with active infections may be at increased risk for perioperative pain crisis or other SCD complications.[5]

Vaso-occlusive episodes occur due to deoxygenation of the hemoglobin molecules. Sickling occurs more in veins than arteries (pH dependent). Vaso-occlusive episodes involve multiple physiological pathways, including vasoconstriction, leukocyte adhesion and migration, platelet activation and adhesion, and coagulation, leading to blood vessel occlusion and tissue ischemia. Sickle cell crises and RBC sickling can be triggered by prolonged exposure to moderate hypoxia, acidosis, stasis, fever, infection, and hypovolemia.

Sickle cell disease is most commonly diagnosed by tests that compare the relative concentrations of hemoglobin variants, including hemoglobin electrophoresis and high-performance liquid chromatography. A positive result can be confirmed with genetic testing. Other tests including solubility tests (which rely on the low solubility of HbS) and peripheral blood smears can be used to screen for sickle cell, but are less accurate and do not differentiate between sickle cell trait and disease. In parts of the world where sickle cell disease and glucose-6-phosphate dehydrogenase (G6PD) deficiency have a high prevalence, a diagnosis of HbSS or HbSc may prompt testing for G6PD deficiency; however, this is not a worldwide recommendation.

Patients with HbSS have the following:

- Sickle cell is not diagnosed using a solubility test. Although it can be screened for with this test, it is not routinely done. Also, it is not recommended that patients diagnosed with sickle cell automatically undergo G6PD deficiency testing because the prevalence is low in most parts of the world. In locations where there is a high co-occurrence, it may be considered.
- While P50 in HbSS patients is higher than normal, it varies depending on the concentration of HbSS, and is closer to 30.

## PERIOPERATIVE CONSIDERATIONS FOR SICKLE CELL DISEASE

### Preoperative

Patients with SCD are at risk for sickle cell crisis, tissue ischemia, bleeding, and infarction during the perioperative period. Patients should be evaluated for SCD complications involving the lungs, spleen, kidneys, brain, and prior blood transfusions. A baseline complete blood count is helpful for assessing the severity of anemia, but it does not predict the risk of perioperative pain crises. Chest x-ray, $SpO_2$, and pulmonary function tests can be used to evaluate the extent of pulmonary involvement. Laboratory tests, including serum urea nitrogen, creatinine, and proteinuria, can be used to evaluate renal involvement. Patients with a history of blood transfusions should have a type and cross done preoperatively.[5]

### Intraoperative

Maintaining adequate oxygenation is critical for patients with SCD. Adequate hydration is also imperative to avoid vaso-occlusive crises and sickling. Blood loss should be monitored and replaced as needed, according to transfusion protocols as discussed previously. Intraoperative thermoregulation is important as hypothermia is associated with perioperative SCD complications. Acidosis may be associated with sickling.[5] Tourniquet use is relatively contraindicated.

### Postoperative

General postoperative care and oxygen supplementation help prevent hypoxemia and SCD complications.[5]

### REFERENCES

1. Kansagra AJ, Stefan MS. Preoperative anemia: evaluation and treatment. *Anesthesiol Clin.* 2016;34(1):127–141.
2. Goodnough LT, Shander A. Patient blood management. *Anesthesiology.* 2012;116(6):1367–1376.
3. Hines RL, Marschall KE. Hematologic disorders. In: *Stoelting's Anesthesia and Co-existing Disease.* Philadelphia, PA: Elsevier; 2018: Chap. 24.
4. Committee on Standards and Practice Parameters; Apfelbaum JL, et al. Practice advisory for preanesthesia evaluation: an updated report by the American Society of Anesthesiologists Task Force on Preanesthesia Evaluation. *Anesthesiology.* 2012;116(3):522–538.
5. Firth PG, Head CA. Sickle cell disease and anesthesia. *Anesthesiology.* 2004;101(3):766–785.

# 171.

# POLYCYTHEMIA

*Victoria Shapiro and Heather Brosnan*

## INTRODUCTION

Polycythemia is defined as an increase in hematocrit and hemoglobin in peripheral blood. Primary polycythemia or polycythemia vera is a myeloproliferative disorder that is due to an acquired mutation in red blood cell (RBC) progenitor cells. Myeloproliferative neoplasm is caused by a JAK2 (Janus kinase 2) mutation due to unknown etiology.[1] Secondary causes of polycythemia are often due to chronic hypoxemia, leading to increased serum levels of erythropoietin (EPO). EPO is a hormone produced mainly by the kidneys as a physiologic response to hypoxia, and it stimulates hematopoietic stem cells to produce new RBCs. Serum EPO levels are elevated in various disease processes, including sleep apnea; obesity hypoventilation syndrome (Pickwickian syndrome); chronic pulmonary disease (i.e., chronic obstructive pulmonary disease [COPD]); exposure to carbon monoxide (chronic smokers, engine exhaust); living or training at high altitude; cyanotic congenital heart defects in infants; EPO-secreting tumors; and renal disease (i.e., renal artery stenosis or following renal transplant).[2] Relative polycythemia can occur with hemoconcentration secondary to dehydration due to diuretics, vomiting, or diarrhea.[2]

Elevated hematocrit can present clinical challenges for multiple reasons. Patients with polycythemia are at increased risk for thrombotic events, including stroke, myocardial infarction, pulmonary embolism, and deep vein thrombosis (DVT), as well as excessive bleeding or bruising.[1,3] The increased hematocrit and hemoglobin lead to hyperviscosity, thereby decreasing blood flow per Poiseille's law. Although a slight increase in hemoglobin and hematocrit can increase the oxygen-carrying capacity of blood, hematocrit levels greater than about 50% can significantly impair microcirculation, resulting in decreased blood flow and net oxygen delivery to tissues. As viscosity and resistance to flow increase, the heart must work harder, leading to cardiac strain. Patients with polycythemia tend to actually be hypervolemic, which benefits the patient by lowering the blood viscosity, but presents a problem in treating these patients as removing red cell mass can also lower the viscosity, leading again to poor oxygen delivery.[2] Polycythemia can also be reflected on pulmonary function tests as an increase in the diffusing lung capacity for carbon monoxide.

## CLINICAL FEATURES

Patients with polycythemia may be asymptomatic, and detection is based on laboratory values; however, when severe enough to cause hyperviscosity with poor oxygen delivery, patients can present with fatigue, headaches, myalgias, cardiovascular symptoms (angina) or cerebral symptoms (confusion), thrombosis (both venous and arterial), and splenomegaly. Hypertension is common in patients with polycythemia and may be attributed to hyperviscosity and increased resistance to flow.[4] Thrombosis is one of the most common presenting symptoms and a significant cause of mortality in polycythemia vera; it can be attributed to not only venous stasis but also altered blood composition impacting normal coagulation.[3,4] Patients with secondary polycythemia tend to present with symptoms specific to the etiology, such as symptoms of sleep apnea (STOP-BANG) or altitude sickness. Neonates can present with elevated hematocrit due to a normal physiological response to intrauterine hypoxia; however, maternal diabetes and delayed cord clamping can lead to detrimentally high hematocrit levels. Clinical symptoms of hyperviscosity can be difficult to detect in infants.[2]

## DIAGNOSIS

Polycythemia is diagnosed based on elevated hemoglobin or hematocrit levels. Polycythemia vera is diagnosed based on World Health Organization (WHO) criteria and includes testing for JAK2 mutations. The following are the 2016 revised WHO criteria for polycythemia vera[1]:

1. Hemoglobin greater than 16 g/dL in women or greater than 16.5 g/dL in men; hematocrit greater than 48% in women or greater than 49% in men; or increased red blood cell mass.
2. Bone marrow tri-lineage proliferation with pleomorphic mature megakaryocytes.
3. Presence of JAK2 mutation.

Laboratory testing for JAK2 mutations is highly sensitive and specific and considered a reliable way to differentiate polycythemia vera from other causes of polycythemia.[1]

## TREATMENT

Treatment for primary polycythemias involves phlebotomy to reduce hematocrit levels below 45% in both males and females and selective use of aspirin. Patients with polycythemia vera can be further risk stratified for thrombotic events: High-risk patients include those over 60 years old and/or those who have a history of a thrombotic event. Low-risk patients with neither risk factor but with microvascular symptoms, cardiovascular risk factors, or leukocytosis can be administered aspirin therapy. Those who are at high risk should be treated with cytoreductive therapy with hydroxyurea and either aspirin (arterial thrombotic history) or systemic anticoagulation (venous thrombosis history). Patients who are resistant or intolerant to hydroxyurea can be treated with pegylated interferon α, busulfan, or ruxolitinib.[1]

Treatment for secondary polycythemias is focused on treating the underlying cause. Once resolved, the patient's hemoglobin and hematocrit levels normalize relatively quickly. For example, treatment with continuous positive airway pressure for obstructive sleep apnea, or weight loss for obesity hypoventilation syndrome tends to result in normalization of hemoglobin and hematocrit values.[2]

## PERIOPERATIVE CONSIDERATIONS

The anesthetic goal is to avoid perioperative complications from thrombosis or hemorrhage.

### PREOPERATIVE

In a patient with elevated hematocrit, phlebotomy can be used to reduce hematocrit levels to 45%. Hemodilution can also be considered, but caution must be exercised as the patient may be hypervolemic. On the contrary, patients with severe hypoxia may need fluid replacement after phlebotomy to maintain adequate volume. For this reason, preoperative fasting should be optimized to minimize dehydration and IV fluids should be continued while fasting. Preoperative platelet count can be a helpful indicator in assessing bleeding risk. Any patient with secondary polycythemia should have a workup for the primary cause since the underlying condition may increase the risk for other anesthetic complications, including those associated with sleep apnea, obesity, COPD, renal disease, and heart defects.[4]

## INTRAOPERATIVE

Intraoperative management should focus on maintaining adequate ventilation to avoid hypoxia as any degree of hypoxia in patients with polycythemia results in a greater total amount of desaturated hemoglobin, thus shortening the time to cyanosis. The anesthesiologist should remain vigilant and replace intraoperative blood loss with intravenous fluid or blood products as indicated to maintain tissue perfusion. DVT prophylaxis should be chosen according to the patient's thrombotic risk and surgical bleeding risk; if a patient is at high risk for thrombosis, heparin infusion can be considered.[4]

## POSTOPERATIVE

Postoperative DVT risk should be mitigated with DVT prophylaxis and early ambulation. Neurological or stroke evaluation should be considered in patients who do not wake up.[4]

## REFERENCES

1. Tefferi A, Barbui T. Polycythemia vera and essential thrombocythemia: 2019 update on diagnosis, risk-stratification and management. *Am J Hematol*. 2019;94(1):133–143. doi:10.1002/ajh.25303
2. Prchal JT. Primary and secondary erythrocytoses. In: Kaushansky K, et al., eds. *Williams Hematology*. 9th ed. McGraw-Hill; 2015.
3. Kwaan HC, Wang J. Hyperviscosity in polycythemia vera and other red cell abnormalities. *Semin Thromb Hemost*. 2003;29(5):451–458. doi:10.1055/s-2003-44552
4. Cundy J. The perioperative management of patients with polycythaemia. *Ann R Coll Surg Engl*. 1980;62(6):470–475.

# 172.

# THROMBOCYTOPENIA AND THROMBOCYTOPATHY

*Victoria Shapiro and Michael Chang*

## INTRODUCTION

Hemostasis and coagulation are parts of a complex process of bleeding cessation requiring a combination of vascular factors, platelets, and plasma coagulation factors. In primary hemostasis, endothelial injury acts as a thrombogenic nidus initiating platelet activation, adhesion, and aggregation, resulting in a hemostatic plug. In secondary hemostasis, the initial platelet plug is stabilized by fibrin, the end product of the blood coagulation cascade. Thrombocytes are biconvex, discoid-shaped cells derived in the bone marrow and play a fundamental role in hemostasis. Disease processes that contribute to thrombocytopenia (platelet count $< 150 \times 10^9/\text{L}$) or thrombocytopathy may lead to significant bleeding tendency.

## HEMOSTASIS

### PRIMARY HEMOSTASIS

In response to an endothelial injury, local vasoconstriction occurs to reduce blood flow. The exposed collagen of the extracellular matrix releases inflammatory mediators and becomes highly thrombogenic, which serves to promote the formation of a hemostatic plug via platelet adhesion, activation, and aggregation. Adhesion is mediated by von Willibrand factor (VWF) that binds to glycoproteins (GP1b) on the platelet surface. Once adhered, platelets become activated and undergo conformational changes to express the GP2b3a glycoprotein in their membrane to promote further platelet adhesion and aggregation. Platelets then degranulate, releasing numerous substances that contribute to hemostasis and coagulation. These substances include serotonin, adenosine diphosphate (ADP), and calcium, among many others.

## SECONDARY HEMOSTASIS

Secondary hemostasis involves interaction of blood proteins or coagulation factors that form cascading enzymatic complexes that result in the conversion of prothrombin to thrombin via the extrinsic pathway. Thrombin then facilitates enzymatic reactions via the intrinsic pathway, which results in the formation of fibrin monomers. These monomers then polymerize and cross-link with the platelet plug, thereby stabilizing it.

# THROMBOCYTOPENIA

## MECHANISM

Platelets are produced by megakarocytes in the bone marrow and removed by macrophages within our spleen. Platelets can also be targeted for destruction once in circulation. Therefore, thrombocytopenia can be classified into three causes: decreased production, increased destruction, and increased splenic sequestration. Platelet production

*Table 172.1* CLASSIFICATION OF
THROMBOCYTOPENIA BY MECHANISM

| DECREASED PRODUCTION | INCREASED DESTRUCTION | SPLENIC SEQUESTRATION |
| --- | --- | --- |
| Aplastic Anemia | DIC | Portal hypertension with splenomegaly |
| MDS | TTP | Cirrhosis with congestive splenomegaly |
| Leukemia | HIT | Gaucher disease |
| DITP | DITP | Myelofibrosis with myeloid metaplasia and splenomegaly |
| ITP | ITP | Viral infections with splenomegaly |

Abbreviations: DIC, disseminated intravascular coagulation; DITP, drug-induced immune thrombocytopenia; HIT, heparin-induced thrombocytopenia; ITP, immune thrombocytopenic purpura; MDS, myelodysplastic syndrome; TTP, thrombotic thrombocytopenic purpura.

Reprinted with permission from Marina Izak and James B. Bussel. Management of Thrombocytopenia. F1000Prime Rep 2014, 6:45. Table 1

deficiencies include bone marrow failure syndromes (e.g., aplastic anemia and myelodysplastic syndrome) and bone marrow–occupying diseases (e.g., leukemia/lymphoma). Ineffective thrombopoiesis is seen in patients with vitamin $B_{12}$ or folate deficiency (alcoholism) and defective folate metabolism. Increased platelet consumption and destruction is secondary to prothrombotic states that commonly occur in the microvasculature (e.g., disseminated intravascular coagulation, heparin-induced thrombocytopenia [HIT], and thrombotic thrombocytopenic purpura [TTP]). Lastly, increased platelet sequestration by the spleen results in splenomegaly. Portal hypertension is a common culprit and causes include heart failure, hepatic vein/vena cava thrombosis, and cirrhosis.

## HEPARIN-INDUCED THROMBOCYTOPENIA

Thrombocytopenia in the setting of heparin therapy or a decrease in platelet numbers by more than 50% from baseline should be investigated for HIT, which typically occurs within 5 to 10 days of initiating therapy. However, patients with a prior HIT history or a recent exposure to heparin can develop clinical symptoms immediately. There are two forms of HIT. HIT1 is clinically benign and does not involve immune complexes. Conversely, HIT2 is immune mediated and disposes the patient to significant risk of hypercoagulability. In this variation, immunoglobulin G antibodies bind to heparin-platelet factor 4 complexes on the platelet surface, resulting in primary hemostasis and thrombosis. Patients suspected of HIT should have heparin therapy discontinued immediately and started on alternative anticoagulation.

## IMMUNE THROMBOCYTOPENIC PURPURA

Immune thrombocytopenic purpura (ITP) is a type of isolated thrombocytopenia with no signs or symptoms of systemic illness, also known as autoimmune idiopathic thrombocytopenic purpura. It is generally a diagnosis of exclusion, and most cases of ITP do not require treatment. Spontaneous remission in children is common. Patients with chronic ITP have platelet counts of $20–100 \times 10^9$/L. In adults, treatment initiation is suggested when platelets are less than $30 \times 10^9$/L while taking clinical factors into consideration (bleeding tendency, comorbidities, etc.). Severe ITP associated with bleeding is a medical emergency and should be treated with high-dose corticosteroids. For patients with intracranial hemorrhage and requiring emergency surgery, intravenous immunoglobulin and platelet transfusion should be administered every 8–12 hours.[1,2]

Patients with chronic ITP and platelet count less than $10–20 \times 10^9$/L may benefit from splenectomy since about half will achieve permanent remission postoperatively.

## THROMBOTIC THROMBOCYTOPENIA PURPURA

Thrombotic thrombocytopenic purpura (TTP) is characterized by microangiopathic hemolysis and formation of platelet-rich thrombi in arterial and capillary microvasculature vessels, leading to multiorgan ischemia/failure. TTP has a high mortality rate. Clinical symptoms include a pentad of fever, hemolytic anemia, thrombocytopenia, renal failure, and neurologic dysfunction. Coagulopathy in these patients should be treated with transfusion of red blood cells and plasma. First-line therapy is plasmapheresis in conjunction with glucocorticoids.

## GESTATIONAL THROMBOCYTOPENIA

Regarding gestational thrombocytopenia, the average platelet count is decreased during pregnancy, most significantly in the third trimester. This is a result of increasing plasma volume leading to hemodilution and elevated thromboxane levels causing increased platelet aggregation. Moderate-to-severe thrombocytopenia may also present with HELLP syndrome, which is named for the triad of hemolysis, elevated liver enzymes, and low platelet count.

## THROMBOCYTOPATHY

Platelets rely on receptor sites on their membranes to facilitate adhesion to the subendothelial injury site as well as to aggregate with other platelets. Therefore, qualitative dysfunctions that impair platelets' ability to adhere and aggregate can cause coagulopathy. Qualitative thrombocytopathy can be either hereditary or secondary to acquired factors such as uremia, liver disease, extracorporeal circulation, and medications (e.g., nonsteroidal anti-inflammatory drugs [NSAIDs], etc.).

## ACQUIRED THROMBOCYTOPATHY

**Chronic Liver Disease:** In addition to increased platelet sequestration as a result of congestive splenomegaly in patients with advanced cirrhosis and chronic liver disease, platelets in this patient population have been shown to be immature (not activated) and have decreased aggregation abilities.[3] Platelet dysfunction resulting from high levels of circulating fibrin degradation products can increase the bleeding tendency.[2] Also, decreased production of factor VII and/or low-grade chronic disseminated intravascular coagulation with increased fibrinolysis can contribute to coagulopathy.

**Uremia:** Uremic toxins in patients with end-stage renal disease cause platelet dysfunction by affecting the glycoprotein that facilitates aggregation, GP2b3a, and by inducing endothelial cell nitric oxide release. Overall, platelet adhesion, activation, and aggregation are abnormal, and thromboxane $A_2$ generation is decreased. Defect in platelet function correlates with the severity of the uremia and anemia. Treatment with desmopressin (DDAVP) or initiation of dialysis is recommended in these patients if they are actively bleeding or about to undergo an invasive procedure.

**Extracorporeal Blood Circulation:** Transient platelet aggregation dysfunction has been observed in patients who have been exposed to extracorporeal blood circulation like hemodialysis, cardiopulmonary bypass, and extracorporeal membrane oxygenation.

**Medication Induced:** Antiplatelet drugs target different elements of platelet function, leading to impairment in coagulation. Aspirin/NSAIDs block the formation of thromboxane $A_2$. Clopidogrel/ticlopidine antagonize ADP receptors. Abciximab antagonizes GP2b3a receptors.

## HEREDITARY THROMBOCYTOPATHY

**Bernard-Soulier Syndrome:** Bernard-Soulier syndrome is an autosomal recessive disorder with an abnormality of the GP1b receptor, leading to impairment of platelet adhesion to VWF at the site of endothelial injury.

**Glanzmann's Thrombasthenia:** Glanzmann's thrombasthenia is an autosomal recessive disorder with a defect in the platelet integrin Gp2b/3a receptor, impairing platelet aggregation.

**Von Willibrand's Disease (VWD):** von Willibrand's disease is the most common hereditary bleeding disorder, with a prevalence of 1% in the general population. VWF is a large multimeric protein that facilitates platelet adhesion to the subendothelium through interaction with the GP1b receptor on the surface of the platelet. VWF also serves as a stability complex for factor VIII and helps localize it to the site of injury. There are three types of VWD. Types 1 and 3 are quantitative deficiencies of VWF, with type 3 being the most severe and rare. Type 2 describes qualitative dysfunction of VWF and can be further classified depending on the functional deficit. Management of patients depends on the type of VWD, its severity, and surgical procedure. First-line treatment of VWD is DDAVP. Antifibrinolytics and VWF/factor VIII concentrates may be required for those who do not respond to DDAVP.

## ANESTHETIC CONSIDERATIONS

### PREOPERATIVE

Preoperatively, it is recommended to bring the platelet count greater than $50 \times 10^9$/L. Patients undergoing ocular or neurosurgery should maintain platelets greater than $100 \times 10^9$/L.[4]

### INTRAOPERATIVE

Patients with thrombocytopenia are at a higher intraoperative risk of surgical hemorrhage/bleeding. The transfusion threshold for the actively bleeding surgical patient is $50 \times 10^9$/L. During massive transfusions, the suggested platelet transfusion threshold is $75 \times 10^9$/L to combat the hemodilution that occurs as a result of the large volume of transfused red cells.[4]

Thrombocytopathy may also occur secondary to extracorporeal circulation, such as dialysis or cardio-pulmonary bypass. If bleeding is observed to be out of proportion to the preoperative platelet level, qualitative deficiency of platelets should be suspected and platelet transfusion initiated.

## REFERENCES

1. Izak M, Bussel JB. Management of thrombocytopenia. *F1000Prime Rep.* 2014;6:45.
2. Hines RL, Marschall KE. Hematologic disorders. In: *Stoelting's Anesthesia and Co-existing Disease.* Philadelphia, PA: Elsevier; 2018: Chap. 24.
3. Witters P, et al. Review article: blood platelet number and function in chronic liver disease and cirrhosis. *Aliment Pharmacol Ther.* 2008;27(11):1017–1029.
4. Liumbruno G, et al.; Italian Society of Transfusion Medicine and Immunohaematology (SIMTI) Work Group. Recommendations for the transfusion of plasma and platelets. *Blood Transfus.* 2009;7(2):132–150.

# 173.

# CONGENITAL AND ACQUIRED FACTOR DEFICIENCIES

*Meghan C. Hughes and Alaa Abd-Elsayed*

## INTRODUCTION

Hemophilia A and B both result in lifelong bleeding disorders. Treatment and therapy for these disorders have changed dramatically over time and have led to significantly improved care for individuals. Synthetic factor replacement has allowed for wide availability and access to standard treatment regimens while minimizing the risk of viral illnesses (hepatitis C virus, HIV) related to repetitive blood transfusions. Regardless, treatment for this disease remains complex with a wide range of severity. Optimal management is challenging and requires continual adjustments.

The most common autoantibodies (acquired factor deficiencies) are those formed against the activity of factor VIII. Why someone develops acquired factor deficiencies remains elusive, but it may be linked to the presence of certain gene polymorphisms.[1] What is clear is that there are identifiable risk factors for developing factor deficiencies, which include pregnancy and the postpartum period as well as various autoimmune diseases, such as rheumatoid arthritis and systemic lupus erythematosus.

For any hemophiliac, the goal of care is to treat any bleeding episode with the specific factor replacement as needed. Patients with hemophilia are often on lifelong continuous factor therapy. Factor replacement is extremely expensive and can be an obstacle to treatment. For instance, the cost of maintenance therapy for a pediatric patient has been estimated to be over $100,000 per year, and this cost is ever increasing since these therapies are dosed by weight.

## CLINICAL FEATURES

Clinical manifestations of congenital or acquired factor deficiencies all relate to bleeding from impaired homeostasis, manifestations from bleeding itself, or complications related to factor infusions. The severity of the disease largely dictates the presentation of the patient.

Patients with the more severe hemophilia are more likely to have spontaneous and severe bleeding as well as an earlier age of their first bleeding episode. Bleeding episodes can occur as early as birth[2] and are often seen with procedures such as circumcision. In all patients with factor deficiencies, immediate and delayed bleeding are possible. This bleeding can be unpredictable and insidious in nature. Due to the increased use of prophylactic factor administration, there has been a general decline of bleeding to the point where some patients with severe disease may never actually experience a severe bleeding event if managed appropriately with access to correct medications.

The hallmark sign of acquired factor VIII antibodies is bleeding, which is first noted after a surgical procedure. Newly symptomatic patients will present with large hematomas, severe mucosal bleeding, or extensive ecchymosis of unknown causes. Patients with acquired factor deficiencies are less likely to experience hemoarthrosis.

Although intracranial hemorrhage is rare when compared to other sites of bleeding in patients with hemophilia, it is one of the most dangerous and life-threatening events in these individuals. It can occur in any individual suffering from congenital or acquired factor deficiencies, at any age, spontaneously or after trauma.

## DIAGNOSIS

The diagnosis of any factor deficiency disorder should begin with clinical observations. Hemophilia is an X-linked disorder and therefore much more common in men. Hemophilia should be suspected in any male with a bleeding history and positive family history. This clinical suspicion must then be supported by codified diagnostic criteria.

Recall that factor VIII is part of the intrinsic pathway of the clotting cascade and directly affects factor X when activated. The position of factor VIII in the clotting cascade will cause the hemophiliac to have prolonged partial thromboplastin time (PTT) and normal prothrombin (PT). Barring other pathology, platelet levels should be within normal limits.

**Hemophilia A (VIII Deficiency):** Factor VIII activity level must be below 40% of normal and/or a pathogenic factor VIII gene mutation must be identified. A normal von Willebrand factor (VWF) antigen should also be documented to eliminate the possibility of some form of von Willebrand disease as this stabilizes factor VIII, and dysfunction with VWF could lead to dysfunction with VIII. A laboratory test will show an increased PTT with normal international normalized ratio (INR).

**Hemophilia B (IX deficiency):** Hemophilia B requires confirmation of factor IX activity level below 40% or normal and/or pathogenic factor IX gene mutation. Keep in mind that newborns will naturally have a lower range for factor IX since it is a vitamin K–dependent factor. Laboratory tests will show an increased PTT with normal INR.

Suspicion for acquired factor VIII inhibitors (acquired hemophilia) should be high when any older individual shows up with sudden, large hematomas or extensive ecchymosis in the setting of no significant trauma or known bleeding disorder. Once clinical suspicion has been aroused, the patient should be evaluated using activated partial thromboplastin time (aPTT) and PT. In the case of acquired hemophilia, the aPTT should be prolonged and the PT should be normal. The presence of heparin use must be excluded in these patients by review of home medications and/or a blood test for this drug itself.

## ANESTHESIA CONSIDERATIONS

Any patient with a congenital or acquired factor deficiency is at a high risk for perioperative bleeding.

### PREOPERATIVE

Preoperative testing should allow for high risk of perioperative bleeding. Factor optimization via replacement or supplementation must be obtained prior to actual surgery and will be critical for surgical hemostasis. Management of factor replacement by a hematologist is recommended. These patients may be contraindicated for neuraxial anesthesia.

### INTRAOPERATIVE

Be aware that these patients can bleed into enclosed spaces: joints, intracranial, pericardium, or thorax. Vital signs should be monitored closely intraoperatively. Blood loss should be minimized during any procedure, and blood conservation strategies should be utilized. Adequate factor replacement should be maintained to ensure hemodynamic stability.

Caution has been issued in respect to induction with succinylcholine as fasciculations could precipitate bleeding.[3] Ensuring adequate depth of anesthesia to avoid airway trauma is also of critical importance. World Federation of Hemophilia guidelines recommend avoiding intramuscular injections and treating the veins of a hemophilia patient with extreme care because they are considered their lifeline (administration route of factor replacement).[4] Utilization of ultrasound should be done early and often since avoiding multiple punctures is pragmatic. Intraoperative management of anesthesia should be focused on minimizing hypertension and tachycardia to subsequently minimize bleeding.[5]

### POSTOPERATIVE

The risk of delayed bleeding at the surgical site is of utmost postoperative concern, and careful monitoring is imperative. The patient's hematologist should be involved in managing the laboratory studies conducted after any procedure so that peak/trough levels of factor VIII are adequate.

## REFERENCES

1. Mahendra A, et al. Do proteolytic antibodies complete the panoply of the autoimmune response in acquired haemophilia A? *Br J Haematol.* 2012;156(1):3–12.
2. Franchini M, et al. Mild hemophilia A. *J Thromb Haemost.* 2010;8(3):421–432.
3. Sethi M, Gurha P. Perioperative management of a patient with haemophilia-A for major abdominal surgery. *Indian J Anesth.* 2017;61(4):354–355.
4. Srivastava A, et al. Guidelines for the management of hemophilia. *Haemophilia.* 2013;19(1):e1–e47.
5. Shah UJ, et al. Anaesthetic considerations in patients with inherited disorders of coagulation. *Contin Educ Anaesth Crit Care Pain.* 2015;15(1):26–31.

# 174.

# DISSEMINATED INTRAVASCULAR COAGULATION

*Gretchen A. Lemmink and Jay Conhaim*

## INTRODUCTION

Disseminated intravascular coagulation (DIC) is an inappropriate, systemic activation of the clotting cascade that leads to diffuse thrombosis and, subsequently, hemorrhage.

## PATHOPHYSIOLOGY

The International Society on Thrombosis and Hemostasis (ISTH) defines DIC as "an acquired syndrome characterized by the intravascular activation of coagulation with loss of localization arising from different causes. It can originate from and cause damage to the microvasculature, which if sufficiently severe, can produce organ dysfunction" (p. 2).[1] The development of DIC cannot occur without an inciting disease process, thus making it a complication of an underlying systemic condition. Identification and treatment of the inciting illness is the linchpin of DIC therapy. Sepsis is the most common inciting condition, with 30%–50% of septic patients manifesting DIC.[2] Additional clinical conditions associated with DIC can be found in Table 174.1. There are two types of DIC, typically classified as latent and overt.[1-3] This review primarily discusses overt DIC, which is a consequence of the failure of clotting factor and platelet synthesis to keep pace with consumption.

Following an initial systemic insult, excessive tissue factor is produced that activates factor VII and the extrinsic clotting pathway. Thrombin is activated and cleaves fibrinogen to fibrin, completing the transition to a prothrombotic state. The resulting fibrin deposition and platelet activation in the absence of endothelial damage leads to diffuse microvascular

*Table 174.1* CLINICAL CONDITIONS OTHER THAN SEPSIS THAT PREDISPOSE A PATIENT TO DEVELOP DIC

| Trauma[a] | • Traumatic brain injury<br>• Burns<br>• Fat embolism |
|---|---|
| Cancers | • Hematologic malignancy (e.g., APL)<br>• Solid tumors (e.g., colorectal, pancreatic, gastric) |
| Obstetrical complications | • Placental abruption<br>• AFE<br>• IUFD<br>• Eclampsia<br>• HELLP syndrome |
| Acute inflammatory conditions | • Acute pancreatitis<br>• Transplant rejection<br>• ABO incompatible transfusion |

APL, acute promyelocytic leukemia; AFE, amniotic fluid embolism; IUFD, intrauterine fetal demise; HELLP, hemolysis, elevated liver enzyme levels, low platelet count.

Adapted from References 2 and 3.

[a]ANY traumatic tissue injury (including surgery) can lead to DIC.

thrombi and diminished end-organ perfusion.[2] As abnormal clotting progresses, fibrin degradation products form that further compromise the function of a dwindling platelet reserve. Excessive thrombin activation also acts as an immunologic stimulant, leading to increased cytokine production (e.g., tumor necrosis factor $\alpha$, interleukins 1 and 6). Proinflammatory cytokines have a further inhibitory effect on circulating platelets, worsening existing bleeding despite the overall prothrombotic state.[1,2] This systemic inflammation also stifles the function of endogenous anticoagulants such as antithrombin, protein C, and tissue factor pathway inhibitor. Such unrestrained factor consumption coupled with diminished platelet function manifests as hemorrhage from multiple distant sites. In acute DIC, hemorrhage is often the initial clinical symptom leading to diagnosis.[2]

## DIAGNOSIS

No gold standard laboratory test exists for the diagnosis of DIC.[2,3] A decline in platelet number and function is the most common laboratory feature of DIC.[4] While DIC can result in severe thrombocytopenia with platelets less than $50 \times 10^3/$ $\mu$L, it can also manifest a much milder form of thrombocytopenia, with some patients maintaining platelet numbers in the normal range.[2,3] Overall, it is the platelet trend that is significant and not necessarily the absolute value. Other markedly abnormal laboratory values (e.g., prothrombin time [PT], activated partial thromboplastin time [aPTT], serum fibrinogen, and fibrin degradation markers such as D-dimer) can be present; however, these assays may also be only slightly anomalous despite ongoing, worsening DIC.[2]

Due to the heterogeneity of laboratory values associated with DIC, the ISTH established a scoring algorithm to aid in the diagnosis. The algorithm is predicated on the patient having a disease process that is known to result in DIC (see Table 174.2). If a patient has a score of 5 or greater, then their clinical and laboratory data are compatible with overt DIC.[1,3] A score of less than 5 does not rule out DIC, and if there is a high clinical suspicion,

then ongoing evaluation of global coagulation tests is warranted. The use of thromboelastography (TEG; or rotational thromboelastometry) in the diagnosis of DIC is not validated; however, practitioners facile in the interpretation of TEG may find the diagnostic modality a useful addition to the screening assays for DIC found in Table 174.2. In DIC secondary to sepsis, a reduction in cascade factors will result in prolonged clot formation time, fibrinogen consumption will decrease the $\alpha$-angle, and platelet consumption with inhibition will decrease the maximum amplitude/maximum clot firmness.[5]

## TREATMENT

Successful treatment of DIC requires both swift identification of the coagulation aberrancy and simultaneous diagnosis and treatment of the underlying inciting disease. If progression of the underlying illness is halted, the associated DIC may spontaneously resolve. In overt DIC associated with active hemorrhage, the transfusion of blood products plays an important role in management. Thresholds for transfusion are based on guideline recommendations in patients who are actively bleeding or at high risk to do so. Prophylactic use of blood component therapy in DIC based on laboratory values alone is not advised. Platelets should be transfused to a threshold greater than $50 \times 10^3/\mu$L in a patient who is at risk for or who is actively bleeding and to a threshold greater than $20 \times 10^3/\mu$L if bleeding risk is low.[2] If fresh frozen plasma (FFP), cryoprecipitate, or packed red blood cells are indicated based on bleeding risk and laboratory evaluation, then they should also be administered.[2] Prothrombin complex concentrates can be considered in situations where FFP transfusion is ill-advised; however, they may increase the risk of thrombotic complications. Any use of blood component therapy in DIC requires ongoing serial coagulation assays to assess treatment success/failure.

Use of anticoagulants in patients with DIC dominated by thrombosis is advised at therapeutic doses and should be considered in these patients without signs of active bleeding.

*Table 174.2* INTERNATIONAL SOCIETY ON THROMBOSIS AND HEMOSTASIS SCORING SYSTEM FOR EVALUATION OF DIC

| PLATELET COUNT | D-DIMER | PROTHROMBIN TIME | FIBRINOGEN LEVEL |
|---|---|---|---|
| >100 × 10³/μL = 0 | No increase = 0 | <3 seconds = 0 | >1.0 g/L = 0 |
| <100 × 10³/μL = 1 | Moderate increase = 1 | >3 seconds = 1 | <1 g/L = 1 |
| <50 × 10³/μL = 2 | Strong increase = 2 | >6 seconds = 2 | |

The numerical score is additive, and a sum greater than or equal to 5 can support the diagnosis of DIC when used in the appropriate clinical context.

Adapted from Reference 2.

Low-molecular-weight heparin is the preferred agent.[2,3] Anticoagulant effect should be closely monitored with drug-specific anti-Xa levels.[2] Inhibition of the coagulation cascade through administration of natural anticoagulants (antithrombin or activated protein C) has not been shown to improve patient outcomes in multiple trials.[2] Finally, the utilization of antifibrinolytics is not recommend in DIC.[3]

## ANESTHETIC CONSIDERATIONS

Preoperative screening assays (e.g., aPTT/PT, fibrinogen, and D-dimer) should be obtained in any patient presenting to the operating theater with an underlying disorder that places them at elevated risk for developing either overt or latent DIC. Coagulopathy should be corrected with blood component therapy as time permits prior to proceeding to the operating room. Ongoing transfusion and evaluation of the patient's coagulopathy will be required throughout surgery. Postoperatively, these patients will have an elevated risk for hemorrhage.

## REFERENCES

1. Taylor FB Jr, et al. Scientific Subcommittee on Disseminated Intravascular Coagulation (DIC) of the International Society on Thrombosis and Haemostasis (ISTH). Towards definition, clinical and laboratory criteria, and a scoring system for disseminated intravascular coagulation. *Thromb Haemost.* 2001;86(5):1327–1330.
2. Papageorgiou C, et al. Disseminated intravascular coagulation: an update on pathogenesis, diagnosis, and therapeutic strategies. *Clin Appl Thromb Hemost.* 2018;24(9 suppl):8S–28S.
3. Wada H, et al. Guidance for diagnosis and treatment of DIC from harmonization of the recommendations from three guidelines. *J Thromb Haemost.* 2013;10.1111/jth.12155.
4. Levi M, Meijers JC. DIC: which laboratory tests are most useful. *Blood Rev.* 2011;25(1):33–37.
5. Sivula M, et al. Thromboelastometry in patients with severe sepsis and disseminated intravascular coagulation. *Blood Coagul Fibrinolysis.* 2009;20(6):419–426.

# 175.

# FIBRINOLYSIS

*Colby B. Tanner and Elaine A. Boydston*

## PHYSIOLOGY OF CLOT FORMATION AND DEGRADATION

Clot formation, maintenance, and degradation is a tightly regulated physiologic process that controls hemostasis. Following vascular endothelial injury, the intrinsic and extrinsic coagulation pathways are initiated, ultimately leading to conversion of coagulation factor X to Xa. Once formed, factor Xa forms a component of the prothrombinase complex, resulting in the conversion of prothrombin to thrombin. Following its formation, thrombin functions to enzymatically convert fibrinogen into fibrin, ultimately leading to fibrin clot formation. As a counterbalancing measure, thrombin also stimulates release of tissue plasminogen activator (tPA), a serine protease predominantly found in vascular endothelial cells. Once released, tPA cleaves plasminogen into the enzymatically active protein plasmin, which ultimately serves to degrade fibrin. Under normal physiologic circumstances, the balance of clot formation and degradation is well maintained. However, in certain circumstances such as with increased physiologic stress induced by trauma, surgery, heparin administration, and use of cardiopulmonary bypass, increased plasmin activity leads to systemic fibrinolysis. This state, often termed hyperfibrinolysis, can lead to pathologic bleeding and difficulty in obtaining hemostasis.

## ASSESSMENT OF FIBRINOLYSIS

While there is no gold standard for testing for fibrinolysis, the most commonly used tests in clinical practice are thromboelastography (TEG) and rotational thromboelastometry (ROTEM). TEG is performed with a cylindrical cup containing whole blood that oscillates while a pin on a torsion wire is suspended in the blood. As the clot forms, rotational force is transmitted to the pin and subsequently the torsion wire, which is transduced electromagnetically.[1,2] Similarly, ROTEM functions via a pin suspended in a cylindrical cup of whole blood. However, in ROTEM the pin rotates rather than the cup. As the strength of the clot increases, the rotation of the pin is impeded, which is detected by an optical sensor.[2] Both tests generate an output graph that demonstrates clot initiation, propagation, stabilization, and lysis, as seen in Figure 175.1. Fibrinolysis is depicted as a tapering of the amplitude over time. Tapering greater than 3% indicates fibrinolysis is occurring and antifibrinolytic therapy may be indicated, while tapering greater than 15% is indicative of hyperfibrinolysis.[3]

## ANTIFIBRINOLYTIC THERAPY

### APROTININ

Aprotinin is a protease inhibitor that reversibly binds and inhibits trypsin, kallikrein, and plasmin and is the most potent antifibrinolytic agent. Fibrinolysis is inhibited by reduced activation of plasminogen and its subsequent conversion to plasmin, as well as by decreased activation of kallikrein. Aprotinin was withdrawn from the market worldwide due to safety concerns and an association with increased mortality. This suspension was lifted in European markets in 2012, where it is used today only in limited settings.[1]

### AMINOCAPROIC ACID

Aminocaproic acid (Amicar) is a synthetic inhibitor of plasminogen activation. It is rapidly excreted in the urine and thus is generally used as a continuous infusion to maintain adequate concentrations. Side effects include hypotension, renal failure, rhabdomyolysis, and arrhythmias.[1]

### TRANEXAMIC ACID

Tranexamic acid (TXA) is a lysine analogue that binds plasminogen and inhibits its ability to bind other proteins, including fibrin. TXA was evaluated in patients with post-traumatic bleeding in the CRASH-2[4] (see Trauma in the Specific Surgical Associations section for more details). Generalized seizures have been reported in studies of patients receiving high doses of TXA during cardiopulmonary bypass. The proposed mechanism is due to antagonism of inhibitory γ- aminobutyric acid transmission resulting in neuroexcitability. This risk appears to be minimal, however, at doses regularly used in clinical practice, resulting in an otherwise excellent safety profile. Due to its safety and efficacy, TXA use has become common in trauma, cardiac surgery, orthopedic surgery and for treatment of idiopathic menorrhagia.[1]

## RISK OF ANTIFIBRINOLYTICS

Multiple studies have reported that antifibrinolytic therapy may activate platelets and the enzymatic components of the coagulation cascade both in vivo and in vitro,[1] potentially resulting in thrombotic complications.

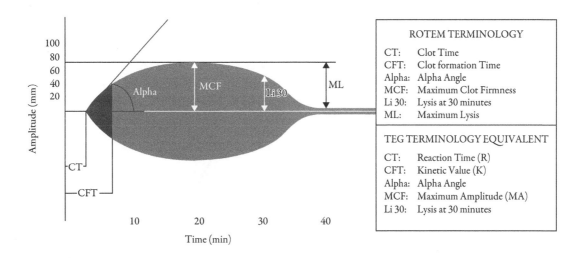

**Figure 175.1** Depiction of a ROTEM output.

Clinical consequences of this theoretical prothrombotic effect of antifibrinolytic therapies have not been demonstrated in clinical trials. This includes trials in high-risk populations such as orthopedic surgery, trauma, and liver transplantation.[1,4,5]

## SPECIFIC SURGICAL ASSOCIATIONS

### CARDIAC SURGERY

Antifibrinolytic therapy has been studied extensively in patients undergoing cardiac surgery, including those procedures performed utilizing cardiopulmonary bypass and those without. Multiple studies have demonstrated that patients who receive antifibrinolytic therapy receive fewer blood product transfusions.[1]

### TRAUMA

Tissue injury from trauma results in fibrinolysis and increased bleeding. The landmark CRASH-2 trial randomized over 20,000 trauma patients to treatment with either TXA or placebo within the first 8 hours of trauma. TXA administration was associated with improved 28-day mortality (14.5% in the TXA group vs. 16% in placebo group). No difference was noted in transfusion requirements between the two groups, however. The mechanism surrounding the survival benefit therefore remains unclear.[1,4]

### LIVER DISEASE

End-stage liver disease and cirrhosis are associated with alterations in coagulation, thrombocytopenia, and increased risk of bleeding, especially during liver transplantation and hepatic resections. Hyperfibrinolysis is frequently noted in patients undergoing liver transplantation by alterations in TEG or ROTEM. Studies of patients undergoing liver transplantation have demonstrated patients treated with tranexamic acid receive fewer blood transfusions versus placebo. The same benefit was not, however, demonstrated in studies of patients undergoing hepatic resections.[1]

### ORTHOPEDIC SURGERY

Antifibrinolytic therapy is routinely used in orthopedic surgery, including during total hip arthroplasty, total knee arthroplasty, and spine surgery. Generally, TXA is the medication of choice during orthopedic surgery and thus has been more extensively studied. Multiple meta-analyses have demonstrated that intraoperative TXA administration during joint replacement and spine surgery is associated with decreased blood loss and decreased blood transfusion requirements as compared to placebo. Analysis of postoperative administration of TXA demonstrated no difference in outcomes versus placebo.[1,5]

## REFERENCES

1. Levy JH, et al. Antifibrinolytic therapy and perioperative considerations. *Anesthesiology*. 2018;128(3):657–670.
2. Whiting D, Dinardo JA. TEG and ROTEM: technology and clinical applications. *Am J Hematol*. 2014;89(2):228–232. doi:10.1002/ajh.23599
3. Ilich A, et al. Global assays of fibrinolysis. *Int J Lab Hematol*. 2017;39(5):441–447.
4. Roberts I, et al. The CRASH-2 trial: a randomised controlled trial and economic evaluation of the effects of tranexamic acid on death, vascular occlusive events and transfusion requirement in bleeding trauma patients. *Health Technol Assess (Rockv)*. 2013;17(10):1–80.
5. Sukeik M, et al. Systematic review and meta-analysis of the use of tranexamic acid in total hip replacement. *J Bone Jt Surg Ser B*. 2011;93(B(1)):39–46.

# 176.

# ANTICOAGULANTS AND ANTAGONISTS

*Suhas Devangam and Gretchen A. Lemmink*

## ANTIPLATELET AGENTS

Antithrombotic agents exist to thwart platelet activation, which plays a key role in coronary and cerebral thrombosis. The first, and most ubiquitous, of these agents is aspirin (ASA), an antagonist of cyclooxygenase 1 (COX1) that inhibits platelet function for 7 to 10 days.[1] Despite this inhibition, ASA administration in the perioperative period is not associated with significant bleeding or with increased mortality.[1] ASA is often continued in the perioperative period in all procedures except those associated with highest risk for bleeding (e.g., intracranial surgery).

Oral P2Y$_{12}$ receptor antagonists (e.g., clopidogrel, prasugrel, and ticagrelor) inhibit platelet aggregation dependent on adenosine diphosphate (ADP).[2] Platelet function may not normalize for more than 7 days after drug discontinuation. The parenteral ADP receptor inhibitor cangrelor has a short half-life, and platelet function recovers within minutes of drug cessation.[1] Glycoprotein IIb/IIIa antagonists (e.g., eptifibatide, tirofiban) comprise the final class of antiplatelet agents. They are reserved for patients undergoing active percutaneous coronary intervention (PCI) and are not routinely encountered perioperatively.[1]

Patients presenting for surgery on antithrombotics may benefit from rapid measurement of platelet function using ASA and P2Y$_{12}$ response assays. Literature suggests a subset of patients prescribed these medications lack therapeutic response and may not exhibit clinically significant anticoagulation despite routine use.[3] In emergent situations requiring rapid antithrombotic reversal, platelet transfusion is required to reverse drug inhibitory effect.[2]

## HEPARINOIDS

Unfractionated heparin (UFH) indirectly inhibits thrombin and factor Xa by potentiating the activity of antithrombin (AT; formerly ATIII). Patients deficient in AT will have marked resistance to heparin and may require exogenous AT administration for anticoagulant effect. Common indications for UFH include treatment of acute coronary syndrome, prophylaxis and treatment of venous thromboembolism (VTE) and stoke prevention in atrial fibrillation (AF). After parenteral administration, clinical effect is monitored by activated partial thromboplastin time (aPTT) or anti–factor Xa.[2] Low-molecular-weight heparins (LMWHs), derivatives of UFH administered subcutaneously, have more specific inhibition of factor Xa.[2] Common preparations include enoxaparin and dalteparin. LMWHs have a longer duration of anticoagulant effect when compared to UFH, thus permitting outpatient administration.

Patients who present for surgery receiving therapeutic heparinoids may require reversal on an individualized basis considering the degree of preexisting anticoagulant effect as well as the risk of bleeding associated with the procedure. Protamine is a cationic protein that inactivates anionic heparin and can be administered after heparin discontinuation.[2] Dosing is based on time elapsed since last heparin dose and dose amount. It may not reliably reverse the anticoagulant effect of LMWH.[2] Protamine carries a black box warning regarding risk of anaphylaxis and cardiovascular collapse; thus, administration should be closely monitored in an intensive care unit or perioperative setting.[2]

## VITAMIN K ANTAGONISTS

The most abundant oral vitamin K antagonist (VKA) used in clinical practice today is warfarin, which acts by inhibiting synthesis of vitamin K–dependent clotting factors (e.g., II, VII, IX, and X).[2] Common indications for its use include mechanical heart valves and stroke prevention in AF. Warfarin's anticoagulant effect is monitored by the international normalized ratio (INR). Diet, polypharmacy, and hepatic insufficiency can all influence warfarin's dose-response relationship. This, coupled with warfarin's narrow therapeutic window, can make it a challenging outpatient therapy for many patients.[4]

Patients who present for major surgery with an elevated INR secondary to warfarin will require anticoagulation reversal. The optimal preoperative INR is dependent on

**Table 176.1** MECHANISM OF ACTION (MOA) AND PHARMACOKINETIC PROPERTIES OF DIRECT ORAL ANTICOAGULANTS

| | DABIGATRAN | APIXABAN | BETRIXABAN | RIVAROXABAN | EDOXABAN |
|---|---|---|---|---|---|
| MOA | DTI | Xa inhibitor | Xa inhibitor | Xa inhibitor | Xa inhibitor |
| Time to peak anticoagulant effect (min) | 120 | 180 | 180 | 120–240 | 60–120 |
| Half-life (h) | 12–17[a] | 12 | 19–27 | 5–13[a] | 10–14[a] |

DTI, direct thrombin inhibitor

[a]DENOTES drug has greater than 50% renal clearance; thus, half-life will be prolonged in patients with abnormal renal function.

From References 2 and 5.

the surgical procedure and risk of bleeding and must be determined on an individualized basis. Patients presenting for elective or less urgent surgeries that permit delay for 24 hours may receive oral or parenteral vitamin K after warfarin discontinuation. This will allow regeneration of the absent clotting factors and a normalization of the INR.[2] For life-threatening bleeding or emergent surgery, vitamin K alone is not sufficient for reversal. In these instances, the patient will require infusion of the absent factors either in the form of fresh frozen plasma (FFP) or using a four-factor prothrombin complex concentrate (PCC). Reversal with FFP may be complicated by hypervolemia and transfusion reactions and has been shown to result in a slower time to INR correction compared with reversal using PCCs.[2,4]

## DIRECT ORAL ANTICOAGULANTS AND PARENTERAL DIRECT THROMBIN INHIBITORS

When compared to warfarin, the direct oral anticoagulants (DOACs) (Table 176.1) have a more rapid onset of anticoagulant activity, have a considerably shorter half-life (averaging 12 hours), and do not require outpatient drug monitoring.[5] Several DOACs are approved for deep vein thrombosis/pulmonary embolism prophylaxis after orthopedic surgery, stroke prophylaxis in AF, and VTE treatment.[5] Rapidly measuring the anticoagulant effect of these drugs in the perioperative setting is challenging. Drug-specific assays are not widely available, and routine clinical coagulation studies such as aPTT, thrombin time, and anti-Xa levels have limited correlation with clinically relevant drug effect.[5]

Patients who have recently taken a DOAC and present for an urgent/emergent procedure associated with a high risk of bleeding may require administration of a reversal agent. For emergency dabigatran reversal, the monoclonal antibody idarucizumab is approved by the Food and Drug Administration (FDA) and binds the drug with high affinity, removing it from circulation.[5] The oral Xa inhibitors rivaroxaban and apixaban can be antagonized using andexanet alfa, which acts as a decoy molecule, binding and sequestering the anticoagulant drug. It is important to note this drug is not yet approved for anticoagulation reversal before surgery but instead holds FDA approval only for reversal in patients experiencing life-threatening bleeding. If andexanet alfa is not available, a four-factor PCC is recommended.[2,5]

Finally, parenteral direct thrombin inhibitors (DTIs; e.g., argatroban, bivalirudin) are used clinically in patients with a contraindication to heparin (e.g., heparin-induced thrombocytopenia) or as an alternate to heparin in PCI. They inactive both circulating and clot-bound thrombin, and their direct action confers a more predictable anticoagulation response when compared to heparin.[2] These agents enjoy relatively short half-lives; however, they must be used judiciously in patients with an elevated risk of bleeding as there is no reversal therapy available. In the perioperative period, discontinuing the agent and allowing time for drug clearance is the only method to assuage their anticoagulant effect.[2]

## REFERENCES

1. Oprea AD, Popescu WM. Perioperative management of antiplatelet therapy. *Br J Anaesth.* 2013;111(suppl 1):i3–i17.
2. Gordon JL, et al. Anticoagulant and antiplatelet medications encountered in emergency surgery patients: a review of reversal strategies. *J Trauma Acute Care Surg.* 2013;75(3):475–486.
3. Parry PV, et al. Utility of the aspirin and P2Y12 response assays to determine the effect of antiplatelet agents on platelet reactivity in traumatic brain injury. *Neurosurgery.* 2017;80(1):92–96.
4. Schulman S, Bijsterveld NR. Anticoagulants and their reversal. *Transfus Med Rev.* 2007;21(1):37–48.
5. Langer A, Connors JM. Assessing and reversing the effect of direct oral anticoagulants on coagulation. *Anesthesiology.* 2020;133(1):223–232.

# 177.

# COAGULOPATHY IN TRAUMA PATIENTS

*Timothy Ford and Alaa Abd-Elsayed*

## PATHOPHYSIOLOGY

The coagulation system consists of a balance between hemostatic and fibrinolytic processes that work to maintain hemostasis in the setting of vascular injury. The physiologic insult of trauma disrupts this balance through numerous mechanisms, resulting in potentially devastating coagulopathy.

## LETHAL TRIAD

The lethal triad of trauma refers to the positive-feedback relationship exhibited by disturbances in three physiologic parameters exhibited in trauma patients: acidosis, hypothermia, and hemodilution coagulopathy. Lactic acidosis occurs secondary to inadequate tissue perfusion in the setting of hemorrhagic shock. It is augmented by excessive chloride and component blood administration. Experimental models demonstrate interference in calcium-dependent steps of the coagulation cascade. Indeed, acidosis correlates with reduction in multiple coagulation factor activity in a concentration-dependent manner. Hypothermia is due to a combination of cold exposure at the time of trauma, transport, exposure for trauma examination, and resuscitation with hypothermic intravenous fluids. Hypothermia is graded as mild (34°C–36°C), moderate (32°C–34°C), or severe (<32°C). Effects of hypothermia on hemostasis include platelet dysfunction and impaired enzymatic dysfunction in the coagulation cascade. It is important to note that acidosis and hypothermia are synergistic when present together. Resuscitation-associated coagulopathy is caused by a large volume of intravenous fluids and improperly balanced transfusion resuscitation.

## DISSEMINATED INTRAVASCULAR COAGULATION

In trauma patients, tissue factor is exposed in the setting of tissue injury with subsequent activation of the extrinsic coagulation cascade in proportion to injury severity. Severe traumas can result in disseminated intravascular coagulation (DIC). DIC is a systemic disorder characterized by diffuse microvascular thrombosis resulting in a consumptive coagulopathy depleting coagulation factors and augmenting hemorrhage.[1,2]

## PLATELET DYSFUNCTION

Platelets are integral to hemostasis after trauma. Both quantitative and qualitative platelet dysfunction have been identified in trauma patients. Platelet count inversely correlates with transfusion and early mortality in trauma patients. Qualitative assessment utilizing platelet aggregometry demonstrated primary platelet dysfunction in 50% of trauma patients on admission and 90% of patients at some point during their hospitalization.

## TRAUMA-INDUCED COAGULOPATHY

Trauma-induced coagulopathy (TIC) is a complex and incompletely understood disorder caused by a combination of tissue injury and shock that result in hemostatic failure that occurs independent of the lethal triad. Innate integration between coagulation and inflammation mediates its widespread adverse downstream consequences. It is thought to be mediated primarily by the thrombomodulin–protein C system. Molecular and physiologic perturbations ultimately manifest as uncontrolled hemorrhage, thromboembolic complications, organ dysfunction, and death. Clinically, it is associated with hypotension, increased early transfusion requirements, high injury severity score, worsening base deficit, and head injury. Coagulopathy occurs in the absence of thrombocytopenia and hypofibrinogenemia, likely making it an overlapping but mechanistically distinct process from DIC. It is currently unknown whether TIC might exist in patients with normal-range values of standard coagulation testing, and thus it is not sufficiently characterized by these measures.[1-3]

## ANESTHETIC CONSIDERATIONS: DIAGNOSIS

Understanding a patient's current coagulopathic state requires a thorough clinical evaluation of the trauma patient's injuries and a thorough laboratory evaluation, including complete blood count, complete metabolic panel, arterial blood gas analysis, standard coagulation tests, fibrinogen, fibrin degradation products, and viscoelastic coagulation assessment. Laboratory studies provide an assessment of acidosis, hemodilution, and severity of shock and as a guide for specific component transfusion administration and as a baseline for assessment of ongoing hemorrhage.

### STANDARD COAGULATION STUDIES

Diagnostic criteria for coagulopathy in trauma patients have been derived from clinical studies. Prothrombin time greater than 18 seconds, international normalized ratio (INR) greater than 1.5, activated partial thromboplastin time greater than 60 seconds, or any of these values greater than 1.5 times baseline are diagnostic of coagulopathy in trauma patients. The prevalence of prolonged prothrombin time is higher, but prolongation of partial thromboplastin time is more specific.

### PLATELET ASSESSMENT

Decreased platelet count and platelet dysfunction contribute to coagulopathy and are associated with poor outcomes in trauma patients, as previously discussed. Platelet assessment includes platelet count, thromboelastography (TEG), platelet function analysis, and platelet aggregometry. TEG serves in part as a holistic assessment of clot formation and reflects platelet count and function. It may be modified to investigate platelet function specifically. Platelet function analysis and whole blood aggregometry have not been evaluated in the setting of trauma and resuscitation.[1-3]

### VISCOELASTIC ASSESSMENT: THROMBOELASTOGRAPHY

Thromboelastography is an important tool in the evaluation of trauma patients because it can identify TIC and facilitates real-time monitoring of ongoing resuscitation efforts. Indeed, TEG parameters have been validated against laboratory tests and provide meaningful diagnostic information with respect to abnormalities, including primary fibrinolysis, secondary hyperfibrinolysis, thrombocytopenia, clotting factor consumption, and hypercoagulability. Additionally, it can be used to guide both transfusion and pharmaceutical therapy for coagulopathy in trauma.

### OTHER COAGULATION LABORATORY TESTS

Fibrinogen is the terminal substrate of the coagulation cascade, and its acquired deficiency in trauma is associated with hemorrhage and mortality. Thus, measurement of fibrinogen levels to guide transfusion therapy is important.

Elevated fibrin degradation products are associated with severity of tissue damage, hyperfibrinolysis, and fibrinogen depletion early after injury. High levels of fibrin degradation products (e.g., D-dimer) in admitted trauma patients was a strong predictor of early death and requirement for massive transfusion, even with high fibrinogen levels.

### CLINICAL SCORING SYSTEMS

Three clinical scoring systems have been developed to help stratify patients who will require massive transfusion: Trauma-Associated Severe Hemorrhage score, McLaughlin score, and Assessment of Blood Consumption scores. While each scoring system demonstrated differences in scoring between patients who required massive transfusion and those who did not, there were no significant predictive differences identified between these scores for each scoring system. Furthermore, none of these scoring systems has been studied with respect to their ability to reduce mortality.

## ANESTHETIC CONSIDERATIONS: TREATMENT

### EMPIRIC TRANSFUSION STRATEGIES

Empiric transfusion strategies implement a protocol with a predetermined ratio of packed red blood cells to plasma to platelets in the setting of hemorrhagic shock. While there is variation between trauma centers with respect to these ratios, multiple studies have demonstrated that ratios that approach that of whole blood, namely 1:1:1, overall result in better outcomes than those that diverge further from that of whole blood. This therapy is beneficial in high-acuity patients. However, empiric transfusion therapy is not without risks, which include the potential for transfusion-related lung injury. Thus, in patients without risk factors for massive transfusion based on injury severity and shock, abnormal coagulation should be corrected in response to specific laboratory deficits.

## THROMBOELASTOGRAPHY-GUIDED TRANSFUSION

Thromboelastography is an important tool in guiding transfusion therapy because of its rapid turnaround and holistic assessment of the coagulation system. Studies are ongoing to assess the utility of TEG as the standard for guiding massive transfusion in trauma patients.

## PHARMACEUTICAL THERAPIES

There are multiple pharmaceutical agents available as adjunct therapy to transfusion for the treatment of severe coagulopathy in trauma patients. Tranexamic acid is the best studied antifibrinolytic agent in the trauma population and has demonstrated mortality benefit. Other pharmacological therapies include recombinant factor VIIa, prothrombin complex concentrate, desmopressin, and other antifibrinolytic agents, including aminocaproic acid and aprotinin. While these agents offer theoretical benefit, they all lack thorough clinical evaluation in trauma patients.[1-3]

## REFERENCES

1. Kutcher M, Chohen M. Coagulopathy in trauma patients. In: Post T, ed. *UpToDate*. Waltham, MA: UpToDate; 2020. http:/www.uptodate.com
2. Kornblith LZ, et al. Trauma-induced coagulopathy: the past, present, and future. *J Thromb Haemostasis*. 2019;17(6):852–862.
3. Peng N, Su L. Progresses in understanding trauma-induced coagulopathy and the underlying mechanism. *Chin J Traumatol*. 2017;20(3):133–136.

# 178.

# HEMOGLOBINOPATHIES AND PORPHYRIAS

*Elizabeth Haynes and Nasir Hussain*

## INTRODUCTION

Hemoglobinopathies are genetic blood disorders that include α- and β-thalassemia as well as diseases that cause abnormal hemoglobin structure. The structural variants of clinical significance include hemoglobin (Hb) S, HbC, and HbE. Based on which hemoglobinopathy is present, patients may exhibit highly variable presentations, ranging from mild anemia to the need for frequent blood transfusions. Porphyrias also encompass a group of metabolic disorders that interfere with the body's normal hemoglobin production by altering heme synthesis. The type of porphyria is determined by which enzyme is deficient in the heme synthesis pathway. The enzyme deficiencies cause an accumulation of heme precursors in erythropoietic cells or the liver, creating various presentations and involvement of multiple body systems.[1-4]

## CLINICAL FEATURES

### HEMOGLOBINOPATHIES

Table 178.1 can be viewed for the common clinical features associated with hemoglobinopathies.

### PORPHYRIAS

The acute hepatic (acute intermittent porphyria, hereditary coproporphyria, variegate porphyria, and ALA-dehydratase deficiency porphyria), hepatic cutaneous (porphyria cutanea tarda), and erythropoietic cutaneous (congenital erythropoietic porphyria, erythropoietic protoporphyria, X-linked protoporphyria) categories of porphyrias vary significantly from one another and have mild-to-severe presentations. Erythropoietic cutaneous porphyrias

*Table 178.1* COMMON PRESENTATIONS OF HEMOGLOBINOPATHIES

| DIAGNOSIS | PRESENTATION |
|---|---|
| Heterozygous α⁺-thalassemia, -α/αα | Mild hypochromia/asymptomatic. |
| Heterozygous α⁰-thalassemia, -/αα, or homozygous α⁺-thalassemia, -α/-α | Mild anemia, hypochromia, microcytosis. |
| HbH disease (compound heterozygous α⁺/α⁰-thalassemia with three inactive α-genes, -/-α) | Moderate hypochromic hemolytic anemia, splenomegaly. Anemic crises with virus or drugs. Cardiac problems, gallstones, folic acid deficiency |
| Hb Bart's hydrops fetalis (homozygous α⁰-thalassemia) | Hemolytic anemia in utero with hydrops and ascites. Fatal if not treated. |
| +Thalassemia minor (heterozygous β-thalassemia) | Mild, microcytic hypochromic anemia. |
| Thalassemia intermedia (mild homozygous or mixed heterozygous β-thalassemia) | Variable symptoms and need for transfusions, skeletal abnormalities. |
| Thalassemia major (severe homozygous or mixed heterozygous β-thalassemia) | Severe anemia, transfusion dependence, skeletal abnormalities, risk of iron overload/multiorgan involvement. |
| Sickle cell disease (HbSS) | Sickle cell/pain crisis exacerbated by low oxygen, dehydration, infection; chronic hemolytic anemia, vascular occlusions. |
| HbC disease (HbCC) | Variable hemolytic anemia. |
| HbE disease (HbEE) | Mild anemia, hemolytic anemia with infection/drugs. |

From Reference 4.

manifest as photosensitivity and friable, thickened skin with bullae and lesions on sun-exposed areas. Porphyrins may accumulate in areas of bone and teeth and cause hemolytic anemia as well as splenomegaly. The hepatic porphyrias are associated with acute neurologic attacks consisting of a wide array of symptoms. Cramping abdominal pain is common in addition to nausea, vomiting, constipation, headache, confusion, chest pain, tachycardia, hypertension, tremors, sweating, and diarrhea. Acute attacks are provoked by factors that include hormones, medications, fasting, stress, alcohol, infection, and diet.[2]

## DIAGNOSIS

If a hemoglobinopathy is suspected, a series of blood tests are used to confirm the diagnosis. This includes a full blood count to measure red blood cell count as well as erythrocyte indices, including mean corpuscular volume and mean corpuscular hemoglobin. The next step involves running a hemoglobin electrophoresis and/or chromatography. Last, a DNA test may be needed if the diagnosis cannot be determined.[4]

In contrast, porphyrias are often difficult to diagnose because of their varied presentations and nonspecific symptoms. Patients who are having acute attacks will have increased porphobilinogen and sometimes aminolevulinic acid (porphyrin precursors) in their urine. Cutaneous porphyrias similarly cause urinary excretion of porphyrin precursors. These often include uroporphyrin and either carboxylate porphyrin or coproporphyrin. Further analyses of porphyrins in the urine and feces help determine the type of porphyria. The diagnosis is confirmed by molecular studies involving an analysis of the gene mutation.[2]

## TREATMENT

The medical therapies for both hemoglobinopathies and porphyrias focus less on curative treatments and aim to provide symptomatic management. Hematopoietic stem cell transplants are potential curative measures for β-thalassemia major and sickle cell anemia, but these are usually not available options.[4] Depending on the severity of thalassemia, patients may require regular transfusions and iron chelation therapy. Prevention of the number and severity of acute pain crises is one of the main goals in sickle cell anemia management. This can be accomplished with the use of hydroxyurea.[4]

When an acute sickle cell crisis does occur, adequate pain medication and intravenous fluids are given for symptomatic treatment.[4] Similarly, acute attacks in porphyrias are managed with therapies such as analgesics, antiemetics, and additional measures to alleviate symptoms. Intravenous glucose (at least 300 g/d) can be effective in relieving mild attacks. For those with refractory symptoms or severe attacks, 3–4 mg of heme (hematin, heme albumin, or heme arginate) should be given daily for 4 days. A liver transplant can be considered as a last resort approach for those with frequent and severe attacks. Cutaneous porphyrias are managed with phlebotomy or the use of hydroxychloroquine or chloroquine to decrease the amount of iron or porphyrins in the liver, respectively.[2]

## ANESTHESIA CONSIDERATIONS

### HEMOGLOBINOPATHIES
#### Preoperative

Patients with hemoglobinopathies should have a detailed history and physical examination to assess pathologies related to a history of numerous blood transfusions or their underlying disorder. This includes discussing the frequency of sickle cell crises and their transfusion history. Transfusion-dependent patients may have cardiomyopathy with resultant pulmonary hypertension or hepatic dysfunction. Exercise tolerance should be evaluated as well as consideration of echocardiography if indicated.[1] A pulmonary examination is performed to assess for baseline dyspnea. A thorough airway examination is needed to determine facial deformities contributing to a difficult airway.[5] Preoperative laboratory tests may be needed to evaluate renal and hepatic function as well as baseline hemoglobin. Consider giving a blood transfusion or exchange transfusion if the patient's hemoglobin is less than 10 g/dL on an individualized basis.[1] Prolonged fasting and anxiety should also be avoided as these can trigger a sickle cell crisis.

### Intraoperative

Prevention of hypoxemia, hypercapnia, acidosis, hypothermia, and hypovolemia is especially important in sickle cell anemia patients to prevent sickling of hemoglobin, acute crisis, and vaso-occlusion. Hypotonic intravenous solutions are usually preferred.[1] Patients with skeletal abnormalities should be positioned carefully intraoperatively due to an increased risk of pathological fractures.[5] It is also important to minimize venous stasis during the procedure.[1]

### Postoperative

Sickle cell anemia patients in particular are at risk for postoperative complications. Incentive spirometry, early ambulation, and avoidance of fluid overload help to maintain adequate ventilation and reduce the risk of acute chest syndrome. Adequate pain control may be an issue in opioid-tolerant patients. Multimodal pain regimens should be utilized with care to avoid respiratory sedation. Patients are also at increased risk of infections, and postoperative fever requires careful evaluation. Deep vein thrombosis prophylaxis should also be administered after major surgeries.[1]

## PORPHYRIAS

### Preoperative

It is important to determine the severity of the patient's disease. Careful attention should be given to the neurologic assessment to evaluate for neuropathies or disturbances in motor function or strength. A cardiovascular examination should assess for autonomic instability or signs suggesting an acute, crisis such as tachycardia or hypertension. Preoperative fasting should be limited while still maintaining fasting guidelines. Dextrose-saline intravenous fluids can be given if prolonged periods of fasting are needed. Preoperative anxiety should also be avoided as this can precipitate an acute crisis. Some benzodiazepines, such as diazepam, have been associated with triggering an acute attack, and they should be used with caution.[3]

### Intraoperative

Many anesthetic medications have the potential to trigger an acute crisis and should be avoided or used with caution. An arterial line should be considered for continuous blood pressure monitoring if hemodynamic lability is anticipated. Hemodynamic instability may also limit the use of regional anesthesia, but porphyrias alone are not an absolute contraindication. Prilocaine and bupivacaine appear to be safe for use. Propofol has been suggested as a safe induction option, while ketamine is classified as unsafe, and etomidate's safety is undetermined. Thiopental is also considered unsafe. All inhaled agents are classified as safe for use except for sevoflurane, which is labeled unsafe. Other unsafe drugs that are porphyrinogenic or possibly porphyrinogenic include oxycodone, diclofenac, rifampicin, erythromycin, and ephedrine.[3]

### Postoperative

Patients should be monitored postoperatively for signs or symptoms of an acute crisis. Cardiac monitoring should continue in the early postoperative period.[3]

## REFERENCES

1. Adjepong KO, et al. Perioperative management of sickle cell disease. *Mediterr J Hematol Infect Dis*. 2018;10(1):e2018032.
2. Balwani M, Desnick RJ. The porphyrias: advances in diagnosis and treatment. *Blood*. 2012;120(23):4496–4504.
3. Findley M, et al. Porphyrias: implications for anaesthesia, critical care, and pain medicine. *Contin Educ Anaesth Crit Care Pain*, 2012;12(3):128–133.
4. Kohne E. Hemoglobinopathies: clinical manifestations, diagnosis, and treatment. *Dtsch Arztebl Int*. 2011;108(31–32):532–540.
5. Staikou C, et al. A narrative review of peri-operative management of patients with thalassaemia. *Anaesthesia*. 2014;69(5):494–510.

# 179.

# TRANSFUSION INDICATIONS AND REACTIONS

*Courtney L. Scott and Elaine A. Boydston*

## INTRODUCTION

The risks and benefits of blood transfusion must always be weighed carefully.

## TRANSFUSION INDICATIONS

### PACKED RED BLOOD CELLS

In the past, it was thought higher hemoglobin levels (target hemoglobin 10 g/dL) would improve outcomes by increasing oxygen delivery. Recent evidence shows a more conservative transfusion strategy is beneficial. Transfusion of packed red blood cells (pRBCs) is typically indicated when the hemoglobin is less than 7 g/dL, and not when it is greater than 10 g/dL (unless hemodynamically unstable with ongoing bleeding).[1] According to the Society of Thoracic Surgeons and Society of Cardiovascular Anesthesiologists, when the hemoglobin level is 7–10 g/dL, transfusion is recommended for evidence of "critical noncardiac end-organ ischemia," active ongoing blood loss, or signs of tissue hypoxia.[1] These may include hypotension, a central venous oxygen saturation of less than 50% (indicating high oxygen extraction by the body), lactate greater than 2 mmol/L, and signs of organ dysfunction, including decreased urine output or cardiac wall motion abnormalities.[2,3] With hemoglobin greater than 10 g/dL, pRBC transfusion typically will not result in improved tissue oxygenation; thus, transfusion is not indicated.[1]

### FRESH FROZEN PLASMA

Fresh frozen plasma (FFP) is the acellular fluid portion of whole blood that contains all the coagulation factors necessary for secondary hemostasis. FFP is indicated for microvascular bleeding in the setting with international normalized ratio (INR) greater than 2, urgent warfarin reversal, or correction of a known factor deficiency when specific concentrates are not available. Other indications include fixed ratios as part of a massive transfusion protocol (MTP) and heparin resistance (e.g., antithrombin III deficiency) for patients requiring heparainization.[4] Table 179.1 summarizes other indications for FFP transfusion.

### PLATELETS

Platelet transfusion is indicated to correct thrombocytopenia, depending on bleeding risk, anticipated invasive procedures, or signs of microvascular bleeding.[5] Other indications include correction of platelet defects such as reversal of antiplatelet medications or platelet dysfunction following cardiopulmonary bypass.[5] Platelets are also given in fixed ratios as part of an MTP.[3] Table 179.1 summarizes other indications for platelet transfusion. Platelets are stored at room temperature on racks that move slowly to increase mixing of the platelets with oxygen passing through the platelet pack. Bacteria can proliferate in platelet concentrates as they are stored at room temperature, increasing the risk of infection.

### CRYOPRECIPITATE

Cryoprecipitate is the fraction of plasma that precipitates when FFP is thawed, and it contains fibrinogen, fibronectin, von Willebrand factor, factor VIII, and factor XIII.[3] Cryoprecipitate is indicated for microvascular bleeding when fibrinogen is less than 150 g/dL, treatment or prophylaxis in patients with hemophilia A, von Willebrand's disease, or congenital fibrinogen deficiencies (when specific factor concentrates are not available) and in fixed ratios as part of an MTP.[3]

## TRANSFUSION REACTIONS

### NONHEMOLYTIC TRANSFUSION REACTIONS

Febrile nonhemolytic transfusion reactions (FNHTRs) and urticarial reactions are the most common transfusion reactions.[2] FNHTRs are due to recipient antibodies (formed after a previous transfusion or pregnancy) against donor white blood cells causing release of pyogenic cytokines.[1] Symptoms are self-limited, occur within 4 hours of transfusion, and include an increase in temperature of

*Table 179.1* INDICATIONS FOR TRANSFUSION OF FFP AND PLATELETS

| BLOOD PRODUCT | CLINICAL SETTING | INDICATIONS |
|---|---|---|
| Fresh frozen plasma (FFP) | | |
| | Massive transfusion | • Correct dilutional coagulopathy |
| | | • Signs of microvascular bleeding |
| | Correction of congenital or acquired deficiencies of clotting factors | • When specific factor concentrates are unavailable |
| | Liver disease resulting in elevated INR | • If active bleeding |
| | | • In preparation for surgery or invasive procedures |
| | Reversal of anticoagulant therapy | • In the presence of major bleeding/intracranial hemorrhage |
| | | • In preparation for surgery that cannot be delayed |
| | Active bleeding in DIC | • Correct consumptive coagulopathy |
| | Reconstitution of whole blood for exchange transfusions | |
| | Replacement fluid for apheresis in thrombotic microangiopathies | • Thrombotic thrombocytopenic purpura |
| | | • Hemolytic uremic syndrome |
| Platelets | | |
| | Thrombocytopenia | • If no signs of bleeding, if platelets < 10,000 |
| | | • If elevated risk of bleeding, if platelets < 20,000 |
| | | • Prior to surgery, if platelets < 50,000 |
| | Platelet dysfunction with bleeding | • Reversal for antiplatelet medications |
| | | • After cardiopulmonary bypass |
| | | • Trauma |
| | Massive transfusion | • One unit of platelets for every 2–5 units of pRBCs |

From References 4 and 5.

1°C–2°C, chills, rigors, myalgias, and headache. Urticarial reactions (without fever) occur due to recipient reaction against plasma proteins in the donor blood, triggering mast cell and basophil degranulation.

Anaphylactic reactions are the most severe form of nonhemolytic transfusion reactions. These most commonly occur when individuals deficient in immunoglobulin (Ig) A receive a blood transfusion containing IgA.[2] Anaphylaxis occurs within minutes, and treatment is supportive. To avoid this response, IgA-deficient patients should only receive blood products from IgA-deficient donors or products that have been washed to remove plasma proteins.[1]

## TRANSFUSION-RELATED ACUTE LUNG INJURY AND TRANSFUSION-ASSOCIATED CIRCULATORY OVERLOAD

Transfusion-related acute lung injury and transfusion-associated circulatory overload are discussed in another chapter.

## HEMOLYTIC TRANSFUSION REACTIONS

Hemolytic transfusion reactions are due to recipient antibodies against donor red blood cells, causing hemolysis. There are two types of reactions, acute and delayed.

1. **Acute hemolytic reactions** are due to ABO incompatibility where complement-fixing antibodies cause immediate intravascular hemolysis.[2] Symptoms include fever, flank pain, and hematuria and can often be missed in patients under anesthesia. Treatment includes stopping the transfusion, circulatory support to maintain blood pressure, renal support with mannitol, Lasix, and bicarbonate (to alkalinize urine and maintain urine output) and management of possible disseminated intravascular coagulation (DIC).[3]

2. **Delayed hemolytic transfusion reactions** present with microvascular hemolysis (malaise, jaundice, fever) 2–21 days after a transfusion.

They occur in recipients previously sensitized to minor red blood cell antigens (following prior transfusion or pregnancy). Reexposure to the antigen results in an anamnestic response, leading to extravascular hemolysis via the reticuloendothelial system.[2]

## INFECTIOUS COMPLICATIONS

Blood products have the potential to transmit pathogens, including viruses, parasites, and bacteria. Today, donor blood is screened for several viruses, leading to a drastic reduction in transmission of these illnesses. Bacterial contamination accounts for the greatest number of transfusion-related infections, with the greatest risk attributable to platelets given their storage at room temperature.[1] Table 179.2

*Table 179.2* RATES OF INFECTIOUS COMPLICATIONS DUE TO BLOOD TRANSFUSION

| PATHOGEN | RISK OF TRANSMISSION |
|---|---|
| HIV | 1/2.3M |
| Hepatitis B | 1/280,000–352,000 |
| Hepatitis C | 1/1.8M |
| Cytomegalovirus | 1%–3% or |
|  | 0.02% if products are leukoreduced |
| Bacterial contamination | 1/3000 |

From Reference 1.

describes the rate of transmission of bloodborne pathogens during blood transfusion.

## MASSIVE TRANSFUSIONS AND ELECTROLYTE ABNORMALITIES

Several complications from blood transfusion occur primarily when large amounts of blood products are transfused due to effects of preservatives or metabolic changes in stored blood. Citrate toxicity causes hypocalcemia, resulting in hypotension and cardiac electrical changes. Hyperkalemia and acidosis may occur due to extracellular accumulation of potassium and the large amounts of lactate and free hydrogen ions produced as red blood cells are stored.[3] If cold blood products are not warmed, hypothermia may also result. Together, these derangements can cause significant metabolic acidosis and hypothermia, worsening tissue hypoxia and coagulopathy.

## REFERENCES

1. Barash PG. *Clinical Anesthesia*. Philadelphia, PA: Wolters Kluwer; 2017.
2. Faust RJ, Cucchiara RF. *Anesthesiology Review*. New York, NY: Churchill Livingstone; 2002.
3. Gropper MA, Miller RD. *Miller's Anesthesia*. Philadelphia, PA: Elsevier; 2020.
4. Liumbruno G, et al.; Italian Society of Transfusion Medicine and Immunohaematology (SIMTI) Work Group. Recommendations for the transfusion of plasma and platelets. *Blood Trans.* 2009;7(2): 132–150.
5. Squires JE. Indications for platelet transfusion in patients with thrombocytopenia. *Blood Trans.* 2015;13(2), 221–226.

# 180.

# COMPLICATIONS OF TRANSFUSION

*Courtney R. Jones and Maggie W. Mechlin*

## INTRODUCTION

While transfusion of whole blood, red cells, and other blood components can be a life-saving intervention, it comes with significant risks to the patient that must be weighed.

## TRANSFUSION-ASSOCIATED CIRCULATORY OVERLOAD

Transfusion-associated circulatory overload (TACO) is hydrostatic, protein-poor pulmonary edema that occurs within 6 hours of a transfusion and must meet three or more of the following criteria from the National Healthcare Safety Network 2016 definition of TACO: (1) acute respiratory distress (dyspnea, orthopnea, and cough); (2) evidence of positive fluid balance; (3) elevated brain natriuretic peptide; (4) radiographic evidence of pulmonary edema; (5) evidence of left heart failure; or (6) elevated central venous pressure.[1] TACO is the most frequent cause of pulmonary complications related to transfusion and increases hospital mortality. The incidence of TACO ranges between 1% and 11% depending on the patient population, with elderly and critically ill patients having the highest risk. TACO appears to occur via a two-hit model, with the first hit being a volume-overloaded state from medical comorbidities such as heart failure, renal failure, or being volume overloaded in general, followed by a second hit of excessive transfusion combined with inability to control the patient's volume status. The blood product itself may contribute to the risk as the incidence decreases with leukoreduced product. TACO is a leading cause of transfusion-associated mortality and is responsible for 30%–44% of transfusion fatalities. Patients can have rapid improvement with supportive care and diuretics.[1]

## TRANSFUSION-RELATED ACUTE LUNG INJURY

Transfusion-related acute lung injury (TRALI) is non-cardiogenic, protein-rich pulmonary edema that results from a capillary leak that occurs within 6 hours of transfusion, resulting in new acute lung injury (ALI). In clinical practice, difficulty arises in assessing whether the transfusion was causal or coincidental in the development of ALI, especially when risk factors for ALI are already present. The risk of TRALI per unit transfused is low at less than 1.12%, but, along with TACO, it is another significant cause of transfusion-related fatalities with 4%–34% of those deaths attributed to TRALI.[1] TRALI can occur with any blood component.[2] The full pathophysiology of TRALI is not well understood, but it also appears to involve a two-hit process. Risk factors for the first hit include alcohol abuse, smoking, volume overload, high peak airway pressures, systemic inflammation, liver surgery, and low interleukin 10 levels. In approximately 80% of cases of TRALI, the second hit is thought to be anti-HLA class I or II antibodies in the plasma-containing product; the remaining cases of TRALI appear to be non–antibody mediated.[1] The incidence of TRALI is significantly higher when the blood donor is female, especially a female with previous pregnancies. Mitigation efforts have led to significant improvements in the incidence of TRALI by screening the blood supply for female donors with specific antibodies.[2] A small number of patients with TRALI develop a mild leukopenia, and thrombocytopenia is more common in these patients. TRALI is treated with supportive care, but critically ill patients have especially high mortality.[1]

## FEBRILE, ALLERGIC, AND HYPOTENSIVE TRANSFUSION REACTIONS

Febrile, allergic, and hypotensive reactions were among the most common reported reactions associated with transfusion morbidity (but not mortality) in 2019 in the United Kingdom.[3] A febrile reaction is graded in severity from mild to severe and requires at least a temperature rise of 1°C or greater to a temperature of 38°C or greater. Greater degrees of temperature rise accompanied by systemic symptoms such as rigors, chills, myalgias, or nausea increase the severity of the reaction. If systemic symptoms present, bacterial contamination or a hemolytic reaction is possible.[3,4] Febrile reactions should be treated with acetaminophen alone, and more severe reactions may require stopping the transfusion and sending blood cultures. The risk of a future febrile reaction can be minimized by pretreating the patient with acetaminophen an hour before subsequent transfusions.

A mild allergic reaction is classified by transient flushing or urticaria, and a moderate reaction is classified by wheezing or angioedema with or without skin manifestations. The presence of respiratory or circulatory compromise, as evidenced by reactions such as bronchospasm, stridor, or anaphylaxis, classify as a severe allergic type reaction. Under anesthesia, this may manifest as rising peak airway pressures, tachycardia, and hypotension. The index of suspicion must be high when the patient is under anesthesia as one may not see urticaria with the patient covered by drapes and the differential diagnosis for hemodynamic changes is broad intraoperatively. Allergic reactions should be treated with antihistamines and albuterol. Epinephrine must be added if anaphylaxis is present, but steroids should not be given as a matter of routine practice. The patient can be pretreated with antihistamines before future transfusions to reduce the risk of a repeated allergic reaction. Additional interventions include washed platelets or packed red blood cells, solvent-detergent–treated plasma, and pooled platelets suspended in platelet additive solution (PAS) to reduce the incidence of allergic reactions.[3,5] Immunoglobulin (Ig) A levels should be checked in patients with moderate-to-severe allergic reactions as patients with IgA deficiency may be more susceptible to anaphylaxis when anti-IgA antibodies are present in the product transfused.[4]

Hypotensive reactions are also further characterized as moderate or severe. Moderate hypotensive reactions require minimal or no additional treatment and are defined by a drop in systolic blood pressure by 30 mm Hg or greater to a systolic blood pressure of 80 mm Hg or less without allergic symptoms. A severe hypotensive reaction causes a shock state and requires intervention.[3] Following a hypotensive transfusion reaction, patients can attempt a transfusion with washed packed red blood cells or platelets suspended in PAS. There are also rare occurrences of significant hypotension that occur with transfusions in patients on angiotensin-converting enzyme inhibitors (ACEIs)

mediated by bradykinin release. These patients may benefit if the ACEI is held prior to transfusion.[4]

## HEMOLYTIC TRANSFUSION REACTIONS

Hemolytic transfusion reactions fall into three categories: acute hemolytic transfusion reaction (AHTR), delayed hemolytic transfusion reaction (DHTR), and hyperhemolysis. AHTR occurs within 24 hours of a transfusion, with DHTR occurring more than 24 hours posttransfusion. Hyperhemolysis can be acute (within 7 days of transfusion) or delayed (>7 days following transfusion) and results in more significant hemolysis. Hyperhemolysis results in the destruction of *both* the patient's and the transfused red cells, with the hemoglobin often falling below pretransfusion levels. This may be triggered by an undetectable red cell antibody and is seen most often in sickle cell patients. Clinical symptoms of hemolysis are more common in AHTR and include dyspnea, tachycardia, rigors, fever, pain, and hemoglobinuria. Laboratory indicators of hemolysis include a decrease in hemoglobin, an increase in bilirubin and lactate dehydrogenase, and a positive direct antiglobulin test (depending on the type of hemolysis). A DHTR will often be accompanied by an incompatible crossmatch that was not able to be identified pretransfusion.[3] If hemolysis occurs while the transfusion is infusing, it should be stopped immediately and the patient treated with supportive care and aggressive hydration to minimize the risk of kidney injury. Hemolysis occurring with transfusion should be evaluated for a clerical error in labeling, product selection, or administration.

## REFERENCES

1. Semple JW, et al. Transfusion-associated circulatory overload and transfusion-related acute lung injury. *Blood.* 2019;133(17):1840–1853.
2. Toy P, et al. Transfusion-related acute lung injury: incidence and risk factors. *Blood.* 2012;119(7):1757–1767.
3. *Annual Serious Hazards of Transfusion (SHOT) Report 2019.* Accessed August 17, 2020. https://www.shotuk.org/wp-content/uploads/myimages/SHOT-REPORT-2019-Final-Bookmarked-v2.pdf
4. Tinegate H, et al. Guideline on the investigation and management of acute transfusion reactions. Prepared by the BCSH Blood Transfusion Task Force. *Br J Haematol.* 2012;159(2):143–153.
5. Estcourt LJ, et al. Guidelines for the use of platelet transfusions. *Br J Haematol.* 2017;176(3):365–394.

# 181.

# TRANSFUSION THERAPY FOR MASSIVE HEMORRHAGE

*Colby B. Tanner and Elaine A. Boydston*

## INTRODUCTION

Massive hemorrhage has historically been defined as hemorrhage requiring transfusion equivalent to an entire blood volume in 24 hours. This definition has since been expanded to consider the rate of transfusion, volume of blood products besides packed red blood cells (pRBCs) and changes in laboratory values, including hemoglobin and hematocrit.[1,2] Although individually distinct, each indicator of massive hemorrhage attempts to identify patients with physiologic changes related to massive blood loss. This allows for the restoration of intravascular volume while balancing oxygen delivery needs and maintaining adequate levels of coagulation factors for hemostasis.

## PHYSIOLOGY OF COAGULATION AND COAGULOPATHY IN HEMORRHAGE

The coagulation cascade and formation of a thrombin clot are tightly regulated processes that may be disturbed during massive hemorrhage. Several physiologic derangements may result from and contribute to hemorrhage and must be considered during resuscitation measures.

### HEMODILUTION

During initial resuscitation of hemorrhaging patients, crystalloid and colloid solutions administered can result in a dilutional coagulopathy. Although the exact etiology is unknown, contributing factors may include decreased thrombin generation, dilution of procoagulant factors, and alterations in fibrinolysis.[2]

### HYPOTHERMIA AND ACIDOSIS

Exposure and resuscitation with room temperature fluids often causes hypothermia and acidosis with associated metabolic derangements. Platelet adhesion and procoagulant enzyme function are altered, resulting in coagulopathy and delayed clot formation.[3]

### HYPERFIBRINOLYSIS

Fibrinolysis is important for maintaining homeostasis of the coagulation system; however, hyperfibrinolysis can result in excessive blood loss in trauma, post–cardiopulmonary bypass, and liver disease. Early initiation of antifibrinolytic therapies such as tranexamic acid in the treatment of trauma patients has been found to decrease transfusion requirements by up to one-third and has improved mortality.[4]

## RESUSCITATION DURING MASSIVE HEMORRHAGE

Damage control resuscitation (DCR) is a term and strategy coined by the military for use in the treatment of hemorrhagic shock. DCR is a comprehensive strategy of resuscitation with the major goal of restoring intravascular volume while managing homeostatic imbalances that occur in the setting of massive hemorrhage and massive transfusion.[4] The following are the major components of DCR.

### PATIENT EVALUATION AND DETECTION OF HEMORRHAGIC SHOCK

Rapid detection of patients who are at risk of massive hemorrhage decreases the time to initiation of DCR. As only 1%–3% of trauma patients presenting to major trauma centers will require massive transfusion, several tools help stratify the risk of massive hemorrhage by looking at factors such as presence of penetrating trauma, systolic blood pressure less 90 mm Hg, heart rate greater than 120 beats per minute, focused abdominal sonography in trauma examination results, and laboratory values, including hemoglobin and base excess. These tools have high sensitivity and specificity for detecting patients at risk for massive hemorrhage.[4,5]

## MINIMIZATION OF CRYSTALLOID PRODUCTS

In the 1980s, the initial response to massive hemorrhage was to administer large volumes of crystalloid solutions to increase cardiac preload and maintain cardiac output to augment oxygen delivery.[5] Subsequent studies showed large volumes of crystalloid caused increased intracellular edema and dysfunction of pancreatic insulin synthesis and secretion, hepatocyte glucose metabolism, and cardiac myocyte excitability, among other complications. In the intraoperative setting, studies have demonstrated restrictive crystalloid fluid regimens are associated with reduced incidence of postoperative ileus and decreased cardiopulmonary and wound healing complications versus fluid liberal regimens.[4,5]

## OPTIMAL TRANSFUSION OF BLOOD PRODUCTS

Studies including the major multicenter PROMMTT (Prospective, Observational, Multicenter, Major Trauma Transfusion) study have shown balanced transfusion with high ratios of fresh frozen plasma (FFP) and platelets relative to pRBCs improves survival. PROMMTT demonstrated that a 1:1 (PRBC-to-FFP) transfusion ratio improved survival compared to 1:2 ratio and greater when given in the first 6 hours of hemorrhage.[1] Many other studies have been conducted to look at optimal ratios of blood product transfusion, and while many different ratios have been considered, nearly all studies demonstrated improved survival with lower transfusion ratios (closer to 1:1).[4,5]

## PERMISSIVE HYPOTENSION

During DCR, the primary hemodynamic goal is to maintain adequate blood pressure to ensure perfusion of vital organs. However, blood pressure should not be so high that it exacerbates hemorrhage while attempts are being made to achieve hemostasis.[4,5]

## MANAGEMENT OF HEMOSTASIS

Prothrombin time (PT) and activated partial thromboplastin time are the most common screening tests for coagulopathy in the setting of massive hemorrhage. PT prolongation is presumed to be a result of hemodilution or loss of coagulation factors during massive hemorrhage. A PT of 1.5 times normal is both sensitive (0.88) and specific (0.88) for at least one nonhemostatic factor after trauma[2] and may signal that FFP transfusion is indicated. Additional laboratory tests include measuring a fibrinogen level (which generally is corrected via cryoprecipitate transfusion to maintain levels greater than 200 mg/dL) and D-dimer.[3] As these conventional laboratory tests may be associated with frequent delays, point-of-care assays, including thromboelastography

(TEG) and rotational thromboelastometry (ROTEM), can be useful. TEG and ROTEM offer the advantages of giving a more a comprehensive analysis of clot formation as well as a detection of fibrinolysis, allowing for targeted therapies.[3] Strategies to correct coagulopathy and defects in clot formation include utilization of coagulation factor concentrates, fibrinogen repletion, desmopressin administration, and reversal of any anticoagulants.[3]

## FREQUENT SETTINGS OF MASSIVE HEMORRHAGE

### TRAUMA

Much of the above data regarding DCR have been developed from the study of trauma patients. These patients can have significant microvascular and macrovascular hemorrhage associated with traumatic injury. Stabilization of trauma patients to allow operative repair of vascular damage is the major goal of DCR.[3-5]

### LIVER DISEASE AND LIVER TRANSPLANT

End-stage liver disease (ESLD) is associated with reductions of both pro- and anticoagulant proteins. This results in a propensity for both bleeding and intravascular thrombus formation. The major causes of bleeding in ESLD patients include portal hypertension–induced gastrointestinal bleeding, reduced hepatic synthetic function causing coagulopathy, hyperfibrinolysis, and massive hemorrhage during liver transplantation.

### CARDIAC SURGERY

Cardiac surgical patients are often taking medications that may promote bleeding, including antiplatelet therapies and anticoagulants. Additionally, use of cardiopulmonary bypass during cardiac surgery increases the propensity for hyperfibrinolysis and coagulopathy.[3]

## REFERENCES

1. Holcomb JB, et al. The prospective, observational, multicenter, major trauma transfusion (PROMMTT) study: comparative effectiveness of a time-varying treatment with competing risks. *JAMA Surg.* 2013;148(2):127–136.
2. Bolliger D, et al. Pathophysiology and treatment of coagulopathy in massive hemorrhage and hemodilution. *Anesthesiology.* 2010;113(5): 1205–1219.
3. Ghadimi K, et al. Perioperative management of the bleeding patient. *Br J Anaesth.* 2016;117:iii18–iii30.
4. Pohlman TH, et al. Damage control resuscitation. *Blood Rev.* 2015;29(4):251–262.
5. Chang R, Holcomb JB. Optimal fluid therapy for traumatic hemorrhagic shock. *Crit Care Clin.* 2017;33(1):15–36.

# 182.

# TRANSFUSION RATIOS

*Albert Lee and Nathan Schulman*

## INTRODUCTION

With regard to massive transfusion scenarios, there has been much interest regarding ideal transfusion ratios for packed red blood cells (pRBCs) and fresh frozen plasma (FFP). On the one extreme, transfusing only pRBCs will eventually create a spiraling iatrogenic coagulopathy. Conversely, transfusing only plasma will do nothing to improve the blood's oxygen-carrying capacity.

Transfusions historically had been conducted with whole blood, but by the 1980s, blood was split into various components and transfused accordingly to—in part—improve resource utilization. The resulting infrastructure was aimed toward correcting specific hematologic deficits with the assistance of laboratory testing and guidance. Component therapy then quickly spurred the development of massive transfusion protocols. Early protocols and policies determining optimal transfusion ratios were based largely on anecdotal evidence, and despite a multitude of trials, the ideal ratio remains highly controversial.

## EVIDENCE

It is important to note that the overwhelming majority of investigations regarding optimal transfusion ratios discussed below are nonrandomized observational studies, both prospective and retrospective (aside from the PROPPR trial, discussed below). This predisposes the discussed findings to both survival and length-of-time bias. In addition, a majority of studies defined massive transfusion as more than 10 units of pRBCs in a 24-hour period, which not only predisposes to heterogenous patient populations requiring transfusion, but also may potentially confound studies with evolving and dynamic indications for transfusion different from the initial issue on presentation.

The PROMMTT (Prospective, Observational, Multicenter, Major Trauma Transfusion) trial (2013) was a multicenter, prospective, observational study largely focused on evaluating the effects of early transfusion and exploring plasma-to–red blood cell (RBC) and platelet-to-RBC ratios in the hopes of laying a foundation for future randomized controlled trials (RCTs). Within the first 6 hours, individuals receiving FFP to RBC and platelet to RBC 1:2 ratios were three to four times more likely to die than those receiving ratios of 1:1 or greater. This transfusion ratio survival benefit extended in the FFP-to-RBC population up to 24 hours. Outside the first 24 hours, there were no observable extended benefits associated with any transfusion ratio.[1]

The PROPPR trial (2015) remains as one of the only multicenter RCTs successfully conducted that analyzed transfusion ratios. A FFP-to-platelet-to-RBC ratio of 1:1:1 was compared to a 1:1:2 ratio in 680 patients with severe hemorrhagic shock. No survival difference was noted between the two groups at primary outcome endpoints at 24 hours or 30 days. Of note, onset of clinical hemostasis was noted to be earlier, and there was a notable decrease in death secondary to exsanguination in the 1:1:1 cohort.[2]

Of the more recent meta-analyses, Rahouma et al. (2018) provided a review of a total of 36 studies, about 16,000 trauma patients, and about 600 nontrauma patients. Survival at 24 hours and 30 days was improved with a higher FFP-to-RBC transfusion ratio. Observed data suggested this applied to both trauma and nontrauma cohorts. Of the available acute respiratory distress syndrome (ARDS) and acute lung injury data, there was no significant difference in incidence between transfusion ratio cohorts.[3]

As noted previously, massive transfusion is largely defined as 10 units pRBCs or more over 24 hours. To potentially target a more homogeneous patient population and account for likely changes in transfusion strategies over 24 hours, Roquet et al. (2019) classified severe bleeding as a massive transfusion requiring 4 units within the first 6 hours of presentation. Retrospective analysis of a French trauma registry revealed an increased 30-day survival in individuals requiring massive transfusion receiving a high-ratio transfusion strategy of 1:1.5 or greater FFP-to-RBC ratio. This perceived survival benefit appeared to persist after correcting for possible survivorship bias.[4]

## RISKS AND CONSIDERATIONS

Among the many known risks and considerations of transfusion, there exist several that must always be kept in mind that remain specific to individuals receiving large quantities of blood products.

In large quantities, the anticoagulant citrate and supernatant potassium present in pRBCs can elicit cardiac dysfunction, arrhythmia, and arrest. The temperature of refrigerated pRBCs can also contribute to patient hypothermia (cold toxicity), resulting in additional risk of cardiovascular collapse, impairment of drug metabolism, and coagulopathy/platelet dysfunction in a patient with massive transfusion requirements. Frequent measurements of serum calcium and potassium, appropriate electrolyte management, and optimizing infusate and patient temperature with appropriate warmers are prudent measures to avoid complications.[5]

Transfusion-associated circulatory overload appears to be directly related to an excess volume of transfused blood, resulting in hydrostatic pulmonary edema and other symptoms of congestive heart failure. Treatment is largely supportive, and though diuretics have not been explicitly studied, they may be reasonable therapies to pursue.[5]

Transfusion-associated lung injury is characterized by noncardiogenic pulmonary edema in the setting of transfusion and is thought to have a significant immune-mediated/neutrophil-driven component, although the mechanism is incompletely understood. Though preventive measures can be optimized, such as prioritizing for male plasma donors and attempting to utilize restrictive transfusion strategies, treatment is largely supportive.[5] After immediate discontinuation of the transfusion, supplemental oxygen with mechanical ventilation with restrictive tidal volume and fluid strategies may be helpful, similar to strategies used to treat ARDS.

One major consideration to keep in mind is the constitution of hematocrit, platelets, and coagulation factors in whole blood versus that of a 1:1:1 transfusion strategy. Whole blood (fresh or stored) contains a hematocrit of approximately 38%–39%, platelet counts of 150,000–200,000/μL, and a coagulation factor concentration of about 85% of predonation levels. However, component therapy reconstituted to a 1:1:1 ratio suffers from significant hemodilution with additive solutions and anticoagulants. This yields an overall hematocrit of about 29%, a platelet count of about 90,000/μL, and a coagulation factor concentration of about 62% of predonation levels.

In all, massive transfusion strategies remain highly controversial, and there remains a lack of robust, randomized clinical evidence to support specific strategies or ratio thresholds. Current available evidence seems to favor transfusion ratios that approach the composition of whole blood, and many institutions have adopted whole-blood, early-transfusion strategies for patients stratified at risk for massive hemorrhage.

## REFERENCES

1. John H, et al. The Prospective, Observational, Multicenter, Major Trauma Transfusion (PROMMTT) study: comparative effectiveness of a time-varying treatment with competing risks. *JAMA Surg.* 2013;148(2):127–136.
2. Holcomb JB, et al. Transfusion of plasma, platelets, and red blood Cells in a 1:1:1 vs a 1:1:2 ratio and mortality in patients with severe trauma: the PROPPR randomized clinical trial. *JAMA.* 2015;313(5):471–482.
3. Mohamed R, et al. Does a balanced transfusion ratio of plasma to packed red blood cells improve outcomes in both trauma and surgical patients? A meta-analysis of randomized controlled trials and observational studies. *Am J Surg.* 2018;216(2):342–350.
4. Florian R, et al. Association of early, high plasma-to-red blood cell transfusion ratio with mortality in adults with severe bleeding after trauma. *JAMA Network Open.* 2019;2(9):e1912076. doi:10.1001/jamanetworkopen.2019.12076
5. Meghan D, et al. Transfusion reactions: prevention, diagnosis, and treatment. *Lancet.* 2016;388(10061):2825–2836.

# 183.

## USE OF UNCROSSMATCHED PRODUCTS

*Christina Stachur*

### INTRODUCTION

Usually, crossmatched blood is available for patients requiring transfusion within an hour of the blood bank receiving a proper sample. However, certain clinical situations, such as massive hemorrhage, necessitate transfusion of blood products before crossmatched blood is available.

### TRANSFUSION OF UNCROSSMATCHED PACKED RED BLOOD CELLS

Uncrossmatched products are used in situations where a patient's ABO blood group is unknown, and they require a life-saving transfusion that cannot wait for crossmatched blood to be prepared. The issued uncrossmatched packed red blood cells (pRBCs) are type O. These erythrocytes have neither antigen A nor antigen B and are therefore compatible with anti-A and anti-B antibodies that may be found in the recipient's plasma.

#### ABO BLOOD GROUP REFRESHER

**Blood type A** has antigen A on the erythrocyte and anti-B antibodies in the plasma. These patients cannot receive B or AB pRBCs but can receive A or O pRBCs. They can receive A or AB plasma.

**Blood type B** has antigen B on the erythrocyte and anti-A antibodies in the plasma. These patients cannot receive A or AB pRBCs but can receive B or O pRBCs. They can receive B or AB plasma.

**Blood type AB** has both antigens A and B on the erythrocyte and neither antibody in the plasma. These patients can receive all types of pRBCs since their plasma does not contain either antibody. They can only receive AB plasma.

**Blood type O** has neither A nor B antigen on the erythrocyte and both anti-A and anti-B antibodies in the plasma. These patients can only receive type

O pRBCs. They are the universal donor. They can receive A, B, AB, and O plasma.

Transfusing type O pRBCs to unknown ABO blood group patients prevents acute intravascular hemolytic reactions from occurring, which can be life threatening. The mechanism involves the destruction of donor RBCs by antibodies in the recipient's plasma. The destruction of these cells leads to activation of the coagulation cascade and complement cascade, promoting the release of inflammatory cytokines. The clinical signs of this type of hemolytic reaction include fever, chills, abdominal pain, flank pain, chest pain, shortness of breath, hypotension, and hemoglobinuria and can even progress to shock, disseminated intravascular coagulation, and death.

### TRANSFUSION OF UNCROSSMATCHED PLASMA

Transfusing type AB plasma is the safest type of plasma to transfuse during massive hemorrhage as it does not contain anti-A or anti-B antibodies. Unfortunately, only 2%–3% of blood donors are group AB, and therefore the AB plasma inventory alone is not enough to meet hospital demands for uncrossmatched products. Since roughly 85% of Caucasians are type A or O, type A plasma would also be compatible for transfusions. Therefore, a majority of trauma centers now issue type A plasma in cases of massive hemorrhage when a patient has an unknown ABO group.

### TRANSFUSION OF UNCROSSMATCHED WHOLE BLOOD

If transfusion begins with type O *whole* blood and more than 2 units have been infused, only type O blood should continue to be used. This is because type O *whole* blood contains anti-A and anti-B antibodies, which can cause hemolytic reactions with type A and type B blood cells if given in significant quantities. Patients should not go on to receive type-specific blood until the blood bank determines that the transfused anti-A and anti-B antibody levels have fallen low enough. This usually takes approximately 2 weeks.

## CONCERNS REGARDING THE USE OF UNCROSSMATCHED RBCS

While using type O uncrossmatched pRBCs prevents an acute intravascular hemolytic reaction, there is still the potential risk of a less severe type of hemolytic reaction from other erythrocyte antigens. These antigens (e.g., D, E, Kell, Duffy, etc.), if present on the donor pRBCs, can potentially react with antibodies in the recipient's plasma. These reactions are usually less severe since they are mediated by immunoglobulin (Ig) G antibodies (as opposed to IgM) and cause erythrocytes to be destroyed in the liver and spleen. This type of extravascular hemolysis, while usually not life threatening, removes the newly transfused erythrocytes from circulation, thereby decreasing the effectiveness of therapy.

The overall rate of having a patient with a hemolytic reaction (verified by either laboratory testing or clinical observation) is very low, approximately 0.1%. The risk increases in proportion to the patient's risk of having been exposed to foreign erythrocytes in the past (e.g., pregnancy or prior blood transfusion). Clinical markers suggestive of hemolysis include but are not limited to jaundice, hematuria, fever, elevated lactate dehydrogenase, and elevated bilirubin. Despite the low risk of a hemolytic reaction, uncrossmatched products should not be used for clinically stable patients who can wait for crossmatched products to become available.

## THE EFFECT OF RHESUS STATUS

Erythrocytes may also express another antigen, the D antigen, on their surface. This antigen is part of the Rh blood group system and is the second most important blood group system after the ABO system. Those with the D antigen are RhD positive and those without are RhD negative. Antibodies to RhD antigens can be involved in hemolytic transfusion reactions. Most people are RhD positive.

During massive hemorrhage, uncrossmatched products are typically RhD negative for all females of childbearing age (<50 years old) or those whose RhD status is unknown. If an RhD-negative female receives RhD-positive blood, she may mount an immune response to the donor antigens. If she later becomes pregnant with an RhD-positive child, the RhD alloimmunization could lead to hemolytic disease of the fetus and newborn. In situations of massive hemorrhage, when RhD-negative patients are transfused with RhD-positive blood, the rate of RhD alloimmunization is approximately 10%–25%. To prevent RhD alloimmunization, Rh immunoglobulin (RhIg; RHoGAM; WinRho) can be administered to neutralize the donor erythrocytes.

## ANESTHETIC CONSIDERATIONS

- Type O RhD-negative pRBCs may be safely transfused to recipients of any ABO RhD type, which has led to a high demand for this limited resource.
- Type O RhD-negative pRBCs should be reserved for three cohorts of females of childbearing potential: those who are type O RhD negative, those who are RhD negative requiring transfusion when type-specific blood is unavailable, and those of unknown blood type who require pRBCs before the completion of pretransfusion testing. All others, including males, should receive RhD-positive erythrocytes.
- Whereas previously only type AB plasma was used for traumatically injured patients of unknown ABO blood type requiring massive transfusion, emerging evidence suggests that it is safe to transfuse type A plasma as well.
- If transfusion begins with type O *whole* blood and more than 2 units have been infused, only type O blood should continue to be used.
- The overall risk of hemolysis following the transfusion of uncrossmatched erythrocytes to patients needing an emergency transfusion is 0.1%. Despite this low risk, uncrossmatched pRBCs should not be used in otherwise stable patients who can wait until crossmatched units become available.

## REFERENCES

1. American Association of Blood Banks. Recommendations on the use of group O red blood cells. AABB Association Bulletin #19-02. June 26, 2019.
2. Yazer MH. Use of uncrossmatched erythrocytes in emergency bleeding situations. *Anesthesiology.* 2018;128(3):650–656.
3. Yao FS, et al., eds. *Yao & Artusio's Anesthesiology: Problem-Oriented Patient Management.* Lippincott Williams & Wilkins; 2008.

# Part 16

# ENDOCRINE AND METABOLIC SYSTEMS

# 184.

# ANATOMY OF THE ENDOCRINE SYSTEM

*Ruzanna Nalbandyan and Nawal E. Ragheb-Mueller*

## INTRODUCTION

The endocrine system consists of a collection of glands that secrete a variety of hormones. These hormones travel to target organs via the bloodstream and regulate vital functions, including metabolism, reproduction, growth and development, as well as response to injury, stress, and mood. The integral components are discussed below.

**Hypothalamus:** The hypothalamus is considered part of the diencephalon (forebrain). It is located below the thalamus and forms the floor and lower lateral walls of the third ventricle. Anteriorly, it extends up to the optic chiasma. The hypothalamus is composed of fiber tracts and nuclei situated symmetrically about the third ventricle. The nuclei are organized into three subdivisions and derived primarily from the hypothalamic blood supply[1]:

- *Anterior (or chiasmatic) region*—extends between the lamina terminalis and the anterior infundibular recess
- *Median (or tuberal) region*—proceeds to the anterior column of the fornix
- *Posterior (or mammillary) region*—stretches to the caudal mammillary bodies

The endocrine hypothalamus secretes neurohormones into the hypophyseal portal blood to act on the anterior pituitary. Hypothalamic arcuate nuclei produce releasing hormones that act on the anterior pituitary (adenohypophysis) and regulate its activity. The hypothalamus releases the following: gonadotropin releasing, thyrotropin releasing), corticotropin releasing, growth hormone releasing, and prolactin releasing hormones.

One of the major efferent pathways from the hypothalamus is the hypothalamic-neurohypophyseal tract, which connects the paraventricular and supraoptic nuclei of the hypothalamus to the nerve terminals in the posterior pituitary. The paraventricular nucleus releases primarily oxytocin and some antidiuretic hormone (ADH), while the supraoptic nucleus releases mostly ADH and some oxytocin, directly into the bloodstream.[2] Hypothalamic neuroendocrine cells are regulated by feedback signals from the endocrine glands and other circulating factors.

**Pituitary Gland:** The pituitary is a pea-sized gland (weighing 0.5 g) enveloped by dura; it sits within the sella turcica of the sphenoid. The sella turcica is a saddle-shaped depression surrounding the inferior, anterior, and posterior aspects of the pituitary. The pituitary's superior aspect is covered by the diaphragm sellae, a fold of dura mater that separates the cerebrospinal fluid–filled subarachnoid space from the pituitary. The infundibulum pierces the diaphragm sellae to connect the pituitary to the hypothalamus. The pituitary's lateral aspects lie adjacent to the cavernous sinuses. From superior to inferior, the cavernous sinus contains cranial nerves III (oculomotor), IV (trochlear), VI (abducens), V1 (ophthalmic branch of trigeminal nerve), and V2 (maxillary branch of trigeminal nerve). The internal carotid artery also courses through the cavernous sinus, medial to these nerves. The pituitary is composed of two functionally distinct structures that differ in embryologic development and anatomy: adenohypophysis (anterior pituitary) and the neurohypophysis (posterior pituitary).

- *Adenohypophysis*—develops from Rathke's pouch, an upward invagination of oral ectoderm from the roof of the mouth.[3] It produces, stores, and releases eight hormones: corticotropin (adrenocorticotropic hormone, ACTH), thyroid-stimulating hormone, follicle-stimulating hormone, luteinizing hormone, growth hormone, insulin-like growth hormone, melanocyte-stimulating hormone, and prolactin.
- *Neurohypophysis*—develops from the infundibulum, a downward extension of neural ectoderm from the diencephalon floor. It stores two hormones (oxytocin and vasopressin) produced in the hypothalamus.

**Pineal Body:** The pineal, or epiphysis, is located in the middle of the brain below the corpus callosum and produces melatonin, which regulates circadian rhythm.

**Thyroid Gland:** The thyroid is a two-lobe endocrine gland connected by an isthmus. It spans the C5-T1 vertebrae and lies behind the sternohyoid and sternothyroid muscles. It wraps around the cricoid cartilage and superior tracheal ring, inferior to the thyroid cartilage of the larynx. The gland consists of follicular and parafollicular cells. Follicular cells produce thyroxine (T4) and triiodothyronine (T3), water-soluble tyrosine-based hormones, primarily responsible for regulation of metabolism. Parafollicular cells are responsible for calcitonin production, a water-soluble polypeptide, which decreases calcium concentration in the body by inhibiting renal absorption of calcium; decreasing the amount of calcium absorbed in the intestines; and increasing bone absorption.

**Parathyroid Glands:** The parathyroids are a group of four small, pea-sized structures, located behind the thyroid, that regulate calcium balance. They produce parathyroid hormone (PTH), which antagonizes calcitonin. PTH increases serum calcium by increasing bone resorption and increasing calcium and phosphorus absorption in the gastrointestinal tract. This promotes synthesis of active vitamin D, increases calcium reabsorption in the renal tubules, and decreases phosphorus reabsorption.

**Adrenal Glands:** The adrenal glands are paired, triangular-shaped organs (each weighing 4–5 g) located on the superior aspect of each kidney. They secrete several vital hormones that regulate the immune system, body metabolism, and salt/water balance and aid stress responses. The adrenals are composed of two distinct tissues: the outer, much larger, cortex and the inner, smaller, medulla. The cortex comprises three distinct zones:

- *Zona glomerulosa (outer layer)*—The zona glomerulosa is responsible for the synthesis of mineralocorticoids, the most important of which, aldosterone, plays a role in electrolyte balance and blood pressure regulation.
- *Zona fasciculata (middle layer)*—The zona fasciculata produces glucocorticoids, of which the predominant hormone is cortisol. Cortisol regulates blood glucose via gluconeogenesis and modulates the immune system as well as the metabolism of lipids, proteins, and carbohydrates. Cortisol secretion is under the regulation of ACTH.
- *Zona reticularis (inner zone)*—The zona reticularis produces androgens and influences development of secondary sexual characteristics. The primary androgen it produces is dehydroepiandrosterone, a precursor for synthesis of progesterone, estrogen, cortisol, and testosterone.

The adrenal medulla synthesizes catecholamines. It is in the medulla, for example, where the enzyme phenylethanolamine *N*-methyltransferase (PNMT) is found.[4] PNMT is responsible for converting norepinephrine to epinephrine.

**Pancreas:** The endocrine pancreas consists of pancreatic islets (formerly islets of Langerhans). These islets contain

- $\alpha$-Cells (20% of each islet) produce glucagon, which is released in response to low glucose levels.
- $\beta$-Cells (75%) produce insulin. Elevated glucose levels stimulate insulin release.
- $\delta$-Cells (4%) secrete somatostatin, which inhibits glucagon and insulin release.
- Pancreatic polypeptide (PP) cells (1%) secrete PP hormone. This hormone influences appetite and regulation of pancreatic exocrine and endocrine secretions. PP hormone released following a meal may reduce further food consumption but is also released in response to fasting.

## REFERENCES

1. Carpenter MB. *Core Text of Neuroanatomy*. 4th ed. Baltimore, MD: Williams and Wilkins; 1991.
2. Braak H, Braak E. Anatomy of the human hypothalamus (chiasmatic and tuberal region). *Prog Brain Res*. 1992;93:3–14; discussion 14–16.
3. Solov'ev GS, et al. Embryonic morphogenesis of the human pituitary. *Neurosci Behav Physiol*. 2008;38(8):829–833.
4. Randall DC. Discovering the role of the adrenal gland in the control of body function. *Am J Physiol Regul Integr Comp Physiol*. 2004; 287(5):R1007–R1008.

# 185.

# HYPOPITUITARY DISEASE

*Ruzanna Nalbandyan and Nawal E. Ragheb-Mueller*

## INTRODUCTION

Hypopituitarism refers to deficient secretion of one or more pituitary hormones, which results from diseases of the pituitary or hypothalamus. Hypopituitarism is a rare disorder and arises from tumors (pituitary 44%, nonpituitary 6%) and other causes (50%).[1]

## ETIOLOGY

The many possible causes span pituitary disorders and hypothalamic disorders.

### PITUITARY DISORDERS

1. Nonfunctioning pituitary adenomas—These are benign, non–hormone-secreting tumors, most commonly associated with hypopituitarism. Clinical presentation results from the growing tumor's mass effect on the anterior pituitary.
2. Mass lesions—Pituitary cysts, craniopharyngiomas, metastatic cancers (germ cell tumors), meningiomas, pituitary abscesses, and other lesions can cause temporary or permanent damage by exerting constant pressure on pituitary cells. The clinical picture depends on the rapidity with which the pathology arises. Patients in whom the hypopituitarism is due to a sellar mass will present with symptoms (e.g., headache, hemianopia, diplopia, or visual loss) specific to its location.
3. Pituitary infarction (Sheehan syndrome)—Excessive peripartum blood loss may lead to severely low blood pressure and cause infarction and necrosis of the pituitary.[2] Clinical features include lethargy, anorexia, fatigue, weight loss, failure of postpartum lactation, and failure to resume menses in the ensuing months.
4. Pituitary apoplexy—Pituitary apoplexy is a rare endocrine emergency that results from sudden hemorrhage into the pituitary. This most commonly involves a pituitary adenoma and may be its initial manifestation. Apoplexy clinically presents with acute onset of excruciating headache, vomiting, altered sensorium, visual defects (involving CN III or IV) and endocrine dysfunction.[3]

### HYPOTHALAMIC DISORDERS

1. Tumors—Tumors include benign tumors that arise in the hypothalamus (craniopharyngiomas) and malignancies that metastasize there (e.g., lung and breast carcinomas).
2. Traumatic brain injury—Severe head trauma to the skull base can cause hypothalamic hormone deficiencies, specifically hormones of the anterior pituitary and vasopressin.[4]
3. Infiltrative lesions—Langerhans cell histiocytosis and sarcoidosis can cause diabetes insipidus and deficiencies in anterior pituitary hormones.

## CLINICAL MANIFESTATIONS OF HYPOPITUITARISM

The clinical presentation of hypopituitarism depends on which anterior pituitary hormones are involved. Damage to the gland can affect the secretion of one, several, or all of its hormones. The clinical presentation will depend on the rapidity with which the pathology develops, the severity of the hormonal perturbations, and the hormones involved.

**ACTH Deficiency:** The adrenocorticotropic hormone (ACTH, corticotropin) deficiency will result in cortisol deficiency and secondary adrenal insufficiency. Chronic ACTH deficiency will manifest with lassitude, fatigue, anorexia, weight loss, decreased libido, postural hypotension, hypoglycemia, and eosinophilia. In acute and severe cases, ACTH deficiency can lead to profound vascular collapse and death.

There are two important clinical distinctions between primary adrenal insufficiency and ACTH deficiency (secondary insufficiency).

1. As opposed to primary adrenal insufficiency, ACTH deficiency *does not* result in hyperpigmentation.
2. ACTH deficiency *does not* cause salt wasting, volume contraction, and hyperkalemia because it does not result in deficiency of aldosterone.

**Thyroid-Stimulating Hormone Deficiency:** Deficiency of thyroid-stimulating hormone (TSH) results in secondary hypothyroidism. Unlike primary hypothyroidism (hypothyroidism caused by the thyroid itself), in secondary hypothyroidism both serum TSH and serum free $T_4$ levels are low. Manifestations include fatigue, cold intolerance, weight gain, decreased appetite, constipation, dry skin, myxedema, menorrhagia or secondary amenorrhea, bradycardia, and delayed relaxation of deep tendon reflexes.

**Growth Hormone Deficiency:** Deficiency of growth hormone (GH) presents as short stature, growth failure, younger looking face, prominent forehead, impaired hair growth, and delayed puberty in children. In adults, it manifests as changes in body composition (increase in fat, decrease in lean body mass), decreased bone mineral density, anxiety, depression, decreased sexual function and interest, dyslipidemia, and cardiovascular disease.

**Gonadotropins Deficiency:** Deficient secretion of follicle-stimulating hormone (FSH) and luteinizing hormone (LH) results in hypogonadotropic hypogonadism (secondary hypogonadism). In women, this presents as ovarian hypofunction and decreased estradiol secretion and manifests similarly to primary ovarian insufficiency (premature ovarian failure). Premenopausal women present with irregular periods or amenorrhea, anovulatory infertility, hot flashes, vaginal atrophy, and decreased bone mineral density. In men, hypogonadism presents with testicular hypofunction and decreases in testosterone production, muscle mass, bone mineral density,[5] libido, and fertility.

**Antidiuretic Hormone Deficiency:** Antidiuretic hormone (ADH, arginine vasopressin) deficiency causes central diabetes insipidus, which manifests with polyuria, polydipsia, and nocturia.

## ANESTHETIC CONSIDERATIONS

### PREOPERATIVE

All patients with hypopituitarism require thorough evaluation before surgery. This includes a complete history and physical to determine disease duration and severity. Proper preoperative laboratory workup includes a complete blood count and basic metabolic profile to evaluate possible electrolyte and metabolic abnormalities. Endocrine evaluation should include a complete thyroid panel, serum levels of cortisol, ACTH, GH, insulinlike growth factor 1, FSH, LH, prolactin, and testosterone levels. Women of childbearing age with secondary amenorrhea should have a pregnancy test before an elective procedure. Depending on the deficiency, preoperative replacement therapy of hydrocortisone, thyroxine, and/or desmopressin (DDAVP) may be indicated.

### INTRAOPERATIVE

Intraoperative management can be challenging. Patients with secondary adrenal insufficiency, secondary hypothyroidism, and/or central diabetes insipidus may require perioperative stress dose hydrocortisone and/or intranasal or subcutaneous DDAVP. Intravenous access with two large-bore peripheral catheters is a necessity; central access should be considered. An arterial line should be placed for continuous hemodynamic and electrolyte monitoring.

An *Addisonian crisis* can occur perioperatively in undiagnosed or poorly managed patients with secondary adrenal insufficiency; this is a life-threatening state in which glucocorticoid and mineralocorticoid requirements exceed endogenous release. Perioperative stress, anxiety, and pain may provoke it. Acute Addisonian crisis manifests with severe weakness, abdominal pain, vomiting, refractory hypotension, and hypoglycemia. Quick identification and prompt treatment with intravenous fluids and steroids reduces morbidity and mortality.

*Myxedema coma* is a rare, but life-threatening, complication that may occur intraoperatively in patients with hypopituitarism and long-standing neglected secondary hypothyroidism. Myxedema coma causes a drastic decrease in metabolic rate with hypotension, bradycardia, hypothermia, hypoventilation, and decreased cardiac output progressing to coma. Mortality in untreated, unrecognized cases approaches 100%. Treatment consists of empirical steroids, intravenous thyroid hormone supplementation, and supportive therapy.

### POSTOPERATIVE

Patients require close postoperative monitoring for hemodynamic stability as well as signs and symptoms of life-threatening complications, such as Addisonian crisis, myxedema coma, and central diabetes insipidus. Hormone replacement therapy is continued postoperatively; stressors, such as pain and anxiety, should be properly treated.

### REFERENCES

1. Tanriverdi F, et al. Etiology of hypopituitarism in tertiary care institutions in Turkish population: analysis of 773 patients from pituitary study group database. *Endocrine*. 2014;47:198
2. Barkan AL. Pituitary atrophy in patients with Sheehan's syndrome. *Am J Med Sci*. 1989;298:38.
3. Capatina C, et al. Management of endocrine disease: pituitary tumor apoplexy. *Eur J Endocrinol*. 2015;172:R179.
4. Edwards OM, Clark JD. Post-traumatic hypopituitarism. Six cases and a review of the literature. *Medicine (Baltimore)*. 1986;65:281.
5. Stepan JJ, et al. Castrated men exhibit bone loss: effect of calcitonin treatment on biochemical indices of bone remodeling. *J Clin Endocrinol Metab*. 1989;69:523.

# 186.

# THYROID GLAND

*Evgenev Romanov and Edward Noguera*

## INTRODUCTION

The thyroid gland is in the neck in front of the thyroid cartilage. It consists of two lobes connected by the isthmus. Up to 30% of the population has a pyramidal lobe originating from the isthmus. Each lobule is filled with microscopic follicles, which are the functional units of the thyroid gland. The thyroid gland secretes thyroid hormones, which play a major role in the regulation of metabolism, development, growth, and brain development.[1]

## BLOOD SUPPLY

Left and right superior thyroid arteries originate from the external carotid artery; the left and right inferior thyroid arteries originate from the thyrocervical trunk; and the single thyroid ima artery originates from the aortic arch or brachiocephalic trunk.

## NERVE SUPPLY

The sympathetic nerve supply is the superior, middle, and inferior cervical ganglion of the sympathetic trunk. The parasympathetic nerve supply is the superior laryngeal nerve and recurrent laryngeal nerve.

## THYROID PHYSIOLOGY

The thyroid hormones triiodothyronine ($T_3$) and thyroxine ($T_4$), regulate major metabolic processes and are responsible for normal cardiac, pulmonary, and neurologic function.

Dietary iodine is taken up by the thyroid gland, coupled by thyroid peroxidase with tyrosine, and attached to thyroglobulin as $T_3$ or $T_4$, which detach from the thyroglobulin on demand and enter the bloodstream.

Thyroid-stimulating hormone (TSH) is synthesized in the anterior pituitary. TSH stimulates iodide uptake and proteolytic release of $T_3$ and $T_4$. Most of the circulating thyroid hormones bind to plasma thyroxine-binding globulin, whereas only a small portion exists in plasma as a free fraction.[1]

## PATHOLOGY OF THE THYROID GLAND

### HYPERTHYROIDISM

Graves' disease and multinodular diffuse goiter are the most common causes of hyperthyroidism (Table 186.1).

**Symptoms:** Symptoms are anxiety and insomnia, palpitations, heat intolerance, increased perspiration, and weight loss without increased appetite.

**Clinical Findings:** Clinically, there is goiter on examination, hypertension, tremors involving fingers/hands, hyperreflexia, proximal muscle weakness, and lid lag.

**Cardiovascular Manifestations:** The cardiovascular manifestations are increased left ventricular contractility and ejection fraction, tachycardia, and elevated systolic blood pressure. The elderly may present with heart failure, atrial fibrillation, or other arrhythmias.

**Management:** Make the patient euthyroid before surgery. Propylthiouracil and methimazole take too long to take effect (6–8 weeks). Potassium iodide inhibits thyroid peroxidase and reduces the size and vascularity of the thyroid. Because of the risk of thyrotoxicosis, the patient must be pretreated with propylthiouracil or methimazole prior to potassium iodide. The β-antagonist propranolol both alleviates excessive adrenergic stimulation and decreases peripheral conversion of $T_4$ to $T_3$. The combination of propranolol (titrated to effect) and potassium iodide (2 to 5

*Table 186.1* **CLASSIFICATION OF DIFFERENT THYROID DISEASES**

| GOITER LIKELY (MAY COMPROMISE AIRWAY) | GOITER UNLIKELY |
|---|---|
| – Graves' disease (80% cases)<br>– Multinodular toxic goiter (15% of cases)<br>– Hashimoto thyroiditis and subacute granulomatous thyroiditis (can cause transient hyperthyroidism)<br>– Thyroid cancer (usually euthyroid) | – Toxic thyroid adenoma<br>– Postpartum thyroiditis<br>– Iodine-induced hyperthyroidism<br>– Iatrogenic (excessive doses of levothyroxine)<br>– Struma ovarii |

drops every 5 hours) is used for 7–14 days to prepare a patient for surgery.[2]

## Hyperthyroid Patients Who Need Emergency Surgery

Consider β-adrenergic blockade to achieve a heart rate less than 90 beats per minute. β-Blockers do not prevent thyroid storm. Dexamethasone (2 to 12 mg/d) decreases the release of thyroid hormones and prevents conversion of $T_4$ to $T_3$.

## Hypothyroid Patients Who Need Emergent Surgery

The main clinical concern for hypothyroid patients who need emergent surgery is the increased likelihood of developing myxedema coma postoperatively. Clinically, a patient with myxedema coma is a patient who is very hypoactive, delirious, or obtunded; has a decreased cardiac output; is hypotensive, hypothermic, hypoglycemic, with delayed deep tendon reflexes; and has a high risk of aspiration postoperatively. Patients with myxedema coma cannot be liberated from mechanical ventilation easily. Myxedema coma requires admission to the intensive care unit and carries a high mortality (~50%). The pharmacological treatment of myxedema coma includes intravenous thyroxin and steroids. Steroids are used for adrenal insufficiency that is related to myxedema coma (hydrocortisone 50 mg IV every 6 hours). Intravenous thyroxin is also known as levothyroxine or $T_4$ (Synthroid*). The dose of levothyroxine for myxedema coma is 200–400 µg IV in 5–10 minutes and then 100 µg IV daily (1.6 µg/kg/d). If there is no improvement within 24 hours, $T_3$ can be considered. Liothryronine or $T_3$ (Cytomel*) is more potent than $T_4$; the dose in myxedema coma is 5–20 µg (~0.2 µg/kg) every 6 hours; the onset of liothyronine is 6–24 hours. Once clinical improvement is noticed, $T_3$ can be discontinued and $T_4$ is used as maintenance.[3] A very strict search for precipitating events of myxedema coma is mandatory. Sepsis is a common cause; thus, liberal use of antibiotics is acceptable.

An endocrinologist should be involved in the management of myxedema coma as therapy should be monitored closely concerning TSH levels and clinical signs. The combination of $T_3$ and $T_4$ has been associated with myocardial ischemia in patients with coronary artery disease.

## ANESTHESIA CONSIDERATIONS FOR HYPERTHYROID PATIENTS

**Preoperative:** Achieving a euthyroid state for elective surgeries is associated with improved patient outcomes. Antithyroid medications should be continued through the morning of surgery.

**Intraoperative:** Intraoperatively, there should be a smooth anesthesia induction to achieve adequate depth of surgical anesthesia that does not provoke excessive sympathetic stimulation.

**Muscle Relaxants:** Consider decreasing initial dosing of muscle relaxants. Careful titration of muscle relaxant depth is also clinically important. Hyperthyroid patients can present with concomitant myasthenia gravis.

**Cardiovascular Considerations:** Hypotension during surgery should be managed with direct-acting vasopressors, rather than medications that stimulate catecholamine release.[1,2] Regional anesthesia is an excellent choice when appropriate. Be aware of a test dose containing epinephrine triggering excessive sympathetic stimulation and thyroid storm, especially in patients who are not euthyroid. If a patient has a history of hyperthyroidism, the basal heart rate (HR) should be assessed. A patient is considered euthyroid if the HR is less than 90 beats per minute and there are minimal symptoms of hyperthyroidism.

## THYROID STORM

**Mechanism:** Thyroid storm is a life-threatening exacerbation of hyperthyroidism. It most commonly occurs in an undiagnosed or untreated hyperthyroid patient.

**Clinical Presentation:** The the thyroid storm presents with hyperthermia, tachycardia, dysrhythmias, myocardial ischemia, congestive heart failure, agitation, and confusion.

## Management of Thyroid Storm

- Intravenous fluids.

- Sodium iodide, 250 mg or IV every 6 hours.

- Propylthiouracil, 200–400 mg oral or via nasogastric tube every 6 hours.

- Hydrocortisone, 50–100 mg IV every 6 hours.

- β-Blockade: Propranolol, 10–40 mg oral every 4–6 hours or esmolol to treat hyperadrenergic signs.

- Temperature management: Cooling blankets, acetaminophen, and meperidine (25–50 mg) IV every 4–6 hours may be used to prevent shivering.

- Unstable supraventricular tachycardia or atrial fibrillation: Electrical cardioversion, rate control (β-blockers, calcium channel blockers, digoxin) versus rhythm control. Consider diuresis if there are signs of decompensated heart failure.

- Remove or treat the precipitating event.[1,2]

## ANESTHESIA FOR THYROID SURGERY

Indications for thyroid surgery are failed medical therapy, underlying cancer, and symptomatic goiter.

## ANESTHETIC MANAGEMENT

General anesthesia is considered the best anesthesia technique. Regional techniques have very limited clinical use. Specialized endotracheal tubes may be considered to assess vocal cord function and nerve-sparing techniques during surgical dissection (the recurrent laryngeal nerve especially). Nasal intubation is required for a transoral approach.

## PREOPERATIVE

A detailed physical examination focused on airway assessment is critical preoperatively. Large goiters or massive thyroid cancer can cause alterations in normal anatomy, leading to difficulty visualizing tracheal structures due to tracheal deviation or airway obstruction. Neck imaging studies should be reviewed before manipulation of the airway. Mass extension and mass effect should be assessed. Pulmonary function tests can help understand the extension and type of obstruction (intra- vs. extrathoracic). Depending on the severity of the mass effect on mediastinal structures, extracorporeal membrane oxygenation cannulation may be considered if the airway is compromised in such a way that the patient is unable to tolerate the decubitus position or even if an awake trach is impossible to be safely performed. A thorough review of the medical record is of paramount importance for knowledge of the clinical comorbidities, review of symptoms, history of radiation or chemotherapy, cardiovascular status, and airway and vocal cord assessment.

## INTRAOPERATIVE

Surgery for thyroid pathology is not usually a procedure associated with large blood loss intraoperatively. Aside from American Society of Anesthesiologists standard monitors, invasive monitors can be considered based on a patient's comorbidities (i.e., coronary artery disease, severe chronic obstructive pulmonary disease, diabetes, and others).

Hypothyroidism is related to decreased minimum alveolar concentration (MAC), delayed emergence, increased sensitivity to respiratory depressants, and potential development of myxedema coma postoperatively.

Hyperthyroidism is related to increased use of medications to control both heart rate and blood pressure; MAC is not affected, and stimulants are to be avoided.

## POSTOPERATIVE

Postoperatively, there may be recurrent laryngeal nerve damage (unilateral compromise leads to hoarseness; bilateral compromise leads to aphonia).[1]

**Neck Hematoma and Tracheal Compression:** Neck hematomas can become a medical and, often, a surgical emergency. Signs of airway obstruction include changes in phonation, moderate-to-severe respiratory distress, hypoxemia, and rapid changes in mental status in the setting of expanding mass in the neck. Neck hematomas compromise venous drainage, leading to engorgement of several structures and airway compromise. Soft tissue in the oropharynx can rapidly lead to airway distortion and displacement. A proactive approach with early tracheal intubation is highly recommended when expanding hematoma is noticed on examination. Reopening of surgical wounds can be considered to alleviate compression of airway structures; however, effective hemostasis is difficult to achieve and external compression of the neck can hinder attempts at tracheal intubation. Urgent or emergent surgical exploration in the operating suite is advised.

**Hypocalcemia Due to Damage of Parathyroid Glands During Surgery:** Parathyroid gland damage during surgery may provoke hypocalcemia and may cause *laryngospasm* because of hypocalcemic tetany. Calcium supplementation with intravenous calcium chloride or calcium gluconate is necessary.[2] Airway monitoring is necessary in severe cases of obstruction. Laryngospasm could become an airway emergency if severe airway obstruction ensues. Positive pressure via bag mask is the first maneuver to attempt. Clinical monitoring of ventilation via physical examination and continuous monitoring of pulse oximetry are required. If obstruction is severe, tracheal intubation should be considered early. Negative pressure pulmonary edema can be caused by increased respiratory efforts in the setting of severe laryngospasm. Severe hypoxemia is the clinical hallmark. Increased frothy pulmonary secretions can obscure emergent laryngoscopy.

## REFERENCES

1. Barash P, et al. *Clinical Anesthesia.* 8th ed. Lippincott, Williams & Wilkins; 2017.
2. *Stoelting's Anesthesia and Coexisting Disease.* 7th ed. Elsevier; 2017.
3. Jonklaas J, et al. Guidelines for the treatment of hypothyroidism. Prepared by the American Thyroid Association Task Force on Thyroid Hormone Replacement. *Thyroid.* 2014;24:1670–1751.

# 187.

# PARATHYROID DISEASE

*Karel T. S. Valenta and Kenneth S. Toth*

## INTRODUCTION

We have four parathyroid glands; these glands contain chief cells that produce the parathyroid hormone (PTH). PTH plays an important part in control of calcium levels. PTH increases calcium levels in the body via bone resorption, gut absorption indirectly via increased vitamin D [1,25(OH)$_2$D$_3$], increased phosphate secretion, and calcium reabsorption in the renal system. Phosphate binds to calcium to make hydroxyapatite, a crystal that forms our bone structure; by resorbing bone and eliminating phosphate via the kidneys, we are left with more free calcium.[1]

## HYPERPARATHYROIDISM

Primary hyperparathyroidism has an estimated incidence of 25 per 100,000. Primary causes of hyperparathyroidism include adenomas (80%), parathyroid hyperplasia (10%–20%), and rarely carcinomas.[1] Chronic renal failure often leads to a secondary hyperparathyroidism due to chronic hypocalcemia. Parathyroid-like–producing hormone can also be found in certain carcinomas, typically lung cancers.

Signs and symptoms are related to hypercalcemia and include hypertension, arrhythmias, fatigue, mental status changes, constipation, and depression. Diagnosis is suspected with high serum calcium levels and is confirmed with an elevated PTH level. Very high calcium levels, usually greater than 14, should lead providers to suspect malignancy rather than adenomas or hyperplasia. Thorough evaluation by an endocrinologist is important to exclude secondary causes of hyperparathyroidism, such as vitamin D deficiency or renal failure.

Treatment of hyperparathyroidism will depend on its cause. Bisphosphonates and calcitonin can be used, and in primary hyperparathyroidism, surgical excision is also a common treatment.

## HYPOPARATHYROIDISM

Hypoparathyroidism is most commonly iatrogenic secondary to parathyroidectomy or total thyroidectomy. Other causes of low PTH levels include congenital or autoimmune hypoparathyroidism and hypomagnesemia. Clinical features of hypoparathyroidism align with hypocalcemia and include perioral numbness, mental status changes, QT prolongation, tetany, muscle weakness, and difficulty breathing. Hypotension and heart failure can also be seen. Treatment consists of supplementation with calcium and vitamin D.

## ANESTHETIC CONSIDERATIONS

### PREOPERATIVE

When assessing a patient with hyperparathyroidism preoperatively, it is important to know the cause and if there are any associated disorders, such as multiple endocrine neoplasia. It is also important to know the patient's calcium levels as patients with significantly elevated calcium levels may require treatment prior to surgery. In patients with hypoparathyroidism, it may be prudent to obtain an electrocardiogram to look for QT prolongation. If patients do have QT prolongation, ondansetron, macrolides, and quinolones should be avoided.[2]

### INTRAOPERATIVE

Parathyroid resections can be performed under general anesthesia or with a cervical block. Conversion from regional to general anesthesia has been described at 10.6%.[3] Intraoperatively, during parathyroid resections, an arterial line is often utilized for blood draws to monitor PTH levels at 5 and 10 minutes postexcision to ensure the surgeon has taken out the correct structure. On occasion, three and a half parathyroids are removed by the surgeon when there is no identifiable single parathyroid causing the issue. These cases are more likely to have nerve damage and hypocalcemia postoperatively. It is also important to note that the operating surgeon can damage the recurrent laryngeal nerve, and intraoperative nerve monitoring with a special endotracheal tube can be performed. Generally, these endotracheal tubes are placed under videoscope guidance to ensure placement of the nerve monitor at the level of the vocal cords.

In patients who have hypoparathyroidism undergoing surgery, it is important to avoid further hypocalcemia. Products such as albumin or blood-containing citrate can further cause hypocalcemia, leading to hypotension and arrhythmias.

## POSTOPERATIVE

The anesthesia provider should look for signs and symptoms of unilateral or bilateral recurrent laryngeal nerve injury or stunning postoperatively. Unilateral recurrent laryngeal nerve injury will present with hoarseness without breathing difficulty. Bilateral nerve injury will present as stridor and difficulty breathing with impending respiratory failure due to inability to abduct the vocal cords, requiring emergent intubation. Temporary recurrent laryngeal nerve injury has been described as occurring in 10% of parathyroidectomies and permanent injury in 1.1% of cases.[4]

Patients are often observed overnight if several parathyroids are removed due to concern for postoperative hypocalcemia. Attention should be taken to ensure the patient has no signs or symptoms of hypocalcemia prior to discharge from the recovery area. Patients and nursing staff should be given instructions on what signs and symptoms to look out for as hypocalcemia can occur for several weeks postoperatively. Typically, the first symptom is a tingling sensation on the lips or tongue. Patients may also have weakness, difficulty breathing, and mental status changes. Progression to tetany can be demonstrated with Chvostek's and Trousseau's signs. If there is any suspicion, ionized calcium levels should be checked and the patient treated appropriately. It is important to distinguish recurrent laryngeal nerve injury versus hypocalcemia as both can cause respiratory compromise.

## REFERENCES

1. Mihai R, Farndon J. Parathyroid disease and calcium metabolism. *Br J Anaesth*. 2000;85(1):29–43.
2. Bajwa SJ, Sehgal V. Anesthetic management of primary hyperparathyroidism: a role rarely noticed and appreciated so far. *Indian J Endocrinol Metab*. 2013;17(2):235.
3. Carling T. Minimally invasive parathyroidectomy using cervical block. *Arch Surg*. 2006;141(4):401.
4. Joliat G-R, et al. Recurrent laryngeal nerve injury after thyroid and parathyroid surgery. *Medicine*. 2017;96(17):e6674.

# 188.

# ADRENAL DISEASE

*Allison K. Dalton*

## INTRODUCTION

The adrenal gland is composed of the medulla and cortex. The adrenal medulla secretes catecholamines, including epinephrine, norepinephrine, and dopamine. The adrenal cortex is responsible for the secretion of androgens, mineralocorticoids (i.e., aldosterone), and glucocorticoids. When there are alterations in the normal secretion of adrenal hormones, patients can experience electrolyte abnormalities, changes in glucose tolerance, hypertension, tachycardia, cardiac arrhythmias, and even death.

## CUSHING SYNDROME

Cushing syndrome is characterized by chronic hypercortisolemia, which results in multiple signs and symptoms, as described in Table 188.1. After exogenous use of glucocorticoids, Cushing disease, which is caused by a pituitary tumor secreting corticotropin (ACTH, adrenocorticotropin), is the most common cause of hypercortisolemia.[1] Cushing syndrome can also be caused by other metabolically active tumors that secrete ACTH, cortisol, or, rarely, corticotropin-releasing hormone. Treatment includes surgical excision for tumors. For unresectable masses, therapy involves radiation, chemotherapy, and/or medications to decrease cortisol production (i.e., cabergoline, pasireotide, metyrapone, etomidate).

## ADRENAL INSUFFICIENCY

In acute adrenally insufficiency states, patients present with signs and symptoms of shock but may exhibit subtle symptoms when chronic (Table 188.1). If left untreated, adrenal insufficiency can be fatal. Primary adrenal insufficiency, also known as Addison disease, is most commonly the result of autoimmune destruction of the adrenal cortex, but it may also occur as a result of infection, metastasis, adrenal hemorrhage or infarction, or drugs (Table 188.2). Patients on long-term, high-dose glucocorticoids may exhibit signs and symptoms of adrenal insufficiency on tapering or discontinuing therapy. Critically ill patients may experience relative adrenal insufficiency due to subnormal corticosteroid production. Diagnosis is typically made following an early morning cortisol level and/or cosyntropin stimulation test. Patients with adrenal insufficiency require treatment with glucocorticoids, and most patients with chronic insufficiency will need mineralocorticoids as well. During times of physiologic stress (i.e., critical illness, trauma, surgery), patients with adrenal insufficiency may require additional supplementation with glucocorticoids (i.e., stress dose steroids).

## HYPERALDOSTERONISM

Under normal physiologic conditions, aldosterone is an end product of the renin-angiotensin system. After conversion of angiotensin I to angiotensin II in the lung, angiotensin II stimulates secretion of aldosterone from the zona glomerulosa of the adrenal cortex. ACTH and potassium can also stimulate aldosterone release. Primary aldosteronism occurs with excess secretion of aldosterone. Conn syndrome is the result of an aldosterone-secreting adrenal tumor. Secondary aldosteronism can be the result of renin-angiotensin system alterations due to comorbid disease states. Hyperaldosteronism leads to hypertension and hypokalemia by increasing sodium channel expression in the kidney, leading to resorption of water and sodium and excretion of potassium in the distal tubule. Aldosterone acts as a pro-inflammatory mediator in cardiac and renal tissue, leading to fibrosis, chronic kidney disease, left ventricular hypertrophy, arrhythmias, and heart failure. Treatment of aldosteronomas includes medical treatment

*Table 188.1* MANAGEMENT OF ADRENAL DISEASE

| | CAUSES | SIGNS AND SYMPTOMS | ANESTHETIC CONCERNS |
|---|---|---|---|
| Cushing syndrome | Exogenous glucocorticoids<br>Cushing disease<br>Ectopic secretory tumors<br>(ACTH, cortisol, CRH) | Obesity<br>Hypertension<br>Glucose intolerance<br>Hirsuitism<br>Osteoporosis<br>Proximal muscle weakness<br>Increased abdominal girth<br>Striae<br>Moon faces<br>Dorsocervical fat pads<br>Depression | *Cardiovascular*<br>Hypertension<br>Myocardial ischemia<br>Stroke<br>Thromboembolism: consider preoperative LE<br>Doppler<br>*Respiratory*—Sleep apnea: consider preoperative<br>sleep study and postoperative CPAP<br>*Endocrine*<br>Obesity: potentially difficult BMV/intubation<br>Hyperglycemia<br>Adrenal insufficiency: may require supplemental<br>steroids perioperatively |
| Adrenal insufficiency | See Table 188.2 | Shock<br>Hypotension<br>Nausea<br>Vomiting<br>Abdominal pain/tenderness<br>Weakness<br>Fatigue<br>Skin hyperpigmentation<br>Fever<br>Altered mental status<br>Coma | *Cardiovascular*—Hypotension, shock<br>*Gastrointestinal*—Aspiration risk (nausea,<br>vomiting, AMS)<br>*Hematologic*—Anemia<br>*Endocrine*<br>Stress dose steroid administration<br>Hypoglycemia<br>*Electrolytes*—Hyponatremia, hyperkalemia |
| Hyperaldosteronism | Conn syndrome<br>Secondary:<br>    Heart failure<br>    Cirrhosis<br>    Nephrotic syndrome<br>    Renal artery stenosis<br>    Bartter syndrome<br>    Bulimia<br>    Excess diuretic therapy | Hypertension<br>Hypokalemia<br>Metabolic alkalosis | *Cardiovascular*<br>Hypertension<br>Arrhythmias: Electrocardiogram<br>Heart failure: TTE, stress testing as appropriate<br>*Renal*<br>Evaluate renal function<br>Metabolic alkalosis<br>*Hepatic*<br>Hepatic function<br>Coagulation status<br>Evaluate for cirrhosis<br>*Electrolytes*—Hypokalemia |
| Pheochromocytoma | Adrenal tumor<br>Sympathetic chain tumor<br>(paraganglioma) | Hypertension (chronic or<br>episodic)<br>Orthostatic hypotension<br>Tachycardia<br>Palpitations<br>Headache<br>Tremor<br>Diaphoresis<br>Flushing<br>Hyperglycemia<br>Weakness and fatigue | *Cardiovascular*<br>Hypertension: preoperative α-antagonism,<br>intraoperative antihypertensive medications<br>Tachycardia: preoperative and intraoperative<br>β-blockade<br>Risk for catecholamine-induced<br>cardiomyopathy: preoperative TTE, consider<br>intraoperative TEE<br>*Endocrine*<br>Hyperglycemia (preoperative and intraoperative)<br>Hypoglycemia (postoperative) |

ACTH, corticotropin; AMS, altered mental status; BMV, bag mask ventilation; CPAP, continuous positive airway pressure; CRH, corticotropin-releasing hormone; LE, lower extremity; TEE, transesophageal echocardiography; TTE, transthoracic echocardiography.

**Table 188.2** CAUSES OF ADRENAL INSUFFICIENCY

| TYPE | CAUSES | SPECIFIC ETIOLOGIES |
|------|--------|---------------------|
| Primary | Autoimmune adrenalitis | Antibodies to the steroidogenic enzymes |
| | Infection | Tuberculosis |
| | | Fungal infections |
| | | Cytomegalovirus |
| | | *Mycobacterium avium-intracellulare* |
| | | Syphilis |
| | | Trypanosomiasis |
| | Bilateral adrenal hemorrhage/infarction | Infection |
| | | Meningococcus, *Pseudomonas aeruginosa, Streptococcus pneumoniae, Neisseria gonorrhoeae, Escherichia coli, Haemophilus influenzae, Staphylococcus aureus* |
| | | Anticoagulation |
| | | Hypercoagulable states |
| | | Surgery |
| | | Trauma |
| | | Sepsis |
| | | Stress |
| | Metastatic disease | Lung cancer |
| | | Breast cancer |
| | | Stomach cancer |
| | | Colon cancer |
| | | Melanoma |
| | | Lymphoma |
| | Drugs | Cortisol inhibitors |
| | | Etomidate, ketoconazole, fluconazole |
| | | Cortisol metabolizers |
| | | Phenytoin, barbiturates, rifampin |
| Secondary | ACTH deficiency | Exogenous glucocorticoids |
| | | Critical illness |
| Tertiary | Pituitary dysfunction | Pituitary apoplexy/infarction |
| | | Pituitary tumor |

with mineralocorticoid receptor antagonists (i.e., spironolactone, eplerenone) and surgical resection.

# PHEOCHROMOCYTOMA

Pheochromocytomas are rare catecholamine -secreting tumors that originate from the chromaffin cells of the adrenal medulla. Chromaffin cells along the sympathetic chain give rise to similarly active paragangliomas. Classic signs and symptoms of pheochromocytoma include headache and hypertension due to excess secretion of norepinephrine, epinephrine, and/or dopamine. Diagnosis is confirmed by 24-hour urine collection for fractionated metanephrines or via plasma free metanephrines. Tumor location should be confirmed via computed tomography or magnetic resonance imaging. Biopsy should be avoided as it may precipitate acute pheochromocytoma crisis, which may be characterized by severe hypertension and tachycardia, arrhythmias, myocardial ischemia, and stroke.[2,3]

## ANESTHETIC MANAGEMENT

### PREOPERATIVE

Preoperatively, focus on patient comorbidities, electrolyte derangements, and glucose abnormalities. Laboratory testing should evaluate for sodium, potassium, glucose, and hormonal abnormalities. Renal and hepatic function should be evaluated for patients with hyperaldosteronism and pheochromocytoma. For patients with tachycardia or palpitations, an electrocardiogram should be performed. Echocardiography is indicated for patients with symptoms of cardiac ischemia, heart failure, or a diagnosis of pheochromocytoma.

Patients with pheochromocytoma require preoperative preparation with α-blockade and volume expansion with electrolyte-rich oral fluids. Phenoxybenzamine is a noncompetitive, long-acting, nonspecific α-antagonist. Alternatives include the selective, competitive, shorter acting α-blockers (i.e., doxazosin, prazosin, terazosin). The α-blockers are uptitrated to achieve orthostatic blood pressure and heart rate changes, which signify vascular resistance to catecholamine secretion. In order to avoid unopposed α-stimulation, β-blockers should be added only after adequate α-blockade has been achieved.

## INTRAOPERATIVE

Adrenal surgery is typically performed under general anesthesia with regional (i.e., epidural, transversus abdominis plane blocks) adjuncts for open procedures. Intraoperatively, stress dose steroids should be administered to patients who have been taking more than 20 mg/d of prednisone (or equivalent) for more than 3 weeks over the past year or for those with clinical Cushing syndrome, but should be held for patients using less than 5 mg/d, steroids for less than 3 weeks over the past year, or for minor procedures. Patients who have taken 5–20 mg/d of prednisone for more than 3 weeks over the preceding year may require additional testing to determine adrenal insufficiency risk.[4]

Patients with pheochromocytoma may exhibit significant heart rate and blood pressure variability intraoperatively despite preoperative α-blockade. Arterial line placement is indicated for invasive blood pressure management and monitoring of glucose. Adequate venous access is required, and central venous access may be necessary. Intraoperatively, acute pheochromocytoma crisis occurs during induction of anesthesia, intubation, surgical incision, and abdominal insufflation and during manipulation of the tumor. Clevidipine, esmolol, nitroprusside, and nitroglycerin have been utilized successfully in pheochromocytoma intraoperative management.[5] Due to excess catecholamine secretion, significant hyperglycemia may occur intraoperatively but should be treated with caution due to postoperative risk of hypoglycemia.

## POSTOPERATIVE

Continue to monitor electrolytes, glucose, and renal function postoperatively. Functional hormone levels (i.e., aldosterone, metanephrines) should be assessed postoperatively to ensure resolution of abnormalities. Following aldosteronoma resection, patients may experience hyperkalemia. Patients with pheochromocytoma and adrenal insufficiency may experience hypoglycemia and hypotension, which may require postoperative intensive care unit admission and treatment with glucose or vasoactive infusions.

## REFERENCES

1. Lacroix A, et al. Cushing's syndrome. *Lancet.* 2015;386(9996): 913–927.
2. Radtke WE, et al. Cardiovascular complications of pheochromocytoma crisis. *Am J Cardiol.* 1975;35:701–705.
3. Vanderveen KA, et al. Biopsy of pheochromocytomas and paragangliomas: potential for disaster. *Surgery.* 2009;146(6): 1158–11566.
4. Liu MM, et al. Perioperative steroid management: approaches based on current evidence. *Anesthesiology.* 2017;127:166–172.
5. Naranjo J, et al. Perioperative management of pheochromocytoma. J Cardiothorac Vasc Anesth. 2017;31(4):1427–1439.

# 189.

# CARCINOID SYNDROME

*Sabrina S. Sam and Nawal E. Ragheb-Mueller*

## INTRODUCTION

Carcinoid syndrome is a paraneoplastic syndrome secondary to vasoactive substances secreted by carcinoid tumors and occurs in 19% of carcinoid tumors.[1,2] A carcinoid tumor is a slow-growing neuroendocrine tumor that predominantly affects women in their 50s–70s and is the most common malignant tumor of the appendix.[2] The tumor alone is usually asymptomatic because its metabolic products are secreted into the portal circulation and metabolized by the liver before systemic effects occur. However, when the tumor is found in the lungs or hepatic metastases are present, the vasoactive substances are able to bypass or overwhelm hepatic degradation, leading to carcinoid syndrome.[1] The most common vasoactive substances secreted are serotonin, histamine, and kinins.[3]

## CLINICAL FEATURES

The most common manifestations of carcinoid syndrome are cutaneous flushing, diarrhea, and bronchospasm. Flushing is the hallmark of the disorder and occurs in up to 78%–94% of cases.[1-3] Serotonin, histamine, bradykinin, and substance P are all thought to cause flushing. Diarrhea is caused by serotonin and prostaglandins and arises in 60%–80% of cases.[1-4] Bronchospasm is presumed to be secondary to serotonin and histamine and occurs in 15%–19% of patients.[1,3] Other signs and symptoms include vomiting, abdominal pain, hepatomegaly, tachycardia, hypotension/hypertension, and hyperglycemia.

Carcinoid heart disease presents as fibrous plaques on the tricuspid or pulmonic valves, leading to tricuspid regurgitation or pulmonic stenosis and eventually right-side heart failure. Left-side valves are usually spared, which indicates the ability of the lung to inactivate vasoactive substances. Uncontrolled levels of serotonin can lead to deficiencies of niacin and tryptophan.[4] A deficiency in niacin can lead to pellagra, which is characterized by dermatitis, diarrhea, and dementia. A deficiency in tryptophan can lead to neurocognitive disorders, such as depression, anxiety, and confusion.

Unchecked rapid release of vasoactive substances can lead to carcinoid crisis, which is a possible life-threatening situation. Carcinoid crisis is characterized by severe bronchospasm, flushing, tachycardia, and blood pressure instability. Arrhythmias and neurologic symptoms may also be present.

## DIAGNOSIS

Carcinoid syndrome is suspected clinically, and diagnosis is confirmed by serotonin metabolites, such as a 24-hour urine sample with 5-hydroxyindoleacetic acid (5-HIAA) levels greater than 25 mg.[3] 5-HIAA is 73%–91% sensitive and 100% specific for carcinoid tumors; these levels are also used to monitor tumor activity.[2,5] Recently, plasma levels of 5-HIAA have been used in place of urine tests and have a sensitivity of 91%–92%.[2] Results, however, can be affected by kidney function, and 5-HIAA levels can be absent when the carcinoid tumor primarily involves the lungs. Diagnosis should also be suspected when chromogranin A is increased; this is 80% sensitive and 95% specific for carcinoid tumors.

Imaging with computed tomography is used to detect the location of the tumor as well as metastases.[5] An octreoscan, which consists of somatostatin receptor scintigraphy using indium 11–labeled octreotide, is used to detect tumors expressing somatostatin receptors. Echocardiography is recommended to screen for cardiac involvement.

## TREATMENT

Treatment for carcinoid syndrome includes therapies aimed at symptom relief and definitive therapy. Octreotide, a somatostatin analogue that decreases the secretion of serotonin, is the mainstay of treatment for controlling symptoms related to serotonin.[4] Telotristat ethyl is an adjunct to octreotide that reduces serotonin production.

Peptide receptor radionuclide therapy is used in patients whose symptoms progress despite treatment with somatostatin analogues.

Definitive therapy is provided with surgical resection when criteria for complete resection are met.[5] Chemotherapy with 5-fluorouracil and doxorubicin has been used, as has chemoembolization of liver lesions.

## ANESTHETIC CONSIDERATIONS

### PREOPERATIVE

It is important to determine the presence and severity of signs and symptoms preoperatively. Laboratory testing should include a complete blood count, basic metabolic profile, liver function tests, and a 24-hour 5-HIAA assessment. Cardiac involvement should be investigated with an electrocardiogram and transthoracic echocardiography. Imaging to determine the presence of metastases is needed to ensure the patient is a surgical candidate.

Immediately prior to surgical intervention, chemoprophylaxis is given. No single octreotide dosing regimen has been shown to be superior, and institutional dosing guidelines should be followed. Proper premedication for anxiolysis is important as anxiety is a trigger.[3]

### INTRAOPERATIVE

Preparation for emergency situations is essential intraoperatively, and proper intravenous access with two large-bore peripheral catheters and possibly a central line should suffice. An arterial line should be used for blood pressure monitoring. Depending on the severity of heart disease and the surgery, a transesophageal echocardiograph might be useful.

Avoidance of surgical and anesthetic triggers that lead to the release of vasoactive substances is also essential as these can lead to carcinoid crisis. Pharmacological triggers include histamine-releasing drugs (atracurium, morphine, and meperidine); vasoactive drugs (norepinephrine, epinephrine, ephedrine); and succinylcholine.[5] Mechanical triggers consist of tumor manipulation and tracheal manipulation. Physiologic triggers include hypovolemia, hypoxia, hypothermia, and hypercarbia, pain, and anxiety. If the procedure permits, regional anesthesia is a feasible option to avoid multiple triggers.

Carcinoid crisis should be treated as an emergency should it occur, and tumor manipulation should be discontinued.[2] An octreotide bolus followed by an infusion, corticosteroids, and histamine antagonists should be given. If inotropic support is necessary for ventricular dysfunction, dopamine can be used. Avoid drugs or situations that increase pulmonary vascular resistance if tricuspid insufficiency is present.

In cases of hemodynamic instability, care needs to be taken to avoid paradoxical reactions that can occur with vasopressors such as norepinephrine and epinephrine.[4] Hypotension should be treated with phenylephrine or vasopressin as first-line agents.[5] Hypertension should be treated with α- and β-adrenergic receptor blockers, such as phenoxybenzamine and propranolol, respectively.

### POSTOPERATIVE

Postoperatively, patients should be taken to an intensive care unit for monitoring for hemodynamic stability as well as for signs and symptoms of vasoactive substance release.[5] Octreotide should be continued until the taper is complete. Many providers place an epidural preoperatively or use a hydromorphone patient-controlled anesthesia postoperatively as pain can trigger a crisis.

## REFERENCES

1. Ferrari AC, et al. Carcinoid syndrome: update on the pathophysiology and treatment. *Clinics.* 2018;73(suppl 1):e490s.
2. Ito T, et al. Carcinoid-syndrome: recent advances, current status and controversies. *Curr Opin Endocrinol Diabetes Obes.* 2018;25(1):22–35.
3. Prakash S. Perioperative management of carcinoid syndrome—an anaesthesiologist's perspective. *J Anesth Clin Res.* 2016;7:9.
4. Clement D, et al. Update on pathophysiology, treatment, and complications of carcinoid syndrome. *J Oncol.* 2020;2020:8341426.
5. Powell B, et al. Carcinoid: the disease and its implications for anaesthesia. *Cont Ed Anaesth Crit Care Pain.* 2011;11(1):9–13.

# 190.

# DIABETES MELLITUS

*Benjamin B. G. Mori and Piotr Al-Jindi*

## INTRODUCTION

Diabetes mellitus (DM) affects roughly 9% of American adults.[1] It is characterized by elevated blood glucose (BG) concentrations secondary to a relative lack of endogenous insulin.[1] DM is classified into type 1 (T1DM) and type 2 (T2DM), which differ in their pathogenesis. T1DM (5%–10% of cases) is characterized by an absence of insulin production due to the autoimmune destruction of pancreatic β-cells.[1] T2DM (90% of cases) is strongly associated with obesity, begins with end-organ insulin resistance with late progression to β-cell failure. Gestational diabetes, a third main form of DM (5% of cases), occurs when pregnant women without a previous history of DM develop high BG levels.[1] The diagnosis of DM is laboratory based, and the diagnostic criteria are summarized in Table 190.1.

*Table 190.1* SUMMARY OF THE DIAGNOSTIC CRITERIA FOR DM BY DIFFERENT LABORATORY-BASED TESTS

| LABORATORY TEST | DIAGNOSTIC CRITERIA TO ESTABLISH THE DIAGNOSIS OF DM |
| --- | --- |
| Glycated hemoglobin (HbA$_{1c}$) test | Hb$_{A1c}$ ≥ 6.5%. |
| Random blood glucose test | BG ≥ 200 mg/dL (11.1 mmol/L) in a patient with classic symptoms of hyperglycemia or hyperglycemic crisis |
| Fasting blood glucose test | BG > 126 mg/dL (7.0 mmol/L); fasting is defined as no caloric intake for at least 8 hours |
| Oral glucose tolerance test | BG ≥ 200 mg/dL (11.1 mmol/L), after OGTT. |

Long-standing DM is associated with numerous complications secondary to hyperglycemia-associated micro- and macroangiopathy. DM is a well-established risk factor for coronary artery disease, renal failure, visual impairment, gastroparesis, and neuropathy.[1]

Table adapted from the American Diabetes Association. Standards of medical care in diabetes 2011. *Diabetes Care.* 2011;34:S11.

## PHARMACOLOGICAL MANAGEMENT AND MONITORING

The mainstay of DM management revolves around glycemic control. The importance of lifestyle modification cannot be understated; however, most diabetics require some form of pharmacotherapy.

Insulin analogues are categorized by their duration of action. In general, rapid- and short-acting insulins are used to mitigate postprandial BG spikes, where intermediate- and long-acting insulins are given to provide basal BG control throughout the day. Figure 190.1 illustrates the relative insulin effect over time of each insulin subtype. Intensive insulin therapy is needed in T1DM to control BG and prevent ketoacidosis, often involving multiple basal and prandial injections daily or a subcutaneous (SC) insulin infusion device.[1]

Metformin reduces hepatic glucose production and is the preferred initial pharmacological therapy for T2DM. Glucagon-like peptide 1(GLP-1) agonists and/or insulin therapy are recommended as second-line therapies.

Glycemic control can be monitored by measuring glycated hemoglobin (HbA$_{1c}$) levels. During hyperglycemia, glucose binds hemoglobin to form HbA$_{1c}$. Since erythrocytes have a 120-day life span, HbA$_{1c}$ levels are reflective of an individual's average BG control over the past 3-month period. A normal HbA$_{1c}$ level is less than 6%, and the risk of DM-associated complications increases with higher HbA$_{1c}$ levels.[1]

## ANESTHETIC CONSIDERATIONS

Perioperative hyperglycemia is associated with adverse outcomes. The stress of fasting, surgery and anesthesia stimulates secretion of counterregulatory hormones (i.e., catecholamines, cortisol, glucagon, growth hormone) and inflammatory mediators (i.e., tumor necrosis factor α, interleukin 6, interleukin 1β), which culminates in increased hepatic glucose production, insulin resistance, and, ultimately, hyperglycemia. Perioperative hyperglycemia is reported in 20%–40% and 80% of patients undergoing general and

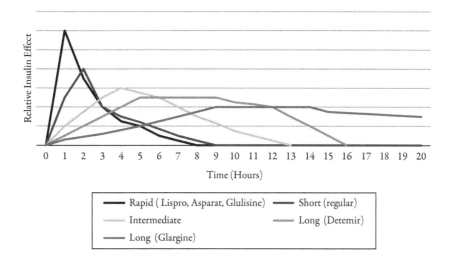

**Figure 190.1** Graph depicting the relative insulin effect of rapid (e.g., Lispro, Aspart, Glulisine); short (e.g., regular); intermediate (e.g., NPH); and long-acting (e.g., Detemir, Glargine) exogenous insulin over time. Source information obtained from Lehmann ED, Tarín C, Bondia J, Teufel E, Deutsch T. Incorporating a generic model of subcutaneous insulin absorption into the AIDA v4 diabetes simulator. 3. Early plasma insulin determinations. J Diabetes Sci Technol. 2009;3(1):190–201.

cardiac surgery, respectively. Substantial evidence supports the use of insulin to correct perioperative hyperglycemia to reduce complications and mortality.[2]

## PREOPERATIVE

Poor preoperative glycemic control is associated with an increased complication rate and reduced survival after surgery. Prolonged fasting should be avoided in DM as it is associated with worse perioperative glycemic control. Carbohydrate loading 2 hours preoperatively, as part of the Enhanced recovery after colorectal surgery (ERAS) protocol, counteracts insulin resistance associated with stress and starvation, decreases postoperative hyperglycemia, and reduces hospital length of stay, particularly in patients undergoing major abdominal surgery.[2] Most oral antidiabetic agents are safe to take up to the day before surgery, with certain medications being safe to continue on the day of surgery.[1,2] Table 190.2 summarizes the recommended use of oral antidiabetic agents leading up to surgery.

For those patients taking insulin, a dose reduction the day before and day of surgery is typically recommended to avoid hyperglycemia associated with fasting.[1,2] The recommended preoperative insulin dosing adjustments can be found summarized in Table 190.3.

## INTRAOPERATIVE

Most investigations into the effects of intraoperative BG control and outcomes have focused on the cardiac surgery population, which demonstrated increased complication rates and mortality with both intraoperative hyperglycemia (>200 mg/dL) and intensive insulin therapy to achieve lower BG targets

(between 80 and 100 mg/dL).[2] As such, intraoperative BG levels should be maintained below 180 mg/dL, where hyperglycemia is treated with rapid-acting insulin analogues or with a regular insulin infusion.[2] Less stringent BG targets (<200 mg/dL) can be considered depending on risk of hypoglycemia and also in the general patient population given the lack of evidence to support more rigorous targets.[3] BG monitoring should be performed every 1–2 hours, with even shorter intervals if BG levels are less than 100 mg/dL or if the rate of fall is rapid, suggesting impending hypoglycemia. Fingerstick glucose levels are less reliable in patients who are critically ill, hypotensive, or on vasopressors. In these cases, venous or arterial blood testing should be used.[4]

## POSTOPERATIVE

During recovery in the postanesthesia care unit, BG checks should continue at least every 2 hours for all DM patients, with rapid-acting insulin used to treat hyperglycemia (>180 mg/dL). For same-day surgery, a patient's preoperative diabetes treatment regimen may be reinstated once the patient is discharged and able to tolerate oral intake. For those patients admitted to the surgical/medical ward, glycemic control (BG < 180 mg/dL) is best achieved with a combination of basal and prandial insulin dosing, often referred to a "basal-bolus" insulin regimen. Subcutaneous insulin dosing can be calculated based on the patient's weight, home insulin requirements, or insulin infusion dose, while adjusting for the patient's nutritional intake and renal function. Of note, the use of oral antidiabetic agents is not recommended in hospitalized patients due to the limited data on their safety and efficacy in this population. Those patients requiring intensive care unit level care should have

*Table 190.2* SUMMARY OF THE RECOMMENDED USE OF ORAL ANTIDIABETIC AGENTS THE DAY BEFORE AND THE DAY OF SURGERY

| ORAL MEDICATION FOR ELECTIVE SURGERY | DAY BEFORE SURGERY | DAY OF SURGERY IF (1) NORMAL ORAL INTAKE ANTICIPATED SAME DAY AND (2) MINIMALLY INVASIVE SURGERY | DAY OF SURGERY IF (1) REDUCED POSTOPERATIVE ORAL INTAKE OR (2) EXTENSIVE SURGERY, ANTICIPATED HEMODYNAMIC CHANGES AND/OR FLUID SHIFTS |
|---|---|---|---|
| Secretagogues | Take | Hold | Hold |
| SGLT-2 inhibitors | Hold | Hold | Hold |
| Thiazolidinediones | Take | Take | Hold |
| Metformin[a] | Take | Take | Hold |
| DPP-4 inhibitors | Take | Take | Take |

[a]Metformin may be taken the day before surgery and restarted on the day of surgery when a normal diet is resumed. Some guidelines allow metformin to be continued on the day of surgery for patients who only missed one meal, unless the surgical procedure involves the use of contrast dye, there is an expected long surgical time, or the patient has impaired renal function (glomerular filtration rate < 45 mL/min) since these factors may increase the risk of metformin-induced lactic acidosis.[2]

SGLT-2 inhibitors (Sodium-glucose contransporter-2 inhibitors

DPP-4 inhibitors (Dipeptidyl peptidase-4 inhibitor

Table adapted from Duggan EW, Carlson K, Umpierrez GE. Perioperative hyperglycemia management: an update. *Anesthesiology*. 2017;126(3):547–560.

*Table 190.3* SUMMARY OF THE RECOMMENDED PREOPERATIVE INSULIN DOSING ADJUSTMENTS

| DAY BEFORE SURGERY | GLARGINE DETERMIR | | NPH 70/30 INSULIN | | LISPRO ASPART GLULISINE REGULAR | |
|---|---|---|---|---|---|---|
| | AM DOSE | PM DOSE | AM DOSE | PM DOSE | AM DOSE | PM DOSE |
| Normal diet until midnight (including clear liquids until 2 hours prior to surgery) | Usual dose | 80% of usual dose | 80% of usual dose | 80% of usual dose | Usual dose | Usual dose |
| Bowel prep and/or clear liquids only 12–24 hours prior to surgery | Usual dose | 80% of usual dose | 80% of usual dose | 80% of usual dose | Usual dose | Usual dose |
| Day of surgery[a] | 80% of usual dose if patient uses twice daily basal therapy | | 50% of usual dose if BG ≥ 120 mg/dL (hold if BG < 120 mg/dL) | | Hold | |

[a]Patients with T1DM undergoing surgery require insulin during the perioperative period to prevent severe hyperglycemia or ketoacidosis. These patients should receive 80% of basal insulin dose the evening before surgery and on the morning of surgery in order to prevent hypoglycemia.

Table adapted from Duggan EW, Carlson K, Umpierrez GE. Perioperative hyperglycemia management: an update. *Anesthesiology*. 2017;126(3):547–560.

all subcutaneous insulin stopped and an intravenous insulin drip started for BG above 180 mg/dL.[2]

## REFERENCES

1. Robertson AC, Furman WR. Nutritional, gastrointestinal, and endocrine disease. In: Miller RD. *Basics of Anesthesia*. 7th ed. Philadelphia, PA: Churchill Livingstone/Elsevier; 2018:501–502.

2. Duggan EW, et al. Perioperative hyperglycemia management: an update. *Anesthesiology*. 2017;126(3):547–560.
3. American Diabetes Association. 14. Diabetes care in the hospital: standards of medical care in diabetes—2018. *Diabetes Care*. 2018;41(suppl 1):S144–S151.
4. Joshi GP, et al.; Society for Ambulatory Anesthesia. Society for Ambulatory Anesthesia consensus statement on perioperative blood glucose management in diabetic patients undergoing ambulatory surgery. *Anesth Analg*. 2010;111(6):1378–1387.

# 191.

# PANCREAS TRANSPLANTATION

*Gorneva Maria and Tzonkov Anna*

## INTRODUCTION

Pancreas transplantation is a surgical treatment for complicated cases of diabetes mellitus type 1 and, in selected cases, type 2. Patients with a history of frequent, severe metabolic complications (marked hypoglycemia or hyperglycemia, ketoacidosis) and failing insulin management are typical candidates. The procedure was first performed in humans in 1966. Now, due to development of better immunosuppressive agents (specifically cyclosporine and anti–T-cell antibodies), advanced surgical techniques, and better patient selection more than 700 various types of pancreatic transplants are performed yearly in the United States alone. Most patients receive a pancreas from a cadaver donor; however, donation by a living-related donor is also possible.

The goals of transplantation are to restore glucose-regulated endogenous insulin secretion, arrest the progression of the complications of diabetes, and improve quality of life.[1] There are several types of such treatment: pancreas transplant alone, simultaneous pancreas-kidney transplant (SPK), pancreas after kidney transplant (PAK), and islet transplant (developing technology). SPK is the most common type of transplant; it is performed on patients with diabetes type 1 complicated by end-stage renal disease. These patients tend to have better outcomes than isolated transplants.[2] The most common reason for graft failure is immunologic rejection; therefore, immunosuppression therapy is required for every transplant. The average graft life expectancy in absence of complications is a decade or longer.

## BENEFITS

Almost immediately post transplantation the metabolic effects for the recipient are tremendous and may render these patients "ex-diabetic." A functioning pancreas transplant is the single most effective way of achieving normoglycemia long term for a diabetic patient. Depending on the type of pancreas transplant, the expectation is that 80% to 90% of recipients will be rendered completely insulin free at 1 year posttransplant.[3] In addition, successful pancreas

transplantation may improve the lipid profile and symptoms of peripheral and autonomic diabetic neuropathy and could possibly reverse established lesions of diabetic nephropathy. There are controversial reports on diabetic retinopathy, with some studies reporting stabilization or even regression of retinal lesions after successful pancreas transplantation (unless retinopathy is advanced at the time of procedure).

## ANESTHETIC CONSIDERATIONS

### PREOPERATIVE

Patients receiving a pancreas transplant are normally relatively young and therefore typically have few comorbidities. Nevertheless, having long-standing diabetes, these patients inevitably carry a certain degree of microcirculatory dysfunction with possible underlying cardiovascular disease. A candidate's functional status must be assessed carefully preoperatively. Since atypical angina is common among diabetics, it is highly important to suspect unrecognized coronary artery disease. There are no formal guidelines for preoperative cardiovascular evaluation of the SPK or isolated pancreas transplant candidate, but it is reasonable to perform a 12-lead electrocardiogram and noninvasive stress testing.[2] Additionally, each candidate should be checked for end-organ dysfunction typical for diabetes, such as gastroparesis, peripheral vascular disease, peripheral neuropathy, and nephropathy. Active infection, malignancy, and in some cases HIV infection are among absolute contraindications for this procedure. Patients with morbid obesity, significant cardiovascular disease, advanced age, limited life expectancy, or significant psychosocial issues may be poor candidates for transplant; therefore, risks and benefits have to be weighed extra carefully in this case.

### INTRAOPERATIVE

The pancreas is transplanted heterotopically with the recipient's own pancreas left in place, and surgical access is through laparotomy. The intraoperative exact location may vary depending on surgical technique and whether the kidney is transplanted simultaneously. Graft function strictly depends on perfusion, and limiting total ischemic time is the key. Traditionally, the bladder was the most frequent site of exocrine duct anastomosis. Due to the complication of chronic metabolic acidosis from loss of bicarbonate-rich secretions, enteric exocrine anastomosis has gained popularity. As for the vascular anastomotic options, it can be performed via systemic versus portal circulation. The former results in high systemic concentrations of insulin postoperatively. Although systemic hyperinsulinemia has been associated with the metabolic syndrome and other complications in the nontransplant setting, there is no evidence to date to suggest that this contrived hyperinsulinemia associated with systemic venous drainage of a pancreas transplant is related to any unique morbidity.[3]

Serum glucose level both intraoperatively and postoperatively is a reflection of the graft's viability; therefore, strict monitoring of glycemic variation is a cornerstone of anesthetic care. Perioperative delayed onset of normoglycemia can reflect a dysfunctional graft, pancreatitis, acute rejection, or insufficient graft size for the recipient's needs and should be communicated to the surgeon promptly.[2] Hemodynamic stability also must be established to ensure stable perfusion of the graft.

Due to the high risk of rejection, most transplant centers advocate for induction of immunosuppression intraoperatively. The most commonly used agents for induction are as follows:

- T-cell–depleting antibodies (e.g., polyclonal rabbit antithymocyte globulin–thymoglobulin [multidose] and monoclonal alemtuzumab [anti-CD52 antibody, single dose]). These two agents are most commonly used, reportedly in 85% of cases.
- nondepleting antibodies such as interleukin 2 receptor antibodies (monoclonal basiliximab).[4]

## POSTOPERATIVE

The graft function is evaluated and classified postoperatively based on the level of glycated hemoglobin ($A_{1c}$), severe hypoglycemic events, insulin requirements, and C-peptide production. Both pancreas and islet transplantation require lifelong immunosuppression to prevent rejection of the graft. Most patients receive monoclonal or polyclonal anti–T-cell antibodies at the time of surgery and a combination of tacrolimus and mycophenolate mofetil for chronic immunosuppression therapy.

Complications following pancreas transplant occur more frequently than in other abdominal solid-organ transplants. Although major complications following pancreas transplant are uncommon, several, including pancreatitis, exocrine duct leaks, and pancreatic pseudocysts, are unique to this transplant.[2] The graft loss is classified based on the time of occurrence into early (within hours or days postsurgery) and late. The former is normally due to "technical failures," such as bleeding, thrombosis, infection, and leaks. The late graft loss is due to rejection, and it is the most common reason. Vascular thrombosis can occur as the result of technical error or may be a symptom of rejection. Technical issues are most rare if the combined SPK procedure is performed; also, failure rates are lower in exocrine duct to bladder anastomosis versus enteric anastomosis. In terms of outcomes, SPK offers a greater chance of long-term graft survival than isolated pancreas or PAK procedures; however, simultaneous procedures are more limited by organ availability. Generally, isolated pancreas procedures yield an 80% 1-year graft survival compared with 82% in PAK procedures and greater than 90% in SPK.[1]

## MANAGEMENT OF BLOOD GLUCOSE LEVELS

Once a donor organ becomes available, the patient is made to fast. The blood glucose level is checked every 2 hours, and insulin is supplemented as needed, with a goal blood glucose of 100 to 150 mg/dL (the range may vary depending on the individual institution policy). If blood glucose is labile, then an insulin infusion is started. The initial infusion rate is 0.2–0.3 U/kg/h, which is then titrated with blood glucose measurements every 1–2 hours to maintain the blood glucose in the abovementioned range. Essentially the same regimen of infusion is followed intraoperatively with the strict rule to maintain euglycemia. Following graft recirculation, pancreatic β-cells begin secreting insulin within 5 minutes, so careful attention to glucose levels is paramount. Postoperative insulin therapy has two forms of management. The first involves initial full insulin replacement to "rest" the β-cells in the transplanted pancreas for the first few days following surgery. Providing complete replacement of insulin in this case is expected to better preserve β-cells' function and avoid injury from acute stress. After 3–4 days of total insulin replacement, patients are switched to an intermittent regimen with β-cells gradually taking over the primary function of producing insulin. The second approach is to let the transplanted pancreas fully function as soon as blood supply is restored, with the advantage of timely monitoring for graft dysfunction.[5]

## REFERENCES

1. Robertson R. Pancreas and islet transplantation in diabetes mellitus. In: Lee S, ed. *UpToDate*. UpToDate; March 2019.
2. Mittel AM, Wagener G. Anesthesia for kidney and pancreas transplantation. *Anesthesiol Clin*. 2017;35(3):439–452.
3. Alhamad T, et al. Pancreas-kidney transplantation in diabetes mellitus: benefits and complications. In: Lee S, ed. *UpToDate*. UpToDate; February 2019.
4. Alhamad T, et al. Pancreas-kidney transplantation in diabetes mellitus: surgical considerations and immunosuppression. In: Lee S, ed., *UpToDate*. UpToDate; July 2020.
5. Shokouh-Amiri MH, et al. Glucose control during and after pancreatic transplantation. *Diabetes Spectrum*. 2002;15(1):49–53.

# Part 17

# NEUROMUSCULAR DISEASES
# AND DISORDERS

# 192.

# MULTIPLE SCLEROSIS

*Justin L. O'Farrell and Maxim S. Eckmann*

## INTRODUCTION

Multiple sclerosis (MS) is an immune-mediated inflammatory disease leading to the demyelination of axons in the central nervous system (CNS). MS is thought to arise in patients with a combination of a genetic susceptibility to autoimmunity coupled with environmental triggers. The most widely accepted theory names autoreactive lymphocytes as the agents responsible for the pathogenesis of MS.[1] As the disease progresses, the pathology expands to include microglial activation, leading to sclerosis and chronic neurodegeneration.

There are multiple patterns of disease seen in MS with differing rates of progression and associated prognoses. Common disease patterns include relapsing-remitting MS (RRMS), secondary progressive MS (SPMS), and primary progressive MS (PPMS).[2] The management of MS will include long-term care through neurology for disease-modifying treatment; however, acute exacerbations will require additional interventions. Attacks of MS are defined as episodes of focal neurologic disturbance that last for no longer than 24 hours that follow a period of clinical stability.

## CLINICAL FEATURES

Multiple sclerosis is a progressive disease with a relapsing-remitting pattern of symptoms. Symptoms tend to develop over the course of hours to days and then remit slowly over weeks to months. There are cases in which remission is not complete.

Charcot's neurologic triad describes the dysarthria, nystagmus, and intention tremor that are seen in patients with MS. Dysarthria manifests with difficult or unclear speech that occurs due to the development of plaques in the brainstem after demyelination. Nystagmus is defined as involuntary and rapid eye movements. Plaques on the optic nerve can cause loss of vision or painful optic neuritis, while plaques on CN III, IV, and VI can cause pain and double vision. The development of intention tremor is due to plaque development along motor pathways leading to muscle weakness and spasms, tremors, ataxia, and paralysis.

Patients with RRMS experience well-defined exacerbations of disease activity after which there may either be full or incomplete recovery. SPMS is characterized by an initial RRMS disease course with the distinction that the disease continues to progress even between the acute exacerbations. The third type of MS is PPMS, which is characterized by steady progression of disability through a patient's lifetime. Due to the steady progression, patients with PPMS have a worse prognosis than patients with RRMS.

## DIAGNOSIS

The diagnosis of MS is made based on clinical, magnetic resonance imaging (MRI), and/or cerebrospinal fluid (CSF) findings based on the McDonald criteria. The characteristic findings include optic neuritis, fatigue, internuclear ophthalmoplegia, onset between ages 15 and 50 years, as well as a relapsing and remitting pattern of symptoms. Clinicians should take a detailed clinical history to rule out prior attacks mirroring the presenting symptoms.

Magnetic resonance imaging is the gold standard test to support the diagnosis of MS. Lesions seen on MRI that are indicative of MS are found in white matter areas such as the periventricular and juxtacortical regions, infratentorial regions, the spinal cord, and the corpus callosum. The lesions are hyperintense on T2-weighted imaging and appear to have an ovoid shape. Acute lesions are usually larger and have more ill-defined borders than chronic MS lesions.

## TREATMENT

Patients diagnosed with MS are recommended to begin disease-modifying therapy as soon as possible as there are multiple immunomodulatory agents that have shown a decreased relapse rate as well as a slower accumulation of brain lesions seen on MRI. Studies have shown that natalizumab, ocrelizumab, and alemtuzumab infusions have the highest level of effectiveness of relapse reduction for patients with MS.[3] Oral therapy includes dimethyl fumarate, teriflunomide, fingolimod, or cladribine. Patients on these therapies have a risk of developing severe lymphopenia. Injection therapy is indicated for patients who value safety over the highest level of effectiveness. In the setting of an acute exacerbation of disease activity, glucocorticoids are the treatment of choice.

## ANESTHETIC CONSIDERATIONS

Preoperative evaluation will require an in-depth history to determine the type of MS that the patient has, whether or not they are experiencing an acute exacerbation, medications currently in use, and the degree of neurologic damage. Patients with any perceived compromise of diaphragmatic and intercostal muscle power are at increased risk of requiring postoperative ventilation due to the respiratory depressant effects of sedative/hypnotics, opioids, and neuromuscular-blocking agents. Consider subspecialty for elective surgery if home oxygen dependence, dyspnea, or other related historical findings are seen.

Pain management can be complicated in the MS patient with advanced disease that is at risk for respiratory impairment. Nonopioid, nonsedating analgesic systemic therapy, provided no contraindications, should be a mainstay of initial therapy. These include primarily the nonsteroidal anti-inflammatory drugs/acetaminophen and subanesthetic ketamine. Opioids, membrane-stabilizing drugs in the antiseizure class, antispasmodics, and antidepressants have a potential sedating effect when initiated.

Concern surrounding neuraxial techniques is based on analysis of the pathophysiological mechanisms of damage within the CNS. Local anesthetics share similar physiological properties to the oligopeptides that are seen in the CSF of patients with MS, which may lead to an exacerbation of MS symptoms if used for central or subarachnoid blocks.[4] Intravenous lidocaine has been associated with worsening MS symptoms, especially symptoms that involve the eye.[5] Extreme caution should be used to avoid intravenous absorption, which may cause additional imbalance in neuronal impulses.

## REFERENCES

1. Weiner HL. Multiple sclerosis is an inflammatory T-cell-mediated autoimmune disease. *Arch Neurol.* 2004;61(10):1613–1615.
2. Zakzanis KK. Distinct neurocognitive profiles in multiple sclerosis subtypes. *Arch Clin Neuropsychol.* 2000;15(2):115–136.
3. Tramacere I, et al. Immunomodulators and immunosuppressants for relapsing-remitting multiple sclerosis: a network meta-analysis. *Cochrane Database Syst Rev.* 2015;(9):CD011381.
4. Brinkmeier H, et al. An endogenous pentapeptide acting as a sodium channel blocker in inflammatory autoimmune disorders of the central nervous system. *Nat Med.* 2000;6(7):808–811.
5. Sakurai M, et al. Lidocaine unmasks silent demyelinative lesions in multiple sclerosis. Neurology. 1992;42(11):2088–2093.

# 193.

# MOTOR NEURON DISEASES

*Allison K. Dalton*

## INTRODUCTION

Upper motor neurons (UMNs) originate in the primary motor cortex and have axons that form the corticospinal and corticobulbar tracts. Upper motor disorders result in weakness, hyperreflexia, and spasticity. Lower motor neurons (LMNs) originate in the motor nuclei of the brainstem and anterior horn of the spinal cord and directly innervate skeletal muscles. LMN disorders are identified by weakness, atrophy, fasciculations and muscle cramps.

## AMYOTROPHIC LATERAL SCLEROSIS

Amyotrophic lateral sclerosis (ALS) is the most common form of motor neuron disease. It is a rare, fatal, progressive neurodegenerative disorder affecting neurons in the corticospinal tracts and anterior horn of the spinal cord. Most cases are diagnosed in the third to fifth decade of life, and median survival is only 3 to 5 years.

Amyotrophic lateral sclerosis presents as a combination of UMN and LMN signs and symptoms. Classic presentation includes asymmetric limb weakness, fasciculations, and muscle atrophy. Bulbar symptoms include dysphagia and dysarthria. Patients may experience pseudobulbar affect, which manifests as inappropriate laughing, crying, or yawning. Extrapyramidal features may occur, including facial masking, tremor, bradykinesia, and postural instability. ALS may be associated with deficits in executive function and language. Behavior changes, including apathy, disinhibition, and perseveration have also been observed. Patients with advanced ALS may experience autonomic symptoms, including diaphoresis, impaired gastrointestinal motility, urinary urgency, and sympathetic hyperactivity significant enough to result in cardiac arrest.[1]

## PRIMARY LATERAL SCLEROSIS

Primary lateral sclerosis (PLS) is a rare progressive disease that is characterized by UMN symptoms of weakness, gait changes, spasticity, and hyperreflexia. Symptoms typically begin in the lower extremity. Given that many patients initially diagnosed with PLS develop LMN disease in the years following diagnosis, PLS is also known as UMN-onset ALS. PLS has slower progression and longer survival than ALS.

## HEREDITARY SPASTIC PARAPLEGIA

Hereditary spastic paraplegia (HSP or Strumpell-Lorrain disease) is a genetically heterogenous disease that results in progressive degeneration of the corticospinal tract, resulting in leg weakness and spasticity. HSP may be inherited by autosomal dominant, autosomal recessive, or X-linked patterns. Patients commonly have bladder dysfunction in addition to the UMN findings. In the complex forms of the disorder, paraplegia coexists with other manifestations as listed in Table 193.1.

## PROGRESSIVE BULBAR PALSY

Progressive bulbar palsy (PBP) is a progressive degenerative UMN and LMN disorder affecting the motor nuclei of the medulla. Initial symptoms result from the degeneration of the glossopharyngeal, vagus, and hypoglossal nerves, leading to atrophy and fasciculations of the lingual muscles as well as dysarthria and dysphagia. This disorder is commonly believed to be a subset of ALS (bulbar-onset ALS) as many patients develop nonbulbar manifestations as the disease progresses.

## SPINAL MUSCULAR ATROPHY

Spinal muscular atrophy (SMA) is a large group of degenerative disorders of the α-motor neurons in the anterior horn of the spinal cord. SMA occurs as the result of a protein (SNM) deficiency due to a chromosomal mutation of the *SMN1* gene on chromosome 5. There are four phenotypic groupings

**Table 193.1 MOTOR NEURON DISEASES**

| | MOTOR NEURONS AFFECTED | SIGNS AND SYMPTOMS |
|---|---|---|
| Amyotrophic lateral sclerosis (ALS) | Upper and lower | Muscle weakness, spasticity, trismus, laryngospasm, sialorrhea, atrophy, fasciculations, dysarthria, dysphagia, respiratory muscle weakness, pseudobulbar affect, parkinsonism, tremor, bradykinesia, masked faces |
| Primary lateral sclerosis (PLS) | Upper | Weakness, spasticity |
| Hereditary spastic paraplegia (HSP) | Upper | Lower extremity weakness, atrophy, spasticity, bladder dysfunction, peripheral neuropathy, mental retardation, dementia, ataxia, extrapyramidal symptoms, hearing/vision loss, dysarthria, epilepsy |
| Progressive bulbar palsy (PBP) | Upper and lower | Tongue atrophy and fasciculations, dysarthria, dysphagia |
| Spinal muscular atrophy (SMA) | Lower | Muscle weakness and atrophy |
| X-linked spinobulbar muscular atrophy (SBMA) | Lower | Bulbar, facial, and limb weakness; androgen insensitivity |

based on age of onset and symptom severity, which typically decreases with older age at diagnosis (Table 193.2).

## X-LINKED SPINOBULBAR MUSCULAR ATROPHY (KENNEDY DISEASE)

Spinobulbar muscular atrophy (SBMA) is an X-linked disorder characterized by progressive weakness and atrophy. This LMN disorder is the result of an unstable cytosine-adenine-guanine (CAG) expansion repeat on the androgen gene of chromosome Xq11-12. Facial, limb, and bulbar muscles are affected. Patients may also have gynecomastia and androgen resistance later in the disease course.

## ANESTHETIC MANAGEMENT

Patients with motor neuron disease may present for anesthetic care for a variety of surgical conditions. Early in the disease course, patients may present for elective procedures unrelated to their diagnosis. In advanced disease, however, procedures are typically limited to those related to symptom management (i.e., tracheostomy or feeding access) or emergency surgery. Worldwide, up to 30% of patients with ALS will opt for a tracheostomy to facilitate ventilatory support in advanced disease.[2]

### PREOPERATIVE

Patients with motor neuron disease require preoperative assessment of skeletal muscle and respiratory muscle strength. While cardiac function is not typically affected by motor neuron diseases, one will be unable to accurately determine cardiac function based on exercise tolerance. Patients at high risk for cardiac comorbidities may require additional preoperative cardiac testing. Pulmonary function testing (PFT) quantifies the severity of respiratory dysfunction and possible need for respiratory support with continuous positive airway pressure or bilevel ventilation.

**Table 193.2 TYPES OF SPINAL MUSCULAR ATROPHY**

| SMA TYPE | EPONYMOUS NAME | AGE OF ONSET | SIGNS AND SYMPTOMS |
|---|---|---|---|
| I | Werdnig-Hoffman disease | <6 months | Generalized muscle weakness<br>Weak cry<br>Respiratory muscle weakness |
| II | Dubowitz disease | 3–15 months | Proximal muscle weakness (lower > upper extremity) |
| III | Kugelberg-Welander disease | 18 months–adulthood | Proximal muscle weakness<br>Difficulty climbing stairs<br>Foot deformities<br>Scoliosis<br>Respiratory muscle weakness |
| IV | | >30 years | Mild weakness |

Patients with advanced disease are also at risk for aspiration due to dysphagia, pharyngeal muscle weakness, and excess oral secretions. Vocal changes may be an indicator of dysfunctional swallowing and aspiration risk.[3] Patients with advanced disease may present to the operating room or procedure suite with advance directives (i.e., do not intubate/do not resuscitate), which should be thoroughly discussed with the patient prior to surgery.

## INTRAOPERATIVE

Intraoperatively, in advanced motor neuron disease with respiratory dysfunction, general anesthesia should be avoided if possible to avoid postoperative intubation and need for tracheostomy. ALS may predispose patients to laryngospasm, trismus, and sialorrhea, which may complicate intubation. Succinylcholine is best avoided in advanced motor neuron disease due to upregulation of acetylcholine receptors and risk for significant hyperkalemia. Epidurals can provide adequate surgical anesthesia while attempting to preserve respiratory muscle function for lower abdominal pelvic and lower extremity procedures. Minor procedures can be performed with administration of local anesthesia and respiratory-sparing sedatives (i.e., dexmedetomidine or ketamine).

## POSTOPERATIVE

Postoperatively, patients should be monitored for respiratory insufficiency. Postoperative intubation or noninvasive positive pressure ventilation may necessitate intensive care unit admission. Patients with ALS and other motor neuron disorders may be at increased risk for significant postoperative pain, which is the result of reduced mobility and preexisting muscle cramps and spasticity.[4] Skin breakdown due to impaired mobility may also contribute. A subset of patients with ALS experience paresthesias, allodynia, and hyperalgesia especially in the late stages of the disease.

## REFERENCES

1. Shimizu T, et al. Autonomic failure in ALS with a novel SOD1 gene mutation. *Neurology*. 2000;54(7):1534–1537.
2. Veronese S, et al. The last months of life for people with amyotrophic lateral sclerosis in mechanical invasive ventilation: a qualitative study. *Amyotroph Lateral Scler Frontotemporal Degener*. 2014;15(7–8):499–504.
3. Da Costa Franceschini A, Mourao LF. Dysarthria and dysphagia in amyotrophic lateral sclerosis with spinal onset: a study of quality of life related to swallowing. *NeuroRehabilitation*. 2015;36(1):127–134.
4. Chiò A, et al. Pain in amyotrophic lateral sclerosis. *Lancet Neurol*. 2017;16(2):144–157.

# 194.

# GUILLAIN-BARRÉ SYNDROME

*Justin L. O'Farrell and Maxim S. Eckmann*

## INTRODUCTION

Guillain-Barré syndrome (GBS), also referred to as acute idiopathic polyneuritis, is an umbrella syndrome with several phenotypic forms. It is an acute immune-mediated paralytic neuropathy resulting from a previous infection that, due to molecular mimicry, affects the peripheral nervous system. The onset of symptoms is typically first noted in the lower extremities prior to progression up to the trunk and upper extremities. GBS has a slight preference for males than for females. The primary subtypes of GBS can be divided into four groups: acute motor axonal neuropathy (AMAN), acute motor and sensory axonal neuropathy (AMSAN), acute inflammatory demyelinating polyradiculoneuropathy (AIDP), and Miller Fisher syndrome (MFS).

## CLINICAL FEATURES

Common presenting symptoms of patients with GBS include weakness that begins caudally and progresses cephalad as well as areflexia. Facial nerve palsies, oropharyngeal weakness, and oculomotor weakness are among other symptoms seen. GBS disease progression occurs bilaterally and rapidly over approximately 2 weeks. The clinical course of progression may last to up to 4 or even 6 weeks after onset in rare and severe cases. Symptoms then resolve, with complete recovery occurring in weeks or it may take longer with some degree of permanent paralysis.

All variants of GBS have distinguishing pathophysiologic and clinical features. AIDP is the most common variant of GBS. In AIDP, the target of the immune attack is the myelin of peripheral nerves. This process of demyelination is responsible for the resultant symptoms, including myalgias and muscle weakness. The second variant is acute motor axonal neuropathy (AMAN), which progresses more rapidly than AIDP but does not affect sensory nerves. AMSAN is the more severe variant as compared to AMAN as this variant targets the axons of sensory nerves in addition to the motor nerves. MFS typically presents with ophthalmoplegia with ataxia and areflexia. There are several other uncommon variants of GBS.

## DIAGNOSIS

Cerebrospinal fluid (CSF) analysis shows albuminocytologic dissociation (elevated CSF protein with a normal white blood cell count) in up to 66% of patients with GBS 1 week after the onset of symptoms.[1] The elevation in protein may be correlated to the degree of increased permeability at the blood-nerve barrier at the proximal nerve roots. Electromyography and nerve conduction studies may be performed to distinguish between variants of GBS. A diagnosis of axonal variants of GBS can be supported by distal motor and sensory amplitudes.[2] The only variant of GBS in which testing for serum antibodies is useful is in the diagnosis of MFS. If there is suspicion for MFS, serum immunoglobulin (Ig) G antibodies to GQ1b have a sensitivity of 85% to 90%.[3]

## TREATMENT

The primary treatment for GBS is symptomatic management and supportive care. These patients are often managed in the intensive care unit due to the associated risk of respiratory failure and autonomic system dysfunction. Close monitoring of these patients is required due to the rapid progression of muscle weakness. The dysautonomia that occurs along with GBS also requires careful monitoring of blood pressure, fluid status, and cardiac rhythm. These measures are also helpful to monitor for cardiovascular complications of GBS.

Disease-modifying treatment for GBS includes plasmapheresis and intravenous immunoglobulin (IVIG). The mechanism of action for IVIG in the context of GBS is unknown. Plasmapheresis is effective through the removal of circulating immunologic factors, including antibodies, complement, and soluble biological response modifiers. Of particular note, glucocorticoids have been shown to be ineffective in the management of GBS.

## ANESTHETIC CONSIDERATIONS

The risk of absent cardiovascular compensatory responses may require increased monitoring and maintenance of intravascular volume, particularly during positive pressure ventilation, changes in posture, or blood loss. If opting for plasmapheresis for disease-modifying management, be aware that plasma exchange may cause hypotension and electrolyte disturbances.[4] Drugs that can cause hypotension, including most anesthetic agents, should be used with caution in patients with GBS.

Respiratory status is a critical factor in assessing and defining perioperative risk for the patient with GBS. Patients with compromise of diaphragmatic and intercostal muscle power are at increased risk of requiring postoperative ventilation due to the respiratory depressant effects of sedative/hypnotics, opioids, and neuromuscular blocking agents. Theoretically, inadvertent cephalad spinal blocks or subdural neuraxial blocks could impair intercostal and diaphragmatic function, leading to unanticipated respiratory failure.[5] Preoperative respiratory status may require specialist assessment prior to undergoing planned surgery if substantial respiratory impairment is suspected.

Regional anesthesia should be considered for amenable operative sites. For example, performance of upper extremity surgery under brachial plexus blockade can avoid the need for general anesthesia, advanced airway management, and mechanical ventilation. However, regional anesthesia that can impair respiratory function, namely, interscalene blockade and the side effect of diaphragmatic paresis, should be considered carefully prior to application.

Pain management can be complicated in the GBS patient at risk for respiratory impairment. Nonopioid, nonsedating analgesic systemic therapy, provided no contraindications, should be a mainstay of initial therapy. These include primarily the nonsteroidal anti-inflammatory drugs/acetaminophen and subanesthetic ketamine. Opioids, membrane-stabilizing drugs in the antiseizure class, antispasmodics, and antidepressants have a potential sedating effect when initiated. Consider perioperative capnography if available during administration parenteral opioid analgesia.

## REFERENCES

1. Yuki N, Hartung HP. Guillain-Barré syndrome. *N Engl J Med.* 2012;366(24):2294–2304.
2. Hadden RD, et al. Electrophysiological classification of Guillain-Barré syndrome: clinical associations and outcome. Plasma Exchange/Sandoglobulin Guillain-Barré Syndrome Trial Group. *Ann Neurol.* 1998;44(5):780–788.
3. Chiba A, et al. Serum anti-GQ1b IgG antibody is associated with ophthalmoplegia in Miller Fisher syndrome and Guillain-Barré syndrome: clinical and immunohistochemical studies. *Neurology.* 1993;43(10):1911–1917.
4. Raphaël JC, et al. Plasma exchange for Guillain-Barré syndrome. *Cochrane Database Syst Rev.* 2012;(7):CD001798.
5. Warren J, Sharma SK. Ventilatory support using bilevel positive airway pressure during neuraxial blockade in a patient with severe respiratory compromise. *Anesth Analg.* 2006;102(3):910–911.

# 195.

# CHARCOT-MARIE-TOOTH DISEASE

*Anthony Fritzler*

## INTRODUCTION

Charcot-Marie-Tooth (CMT) disease was first described in the year 1886 by three physicians: Jean-Martin Charcot and Pierre Marie of France and Howard Henry Tooth of England.[1] It is the most common inherited neuromuscular disease, with a prevalence of approximately 1:2500. The disease has also been known as hereditary motor and sensory neuropathy. Multiple types of CMT disease exist, including the following: (1) type 1 (CMT1; hypertrophic or demyelinating); (2) type 2 (CMT2; neuronal or axonal); (3) type 3, reserved for Dejerine-Sottas disease or patients with severe forms of hypomyelinating CMT; (4) X chromosome–linked forms; and (5) complex forms.[1] CMT1 is the most common, of which 70% are CMT1A.[1] The key characteristics of CMT are genetic heterogeneity, age-dependent penetrance, and variable expressivity.[2]

## ETIOLOGY

Mutations in over 30 genes have been attributed to the development of CMT. Autosomal dominant (AD), autosomal recessive, and X-linked patterns of inheritance have been observed throughout families with CMT disease. However, it is estimated that approximately one-third of point mutations and 5%–24% of the duplication mutations may occur de novo.[2] Generally, mutations occur in genes responsible for encoding proteins that are essential to the normal structure and function of the peripheral nerve axon or myelin sheath. CMT1 represents the demyelinating form and CMT2 the axonal form. CMT1A possesses AD inheritance and is caused by a duplication of chromosome 17 containing the peripheral myelin protein 22 (*PMP 22*) gene.[3] This duplication results in excess gene expression, which is thought to cause overproduction of *PMP 22* and accumulation in Schwann cells, inducing stress on the endoplasmic reticulum and subsequent cell death.[1] CMT2A, the most common form of AD CMT2, is caused by mutations in Mitofusin 2 (*MFN2*), a protein associated with mitochondrial fusion.[4]

## DIAGNOSIS

The diagnostic approach to any patient suspected of having CMT disease begins with a standard history and physical examination, including a thorough family history and musculoskeletal/neurological examination. The physical manifestations of CMT disease usually become evident by the first or second decade of life.[2] Symptoms such as skeletal muscle weakness and atrophy and loss of tendon reflexes typically begin in the feet and progress proximally throughout the lower extremities. The hands and upper extremities can also be affected later in the disease. Pes cavus (high-arched feet) and hammertoes are hallmarks of CMT disease. Sensory system involvement is observed in 70% of cases and manifests as loss of vibration and joint position, followed by decreased pain and temperature sensation in a stocking-and-glove distribution.[2] Clinical features alone do not allow for differentiation of the demyelinating or axonal types.[2]

The next step in the diagnostic approach is to perform nerve conduction studies. Upper limb motor conduction velocities (MCVs) are performed to differentiate between CMT1 (demyelinating) and CMT2 (axonal). CMT1 is defined as MCVs less than 38 m/s and CMT2 as MCVs greater than 38 m/s.[3] Results from these studies assist in guiding genetic testing and ascertaining an accurate molecular diagnosis.

Invasive diagnostic studies, such as sural nerve biopsy, are seldom needed and are reserved for when genetic studies are inconclusive, patients have atypical presentations, or patients who are suspected of having an inflammatory neuropathy.[2] When a nerve biopsy is performed, the classic histological finding with CMT1 is onion bulb formation. Onion bulb formations represent axons surrounded by layers of demyelinating and remyelinating Schwann cells.[4] With CMT2, axonal loss is evident; however, onion bulbs are rare or absent, and there is no evidence of demyelination.[2]

## TREATMENT

Charcot-Marie-Tooth disease is a lifelong disease and despite the potential for long-term disability, individuals are generally expected to live a normal life span. There is no specific treatment for the disease. Treatment is largely supportive and focuses on the management of symptoms through physical and occupational therapy, braces, analgesic medications, and orthopedic surgical interventions when necessary. Nonetheless, symptomatic treatment can significantly improve quality of life.

Nonsteroidal anti-inflammatory drugs can be used to treat musculoskeletal pain. Antiepileptic drugs (gabapentin, pregabalin, topiramate) and tricyclic antidepressants (amitriptyline) can be used for neuropathic pain.[2] Caffeine and nicotine should be avoided, as they can aggravate the fine intentional tremor associated with CMT disease.[2] Any neurotoxic drugs, including alcohol, should be avoided.

Research related to treatment is ongoing. Promising areas of research include gene therapy and the use of trophic factors or nerve growth factors to prevent nerve degeneration.[4]

## ANESTHETIC CONSIDERATIONS

### PREOPERATIVE

Preoperatively, one should be cognizant of potential cardiopulmonary anomalies associated with CMT disease. Cardiac conduction anomalies, including long QT syndrome, paroxysmal atrial flutter, cardiomyopathy, and atrioventricular block have been anecdotally reported; however, findings have not been consistent. An increased incidence of mitral valve prolapse has also been reported in some studies. In later stages of CMT disease, pulmonary function may become impaired. Proximal arm weakness could be a predictor of respiratory muscle impairment.[5]

### INTRAOPERATIVE

General, neuraxial, and regional anesthesia have all been performed safely and successfully in patients with CMT disease. In general, the anesthetic should be tailored to the needs of the patient. CMT disease is considered to be a condition of chronic denervation. Therefore, concerns have arisen regarding the use of succinylcholine and associated hyperkalemia as well the possibility of malignant hyperthermia (MH) with triggering agents. Overall, succinylcholine use appears to be well tolerated with CMT patients. Nevertheless, it is reasonable to avoid its use out of theoretical concerns for a hyperkalemic response in patients with neuromuscular disease.[6] Drugs known to trigger malignant hyperthermia have been used widely and safely. There has been one case report of MH in a patient with CMT1A; however, this occurrence most likely represents a chance phenomenon independent of CMT1A.[6] Nondepolarizing neuromuscular blocking drugs have been widely used and responses overall appear predictable without prolonged blockade. Continuous intraoperative monitoring of blockade should be performed. Monitoring of facial nerves may be more appropriate secondary to the effects of CMT disease on the extremities.[5] While neuraxial and regional anesthesia can be performed safely, it is important to document any preexisting neurological abnormalities.

### POSTOPERATIVE

If respiratory impairment is suspected or known preoperatively, it is important to be vigilant in monitoring for complications related to this in the postoperative recovery period. Opioid analgesics should also be cautiously dosed in those with impaired pulmonary function.

### REFERENCES

1. Berciano J, et al. Charcot-Marie Tooth disease: a review with emphasis on the pathophysiology of pes cavus. *Rev Esp Cir Ortop Traumatol.* 2011;55(2):140–150.

2. Szigeti K, Lupski JR. Charcot-Marie-Tooth disease. *Eur J Hum Genet*. 2009;17:703–710.
3. Reilly MM, et al. Charcot-Marie-Tooth disease. *J Peripher Nerv Syst*. 2011;16:1–14.
4. NIH: National Institute of Neurological Disorders and Stroke. Charcot-Marie-Tooth disease fact sheet. Updated March 13, 2020.

https://www.ninds.nih.gov/Disorders/Patient-Caregiver-Education/Fact-Sheets/Charcot-Marie-Tooth-Disease-Fact-Sheet
5. Kim JW, et al. Anesthetic management of Charcot-Marie-Tooth disease. *Arch Clin Med Case Rep*. 2020;4(1):138–152.
6. Pasternak JJ, Lanier WL. Spinal cord disorders. In: Hine RL, Marschall KE, eds. *Stoelting's Anesthesia and Co-existing Disease*. 5th ed. Philadelphia, PA: Churchill Livingstone; 2008:254.

# 196.

# MUSCULAR DYSTROPHIES

*Maura C. Berkelhamer*

## DUCHENNE MUSCULAR DYSTROPHY

Duchenne muscular dystrophy (DMD) is pseudohypertrophic *progressive* muscular dystrophy. It is inherited as a recessive X-linked disorder with an incidence of 1 in 3300 male births. The mutation in the dystrophin gene on the X chromosome (Xp21) causes an *absence* of dystrophin protein on the cell membrane of muscle fibers. Lack of dystrophin creates an unstable membrane. Females who are carriers of the mutation are rarely affected; only 20% will show symptoms of DMD, including muscle weakness and cardiac abnormalities. Diagnosis is made with genetic testing, muscle biopsy for dystrophin studies, and elevated blood creatine kinase levels.

Boys with DMD exhibit motor delays by 1 year of age. Affected boys demonstrate pseudohypertrophy of their calf muscles and weakness of pelvic and leg muscles as those muscles atrophy. Gowers sign indicates weakness of proximal leg muscles in the hip and thigh. By early adolescence, most individuals require a wheelchair. Muscular weakness causes skeletal deformities that contribute to restrictive lung disease. Large tongues and weakness of thoracic muscles impair coughing and create upper airway obstruction. Muscle wasting slows in adolescents with DMD, but cardiomyopathy continues to progress. Impaired myocardial contractility and conduction disturbances are a feature of DMD patients in their teens. Some degree of cognitive impairment is noted in 30%–50% of patients with DMD. Respiratory failure is common by age 20. Few males with DMD survive beyond their 30s.

Treatment is symptomatic and aimed at maintaining respiratory parameters and cardiac function, including aggressive management of dilated cardiomyopathy with anticongestive medications and ventilatory assistive devices as DMD progresses, especially during sleep. Prednisone can improve strength. Scoliosis surgery can improve respiratory mechanics.

## BECKER MUSCULAR DYSTROPHY

Becker muscular dystrophy (BMD) is pseudohypertrophic *benign* muscular dystrophy. It is inherited as a recessive X-linked disorder with an incidence of 1 in 20,000 male births. The mutation in the dystrophin gene on the X chromosome (Xp21.2) causes an *altered size and quantity* of dystrophin protein on the cell membrane of muscle fibers. BMD muscle weakness presents much later in childhood and worsens at a much slower rate than DMD. Impaired myocardial contractility and conduction disturbances affect BMD patients in their teens. Cognitive impairment is noted in patients with BMD. Males with BMD remain able to walk. They can survive into their 40s or beyond. Respiratory muscle weakness and dysphagia predispose patients with BMD to aspiration and pulmonary infections.

## EMERY-DREIFUSS MUSCULAR DYSTROPHY

Emery-Dreifuss muscular dystrophy (EDMD) is a syndrome of progressive muscle weakness. It has several genetic patterns of inheritance: X linked, autosomal dominant, and autosomal recessive. They have similar signs and symptoms, although a small percentage of people with the autosomal dominant form do not experience weakness or wasting of skeletal muscles. Abnormalities in the nuclear envelope and cell signaling in skeletal and cardiac muscle underlie EDMD. The progression of muscle weakness is usually slow through young adulthood. Muscle symptoms may begin to progress more rapidly in the fourth decade of adulthood. Most people with EDMD remain able to walk. Cardiomyopathy and arrhythmias are progressive in EDMD. These problems arise around the second decade of life (age 10 to 19) and increase the risk of sudden death.[1]

## MYOTONIC DYSTROPHY (DM1 AND DM2)

Myotonic dystrophy (DM) is associated with persistent contraction of skeletal and bulbar muscles (myotonic episodes) with delayed relaxation. Myotonic dystrophy type 1 (DM1; Steinert Disease) and type 2 (proximal myotonic myopathy) results from expansion of a CTG-trinucleotide repeat that causes an abnormality in the *DMPK* gene for DM1, while DM2 results from mutations in the *CNBP* gene. The protein produced from the *DMPK* gene likely plays a role in communication within cells. Alterations in chloride and sodium channels exist in cell membranes. DM1 has autosomal dominant inheritance with anticipation. The repeat count of CTG-trinucleotide increases over successive generations, causing subsequent generations to manifest symptoms earlier in life. Diagnosis is made through genetic testing and electromyographic analysis. Creatine kinase is mildly elevated.[2]

Myotonic dystrophy type 1 has three clinical subtypes. Congenital DM1 presents in the neonatal period. Childhood DM1 manifests symptoms by age 10. Classic DM1 and DM2 present in adulthood. DM is characterized by progressive muscle wasting and weakness. The DM subtypes also cause hypotonia, cognitive impairment, cataracts, cardiac arrhythmias and cardiomyopathy, and insulin resistance. Cardiac arrhythmias, particularly conduction defects, are a prominent feature in young adults, with DM subtypes predisposing them to sudden cardiac death. People affected by DM have prolonged muscle contractions (myotonia, myotonic episodes) and are not able to relax muscles after use.

## RHABDOMYOLYSIS AND MUSCULAR DYSTROPHIES

The lack of dystrophin or an altered dystrophin protein (DMD, BMD) and defects in cell membrane ion channels (EDMD, DM1, DM2) create unstable muscle membranes. Volatile anesthetic agents further destabilize the muscle membranes releasing myoglobin and potassium from the muscle cells.[3] Succinylcholine also triggers rhabdomyolysis in patients with muscular dystrophies, resulting in hyperkalemia, leading to cardiac arrest. Patients with DMD, BMD, and EDMD should not receive anesthetic medications that trigger rhabdomyolysis, hyperkalemia, and myoglobinuria, such as volatile anesthetics and succinylcholine. Patients with the myotonic myopathy subtypes (DM1, DM2) and mitochondrial myopathies should not receive succinylcholine, which precipitates rhabdomyolysis, leading to hyperkalemic arrest. Patients with the DM subtypes can tolerate carefully titrated volatile anesthetics sevoflurane and desflurane.[2] Most patients with a muscular dystrophy have an elevated serum creatine kinase. Muscular dystrophies are *not* associated with a risk of malignant hyperthermia (MH) greater than the general population. Only King-Denborough syndrome and central core are associated with MH. The Malignant Hyperthermia Association of the United States recognizes that mutations in the ryanodine (*RYR1*) gene make patients susceptible to MH.

## ANESTHETIC CONSIDERATIONS

Patients with muscular dystrophies have heightened sensitivity to the effects of all categories of anesthetic agents as well as prolongation of these effects with the interaction of sedatives and analgesics. Muscle wasting predisposes to hypothermia. Respiratory muscle weakness predisposes patients to restrictive lung disease and ineffective cough.[2] Arterial hypoxemia and a diminished ventilatory response to hypoxia and hypercapnia occur. Preoperative assessment of decreased vital capacity indicates the need for initiation of noninvasive ventilation (continuous positive airway pressure/bilevel positive airway pressure [CPAP/BiPAP]) prior to surgery and intensive care unit monitoring in the postoperative period.[4] Reduced level of consciousness, pharyngeal dysfunction and aspiration, and gastrointestinal dysmotility are also prolonged in the postoperative period. These risks can be mitigated by sustained monitoring and noninvasive ventilatory assistance into the postoperative period. A multidisciplinary approach to the perioperative care of patients with muscular dystrophies is a necessary paradigm.

Regional, spinal, and combined anesthetic techniques are a reasonable approach to minimize the amounts of

**Table 196.1** ANESTHETIC CONSIDERATIONS FOR DIFFERENT MUSCULAR CONDITIONS

| | MITOCHONDRIAL MYOPATHY | MUSCULAR DYSTROPHIES | MYOTONIC DYSTROPHY | UNDIAGNOSED HYPOTONIA |
|---|---|---|---|---|
| TIVA versus volatile | Sevoflurane | TIVA | Either | TIVA[a] |
| Muscle disorder | Rhabdomyolysis | Rhabdomyolysis | Contracture | |
| Succinylcholine | Avoid | Avoid | Avoid | Avoid |
| MH risk | No | No | No | Possibly[b] |
| Creatine kinase | Mild ↑ | ↑↑ | Mild ↑ | Variable |
| Postoperative complications | Respiratory and central nervous system depression | Respiratory insufficiency Cardiac collapse | Rigidity Respiratory insufficiency | Weakness Dysphagia Aspiration |

[a]Short duration.

[b]KING-DENBOROUGH syndrome, central core disease, ryanodine receptor defects.

Berkelhamer MC. 2020.

intraoperative anesthesia and analgesic agents used and manage postoperative pain with opioid sparing. This can lessen sedation and depression of cough and respiratory parameters.

Patients with DMD are at high risk for postoperative airway obstruction and respiratory insufficiency, leading to acute respiratory distress syndrome. Preoperative evaluation to initiate CPAP/BiPAP and cough assist therapy should occur several weeks before surgery. Noninvasive ventilator support modalities to transition from mechanical ventilation to spontaneous ventilation is necessary in DMD patients.[4] Aggressive optimization of cardiac function should be undertaken prior to anesthesia for surgery. They are also at high risk for life-threatening cardiac complications through postoperative day 3. DMD patients have large tongues, hypotonic pharyngeal muscle, and a body habitus affected by obesity and scoliosis. These factors can create conditions for difficult mask ventilation and difficult intubation.

Patients with DM1 and DM2 have prolonged muscle contractions with several perioperative triggers, including hypothermia, depolarizing muscle relaxants (succinylcholine), acetylcholinesterase inhibitors (neostigmine), electrocautery, nerve stimulators, and shivering. Paradoxically, succinylcholine can cause laryngospasm in patients with DM. Myotonic contractions make ventilation difficult. DM1 patients also have narrow faces, high-arched palates, and a limited mouth opening, complicating intubation. Treatment for myotonic contractions include phenytoin, procainamide, and benzodiazepines. Redosing muscle relaxants or intravenous anesthetic agents do not relax myotonic contractions. Muscle weakness and chronic and acute aspiration contribute to respiratory insufficiency in DM patients. Arrhythmias and heart block should be identified preoperatively and monitored closely.

## ANESTHETIC APPROACH TO UNDIAGNOSED HYPOTONIA

When planning the perioperative course for patients with hypotonia requiring diagnostic skin and muscle biopsies, continue anticonvulsant therapy, avoid lactated Ringer solution, and use glucose-containing intravenous fluids. If a diagnosis is known, the anesthetic choices differ. When undiagnosed,[5] consider total intravenous anesthesia (TIVA) with propofol for a short duration or other intravenous hypnotic and analgesic alternatives; titrate anesthetic dosing with a bispectral index monitor[6] (Table 196.1).

## REFERENCES

1. National Institute of Health Genetic and Rare Diseases Information Center. Emery-Dreifuss muscular dystrophy. https://rarediseases.info.nih.gov/diseases/6329/emery-dreifuss-muscular-dystrophy#:~:text=Summary,-Listen&text=Emery%2DDreifuss%20muscular%20dystrophy%20is,worsening%20muscle%20weakness%20and%20wasting
2. Myotonic Dystrophy Foundation. Ferschl M, et al. Practical suggestions for the anesthetic management of a myotonic dystrophy patient. November 5, 2019. https://www.myotonic.org/sites/default/files/pages/files/Myotonic-Anesthesia-DM1-2019-11-05.pdf
3. Lerman J, et al. Induction, maintenance, and emergence from anesthesia. In: Gregory GA, Andropoulos DB, eds. *Gregory's Pediatric Anesthesia*. 5th ed. Hoboken, NJ: Wiley-Blackwell; 2012:334.
4. Harper CM, et al. The prognostic value of preoperative predicted forced vital capacity in corrective spinal surgery for Duchenne's muscular dystrophy. *Anaesthesia*. 2004;59:1160–1162.
5. D'Mello A. Mitochondrial disease. In: Lalwani K, ed. *Pediatric Anesthesia: A Problem Based Learning Approach*. New York, NY: Oxford University Press; 2018:419–423.
6. Kinder RA. Muscular dystrophy versus mitochondrial myopathy: the dilemma of the undiagnosed hypotonic child. *Pediatr Anesth*. 2007;17:1–6.

# 197.

# MITOCHONDRIAL MYOPATHIES

*Maura C. Berkelhamer*

## MITOCHONDRIAL FUNCTION

Mitochondria produce adenosine triphosphate (ATP) by oxidative phosphorylation by the transport of electrons from the products of the Krebs cycle (NADH [reduced nicotinamide adenine dinucleotide]) and fatty acid oxidation (NADH and reduced flavin adenine dinucleotide [$FADH_2$]) via an electron transport chain formed by five enzyme/protein complexes on the inner mitochondrial membrane: Complex I (NADH dehydrogenase), complex II (succinate dehydrogenase), coenzyme Q, complex III, reduced cytochrome c, complex IV (cytochrome c oxidase), and complex V. This process of oxidative phosphorylation produces the essential cellular energy substrate ATP as well as oxygen free radicals. Abnormalities in these complexes and cofactors in the electron transport chain disrupt ATP production and cause the clinical presentations of decreased organ bioenergetic capacity, including myopathies and encephalopathies. Acidosis results from an overproduction of lactate and pyruvate when glycolysis is upregulated in the face of low levels of ATP.

## GENETICS AND VARIED CLINICAL PRESENTATIONS

Cellular mitochondria are a maternal contribution to the organism from the cytoplasm of the ova. Inheritance of mitochondrial disorders is usually maternal but can be sporadic. The concept of *heteroplasmy* best explains the varied clinical expressions and onset of mitochondrial disorders. The genetic sequences for the five enzyme/protein complexes are encoded by the nuclear genome of the cell (nDNA) *and* the mitochondrial genome found in the mitochondria itself (mtDNA). If a mutant form of mtDNA arises, it exists with the normal type of mtDNA. These two forms of DNA are distributed in different proportions to the cells throughout embryogenesis. The random complements of normal and mutant mtDNA in an organ create the severity of clinical dysfunction and the onset of pathology from birth through adulthood.

## MITOCHONDRIAL DISORDERS

Mitochondria are central to a wide variety of metabolic and cell regulatory functions. Because mitochondria are in every cell of the body, mitochondrial disorders can affect every organ system. Mitochondria are involved in the synthesis of heme and phospholipids. In hepatic cells, mitochondria detoxify ammonia. In neurons, mitochondria are essential for the synthesis of neurotransmitters. Mitochondrial membranes host the electron transport chain complexes responsible for cellular energy production. Deficiencies in the respiratory chain impact metabolic energy production in the form of ATP and produce excessive levels of "free radical" reactive oxygen species and metabolic acidosis.

The constellation of mitochondrial defects can be categorized as childhood onset, adult onset, and acquired. Childhood onset disorders are identified during infancy and severely impact neurologic development. They present in infants with acute onset of cyanosis, seizures, temperature instability, myopathies, and encephalopathy. The syndrome of *MELAS* (mitochondrial encephalopathy with lactic acidosis and stroke-like episodes) may also include hypertrophic cardiomyopathy. Children with *Leber's hereditary optic neuropathy* may have heart block, preexcitation syndrome, and a dilated cardiomyopathy. Other syndromes of mitochondrial dysfunction are associated with cardiac involvement, such as *Kearns-Sayer* and *MERRF* (myoclonic epilepsy with ragged-red fibers). Mitochondrial disorders present in adults as declining function in organ systems such as the brain and retina, which have higher rates of metabolic activity. Decreased bioenergetic capacity of major organ systems creates weakness and myopathies such as droopy eyelids, limited mobility of the eyes, cardiomyopathies, arrhythmias, dysphagia and gastrointestinal dysmotility, and vomiting.

Diabetes mellitus and growth hormone deficiency present as later onset mitochondrial disorders.

## MALIGNANT HYPERTHERMIA AND RHABDOMYOLYSIS

According to the Malignant Hyperthermia Association of the United States, review of literature *does not* indicate an increased susceptibility to malignant hyperthermia (MH) by most patients diagnosed with mitochondrial myopathy (MM). Volatile agents should not be avoided out of concern for possible MH susceptibility in MM patients. While it is very rare to have mitochondrial myopathies with "multicore" or "minicore" histology, these patients are considered to be at risk for MH when the recessive mutations exist in the skeletal muscle ryanodine receptor *(RYR1)* gene. Avoidance of depolarizing muscle relaxants reduces the risk of MH in these patients with MM. Succinylcholine should be avoided in patients with mitochondrial disorders due to evidence of succinylcholine-induced rhabdomyolysis and hyperkalemia cardiac arrest. However, there is increased sensitivity to nondepolarizing blockade.

## ANESTHETIC CONSIDERATIONS

### PREOPERATIVE

Because mitochondrial disorders can affect many organ systems, inquire about the following during the preoperative evaluation: central nervous system abnormalities, cardiac arrhythmias or shortness of breath, skeletal muscle weakness, hepatic or renal function abnormalities, glucose regulation abnormalities, adverse drug reactions, and prior anesthetics. Avoid hypoglycemia from a prolonged fast by instructing patients with mitochondrial disorders to drink sugary clear liquids greater than 2 hours prior to their operating room time unless they have significantly delayed gastric emptying times from their myopathy. Glucose-containing intravenous fluids should be administered. Lactated Ringer solution is avoided because of the additional lactate load.

Coordinate with the patient's subspecialist to evaluate and optimize cardiac and pulmonary function. Surgical patients with mitochondrial myopathies are at significantly higher risk for adverse outcome from deterioration of neurologic status, seizures, respiratory failure, arrhythmias, and metabolic crisis.

### INTRAOPERATIVE

There is no ideal intraoperative anesthetic for patients with mitochondrial myopathies. Avoidance of acidosis leading to metabolic crisis is the central tenant of perioperative care for patients with mitochondrial disorders. Metabolic crisis is caused by low blood sugar, acidosis, and the buildup of toxic substances in the blood. Symptoms of a metabolic crisis are nausea, vomiting, diarrhea, extreme somnolence, irritable mood, and behavior changes. If not treated promptly, respiratory insufficiency, seizures, coma, and sometimes even death can occur.

All volatile, local, and intravenous anesthetics have depressant effects on mitochondrial energy production.[1] The effects of anesthetic agents are believed to occur at the level of the electron transport chain. It is interesting to suppose that depressed bioenergetic activity in cells may explain the primary effects of anesthetic drugs. These effects are observed to occur in a dose-dependent fashion. Caution is necessary extrapolating to humans as this comes from in vitro study data. In a study of children with MM, the children had significantly increased sensitivity to volatile anesthetic, as reflected by low bispectral index monitoring values.[2] In vitro studies have shown complex I is inhibited by halothane, isoflurane, barbiturates, etomidate, ketamine, and propofol. Propofol additionally depresses mitochondrial function in complex IV, cytochrome c, as well as uncoupling oxidative phosphorylation. Sevoflurane, etomidate, and ketamine have been used safely in patients with mitochondrial disorders when titrated cautiously. The mitochondrial effects of dexmedetomidine are unknown. It should be used with caution in mitochondrial disorder patients with arrhythmias. Local anesthetics disrupt oxidative phosphorylation in an unknown manner. Lidocaine and ropivacaine have less inhibitory effects on mitochondrial function when compared to bupivacaine and are preferred.[3] Maintaining body temperature and acid-base balance is crucial to avoid metabolic crisis from acidosis further depressing mitochondrial and organ function. Frequent blood sampling for analysis of pH, acid-base status, lactate levels, and glucose and monitoring for cardiac arrhythmias are necessary perioperatively.

### POSTOPERATIVE

Mitochondrial myopathy patients with significant muscle weakness are at risk for postoperative hypoventilation and respiratory failure and central nervous system depression in the immediate postoperative period. A comprehensive perioperative evaluation and plan, across specialties, is necessary to avoid acidosis and subsequent metabolic collapse in patients affected by mitochondrial disorders.

## REFERENCES

1. Levy R, Muravchick S. Mitochondrial diseases. In Fleisher L, ed. *Anesthesia and Uncommon Diseases*. 5th ed. Philadelphia, PA: Saunders Elsevier; 2006:455–467.
2. Morgan PG, et al. Mitochondrial defects and anesthetic sensitivity. *Anesthesiology*. 2002;96:1268–1270.
3. D'Mello A. Mitochondrial disease. In: Lalwani K, ed. *Pediatric Anesthesia: A Problem Based Learning Approach*. New York, NY: Oxford University Press; 2018:419–423.

# 198.

# MYASTHENIA GRAVIS

*Michael Morkos and Daniel Cormican*

## INTRODUCTION

Myasthenia gravis is the most common disorder of the neuromuscular junction. It is a chronic autoimmune disease resulting in an antibody (Ab)–mediated functional decrease in acetylcholine receptors (AChRs) of the postsynaptic membrane. Pathognomonic symptoms include fluctuating skeletal muscle weakness exacerbated by activity and improving with rest. This is in contrast to Lambert-Eaton myasthenic syndrome (LEMS), which can be compared in Table 198.1. Ptosis of one or both eyes is often the presenting sign, usually progressing to involve extrabulbar symptoms. The condition is found in 1/7500 people, with a bimodal pattern of distribution dependent on gender; women are often affected in their third or fourth decade of life, while men are typically diagnosed in their sixth decade.[1]

## PATHOPHYSIOLOGY

Myasthenia gravis is caused by the formation of autoimmune Abs directed against the $\alpha$-subunit of nicotinic AChR. The Abs can be detected in roughly 80% of patients' serum and are thought to originate from the thymus gland.[1,2] Increased antibody protein production leads to thymic hyperplasia in this population, with 10%–15% of these individuals diagnosed with thymomas.[2] The autoimmune attack causes a decrease in functional receptors by 70%–80% (Figure 198.1), accounting for the characteristic skeletal muscle weakness and fatigue following repetitive use.[2] Interestingly, neuronal AChRs are unaffected, with destruction only occurring with AChRs at the neuromuscular interface. Muscles innervated by cranial nerves are the most susceptible to motor weakness, explaining the ptosis, diplopia, and dysphagia typically encountered.

## DIAGNOSIS

Recognition of myasthenia gravis requires thorough neurological examination with confirmatory laboratory testing

*Table 198.1* COMPARISON BETWEEN MYASTHENIA GRAVIS AND LAMBERT-EATON SYNDROME

|  | MYASTHENIA GRAVIS | LEMS |
|---|---|---|
| Pathophysiology | Antibodies directed against postsynaptic AChR | Antibodies directed against presynaptic, voltage-gated calcium channels |
| Muscle fatigue | Exacerbated by muscle use | Improves with muscle use |
| Commonly affected areas | Facial, extraocular, and bulbar muscles | Proximal limb muscles |
| Comorbidities | Thymoma | Small cell lung cancer |
| Deep tendon reflexes | Present | Absent or reduced |
| Treatment | Anticholinesterases | Diaminopyridines |
| Depolarizing neuromuscular blocker | Resistant | Sensitive |
| Nondepolarizing neuromuscular blocker | Sensitive | Sensitive |

as needed. As mentioned, the most common initial findings on physical examination are ptosis and diplopia, which worsen with persistent activity. Proximal muscle weakness is often seen as the disease progresses. Blood testing reveal AChR Abs in up to 80% of patients. Definitive confirmation can be done utilizing a short-acting anticholinesterase, typically edrophonium (Tensilon test). Following edrophonium administration, patients demonstrate a brief, but dramatic, increase in strength, verifying the diagnosis of myasthenia gravis.

Differential diagnosis includes Lambert-Eaton syndrome, hypothyroidism, botulism, and compression of the cranial nerves. Clinicians should also be aware that autoimmune conditions such as rheumatoid arthritis,

# Myasthenia Gravis

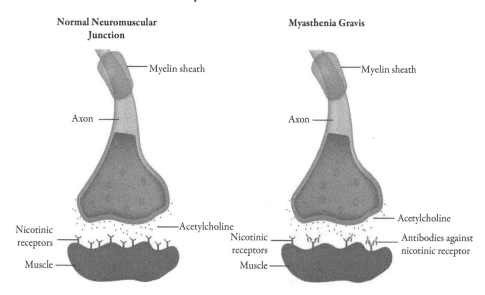

**Figure 198.1** Demonstration of the decreased number of functional receptors present on the postsynaptic membrane of the neuromuscular junction in myasthenia gravis.

systemic lupus erythematosus, and anemia are also often present.

## TREATMENT

First-line treatment for myasthenia gravis includes acetylcholinesterase inhibitors to increase the concentration of acetylcholine (ACh) available in the neuromuscular junction.[3] This class of medication inhibits the enzyme responsible for metabolism of ACh, thereby increasing the amount of the neurotransmitter available to bind receptors. Of these medications, pyridostigmine is the most commonly used. Corticosteroids and immunosuppressants are often used as adjuvant therapy when therapeutic control is inadequate with pyridostigmine.[3]

Plasmapheresis and immunoglobulins may be used as an immediate, but transient, intervention for those experiencing severe symptoms. While plasmapheresis is used to remove circulating Abs from the bloodstream, intravenous immunoglobulin nonspecifically binds antibodies in an attempt to decrease the concentration of functional AChR Abs.[3]

## ANESTHETIC CONSIDERATIONS

### PREOPERATIVE

Continued use of cholinesterase inhibitors throughout the perioperative period is essential in maintaining musculoskeletal strength. Patients must be informed on the increased risk of ventilator dependence postoperatively in the presence of severe risk factors (Table 198.2).

Preoperatively, routine administration of sedatives, including barbiturates and opioids, should not be used to avoid respiratory depression.

### INTRAOPERATIVE

Regional anesthesia can be safely used intraoperatively as it reduces/obviates the need for opioids and paralytics. Amide local anesthetics (ropivacaine, bupivacaine, mepivacaine, lidocaine) should be the agent of choice as esters may be poorly metabolized in the setting of acetylcholinesterase inhibitors. Brachial plexus blocks (particularly interscalene) have a known complication of ipsilateral diaphragmatic paralysis and should be avoided. Neuraxial anesthesia can also be used under the appropriate circumstances. Epidurals have the benefit of prolonged pain control and well-demarcated block level, while spinals are advantageous in using reduced levels of local anesthetic. The threshold for intubation is unavoidably low as accessory muscle paralysis and high spinal spread are well-known complications.

Consideration must be given to the choice of antibiotics as several classes have been known to exacerbate neuromuscular blockade, particularly aminoglycosides and fluoroquionolones.

Neuromuscular blockade must be carefully managed. The decrease in functional AChRs results in a profound sensitivity to nondepolarizing neuromuscular blockade. Dosing is reduced to 0.1–0.2 times the effective dose in 95% of the population ($ED_{95}$) to avoid prolonged respiratory muscle weakness. Sugammadex has provided reliable reversal of neuromuscular blockade in myasthenia gravis. In contrast, patients display a significant resistance to

*Table 198.2* RISK FACTORS FOR VENTILATOR
DEPENDENCE FOLLOWING INTRAOPERATIVE CARE

---

- Duration > 72 months (6 years)
- Daily pyridostigmine dose > 750 mg
- Vital capacity < 2.9 L
- Concomitant respiratory disease

---

depolarizing neuromuscular blockade (succinylcholine), requiring doses of 2.6 times the $ED_{95}$ to provide adequate conditions for intubation.[1] It must be noted in patients taking acetylcholinesterase inhibitors that the duration of action of succinylcholine will be prolonged due to inhibition of pseudocholinesterase.

Volatile agents may be used as the sole induction agent and anesthetic as they contain properties that decrease neuromuscular transmission.[1,5] Maintenance with volatile anesthetics decreases the dose of muscle relaxant required by up to one-half.[5] The administration of magnesium as an adjunct analgesic, antiarrhythmic, or for replacement therapy should not be done as it will exacerbate muscle weakness. Also, chronic corticosteroids may result in adrenocortical suppression, requiring intraoperative stress dose steroids.

## POSTOPERATIVE

Delaying extubation until adequate respiratory function is maintained is essential. Patients with two or more of the criteria given in Table 198.1 have a higher likelihood of difficulty weaning from mechanical ventilation and may need to be monitored postoperatively n an intensive care unit until sufficient muscle function for extubation returns. Immediate postoperative extubation may be deliberated in patients with less than two criteria after giving consideration to pain control, anesthetics administered, and preoperative neuromuscular function. When finally attempting to extubate, thought must be given to the fact that there is a higher risk of aspiration due to pharyngeal muscle weakness and the potential for continued weakness in the hours immediately following.

## REFERENCES

1. Eisenkraft JB, et al. Resistance to succinylcholine in myasthenia gravis: a dose-response study. *Anesthesiology.* 1988;69:760–763.
2. Trouth J, et al. Myasthenia gravis: a review. *Autoimmune Dis.* 2012;2012:874680.
3. Gold R, et al. Progress in the treatment of myasthenia gravis. *Ther Adv Neurol Disord.* 2008;1:36–51.
4. Sanfilippo M, et al. Rocuronium in two myasthenic patients undergoing thymectomy. *Acta Anaesthesiol Scand.* 1997;41:1365–1366.
5. Kiran U, et al. Sevoflurane as a sole anaesthetic for thymectomy in myasthenia gravis. *Acta Anaesthesiol Scand.* 2000;4:351–353.

# 199.

# LAMBERT-EATON MYASTHENIC SYNDROME

*Sabrina S. Sam and Syena Sarrafpour*

## INTRODUCTION

Lambert-Eaton myasthenic syndrome (LEMS) is an autoimmune channelopathy that results in decreased release of acetylcholine (ACh) at the neuromuscular junction secondary to autoantibodies against calcium channels at the presynaptic nerve terminal.[1] At a normally functioning neuromuscular junction, an action potential results in the opening of voltage-gated calcium channels. Calcium ions enter through the channels and then bind to proteins on ACh-containing vesicles, prompting the release of ACh. Once released from presynaptic nerve endings, ACh then diffuses across the neuromuscular junction to the muscle cell. ACh then binds to ACh receptors, resulting in the inward movement of electrical current, which generates muscle contraction. With destruction of the voltage-gated calcium channels, there is not enough ACh to produce normal muscle contraction, thus resulting in muscle weakness.

## EPIDEMIOLOGY

Lambert-Eaton myasthenic syndrome affects approximately 1 in 100,000 individuals, with a slightly higher prevalence in males. Typically, the syndrome affects persons over the age of 40; however, age of onset can vary greatly. When it presents in younger individuals, there is often no associated neoplasm.

Lambert-Eaton myasthenic syndrome is frequently associated with paraneoplastic states, particularly in men.[2] The most common neoplasms are small cell lung cancer and gastrointestinal malignancies. The malignancies themselves are thought to contribute to disease progression; therefore, individuals with LEMS and neoplasm have a more rapid progression of symptoms. This is thought to be secondary to the production of calcium channels similar to those on motor neurons by cancer cells derived from neuroendocrine cells. The immune system produces antibodies against the cancer's calcium channels and inadvertently recognizes the calcium channels on presynaptic nerve terminals, resulting in destruction.[1]

Approximately 40% of individuals with LEMS do not have an associated neoplasm.[2] These patients often develop symptoms earlier in life with slow progression and are more likely to have autonomic symptoms without a shortened life expectancy. Some patients have associated immunologic disorders, including myasthenia gravis (MG), pernicious anemia, diabetes, sarcoidosis, thyroiditis, and celiac disease. It is not linked with thymic abnormalities.

## CLINICAL FEATURES

Patients with LEMS generally have proximal limb muscle weakness that is worse in the lower extremities, contrary to patients with MG, who have weakness that predominantly affects the extraocular and bulbar muscles. However, some degree of weakness around the eyes can be seen, resulting in ptosis or diplopia. In severe disease, patients may have difficulty walking or performing daily activities of self-care. Another distinguishing factor is the improvement in strength with activity and worsening with inactivity in those with LEMS rather than the increasing fatigue seen throughout the day in those with MG. This improvement is secondary to buildup of presynaptic calcium, resulting in increased ability to release ACh.[1] The disease course is typically slowly progressive, with day-to-day fluctuations in

symptoms. Stressors such as stress, heat, and decreased sleep can worsen symptoms.

Lambert-Eaton myasthenic syndrome can be associated with autonomic dysfunction in some patients, particularly those with an associated neoplasm. Typical presentations include dry mouth, gastroparesis, urinary retention, orthostatic hypotension, or erectile dysfunction in men. This potential autonomic dysfunction is not seen in those with MG.

## DIAGNOSIS

Lambert-Eaton myasthenic syndrome is diagnosed via detailed history and physical examination along with electrophysiology. It can be a difficult diagnosis to make given the first complaints are of thigh weakness; therefore, suspicion may be low without an associated malignancy. On physical examination, reflexes are usually decreased, and some patients might have improvement on repeat examination. Electromyography (EMG) results in low nerve responses. In LEMS, the examiner should have the patient exercise for 10 seconds and then repeat the test. When the response increases by more than 60%–100%, the EMG is diagnostic for LEMS.[3] A blood test to detect antibodies against calcium channels on the presynaptic nerve terminal might also be utilized; however, approximately 15% of patients with LEMS will not be positive for antibodies against voltage-gated calcium channels.

Once the diagnosis is confirmed, imaging of the chest should be performed to rule out small cell lung cancer. If computed tomography of the thorax is negative, [18]F-fluorodeoxyglucose–positron emission tomography should be performed. If negative, screening should be repeated at 3–6 months, with follow-up imaging obtained every 6 months for 2 years.

## TREATMENT

In the subtype of LEMS associated with neoplasm, treating the cancer can result in resolution of LEMS. However, there is no cure for LEMS not associated with malignancy; therefore, therapy is targeted at symptom relief. Potassium channel blockers are newer forms of therapy. They allow increased electrical activity at the neuromuscular junction, resulting in increased calcium influx and therefore increased release of ACh.[4] There are currently two potassium channel blockers approved for treatment of LEMS in the United States: Firdapse (3,4-diaminopyridine or 3,4-DAP) and Ruzurgi (amifampridine). Firdapse was approved by the Food and Drug Administration (FDA) in 2018 for treatment of adults with LEMS. Therapeutic dose ranges from 5 to 25 mg three to four times per day. Ruzurgi was approved by the FDA in 2019 for the treatment of LEMS in children aged 6–17. Both of these pharmaceuticals are contraindicated in people with a history of seizures. According to their prescribing information, common side effects include paresthesias, abdominal pain, and nausea.

Cholinesterase inhibitors have been the mainstay of therapy in MG, but can also be used for mild LEMS. They decrease the breakdown of ACh, therefore allowing more ACh to work at the postsynaptic nerve terminal.[5] The most common cholinesterase inhibitor used is pyridostigmine.

Immunosuppression is sometimes used, but this course of therapy has many side effects. The drugs used are similar to those for treatment of MG and include prednisone, azathioprine, mycophenolate mofetil, or cyclosporine. Immune modulation with plasma exchange and intravenous immunoglobulin (IVIG) therapy can also be utilized. Plasma exchange briefly eliminates antibodies from the blood. The benefits of IVIG last longer, with peak benefits at 2–4 weeks. IVIG therapy works by decreasing the immune system's production of antibodies and blocking the binding of antibodies.

Research into new therapies for LEMS is ongoing. A new medication in preclinical development is designed to hold calcium channels open longer. Combined with Firdapse, ACh levels can be returned to normal.

## ANESTHETIC CONSIDERATIONS

### PREOPERATIVE

Patients with LEMS require careful preoperative evaluation for increased risk of postoperative respiratory failure and potential need for prolonged intubation.

### INTRAOPERATIVE

Individuals with LEMS are sensitive to both depolarizing and nondepolarizing neuromuscular blocking drugs. Typically, endotracheal intubation and surgical procedures can be performed with volatile agents unaided by paralyzing agents. If neuromuscular blocking agents are used intraoperatively, smaller doses are required and should be titrated based on vigilant monitoring with a twitch monitor.

Anesthesia providers must be knowledgeable regarding interactions of various medications in patients with LEMS. If patients have been previously treated with Firdapse or pyridostigmine, reversal of neuromuscular blockade may be unsuccessful. Symptoms can be exacerbated by several drugs, including paralytics, aminoglycoside, fluoroquinolone, ofloxacin, magnesium, diltiazem, verapamil, iodinated intravenous contrast, and varenicline.

### POSTOPERATIVE

Monitoring will be needed postoperatively.

### REFERENCES

1. Wirtz PW, et al. Lambert-Eaton myasthenic syndrome has a more progressive course in patients with lung cancer. *Muscle Nerve.* 2005;32(2):226–229.
2. Small S, et al. Anesthesia for unsuspected Lambert-Eaton myasthenic syndrome with autoantibodies and occult small cell lung carcinoma. *Anesthesiology.* 1992;76:142.
3. Titulaer MJ, et al. Screening for tumours in paraneoplastic syndromes: report of an EFNS task force. *Eur J Neurol.* 2011;18(1):19–e3.
4. Roden DM. Pharmacogenetics of potassium channel blockers. *Card Electrophysiol Clin.* 2016;8(2):385–393.
5. Keogh M, et al. Treatment for Lambert-Eaton myasthenic syndrome. *Cochrane Database Syst Rev.* 2011;2011(2):CD003279.

# 200.

# CONGENITAL MYASTHENIC SYNDROMES

*Sabrina S. Sam and Nawal E. Ragheb-Mueller*

## INTRODUCTION

Congenital myasthenic syndromes (CMSs) are rare disorders caused by hereditary mutations affecting the neuromuscular junction. The genetic mutations can affect the synaptic vesicles, acetylcholinesterase, or nicotinic acetylcholine (ACh) receptors, leading to an abnormal response to ACh.[1] CMS is typically inherited in an autosomal recessive manner, with the exception of slow-channel CMS, which is inherited in an autosomal dominant pattern. There are three main categories of CMS: presynaptic, postsynaptic, and synaptic.

Presynaptic CMS comprises mutations on the nerve side of the junction, resulting in inadequate release of ACh. It is the least common type of CMS and typically presents as CMS with episodic apnea. This type manifests during infancy with weakness of the facial muscles, such as ocular and bulbar muscles. It also presents with episodes of apnea.

Postsynaptic CMS involves mutations on the muscle side of the junction and is the most common type of CMS. Postsynaptic CMS is further divided into various subtypes, mostly involving abnormalities in acetylcholine receptors (AChRs).[2] Fast-channel CMS ensues when the AChRs close too soon. Slow-channel CMS arises when the AChRs stay open for too long. AChR deficiency occurs when there are not enough AChRs for ACh to work properly. Inadequate clustering of AChRs is a subtype that is caused by deficiencies in proteins such as RAPSYN and DOK-7. Another subtype is disorders of glycosylation, which involves modification to the shape and function of proteins and is thought to have some crossover with inadequate clustering.

Synaptic CMS encompasses mutations at the gap between the nerve and the muscle, characteristically a deficiency in acetylcholinesterase. This results in severe, early onset weakness resulting in difficulties feeding and ambulating.

## CLINICAL FEATURES

Congenital myasthenic syndrome is characterized by fatigable muscle weakness, but severity and onset of symptoms can vary greatly. Earlier onset of CMS is correlated with increased severity of symptoms.[3] Muscles around the eyes and muscles used for chewing and swallowing are the most commonly affected, although any skeletal muscle can be affected. In infants, weakness can lead to feeding and breathing problems. Infants can suffer from delayed milestones in sitting, crawling, and walking. Onset in adolescence or adulthood is typically mild and features ptosis and fatigue that does not usually interfere with activities of daily living. The prevalence of CMS is unknown. A study from Parr et al. found a prevalence of 9.2 children per million, with equal distribution between genders.[4]

## DIAGNOSIS

Patients with symptoms concerning for CMS are often sent to a neurologist for definitive diagnosis. A detailed history consistent with symptoms, such as ptosis and delayed motor milestones, is the first step. Physical examination may be similar to that of myasthenia gravis, and blood tests to rule out antibodies are usually performed. The next step is typically electrodiagnostic testing. Sometimes a Tensilon test is done. This is where an intravenous injection of edrophonium (Tensilon), a cholinesterase inhibitor, is given and strength is measured afterward. A temporary increase after Tensilon is consistent with CMS.[1] Genetic testing is required to differentiate between the subtypes.[2] This is important given that the therapy varies for different subtypes.

## TREATMENT

Unlike Lambert-Eaton and myasthenia gravis, CMS does not respond to steroids or immune modulation as it is not an autoimmune disorder. The management of CMS is dependent on the genetic mutation.[1] Cholinesterase inhibitors, such as pyridostigmine, have been used in certain types of CMS to increase levels of ACh at the neuromuscular junction. Presynaptic CMS and postsynaptic subtypes, ACh receptor deficiency, and fast-channel CMS, have been managed successfully with pyridostigmine. The postsynaptic CMS subtypes that respond to cholinesterase inhibitors can also be treated with amifampridine-containing drugs, such as Firdapse (3,4-diaminopyridine). Firdapse works by increasing ACh release from prejunctional nerve terminals. Slow-channel postsynaptic CMS does not respond to anticholinesterases and is instead treated with quinidine or fluoxetine. Quinidine and fluoxetine work by stabilizing the AChR in the desensitized state, leading to decreased opening time of the channel. The inadequate clustering subtype is sometimes managed with albuterol or ephedrine. Both stimulate $\beta_2$-adrenergic receptors, resulting in activation of the musculoskeletal system. Synaptic CMS currently has no known therapies.

## ANESTHETIC CONSIDERATIONS

### PREOPERATIVE

The anesthesia provider must be familiar with drugs to treat CMS and know the common interactions with anesthetic medications. As with myasthenia gravis and Lambert-Eaton, patients are often treated with anticholinesterase medications. Preoperative use of pyridostigmine may result in unsuccessful reversal of neuromuscular blockade.

### INTRAOPERATIVE

Congenital myasthenic syndrome can also be exacerbated by paralytics; various antibiotics (aminoglycosides, fluoroquinolone, ofloxacin); magnesium; and calcium channel blockers (diltiazem, verapamil). Intraoperatively, it may be prudent to avoid muscle relaxation for intubation if the surgical procedure allows it.

### POSTOPERATIVE

Additional potential problems are the patient's increased likelihood for aspiration if bulbar weakness is present preoperatively as well as the possible need for noninvasive ventilation postoperatively or prolonged intubation. Multiple case reports exist of patients needing prolonged ventilatory support postoperatively.[5,6]

## REFERENCES

1. Engel AG, et al. Congenital myasthenic syndromes: pathogenesis, diagnosis, and treatment. *Lancet Neurol.* 2015;14(4):420–434.
2. Engel AG. Genetic basis and phenotypic features of congenital myasthenic syndromes. *Handbk Clin Neurol.* 2018;148:565–589. https://ncbi.nlm.nih.gov/pubmed/29478601
3. Wadwekar V, et al. Congenital myasthenic syndrome: ten years clinical experience from a quaternary care south-Indian hospital. *J Clin Neurosci.* 2020;72:238–243.
4. Parr JR, et al. How common is childhood myasthenia? The UK incidence and prevalence of autoimmune and congenital myasthenia. *Arch Dis Child.* 2014;99(6):539–542. doi:10.1136/archdischild-2013-304788. Epub 2014 Feb 5. PMID: 24500997.
5. Koh LKD, et al. Perioperative management of a patient with congenital myasthenia gravis for elective caesarean section. *Singapore Med J.* 2001;42(2):61–63.
6. Maxwell T, et al. Obstetric and anesthetic management of severe congenital myasthenia syndrome. *Anesth Analg.* 2008;107(4):1313–1315.

# 201.

# ION CHANNEL MYOTONIAS, MYOTONIA CONGENITA, AND ACQUIRED NEUROMYOTONIA

*Meghan C. Hughes and Alaa Abd-Elsayed*

## INTRODUCTION

### NONDYSTROPHIC MYOTONIAS: MYOTONIA CONGENITA AND ION CHANNEL MYOTONIAS MYOTONIA CONGENITA

The dysfunction in MC is caused by an abhorrent chloride channel found on chromosome 7 that leads to delayed skeletal muscle relaxation (also known as myotonia). There is significant phenotypic variance within this disease (Thomas and Becker types); it can go unnoticed or lead to severe, disabling myotonia with transient weakness and myopathy.

### ION-CHANNEL MYOTONIAS

Paramyotonia congenita (PMC) and the potassium-aggravated myotonias (PAMs) are both caused by missense mutations of the skeletal muscle voltage-gated sodium channel gene. The mutation associated with PAM leads to myotonia only, while the one causing PMC leads to myotonia plus periodic paralysis.[1]

### ACQUIRED NEUROMYOTONIA

Acquired neuromyotonia causes involuntary and continuous muscle fiber activity, which leads to delayed relaxation and stiffness of the muscles affected. This condition can also lead to ataxia due to poor muscle coordination as well as lack of balance and staggering. The disorder is known for its progressive weakness, stiffness, and muscle cramping. Muscle movement does not stop, not even in sleep, and patients often suffer hyperhidrosis, tachycardia, and weight loss along with chronic pain.

## DIAGNOSIS

### NONDYSTROPHIC MYOTONIAS: MYOTONIA CONGENITA AND ION CHANNEL MYOTONIAS MYOTONIA CONGENITA

Myotonia congenita (MG) can be diagnosed in early infancy to early childhood. It typically begins with a thorough clinical evaluation and family history and is finalized with genetic testing. Electromyography (EMG) will typically demonstrate action potentials after myotonic discharges. Muscle biopsies may be helpful in some individuals but typically only reveal minimal abnormalities.

### ION CHANNEL MYOTONIAS: PMCS AND PAMS

When clinical suspicion is present testing should begin with an EMG. If the disease state is present, the EMG should show rapid repetitive electrical discharges in the muscles in question. EMG may not be conclusive, and genetic testing may be required.

### ACQUIRED NEUROMYOTONIA

The diagnosis of acquired neuromyotonia is made by evidence of continuous muscle contractions, particularly in the face and hands and muscle cramps. Confirmation of the suspected diagnosis is done via an EMG. In addition, serum studies should reveal the presence of an anti–gated potassium channel.

# TREATMENT

## MYOTONIA CONGENITA

Therapy for MG should be addressed on a patient-by-patient basis given the high variability of the disease. Early intervention is paramount in order to help affected individuals reclaim as much of their function as possible. Genetic counseling should be provided to families.

## ION CHANNEL MYOTONIAS

Many patients with PMC and PAM can lead normal lives and symptom treatment can be handled on a day-by-day basis. Individuals with this disease should avoid sudden exposure to the cold as well as sudden heavy physical activity.

Another component to treatment is diet as potassium-rich foods can trigger the disorder. Patients will need to learn how to manage their potassium intake. Pharmaceuticals that affect the sodium channels (mexiletine, lamortrigine, thiazide diuretics) may also benefit these patients .Genetic counseling is recommended for patients and their families.

## ACQUIRED NEUROMYOTONIA

The therapy of choice for acquired neuromyotonia is the use of anticonvulsant drugs (phenytoin or carbamazepine). These drugs will help to stop the abnormal impulses caused by this condition. Plasma exchange and intravenous immune globins have been utilized with limited success, and no long-term, controlled clinical studies have been completed.

# ANESTHETIC CONSIDERATIONS

The anesthesia considerations are largely the same across all of the disease states discussed in this chapter. For this reason, anesthetic considerations are not broken down by disease state but simply by stage (pre-, intra-, and postoperatively).

## PREOPERATIVE

For all of these conditions, neuromuscular monitoring is mandatory, as is the need to maintain normothermia since shivering can induce myotonic reactions. Anticipate that myotonic contraction during surgical manipulation will be a major challenge, and that this myotonia will *not* be responsive to neuromuscular block, reginal block, or peripheral nerve block. Procainamide and phenytoin may be useful in these patients since they are able to stabilize the muscle membranes.[2] In addition, topical anesthetics have proven useful and successful. Familiarity with the malignant hyperthermia protocol and drug placement is essential before attempting any suspected case.[3]

## INTRAOPERATIVE

Perhaps the greatest take away from this chapter should be this: Do not use succinylcholine on these patients intraoperatively as it will provoke severe generalized myotonia and possibly malignant hyperthermia.[3] Although the response to nondepolarizing agents is normal, it should be administered with caution and monitored constantly.[4]

Anticholinesterase drugs may precipitate myotonia as well. If propofol is used, prevention of pain on injection is mandatory because pain can induce a myotonic reaction of the limb or even of the whole body.[5] Neither regional anesthesia nor muscle relaxation can control myotonic contractions. No potassium supplementation should be given as it can also trigger severe myotonia in these patients.

In general, short-acting, non-depolarizing muscle relaxants (e.g., atracurium) should be used when possible.

## POSTOPERATIVE

Normothermia should be maintained in all patients, and EMG should be used to continually monitor muscle activity postoperatively. Patients should be carefully monitored until full, normal muscular functioning has returned.

## REFERENCES

1. Gay S, et al. Severe neonatal non-dystrophic myotonia secondary to a novel mutation of the voltage-gated sodium channel (SCN4A) gene. *Am J Med Genet A*. 2008;146(3):380–383.
2. Geschwind N, Simpson J. Procaine amide in the treatment of myotonia. *Brain*. 1955;78(1):81–91.
3. Russell S, Hirsch N. Anaesthesia and myotonia. *Br J Anaesth*. 1994;72(2):210–216.
4. Azar I. The response of patients with neuromuscular disorders to muscle relaxants: A review. *Anesthesiology*. 1984;61(2):173–187.
5. Milligan K. Propofol and dystrophia myotonica. *Anaesthesia*. 1988;43(6):513–514.

# 202.

# HYPERKALEMIC PERIODIC PARALYSIS

*Brett Simmons and David Matteson*

## INTRODUCTION

Hyperkalemic periodic paralysis (HyperPP) is a hereditary neuromuscular disorder, classified as a skeletal muscle channelopathy, defined by episodes of skeletal muscle weakness associated with elevated potassium levels. It was first described in 1951 and is characterized clinically by flaccid weakness with decreased tendon reflexes during episodes. Between episodes, a mild myotonia that does not hinder voluntary movements may be present. Key anesthetic considerations involve preventing hyperkalemia and hypoglycemia.

## EPIDEMIOLOGY AND GENETICS

The prevalence of HyperPP is estimated to be approximately 1:200,000, which is less common than the related channelopathy, hypokalemic periodic paralysis (HypoPP); see Chapter 203 for more details on this disorder. Males and females are equally affected. The disease is inherited in an autosomal dominant pattern and is caused by one of nine known mutations in the gene encoding the NaV1.4 voltage-gated sodium channel. Signs and symptoms of HyperPP typically begin in the first decade of life.[1]

Genetic testing is the gold standard for diagnosis as testing for all nine mutations is available. Previously, electromyographic exercise testing was a common diagnostic tool. Provocative testing with oral potassium, exercise, and adrenocorticotropic hormone administration may also be utilized.

## PATHOPHYSIOLOGY

The NaV1.4 sodium channel is a large protein consisting of four subunits. When acetylcholine binds to muscle cell receptors, the sodium channel opens to allow an influx of sodium ions, and the resulting depolarization leads to muscle contraction. The sodium channel is closed during the subsequent resting phase. In patients with HyperPP, the sodium channels open normally but fail to appropriately inactivate, allowing sodium to leak into the muscle cell during the resting phase. The prolonged sodium channel current causes longer depolarization, cell membrane desensitization, and loss of excitability; these effects together lead to myotonia and paralysis. The neuromuscular junction is not affected in HyperPP.[2]

Potassium, which is normally concentrated intracellularly, is important in repolarizing the cell and terminating the action potential via potassium efflux from the cell into the bloodstream. Higher levels of extracellular potassium, as seen with hyperkalemia, reduce the potassium gradient and the ability of cells to repolarize. Since muscle cells in patients with HyperPP are already resistant to repolarization due to the prolonged depolarization, hyperkalemia exacerbates the problem and is the major factor contributing to an attack.

## PRESENTATION

Attacks of HyperPP are characterized by hypotonia and generalized skeletal muscle weakness occurring when potassium levels rise above 5.0–5.5 mEq/L. Attacks may occur frequently (several times daily), and the duration of symptoms usually ranges from minutes to an hour, though there are reports of individuals having attacks lasting as long as a month. Compared to HypoPP, hyperkalemic attacks are usually shorter and less severe but occur more frequently. Paralytic attacks decrease in both severity and frequency with age. However, most patients develop a progressive myopathic weakness in their 40s to 60s, which leads to edema, fatty changes, and muscle atrophy.[3]

Between attacks, muscle strength and potassium levels return to normal. Though often subclinical, myotonia (delayed muscle relaxation after contraction) affects approximately half of affected individuals between attacks.

Although generalized weakness is common, focal symptoms affecting single muscle groups or limbs can occur. Some attacks may even be localized to the tongue and eyelids. The respiratory muscles, especially the diaphragm, are usually spared. The central nervous system and consciousness are not affected by attacks.[4]

Hyperkalemia-induced arrythmias are uncommon but have been reported. The presence of peaked T waves on an electrocardiogram (ECG) during an attack can be helpful in diagnosing the disorder.

## PREVENTION

The best way to prevent HyperPP attacks is to avoid common triggers (see Table 202.1). Episodes can be prevented through dietary means (low potassium, high carbohydrate, high salt) and avoidance of strenuous exercise. Medications, particularly carbonic anhydrase inhibitors such as acetazolamide and dichlorphenamide, can be used prophylactically to decrease the frequency and severity of attacks. These drugs help prevent hyperkalemia by promoting renal potassium excretion. Interestingly, acetazolamide is also useful for HypoPP since it causes a non–anion gap acidosis, which helps prevent hypokalemia. Thiazide diuretics may also prevent attacks by lowering serum potassium.[5]

## TREATMENT

Acute, brief attacks often do not require treatment and can often be shortened or stopped with mild activity or glucose-rich food or drink (which triggers insulin secretion, driving potassium intracellularly). Intravenous calcium, inhaled β-agonists, and thiazide diuretics can be used in more severe or longer lasting attacks, which are often accompanied by higher potassium levels.

## ANESTHETIC CONSIDERATIONS

Anesthetic considerations for HyperPP focus on achieving strict homeostasis of blood potassium levels and avoidance of precipitating factors (see Table 202.2).

*Table 202.1* COMMON TRIGGERS FOR HYPERKALEMIC PERIODIC PARALYSIS

| PATIENT RELATED | PERIOPERATIVE |
| --- | --- |
| Exercise, especially strenuous | Hypothermia |
| Fasting | Metabolic acidosis |
| Meals high in potassium | Potassium-rich intravenous fluids |
| Stress | Potassium-raising medications |

*Table 202.2* ANESTHETIC CONSIDERATIONS FOR HYPERKALEMIC PERIODIC PARALYSIS

| PREOPERATIVE | INTRAOPERATIVE | POSTOPERATIVE |
| --- | --- | --- |
| Monitor, optimize potassium level (low-normal) | Monitor potassium and glucose levels | Monitor blood glucose, potassium, patient strength |
| Continue prophylactic medications | Aggressive treatment of hyperkalemia | High-carbohydrate meals |
| Minimize fasting, consider clear carbohydrate drink > 2 hours before surgery | Use caution with potassium-raising medications | |
| | Consider dextrose-containing intravenous fluids | |
| | Judicious dosing of muscle relaxants, acetylcholinesterase inhibitors | |
| | Maintain normothermia | |

### PREOPERATIVE

Carbohydrate depletion is common in the perioperative period due to fasting guidelines and may provoke an attack. Therefore, preoperatively consider allowing a liberal fasting policy for HyperPP patients, for example, clear carbohydrate drinks up to 2 hours before surgery. Prophylactic HyperPP medications should be continued in the perioperative period. Measures to prevent onset of an attack and optimize patient outcomes include consideration of a regional anesthetic technique and decreasing potassium concentrations to below-normal levels. Potassium depletion is usually accomplished with diuretics and glucose-containing fluids.

### INTRAOPERATIVE

The primary goal of anesthetic management intraoperatively is minimizing the risk of precipitating skeletal muscle weakness. During longer procedures, electrolyte monitoring (primarily potassium and glucose) may aid in the acute management of the patient. Dextrose-containing, potassium-free intravenous fluids should be strongly considered. Avoidance of potassium-raising medications, such as succinylcholine, some diuretics, and nonsteroidal anti-inflammatory drugs in sensitive patients is critical. Nondepolarizing muscle relaxants can be safely administered, though caution should be used when administering acetylcholinesterase inhibitors as these drugs can worsen myotonia. Maintaining a normal body temperature is also beneficial.

Signs of hyperkalemia are often first recognized on the ECG, namely, the presence of spiked T waves. Use of intravenous calcium with insulin and glucose, β-agonists, and/or Kayexalate should also be considered if hyperkalemia is identified.

## POSTOPERATIVE

For high-risk patients, potassium levels should continue to be monitored in the postoperative period as surgical stress and fluid shifts can lead to electrolyte imbalances and higher potassium levels. Glycemic monitoring to avoid hypoglycemia is also important. Early oral intake of carbohydrates should be considered. Postoperative ventilation may be required in the setting of prolonged paralysis or myotonia.

## REFERENCES

1. Fontaine B. Periodic paralysis. In: Rouleau G, Gaspar C, eds. *Advances in Genetics*. Vol. 63. San Diego, CA: Elsevier; 2008:3–23.
2. Zhou J, et al. Neuromuscular disorders including malignant hyperthermia and other genetic disorders. In: Gropper MA, ed. *Miller's Anesthesia*. 9th ed. Philadelphia, PA: Elsevier; 2020:1113–1144.
3. Marschall K. Skin and musculoskeletal diseases. In: Hines R, Marschall K, eds. *Stoelting's Anesthesia and Co-Existing Disease*. 7th ed. Philadelphia, PA: Elsevier; 2018:507–537.
4. Gutmann L, Conwit R. Hyperkalemic periodic paralysis. In: Post TW, ed. UpToDate. UpToDate; Updated March 8, 2020. Accessed July 12, 2020. https://www.uptodate.com/contents/hyperkalemic-periodic-paralysis
5. Dierdorf S, et al. Rare coexisting diseases. In: Barash P, et al. *Clinical Anesthesia*. 8th ed. Philadelphia, PA: Wolters Kluwer; 2017:612–643.

# 203.

# HYPOKALEMIC PERIODIC PARALYSIS

*Brett Simmons and David Matteson*

## INTRODUCTION

Hypokalemic periodic paralysis (HypoPP) is a rare hereditary neuromuscular disorder, classified as a skeletal muscle channelopathy, defined by episodes of skeletal muscle weakness associated with low potassium levels. It is characterized by hypokalemia during periods of weakness and normokalemia between episodes. Oliguria, diaphoresis, constipation, and sinus bradycardia may accompany episodes. Key anesthetic considerations for HypoPP include potassium repletion if potassium levels fall below normal and avoiding hypokalemia and known triggers.

## EPIDEMIOLOGY AND GENETICS

Hypokalemic periodic paralysis is relatively rare, with a prevalence of approximately 1:100,000, though it is twice as common as hyperkalemic periodic paralysis (HyperPP).

While most cases are hereditary and inherited in an autosomal dominant pattern, acquired cases associated with hyperthyroidism have been reported. Approximately two-thirds of cases are caused by a defective dihydropyridine-sensitive calcium channel in skeletal muscle (type 1), while the remaining cases are associated with a mutation in the skeletal muscle sodium channel SCN4A (type 2). Penetrance is often incomplete in families with the calcium channel subtype, and the disorder is clinically expressed much more commonly in males.[1]

Diagnosis is complicated as potassium levels return to normal between attacks, which may be relatively infrequent. While genetic testing is the gold standard for diagnostic confirmation, it is not available for all possible mutations. Provocative testing with insulin, an oral glucose bolus, or intense exercise is sometimes employed in an inpatient setting. Electromyography and muscle biopsy are more invasive diagnostic tests and less commonly employed. In cases with an established family history of HypoPP, further diagnostic testing may not be required.

## PATHOPHYSIOLOGY

Type 1 HypoPP is caused by a mutation in a gene encoding the $\alpha_1$-subunit of the dihydropyridine-sensitive calcium channel. The mechanism of how a reduction in calcium current affects potassium flux and/or clinical expression is not completely understood, but the dihydropyridine-sensitive calcium channel may also function as a voltage sensor for excitation-contraction coupling.

In the less common type 2 HypoPP, voltage-sensing changes are caused by mutations in the $\alpha$-subunit of the SCN4A gene, which encodes the NaV1.4 protein. While mutations elsewhere in this gene can produce HyperPP, mutations in the voltage sensor domain lead to a reduced myocyte membrane potential. This causes slower and smaller action potentials, particularly with hypokalemia.[2]

## PRESENTATION

Attacks of HypoPP are characterized by weakness affecting proximal more than distal muscle groups. Lower extremities are more often involved than upper extremities. Affected individuals are conscious during attacks, and involvement of respiratory muscles is rare. Potassium levels during an attack are typically below 3.0 mEq/L and may fall to as low as 1.5 mEq/L. Attacks vary in frequency and duration, typically lasting several hours, with attack-free intervals of weeks to months. They are typically longer in duration and occur less frequently than those of HyperPP. Between attacks, muscle strength and potassium levels return to normal. Myotonia is not a feature of HypoPP.[3]

The onset of symptoms typically occurs in the first or second decade of life. Type 2 HypoPP may be associated with a younger age of onset and more prominent myalgias, as well as a less predictable response to acetazolamide. Similar to HyperPP, attacks decrease in number and severity with age. A progressive proximal myopathy is usually seen after the age of 50, which can be severely disabling.

Hypokalemia-induced arrhythmias are uncommon but may occur during attacks. The presence of ST segment depression and increase in U-wave amplitude on an electrocardiogram can be helpful in diagnosis and management.

## PREVENTION

The best way to prevent HypoPP attacks is to avoid common triggers (see Table 203.1). Episodes of HypoPP can be prevented through dietary means (low carbohydrate intake) and avoidance of vigorous exercise. When attacks are not controlled with nonpharmacological regimens, prophylactic medications and potassium supplementation may be indicated. The carbonic anhydrase inhibitors acetazolamide and dichlorphenamide decrease the frequency and severity of attacks by stimulating calcium-activated potassium channels in skeletal muscle and by producing a non–anion gap acidosis, which protects against hypokalemia. The potassium-sparing diuretics spironolactone and triamterene decrease the incidence and severity of attacks by maintaining higher blood potassium levels.[4]

## TREATMENT

Mild episodes often do not require treatment and can usually be terminated by light exercise. When treatment is necessary, oral or intravenous potassium chloride is the principal therapy. Cardiac monitoring is recommended, and rebound hyperkalemia is common as potassium diffuses extracellularly.

## ANESTHETIC CONSIDERATIONS

Anesthetic considerations for HypoPP involve avoiding and treating low blood potassium levels and minimizing the risk of precipitating factors (see Table 203.2).

## PREOPERATIVE

Prophylactic HypoPP medications should be continued perioperatively unless otherwise contraindicated. Measures to prevent the onset of an attack and optimize patient outcomes include consideration of a regional anesthetic technique and increasing potassium concentrations to high-normal levels. High-carbohydrate meals should be avoided within 24 hours of surgery. Electrolyte levels should be monitored and optimized preoperatively. Potassium repletion can be accomplished with oral or intravenous potassium chloride.[5]

*Table 203.1* COMMON TRIGGERS FOR HYPOKALEMIC PERIODIC PARALYSIS

| PATIENT RELATED | PERIOPERATIVE |
|---|---|
| Alcohol use | Dilutional hypokalemia (excessive intravenous fluids) |
| Carbohydrate-rich meals | Hypothermia |
| High salt (sodium) intake | Metabolic alkalosis |
| Pregnancy | Potassium-lowering medications |
| Strenuous exercise (or cessation of) | |
| Stress | |

**Table 203.2** ANESTHETIC CONSIDERATIONS FOR HYPOKALEMIC PERIODIC PARALYSIS

| PREOPERATIVE | INTRAOPERATIVE | POSTOPERATIVE |
|---|---|---|
| Monitor, optimize potassium level (high-normal) | Monitor potassium levels | Monitor blood glucose, potassium, patient strength |
| Continue prophylactic medications | Aggressive treatment of hypokalemia | Low carbohydrate meals |
| Avoid high-carbohydrate meals | Use caution with potassium-lowering medications | |
| | Judicious dosing of muscle relaxants | |
| | Maintain normothermia | |

## INTRAOPERATIVE

The primary goal of anesthetic management involves reducing the risk of skeletal muscle weakness. This is accomplished intraoperatively by maintaining normothermia, minimizing stress, and avoiding medications that lower potassium. Caution should be employed when administering glucose-containing solutions, β-adrenergic agonists, epinephrine, and insulin as these can cause movement of extracellular potassium into cells and thus lower blood potassium levels. If the operative procedure requires diuresis, mannitol can be administered instead of a potassium-wasting diuretic. Frequent monitoring of serum potassium levels is recommended, and hypokalemia should be aggressively treated with intravenous potassium chloride at a rate of up to 40 mEq/h. Both depolarizing and nondepolarizing muscle relaxants are relatively safe but shorter acting agents are preferred to minimize the effects of cumulative muscle weakness.

## POSTOPERATIVE

For higher risk patients, potassium levels and strength should continue to be monitored in the postoperative period as surgical stress and fluid shifts can lead to electrolyte imbalances and altered potassium levels. Glycemic monitoring may aid in the prevention of hyperglycemia. When oral intake is restarted, low-carbohydrate food and drink are preferred. Postoperative ventilation may be required in the setting of prolonged muscle weakness.

## REFERENCES

1. Jurkat-Rott K, et al. Voltage-sensor sodium channel mutations cause hypokalemic periodic paralysis type 2 by enhanced inactivation and reduced current. *Proc Natl Acad Sci U S A*. 2000;97:9549–9554.
2. Zhou J, et al. Neuromuscular disorders including malignant hyperthermia and other genetic disorders. In: Gropper MA, ed. *Miller's Anesthesia*. 9th ed. Philadelphia, PA: Elsevier; 2020:1113–1144.
3. Fontaine B. Periodic paralysis. In: Rouleau G, Gaspar C., eds. *Advances in Genetics*. Vol. 63. San Diego, CA: Elsevier; 2008:3–23.
4. Dierdorf S, et al. Rare coexisting diseases. In: Barash P, et al., eds. *Clinical Anesthesia*. 8th ed. Philadelphia, PA: Wolters Kluwer; 2017:612–643.
5. Marschall K. Skin and musculoskeletal diseases. In: Hines R, Marschall K., eds. *Stoelting's Anesthesia and Co-Existing Disease*. 7th ed. Philadelphia, PA: Elsevier; 2018:507–537.

# Part 18

# CLINICAL SUBSPECIALTIES

# 204.

# PAINFUL DISEASE STATES

## *Timothy Rushmer and Alaa Abd-Elsayed*

## INTRODUCTION

The International Association for the Study of Pain defines pain as "an unpleasant sensory and emotional experience associated with, or resembling that associated with, actual or potential tissue damage."[1] With such an open definition, it is best to further classify different types of pain and pain states. Frequently, this is done pathophysiologically, etiologically, anatomically, and in terms of duration.

## GENERAL PAIN TERMS

*Allodynia*: pain in response to a nonpainful (nonnoxious) stimulus

*Analgesia*: lack of pain sensation

*Anesthesia*: lack of any sensation

*Dysesthesia*: abnormal or unpleasant sensation, whether from a stimulus or not

*Hyperalgesia*: an increased amount of pain to a stimulus that is normally painful

*Neuralgia*: pain in the distribution of a nerve

*Paresthesia*: abnormal or unpleasant sensation not from a stimulus

*Radiculopathy*: injury or damage to a nerve root as it leaves the spine

*Anesthesia dolorosa*: painful numbness; seen in deafferentation pain syndrome

## NOCICEPTIVE PAIN

Pain sensation serves as a physiologic protective system to warn and prevent contact with noxious or damaging stimuli. Damage to body tissue is detected through nociceptors present on the end of afferent Aδ and C nerve fibers. The transduction and transmission of a noxious signal are the basis for nociceptive pain, which is defined simply as pain generated from nociceptor stimulation. Nociceptive pain can be further divided into somatic and visceral pain. Somatic pain originates from tissue damage such as inflammation, trauma, ischemia, and burns and is transmitted by somatic nerves innervating skin, muscle, bone, and so on. Thus, somatic pain has a precise location and is often described as feeling sharp, burning, aching, or throbbing. Visceral pain originates from visceral organs/structures and is transmitted by sympathetic fibers. It is usually diffuse, difficult to localize, and often described as dull or crampy.

## NEUROPATHIC PAIN

Neuropathic pain is caused by a lesion or dysfunction of the nervous system itself. Neuropathic pain is often broken down into central neuropathic pain and peripheral neuropathic pain based on the location of the lesion or dysfunction. Examples of peripheral neuropathic pain are painful diabetic neuropathy and postherpetic neuralgia (PHN). Examples of central neuropathic pain are poststroke pain and thalamic pain syndrome. Neuropathic pain is frequently described as lancinating or burning. Neuropathic pain often involves allodynia, hyperalgesia, and paresthesias. Treatment of neuropathic pain is multimodal, involving: tricyclic antidepressants (TCAs); serotonin norepinephrine reuptake inhibitor (SNRIs); anticonvulsants (gabapentin, pregabalin, carbamazepine, and oxcarbazepine); and transcutaneous electrical nerve stimulation units. Select patients may benefit from opioids and spinal cord stimulation.

## SYMPATHETICALLY MAINTAINED PAIN

A subtype of neuropathic pain, examples of sympathetically mediated pain include PHN and complex regional pain syndrome (CRPS). The exact role of the autonomic nervous system in these disease states is still unclear. However, these syndromes are at least partially mediated by sympathetic nerve efferent fibers; thus, sympathetic blocks can provide at least short-term analgesia, which in turn can help facilitate physical therapy, occupational therapy, and functional recovery.[2] In the case of CRPS, sympathetically mediated symptoms include alterations in autonomic functions such as blood flow (resulting in changes in skin color and temperature), sweating (usually hyperhidrosis), and trophic changes to hair and nails.

## ACUTE AND CHRONIC PAIN

Acute pain is a term generally used to describe nociceptive pain since it is pain caused by substantial injury or damage to body tissue that activates nociceptors. Examples include pain from a disease process, surgical pain, and obstetric pain. In contrast, chronic pain is pain that continues beyond the typical course of healing for the acute processes (>3 months) described previously. It is pain that stops serving its physiological purpose of warning the body of tissue damage. Chronic pain can be nociceptive, neuropathic, psychological, or other, and frequently has components of several types of pain.

The process of the transition from acute to chronic pain is not fully understood. It involves repeated stimulation of the nociceptive pain pathways, leading to increased sensitivity of nerves to their signaling molecules over time. This leads to phosphorylation of NMDA (N-methyl-d-aspartate) and AMPA (α-amino-3-hydroxy-5-methyl-4-isoxazole propionic acid) receptors and increased expression of sodium channels causing hyperexcitability. The nerves send progressively stronger pain signals in response to the continued nociceptor activation, which is the definition of the term windup. Windup and hyperexcitability lead to changes in the way the nerves of the central nervous system modify the pain signal. This is the basis for the term central sensitization, which is thought to contribute to the development of chronic pain.[3]

## MUSCULOSKELETAL PAIN

Musculoskeletal pain encompasses two of the most common painful disease states: myofascial pain syndrome and fibromyalgia. Myofascial pain arises from localized and palpable trigger points. Trigger points are hyperirritable areas within skeletal muscle, fascia, or associated tendons that cause pain on palpation as well as referred pain in a nondermatomal distribution. Often taut, rope-like bands are felt over the trigger points. Trigger points are associated with stiffness, reduced range of motion, and muscle spasm. Treatment involves physical therapy and stretching to help with stiffness, strengthening, and range of motion. Additionally, needle placement within the hyperirritable point (often causing a characteristic twitch) leads to pain relief and relaxation of the muscle. These trigger point injections are often done with a small volume of local anesthetic for short-term analgesia.

Whereas myofascial pain syndrome is localized/regional pain, fibromyalgia is defined by widespread musculoskeletal and soft tissue pain for at least 3 months.[2,4] Fibromyalgia is often accompanied by somatic symptoms such as fatigue, difficulty sleeping, headache, and cognitive disturbances. It frequently co-occurs in other rheumatic conditions and is more common in women than men. It can mimic many other chronic pain states and thus should frequently be on the differential diagnosis. The pathophysiology of fibromyalgia is unclear, but likely involves sensitization of central pain pathways. Treatment is mostly behavioral: increased physical activity, cognitive behavior therapy, and improved sleep hygiene. Pharmacologic therapy with TCAs, SNRIs, and pregabalin are the next line of therapy and have been shown to help reduce fibromyalgia pain.

## REFERENCES

1. Raja SN, et al. The revised International Association for the Study of Pain definition of pain: concepts, challenges, and compromises. *Pain*. 2020;161(9):1976–1982.
2. Benzon HT, et al. *Essentials of Pain Medicine*. Philadelphia, PA: Elsevier; 2018:223–232.
3. Gropper MA, Miller RD. Management of the patient with chronic pain. In: Gropper MA, ed. *Miller's Anesthesia*. Philadelphia, PA: Elsevier; 2020:1604–1621.
4. Wolfe F, et al. The American College of Rheumatology preliminary diagnostic criteria for fibromyalgia and measurement of symptom severity. *Arthritis Care Res (Hoboken)*. 2010;62(5):600–610.

# 205.

# CANCER PAIN

*Kevin E. Vorenkamp and Alaa Abd-Elsayed*

## INTRODUCTION

The American Cancer Society estimated that more than 1.8 million new cancer cases were expected to be diagnosed in 2020.[1] Over 600,000 Americans were expected to die of cancer in 2020, which translates to about 1660 deaths per day. Cancer is the second most common cause of death in the United States, exceeded only by heart disease. The 5-year relative survival rate for all cancers combined has increased substantially since the early 1960s, from about 35% to nearly 70%. Overall, a recent meta-analysis demonstrated a prevalence rate of moderate or severe pain in 38% of all patients with a cancer diagnosis, but these rates are nearly doubled for patients with advanced, metastatic, or terminal cancer diagnoses.[2] Cancer pain negatively impacts a patient's function, well-being, and overall quality of life. Adequate pain treatment can result in significant improvement in these domains.

## CAUSES OF PAIN AND TREATMENT STRATEGIES

Patients may experience pain arising from direct tumor involvement, cancer-related therapies, and mechanisms unrelated to cancer or its treatment. Cancer pain may be nociceptive, neuropathic, nociplastic, or mixed in nature. Similar to nonmalignant pain, successful treatment, particularly with regard to interventional therapies, relies on accurately identifying the etiology of pain. However, for malignant pain, analgesic treatment should commence while determining etiology. Often, this begins with pharmacological management. The World Health Organization analgesic ladder consists of three tiers of oral medications: (1) nonopioid analgesics and adjuvants, (2) weak opioids, and (3) strong opioids. Overall, the success rate with this approach is reported as 75%–80% of ambulatory patients with cancer. However, treatment with opioids and other pain medications for cancer patients is limited by the same shortcoming as it is for other nonmalignant etiologies. Opioid-related side effects such as nausea and constipation can be particularly bothersome for patients with visceral malignancies. Constipation can aggravate underlying abdominal pain. Additionally, tolerance can develop to opioid analgesics, and further dose escalation can result in opioid-induced hyperalgesia. Although addiction and opioid use disorder is less concerning in patients with terminal illness, care should be taken when selecting cancer patients for systemic opioid therapy since the 5-year survival rate for all cancer patients is approaching 70%. This is particularly true for cancer patients with abuse history when other appropriate options exist to control their pain. Finally, patients with cancer pain may be particularly susceptible to opioid-induced respiratory depression and death, especially if they have other pharmacological (benzodiazepines), metabolic, or neurological (brain tumor or metastasis) conditions.

## TREATMENT

As more oncologists are comfortable treating patients with cancer-related pain, pain medicine physicians often see the patients who experience refractory pain or intolerable side effects with this initial pharmacological approach. Some patients are not able to tolerate oral pain medications and may be considered for other routes of administration, including transdermal, buccal, sublingual, rectal, intravenous, subcutaneous, or neuraxial. Patient-controlled analgesia (PCA) is often used for episodes of acute pain and pain exacerbations requiring hospital admission and for patients with terminal illness. Pharmacological treatment is covered in other sections of this textbook, and the remainder of this chapter focuses on interventional treatments for cancer pain.

Nerve blocks can be utilized when the etiology of a patient's pain is clearly identified and contained to a single nerve or plexus of nerves. If patients receive short-term benefit from an injection of local anesthetic, neurolytic blocks, usually performed with alcohol or phenol, can then be performed to provide longer term benefit. In situations where the pain pattern is well defined, some physicians elect to go directly for the neurolytic block rather than consign the patient to multiple procedures. For patients with pancreatic cancer, proceeding directly to celiac plexus neurolysis has been advocated to avoid repeat procedures and to avoid false-negative results with the initial diagnostic block due to patient discomfort or technical limitations.[3]

## SOMATIC BLOCKS AND NEUROLYSIS

Peripheral nerve or plexus blocks and neurolysis can be considered when there is direct invasion of the relevant nerve. If the nerve or nerve plexus has motor function, then priorities of treatment with the patient should be discussed. For example, if the patient is experiencing refractory pain from brachial plexus invasion, a neurolytic block may be considered. This would be expected to result in motor weakness, although using more dilute solutions may lessen the degree of deficit while still providing pain control.[4] Other reported examples of somatic neurolysis include treatment of the following nerves: intercostal, axillary, suprascapular, trigeminal, femoral, sciatic, pudendal, genitofemoral, and ilioinguinal. Neuraxial blocks have also been described for refractory pain. These include intrathecal neurolysis and transforaminal injection of neurolytic agents.

## VISCERAL BLOCKS AND NEUROLYSIS

There are three great plexuses of the chest and abdomen. These contain visceral afferent and efferent fibers as well as some parasympathetic fibers. The cardiac plexus innervates the thoracic structures. The celiac plexus provides innervation to most of the gut and is the largest of the three great plexuses. The hypogastric plexus supplies the pelvic organs. The celiac plexus is located in the retroperitoneal space at the level of the T12 and L1 vertebrae. The celiac plexus receives its primary innervation from the greater (T5-T9), lesser (T10-T11), and least splanchnic nerves (T12). The plexus innervates most of the abdominal viscera, from the distal esophagus to the transverse colon at the level of the splenic flexure. There are at least two different areas to target for the block. The first involves targeting the deep splanchnic nerves via a retrocrural approach. Traditionally, this involves a bilateral posterior approach, typically at T12. The second involves placing the needle anterior to the aorta at the L1 level in the vicinity of the celiac plexus itself. Celiac plexus neurolysis can provide excellent pain relief and reduce the need for additional analgesics. Meta-analysis showed long-lasting benefit for 70%–90% of patients with intra-abdominal malignancy[5] and is recommended treatment for patients with pancreatic cancer. Superior hypogastric plexus neurolysis has been performed with benefit

for patients with pain arising from pelvic viscera. The ganglion impar consists of a semicircular retroperitoneal median structure, anterior to the coccyx or the sacrococcygeal junction. Its neural network includes nerve fibers of the perineum, distal portion of the rectum, anus, distal urethra, lower third of the vagina, and vulva/scrotum. Ganglion impar neurolysis has been used in the treatment of pelvic-perineal pain with efficacy and rare complications.

## NEURAXIAL INFUSIONS

When patients have persistent pain despite the above approaches, then neuraxial infusions can be considered. Typically, neuraxial opioids are first-line treatment, although other agents, including bupivacaine, clonidine, and ziconotide, can be considered if opioids alone are ineffective. The main advantage with neuraxial opioids over systemic is that a much smaller dose can be delivered to minimize side effects, such as altered mental status and nausea. For morphine, the typical equianalgesic dose is 1 mg intrathecal = 10 mg epidural = 100 mg intravenous = 300 mg oral. Certain side effects, including pruritis and urinary hesitancy, are more common with neuraxial versus systemic therapy. If the patient's life expectancy is less than 90 days, then often an external system might be utilized. This may consist of an epidural or intrathecal catheter that may be tunneled subcutaneously to minimize risk of migration and infection, but connected to an external pump and tubing similar to a PCA. If life expectancy is more than 90 days, then often an intrathecal drug delivery system with pump reservoir is implanted. This involves incisions to secure the catheter and tunnel the catheter to an internal pump, which is typically placed in the abdomen and can hold several months of medicine without requiring external tubing. The intrathecal pump can be reprogrammed to change the rate via telemetry, and the pump can be refilled via a percutaneous approach in the clinic setting. This represents a much more reliable system, but comes with an initial cost of implantation and discomfort with the implantation surgery. The 90-day threshold is based on prior cost analysis, but decisions should consider other patient considerations and desired approach.

## REFERENCES

1. Siegel RL, et al. Cancer statistics, 2020. *CA A Cancer J Clin.* 2020;70:7–30.
2. van den Beuken-van Everdingen MH, et al. Update on prevalence of pain in patients with cancer: systematic review and meta-analysis. *J Pain Symptom Manage.* 2016;51(6):1070–1090.
3. Vorenkamp KE, Dahle NA. Diagnostic celiac plexus block and outcome with neurolysis. *Tech Reg Anesth Pain Manag.* 2011;15:28–32.
4. Mullin V. Brachial plexus block with phenol for painful arm associated with Pancoast's syndrome. *Anesthesiology.* 1980;53(5):431–433.
5. Eisenberg E, et al. Neurolytic celiac plexus block for treatment of cancer pain: a meta-analysis. *Anesth Analg.* 1995;80(2):290–295.

# 206.

# ACUTE AND CHRONIC NECK AND LOW BACK PAIN

*Richard Tennant and Alaa Abd-Elsayed*

## INTRODUCTION

Neck pain is the fourth leading cause of disability with numerous causes.[1,2] It is one of the top five most prevalent chronic pain conditions. The estimated annual cost of combined low back and neck pain is $86.7 billion, third only behind diabetes and heart disease.[2]

## ACUTE NECK PAIN

**Presentations:** Acute neck pain has many arbitrary definitions depending on the source reviewed. One such definition of acute neck pain is pain lasting less than 6 weeks. Subacute pain is pain lasting 3 months or less. Chronic neck pain is defined as pain lasting over 6 months.[1] Duration of pain appears to be inversely correlated to outcomes. Most cases of acute neck pain resolve within 2 months from the initial pain episode. However, neck pain is often recurrent, with the best predictor of an attack of future neck pain being a past medical history of neck pain. The development of chronic neck pain is associated with low work satisfaction, inactivity, female gender, poor posture, headaches, and various psychiatric conditions.[1]

**Causes:** Axial pain has many causes and may include disk herniation, osteophyte formation, uncovertebral changes, cervical facet joint changes, and disk-related issues. Radicular pain is generally neurogenic in nature and most commonly involves C6 and C7 nerve roots.[1] Often, the patients will have "nonspecific" pain when pain cannot be attributed to a specific cause.

## ANESTHETIC CONSIDERATIONS

### Preoperative

Anticipate possible difficult airway and one should carefully evaluate the airway prior to induction of anesthesia. These patients, especially if involved in trauma, may require cervical spine stabilization (e.g., the patient may be in a c-collar), which may make direct laryngoscopy/airway

management more challenging. Additionally, this may affect positioning for regional anesthesia. Preoperatively, consider the mechanism of injury and recent medications/drugs, fasting status, and the like.

### Intraoperative

Intraoperatively, position the spine in a neutral way or in a position of comfort for the patient. Ensure the patient meets extubation criteria prior to extubation, especially in cases involving a difficult airway. Consider initially avoiding long-acting medications that decrease respiratory drive if planning to extubate.

### Postoperative

A patient may have considerable pain postoperatively. Consider use of multimodal analgesia and titrate medication doses to effect to avoid oversedation and respiratory depression.

## CHRONIC NECK PAIN

**Introduction:** Neck pain is often recurrent. As mentioned, the best predictor for chronic neck pain is a past medical history of neck pain. The prognosis of chronic neck pain appears to be inversely related to the duration of the neck pain.[1]

**Presentations:** Neck pain is often recurrent. Chronic neck pain is pain lasting longer than 6 months.[1] These patients may have previous surgical neck stabilization and may also be on several chronic pain medications.

## ANESTHETIC CONSIDERATIONS

### Preoperative

Patients may have previous surgical stabilization of the cervical spine, which may complicate airway management. Preoperatively, carefully evaluate the airway prior to induction of anesthesia. Patients may be on long-term opioid therapy.

## Intraoperative

Position the patient in a position that is comfortable. Intraoperatively, ensure that the patient meets extubation criteria prior to extubation, especially in cases involving a known difficult airway.

## Postoperative

Postoperative pain control may be difficult in these patients, especially if they have been on chronic opioid therapy (may induce hyperalgesia). Consider use of multimodal analgesia to avoid oversedation and respiratory depression.

## LOW BACK PAIN

### INTRODUCTION

Low back pain generally refers to pain over the lumbosacral area.[3] Sciatica is a low back pain that radiates to the lower extremity in a dermatomal pattern and is caused by stimulation of spinal nerves. Since these definitions are very broad, diagnosis and treatment plans should be made as specific as possible. Low back pain is one of the most common medical conditions leading patients to seek medical care.[3] In fact, it is the leading cause of disability worldwide, with a lifetime prevalence of up to 84% in adults.[1] There is evidence that previous low back pain is a predictor of future back pain.

## ACUTE LOW BACK PAIN

### INTRODUCTION

The majority of cases of acute low back pain, with or without radicular pain, resolve without treatment.[3] In fact, 60%–70% of these cases resolve within 6 weeks and up to 80%–90% by week 12. Up to 90% of these patients stop seeing their medical provider for back pain within 3 months of the first visit, which also suggests that most of the cases of low back pain resolve with minimal intervention.[4] Most patients with acute back pain without radiculopathy present with no abnormal physical findings.[3] However, cases lasting longer often have a more uncertain course.

**Causes:** The back is composed of connective tissues (e.g., bone, intervertebral disk, ligaments, fascia); muscles; and nerves, and any of these can be the source of the pain.[1,3] Common sources of pain include the sacroiliac (SI) joints, intervertebral disks, facet joints, and vertebral bodies.[1] However, infection (e.g., with previous neuraxial or surgical interventions, "Potts disease"); inflammatory conditions/ arthropathies; and cancer (especially in patients with known cancer history) must also be ruled out. "Red flag" symptoms include bowel/bladder incontinence; perineal numbness/tingling (also known as "saddle" anesthesia); and progressive neurologic deficits, such as worsening numbness or weakness, should warrant urgent imaging and urgent surgical consultation.[1,3]

## ANESTHETIC CONSIDERATIONS

### Preoperative

Preoperatively, consider the mechanism of injury and recent medications/drugs, fasting status, and the like. Attempt to position the patient in a comfortable position while considering the surgical site and duration of surgery.

### Intraoperative

Intraoperatively, attend to appropriate positioning.

### Postoperative

Consider use of multimodal analgesia postoperatively.

## CHRONIC LOW BACK PAIN

### PRESENTATIONS

**Introduction:** Chronic back pain has many arbitrary definitions depending on the source reviewed, but a common definition is low back pain lasting longer than 3 months, versus acute if the duration is under 3 months.[3] Pain lasting longer than 12 weeks has a long and uncertain course. The duration of the pain and prognosis again appear to be inversely related. Approximately half of patients deemed disabled for 6 months return to work, and for those disabled beyond 2 years it is almost zero. Most patients with low back pain have at least one recurrent episode. Risk factors include increasing age, gender, socioeconomic status, job dissatisfaction, physical activity, depression, education level, and tobacco use.[3]

### CAUSES

Common sources of pain include the SI joints, intervertebral disks/herniated nucleus pulposus (HNP), facet joints, and vertebral bodies.[1] HNP can cause an inflammatory response, which contributes to nerve compression (foraminal or central canal stenosis) and radicular symptoms. HNP is initially treated conservatively as symptoms resolve spontaneously in up to 90% of cases. Persistent radicular pain warrants further investigation with imaging to search for a reversible cause of pain, such as nerve compression, including postsurgical scar tissue formation.[3] However, in up to 90% of cases, an anatomic cause is not defined with certainty.

## ANESTHETIC CONSIDERATIONS

### Preoperative

Preoperatively, because patients may be on long-term opioid therapy; titrate medications to effect.

### Intraoperative

Intraoperatively, provide appropriate positioning.

### Postoperative

Postoperative pain control may be difficult in these patients due to increased opioid use and opioid-induced hyperalgesia.[3] Consider use of multimodal analgesia.

## INTERVENTIONAL TREATMENTS FOR NECK AND LOW BACK PAIN

**Epidural Steroid Injections:** Epidural steroid injections can be used for various types of pain throughout the spine. They are often used when patients present with radicular symptoms.[3] The success rate is often inversely related to duration of pain. These are often performed under fluoroscopic guidance, and spread of contrast seen on x-ray confirms that the medication goes into the epidural space. These injections can also be done in a transforaminal approach, which can block a single spinal nerve for diagnostic and treatment purposes.[3]

**Facet Injections:** For suspected facet joint–mediated pain, the facet joint(s) can be injected with local anesthetic and/or corticosteroids.[3] This can help reduce pain by reducing inflammation in the joint. This can also be used diagnostically to help determine if the facet joint is the cause of the patient's pain.

**Medial Branch Blocks:** The medial branches of the posterior ramus provide innervation to the facet joint. Two branches supply each facet joint, one from the level above and one from the level below.[3] In order to block the pain from this facet joint, both of these must be blocked. These blocks are often performed diagnostically under fluoroscopic guidance with only a short-acting local anesthetic. If the patient gets relief from the block, it is suggestive as the source of the patient's pain. A longer acting local anesthetic is often injected as a "confirmatory" block prior to proceeding with radio-frequency ablation (RFA).

**Radio-Frequency Ablation:** RFA is a minimally invasive procedure that can be performed to ablate the sensory nerves that are suspected to be causing the patient's pain.[5] These are usually performed after diagnostic/confirmatory nerve block testing. RFA can provide longer term pain relief to patients, with pain typically returning in 6–12 months.[3]

**Trigger Point Injections:** If myofascial pain is suspected, trigger point injections may be considered. The muscles are palpated to find tender trigger points. The point is then "needled" and often injected with local anesthetic and/or steroid. These help the muscles to relax and can temporarily reduce myofascial pain.

## REFERENCES

1. Popescu A, Lee H. Neck pain and lower back pain. *Med Clin N Am.* 2020;104:279–292.
2. Cohen S, Hooten WM. Advances in the diagnosis and management of neck pain. *BMJ.* 2017;358:j3221.
3. Miller RD, Pardo MC. *Basics of Anesthesia.* Philadelphia, PA: Saunders Elsevier; 2011.
4. Yang RJ, et al. *Pain Medicine: An Essential Review.* Cham, Switzerland: Springer; 2017
5. Abd-Elsayed A, et al. Radiofrequency ablation for treating headache. *Curr Pain Headache Rep.* 2019;23:18.

# 207.

# NEUROPATHIC PAIN STATES

*Robert H. Jenkinson and Alaa Abd-Elsayed*

## BACKGROUND

The International Association for the Study of Pain defines neuropathic pain as "pain caused by a lesion or disease of the somatosensory nervous system."[1] Therefore, by definition, neuropathic pain can originate from any site of pathology along this neuroanatomic pathway, including within and along peripheral nerves, the spinal cord, brainstem, and cortex. It is often further classified as central (brain and spinal cord) or peripheral (peripheral nerves to nerve root). The specific site may be identified by imaging or other specific testing, but often the underlying cause or site of pathology cannot be determined. Many neuropathic diseases are defined entirely by their clinical presentation or history, as is the case in both trigeminal neuralgia and postherpetic neuralgia.

It is important to remember that neuropathic pain is a clinical description and not a specific diagnosis. Therefore, careful judgment is required to condense the clinical findings for a particular patient to a more specific group of diagnoses or a single diagnosis. Important and common causes of neuropathic pain include lumbar radiculopathy, diabetic neuropathy, trigeminal neuralgia, chronic postsurgical pain, postherpetic neuralgia, poststroke pain, phantom limb pain, and complex regional pain syndrome (CRPS).

## INCIDENCE, FINDINGS, AND MECHANISM

Neuropathic pain presents a significant challenge for healthcare professionals. The underdiagnoses and undertreatment of neuropathic pain conditions leads to decreased quality of life, disability, increased healthcare costs, and unnecessary human suffering. Roughly 10% of the general population suffers from chronic neuropathic pain.[1] Pain may be the primary feature in some disease states, such as trigeminal neuralgia, or may only occur in a subset of patients, as in diabetic peripheral neuropathy. There is a common association between neuropathic pain and coexisting anxiety, depression, and sleep disorders.[2] Neuropathic pain can be continuous (as is often the case in a radiculopathy) or intermittent (as seen with the classic paroxysmal pattern in trigeminal neuralgia). Patients will often have provoked pain on stimulation. Mechanical and thermal hyperalgesia and/or allodynia are commonly found on examination.

It is unclear why the same condition (e.g., chemotherapy-induced peripheral neuropathy, peripheral nerve injury, etc.) can be painful in some patients and painless in others. Patients may present with multiple symptoms and mixed pain states involving both nociceptive and neuropathic pain, raising the possibility that there are multiple mechanisms leading to the experience of neuropathic pain. Several well-characterized mechanisms may be important in the generation and maintenance of neuropathic pain, including ectopic neuronal activity, peripheral sensitization, central sensitization, and impaired inhibitory activity.[2,3] However, no universal theory for the mechanism of neuropathic pain exists.

## DIAGNOSIS AND TREATMENT

The diagnostic process for any pain-related complaint relies primarily on a thorough clinical assessment with a high index of suspicion, as many neuropathic pain diagnoses are simply not recognized. The quality of neuropathic pain is often described as a burning, pins-and-needles, shooting, or electrical sensation, but pain descriptors are not an accurate sole diagnostic feature.[4] The location of discomfort should be neuroanatomically plausible, and neuropathic pain complaints should follow the somatotopic territory of suspected somatosensory pathology. Basic sensory testing, not only to assess for deficits but also to characterize any dysesthesias, is an integral component of the diagnostic process. History and physical examination may be all that is necessary for more straightforward diagnoses, such as postherpetic neuralgia or postsurgical nerve lesions, but more complex presentations may require electromyography, quantitative sensory testing, laboratory testing, or additional imaging studies.[2,4]

A symptom-based approach that accounts for the patient's reported symptoms, suspected underlying disease, and psychosocial aspects of pain remains the mainstay of treatment. The initial focus should be on an assessment of treatable underlying medical conditions, patient education, and reassurance. Multidisciplinary management is often needed and, in some instances (such as physiotherapy for CRPS), may represent the primary component of therapy. Standard analgesic agents, such as acetaminophen or nonsteroidal anti-inflammatory drugs, are typically ineffective. Pharmacological treatment for most neuropathic pain conditions consists of antiepileptic drugs and antidepressants.[5] If a specific underlying condition is suspected, targeted therapeutic options should be optimized (e.g., immunosuppression for multiple sclerosis or glycemic control for diabetic peripheral neuropathy).

## SPECIFIC CONDITIONS

There are a variety of described neuropathic pain conditions, and this section presents only a select group of common or uniquely characterized neuropathic pain states.

### COMPLEX REGIONAL PAIN SYNDROME TYPES I AND II

Complex regional pain syndrome typically develops after an injury or trauma to an upper or lower extremity. CRPS is divided into type 1 (no sign of identifiable nerve damage) and type 2 (evidence of a specific nerve lesion). The primary features of CRPS type 1 and type 2 are the presence of sensory, motor, and autonomic abnormalities (e.g., temperature and skin color asymmetry, edema, sweating, and/or trophic changes in the affected limb). Some patients with CRPS respond to sympathetic blockade via stellate ganglion or lumbar sympathetic block.

### TRIGEMINAL NEURALGIA

Trigeminal neuralgia is clinically distinct in that it is limited to the facial or intraoral territory of the trigeminal nerve, most commonly the maxillary or mandibular branches. Patients experience brief paroxysms of intense lancing pain lasting seconds to minutes that is sometimes triggered by seemingly innocuous stimulation. Pharmacological therapy initially with carbamazepine is the main treatment for idiopathic cases without an identifiable trigeminal nerve lesion or microvascular anomaly.

### POSTHERPETIC NEURALGIA

Postherpetic neuralgia is defined as pain recurring or persisting for 3 months or more after the onset of herpes zoster.[1] There is typically a unilateral distribution of lancing pain, most commonly affecting the thoracic dermatomes or the ophthalmic division of the trigeminal nerve.

### PHANTOM LIMB PAIN

While phantom *sensations* are common after amputation, particularly in the early postoperative period, phantom *pain* is less common and describes the perception of pain in an amputated limb or appendage. Typically, phantom pain is felt most prominently at the distal aspect of the amputated appendage.

### POSTSTROKE PAIN

Central poststroke pain develops in 7% to 8% of patients after a stroke and up to 60% of patients after a spinal cord injury.[2] These patients typically report spontaneous and ongoing pain either at or below the level of their spinal cord lesion or contralateral to the site of their stroke. Those with some preserved sensation will often report some form of hypersensitivity or allodynia in the area of the body with disrupted somatosensory transmission.

### PERIPHERAL NEUROPATHIES

Chronic pain can occur in many polyneuropathies due to metabolic, autoimmune, infectious, or neurotoxic medications or from unknown etiologies. Diabetic peripheral neuropathy is the most common form seen in advanced healthcare systems.

## REFERENCES

1. Scholz J, et al. The IASP classification of chronic pain for ICD-11: chronic neuropathic pain. *Pain*. 2019;160(1):53–59.
2. Gilron I, et al. Neuropathic pain: principles of diagnosis and treatment. *Mayo Clinic Proc*. 2015;90(4):532–545.
3. Cohen SP, Mao J. Neuropathic pain: mechanisms and their clinical implications. BMJ. 2014;348:f7656.
4. Finnerup NB, et al. Neuropathic pain: an updated grading system for research and clinical practice. *Pain*. 2016;157(8):1599–1606.
5. National Institute for Health and Care Excellence. Neuropathic pain in adults: pharmacological management in non-specialist settings (NICE clinical guideline 173). London, England: NICE; 2013. https://www.nice.org.uk/guidance/cg173

# 208.

# COMPLEX REGIONAL PAIN SYNDROME

*Kim Mauer and Alaa Abd-Elsayed*

Complex regional pain syndrome (CRPS) types 1 and 2 are very similar. Most of the clinical characteristics are shared. CRPS, formerly known as RDS or reflex sympathetic dystrophy, is a condition difficult to diagnose and treat. It usually affects an arm or a leg. Overall, CRPS is a relatively uncommon disease state in acute and chronic pain management.

There are two types of CRPS, type 1 and type 2. CRPS type 1 occurs more commonly in females, and its peak occurrence is in the fourth and fifth decades. CRPS presents very differently among patients but almost all would agree that it most commonly presents as a constellation of symptoms.

Complex regional pain syndrome 1 and 2 also occur in children. The diagnosis is less common in children, and when it is diagnosed, it is often diagnosed later in the course of the disease process.[1-4]

One of the most common denominators and often the precipitating event is trauma. Usually, CRPS involves an extremity, and although rarely abdominal CRPS and CRPS of the eyes are rarely seen.

We now know that CRPS 1 and 2 are not likely a neuropathic pain syndrome solely. It is even thought that CRPS type 1 may not be neuropathic as usually a distinct nerve pathology is not identified.[3,4] It was proposed that type 1 is caused by minor nerve injury, while type 2 follows a major nerve injury.

The history of CRPS is an interesting one that started during the American Civil War with the physician Weir Mitchell, who observed the pathology and symptomatology that are so synonymous with the disease process.

Some of the constellation of symptoms involve sudomotor and vasomotor changes, trophic changes, edema, allodynia, spontaneous pain, hyperalgesia, and autonomic dysfunction. We know that treatment is more effective when begun early. Symptoms may change over time and, as mentioned previously, vary from patient to patient.

Further symptom involvement can include the following:

Decreased ability to move the affected body part

Joint swelling and stiffness

Skin texture changes, such as shininess of the skin or skin thinning, dryness

Skin temperature changes

Sensitivity to touch and cold

Muscle tremors, spasms, muscle weakness, muscle atrophy

Changes in hair and nail growth (brittle nails, less hair growth, increased hair growth)

Skin color changes such as red or blue discoloration (usually transient skin color changes)

Swelling of the painful extremity

Complex regional pain syndrome used to be treated and evaluated according to stages. We no longer look at stages of the disease but do monitor progression. CRPS may spread occasionally, most likely to the opposite limb as this disease process usually affects the extremities.

There is no specific test that can confirm CRPS. Diagnosis is mostly based on history of present illness, symptoms, and signs that match a patient's presentation.

We do not have a complete understanding of the cause of CRPS. Most are in agreement that there is an abnormality of the peripheral and central nervous system that contributes to the symptomatology. There are more data emerging that suggest an inappropriate inflammatory response contributes to the pathogenesis of CRPS. In patients with CRPS, we often find peripheral nerve injuries that include small unmyelinated and thin myelinated sensory nerve fibers.

Testing can be done to rule out other pathologies. Conditions that might be ruled out include some of the following:

Small-fiber polyneuropathies

Generalized muscle diseases

Generalized arthritis

Lyme disease

As we mentioned, early treatment allows the disease progression to fare better. The early symptoms of the disease process may appear within hours or days.[1-4]

Some progression of the disease may include

Muscle contracture and tightening

Atrophy of affected tissues

There are no treatments specifically indicated only for CRPS. We often employ treatments that are used for neuropathic pain (e.g., gabapentin, pregabalin, tricyclic antidepressants, and antiseizure medications). Some literature suggests that there are some simple measures that may reduce the risk of developing CRPS. These include taking vitamin C after a fracture (especially a fracture of the wrist), early mobilization after a cerebrovascular accident, and mobilization after any sprain, strain, or fracture of the upper or lower extremity.

Sympathetic nerve blocks can be used. Spinal cord stimulation is a frequent modality employed for treatment of CRPS type 1 and type 2. One could argue that it is one of the most commonly used therapies. Surgical sympathectomy is also a treatment but often saved until all other therapies have failed.[4]

One cannot talk about a chapter on CRPS type 1 and type 2 without discussing the Budapest criteria. The original criteria for complex regional pain syndrome was written in 1994 by the International Association of the Study of Pain (IASP). This criteria was written so that clinicians would have an easier time diagnosing and recognizing the diagnosis. The Budapest criteria were recently written and created to further define the diagnosis and recognition of the syndrome. The IASP criteria had high sensitivity for diagnosis of CRPS but low specificity. There was a set of criteria that preceded the Budapest criteria, and this was called the Orlando criteria.

*Table 208.1* BUDAPEST CRITERIA FOR CRPS

| NO. | CATEGORY | SIGNS/SYMPTOMS |
|-----|----------|----------------|
| 1 | Sensory | Allodynia (pain to light touch and/or temperature sensation and/or deep somatic pressure and/or joint movement) and/or hyperalgesia (to pinprick) |
| 2 | Vasomotor | Temperature asymmetry and/or skin color changes and/or skin color asymmetry |
| 3 | Sudomotor/edema | Edema and/or sweating changes and/or sweating asymmetry |
| 4 | Motor/trophic | Decreased range of motion and/or motor dysfunction (weakness, tremor, dystonia) and/or trophic changes (hair/nails/skin) |

A table for explanation of the Budapest criteria and diagnosis of CRPS is included (Table 208.1).

All of the following statements must be met:

- The patient has continuing pain that is disproportionate to any inciting event.
- The patient has at least one sign in two or more of the categories below.
- The patient reports at least one symptom in three or more of the categories below.
- No other diagnosis can better explain the signs and symptoms.

## REFERENCES

1. Mayo Clinic Organization. https://www.mayoclinic.com
2. Pergolesi JV, et al. The Budapest criteria for complex regional pain syndrome: the diagnostic challenge. *Anaesthesiol Clin Sci Res.* 2018;2(1):1–10.
3. Waldman SD. *Pain Review.* Saunders Elsevier; 2009:328–329.
4. Waldman, SD. *Pain Management.* Saunders Elsevier; 2007:216–217, 283–298.

# 209.

# POSTHERPETIC NEURALGIA

*Alaa Abd-Elsayed and Kim Mauer*

Postherpetic neuralgia can be a troubling diagnosis, but it is also known as a classic example of a neuropathic pain condition and is well studied. It provides a clear example of how a peripheral nerve change can lead to dysfunction of the central nervous system.

Postherpetic neuralgia is the most common complication of shingles. Approximately 20% of people who had herpes zoster continue with pain 3 months after the initial episode in the affected area. Approximately 15% of people continue with pain 2 years after the rash. Shingles, the condition caused by the herpes zoster virus, is related to a common condition: chickenpox or varicella. The thoracic nerve roots are the most common site for the development of acute herpes zoster.[1,2] The condition commonly develops in a single thoracic dermatome or the ophthalmic division of the trigeminal nerve.

It is thought that during the course of primary infection with varicella zoster virus, the virus migrates to the dorsal root of the thoracic nerves. The virus then remains dormant in the ganglia, producing no clinically evident disease, unless the host becomes immunocompromised. We do not know why reactivation occurs in some individuals and does not occur in others. Lymphoma is a condition that seems particularly prone to reactivation with shingles. Because the immune system is so integrally tied to the development of shingles and subsequently postherpetic neuralgia, we see the postherpetic neuralgia condition more often in patients over 60 years of age and rarely in patients under age 20.[3,4]

Shingles is characterized by its classical dermatomal rash. The pain is a classical neuropathic, burning pain that is characterized by lasting long after the rash and blisters have disappeared. It is during the rash and blisters phase that antivirals can be started to lessen the disability and duration of the disease course. As the viral reactivation process begins, ganglionitis and peripheral neuritis cause pain, which is generally localized to the thoracic nerve roots. The pain begins as a dull, aching sensation and moves on to allodynia, dysesthesia, hyperalgesia, and many other neuropathic pain qualities. There are many ways to describe the pain: episodes of severe shooting or electric-like pain and a sensitivity to gentle touch (allodynia). Allodynia has many types, and this type is referred to as mechanical allodynia. There is also hyperalgesia, which is overexaggerated pain to a painful stimuli. You can also experience symptoms such as itching and abnormal sensations.[5]

We often see the pain begin prior to the rash by 3 to 7 days. We often make the diagnosis, not only with the pain, but also when the characteristic lesion begins. At the end of the shingles course, the lesions often crust over. In most people, the pain dissipates when the lesions are healed. In others, the condition in question, postherpetic neuralgia, develops. In some patients, postherpetic neuralgia can be quite mild, whereas in others it can become a debilitating disease process.

One of the most important points we can emphasize is that the earlier the acute phase is treated and "kept in check," the less likely a more severe form of postherpetic neuralgia will develop (if it develops)—at least this is the common thinking of most pain providers.

Causation of postherpetic neuralgia is damage to a peripheral nerve caused by reactivation of the varicella zoster virus (herpes zoster, also known as shingles). After 3 months of pain, we make the diagnosis of postherpetic neuralgia. The rash typically follows a single dermatome, with the ophthalmic division of the trigeminal nerve being the most commonly affected dermatome. The second most affected dermatome is the thoracic dermatome. Usually we see the dermatomal nerve pain occur for approximately 90 days.

Interestingly, the risk of postherpetic neuralgia increases with age. The demographic most affected is people older than age 60. There is no cure but there are many successful treatment courses.

The diagnosis is made by some of the following:

1. No laboratory work is usually necessary.
2. Often cerebrospinal fluid has abnormal findings, but this is not a diagnostic criteria for postherpetic neuralgia.
3. You can do culture studies to differentiate herpes simplex from herpes zoster.

4. Antibodies to herpes zoster can be measured. It is knowing the titer numbers of antibodies that helps determine the diagnosis of postherpetic neuralgia

Some of the successful treatment courses include topical agents such as gabapentin, capsaicin cream (over the counter), lidocaine patches, pregabalin, tricyclic antidepressants, and, of course, over-the-counter medications such as ibuprofen and acetaminophen.

For the acute treatment course, we often recommend sympathetic neural blockade with local anesthetic and steroid via a thoracic epidural approach. The sympathetic properties of the thoracic epidural is thought to produce pain relief by blocking the profound sympathetic stimulation that comes with the viral inflammation. There is some thought that the steroids can reduce neural scarring and further damage to the nerve.

The transition from a nociceptive pain (the pain of the rash from the acute herpes zoster) to a chronic neuropathic pain condition may result from deafferentation of the second-order neurons of the spinothalamic tract because of primary sensory neuronal death. This has not conclusively been shown.

Opioids have a limited role in the management of postherpetic neuralgia. If opioids are used in the management of this condition, one must take care to manage the possible constipation that accompanies opioid administration in some cases.

When we look at therapies such as ice or heat, heat often increases pain, but ice can be relieving. Transcutaneous electrical nerve stimulation has been found to be effective in some patients. The higher dose capsaicin patch, Qutenza (trade name) is approved by the Food and Drug Administration (FDA) for the treatment of postherpetic neuralgia. This is an 8% capsaicin patch compared to the over-the-counter formulations, which are less than 1%. The application of the patch can be painful, so often EMLA or a lidocaine-based topical cream or ointment is applied to the skin before the placement of the capsaicin patch. In addition, Qutenza recently obtained a second FDA approval for pain, and this is for diabetic peripheral neuropathy.[3]

In conclusion, as with all chronic pain condition, one therapy alone is not sufficient for maximal pain relief and return to quality of life. It takes a multimodal approach. Of note, in 1995, the FDA approved the varicella vaccine to prevent chickenpox. Its effect on postherpetic neuralgia is still unknown. The vaccine is made from a weakened form of the varicella zoster virus (chickenpox).

We do know that each year in the United States approximately 1 million individuals develop herpes zoster.

## REFERENCES

1. Johnson RW, Rice AS. Clinical practice. Post herpetic neuralgia. N Engl J Med. 2014;371(16):1526–1533.
2. Shutterstock Web Images. 2003–2020. Shutterstock Inc.
3. Qutenza capsaicin patch website. M-QZA-US-07-20-0065 July 2020.
4. Waldman SD. *Pain Management*. Vol. 1. Saunders Elsevier; 2007:215–217.
5. Waldman SD. *Pain Review*. Saunders Elsevier; 2009:287, 289–290.

# 210.

# PHANTOM LIMB PAIN

## *Kim Mauer and Alaa Abd-Elsayed*

Phantom limb syndrome is defined as the ability to feel sensations and even pain in a limb or limbs that no longer exist.[1] Interestingly, phantom limb is almost a universal condition in the first few days to first month after surgery. In most patients, the phantom limb sensations resolve.[2,3] Phantom limb syndrome can have painful and nonpainful sensations. The most common group of patients to experience phantom limb syndrome is patients who have had amputations. Often phantom limb syndrome occurs in the early months and years after limb loss. It is most common to occur early on after the injury than later on in the course of the disease process.

Some descriptions of the pain of phantom limb are similar to those descriptions of complex regional pain syndrome type 1 or type 2. Descriptions of symptoms such as "pins and needles," twisting, crushing, and electrical shocks are common. Stump pain is reported with a prevalence of up to 50% at times.[4]

These same characteristic symptoms can occur in patients who had not had amputations, and we then refer to that painful syndrome as poststroke syndrome as this syndrome occurs after patients have survived strokes.

Phantom limb syndrome was first described in 1552 by a French surgeon. Dr. Pare operated on wounded soldiers and wrote about his patients who returned after these surgeries with continued pain. Other scientists and other discoverers also wrote about these same patients.[1]

We know that neuroplasticity, the ability of our neuronal pathways to modify and adjust, is likely responsible for some of the characteristics of phantom limb syndrome. We see cortical reorganization occur in this disease process.[1] Thalamic stimulation has taught us reorganization also occurs at the thalamic area.[3]

Overall, the etiology and pathophysiologic mechanisms of phantom pain are not clearly defined. However, we do feel that there is likely a mechanism of both peripheral and central neuronal mechanisms.[4]

Diagnosis relies solely on history taking and physical examination, although physical examination is not that helpful. Sometimes there are trigger points in the stump that can reproduce the stump pain.[4]

There have been many studies looking at prevention of phantom limb syndrome. Pre- and postsurgical epidural blockade are thought to help reduce the intensity of the pain, but there is no preventive therapy. Regional blocks are often employed, as are presurgical neuromodulating agents such as gabapentin and pregabalin. There is also literature suggesting that appropriate psychological preparation of the patient prior to surgery can be preventive for the development of phantom limb syndrome.

There are many therapies used for both phantom limb and poststroke pain, but one of the more unique treatments is mirror box therapy. At one time, mirror box therapy was a unique therapy for these conditions, although now it is mainstay. Descriptions of mirror box therapy can be found in many references.[2]

The idea behind mirror box therapy is that when a patient views the reflection of the intact limb in a mirror, his or her brain will be tricked into "seeing" the phantom limb. When one moves the intact limb, they are able to observe the intact limb's reflection in the mirror and this "fools" the brain into seeing the phantom limb move.[1]

Medication therapies can involve opioids and intravenous lidocaine. In most patients with significant postamputation pain, treatment modalities directed at neuropathic pain are more effective.[3]

## REFERENCES

1. Neuromatrix training. https://www.neurometrix.com. 2020.
2. Britannica.com. https://www.britannica.com/topic/Encyclopaedia-Britannica-English-language-reference-work
3. Science Direct. Copyright 2020 Elsevier B.V. Science Direct is a registered trademark of Elsevier B.V.
4. Waldman SD. *Pain Management*. Saunders Elsevier; 2007:304–312.

# 211.

# PERIPHERAL NEUROPATHIES

*Kim Mauer and Alaa Abd-Elsayed*

## INTRODUCTION

Peripheral neuropathies are disorders of nerve or nerves in the peripheral nervous system, including radiculopathies, mononeuropathies, and polyneuropathies. In this chapter, we discuss common etiologies of peripheral neuropathies seen in the preoperative setting, factors that increase the susceptibility of peripheral nerve injuries, and the pathophysiology of peripheral nerve injury occurring during anesthetic practice.

## PERIPHERAL NERVE ANATOMY

Peripheral nerves have three layers of connective tissue:

Epineurium—This is the outermost layer of connective tissue that is continuous with the dura mater. It also includes the connective tissue in between any fascicles (bundles) within the nerve.

Perineurium—The perineurium is the connective tissue sheath that surrounds a fascicle of axons.

Endoneurium—The endoneurium is the delicate connective tissue fibers that surround individual axons.

## PERIPHERAL NERVOUS SYSTEM

The peripheral nervous system is divided into somatic and autonomic components. The somatic nervous system includes the sensory and motor nerves that innervate the limbs and body wall. Sensory nerve fibers in the peripheral nerves are the peripheral axonal process of neurons in the dorsal root ganglion. The motor axons are the processes of anterior horn cells of the spinal cord.

Nonmyelinated nerves, such as autonomic postganglionic efferent and nociceptive afferent C fibers, contain many axons encased in a single Schwann cell sheath.

All large motor and sensory fibers are enclosed in many layers of myelin, which consists of the plasma membranes of specialized Schwann cells that wrap themselves around the axon during axonal outgrowth.

Much of the neuropathic pain we diagnose in chronic pain management centers revolves around changes to the afferent and efferent fibers as well as the myelin sheath.

in a loose outer sheath called the epineurium. To reach the nerve axon, a local anesthetic molecule must traverse four or five layers of connective tissue, lipid membranous barriers, or both.

## COMMON PREEXISTING PERIPHERAL NEUROPATHIES

This section talks about common preexisting peripheral neuropathies that patients present with preoperatively and their intraoperative anesthetic considerations. Diabetes, one of the most common conditions causing neuropathic pain, can contribute to neuropathic pain in many different areas of the body. Diabetes most commonly produces a peripheral neuropathy that is painful in some cases. We see other neuropathic conditions with diabetes, such as retinopathy, gastroparesis, impotence, and others. However, it is the diabetic peripheral neuropathy that pain providers focus on the most.[1,2]

## INTRAOPERATIVE NEW PERIPHERAL NEUROPATHY AND RISK FACTORS

During surgeries, patients can develop neuropathies such as ulnar neuropathy and common peroneal neuropathy from the stirrups during prolonged positioning. Pain providers will often see these conditions in their pain centers following surgery. Most of the injured lower extremity nerve situations occur following surgeries in the lithotomy position. By far, the common peroneal is the most common, and it is often seen in 78% of these cases. Median nerve neuropathy can occur with brachial arterial line placement, and brachial plexus injuries can occur with arm abduction or stretching.

There are many more nerve injuries we can focus on as these are just a few. Figure 211.1 is a schematic cartoon of a nerve and its anatomy.

The cause of neuropathic pain is a vast topic. When you evaluate neuropathic pain, you begin with the history. This is the most important part of the diagnostic process. You will need to inquire about such items as the duration of the pain, the location of the pain, and, probably most importantly, the description of the pain. A description of burning pain will be classic for neuropathic pain. Other clinical findings of importance include weakness, past medical history, tingling, numbness, and so on[3] (Table 211.1).

Laboratory work is helpful as well in the diagnosis. A basic panel, especially looking at fasting glucose and hemoglobin $A_{1c}$ can be very important in the diagnosis. Impaired glucose tolerance is often an additional diagnostic aid.

As far as imaging, computed tomography and magnetic resonance imaging have revolutionized diagnosis of neuropathic pain, especially when it comes to neuropathic pain caused by disk protrusion, disk extrusion, and moderate and severe spinal stenosis. Magnetic resonance neurography, a growing field, is also playing an important role in the diagnosis of the disease condition.

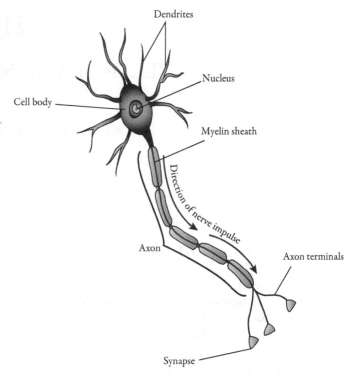

Figure 211.1 Healthy nerve cell.

Table 211.1 CLASSIFICATION OF NERVE INJURY ACCORDING TO SEDDON AND SUNDERLAND WITH CORRESPONDING FINDINGS ON HRUS AND MRI

| SEDDON | SUNDERLAND | DESCRIPTION | MRI | ULTRASOUND |
|---|---|---|---|---|
| Neuropraxia | I | Conduction block | T2 hyperintensity | Decreased echogenicity of nerve (hypoechoic) |
| Axonotmesis | II | Discontinuity of axon with Wallerian degeneration | T2 hyperintensity with increased size | Decreased echogenicity and increased caliber of the nerve |
| | III | Scarring of the endoneurium | Endoneurium cannot be delineated with current MR technique T2 hyperintensity with increased size Hyperintensity in muscles due to denervation | Focal decrease in echogenicity with increase in caliber with change in echotexture of the affected muscles |
| | IV | Neuroma in continuity with formation of scar that blocks nerve regeneration | T1 hypointense, T2 hyperintense focal enlargement with loss of fascicular pattern Hyperintensity in muscles due to denervation | Hypoechoic fusiform lesion in continuity with the nerve with loss of fascicular architecture with altered echogenicity of denervated muscles. |
| Neurotmesis | V | Rupture of the nerve | End neuroma formation at proximal end with denervation changes in muscle | Hypoechoic neuroma at proximal end with local soft tissue edema and denervation changes in muscle |
| | Mackinnon and Dellon type VI | Mixed inquiry | Variable findings with nerve heterogeneity and muscle denervation changes | Hypoechoic enlarged with mixed findings of scarring, discontinuity, or neuroma formation |

HRUS, high-resolution ultrasound; MRI, magnetic resonance imaging.

FROM Reference 10.

This chapter has not focused on some other large neuropathic conditions seen in the pain field, such as facial neuropathy, carpal tunnel syndrome, trigeminal neuralgia, trigeminal neuropathic pain, as well as occipital neuralgia. All of these have their distinct characteristics and treatment protocols.

## REFERENCES

1. Chhabra A, et al. Peripheral nerve injury grading simplified on MR neurography: as referenced to Seddon and Sunderland classifications. *Indian J Radiol Imaging.* 2014;24(3):217–224.
2. Charlson ME, et al. The preoperative and intraoperative hemodynamic predictors of postoperative myocardial infarction or ischemia in patients undergoing noncardiac surgery. *Ann Surg.* 1989;210(5):637–648.
3. Waldman S. *Pain Management.* Saunders Elsevier; 2007:272–274.

# 212.

# POSTOPERATIVE EPIDURAL ANALGESIA

*Timothy Rushmer and Alaa Abd-Elsayed*

## INTRODUCTION

Epidural analgesia is often used in postoperative patients as part of a multimodal analgesic plan. Epidurals are often placed prior to surgery in patients undergoing large incisions and/or expected to have issues with pain control postoperatively. Occasionally, epidurals are placed after surgery. One common situation is patients who develop postoperative ileus and have high opioid requirements; epidurals can facilitate reduced opioid requirements and improvement of the ileus.

## CONTRAINDICATIONS

Just as with any neuraxial technique, absolute contraindications include infection at the injection site, severe coagulopathy (epidural hematoma), conditions causing increased intracranial pressure (concern for herniation), and allergy to medications. Relative contraindications include aortic stenosis or other cardiac output–limiting conditions such as LVOT obstruction, preexisting neurological deficits, sepsis or systemic infection, severe hypovolemia, and severe spinal deformity.[1,2] With the wide variety of anticoagulant and antiplatelet agents patients may be taking in the perioperative setting, it is best to follow

American Society of Regional Anesthesia and Pain Medicine (ASRA) guidelines on the time to wait before neuraxial anesthesia after the last dose of these medications. These time intervals following medication administration are frequently tested (Table 212.1).

## HIGH-YIELD ANATOMY

During midline epidural anesthesia, the spinal needle passes through skin, subcutaneous tissue, supraspinous ligament, interspinous ligament, and ligamentum flavum and into the epidural space. During a paramedian approach, the spinal needle passes through the skin, subcutaneous tissue, paraspinal muscle, ligamentum flavum, and into the epidural space.[3] Caudal epidurals are done through the sacral hiatus at the S4-5 level. The needle travels through the sacrococcygeal ligament just prior to entering the epidural space.

## HIGH-YIELD PHYSIOLOGIC EFFECTS OF EPIDURALS

Blockade of sympathetic fibers usually extends at least two levels beyond the block of sensory fibers. Block of

*Table 212.1* ANTICOAGULANT/ANTIPLATELET AGENTS AND ASRA RECOMMENDED TIME INTERVAL BETWEEN DISCONTINUATION AND SAFE START OF NEURAXIAL ANESTHESIA

| ANTICOAGULANT/ ANTIPLATELET AGENT | TIME FROM DISCONTINUATION UNTIL NEURAXIAL ANESTHESIA |
|---|---|
| Apixaban (Eliquis) | 3 days |
| Clopidogrel (Plavix) | 7 days |
| Heparin SQ PPX, 5000 units two or three times daily | 4–6 hours |
| Heparin intravenous | 4–6 hours + normal coagulation laboratory tests |
| LMWH/enoxaparin twice daily prophylaxis | 12 hours |
| LMWH/enoxaparin therapeutic 1 mg/kg | 24 hours |
| Rivaroxaban (Xarelto) | 3 days |
| Warfarin (Coumadin) | 5 days AND normal INR |

INR, international normalized ratio; LMWH, low-molecular-weight heparin.
FROM Reference 1.

sympathetic fibers leads to decreased systemic vascular resistance through reduction of arterial and venous sympathetic tone. Compensatory vasoconstriction is seen above the level of the block.[2] Vasodilation results in decreased stroke volume. Bradycardia is usually only seen if the block reaches the cardiac accelerator fibers at T1-T4. Respiratory function is largely unchanged except when accessory muscles of respiration are blocked, which can lead to reduced vital capacity and be problematic in obese patients or those with severe respiratory disease. Unopposed parasympathetic tone in the gastrointestinal systems leads to contracted gut and hyperperistalsis, which can lead to nausea.

## FACTORS AFFECTING THE SPREAD OF EPIDURALS

The most important factor affecting epidural spread is the volume administered. A general rule is 1–2 mL of local anesthesia are needed per level being blocked. Increasing age causes increased epidural space and decreased permeability of the dura, both of which lead to increased spread in elderly patients.[2] Pregnant patients have increased epidural spread due to engorgement of epidural veins. Additionally, epidural spread depends on the level of the injection. Injections in the cervical region spread mostly caudal. Injections at the upper thoracic level injections spread equally caudal

and cephalad. Low thoracic and lumbar epidural injections spread primarily cephalad. Patient positioning can play a small role in epidural spread with the patient's dependent side having greater spread.

## EPIDURAL ADDITIVES

Epinephrine increases the density and duration of blocks due to its vasoconstrictive properties; in addition, it helps detect intravascular injection (increase in heart rate will be detected). It may also have analgesic benefit from dorsal horn $\alpha_2$-receptor activation. Other $\alpha_2$-agonists (clonidine, dexmedetomidine) also tend to prolong the block and improve analgesia. Epidural opioids work by crossing the dura and entering the cerebrospinal fluid (CSF). Hydrophilic (less-lipophilic) opioids, such as morphine and hydromorphone, have greater spread in CSF, leading to less systemic absorption and longer duration of action. Lipophilic opioids like fentanyl have greater systemic absorption through surrounding fat and therefore less spread and a shorter duration of action. Bicarbonate may increase the speed of onset of the block due to the increased nonionized form of the local anesthetic.

## COMPLICATIONS OF EPIDURALS

Accidental intrathecal or subdural injection during epidural can lead to high neural blockade, causing hypotension, bradycardia, and respiratory failure; treatment is supportive. Other complications include intravascular injection leading to local anesthetic systemic toxicity, epidural hematoma or abscess, postdural puncture headache, and nerve injury. These complications highlight the importance of a "test dose," usually with a small amount of local anesthetic and epinephrine prior to use of the epidural, to help confirm catheter placement. An increase in systolic blood pressure of 15 mm Hg or an increase in heart rate of 10 beats/min would be concerning for intravascular injection; if the patient is on β-blockers, only the increase in blood pressure would likely be seen. Changes in sensation of the lower extremities would likely represent intrathecal or subdural injection.

## TRANSITION FROM THE OPERATING ROOM TO THE POST ANESTHESIA CARE UNIT AND INPATIENT UNIT

Frequently, epidurals are bolused with local anesthetic and/ or opioids toward the end of surgery so patients have appropriate levels of analgesia on recovery from general anesthesia. Bolusing epidurals at the end of surgical cases lessens the risk of hypotension during potentially critical portions of the operation, when the patient may be losing blood or already hemodynamically tenuous. Continuous infusions and/or patient-controlled epidural anesthesia dosing can be set up for analgesia postoperatively. Typically, longer acting local anesthetics such as ropivacaine and bupivacaine are used. The amount of volume infused, concentration, and opioid additives can be modified to alter spread and density of block.[4]

## REFERENCES

1. Horlocker TT, et al. Regional anesthesia in the patient receiving antithrombotic or thrombolytic therapy: American Society of Regional Anesthesia and Pain Medicine evidence-based guidelines (fourth edition). *Reg Anesth Pain Med.* 2018;43(3):263–309.
2. Spinal, epidural, & caudal blocks. In: Butterworth JF IV, et al., eds. *Morgan & Mikhail's Clinical Anesthesiology.* 6e. McGraw-Hill.
3. Ehab F. Epidural block. In: *Brown's Atlas of Regional Anesthesia.* 6e. Philadelphia, PA: Elsevier; 2021:261–272.
4. Ituk U, Wong CA. Epidural analgesia for postoperative pain. In: Post T, ed. UpToDate. Waltham, MA: UpToDate; 2014. https://www.wolterskluwer.com/en/solutions/uptodate

# 213.

# NEURAXIAL OPIOIDS

*Robert H. Jenkinson and Alaa Abd-Elsayed*

## INTRODUCTION

Neuraxial opioids can be administered to either the epidural or intrathecal space via single-shot injection, through an indwelling catheter, or both for acute and chronic pain management. Epidural and intrathecal opioids can provide profound analgesia in significantly smaller doses than if administered parenterally. Intrathecal drug delivery via an implanted infusion pump and catheter is an additional technique used in both chronic noncancer pain and cancer pain treatment when more conservative therapeutic options have failed. Epidural analgesia has been demonstrated to have superior pain control in the postoperative setting when compared to intravenous patient-controlled analgesia with opioids.[1] Compared to local anesthetic administration, intrathecal opioids do not cause any significant sensory, motor, or sympathetic blockade.[2]

Opioid analgesics exert an effect primarily by binding to opioid receptors in the spinal cord, which ultimately inhibit pre- and postsynaptic neurotransmitter release. Specifically, neuraxial opioids bind to receptors in the dorsal horn of the spinal cord within the substantia gelatinosa, primarily in laminae II.[3] Neuraxial opioids also exert supraspinal effects by either rostral spread in the cerebral spinal fluid (CSF) or vascular absorption and subsequent redistribution in the blood stream.

## CLINICAL PHARMACOLOGY

The most important factor in the bioavailability of opioids in the CSF and spinal cord is lipid solubility. The degree of lipid solubility for each opioid is determined by the octanol and water partition coefficient.[3] Epinephrine is often coadministered with intrathecal opioids and local anesthetics in order to decrease meningeal blood flow, thus decreasing transit out of the intrathecal and epidural space into systemic circulation.[3,4] Opioids are commonly categorized as either hydrophilic, such as morphine, or lipophilic, such as fentanyl and sufentanil. Lipophilic opioids have a rapid onset and a short duration of action due to rapid elimination from the CSF and epidural space. These medications also undergo limited rostral spread when compared to hydrophilic opioids and have a narrower site action in the spinal cord.[3,4] For instance, fentanyl penetrates the spinal cord quickly, undergoes rapid vascular reabsorption, and therefore little distribution in the CSF. This leads to a more segmental effect based on location of administration within the spinal column. Contrast that with morphine, which slowly penetrates the spinal cord but can have considerable spread within the intrathecal space. Morphine does not cause as pronounced of a segmental effect when compared to fentanyl, but has a significantly longer duration of action.[4]

Opioid movement into and within the intrathecal space is primarily dictated by simple diffusion and CSF flow. CSF, and any intrathecal opioids distributed within this space, will ascend cephalad toward the cisterna magna, typically taking 1 to 4 hours following a lumbar injection to reach this point.[2] The bulk movement due to CSF flow is similar for all opioids; however, hydrophilic medications experience significantly more spread due to slower clearance from the CSF.[3] Therefore, medications such as morphine may be a good choice to minimize systemic absorption but may not be as ideal for continuous infusion.[4]

Morphine, typically administered in a range from 100 to 500 μg, provides 18–24 hours of analgesia after intrathecal administration.[4] Fentanyl, which is commonly administered in doses of 5μ25 mcg, provides only 1–4 hours of analgesia after intrathecal administration.[4] The spinal selectivity of a variety of opioids is summarized in Table 213.1.

## ADVANTAGES

Epidural and intrathecal opioids, when compared with local anesthetic agents, possess one major advantage: the ability to produce analgesia without significant motor or autonomic blockade. Patients retain skeletal muscle control with minimal risk of hypotension when neuraxial opioids are used on their own.[4] Substantially smaller doses of opioids are needed to produce equivalent analgesia when administered via epidural or intrathecal injection compared to intravenous administration, thus possibly decreasing the risk of sedation and constipation. Postoperative epidural analgesia with opioids leads to improved pain control at rest and with activity for up to 3 days after surgery when compared to intravenous patient-controlled analgesia alone.[1]

## SIDE EFFECTS

The side effects of neuraxial opioids are dose dependent and include respiratory depression, sedation, nausea and vomiting, pruritus, and urinary retention.[2,4] Intrathecal opioids have a biphasic respiratory depressant effect. The initial period of respiratory depression is due to systemic absorption secondary to vascular uptake and occurs within 1 to 2 hours of initial opioid administration.[2] A delayed respiratory depressant effect can occur after 2 hours, particularly for hydrophilic opioids, due to rostral spread of medication to the respiratory centers of the brainstem. This can occur 6 to 24 hours following neuraxial administration of morphine, and patients should be monitored for delayed respiratory depression for 24 hours after neuraxial morphine administration.[4,5] During continuous infusion via a catheter, the adequacy of patient oxygenation, ventilation, and level of consciousness must be performed regularly during the entire time the infusion is being used.[5] Risk factors for respiratory depression include advanced age, large or repeated neuraxial opioid doses, sleep apnea, obesity, and coadministration of other sedatives.[2,5] Due to this risk of delayed respiratory depression with hydrophilic opioids, there is strong consensus agreement that neuraxial morphine and hydromorphone should not be administered to patients undergoing outpatient surgery.[4,5]

Pruritus is the most common side effect of neuraxial opioid administration and is more likely to occur with intrathecal injection.[2,4] The mechanism of itching is unclear; however, it does not appear to be histaminergic in nature, and therefore antihistamines such as diphenhydramine only seem to be effective due to their sedative properties.[2] Low-dose opioid antagonist administration with naloxone can be helpful.[4] Nausea still occurs with neuraxial opioids and is likely due to direct stimulation of the medullary vomiting center in the area postrema.[2,4] Reduction of sacral

*Table 213.1* DEGREE OF SPINAL SELECTIVITY FOR OPIOIDS BY ROUTE OF ADMINISTRATION

| OPIOID AND LIPID SOLUBILITY | EPIDURAL ADMINISTRATION | INTRATHECAL ADMINISTRATION |
| --- | --- | --- |
| Morphine (hydrophilic) | High | High |
| Hydromorphone (intermediate) | High | High |
| Fentanyl (lipophilic) | Low | Moderate |
| Sufentanil (lipophilic) | Negligible | Moderate |

Adapted from Bernards CM. Understanding the physiology and pharmacology of epidural and intrathecal opioids. *Best Practice & Research: Clinical Anesthesiology.* 2002;16(4):489–505.

parasympathetic outflow results in increased bladder capacity, detrusor muscle relaxation, and urinary retention.[3,4] Placement of an indwelling catheter should be considered for this reason.

## OPIOID CONVERSION

The relative potency and conversion of equianalgesic doses of opioids from intravenous to intrathecal administration has an inverse relationship to lipophilicity.[2] The more hydrophilic medications such as morphine have a higher conversion ratio due to lower rates of systemic absorption. Lipophilic medications like fentanyl undergo more rapid systemic absorption from the intrathecal and epidural space and therefore have a much lower conversion ratio. Intrathecal to intravenous potency ratios for fentanyl are roughly 1:10, while morphine has a much higher ratio of

roughly 1:200, although a 1:300 ratio is also commonly cited.[4]

## REFERENCES

1. Wu CL, et al. Efficacy of postoperative patient-controlled and continuous infusion epidural analgesia versus intravenous patient-controlled analgesia with opioids: a meta-analysis. *Anesthesiology.* 2005;103:1079–1088.
2. Chaney MA. Side effects of intrathecal and epidural opioids. *Can J Anesth.* 1995;42(10):891–903.
3. Bernards CM. Understanding the physiology and pharmacology of epidural and intrathecal opioids. *Best Pract Res Clin Anesthesiol.* 2002;16(4):489–505.
4. Rathmell JP, et al. The role of intrathecal drugs in the treatment of acute pain. *Anesth Analg.* 2005;101:S30–S43.
5. American Society of Anesthesiologists. Practice guidelines for the prevention, detection, and management of respiratory depression associated with neuraxial opioid administration. *Anesthesiology.* 2016;124(3):535–552.

# 214.

# PATIENT-CONTROLLED ANALGESIA

*Robert H. Jenkinson and Alaa Abd-Elsayed*

## INTRODUCTION

Patient-controlled analgesia (PCA) refers to any form of pain control that allows for intermittent, on-demand analgesic administration that is under direct control by patients. Intravenous PCA utilizing a programmable infusion pump is the most common form, but PCA can also be delivered via patient-controlled epidural analgesia and patient-controlled regional analgesia via a peripheral nerve catheter.[1] Although PCA can be achieved utilizing additional routes of transmission, including oral, transnasal and subcutaneous, this chapter focuses on intravenous administration via programmable infusion pumps.

The administration of on-demand opioid doses by machine was first reported in 1971, and in 1976 a commercially available PCA pump was released.[1] PCA devices have

subsequently become the standard of care for inpatient acute pain management.[2] Morphine, hydromorphone, and fentanyl are the most commonly administered opioid analgesics via PCA. It can be an effective and safe method of providing patients with pain relief and allows for a patient to individualize their therapy more easily when compared to conventional methods of analgesic delivery. PCA therapy should be individualized to each patient and requires careful monitoring, particularly during the initiation period. Regular monitoring for adequate analgesia, drug-related side effects, and patient compliance should be conducted. The use of systemic opioid PCA as part of a perioperative pain management strategy was strongly recommended by the most recent 2012 American Society of Anesthesiologists practice guidelines for acute pain management.[3]

## PCA DOSING PRINCIPLES

Effective opioid analgesic administration ideally maintains a relatively stable plasma opioid concentration, avoids peaks and troughs, and titrates the doses to achieve pain relief within an effective concentration range.[1] These goals may be difficult to achieve with as-needed administration of larger and more infrequent doses (Figure 214.1). PCA increases patient satisfaction and is associated with improved pain control when compared to traditional as-needed analgesic regimens.[1,2] Dosing must be individualized for each patient depending on their comorbidities, weight, sex, age, concurrent medications, and clinical situation. For the postoperative period, initial dose finding should be conducted in a highly monitored setting with continuous pulse oximetry and monitoring of ventilation such as a postanesthesia care unit or intensive care unit.[3] This allows for more rapid drug titration and a concurrent assessment of each patient's response to the sedative and respiratory depressant effects of opioids.

The most common modes of PCA administration are demand dosing only (delivery of a fixed dose on patient initiation) and continuous infusion with additional demand dosing.[1,2] The five basic modifiable variables for PCA pumps include a loading dose, demand dose, lockout interval, fixed-rate continuous infusion, and hourly total dose limits. The loading dose is intended to quickly establish an effective serum concentration necessary for adequate analgesia. This dose is activated by the programmer or used for "breakthrough" dosing by inpatient nurses. Subsequent maintenance should be maintained with demand dosing. This demand dose (sometimes called incremental or PCA dose) is the quantity of medication given to the patient on activation of the demand button. To prevent an overdose from continual demand requests, all PCA devices use a lockout interval or delay. The lockout interval is a set length of time after a successful patient demand during which the device will not administer another demand dose (even if the patient pushes the demand button). The background or continuous infusion is a fixed-rate infusion that is administered regardless of whether the patient activates the demand dose. The use of continuous infusion is generally not recommended in adult patients unless undergoing mechanical ventilation. Finally, some devices allow entry of a total dose limit over a 1-hour or 4-hour period.

By regularly monitoring the demand initiation requests (button pushes) relative to number of doses delivered, adjustments can be made to the size of the demand dose and lockout interval to improve analgesia on an individual basis. For example, a patient who has made 20 attempts per hour at initiating the demand dose on an PCA that is only programmed to allow for 1 demand dose every 10 minutes may have inadequate analgesia and may require a higher demand dose or a lower lockout interval (Table 214.1).

## BENEFITS OF PCA

The two primary advantages for patients are, first, a steadier serum concentration of opioid analgesic agents with fewer "peaks and troughs" (see Figure 214.1), and second, more immediate pain control on demand. By allowing for more frequent administration of smaller doses of medication, patients are more likely to remain within an optimal analgesic therapeutic window. Being outside of this analgesic window can lead to sedation or to unnecessary pain, which can limit patient progress with ambulation, pulmonary toilet, and participation with postoperative rehabilitation.[2] A decreased delay between the request for analgesic drug administration and the actual delivery provides a more immediate sense of control and ability for patients to more precisely titrate their desired level of analgesia. PCA is less time intensive for nursing compared to frequent administration of as-needed doses. Although it appears patients have a higher satisfaction with PCA, there are some patients who have reported a fear of addiction, fear of overdose, or

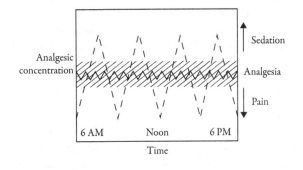

**Figure 214.1** Serum levels of a theoretical opioid analgesic comparing intermittent bolus administration (dashed lines) or frequent small-dose, patient-controlled analgesia (solid line). Adapted from Grass JE. Patient-controlled analgesia. *Anesthesia & Analgesia.* 2005;101:S44–S61.

*Table 214.1* TYPICAL DOSING REGIMEN FOR OPIOID-NAÏVE PATIENTS

| OPIOID | DEMAND DOSE | LOCKOUT | CONTINUOUS BASAL RATE[a] |
|---|---|---|---|
| Morphine | 1–2 mg | 6–10 min | 0–2 mg/h |
| Hydromorphone | 0.2–0.4 mg | 6–10 min | 0–0.4 mg/h |
| Fentanyl | 20–50 µg | 5–10 min | 0–60 µg/h |

[a]Not recommended for initial programming.

Adapted from Grass JE. Patient-controlled analgesia. *Anesthesia & Analgesia.* 2005;101:S44–S61. PCA dose ranges and other details are suggestions only. Protocols will vary by institution and should be individualized for each patient.

simply lack of trust in the machine when offered PCA, and all patients should be thoroughly educated prior to initiation of PCA.[4]

## SAFETY CONCERNS AND LIMITATIONS

The most severe and life-threatening complication of opioid therapy is respiratory depression, and clinicians should always seek to minimize the risk of respiratory depression and overdose. Risk factors for respiratory depression with PCA include pulmonary disease, obstructive sleep apnea, altered mental status, congestive heart failure, neurologic injury, use of a basal infusion, concomitant use of sedative hypnotics, as well as renal and/or hepatic dysfunction.[4] Additional risks inherent to opioid administration include nausea, vomiting, pruritus, and somnolence. Patients require regular evaluation by nursing and/or medical staff to assess for pain control, state of arousal, level of sedation, and vital signs.

Appropriate patients must be alert, be physically able to push the button, and have the capacity to understand the concept of PCA and instructions for device use. A PCA may be less suitable for patients who are cognitively impaired, have difficulty with communicating (e.g., cultural or language barriers), or are critically ill.[3] An additional safety mechanism is simply patient sedation and inability to actually initiate a demand bolus in cases of oversedation. However, this protection is no longer valid when someone initiates the PCA "by proxy," such as a family member initiating bolus doses.[4] Patients, family members, and medical staff all need to be educated on the use of the PCA and risks of overdose with activations by proxy. There always remains the risk of possible device failure, programming error, and human error with setup. Medical staff must stay cognizant of the need for adequate monitoring and adequate education for all personnel involved in PCA initiation and management.[2]

## REFERENCES

1. Grass JE. Patient-controlled analgesia. *Anesth Analg.* 2005;101:S44–S61.
2. Lehmann KA. Recent developments in patient-controlled analgesia. *J Pain Symptom Manag.* 2005;29(5S):S72–S89.
3. American Society of Anesthesiologists. Practice guidelines for acute pain management in the perioperative setting. *Anesthesiology.* 2012;116(2):248–273.
4. Macintyre PE. Safety and efficacy of patient-controlled analgesia. *Br J Anesth.* 2001;87(1):36–46.

# 215.

# SYSTEMIC MULTIMODAL ANALGESIA

*Richard Lennertz and Kristin Bevil*

## INTRODUCTION

Pain management is a focus of Enhanced Recovery After Surgery (ERAS) protocols. It influences patient satisfaction, recovery after surgery, patient outcomes, and cost reduction. While regional anesthesia plays an important role in pain management, this chapter focuses on systemic medications used for analgesia. *Multimodal analgesia* refers to the use of medications with different mechanisms of action to provide analgesia. This approach is currently recommended by the American Society of Anesthesiologists and the American Society for Regional Anesthesia. The central principle of multimodal analgesia is that combining medications provides additive or synergistic analgesia while limiting the side effects from any single medication. Opioids provide potent analgesia and continue to play an important role in pain management. However, concerns regarding the side effects of opioids (namely, respiratory depression and constipation) and the risk of opioid addiction have heightened interest in multimodal analgesia. Many studies support that multimodal analgesia improves pain scores or reduces opioid use. However, other well-designed studies have found no benefit or a benefit only in some types of surgery. Many studies do not adequately assess side effects. Complicating the matter, several different medications (at varying doses) have been used for multimodal analgesia. Acetaminophen and nonsteroidal anti-inflammatory drugs (NSAIDs) are the most broadly supported and accepted medications used in these regimens.[1,2]

## ACETAMINOPHEN AND NSAIDS

Acetaminophen and NSAIDs produce analgesia through inhibition of the cyclooxygenase (COX) 1 and COX-2 enzymes in the prostaglandin synthesis pathway. Common NSAIDs include aspirin, ibuprofen, diclofenac, naproxen, ketorolac, and celecoxib. Acetaminophen and celecoxib are selective for the COX-2 enzyme, while other NSAIDS exhibit less selectivity. The scheduled administration of acetaminophen and NSAIDs provides a continuous level of analgesia and serves as the foundation of most multimodal analgesic regimens. This practice minimizes the risks of side effects, principally renal toxicity, gastritis, and platelet inhibition with NSAIDs and hepatic toxicity with acetaminophen, while reserving other analgesics for breakthrough pain coverage. NSAIDS with greater relative inhibition of COX-1 are more likely to cause gastric ulcers, while NSAIDS with greater inhibition of COX-2 are more likely to cause cardiovascular side effects.

## DEXAMETHASONE

Dexamethasone acts at glucocorticoid receptors to produce potent and long-lasting anti-inflammatory effects. Most often used for its antiemetic effect, dexamethasone has been studied as a component of multimodal analgesia. Systematic review and meta-analysis indicate that its analgesic benefit is relatively small. A single perioperative dose used for analgesia is unlikely to impair wound healing or promote surgical site infection but will increase perioperative glucose.

## DEXMEDETOMIDINE

Dexmedetomidine promotes analgesia by activating $\alpha_2$-receptors in the spinal cord, similar to noradrenergic descending inhibition from the locus coeruleus. Meta-analyses generally supported that dexmedetomidine reduces

postoperative pain, opioid requirements, and nausea.[3] Some studies suggested a reduction in the stress response to surgery. The use of dexmedetomidine may be limited by hemodynamic stability (as it may cause bradycardia) and postoperative sedation.

## GABAPENTINOIDS

Gabapentin and pregabalin modulate neuronal activity by inhibiting voltage-gated calcium channels. Both are antiepileptics as well as effective treatments for chronic neuropathic pain. However, it is unclear whether these drugs reduce acute perioperative pain. Meta-analyses indicated that previously reported analgesic benefit was inflated, and the risk of adverse effects, namely sedation and respiratory suppression, are underreported.[4] Gabapentin does not prevent the development of chronic pain.

## KETAMINE

Ketamine, an $N$-methyl-D-aspartate (NMDA) receptor antagonist, provides analgesia and may lessen hyperalgesia and opioid tolerance. Ketamine has been shown to reduce windup in the dorsal horn of the spinal cord. A recent meta-analysis estimated that intraoperative ketamine reduces pain scores and opioid requirements by 15%–20% across a range of surgeries.[5] Ketamine does not suppress ventilatory drive and maintains cardiovascular stability in patients who are not sympathetically depleted. However, it should be used with caution in patients with coronary artery disease or psychiatric disease or who are at risk for increased intracranial pressure.

## LIDOCAINE (INTRAVENOUS)

Systemic lidocaine infusions may decrease the activity of injured nerves and spinal neurons. At least some meta-analyses supported that lidocaine infusions reduce postoperative pain, opioid consumption, and nausea after abdominal surgery. However, lidocaine infusions have demonstrated little or no benefit in other surgical procedures. There is no clear explanation for this disparity. Few studies have compared lidocaine infusions to epidurals or quadratus lumborum blocks at this time, but clinical practice has favored regional techniques.

## MAGNESIUM

Magnesium also inhibits NMDA receptors, though to a lesser extent than ketamine. Meta-analyses repeatedly showed minimal benefit, and there was no dose-related correlation. Magnesium is highly reliant on dietary intake and is often deficient at the time of surgery. Its supplementation may be all that is necessary to achieve a slight analgesic benefit. Magnesium has a large therapeutic index, and supplementation is unlikely to cause harm.

## ANESTHETIC CONSIDERATIONS

- Preoperative
  - Continue home medications for chronic pain conditions, such as gabapentin.
- Intraoperative
  - Consider multimodal analgesia, particularly for surgeries with significant postoperative pain (e.g., intrathoracic, open abdominal, mastectomy, spine, and amputation surgeries).
  - Consider administering an intravenous NSAID during emergence depending on the type of surgery and renal function.
- Postoperative
  - Incorporate acetaminophen and an NSAID in postoperative pain management.
  - Consider ketamine infusion for inpatients with poor postoperative pain control.

## REFERENCES

1. Chen LL, Mao J. Nonopioid pain medications. In: Gropper MA, et al., eds. *Miller's Anesthesia*. 9th ed. Elsevier; 2019:742–746.e2.
2. Hurley RW, et al. Acute postoperative pain. In: Gropper MA, et al., eds. *Miller's Anesthesia*. 9th ed. Elsevier; 2019:2614–2638.e5.
3. Schnabel A, et al. Is intraoperative dexmedetomidine a new option for postoperative pain treatment? A meta-analysis of randomized controlled trials. *Pain*. 2013;154(7):1140–1149.
4. Fabritius M, et al. Dose-related beneficial and harmful effects of gabapentin in postoperative pain management—post hoc analyses from a systematic review with meta-analyses and trial sequential analyses. *J Pain Res*. 2017;10:2547–2563.
5. Brinck E, et al. Perioperative intravenous ketamine for acute postoperative pain in adults. *Cochrane Database Syst Rev*. 2018;12(12):CD012033.

# 216.

# CONTINUOUS SPINAL AND EPIDURAL ANESTHESIA

*Brook Girma and Alan D. Kaye*

## INTRODUCTION

During the conception of neuroaxial anesthesia, there were reports of permanent neurological damage in the initial stages. Future studies conducted proved that complications were rare when performed with proper technique and with use of safer local anesthetics. Epidural and spinal anesthesia expanded the field of anesthesia, providing alternatives to general anesthesia or even in conjunction with general anesthesia and interventional pain management. Neuroaxial blockade may be performed as a single injection or with a catheter, allowing intermittent or continuous boluses. Some studies have shown that neuroaxial anesthesia was associated with lower postoperative morbidity, diminished surgical stress response demonstrated by decreased hyperglycemia, lower cortisol levels, and lower pro-inflammatory cytokines interleukin (IL) 1β, IL-6, and IL-10.[1] This method of anesthesia is widely used as the primary anesthetic in laboring women or elderly patients, especially those with several comorbities.

## ANATOMY

The spine consists of 7 cervical, 12 thoracic, and 5 lumbar vertebrae as well as the sacrum, which is a fusion of 5 sacral vertebrae. At each level, there are paired spinal nerves that exit the central nervous system, providing sensory, somatic, motor, and autonomic transmission. The spinal canal contains the spinal cord, fatty tissue, and a venous plexus. The spinal cord coverings, or meninges, are composed of three layers: pia mater, arachnoid mater, and dura mater. Cerebrospinal fluid (CSF) is contained between the pia and arachnoid maters in the subarachnoid space. The epidural space is a potential space and defined as the space within the spinal canal that is bounded by the dura and ligamentum flavum. It is important to understand anatomy for the proper administration of neuroaxial blockade to achieve the desired effect.

## MECHANISM OF BLOCKADE

The principal site of action is believed to be at the nerve root initially. Local anesthetics injected into CSF (spinal) or the epidural space bathes the nerve roots. Spinal anesthesia requires smaller doses and volume of local anesthesia to achieve a dense sensory and motor blockade, while epidural anesthesia requires larger volumes to achieve the same blockade. By blocking the afferent transmission of painful stimuli, efferent responses are also terminated. Smaller and myelinated fibers are generally more easily blocked than larger and unmyelinated fibers, which explains the phenomenon of differential blockade. Neuroaxial blockade also interrupts efferent autonomic transmission producing a sympathetic blockade. This autonomic blockade contributes to the variable decreases in blood pressure and decrease in heart rate secondary to the unopposed vagal tone. Blockade of muscles or respiration may lead to a decrease in vital capacity and forced expiration. Vagal dominance also increases gastrointestinal motility and urinary retention.

## DIFFERENCES IN METHODS OF DELIVERY

### CONTINUOUS EPIDURAL ANALGESIA

The current standard for labor analgesia in North America and Europe is local anesthetic in combination with opioid continuous epidural analgesia (CEA). This continuous infusion method allows for improved analgesia and does not allow delay of care, as seen in intermittent epidural boluses. Despite improved analgesia with CEA with or without patient-controlled epidural analgesia compared with nonneuraxial analgesia, local anesthetic doses may be large, with resulting profound motor blockade.[2] Although some studies suggested it does not reduce the second stage

of labor, CEA may cause difficulty in "bearing down" and may increase the duration of the second stage of labor. CEA has been shown to be beneficial in postoperative analgesia in thoracic surgeries and reducing incidence of atelectasis. Also, postoperative CEA decreases the use of systemic opioids, as well as providing a vagal dominance, which hastens the return of gastrointestinal function after open abdominal procedures.

## CONTINUOUS SPINAL ANALGESIA

In 1907, continuous spinal anesthesia (CSA) was first described for anesthesia practice, and now the technique is used in Europe for more cardiovascular stability in high-risk patients undergoing lower limb and lower abdominal surgery. CSA requires smaller doses to achieve the desired effect and provides a denser neuroaxial block.[3] It is important to point out that it takes approximately 25 mL of volume to fill the catheter, and this is an important consideration when dosing. CSA is associated with significant motor blockade and hypotension, largely related to high sympathetic blockade. The key to achieving hemodynamic stability is by giving a small initial bolus, then titrating the block up to the required height.

## ANESTHETIC CONSIDERATIONS

Neuroaxial anesthesia may be used as a primary anesthetic or in combination with general anesthesia. It has proven useful in surgeries performed below the umbilicus as well as for intractable analgesia below the nipples. Absolute contraindications include infection at the site of the injection, lack of consent, coagulopathy or other bleeding disorders, severe hypovolemia, and increased intracranial pressures. Neuroaxial blockade performed in the setting of anticoagulants and antiplatelet agents can be problematic, as this increases the risk of epidural hematoma, although the incidence is reported to be infrequent (1 per 1,000,000). Follow guidelines for discontinuation periods prior to performing neuroaxial anesthesia.

## REFERENCES

1. Epidural hematoma: background, pathophysiology, epidemiology. Accessed August 29, 2020. https://emedicine.medscape.com/article/1137065-overview#a6
2. Bullingham A, et al. Continuous epidural infusion vs programmed intermittent epidural bolus for labour analgesia: a prospective, controlled, before-and-after cohort study of labour outcomes. *Br J Anaesth*. 2018;121(2):432–437.
3. Hassan K, et al. Continuous epidural versus continuous spinal anesthesia for elderly patients undergoing radical cystectomy: a comparative study. 2020. www.zumj.journals.ekb.eg

# 217.

# NEUROLYTIC AND NONNEUROLYTIC BLOCKS IN PAIN MANAGEMENT

*Timothy Rushmer and Alaa Abd-Elsayed*

## INDICATIONS FOR NEUROLYTIC BLOCKS

Neurolytic blocks are high-risk procedures with the potential for devastating complications. Thus, they should be reserved for pain that is severe, unresponsive to medical management, and affecting the patient's functioning or quality of life in a dramatic fashion. The patient's pain should be well localized to a known distribution and should be relieved by a diagnostic block prior to attempting neurolytic block. Neurolytic blocks are not permanent, as nerves regrow over time, but if successful, they provide long-lasting pain relief for up to months at a time. Cancer pain is the most frequent type of pain to meet these indications, especially in patients near the end of life. When performed for cancer pain management, neurolytic blocks are part of the fourth step in the World Health Organization analgesic ladder and are reserved for patients who have failed more conservative therapies.[1] Chemical neurolytic blocks are also done for some chronic pain conditions, such as vascular insufficiency, coccygodynia, neuromas, and trigeminal neuralgia.

## TYPES OF CHEMICAL NEUROLYTIC AGENTS

Alcohol, phenol, and glycerol are all used as chemical neurolytic agents, each with their own unique properties. These properties can be visualized in Table 217.1. Ethyl alcohol in high concentrations leads to demyelination of the nerves. Notably, alcohol can be absorbed into the bloodstream when used in large volumes and interact with other medications. Phenol is used in lower concentrations and often is mixed with glycerin, which leads to limited anatomic spread on injection. Glycerol is mostly used in neurolysis of the gasserian ganglion. Glycerol is viscous and has limited spread, potentially sparing other nearby structures. Glycerol also requires lower concentrations, as it is thought to have a greater effect on nerves that are already damaged, making it a good choice in gasserian ganglion neurolysis for trigeminal neuralgia.[2]

## COMPLICATIONS OF NEUROLYTIC BLOCKS

In addition to complications specific to each type of neurolytic block, all neurolytic blocks have the potential to cause deafferentation pain, which is pain due to loss of sensory input to the central nervous system (CNS), usually due to lesions in the peripheral nervous system. This is because neurolytic blocks cause wallerian degeneration, which is degeneration of the nerve distal to the lesion, thus blocking CNS input. It can be difficult to control the spread of the neurolytic agent, which can result in damage to motor nerves, causing paresis, or autonomic nerves, causing loss of bowel/bladder function or orthostatic hypotension.[3] Accidental neurolysis of adjacent sensory nerves can result in numbness or deafferentation pain in a new distribution. Frequently, neurolytic blocks do not completely relieve patients' pain.

### CELIAC PLEXUS NEUROLYSIS

Celiac plexus neurolysis is most frequently used to treat pain from pancreatic cancer or other upper abdominal malignancies. The most common complications of celiac plexus block are orthostatic hypotension due to resultant splanchnic vasodilation and diarrhea due to blockade of sympathetic fibers.[4]

### SUPERIOR HYPOGASTRIC PLEXUS NEUROLYSIS

Superior hypogastric plexus neurolysis is most commonly used for patients with visceral pelvic pain, specifically

**Table 217.1** PROPERTIES OF CHEMICAL NEUROLYTIC AGENTS

| | ALCOHOL | PHENOL |
|---|---|---|
| Physical properties | Low water solubility | Absorbs water on air exposure |
| Stability at room temperature | Unstable | Stable |
| Concentration | 100% | 4%–8% |
| Diluent | None | Glycerin |
| Relative to cerebrospinal fluid | Hypobaric | Hyperbaric |
| Injection sensation | Burning pain | Painless, warm feeling |
| Onset of neurolysis | Immediate | Delayed (15 minutes) |
| CSF uptake ends | 30 minutes | 15 minutes |
| Full effect of neurolysis | 3–5 days | 1 day |

From Reference 2.

from pelvic malignancies. Notable complications include injury to the bowel or bladder itself and loss of bowel or bladder function, from uncontrolled spread of the neurolytic agent to the nerves that innervate them.

## GANGLION IMPAR NEUROLYSIS

Indications for ganglion impar neurolysis are pain from malignancies in the anus, distal rectum, perineum, or vagina and in patients with coccygodynia who have failed conservative management. Notable complications include perforation of the rectum or anus and infection.

## LUMBAR SYMPATHETIC NEUROLYSIS

Indications for lumbar sympathetic neurolysis can be divided into three categories. First are etiologies of circulatory insufficiency in the leg (peripheral vascular disease, Raynaud disease, Buerger disease, reconstructive vascular surgery). The second etiology involves nonvascular causes of pain such as complex regional pain syndrome (CRPS), phantom pain, stump pain, and renal colic pain. Third are nonpainful, but sympathetically mediated conditions such as hyperhidrosis.[4] Notable complications of lumbar sympathetic block include injury to kidney, viscera, and nerve roots.

## STELLATE GANGLION BLOCK/NEUROLYSIS

Indications for stellate ganglion neurolysis are very similar to lumbar sympathetic neurolysis, but in the upper extremity distribution. Complications can include hematoma, brachial plexus injury, pneumothorax, and hoarseness from laryngeal nerve block.

## NEUROLYSIS OF MEDIAL BRANCHES FOR FACET-MEDIATED PAIN

The facet joints of the spine are innervated by the medial branches of the posterior rami of the spinal nerves above and below the facet joint. These facet joints are a potential source of chronic neck and back pain. Patients who get relief from diagnostic blocks of these nerves may benefit from neurolysis for prolonged pain relief. Neurolysis of medial branches for facet-mediated pain is most often done with radio-frequency ablation under fluoroscopic guidance.

## NEUROLYSIS WITH RADIO-FREQUENCY ABLATION

Radio-frequency ablation is used for neurolysis of several other nerves frequently implicated in chronic pain conditions, such as the greater occipital nerve (migraines) and genicular nerve (osteoarthritis pain of the knee).

## NONNEUROLYTIC BLOCK

Nonneurolytic blocks are based on perioperative regional anesthesia techniques (described in other chapters), but can be used to manage various conditions in the setting of chronic pain. Often, pain relief is experienced for a longer duration than the pharmacological activity of the local anesthetic injected. Suprascapular nerve blocks are an example, as they are used for both acute and chronic pain of the shoulder. Pectoral nerve blocks can be used for not only perioperative pain control, but also management of chronic pain after breast surgery. Ilioinguinal and iliohypogastric nerve blocks are used in patients with neuralgias and nerve entrapment syndromes, as well as patients with chronic postsurgical pain in these nerve distributions.[4] Nonneurolytic sympathetic nerve blocks are performed in series for patients with CRPS to limit pain and allow time for functional recovery.

## REFERENCES

1. Miguel R. Interventional treatment of cancer pain: the fourth step in the World Health Organization analgesic ladder? *Cancer Control.* 2000;7:149–156.

2. Hurley RW, Adams MC. Chemical neurolytic blocks. In: Benzon HT, et al., eds. *Practical Management of Pain.* Philadelphia, PA: Elsevier Mosby; 2014:784–793.

3. Portenoy RK, Copenhaver DJ. Cancer pain management: interventional therapies. In: Post T, ed. UpToDate. Waltham, MA: UpToDate; 2014. Accessed September 6, 2020. https://www.woltersskluwer.com/en/solutions/uptodate

4. Benzon HT, et al., eds. *Essentials of Pain Medicine.* Philadelphia, PA: Elsevier; 2018:647–654, 789–804.

5. Bhatia A, Peng P. Ultrasound-Guided Procedures for Pain Management: Spine Injections and Relevant Peripheral Nerve Blocks. In: Benzon HT, et al., eds. *Essentials of Pain Medicine.* Philadelphia, PA: Elsevier; Chapter 79, 725–736.e1.

# 218.

# WORLD HEALTH ORGANIZATION (WHO) ANALGESIC LADDER

*Robert H. Jenkinson and Alaa Abd-Elsayed*

## BACKGROUND

In 1986, the World Health Organization (WHO) published a report first proposing a comprehensive approach to cancer pain management.[1] Within that report was a three-step "analgesic ladder" summarizing WHO suggestions for a sequential approach to analgesics based on pain severity and response to prior therapy. This milestone publication offered a simple and logical approach to pain control that could be implemented even in underdeveloped countries and low-resource areas. While the analgesic ladder remains largely unchanged in recent reports, the most recently revised WHO guidelines note that the ladder should be used as an educational tool and not as a strict treatment protocol.[2] The 1986 report noted that cancer pain relief was an often-neglected public health issue during a time of more restrictive opioid prescribing. Additionally, a sequential set of goals for cancer pain management was proposed, beginning with increasing the hours of pain-free sleep, then relieving pain while at rest, and finally relieving pain on standing and during activity. The guidelines noted that analgesic drugs

are the mainstay of cancer pain management and, when used correctly, offer effective pain control in greater than 80%–90% of patients.[1,3]

## THE ANALGESIC LADDER

The WHO analgesic ladder specifies treatments based on analgesic strength and pain intensity, beginning with simple analgesics such as non-steroidal anti-inflammatory drugs (NSAIDs) and progressing to strong opioid agonists. As shown in Figure 218.1, there are three progressive steps based on pain intensity and response to prior interventions. In patients having mild pain, NSAIDs and acetaminophen are the mainstay of treatment. In moderate severity pain or pain resistant to nonopioid medications, the addition of codeine or an alternative weak opioid such as tramadol is recommended. Finally, for severe pain or pain resistant to weak opioid therapy, the addition of a strong opioid such as morphine is recommended. At any step along the analgesic ladder, the addition of adjuvant drug therapy, particularly

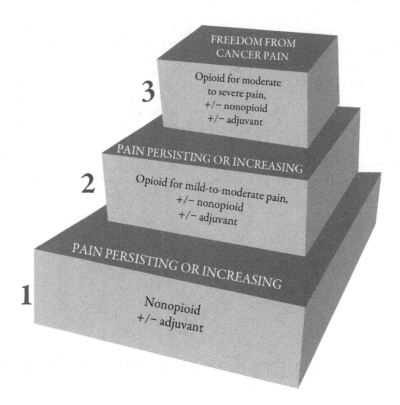

**Figure 218.1** WHO ladder. From World Health Organization, 2018.[2]

for patients with nerve injury or neuropathic pain, is appropriate and recommended by WHO. These medications include antidepressants, anticonvulsants, and corticosteroids. Additionally, though not included on the WHO figure, the report noted that procedural intervention is an important therapeutic option, particularly for pain that does not respond well to opioids.[1]

## PRINCIPLES FOR ANALGESIC PRESCRIBING

In addition to the sequential use of analgesics, several main principles to analgesic management were proposed. The five main principles, summarized below, are titled "by mouth, by clock, by ladder, by individual, and attention to detail."[1] First, whenever possible, the preferred route of administration should be by mouth. Medications should be given by the clock, meaning at fixed intervals to allow for more continuous pain control. By the ladder reinforces the concept of sequential escalation of analgesic medications. By individual refers to determination of the specific medication, optimal dose, and subsequent titration on a case-by-case basis. Finally, attention to detail reiterates the need for not only careful monitoring and systematic treatment of side effects but also assessing response and progress with therapy.[1]

## CRITICISMS AND APPLICATION IN NONCANCER PAIN

Despite being published as an approach to treat cancer pain, the three-step ladder has become commonly used in the treatment of chronic noncancer pain.[4] The opioid epidemic is a complex and multifactorial issue, but a critical factor in the escalation of opioid prescribing has been the application of a primarily pharmacologically based strategy to patients with chronic noncancer pain. The lack of emphasis on a multimodal approach, including psychotherapy, physiotherapy, and interventional treatments, in the management of pain remains one of the strongest criticisms of the WHO analgesic ladder.[3–5] These criticisms have led to the publication of a variety of alternative ladders that place more emphasis on integrative therapies, minimally invasive interventional therapies, and neuromodulation prior to escalation to more potent long-term opioid analgesics.[4] These alternative ladders include integrative therapies in the first step of treatment and typically include interventional procedures and neuromodulation between steps 1 and 2 or 2 and 3, respectively. Additionally, there is now significant evidence that select cancer pain patients have improved analgesia and quality of life with nonoral routes of administration, particularly intrathecal drug delivery systems, which is not addressed in the WHO guidelines.[5]

## REFERENCES

1. World Health Organization. *Cancer Pain Relief.* Geneva, Switzerland: World Health Organization; 1986.
2. World Health Organization. *WHO Guidelines for the Pharmacological and Radiotherapeutic Management of Cancer Pain in Adults and Adolescents.* Geneva, Switzerland: World Health Organization; 2018.
3. Carlson C. Effectiveness of the World Health Organization cancer pain relief guidelines: an integrative review. *J Pain Res.* 2016;9:515–534.
4. Yang J, et al. The modified WHO analgesic ladder: is it appropriate for chronic non-cancer pain? *J Pain Res.* 2020;13:411–417.
5. Brogan SE, Gulati A. The new face of cancer pain and its treatment. *Anesth Analg.* 2020;130(2):286–288.

# Part 19

# PEDIATRIC ANESTHESIA

# 219.

# APPARATUS AND BREATHING CIRCUITS

*Jamie W. Sinton*

## INTRODUCTION

The breathing circuits used in adults can be used for children. This chapter discusses breathing circuits as they apply to neonatal and pediatric patients.

## MAINTENANCE OF HOMEOSTASIS

Maintenance of homeostasis in neonates and infants is discussed with emphasis on those parameters that are impacted by breathing circuits. Breathing circuits impact homeostasis in relation to thermal regulation, humidity, and ventilation specifically via circuit dead space. Infants are especially vulnerable to hypothermia because of their large ratio of body surface area to weight. They produce heat by nonshivering thermogenesis, which requires oxygen to be consumed; therefore, a distressed, hypoxic infant is unable to thermoregulate. In addition, ventilation with cold, dry air increases airway reactivity, creating obstructive ventilation patterns as shown in Figure 219.1, which shows a flow-volume loop of an infant at baseline and then after inhaling cold air.[1]

Therefore heated, humidified breathing circuits are preferred as they reduce heat loss and airway desiccation

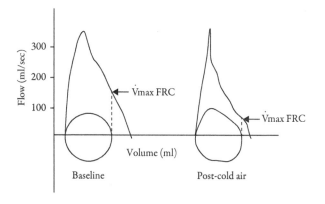

**Figure 219.1** Flow-volume loop of an infant at baseline and then after inhaling cold dry air. FRC, functional residual capacity, $\dot{V}$, maximum expiratory flow at FC.

from evaporation. Dead space is the volume of lung over which gas exchange (ventilation) does not occur. Apparatus dead space may be significant for those children age 0-36 months.[2]

## TUBES

There are no standardized recommendations for sizing of pediatric endotracheal or tracheostomy tubes based on airflow resistance or the cross-sectional area of the inner cannula. According to the Hagen-Poiseuille equation, radius of the tube is the major determinant of airflow resistance. So, while half of a millimeter does not sound significant, airflow resistance may be reduced by almost half by exchanging a 3 millimeter tube for a 3.5 millimeter tube.

## CIRCLE SYSTEM CONSIDERATIONS IN PEDIATRICS

Advantages of the circle system are the same for pediatrics as adults with a few caveats. Smaller diameter, more rigid circle system circuits with one liter volume breathing bags are available for use in pediatrics. The accuracy of the exhaled tidal volume monitor is highly dependent on the circuit compliance, which is a value calculated by the anesthesia machine during the preuse self-test. Tidal volume becomes less accurate if the circuit is compressed during the preuse self-test then stretched during patient care. Other factors affecting tidal volume delivery during pressure control ventilation (PCV) include leak around endotracheal tube or supraglottic device and the use of sidestream capnometry.

Despite the use of modern ventilators and accurate tidal volume (VT) delivery, some anesthesiologists still prefer pressure control ventilation (PCV) in pediatrics. This strategy is for safety in an operating room (OR) in which both pediatric and adult patients receive care. In this way, the child's mechanical ventilation can be initiated without fear of delivering the tidal volume from a previous adult patient; it may be a VT so large that barotrauma, volutrauma or even pneumothoraces are created. In the ICU, neonates can be ventilated equally well with pressure or volume type ventilation strategies.[3]

## PORTABLE DEVICES

### JACKSON-REES MODIFICATION OF THE MAPLESON D CIRCUIT

Mapleson D, E and F circuits are inefficient during spontaneous ventilation requiring fresh gas flow (FGF) of at least 1.5 to 2 times minute ventilation. Other than the Bain modification of the Mapleson D, they also do not conserve heat or humidity. So why are Jackson-Rees circuits so prevalent in pediatric anesthesia? Inspiratory and expiratory resistances, and arterial carbon dioxide tension in infants ventilated with the Jackson-Rees circuit are significantly lower than those ventilated with the pediatric circle system.[4]

### NEONATAL T-PIECE RESUSCITATORS

The neonatal population can be ventilated with infant t-piece resuscitators (ITPRs) (e.g., Neopuff™). Figure 219.2 shows an ITPR; note the lack of breathing bag and therefore dead space. Positive pressure builds in a circuit while the hole (near where a y-piece would be in a circle system) is depressed. This provides the tidal volume to the patient. Release of the operator's finger from the hole allows for exhalation. Limitations of these devices include device-generated inadvertent positive end-expiratory pressure and overdelivery of peak inflating pressure, which are significant, especially in the newborn population.[5]

## BLENDERS

Ventilation of infants with many medical conditions favors or necessitates the use of minimal or no supplemental oxygen (fraction of inspired oxygen, $FiO_2$). Infants with a patent ductus arteriosus (PDA) and PDA-dependent cardiac lesions as well as those with or at risk for retinopathy of immaturity benefit from ventilation with room air or very little supplemental oxygen.

In order to achieve low $FiO_2$ with the ability to deliver small amounts of supplemental oxygen, infants can be ventilated using a circuit and blender. Components of a blender include oxygen and air e-cylinders, flowmeters, and the rotary knob required to adjust $FiO_2$.

## ANESTHETIC CONSIDERATIONS

### PREOPERATIVE

For children requiring respiratory support, the transfer of patients from the intensive care unit to the operating room requires attention to ventilation. Jackson-Rees or ITPR can be used with a blender to adjust the $FiO_2$. An example of transport with bubble continuous positive airway pressure follows in Chapter 256, Respiratory Distress Syndrome.

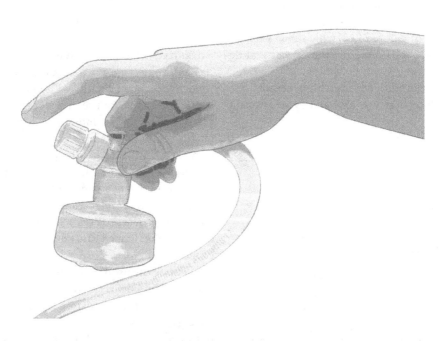

**Figure 219.2** Schematic of an infant t-piece resuscitator (ITPR). The cupped end goes over the nose and mouth of the infant.

## INTRAOPERATIVE

Most pediatric patients undergo inhalation induction of anesthesia. During inhalation induction, speed of induction depends on inspired gas concentration (Fi), the circuit volume, FGF, and circuit absorption. Circle system circuit absorption can be reduced by leaving the circuit compressed.

## POSTOPERATIVE

Opposing priorities often influence emergence and patient transfer to the postanesthesia care unit (PACU). The parental priority is to be present for emergence in the PACU. Meanwhile, the anesthesiologist prefers to ensure safe transfer to the PACU free of breathing complications. Consequently, many children undergo deep extubation and emerge during transport to the PACU. The risk of harm due to laryngospasm is mitigated by the ability to provide positive pressure ventilation and can be achieved via a Jackson-Rees circuit.

## REFERENCES

1. Geller DE, et al. Airway responsiveness to cold, dry air in normal infants. *Pediatr Pulmonol.* 1988;4(2):90–97.
2. Pearsall MF, Feldman JM. When does apparatus dead space matter for the pediatric patient? *Anesth Analg.* 2014;118(4):776–780.
3. Klingenberg C, et al. Volume-targeted versus pressure-limited ventilation in neonates. Cochrane Database Syst Rev. 2017;10(10):CD003666.
4. Nakae Y, et al. Comparison of the Jackson-Rees Circuit, the pediatric circle, and the MERA F breathing system for pediatric anesthesia. *Anesth Analg.* 199683(3):488–492.
5. Hinder M, et al. T-piece resuscitators: how do they compare? *Arch Dis Child Fetal Neonatal Ed.* 2019;104:F122–F127.

# 220.

# ENDOTRACHEAL TUBE SELECTION

*Balazs Horvath and Benjamin Kloesel*

## INTRODUCTION

Endotracheal intubation has been used since the early 1900s in pediatric patients. The size of the endotracheal tube (ETT) has been primarily determined by the age of the infant or child. However, there are other, equally important, factors to consider during pediatric airway management. For decades, ETT selection was influenced by the classical anatomical description of infants and young children. The key points of that are as follows:

- Large occiput
- Position of the larynx C3-4
- Shape of the epiglottis: long, omega shaped, stiff, 45° angle
- Vocal cords angled more anteriorly (vs. perpendicular to the trachea in adults)
- The cricoid ring was considered the narrowest part; glottic inlet and upper trachea form a cone-shaped upper airway

In addition, postintubation complications, most notably stridor, and the development of subglottic stenosis have been important concerns for pediatric anesthesiologists.[1] These complications are explained by the small subglottic diameter of the trachea and the interrupted perfusion of the tracheal mucosa by the pressure of the ETT against the trachea.[1,2] The resulting mucosal swelling after the removal of the ETT presents a larger percentage of narrowing of the pediatric airway, with same degree of edema when compared to that of adults. That increases the resistance to airflow significantly in the pediatric airway according to the Poiseulle's law ($R = 8\eta L/\pi r^4$, where r is the radius of the tracheal lumen, which is significantly diminished by the mucosal swelling). Even a small amount of narrowing in the already small pediatric airway could have severe consequences on respiratory function. That includes increased respiratory rate, increased work of breathing, increased oxygen consumption, and decreased ventilation and hypoxemia. The utilization of the accessory respiratory musculature is ineffective due to either their underdevelopment or fatigue with ensuing severe respiratory distress and insufficiency.[1]

Because of the above concerns and considerations, until fairly recently uncuffed ETTs were selected for infants and children younger than 8 years of age. It was also standard of care to select the ETT size for a patient that allows air leak at 20 cm $H_2O$. The concept behind this practice was the above belief that the narrowest part of the trachea is at the cricoid ring, and that its shape is circular, while the 20 cm $H_2O$ pressure is lower than that of the perfusion pressure of the mucosal circulation.[1-3]

## DISCUSSION

Contemporary imaging results contradicted the classical anatomical concept of the pediatric airway.[4,5] This section reviews the new information that is based on modern airway imaging studies and how the updated information influences ETT selection.

The key differences between the classical and contemporary concepts of the pediatric airway are the following:

- The narrowest part of the trachea is the subglottic area and not the cricoid ring.
- The cricoid ring is still a vulnerable site due to being the only fully enclosed cartilage of the trachea.
- The horizontal cross section of the entire trachea is elliptical shaped (not circular).
- The anteroposterior diameter of the ellipsis is longer than the transverse diameter.
- When a circular, uncuffed ETT is placed in the elliptical airway, it may exert high (>30 cm $H_2O$) pressure on the lateral mucosa, while allowing leakage during the positive airway pressure test anterior and posterior to the ETT at 20–30 cm $H_2O$.
- Conversely, an ETT that has a high-volume/low-pressure cuff can seal the airway with safe (20–30 cm $H_2O$) and equal pressure at all levels.

This new concept of the pediatric airway has led to the utilization of endotracheal cuffs in infants and children at all ages (Table 220.1).[3,4] The safe insertion and maintenance of cuffed ETTs require the selection of the appropriate size ETT that is equipped with a low-pressure cuff, and the inflation pressure of the cuff is measured after endotracheal intubation and during the maintenance of the ETT.[4]

Table 220.1 APPROPRIATE TRADITIONAL CUFFED AND UNCUFFED ETT SIZES BY AGE

| AGE | UNCUFFED | CUFFED |
| --- | --- | --- |
| Preterm, < 1000 g | 2.0–2.5 | — |
| Preterm, > 1000–2500 g | 2.5–3.0 | — |
| Neonate to 6 months | 3.0–3.5 | 3.0 |
| 6–12 months | 3.5–4.0 | 3.0–3.5 |
| 1–2 years | 4.0–4.5 | 3.5–4.0 |
| >2 years | (Age/4) + 4 | (Age/4) + 3–3.5 |

In certain patients, insertion of a cuffed ETT might not be feasible due to either their underlying anatomy or the presence of a mass or other lesion.[2,3] For that reason, familiarity with the age-appropriate size of uncuffed ETTs is still essential. It is also important to emphasize that selecting a smaller inner diameter (ID) ETT than indicated by age may represent significantly increased resistance to air flow. It may result in unsafely elevated airway pressure in the mechanically ventilated patient or demand increase respiratory efforts of a spontaneously breathing patient with resulting respiratory insufficiency. In addition, both the ID and the outer diameter (OD) of the ETT must be considered, especially when a specially shaped or reinforced ETT is required for a given procedure (see below).

There are formulas that help with size selection.[1,2] Below is the most commonly used with modification for cuffed ETTs. When these formulas are used, it is important to keep in mind that they assume normal airway anatomy. It is also a common recommendation to select a cuffed tube that has an 0.5-mm smaller ID than an uncuffed tube that would be selected based on traditional calculations and charts.

$$1 \times ETT = (Age/4) + 4 \text{ (Formula for } uncuffed \text{ tubes)}$$
$$1 \times ETT = (Age/4) + 3\text{-}3.5 \text{ (Formula for } \textbf{cuffed} \text{ tubes)}$$

Modern cuffed ETTs are characterized by high-volume cuffs with low inflation pressure.[4] Modified cuffed ETTs with low inflation pressure are available for neonates and infants. The cuff is made of ultrathin (10-$\mu$m) polyurethane, which allows a safe and effective tracheal seal at pressures that are below the physiological mucosal perfusion pressure. These ETTs have no Murphy eye; instead, the cuff is more distal, allowing a more reliable cuff location below the cricoid ring, which is the most rigid part of the trachea.

Cuff pressure can be measured intermittently using a manometer or continuously by connecting either the manometer to the ETT cuff or the cuff with a pressure transducer to the anesthesia monitor.[4] The cuff pressure

*Table 220.2* MODIFIED ENDOTRACHEAL TUBES WITH THEIR INDICATIONS

| ETT TYPE | INDICATION | NOTE |
|---|---|---|
| Oral RAE tube | Ear, nose, and throat; oral surgery (tonsillectomy, palatoplasty, etc.); ophthalmology | ETT and anesthesia circuit required to be directed away from surgical field |
| Nasal RAE tube | Dental procedures, maxillofacial, mandibular surgery | Free access to surgical area, and as above |
| Wire-reinforced tube | Neurosurgery, head and neck surgery, prone procedures: potential ETT compression/kinking | Obstruction due to external compression or disintegration of the wall of the ETT may occur |
| Microlaryngoscopy tube | Laryngeal diagnostic and therapeutic procedures, including using laser | Small OD facilitates surgical exposure; cuff should be filled with saline to mitigate risk of airway fire should cuff burst |
| Armored tube | Airway procedures involving laser | OD significantly higher than that of standard ETTs; cuff should be filled with saline to mitigate risk of airway fire if laser bursts the cuff |

ETT, endotracheal tube; OD, outer diameter; RAE, Ring-Adair-Elywn.

requires adjustment due to several factors, and that is an especially important consideration during prolonged intubation for long surgical procedures and in the intensive care unit.

Certain procedures or patient positioning require ETTs with a modified shape (RAE [Ring-Adair-Elywn], double lumen), with reinforced wall and built-in sensors for nerve monitoring or with shield to protect them from laser-induced airway fire.[1] Whenever an ETT is selected that is not used routinely, it is recommended to carefully check the recommended tube size for both the age and size of the patient, including both ID and OD parameters (Table 220.2).

# REFERENCES

1. Coté CJ. *A Practice of Anesthesia for Infants and Children.* 4th ed. Edited by CJ. Coté et al. Philadelphia, PA: Saunders; 2009.
2. Bhardwaj N. Pediatric cuffed endotracheal tubes. *J Anaesthesiol Clin Pharmacol.* 2013;29(1):13.
3. Litman SR, Maxwell GL. Cuffed versus uncuffed endotracheal tubes in pediatric anesthesia: the debate should finally end. *Anesthesiology.* 2013;118(3):500–501.
4. Tobias JD. Pediatric airway anatomy may not be what we thought: implications for clinical practice and the use of cuffed endotracheal tubes. *Pediatr Anesth.* 2015;25(1):9–19.
5. Wani TM, et al. Age-based analysis of pediatric upper airway dimensions using computed tomography imaging. *Pediatr Pulmonol.* 2016;51(3):267.

# 221.

# WARMING DEVICES

*Eric Brzozowski and Shelley Ohliger*

## INTRODUCTION

Temperature monitoring and regulation are necessary for any general or regional anesthetic lasting longer than 30 minutes.[1] Pediatric patients are particularly susceptible to intraoperative heat loss.

## WARMING DEVICES

Heat is transferred through four main mechanisms: radiation, conduction, convection, and evaporation. Each of these mechanisms can be a source of intraoperative heat loss as well as a target for warming. Commonly used warming devices and heating strategies are discussed next with regard to their means of heat transfer.

### RADIATION

Radiation occurs when heat is transferred through electromagnetic waves between two objects that do not contact each other. Heat can be transferred between a patient and the room that they are in. Radiation is proportional to the amount of body surface area exposed to the environment. Infants have a larger ratio than adults of body surface area to body mass, so they are more prone to heat loss from radiation.[2] Radiation is the largest source of heat loss in the perioperative period. It accounts for roughly 60% of total heat loss.[2]

Radiant heat loss can be minimized by raising the temperature of the operating room.[3] Overhead radiant warmers are devices that produce infrared radiation to warm the patient. These are highly effective for smaller pediatric patients and neonates. Care must be taken to avoid placing them too close to a patient, which may result in overheating or even burns. Additionally, prolonged use can increase insensible fluid losses.[4]

### CONDUCTION

Conduction is the direct transfer of heat from two objects that are touching. A patient lying on a cold operating room table would lose heat from conduction, and this can

be prevented by prewarming the table. Similarly, an infusion of 1 L of crystalloid at 21°C (room temperature) will lower core temperature by 0.25°C per hour.[4] Intravenous fluid warmers should be considered whenever large fluids volumes or packed red blood cells are required. They function best when the tubing is short to minimize portions of intravenous tubing exposed to room air.

Adding layers of insulation is a passive way to prevent conductive heat loss. By adding a material with low conductivity, the rate of heat transfer between objects is decreased. Insulation also reduces the heat lost through radiation, evaporation, and convection. Blankets and surgical drapes are common forms of insulation used in the perioperative setting. A single cotton blanket can reduce heat loss by 30%.[4] Specific to small infants and neonates with large heads relative to body size, conductive and radiant heat loss can be prevented using hats.

Heating pads and water mattresses can both provide warmth through conduction. Water mattresses are placed under the patient at the start of the case. They provide warmth to the patient's posterior surface. Generally, this is less effective than warming anterior surfaces because body weight compresses surface capillaries.[4] This reduces blood flow to the surface tissue in contact with the warming device. Water garments can be used in a similar fashion to cover anterior surfaces and are more effective.

The single most effective warming method is cardiopulmonary bypass (CPB).[2,4] It can augment temperature by up to 9°C per hour. The CPB circuit warms or cools blood as it passes through the circuit. This can allow for rapid and specific temperature control during cardiac procedures. Similarly, venovenous and venoarterial extracorporeal membrane oxygenation can also provide rapid warming. Except in cases of severe hypothermia, these devices are rarely used solely for their warming capabilities.

### CONVECTION

Convection is the transfer of heat through moving molecules in gases or liquids. The rate of heat transfer depends on the exposed surface area, the speed of the gas or liquid, and the temperature difference between an object and the gas or liquid.

Forced air warmers are the most effective noninvasive way to warm a patient.[4] These devices use electricity to generate a warm air current that flows through a disposable blanket. The blanket can be placed under the body or draped over an exposed area to warm the patient. Warming improves when a larger surface area is covered. Their effectiveness may be limited by a large surgical incision site or sterile field. Of note, forced air warmers have not been shown to increase the rate of infection.[4]

## EVAPORATION

Evaporation is the loss of heat through water vapor. Intraoperatively, most evaporative heat loss occurs through tissue exposure at the incision site. Evaporative heat is also lost through the respiratory tract. Low fresh gas flows can help reduce the amount of evaporative heat loss. Evaporation accounts for 10%–20% of heat loss intraoperatively.[2]

Inhaled air is naturally warmed and humidified by the nasal turbinates. This process is bypassed with intubation. Both active and passive airway humidifiers can reduce evaporative heat loss in an intubated patient. Passive filters are known as heat and moisture exchangers (HMEs). They function by trapping the moisture and heat released during expiration and recycling it for inspiration. HMEs can also help reduce bacterial and viral transmission.[5] Active airway humidifiers vaporize water to add both humidification and heat. Active humidifiers fail to demonstrate clinical benefit when compared to HMEs. These devices can be useful with prolonged ventilation. Adverse effects of adding a humidifier include increasing airway resistance, dead space, and work of breathing.[4,5]

## HYPERTHERMIA

Pediatric patients are particularly susceptible to burns and hyperthermia. Anesthesiologists must remain vigilant whenever using warming devices. Burns can result from direct contact with hot surfaces, such as the hose of a forced air warmer. This can be prevented by placing a blanket under the hose. Iatrogenic overheating can occur, so continuous temperature monitoring is important. Once the

*Table 220.1* CORE TEMPERATURE-MONITORING LOCATIONS

| CORE TEMPERATURE SITES | CONSIDERATIONS |
|---|---|
| Pulmonary artery | Gold standard for accuracy; invasive; potential complications with placement |
| Distal esophagus | Device may enter trachea |
| Tympanic membrane | Perforation is possible |
| Nasopharynx | Bleeding may occur |
| Noncore temperature sites | Considerations |
| Bladder | Invasive; patient must have urine flow to be accurate |
| Rectum | Invasive; measurements often lag behind core temperature |
| Skin | Axilla is most accurate skin site |

patient has reached a core temperature of 37°C, warming devices should be turned down to prevent hyperthermia (Table 220.1). Iatrogenic hyperthermia can result in systemic effects, including increased cardiac output, pulmonary edema, coagulopathy, renal hypoperfusion and acute kidney injury, elevations in aspartate aminotransferase and alanine aminotransferase, cognitive dysfunction, and QT and ST changes.[1]

## REFERENCES

1. Balbi KE, Littman RS. Pediatric hyperthermia. In: Fleisher LA, Rosenbaum SH, eds. *Complications in Anesthesia*. 3rd ed. Philadelphia, PA: Elsevier; 2018:756–757.
2. Sessler DI, Todd MM. Perioperative heat balance. *Anesthesiology* 2000;92(2):578–596.
3. Butterworth JF, et al. *Morgan and Mikhail's Clinical Anesthesiology.* 5th ed. New York, NY: McGraw-Hill; 2013:1183–1191.
4. Deutsch N. Body warming devices. In: Freeman BS, Berger JS, eds. *Anesthesiology Core Review: Part One Basic Exam*. New York, NY: McGraw-Hill; 2014:81–82.
5. Wilkes AR. Heat and moisture exchangers and breathing systems: their use in anaesthesia and intensive care. *Anaesthesia*. 2011;66:40–51.

# 222.

# PREMEDICATIONS

*Natalie R. Barnett and Ilana R. Fromer*

## INTRODUCTION

Surgery and general anesthesia can generate significant stress for both children and their caregivers, starting even before the day of surgery and culminating in the postoperative period. Factors such as separation from parents, anticipation of upcoming surgical procedure, and unfamiliar environment and people can all heighten preoperative anxiety.[1] However, the stress from the experience may remain long after the surgery and anesthetic have ended. It is essential to identify characteristics of children at risk for increased perioperative anxiety: age, prior experiences, parents/caregivers, family dynamics, and environment.

There are both short- and long-term sequelae associated with perioperative anxiety. These sequelae include a difficult induction of anesthesia, breath holding with risk of laryngospasm, increased pain, negative postoperative behavioral changes, and the potential for long-term psychological stress.[1,2] Typical points of increased anxiety in the perioperative period for pediatric patients include peripheral intravenous line (PIV) placement and mask induction of anesthesia. Topical anesthesia can aid in alleviating anxiety associated with PIV placement, whereas premedication, parental presence, and distraction can aid with anxiety associated with the surgical procedure/general anesthesia.[1,3]

## TOPICAL ANESTHESIA

In order to effectively lessen anxiety associated with PIV placement , the ideal local/topical anesthetic would be fast acting, painless/minimally invasive, and effective. Topical anesthetics such as EMLA (eutectic mixture of local anesthetics; 5% lidocaine and prilocaine in 1:1 aqueous emulsion) or ELA-Max cream (4% liposomal lidocaine) can potentially alleviate anxiety surrounding PIV placement by minimizing the pain response. However, these topical anesthetics typically require 30–60 minutes for optimal effect. In contrast, jet injection of 1% buffered lidocaine (J-tip injector) can provide effective topical anesthesia for PIV catheter placement but with a time of onset of about 1 minute.[3]

## PREMEDICATION

Premedication can be administered via oral, nasal, rectal, buccal, intravenous, or intramuscular routes. Considerations for the route of delivery include drug characteristics, desired drug effect, and the readiness of the child to accept a medication from the proposed route. Moreover, the "ideal" premedication would have a rapid onset, a short duration of action, simple administration, easy acceptance by the child, minimal side effects, and analgesic properties and work as a supplement to the anesthetic plan.

The general goals of premedication should provide anxiolysis and facilitate induction. Perioperative anxiety can lead to postoperative psychological trauma.[1] Parental anxiety is also assuaged when premedication effectively calms their child.[4] Despite countless studies of premedication, there is no one-size-fits-all medication(s) or route of delivery. Potential medications include barbiturates, benzodiazepines, ketamine, α-adrenergic agonists, and opioids. For this review chapter, the focus is on the most commonly utilized premedications: midazolam, dexmedetomidine, and ketamine.

## MIDAZOLAM

The most commonly used medication for pediatric premedication is midazolam, a benzodiazepine. Midazolam is frequently utilized due to its relatively fast onset following oral administration (10–30 minutes), short duration of action (about 2 hours), its effectiveness at decreasing anxiety associated with parental separation and anesthesia induction, as well as its minimal effect on recovery times.[4,5] It can be given orally, intranasally, rectally, intravenously, intramuscularly, or sublingually. Most pediatric anesthesiologists prefer the most noninvasive and least painful and anxiety-provoking routes. Intranasal midazolam has a very quick onset, but it can cause significant discomfort and crying when administered. Rectal midazolam can also be reliably administered and although not painful may still cause distress to both parents and children. Because of this, the oral route remains the most common,[5] although it also requires the child's cooperation.

Midazolam is not without side effects, and some children experience a paradoxical drug reaction with agitation.[5] Another potential negative for midazolam as a premedication is its inability to prevent emergence delirium.[4] In light of these negative side effects, other medications have become popular in recent years.

## KETAMINE

Ketamine is a phencyclidine derivative that acts as an NMDA (N-methyl-D-aspartate) antagonist. It acts as both a sedative and an analgesic. It can be given orally, intramuscularly, intranasally, rectally, and intravenously. Because of its rapid onset when given intramuscularly, it is commonly used for noncooperative and/or aggressive patients unable or unwilling to take an oral premedication. It is also helpful when combined with midazolam as an oral premedication for larger patients cooperative enough to take an oral medication. Unfortunately, it is commonly associated with side effects, such as excessive salivation, psychiatric disturbances, postoperative delirium, and nausea/vomiting. In contrast to midazolam or dexmedetomidine, ketamine causes a dissociative amnesia and analgesia.[5]

## DEXMEDETOMIDINE

Dexmedetomidine is a short-acting $\alpha_2$-adrenergic agonist.[5] It typically creates a cooperative and arousable sedation without an associated respiratory depression. It can be given via many different routes, most commonly intranasally or orally.[4] Dexmedetomidine also has potential analgesic effects and causes a dose-dependent depth of sedation. Potential side effects include bradycardia and hemodynamic fluctuations; therefore, patients receiving dexmedetomidine should still be routinely monitored[5] (Table 222.1).

## PARENTAL PRESENCE

The utility of parental presence during induction of anesthesia for anxiolysis in the pediatric patient is not well supported by the literature; however, it is common for hospitals and ambulatory care centers to offer the option to parents. The success of the technique is improved if there is adequate education and preparation for the parent or caregiver as the anxiety level of the parent can adversely affect the anxiety of the child. Most studies looking at parental presence versus distraction techniques or premedication find that the distraction technique or premedication is more effective at anxiety reduction at the time of anesthesia induction than parental presence alone. However, parental presence plus the distraction technique or premedication seem to have superior results for anxiety reduction.[2]

## NONPHARMACOLOGICAL INTERVENTIONS

For nonpharmacological interventions, distraction techniques such as music therapy, video games, or cartoons/handheld devices have been employed as an anxiety

*Table 222.1* PREMEDICATIONS

| MEDICATION | ACTION | ROUTE OF ADMINISTRATION/ DOSING (MG/KG) | PROS | CONS |
|---|---|---|---|---|
| Midazolam | GABA$_A$ receptor agonist | IV: 0.05–0.15 IM: 0.1–0.2 Oral: 0.5–0.75 Intranasal: 0.2 Rectal: 0.5–1 | Fast onset Short duration Sedative Anxiolysis Anterograde amnesia | Potential paradoxical reaction Behavior changes Maintains implicit memory Dose dependent respiratory depression Potential for emergence delirium |
| Ketamine | NMDA antagonist | IV: 1–2 IM: 2–10 Oral: 3–6 Intranasal: 6 Rectal: 5 | Fast onset Sedative Analgesia No respiratory depression | Excessive salivation Psychiatric complications/ hallucinations Nausea/vomiting Postoperative delirium |
| Dexmedetomidine | $\alpha_2$-Agonist | Oral: 2–4 Intranasal: 1–2 (dose in μg/kg) | Short duration Sedative Anxiolysis Analgesia No respiratory depression | Potential for delayed emergence Bradycardia Hemodynamic fluctuations Can take 30 minutes for onset intranasally |

GABA, γ-aminobutyric acid; IM, intramuscular; IV, intravenous.

reduction technique in the perioperative period. The appeal of distraction techniques includes minimal cost and side effects as well as ease of administration. Animated cartoons are easily accessible to the pediatric anesthesiologist and can hold the interest of children across many age groups. Moreover, viewing cartoons can be all encompassing for young children, allowing for more total distraction and anxiety alleviation during the perioperative period.[1] Distraction techniques should be considered as an adjunct to, or even as a replacement for, the more commonly utilized premedication and/or parental presence.

## REFERENCES

1. Lee J, et al. Cartoon distraction alleviates anxiety in children during induction of anesthesia. *Anesth Analg.* 2012;115(5):1168–1173.
2. Scully SM. Parental presence during pediatric anesthesia induction. *AORN J.* 2012;96(1):26–33.
3. Spanos S, et al. Jet injection of 1% buffered lidocaine versus topical ELA-Max for anesthesia before peripheral intravenous catheterization in children. *Pediatr Emerg Care.* 2008;24(8):511–515.
4. Pasin L, et al. Dexmedetomidine vs midazolam as preanesthetic medication in children: a meta-analysis of randomized controlled trials. *Pediatr Anesth.* 2015;25(5):468–476.
5. Khurmi N, et al. Pharmacologic considerations for pediatric sedation and anesthesia outside the operating room: a review for anesthesia and non-anesthesia providers. *Pediatr Drugs.* 2017;19(5):435–446.

# 223.

# AGENTS, TECHNIQUES, AND MAPLESON CIRCUITS

*Jamie W. Sinton*

## INTRODUCTION

Children have very elastic blood vessels, higher body water content, shorter stature, and therefore lower blood pressure than adults due to the effects of scaling. Hemodynamic effects of inhaled, intravenous, and awake spinal anesthetics are examined. Next, this chapter contrasts types of Mapleson breathing circuits and describe their uses.

## HEMODYNAMIC IMPACT OF ANESTHETIC CHOICE

The hemodynamic impact of the anesthetic in a healthy child varies by technique, and most are well tolerated. Impacts of inhalational, intravenous, and awake spinal anesthetics are unique and presented here, often with cardiac catheterization laboratory studies where hemodynamics can be assessed with gold standard measurement techniques. As catheterization procedures are not very stimulating following vascular access, the anesthetic doses studied are often small.

## INHALATIONAL ANESTHETICS

Nitrous oxide has no impact on pulmonary vascular resistance (PVR) in infants, in contrast to adults.[1] Potent inhalation agents, of course, not only decrease systemic vascular resistance (SVR) but also, in infants, decrease PVR.[1]

## INTRAVENOUS ANESTHETICS

Pediatric total intravenous anesthesia (TIVA) has widespread use in children for reduction of respiratory complications and reduction of emergence delirium.[2] Certainly these advantages maintain hemodynamic stability; for example, if hypoxia is avoided, usually then is bradycardia. The opioids, fentanyl, remifentanil, and morphine uniformly decrease SVR but have no impact, decrease, and increase PVR, respectively.[1]

Ketamine can even be used safely in children with pulmonary hypertension as long as normocarbia is maintained.[1,3] Propofol has no impact on PVR, while dexmedetomidine decreases PVR and increases SVR.[1]

## AWAKE SPINAL

While placement of regional analgesic injections is safe postinduction,[4] awake spinals also show hemodynamic benefits. Less hypotension has been observed in young infants undergoing pyloromyotomy compared to inhaled anesthetics.[5] The additional benefit of lower extremity insensation and venodilation facilitate intravenous placement, although not neurologic benefit, over inhaled agents. Yes, that is correct: A spinal anesthetic can be placed in an infant prior to intravenous placement.[6,7] Note the contrast in hemodynamic response to spinal anesthetics in infants and in adults.

## MAPLESON CIRCUITS

Types of breathing systems used in children are discussed in Chapter 219, Apparatus and Breathing Circuits. Mapleson circuits specifically comprise a fresh gas inlet, adjustable pressure limiting (APL) valve, and reservoir bag as shown in Figure 223.1.

Mapleson circuits offer advantages over draw-over systems, and open drop and insufflation anesthesia because fresh gas flow (FGF) can be controlled; there is slightly more ability to regulate inspired gas concentration, as well as the ability to assist or control ventilation. The reservoir bag adds additional protection from barotrauma if the APL valve is accidently left closed. The reservoir bag begins to fill to its (usually 1 or 3 L) capacity; at this point, the bag distends, and once maximally distended, the pressure in the bag decreases. In this way, barotrauma is prevented.

The use of Mapleson circuits during spontaneous ventilation requires FGF of at least twice minute ventilation, and scavenging is difficult. The *Mapleson A* circuit is most efficient for use in spontaneous ventilation as it is the only circuit that can accomplish spontaneous ventilation with FGF equal to minute ventilation. The primary advantage of a *Mapleson D* circuit is warmth and humidity as FGF flows around the exhaled gas; this is especially useful in infants, who are prone to hypothermia and dehydration. The Bain system is a modification of the Mapleson D system; it delivers FGF through a small tube fixed inside a larger expiratory tube. A *Mapleson E* circuit has no reservoir and is in that way the simplest circuit. If exhalation tubing volume is less than minute ventilation, rebreathing is permitted. This may be useful in the case of emergence

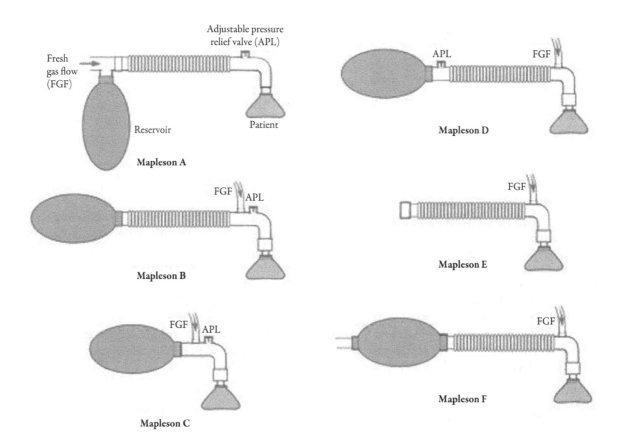

**Figure 223.1** Diagram of the common Mapleson circuits. Note that the Mapleson A circuit is also called a Magill attachment, Mapleson C is a Waters' to and fro, Mapleson D is the Bain modification, Mapleson E is the Ayre's t-piece, and Mapleson F is the Jackson-Rees modification.

and support of a patient who is returning to spontaneous ventilation following an anesthetic. *Mapleson F* circuits are widely used in pediatric anesthesia, especially for transport to the postanesthetic care unit. This circuit supports emergence in pediatrics with the use of FGF two to three times minute ventilation for redistribution and exhalation of inhaled agents as well as readily accessible treatment of airway complications, which are so common in pediatric anesthesia. Overall, rebreathing happens in a circuit system if valves are incompetent or absent.

The Mapelson breathing circuits in order of increasing rebreathing are

- During spontaneous ventilation: Mapleson A < D < C < B
- During controlled ventilation: Mapleson D < B < C < A

## REFERENCES

1. Lam JE, et al. Anesthesia and the pediatric cardiac catheterization suite: a review. *Paediatr Anaesth.* 2015;25(2):127–134.
2. Lauder GR. Total intravenous anesthesia will supercede inhalational anesthesia in pediatric anesthetic practice. *Paediatr Anaesth.* 2015;25(1):52–64.
3. Robert H, et al. Hemodynamic response to ketamine in children with pulmonary hypertension. *Pediatr Anesth.* 2016;26:102–108.
4. Taenzer AH, et al. Asleep versus awake: does it matter? Pediatric regional block complications by patient state: a report from the Pediatric Regional Anesthesia Network. *Reg Anesth Pain Med.* 2014;39(4):279–283.
5. Ing C, et al. Differences in intraoperative hemodynamics between spinal and general anesthesia in infants undergoing pyloromyotomy. *Paediatr Anaesth.* 2017;27(7):733–741.
6. Ebert KM, et al. Benefits of spinal anesthesia for urologic surgery in the youngest of patients. *J Pediatr Urol.* 2019;15(1):49.e1–49.e5.
7. Davidson AJ. Neurodevelopmental outcome at 2 years of age after general anaesthesia and awake-regional anaesthesia in infancy (GAS): an international multicentre, randomised controlled trial. *Lancet.* 2015;387(10015):239–250.

# 224.

# INDUCTION TECHNIQUES

*Sadiq S. Shaik and Lydia C. Boyette*

## INTRODUCTION

Induction of general anesthesia in children can be safely performed using multiple techniques. The technique depends on age of the child, their level of cooperation, surgical procedure, medical history, plan for discharge, and preference of the anesthesiologists, family, and the patient. The techniques of induction include inhalational, intravenous (IV), intramuscular (IM), rectal, and combinations of the aforementioned modalities.

## PARENTAL PRESENCE

- *Communication*: It is imperative to communicate and reassure parents about the process. Parents should be informed of the signs children may exhibit during various phases of a normal induction.

- *Evidence:* There is no clear benefit of decreasing patient anxiety with parental presence as compared to premedication with midazolam, and the practice may depend on institutional preference.
- *Appropriate parental presence*: It is reserved for elective procedures and children that have stranger and separation anxiety. It is best avoided in patients with risk for malignant hyperthermia, risk for aspiration, critically ill patients, emergency surgeries, and in parents who are extremely anxious.

## INHALATIONAL INDUCTION

- *Indications:* Inhalational induction is the most commonly performed technique due to its noninvasive nature.

- *Techniques*: Inhalational induction is best achieved by establishing a calm environment with the child either premedicated or awake in a sitting or lying down position, with or without a distraction strategy and in the presence or absence of a parent.[1]
- *Preparation and induction:* The lightly scented mask is placed gently on the face by either the anesthesia provider or parent and in some cases by the child themselves. Distraction techniques can include storytelling, singing, and conversation. For the first 2 minutes, a nitrous oxide–oxygen mixture in a 2:1 ratio can cause a sedative effect. Thereafter, incremental concentrations of sevoflurane can be titrated to induce general anesthesia. The peak of onset for sevoflurane depends on the level of anxiety and cooperation of the child.[2]

## INTRAVENOUS INDUCTION AGENTS

- *Introduction*: Intravenous induction is safe and efficient and should be considered in older children, emergency surgeries, and patients with risk of aspiration. Patients at risk for malignant hyperthermia and Duchene muscular dystrophy are candidates because inhalational agents are contraindicated. Disadvantages include pain, fear, anxiety, parental discomfort, and difficulty associated with the procedure.[1,2]
- *Propofol*: At induction doses, propofol can reduce systemic vascular resistance, blood pressure, and cardiac output.
  - Dose: Usually 2–3 mg/kg, but a higher dosage may be required for children less than 3 years. Compared to adults, the higher dose requirement of propofol is attributed to greater volume of distribution, rapid redistribution to vessel-rich organs, and rapid clearance.[3]
  - Egg allergy: Most patients are specifically allergic to the albumin component of the egg. Even though lecithin is derived from egg yolk, patients do not experience an allergic reaction to its presence in propofol. Therefore, unless a patient has an anaphylactic egg allergy, it is usually safe to use propofol.
- *Ketamine:* Apart from being an induction agent, it has analgesic properties and bronchodilating effects, which may have benefit in asthmatics. Ketamine also produces sympathomimetic effects of increased heart rate, blood pressure, and cardiac output.
  - Dose: 1–2 mg/kg.
  - Indications: Ketamine maintains systemic vascular resistance and is a preferred induction agent in tetralogy of Fallot, aortic stenosis, and cardiac tamponade and with hemodynamic instability.
  - Administration of midazolam is recommended to avoid psychomimetic side effects.
- *Etomidate*
  - Dose: 0.2 to 0.3 mg/kg.

- Indications: It is a useful agent to provide cardiovascular stability in patients with hemodynamic instability and cardiac failure.
- Side effects: Etomidate can cause pain on injection, myoclonic movements, postoperative nausea and vomiting, and potential adrenal suppression.

## NONINTRAVENOUS INDUCTION AGENTS

- *Indications for nonintravenous induction agents*: Nonintravenous agents are for patients who are uncooperative, cognitively handicapped, and refuse all modes of sedation.
- *Intramuscular agent:* Ketamine is used in doses of 2–3 mg/kg to achieve sedation and 5–6 mg/kg for induction. Onset of action is approximately 4–6 minutes, and the effects last 45–60 minutes.
- *Rectal induction:* This form of induction is a last resort in such an uncooperative patient.
  - Limitations: Children 5 years or younger due to dose limitations.
    - Agents: Methohexital 20–25 mg/kg, ketamine 5 mg/kg, or midazolam 1 mg/kg.
      - Disadvantages: Poor drug availability due to unpredictable drug absorption and delayed recovery after surgery.

## ANESTHETIC INDUCTION COMPLICATIONS

- *Upper airway obstruction:* The most common provider-induced error during mask ventilation is compression of soft tissue below the mandibular ridge that occludes the airway.
  - Recognition and treatment: It is important to recognize upper airway obstruction with greater depths of anesthesia. Typical maneuvers to relieve the airway obstruction are jaw thrust, neck extension, and applying continuous positive airway pressure (CPAP) of at least 10–15 cm $H_2O$.
  - Laryngospasm: Laryngospasm is suspected with an inability to provide positive pressure ventilation after mask readjustment, positioning, and oral airway placement. If not recognized early, it can lead to hypoxemia, bradycardia, and cardiac arrest.
  - Risk factors: Younger age, recent upper respiratory tract infection, history of asthma or lung irritation such as secondhand smoke inhalation, and airway surgeries.
  - Triggers: Commonly, insufficient depth of anesthesia is a trigger; others include blood or secretions in the airway or mechanical airway stimulation.
  - Treatment: Positive pressure ventilation with CPAP needs to be continued along with a jaw thrust. If this

fails, the anesthetic plane should be deepened, and sometimes depolarizing muscular blockers may need to be used to enable ventilation.[4]

- *Bronchospasm:* Bronchospasm is recognized by increased airway pressures, slow upslope of end-tidal $CO_2$ waveform, and hypoxemia.
  - Risk factors: Reactive or obstructive airway diseases, recent or recurrent upper respiratory tract infection, secondhand smoke exposure, and gastroesophageal reflux disease are risk factors.
  - Treatment: Inhaled β-adrenergic agonists with or without a small dose of intravenous epinephrine and increasing the depth of anesthesia are treatments.
- *Cardiovascular adverse effects of induction:*
  - Agents: At higher concentrations of sevoflurane, myocardial depression, depressed respirations, and decreased systemic vascular resistance can occur.

- At higher concentrations of sevoflurane, patients can experience decreases of myocardial activity, respirations, and systemic vascular resistance. Children with Down's syndrome have a higher incidence of bradycardia during inhalational induction.[1]

## REFERENCES

1. Lerman J, et al. The pharmacology of sevoflurane in infants and children. *Anesthesiology.* 1994;80(4):814–824.
2. Dubois MC, et al. Comparison of three techniques for induction of anaesthesia with sevoflurane in children. *Paediatr Anaesth.* 1999;9(1):19–23.
3. Hannallah RS, et al. Propofol: effective dose and induction characteristics in unpremedicated children. *Anesthesiology.* 1991;74(2):217–219.
4. Hampson-Evans D, et al. Pediatric laryngospasm. *Paediatr Anaesth.* 2008;18(4):303–307.

# 225.

# ANESTHETIC ACTIONS DIFFERENT FROM ADULTS

*Christopher O. Fadumiye*

## INTRODUCTION

One of the biggest differences between adults and neonates/infants is oxygen consumption. In neonates, it may be as high as 6 mL/kg[-1], which is roughly about twice in adults; thus, to attain this increase in demand there are a few cardiac and pulmonary changes present in neonates that distinguish them from adults.[1]

## CARDIOVASCULAR AND PULMONARY DIFFERENCES

The myocardial structure of the heart is vastly less developed in neonates than in adults, which leads to a leftward shift of the cardiac function curve. Coupled with the increase in oxygen requirements, which further shifts the oxygen dissociation curve to the left. The neonate compensates with the presence of fetal hemoglobin and an increase in cardiac output. These two important factors, an increased oxygen requirement and myocardial immaturity, account for the increased sensitivity to volume loading and a heart rate–dependent cardiac output in the neonate.[2]

Alveolar ventilation is doubled in neonates to help achieve increased oxygen requirements. Another important factor is the makeup of intercostal and diaphragmatic muscles, which do not possess type 1 muscle fibers until approximately 2 years of age. This in turn can lead to fatigue with the increased work of breathing. Fatigue subsequently leads to apnea and respiratory failure. Central nervous system regulation of ventilation is immature in neonates, and hence their response to hypoxia is less predictable. Last, neonates have been described as obligate nasal breathers; nonetheless, about 8% of premature neonates and 40% of term newborns can convert to oral breathing in the presence of nasal obstruction.[2]

## OTHER PHYSIOLOGIC DIFFERENCES

**Temperature Regulation:** Maintaining normal body temperature in infants is more challenging than for adults. Infants keep their body temperature by moving vigorously and by metabolizing brown fat. It is even more challenging compared to adults because of a large ratio of surface to volume and increased metabolism.[1] These factors underscore the necessity of minimizing heat loss infants and neonates.

**Renal:** The presence of low perfusion pressure and an immature glomerular function in infants means their renal function is diminished. Complete maturation does not occur until around 2 years of age.[2] This is important to consider when administering medications and volume as the ability to metabolize and excrete administered medications might be diminished.

## PHARMACOLOGICAL DIFFERENCES IN INFANTS AND NEONATES

Neonates and infants respond differently to medications; this is particularly the case because of their relative size, immature liver and kidneys, differences in extracellular fluid volume and metabolic rate.

**Inhaled Anesthetics:** Due to the smaller functional residual capacity per body weight, the rate of induction of volatile anesthetics is lessened in neonates and infants. Full-term neonates require a lower concentration of volatile anesthetics than infants.[2]

**Intravenous Anesthetic:** Neonates also require a lower dose of intravenous anesthetic medications (hypnotics) to produce required pharmacologic effects. This can be attributed to an immature blood-brain barrier, and a decreased ability to metabolize these medications.

**Muscle Relaxants:** Neonates and infants are also more sensitive to neuromuscular blockers. Immaturity of the hepatic and renal system could lead to prolongation of neuromuscular blockade, especially for medications that are dependent on these systems for clearance. Increased succinylcholine doses are required in neonates and infants than adults to attain muscle paralysis.[1]

## ANESTHETIC CONSIDERATION AND APPROACH

Anesthetic administration for neonates and infants varies vastly depending on the medical condition and the planned surgical procedure, the emotional and psychological makeup of the parent, and overall safety of the proposed approach. It is essential to review the patient's medical profile and establish an anesthetic plan before proceeding with the surgical procedure. A key role of the anesthesiologist is to play a reassuring figure in ensuring the neonate/infant and their parents are comfortable with the whole process.

Mask inductions are usually used in infants and neonates, while an intravenous access is secured postinduction. It is important to rapidly reduce the concentration of volatile anesthetic until the intravenous access is secured. It is also prudent to administer heated and humidified gases to neonates to decrease intraoperative heat loss and decrease body temperature, which can be detrimental to the neonate or infant.

## COMMON MEDICAL AND SURGICAL DISEASES THAT AFFECT PEDIATRIC PATIENTS

**Spells of Apnea:** Stoppage of breathing lasting greater than 20 seconds (apnea) in neonates and infants is not uncommon. It occurs in roughly 20% to 30% of neonates.[1] It can be further exacerbated following administration of general anesthetics; it is thus recommended to have appropriate monitoring devices and rescue equipment if hemodynamic instability, bradycardia, or hypoxemia occurs as a result of an apneic spell.

**Epiglottitis:** An inflammatory infection of the epiglottis or the supraglottic soft tissues by *Haemophilus influenza* (most common causative bacteria) potentially can lead to complete airway obstruction. Classic presentation of fever, inspiratory stridor, and pain with swallowing are crucial in helping alert the caregiver to the diagnosis of epiglottitis. Visualization and securing the airway should not be attempted until the child is in the operating room. Airway intubation and administration of antibiotics are the mainstay of treatment. Extubation should only be attempted once direct visualization confirms resolution of the epiglottic swelling.

**Retinopathy of Prematurity:** Retrolental fibroplasia reflects suboptimal vascularization and scarring of retinal vessels, leading to visual impairments. A significant risk factor is prematurity and arterial hyperoxia. It is thus essential to maintain inhaled concentration of oxygen to a $PaO_2$ between 60 and 80 mm hg[1] during administration of general anesthesia.

**Malignant Hyperthermia:** Malignant hyperthermia is an inherited disease that affects calcium release channels in skeletal muscles, leading to persistent muscle contractions when exposed to triggering agents. It is unusually more common in infants and neonates with an incidence that approaches 1:12,000 pediatric cases.[1] Genetic identification in the presence of a family history and avoidance of triggering agents (succinylcholine, volatile anesthetic) are the mainstays of prevention. Management with intravenous dantrolene (up to 10 mg/kg)[1] along with hemodynamic supportive measures (cooling blankets, intensive care unit monitoring) are the mainstays of treatment.

**Pyloric Stenosis:** Narrowing of the opening from the stomach to the first part of the small intestine (pylorus) occurs in about 1 to every 500 live births and is mostly common in males.[1] Presenting symptoms include projectile vomiting right after the baby is fed. Risk factors include cesarean delivery and preterm birth. Attention should be paid to correcting potential electrolyte derangement (hypokalemic, hypochloremic metabolic acidosis) that can occur with prolonged vomiting. The mainstay of management is correcting the electrolyte instability before proceeding to surgery; thus, pyloric stenosis is never a surgical emergency. Last, care must be taken to empty the stomach before induction of general anesthesia to avoid significant aspiration.

## REFERENCES

1. Stoetling RK, Miller RD. Pediatrics. In: *Basics of Anesthesia*. 3rd ed. New York, NY; 381–383, 390–392.
2. Cote CJ, Miller RD. Pediatric anesthesia. In: *Miller's Anesthesia*. 4th ed. Philadelphia, PA; 2102–2103:2108–2109.

# 226.

# DRUG TOXICITIES PREFERENTIALLY OCCURRING IN CHILDREN

*Caylynn Yao and Elisha Peterson*

## INTRODUCTION

Neonates, infants, and children have unique considerations in their pharmacokinetics and pharmacodynamics that increase the risk of drug toxicity. Underlying these considerations are developmental changes in organ function, protein binding, and body composition. Most drugs are hepatically metabolized and renally cleared. Neonates and infants have vulnerability in both the metabolization and clearance of drugs due to the immaturity of hepatic enzymes, decreased amount of plasma proteins, and functionally immature kidneys which require decreased dosing and decreased frequency of drug administration as seen in amide local anesthetics. Genetic heterogeneity in the cytochrome P450 (CYP450; also CYP) enzymes render children vulnerable to toxicity in drugs such as codeine that rely on these enzymes for conversion to an active drug. Reyes syndrome and propofol infusion syndrome (PRIS), which primarily occurs in children and have been theorized to be due to underlying mitochondrial failure; the exact mechanisms have yet to be elucidated.

## CODEINE

Codeine is used to treat pain and suppress cough; it is a prodrug- the drug must be metabolized to an active compound to exert its desired effect. Codeine undergoes hepatic metabolism via cytochrome P450 (CYP) 2D6 into morphine. Genetics dictate the degree of CYP activity. Codeine administered at the same dose in 2 different patients can yield varying responses. Patients with deficient CYP2D6 enzymes receive little to no analgesic benefit from codeine as little is metabolized into morphine, whereas patients with high CYP2D6 enzyme activity, known as "ultrametabolizers," convert more codeine, resulting in high amounts of morphine, thus leading to respiratory depression and in some cases death.[1]

A review of 50 years of Food and Drug Administration (FDA) adverse event reports in children for codeine demonstrated over 60 cases of significant respiratory depression and over 20 cases of death. A case series identified 10 deaths in children from codeine, where the majority occurred postoperatively from tonsillectomy and/or adenoidectomy.

Many children undergo these otolaryngology procedures for obstructive sleep apnea, for which opioids worsen sleep disordered breathing postoperatively[1]; superimpose this increased opioid sensitivity with a child with a potentially high CYP2D6 activity, and opioid overdose is highly likely in this setting. A FDA black box warning was added to codeine to avoid its use in children for postoperative pain after tonsillectomy or adenoidectomy.[1] Naloxone and supportive respiratory measures are indicated in the setting of a suspected codeine overdose akin to all opioid overdoses.

## SALICYLATES AND REYE SYNDROME

Salicylates are commonly used as analgesics, antipyretics, anti-inflammatories, and inhibitors of platelet aggregation. Aspirin has been strongly associated with Reye syndrome. Reye syndrome has two phases. The first phase is a viral illness; days to weeks after a viral infection there is protracted vomiting and mental status changes. It is characterized by acute encephalopathy with hepatic dysfunction and is more common in children than adults. A pathologic feature of Reye syndrome is microvesicular fatty accumulation in the liver and other organs due to a failure of fatty acid oxidation, particularly in long-chain fatty acids from mitochondrial dysfunction.[2] Clinical presentation of Reye syndrome includes vomiting, dehydration, headache, altered mental status, and seizures. Treatment includes supportive care in the intensive care unit with hydration and restoration of electrolyte disturbances.

## LOCAL ANESTHETICS

Local anesthetics are increasingly used in children as advances in regional anesthetic techniques are applied in pediatric patients. Local anesthetics exert their effects through action on voltage-gated sodium channels. They are structurally divided into ester and amide local anesthetics. Ester local anesthetics are short acting and metabolized by nonspecific tissue esterases and pseudocholisterase, which are rich in number and function in neonates. However, amide local anesthetics are hepatically metabolized through CYP and predominantly bound by $\alpha_1$ acid glycoprotein (AAG); at birth, neonates have immature hepatic enzymes and less than 50% AAG in plasma compared to an adult.[3] Levels of AAG reach adult levels by 1 year of age.[4]

Amide local anesthetics are most used in regional anesthetics due to their longer duration of action. Because neonates have decreased function of their hepatic enzymes as well as a quantitative decrease in AAG plasma protein, they are at risk for local anesthetic toxicity as this results in higher amounts of unbound drug in the blood stream. Local

*Table 226.1* CLINICAL MANIFESTATIONS OF PRIS

| ORGAN SYSTEMS AFFECTED | SIGNS AND SYMPTOMS |
| --- | --- |
| Cardiovascular | Myocardial depression, hypotension, electrocardiographic changes (i.e., bradyarrhythmia) |
| Gastrointestinal | Hepatomegaly, increased aspartase aminotransferase/alanine aminotransferase |
| Musculoskeletal | Rhabdomyolysis |
| Renal | Increased blood urea nitrogen/creatinine, oligoanuria |
| Fluids/electrolytes/ nutrition | Metabolic acidosis, hyperkalemia |

anesthetic toxicity has central nervous system and cardiac manifestations. Signs of local anesthetic systemic toxicity (LAST) are difficult to ascertain in neonates as they cannot report tinnitus or metallic taste in mouth. Seizures and/or arrhythmias would be the presenting symptom for LAST in neonates. The treatment of local anesthetic toxicity is with 20% lipid emulsion; although propofol is dissolved in a lipid emulsion, its use is discouraged in the treatment of LAST due to the myocardial depressant effects of propofol.[4]

## PROPOFOL INFUSION SYNDROME

Propofol is one of the most used hypnotic agents in general anesthesia. PRIS describes a constellation of findings primarily effecting cardiac and skeletal muscle: metabolic acidosis, bradyarrhythmias, and rhabdomyolysis that can result in renal failure, as seen in Table 226.1. Death from PRIS is rare[5] and can manifest in both children and adults, with increased vulnerability in children.[4] In a review of 44 children with PRIS, the average rate and duration of propofol infusion was 7 mg/kg/h over 2.7 days.[5] The underlying cellular mechanisms of PRIS have yet to be elucidated; mitochondrial dysfunction is central to many theories, such as propofol results in the uncoupling in the electron transport chain or causes impairments in fatty acid oxidation- particularly long-chain fatty acids. The treatment is hemofiltration,[5] which clears the lactic acid and reverses the cardiac depression and metabolic derangements.

## REFERENCES

1. Tobias JD, et al.; Section on Anesthesiology and Pain Medicine, Committee on Drugs. Codeine: Time to Say "No." *Pediatrics.* 2016;138(4):e20151648.

2. Glasgow JF, Middleton B. Reye syndrome—insights on causation and prognosis. *Arch Dis Child.* 2001;85(5):351–353.
3. Wilder RT. Local anesthetics for the pediatric patient. *Pediatr Clin North Am.* 2000;47(3):545–558. doi:10.1016/S0031-3955(05)70225-X
4. Charles C, et al. *A Practice of Anesthesia for Infants and Children.* 6th ed. Elsevier, Inc; 2018.
5. Hemphill S et al. Propofol infusion syndrome: a structured literature review and analysis of published case reports. *Br J Anaesth.* 2019;122(4):448–459.

# 227.

# OPIOID DOSING AND SENSITIVITY—PEDIATRICS

*Rewais B. Hanna and Alaa Abd-Elsayed*

## INTRODUCTION

Children are at an increased risk of adverse effects of opioids for a variety of reasons, including inaccurate pain assessment, immature metabolism, and incorrect age-appropriate dosing, among other factors. Moreover, the negative side effects of inappropriate dosing (nausea, pruritis, ileus, urinary retention, sedation, and respiratory depression) can be exceedingly difficult on pediatric patients and their families. Because of this, close monitoring and vigilance are required for these susceptible patients. Additionally, patient-controlled analgesia (PCA) can be difficult to administer to pediatric patients, who may be unable to operate it. Therefore, the importance of opioid dosing cannot be overstated. The most commonly prescribed opioids for children are codeine, hydrocodone, oxycodone, and morphine.[1] This changes for parenteral opioids, which are most commonly fentanyl and morphine.

## PAIN ASSESSMENT

One of the most important concepts of opioid dosing for children is correctly identifying the severity of pain. The assessment of pain depends on type of pain, location, and severity. Beginning with types of pain, this can be separated into two categories: nociceptive and neuropathic. Nociceptive pain is that of tissue injury and inflammation causing either somatic (well-localized) or visceral (poorly localized) pain and is generally described as stabbing or

sharp pain. Neuropathic pain is that caused by abnormal functioning of damaged sensory nerves and is generally described as numbness, tingling, or shooting pain. The next step is to decipher the location of the pain, which can be gleaned from having a child color on a picture the location of their pain. Last, evaluating the severity of the pain is likely the most difficult part in adolescents. Under the age of 11, this is commonly assessed using visual analogue pain scales.[2,3] This is exceedingly difficult in those under 3 years of age, where parental involvement can be helpful.

## OPIOID DOSING

Opioids in the perioperative period are held for pain that is refractory to nonopioid analgesic modalities. Efforts should be made to administer acetaminophen and nonsteroidal anti-inflammatory drugs prior to opioids. Choosing which type of opioid should depend on severity, location, and duration of pain. When a clinician decides opioids are the appropriate modality for pain management in children, dosing can be a difficult proposition. Generally, opioid administration should begin in low doses and increase in small increments. Past medical history should be considered, including age, prematurity, history of apnea, or other underlying pathologies. Other important concepts are to avoid opioid infusions, respiratory depressants, and use of opioids in high-risk individuals such as those who suffer from seizures or spasticity. As-needed dosing for breakthrough pain is preferred in children with frequent monitoring. It is important to observe for sedation and respiratory depression. Meperidine should be avoided in all children. Last, short-acting oral opioids are preferred for acute pain perioperative in children over continuous PCA infusions. Oral opioids are also preferred because other forms, such as intravenous, can be painful to administer to children. The following doses are for children over the age of 6 months:

## MORPHINE

Orally, the recommended dosage is 0.3 mg/kg every 3–4 hours.

Intravenously, the recommended dosage is 0.1 mg/kg every 2–3 hours.

## CODEINE

Orally, the recommended dosage is 0.5–1.0 mg/kg every 3–4 hours.

Intramuscularly, the recommended dosage is 0.3–0.5 mg/kg every 4–6 hours.

## FENTANYL

Intravenously, the recommended dosage is 0.5–1.0 µg/kg every 1–2 hours.

Intranasally, the recommended dosage is 1.5 µg/kg and repeat once at 10 minutes.

Second dose intranasally; the recommended dosage is 0.75–1.5 µg/kg.

## HYDROCODONE

Orally, the recommended dosage is 0.1–0.15 mg/kg every 3μ4 hours.

## HYDROMORPHONE

Orally, the recommended dosage is 40–80 µg/kg every 3–4 hours.

Intravenously, the recommended dosage is 10–20 µg/kg every 2–4 hours.

## OXYCODONE

Orally, the recommended dosage is 0.1–0.2 mg/kg every 3–4 hours.[1,4]

## OPIOID INTOXICATION AND MANAGEMENT

History and physical examination are important parts of diagnosing opioid intoxication. The first step is to identify specific drug, dose, and formulation to which the patient was exposed, the presence of nonopioid coexposures, including drug-drug interactions, and the patient's prior history of opioid use.[5] On physical examination, you may see miosis, central nervous system depression, respiratory depression, hyporeflexia, hypothermia, flushing, pruritus, bradycardia, hypotension, or decreased bowel sounds. The most predictive physical examination finding of opioid intoxication is respiratory depression.

## MANAGEMENT

The keys to managing opioid intoxication or toxicity are supportive care, body packers and stuffers, gastrointestinal decontamination, and naloxone. Beginning with supportive care, 100% oxygen and bag mask ventilation or even endotracheal intubation, depending on the severity, should be utilized. For gastrointestinal decontamination, it is recommended to administer activated charcoal (1 g/kg orally or by nasogastric tube with a maximum of 50 g) to alert young children and adolescents within 1 hour of oral overdose.[5]

## NALOXONE DOSAGE

Children under 20 kg should receive naloxone 0.1 mg/kg IV (maximum 2 mg per dose).

- Children 20 kg or greater should receive naloxone 2 mg IV.
- Adolescents suspected of opioid addiction may receive lower incremental doses of naloxone (0.04 mg or 0.4 mg per dose), with repeat doses every 3 to 5 minutes titrated to patient response to avoid iatrogenic opioid withdrawal.
- Naloxone should be repeated every 3 minutes until improvement in respiratory depression is noted. Cumulative doses of naloxone great than 10 mg in the first half hour are unlikely to yield additional benefit. Larger than customary doses of naloxone may be required to reverse the effects of drugs with higher receptor affinity than morphine.
- If respiratory depression of unknown etiology has failed to improve with a cumulative dose of 10 mg of naloxone, then isolated opioid toxicity is unlikely.[5]

## REFERENCES

1. O'Donnell FT, Rosen KR. Pediatric pain management: a review. *Mo Med.* 2014;111(3):231–237.
2. Wong DL, Baker CM. Pain in children: comparison of assessment scales. *Pediatr Nurs.* 1988;14:9.
3. Tomlinson D, et al. A systematic review of faces scales for the self-report of pain intensity in children. *Pediatrics.* 2010;126:e1168.
4. Greco C, Berde C. Pain management for the hospitalized pediatric patient. *Pediatr Clin North Am.* 2005;52:995.
5. Chamberlain JM, Klein BL. A comprehensive review of naloxone for the emergency physician. *Am J Emerg Med.* 1994;12:650.

# 228.

# NEUROMUSCULAR BLOCKERS

*Harsh Nathani and Chike Gwam*

## INTRODUCTION

Neuromuscular blocking agents are used to facilitate tracheal intubation, relax abdominal muscles, maintain immobility during surgery, and facilitate mechanical ventilation. Neuromuscular blockers are generally divided into two subcategories: depolarizing and nondepolarizing agents. They have their effect on the nicotinic acetylcholine receptors at the neuromuscular junction. Depolarizing agents such as succinylcholine are significantly more resistant to degradation by acetylcholinesterase present in the neuromuscular junction, leading to persistent depolarization of the motor end plate and paralysis. Nondepolarizing agents are competitive antagonists at the same receptors and impair the ability of acetylcholine to cause depolarization of the motor end plate. Clinicians should consider the physiological and pharmacological differences between children and adults when using these agents in the pediatric populations to better titrate neuromuscular blockade when indicated.

The maturation of the neuromuscular transmission likely occurs at 2 months of age, and the neuromuscular junction is not completely developed at birth. This leads to an increased sensitivity to neuromuscular blockade in a neonate, resulting in a lower required plasma concentration of neuromuscular blocker to achieve the desired level of blockade. Furthermore, the maturational changes of organ function also impact the clearance of drugs and may lead to longer elimination half-life in the younger patient, suggesting that lower doses are required to maintain neuromuscular blockade.[1]

On the other hand, infants have a much larger volume of distribution due to a higher percentage of extracellular fluid space of total body water, meaning that these patients may require larger doses of neuromuscular blockers. Another consideration is the composition of muscle mass in the patient—type 1 muscle fibers are more sensitive to blockade, and in preterm neonates, this consists only of 10% of the fibers present in the diaphragm.[1] This may lead to faster recovery of the diaphragm, suggesting that more frequent redosing of neuromuscular blockade is required.

## DEPOLARIZING AGENTS

Succinylcholine is a popular depolarizing neuromuscular blocker used in both pediatric and adult anesthesia practice and desired for its rapid onset and short duration of action. There is a role for the use of succinylcholine in situations requiring rapid emergent airway management and management of laryngospasm. Furthermore, it can be injected intramuscularly and is effective at creating intubating conditions with doses of 4 mg/kg IM within 4 minutes. However, due to many issues encountered in clinical practice with its use, there are many advocates for its elimination from pediatric practice. Historically, with concurrent use of halothane and succinylcholine, there were many reports of cardiac arrest secondary to massive muscle breakdown and hyperkalemia in the pediatric population, particularly in young male patients with silent muscular dystrophies, leading to a black box warning on its use by the Food and Drug Administration. Malignant hyperthermia is also of concern, especially when an inhalational induction has been performed prior to the use of succinylcholine—as is common practice in the United States. Masseter muscle rigidity is a less severe but more frequently occurring complication of succinylcholine use. In the pediatric population, succinylcholine may also trigger a profound vagal response, leading to bradycardia and cardiac arrest, and this phenomenon is more common if repeated doses of succinylcholine are administered. Exaggerated increases in serum potassium levels occur in patients with burn injuries, prolonged immobility, neuromuscular diseases, and certain motor-neuron lesions; however, patients with myelomeningocele and cerebral palsy do not exhibit this phenomenon.[2]

## NONDEPOLARIZING AGENTS

There are many nondepolarizing agents available for use in the pediatric population, and all have variable onset, duration of action, metabolism, and adverse effects. Commonly used medications include rocuronium, vecuronium, cisatracurium, pancuronium, and mivacurium.[1]

## ROCURONIUM

Rocuronium has the fastest onset of the nondepolarizing muscle relaxants and can be used for rapid sequence intubation. The dose commonly used for intubation is 0.6 mg/kg and produces intubating conditions at approximately 0.8–1.3 minutes and has a duration of action that lasts approximately 27 minutes. It can also be used for rapid sequence intubation at a dose of 1.2 mg/kg. It is metabolized primarily through the liver and is excreted renally. It is also readily reversed with sugammadex.[3]

## VECURONIUM

The intubating dose for vecuronium is 0.1 mg/kg; however, it has a relatively slower onset. Increasing the dose to 0.4 mg/kg increases the onset time to one comparable to succinylcholine; however, the duration of action increases significantly with doses exceeding 150 µg/kg. Vecuronium offers the benefit of a minimal increase in heart rate, which can be seen with injection of rocuronium.[1]

## CISATRACURIUM

Cisatracurium offers the benefit of having metabolism that does not depend on the hepatic or renal systems and can be safely given in patients with kidney or liver failure.[3]

## PANCURONIUM

Pancuronium is a long-acting, nondepolarizing agent that is primarily excreted renally. Injection is associated with tachycardia secondary to decreased presynaptic uptake of norepinephrine.[1]

## MIVACURIUM

Mivacurium is a nondepolarizing agent that is rapidly cleared from the blood by plasma cholinesterase and offers rapid spontaneous recovery of blockade. It is, however, associated with histamine release and can cause cutaneous flushing and hypotension on injection. Furthermore, a deep blockade with mivacurium has variable reversibility with acetylcholinesterase inhibitors due to the activity of these drugs on plasma cholinesterase.[3]

## ANTAGONISM OF NEUROMUSCULAR BLOCKADE

The use of acetylcholinesterase inhibitors to reverse the actions of nondepolarizing neuromuscular blockade is well studied. Commonly used agents include neostigmine at doses of 0.07 mg/kg after being pretreated with an antimuscarinic agent such as glycopyrrolate or atropine. Reversal with these agents is appropriate when there is evidence of recovery demonstrated with at least three to four responses in TOF stimulation.[3]

Sugammadex has also been used to reverse rocuronium and vecuronium, and there is research suggesting it is a safe alternative to acetylcholinesterase-based reversal in the pediatric population. Sugammadex is a selective binding agent that encapsulates a neuromuscular blocker, thus rendering it ineffective. In children aged greater than 2 years it has been used at doses ranging from 2 to 16 mg/kg; however, this evidence has not been substantiated by the Food and Drug Administration and is currently not approved for use within the United States in the pediatric population.[4]

## REFERENCES

1. Cote′ CJ, et al. *Practice of Anesthesia for Infants and Children*. 6th ed. Elsevier; 2018.
2. Fisher D. Neuromuscular blocking agents in paediatric anaesthesia. *Br J Anaesth*. 1999;83(1):58–64.
3. Brandom B. Neuromuscular blocking drugs in pediatric anesthesia. Semin Anesth Periop Med Pain. 1995;14(1):16–25.
4. Liu G, et al. The efficacy and safety of sugammadex for reversing postoperative residual neuromuscular blockade in pediatric patients: a systematic review. *Sci Rep*. 2017;7(1):5724.

# 229.

# REGIONAL ANESTHESIA

*Cassandra Hoffmann and Tiffany Frazee*

## INTRODUCTION

Many differences exist between pediatric and adult regional anesthesia procedures, including differing neurocognitive states, anatomy, physiology, and pharmacodynamics. Pediatric regional techniques leave little room for error, and dosing of local anesthetics is closer to the toxic threshold. The volume of local anesthetic is often limited by the patient's maximum allowable dose. Regional anesthesia can result in improved postoperative analgesia, improved postoperative respiratory function, decreased intraoperative anesthetic requirements, and decreased opioid requirements.

## ANESTHETIC CONSIDERATIONS

### PREOPERATIVE: AWAKE VERSUS ASLEEP AND SELECTING THE LOCAL ANESTHETIC

General anesthesia is often induced in pediatric patients prior to block placement because many children and infants will not tolerate awake procedures. The pediatric literature describes that performing regional blocks under general anesthesia is safe and potentially safer than awake or sedated blocks.[1] The use of ultrasound guidance allows direct visualization of anatomical structures and the deposition or spread of local anesthetic, thus improving block success and dosing. The use of ultrasound guidance has become standard of care for pediatric regional procedures. Ultrasound can be used to troubleshoot difficult neuraxial block placement by gauging depth to target structures and direction for needle placement. The indication for pediatric regional procedures is often surgery. Contraindications to regional block placement include infection at the block site; coagulopathy (if not currently coagulopathic, will they be at risk to become so postprocedure?); anatomical difficulty or congenital anomaly involving the block site; and sepsis (particularly if neuraxial).[2]

The pharmacodynamics of local anesthetics in pediatric patients are affected by decreased levels of $\alpha_1$-glycoprotein, which result in decreased protein binding of local anesthetics and can increase toxicity risk. Immature hepatic function may decrease metabolism of local anesthetics and prolong block duration. These differences make careful selection of local anesthetic of utmost importance. Pediatric regional techniques leave little room for error, and dosing of local anesthetics is often closer to toxic threshold. Bupivacaine is known for cardiotoxicity, and many providers select ropivacaine as the local anesthetic of choice due to a higher safety profile. The volume of local anesthetic is limited by the patient's maximum allowable dose. The maximum allowable dose of bupivacaine is 2.5 mg/kg, and ropivacaine's is 3 mg/kg.[2] Pediatric patients have multiple factors that increase the risk of local anesthetic systemic toxicity. The maximum dose of local for the regional procedure should be calculated in advance, including all other forms of local anesthetic agents (surgical infiltration or intravenous dosing on induction). It is important to use incremental injection and monitor for T-wave changes, indicating intravascular injection. If local anesthetic systemic toxicity is suspected, give an initial bolus of intralipid of 1.5 mL/kg over 1 minute and start infusion of intralipid at 15 mL/kg/h.[2]

### INTRAOPERATIVE: NEURAXIAL AND PERIPHERAL BLOCKS

A pediatric spinal or subarachnoid block is primarily used in infants undergoing urological or hernia surgery. Infants experience minimal hemodynamic lability with spinal anesthesia; heart rate, blood pressure, and respirations are preserved. Under spinal anesthesia, infants often get sleepy and do not require further sedation. This is thought to occur due to loss of sensory input from skin, resulting in decreased renin-angiotensin system activity. Avoidance of systemic anesthetic agents was thought to potentially decrease the incidence of postoperative apnea in ex-premature infants, but data have not supported this theory. Infants have a high dose requirement to achieve blockade, a short duration secondary to increased volume of cerebrospinal fluid to body surface area, and a high rate of cerebrospinal fluid turnover. The conus medullaris lies lower in infants (L3) compared to adults (L1), and spinal blocks should not be attempted higher than L3-4.[2]

Caudal anesthesia is the most common block performed in pediatric patients, and the incidence of complications is low.[3] Caudal injection is performed through the sacral hiatus by piercing the sacrococcygeal ligament to access the caudal epidural space. Data for proper dosing and dermatome level vary, but injections between 0.5 and 1 mL/kg are often recommended. Dermatome level usually does not exceed the midthoracic region, and care should be taken not to exceed the maximum allowable dosing. Hemodynamic changes are not expected after injection in pediatric patients. A test dose should include both local anesthetic and epinephrine to be reliable to detect potential intravascular injection. Careful aspiration and slow injection should be performed to watch for electrocardiographic changes (T-wave changes), which indicate intravascular injection. Advancing the needle too far during a procedure can result in inadvertent dural puncture.[2]

Peripheral nerve blocks can be performed similarly to adult nerve blocks with the use of ultrasound, but toxicity remains a concern. In children, the volume of local is limited by the maximum allowable local anesthetic dose and may be closer to the toxic threshold. The supraclavicular block is the most commonly performed upper extremity block in pediatric patients.[3] It provides anesthesia for the entire arm, and the plexus is easily visible as an anechoic grouping. There is an increased risk of pneumothorax due to the high apex of lung in pediatric patients. The fascia iliaca block is a favored lower extremity block for pediatric regional procedures because it covers both the femoral and lateral femoral cutaneous nerves and has a high success rate. The sciatic nerve is often blocked via the popliteal approach.[3]

Truncal blocks (quadratus lumborum, erector spinae) are gaining favor in pediatric patients due to ease of placement and injection in the fascial plane. These blocks can have a longer duration than a caudal block and result in longer duration of postoperative analgesia.[4] The erector spinae plane block has unique property of providing high thoracic analgesia and has been safely described in children.[5] The rectus sheath block is used for umbilical hernia procedures and blocks T9-11 intercostal nerves.[2]

## POSTOPERATIVE: ENHANCED RECOVERY AFTER SURGERY

Emerging initiatives suggest that regional anesthesia is a key component to enhanced recovery after surgery protocols in addition to multimodal analgesia, early mobilization, and optimization of nutrition. Many children's hospitals have a pediatric pain service to provide postoperative management of regional blocks or catheters and recommendations for multimodal pain management.

## REFERENCES

1. Taenzer AH, et al. Asleep versus awake: does it matter? *Reg Anesth Pain Med.* 2014;39:279–283.
2. Flack S. Regional anesthesia. In: Davis PJ, et al. *Smith's Anesthesia for Infants and Children.* 8th ed. St. Louis, MO: Mosby; 2011:452–510.
3. Benjamin J, et al. Complications in pediatric regional anesthesia: an analysis of more than 100,000 blocks from the Pediatric Regional Anesthesia Network. *Anesthesiology.* 2018;129:721–732.
4. Sato M. Ultrasound-guided quadratus lumborum block compared to caudal ropivacaine/morphine in children undergoing surgery for vesicoureteric reflex. *Paediatr Anaesth.* 2019;29(7):738–743.
5. Holland EL, Bosenberg AT. Early experience with erector spinae plane blocks in children. *Pediatr Anesth.* 2020;30:96–107.

# 230.

# FLUID THERAPY AND BLOOD REPLACEMENT

*Iana Bilga and Anna Tzonkov*

## INTRODUCTION

Neonates, infants, and young children are more susceptible to overhydration and dehydration in the perioperative period than adults. Fluid management in the pediatric population continues to be based on the replacement of fluid deficit, maintenance requirement, and intraoperative losses. Fluid administration and transfusion of blood products require meticulous attention intraoperatively as well as in the postoperative period in pediatric patients due to physiological age group differences, immaturity, and small reserve.

## PHYSIOLOGICAL ASPECTS

The body consists of two fluid compartments: the intracellular fluid (ICF) and the extracellular fluid (ECF). The ICF comprises two-thirds of the total body water (TBW), while the ECF accounts for the remaining third. The ECF is further divided into the interstitial fluid (75%) and plasma (25%). The TBW in infants composes approximately 70% of body weight, 65% in children, and 60% in adults.

Infants and young children have higher body water content, along with higher metabolic rates and increased index of body surface area to mass. This contributes to their faster exchange of fluids and solute. Besides, up to 1 year of age patients' more immature renal tubules have a decreased ability to absorb and excrete sodium, potassium, bicarbonate, glucose, amino acids, and phosphates, which makes them more susceptible to overhydration, dehydration, and metabolic acidosis. The inability to respond fully to aldosterone results in obligatory sodium loss in the urine, which necessitates intraoperative administration of sodium-containing fluids.[1]

## FLUID ADMINISTRATION

Fluid therapy in pediatric patients is focused on three main targets: replacement of preoperative deficit, maintenance fluids, and ongoing intraoperative losses.

Replacement of preoperative fluid deficit is classically calculated by multiplication of the number of the hours the patient received nothing by mouth before the surgery by the hourly fluid maintenance requirement of the patient. At the same time, the hourly fluid requirement is calculated by the 4–2–1 rule. If the patient is less than 10-kg, fluid requirement is 4 mL/kg. After that 2 mL/kg from 11to 20 kg, 1 mL/kg for more than 20 kg (to calculate hourly fluid maintenance requirements for 27 kg, we need to use 40 + 20 + 7 mL, which equals 67 mL/h). Generally, the first half is given during the first hour of anesthesia, and the rest is replaced during the following 2 hours.

Maintenance fluids are calculated based on the 4–2–1 rule and are given in addition to the preoperative deficit and intraoperative losses.

Replacement of intraoperative losses can be defined as whole blood loss, evaporation, and third-space redistribution. The 3:1 ratio is used to replace the whole blood loss when crystalloid or colloid solutions are used. Evaporation and third-space restoration is calculated based on the type of surgery: 0–2 mL/kg/h for noninvasive, 2–4 mL/kg/h for mildly invasive, 4–10 mL/kg/h for moderately invasive, and more than 10 mL/kg/h for significantly invasive surgery.

Treatment of hypovolemia is based on hemodynamic variables. Tachycardia, hypotension, decreased urine output, as well as central venous pressure variations all can suggest significant hypovolemia. Replacement is accomplished with 10–20 mL/kg fluid bolus.[1,2]

## TYPE OF FLUID

Crystalloids are fluid solutions that contain ion salts and other low-molecular-weight substances. Colloid solutions contain macromolecules suspended in electrolyte solutions. Albumin is produced from human blood and is suspended in saline.

The selection of fluid in pediatric patients depends on age and settings. The 0.2% normal saline with added dextrose and potassium is a maintenance fluid of choice preoperatively. Intraoperatively, isotonic non–glucose-added solutions such as Lactated Ringer and Plasma-Lyte are recommended. Glucose is not recommended in patients older than 1 year for maintenance intraoperatively due to stress from surgery, and subsequent catecholamine release usually prevents hypoglycemia. On the other hand, due to immature responses, glucose is given to patients younger than a year old or less than 10 kg. In this case, 5%–10% glucose solution can be administered for maintenance fluid intraoperatively. Neonates have decreased glycogen stores and are prone to significant hypoglycemia, withe preterm neonates at even greater risk. Glucose replacement is essential intraoperatively and is given at 3–5 mL/kg/min in term and 5–6 mg/kg/min in preterm neonates. However, in any case, it is not recommended to administer boluses of glucose or potassium-containing fluids.[1,2]

## TRANSFUSION THERAPY

Indications for blood component therapy in pediatric patients is not always consistent. The decision must be based on not only estimated blood loss but also the patient's blood volume, preoperative hematocrit, underlying medical conditions, nature of the surgical procedure, and risks versus benefits of transfusion. Blood loss needs to be estimated very accurately, and any intraoperative losses need to be replaced in a timely manner to maintain intravascular volume. Pediatric patient blood management may include the following measures: timely preoperative anemia diagnosis and management, minimizing blood draw and sample size, use of restrictive blood transfusion algorithms, surgical techniques to minimize blood loss, avoidance of hemodilution by careful fluid management, use of a massive hemorrhage protocol to guide goal-directed treatment of bleeding, and cell salvage.[3]

Before any procedure that carries the potential risk of bleeding, anesthesiologists should calculate the maximum allowable blood loss (MABL). MABL equals patient hematocrit minus minimum acceptable hematocrit divided by patient hematocrit and then multiplied by estimated blood volume (EBV). The EBV depends on the child's age.

Intraoperative blood loss was initially replaced by boluses of crystalloids or colloids in 1:3 ratios. When hematocrit reaches a minimum acceptable hematocrit, a MABL blood product transfusion is initiated in a 1:1 ratio.

Red blood cell transfusion of 10–15 mL/kg can increase hemoglobin concentration up to 2–3 g/dL. Platelet administration of 5–10 mL/kg should increase the platelet count 50,000/dL to 100,000/dL. Fresh frozen plasma (FFP) is given to correct coagulopathy due to insufficient coagulation factors. Transfusion of 10–15 mL/kg of FFP increases coagulation factors by 15%–20%. Cryoprecipitate consists of fibrinogen, factor VIII, factor XIII, and in the general administration of 1 U (10–20 mL) per every 5 kg up to 4 U total, usually enough to correct coagulopathy. Transfusion of red blood cells and FFP should be 2:1. Transfuse blood and blood products through a fluid wormer to avoid hypothermia. Hypothermia causes platelet dysfunction even with a normal count.[1,2]

## REFERENCES

1. Pardo M, Miller RD. *Basics of Anesthesia*. 7th ed. Philadelphia, PA: Elsevier–Health Sciences Division; 2017.
2. Barash PG, et al., eds. *Clinical Anesthesia*. 6th ed. Philadelphia, PA: Lippincott, Williams and Wilkins; 2009.
3. Klein MJ. Pediatric blood transfusion therapy and patient blood management. *SPA News*. 2019;32(2). Accessed August 20, 2020. https://www2.pedsanesthesia.org/newsletters/2019fall/blood%20 transfusion.html

# 231.

# NPO GUIDELINES FOR PEDIATRIC PATIENTS

*Jonathan W. Klein*

## NPO GUIDELINES

The American Society of Anesthesiologists has long-established fasting guidelines in regard to its patient population; however, these may be modified to either institutional policies or specific patient situations. These recommendations are based on best practice for the safety and well-being of patients undergoing elective surgery. Nil per os or NPO (nothing by mouth; fasting) guidelines are directed toward reducing the risk of pulmonary aspiration. Perioperative pulmonary aspiration is the aspiration of gastric contents in any phase of the anesthetic, whether it be during the induction, intraoperatively, or immediate postoperatively. Fasting guidelines are based on gastric physiology and various clinical trials and are geared toward minimizing gastric content at the time of surgery. These recommendations are applied to healthy patients who are undergoing elective procedures requiring general anesthesia, regional anesthesia, or procedural sedation and analgesia.[1] The fasting recommendations set forth by the ASA are as follows:

### NPO Guidelines

| Type of Food Source | Hours Stopped Prior to Surgery |
| --- | --- |
| Clear liquids | 2 hours |
| Breast milk | 4 hours |
| Infant formula | 6 hours |
| Nonhuman milk | 6 hours |
| Light meal | 6 hours |
| Large meal/fried fatty foods/meat | 8 hours |

Source: American Society of Anesthesiologists Task Force on Preoperative Fasting.

In regard to clear liquids, these may include water, pulp-free juices, coffee or tea, and carbohydrate drinks.[1] However, the Canadian Pediatric Anesthesia Society and the European Society of Anesthesiology allow pediatric patients to consume clear liquids up to 1 hour prior to their planned procedure.[2,3] This practice has not been adopted by the ASA. Clear liquids do not pertain to alcohol and should not be consumed by the patient prior to any form of anesthetic. Enteral feeds or tube feeds are another consideration. These feeds often have a large fat, protein, and carbohydrate content and therefore are considered a large meal and should be discontinued 8 hours prior to surgery.[1]

Special consideration should be taken for various patient populations who may exhibit delayed gastric emptying. These individuals are considered to be laboring patients, the elderly, and diabetics with a history of gastroparesis. As for solids, the gastric-emptying time is delayed by increased food weight, caloric density, and fat content, and therefore the NPO guidelines for these various patient populations may need to be altered to promote patient safety.[4] Various pharmacological agents should be considered to reduce the risk of pulmonary aspiration.

### Factors That Increase Gastroparesis

<u>Endocrine</u>: Diabetes, hyperthyroidism, hypothyroidism

<u>Diseases Affecting the Nervous System</u>: Parkinson disease, multiple sclerosis, brainstem stroke or tumor, amyloid neuropathy

<u>Connective Tissue Disorder</u>: Scleroderma

<u>Immune Disorders</u>: Human immunodeficiency virus and acquired immune deficiency syndrome (HIV/AIDS)

<u>Medications</u>: Narcotics, $\alpha_2$-adrenergic agonists, tricyclic antidepressants, calcium channel blockers, dopamine agonists, muscarinic cholinergic receptor antagonists, glucagon-like peptide 1, octreotide

<u>Surgical Procedures</u>: Surgeries of the abdomen and esophagus

<u>Infections</u>: Viral pathogens

Source: Gastroparesis: definitions and diagnosis.

In regard to gum chewing, according to a statement released by the ASA in 2014, "Although chewing gum significantly increases the volume of liquids in the stomach, it is safe to administer sedatives or anesthesia to patients who have chewed gum while fasting before surgery."[5] This statement is based on a study performed at the Perelman School of Medicine at the University of Pennsylvania, Philadelphia. The researchers concluded that the gastric volume was indeed larger in the group that had chewed gum; however, the pH of either group was not significantly different.[5] Notwithstanding, if a patient has swallowed the gum, then this would be considered a solid and should wait the appropriate 6 hours.

Information garnered during the preoperative examination is a valuable tool in the anesthesiologist's armament, which includes the patient's NPO status. This information allows the anesthesia practitioner to provide a safe and effective anesthetic.

## REFERENCES

1. American Society of Anesthesiologists. Practice guidelines for preoperative fasting and the use of pharmacologic agents to reduce the risk of pulmonary aspiration: application to healthy patients undergoing elective procedures: an updated report by the American Society of Anesthesiologists Task Force on Preoperative Fasting and the Use of Pharmacologic Agents to Reduce the Risk of Pulmonary Aspiration. *Anesthesiology*. 2017;126:376–393.
2. Rosen D, et al. Canadian Pediatric Anesthesia Society statement on clear fluid fasting for elective pediatric anesthesia. *Can J Anaesth*. 2019;66:991–992.
3. Smith I, et al. Perioperative fasting in adults and children: guidelines from the European Society of Anaesthesiology. *Eur J Anaesthesiol*. 2011;28:556–569.
4. Pasriche PJ, Parkman HP. Gastroparesis: definitions and diagnosis. *Gastroenterol Clin North Am*. 2015;44(1):1–7.
5. American Society of Anesthesiologists. Statement: chewing gum while fasting before surgery is safe, study finds. 2014. https://www.asahq.org/about-asa/newsroom/news-releases/2014/10/chewing-gum-while-fasting-before-surgery-is-safe-study-finds

# 232.

# PROBLEMS IN INTUBATION AND EXTUBATION

*Balazs Horvath and Benjamin Kloesel*

## INTRODUCTION

Nearly three-quarters of perianesthesia critical incidents and a third of cardiac arrests in children are associated with perioperative respiratory adverse events (PRAEs).[1]

Specific coexisting conditions require knowledge and skills in evaluating and managing the airway of neonates, infants, and children. Meticulous attention to the steps and anticipating potential pitfalls of airway management from the first moment of encountering the patient until discharge from the recovery room are keys to safe patient care. Familiarity with proper sedation techniques as well as effective maintenance of oxygenation during airway manipulation are imperative.[2]

## DISCUSSION

When an endotracheal tube (ETT) placement is deemed necessary, a structured approach ensures an increased success rate and decreased incidence of complications, and it addresses the timing and method of endotracheal extubation.[2] It is important to differentiate difficult intubation from difficult ventilation and identify the risk of their presence in every patient. Implementing one of the pediatric difficult airway algorithms, repetitive education and training, as well as preparedness for the recommended steps are imperative for every institution that takes care of pediatric patients.

Craniofacial disorders, chromosomal abnormalities, and metabolic diseases are common causes of upper airway obstruction and difficult airway scenarios. Congenital and acquired anatomical changes that impair both tongue and soft tissue displacement and flexion and extension during laryngoscopy predict difficult airway management (Table 232.1).

Dentition must be carefully assessed, especially when a difficult laryngoscopy is anticipated. Loose decidual teeth are normally present in 6- to 12-year-old children. Those, and preexisting poor dentition, as well as difficult laryngoscopy increase the risk of dental injury. Misaligned

*Table 232.1* MOST RELEVANT CONGENITAL SYNDROMES AND MALFORMATIONS THAT INFLUENCE AIRWAY MANAGEMENT

| SYNDROME | FEATURES | IMPACT ON AIRWAY MANAGEMENT | RECOMMENDATIONS/NOTES |
|---|---|---|---|
| Pierre-Robin sequence | Micrognathia<br>Glossoptosis<br>Airway obstruction | Potential difficult mask ventilation<br>Difficult intubation | Evaluate history and assess patient if mask ventilation is feasible.<br>Reconstructive surgery may improve airway conditions. |
| Treacher-Collins syndrome | Hypoplastic maxilla, zygomatic, mandible<br>Small mouth, high-arched palate<br>Laterally sloping palpebral fissures, notched lower eyelids, coloboma, and hearing loss<br>Variable association with cleft palate and velopharyngeal incompetence | Severe airway obstruction<br>Difficult mask ventilation<br>Difficult intubation | Flexible bronchoscopy.<br>Supraglottic airway device.<br>Low threshold for surgical airway access—otolaryngologist informed and readily available.<br>Progressively worsening airway condition. |
| Crouzon syndrome | A type of craniosynostosis<br>Midface hypoplasia<br>Hypertelorism<br>Proptosis<br>Normal size mandible, but appears to be relatively prognathic secondary to midface hypoplasia<br>High-arched palate<br>Nasal passages are small with some degree of choanal stenosis<br>Primarily mouth breathers<br>Obstructive sleep apnea—may require tracheostomy<br>Vertebral abnormalities that may limit neck motion<br>Tracheal ring abnormalities | Difficult-to-impossible mask ventilation<br>Intubation may be easy or difficult | Mask fitting and adequate seal maybe difficult because of the small midface and proptosis.<br>Closure of the mouth occludes oropharynx as the tongue fills the smaller oral cavity.<br>Small nares and choanal stenosis create resistance to airflow via the nasal route.<br>Helpful maneuvers:<br>1. Keeping the mouth open during induction and press down on the mask to obtain a good seal.<br>2. Oropharyngeal topical anesthetic application allows placement of an oropharyngeal airway before deep anesthesia achieved.<br>Intubation may be difficult if neck mobility is impaired.<br>Smaller-than-expected ETT recommended due to tracheal abnormalities.<br>Nasal intubation may also require a smaller ETT. |
| Goldenhar syndrome | Hemifacial microsomia<br>Varying degree of mandibular hypoplasia<br>Auricular abnormalities<br>Overlying soft tissue loss<br>Facial nerve weakness<br>May present bilaterally<br>Macrostomia<br>Vertebral bone abnormalities | Possible difficult ventilation<br>Difficult intubation | Flexible bronchoscopy.<br>Intubation can be more difficult after temporomandibular joint and jaw reconstruction due to ensuing soft tissue contractures that restrict mouth opening. |
| Hurler syndrome | Mucopolysaccharide deposits progressively lead to tongue enlargement<br>Thickening and redundancy of the soft tissue mucosa of the oropharynx<br>Blockage of nasal passages | Difficult mask ventilation<br>Difficult intubation | Indirect (video) laryngoscopy.<br>Flexible bronchoscope.<br>Reduced ETT size for age.<br>Bone marrow transplantation may reverse the airway changes. |

teeth alone or in combination with other craniofacial malformations may make laryngoscopy difficult.

Both endotracheal intubation and extubation carry the risk of multiple complications and adverse events.[3] Those are especially common in neonates and infants.[2] The above structural malformations, chronic and acute respiratory diseases,[4] emergency, and impaired gastric emptying[5] increase the incidence of PRAEs.

Table 232.2 lists the common problems during intubation, including the etiology and recommended

management. We chose to divide the potential problems during intubation into two categories. The first category is related to patient and anesthesiologist factors (i.e., "what we do to the endotracheal tube").

The second category lists the complications that follow a successful ETT placement (i.e., "what the ETT does to the patient").

There are patient-related factors that predict postintubation problems (e.g., bronchospasm in patients with asthma). However, following the flow of events step

*Table 232.2* COMMON PROBLEMS DURING INTUBATION, INCLUDING ETIOLOGY AND RECOMMENDED MANAGEMENT

| | PATIENT-RELATED FACTORS | ANESTHESIOLOGIST-RELATED FACTORS | PREVENTION/PREPARATION MANAGEMENT |
|---|---|---|---|
| **Preintubation Events** | | | |
| Difficult laryngoscopy | - Age < 1 year<br>- Congenital malformations<br>- Metabolic diseases<br>- Morbid obesity<br>- Limited mouth opening<br>- Limited neck range of motion<br>- Maxillofacial trauma | Inadequate assessment<br>Inadequate preparation<br>Inexperience<br>Emergency | Thorough evaluation and preparation<br>Advanced airway devices<br>Intubation by the most experienced anesthesiologist |
| Difficult ETT advancement | - As above<br>- Subglottic stenosis<br>- History of reconstructive airway surgery | As above | History of previous intubations<br>Advanced airway devices<br>Ear, nose, throat specialist availability (rigid bronchoscopy) |
| Aspiration during laryngoscopy | - Full stomach<br>- Emergency<br>- Major trauma<br>- Severe pain<br>- Preoperative opioids<br>- Diabetes | Not following RSI when indicated<br>Suboptimal anesthesia depth resulting in gag response to DL<br>Emergency<br>Hypoxemia during RSI requiring bag/mask ventilation | Thorough history of NPO status<br>Assessment of conditions resulting in delayed gastric emptying<br>Proper sequence of RSI<br>Adequate anesthetic depth or awake flexible bronchoscopic intubation when indicated and feasible |
| Dental, oropharyngeal injury | - Preexisting dental pathology<br>- Limited mouth opening<br>- Prominent upper incisors, significant overbite | Emergency intubation<br>Inexperience<br>Inadequate choice of laryngoscopy | Dental guard<br>Advanced airway device |
| Hypoxemia | - Morbid obesity<br>- Chronic lung disease<br>- Difficult ventilation due to patient factors<br>- Difficult laryngoscopy (see causes above) | Lack of adequate preoxygenation<br>Emergency<br>Inexperience | Adequate preoxygenation/denitrogenating<br>$O_2$ via high-flow nasal cannula during airway manipulation<br>Awake airway management if feasible when difficult mask ventilation anticipated |
| Hypercapnia | - Morbid obesity<br>- Chronic obstructive lung disease<br>- Obstructive sleep apnea | Inadequate ventilation<br>Emergency | Positioning<br>Bronchodilators<br>Avoid preoperative sedatives and opioids |
| Increased sympathetic tone, dysrhythmia, hypertension | - Pheochromocytoma<br>- Hyperthyroidism | Inadequate anesthesia depth during DL | Adequate patient preparation for the procedure<br>Adequate planning for induction of anesthesia<br>Emergency medications readily available |
| Esophageal intubation | - Difficult laryngoscopy (see causes above) | Inexperience<br>Emergency | Proper equipment for airway management<br>Early detection and correction of ETT placement |
| **Postintubation Events** | | | |
| Mainstem intubation | - Age < 1year<br>- Short trachea<br>- History of reconstructive airway surgery | Inadequate depth of ETT<br>Inadequate positioning/neck anteflexion<br>Inexperience | Understanding age-related anatomy of neonates, infants, and children<br>Proper positioning |

*(continued)*

*Table 232.2* CONTINUED

| | PATIENT-RELATED FACTORS | ANESTHESIOLOGIST-RELATED FACTORS | PREVENTION/PREPARATION MANAGEMENT |
|---|---|---|---|
| Hypoxemia | - Chronic lung disease of prematurity<br>- Severe reactive airway disease<br>- Severe bronchospasm<br>- $O_2$ dependence<br>- Increased $O_2$ consumption | Inexperience<br>Inadequate preparation<br>Emergency | Adequate control of underlying lung disease<br>Adequate airway management technique<br>Regional anesthesia when feasible |
| Palatopharyngeal injury | - Difficult laryngoscopy (see causes above)<br>- Palatopharyngeal pathology<br>- Limited mouth opening<br>- Macroglossia | Emergency<br>Inexperience<br>Tip of rigid stylet is beyond the tip of ETT<br>Eyes on screen while inserting ETT during video laryngoscopy | Optimizing training, including eye-hand coordination<br>Proper preparation of equipment |
| Epistaxis (nasal intubation) | - History of frequent nose bleed<br>- Bleeding diathesis<br>- Hypertrophic mucosa, nasal polyps<br>- Hypertrophic adenoids | Incomplete patient evaluation<br>Lack of nasal decongestant use<br>Lack of dilation of nasal passage and using proper ETT size<br>Inexperience | Rule out presence of increased risk of bleeding<br>Judicious use of nasal decongestant<br>Lubricant<br>Use of nasopharyngeal airway with size increments to dilate the nasal cavity<br>Understand the anatomy of the nasal passage<br>Appropriate size ETT |
| Laryngeal injury | - Laryngeal cleft<br>- Prior laryngeal surgery<br>- Radiation of head and neck | Large ETT for the patient<br>Excess force<br>Inexperience | Avoid excess force, downsize ETT when not passing between vocal cords |
| Laryngospasm | - Recent upper respiratory tract infection<br>- Smoking exposure | Inadequate depth during anesthesia induction when intubating without muscle relaxant | |
| Bronchospasm | - Chronic lung disease of prematurity<br>- Reactive airway disease<br>- Asthma<br>- Bronchiolitis | Emergency | Optimize/treat underlying lung disease |
| Tracheal mucosa necrosis | - Tracheomalacia<br>- Tracheobronchitis<br>- Recent intubation<br>- History of reconstructive surgery | Large-for-size ETT<br>ETT cuff inflation pressure > 20–30 cm $H_2O$ | Proper size ETT<br>Monitor cuff pressure |
| Tracheal perforation | - Tracheal stenosis<br>- History of prolonged/ frequent intubations<br>- History of reconstructive airway surgery | Large-for-size ETT<br>ETT cuff inflation pressure > 30 cm $H_2O$<br>Rigid stylet tip beyond the tip of ETT<br>Excessive force<br>Inexperience | Proper size ETT<br>Monitor cuff pressure<br>Proper equipment preparation |

*Table 232.3* COMMON PROBLEMS DURING "DEEP" AND "AWAKE" EXTUBATION, INCLUDING ETIOLOGY AND RECOMMENDED MANAGEMENT

| | PATIENT-RELATED FACTORS | ANESTHESIOLOGIST-RELATED FACTORS | MANAGEMENT |
|---|---|---|---|
| | Awake Extubation | | |
| Laryngospasm | - Recent upper respiratory infection (URI)<br>- Smoking exposure | Premature ETT removal<br>Secretion | Oropharyngeal suctioning<br>100% O$_2$<br>Bag/mask ventilation<br>Propofol<br>Succinylcholine |
| Bronchospasm | - Reactive airway disease<br>- Bronchiolitis | | Inhaled $\alpha_2$-agonist bronchodilator<br>Subcutaneous or intravenous low-dose epinephrine |
| Stridor | - Preexisting tracheal stenosis<br>- Recent URI | Large-for size-ETT<br>ETT cuff inflation pressure<br>   > 30 cm H$_2$O | Proper size ETT<br>Monitor cuff pressure<br>Racemic epinephrine |
| | Deep Extubation | | |
| Upper airway obstruction | - Morbid obesity<br>- Tonsillar-adenoid hypertrophy | Failure to reverse muscle<br>   relaxant<br>Lack of maintaining patent<br>   airway | Ensure that all extubation criteria met<br>Place oropharyngeal or nasopharyngeal airway |
| Laryngospasm | - Recent URI<br>- Smoking exposure | Secretion/bleeding | 100% O$_2$<br>Bag/mask ventilation<br>Propofol<br>Succinylcholine |
| Bronchospasm | - Reactive airway disease<br>- Bronchiolitis | | Inhaled $\alpha_2$-agonist bronchodilator<br>Subcutaneous or intravenous low-dose epinephrine |
| Stridor | - Preexisting tracheal stenosis<br>- Recent URI | Large-for-size ETT<br>ETT cuff inflation pressure<br>   > 30 cm H$_2$O | Proper size ETT<br>Monitor cuff pressure<br>Racemic epinephrine |
| Aspiration | - Residual gastric content | Deep extubation despite<br>   increased aspiration risk<br>   (see above) | Deep extubation only when appropriate |

by step during airway management may help remember the potential pitfalls, thereby reducing the incidence of preventable complications (Table 232.3).

# REFERENCES

1. Drake-Brockman T, et al. The effect of endotracheal tubes versus laryngeal mask airways on perioperative respiratory adverse events in infants: a randomised controlled trial. *Lancet*. 2017;389(10070):701–708.
2. Engelhardt T, et al. A framework for the management of the pediatric airway. *Paediatr Anaesth*. 2019;29(10):985–992.
3. Von Ungern-Sternberg B, et al. Risk assessment for respiratory complications in paediatric anaesthesia: a prospective cohort study. *Lancet*. 2010;376(9743):773–783.
4. Regli A, et al. An update on the perioperative management of children with upper respiratory tract infections. *Curr Opin Anesthesiol*. 2017;30(3):362–367.
5. Griesdale D, et al. Complications of endotracheal intubation in the critically ill. *Intens Care Med*. 2008;34(10):1835–1842.

# 233.

# NEONATAL PHYSIOLOGY

*Nupur Dua and Ilana R. Fromer*

## INTRODUCTION

Children are not little adults; infants are not little children, and neonates are not little infants. There are essential differences between children, infants, and neonates, and physiological changes do not occur in a linear manner.[1]

## RESPIRATORY SYSTEM

### DEVELOPMENT, ANATOMY, AND SURFACTANT

Lung development has five stages:

1. The embryonic stage (4–6 weeks of gestation), when early upper airways appear.
2. The glandular stage (7–16 weeks), when the lower conducting airways form.
3. The canalicular phase (17–28 weeks), when acini and capillaries develop.
4. The terminal sac period (29–36 weeks), when the first respiratory units for gas exchange (terminal sacs and surrounding capillaries) make their appearance.
5. The alveolar phase, when alveoli develop; begins at about 36 weeks and continues until at least 18 months of age.[2]

In general, extrauterine viability increases after 26 weeks because respiratory saccules have developed, and capillaries are in close approximation to the developing distal airways, allowing alveolar exchange.

The surfactant is produced by type II pneumocytes. The synthesis begins at around 25 weeks of gestation but is not secreted into the alveoli until 34–36 weeks. The surfactant is necessary to stabilize the lung during expiration; hence, infants born before 34 weeks will have "collapsed alveoli" during expiration and develop respiratory distress syndrome.

## PULMONARY FUNCTION

There are several differences that make respiration less efficient in neonates:

1. Smaller diameter of the airways, which increases resistance to airflow.
2. Lower lung volumes in relation to body size.
3. Chest walls of neonates are highly compliant as they are poorly supported by surrounding structures; negative intrathoracic pressure is poorly maintained, decreasing functional residual capacity and increasing atelectasis.
4. Oxygen consumption is two to three times higher than adults.
5. Composition of the diaphragmatic and intercostal muscles: The muscles do not achieve the adult configuration of type I muscle until the child is approximately 2 years old. Because type I fibers provide the ability to perform repeated exercise, any factor that increases the work of breathing contributes to early fatigue of respiratory muscles of neonates.[3]

Hence, neonates are prone for rapid hypoxia with apnea.

## DIFFERENCE BETWEEN INFANT AND ADULT AIRWAYS

1. The large size of the tongue in relation to the oropharynx increases the likelihood of airway obstruction and difficulty with laryngoscopy.
2. More cephalad and anterior location of the larynx make straight blades more useful than curved ones.
3. Epiglottis is floppy, omega shaped, adding to difficulty with laryngoscopy.
4. Narrowest portion in infant larynx is the cricoid. An endotracheal tube that passes through the vocal cord may be tight in the subglottic region. Therefore,

it is important to ascertain a leak around the cuff to avoid tracheal mucosal injury.

## PULMONARY OXYGEN TOXICITY

Hyperoxia can lead to a surplus of free radicals that induce inflammation and damage cellular structure. It also inhibits synthesis of surfactant and increases pulmonary reactivity. It is specifically harmful in premature infants with immature lungs and with inadequate systems to protect against oxygen-induced injury. Therefore, it is advised to use the minimal oxygen concentration to achieve the target oxygen saturation in neonates.

# CARDIOVASCULAR SYSTEM

### The Fetal Circulation

Desaturated blood from the superior vena cava preferentially flows into the right ventricle, into the pulmonary artery, across the ductus arteriosus, and to the descending aorta to the placenta. Relatively well-saturated blood from the ductus venosus enters the inferior vena cava and preferentially crosses the foramen ovale to the left atrium, the left ventricle, and into the cerebral circulation.

## HALLMARKS OF FETAL CIRCULATION

The following are hallmarks of fetal circulation: increased pulmonary vascular resistance (PVR), decreased pulmonary blood flow, decreased systemic vascular resistance (SVR), and blood flow from left to right through a patent ductus arteriosus and the foramen ovale (Figure 233.1).

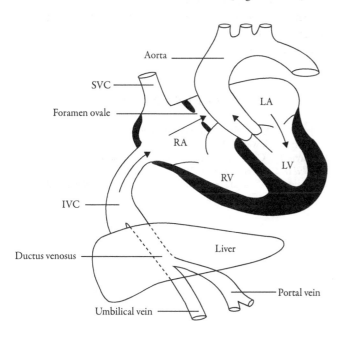

Figure 233.1 Fetal circulation. IVC, inferior vena cava; LA, left atrium; LV, left ventricle; RA, right atrium; RV, right ventricle.

## TRANSITION FROM FETAL TO ADULT CIRCULATION

1. As the placenta is removed from the circulation, the portal pressure falls, which causes closure of the ductus venosus.
2. Lung expansion and onset of breathing causes oxygenation of blood through the lungs. Exposure of the ductus arteriosus to oxygenated blood induces ductal closure. Functional closure of the ductus arteriosus occurs within 24 hours; however, anatomic closure occurs after several days.
3. PVR decreases, while SVR increases.
4. Pulmonary blood flow increases as PVR decreases, raising both the volume and pressure of the left atrium, mechanically closing the foramen ovale.

## PERSISTENT FETAL CIRCULATION/ PERSISTENT PULMONARY HYPERTENSION OF THE NEWBORN

Arterial hypoxemia, acidosis, or exposure to cold causes pulmonary arterial vasoconstriction and decreased pulmonary blood flow. The resultant increase in right atrial pressure reestablishes right-to-left shunting of deoxygenated blood through the foramen ovale and ductus arteriosus. This may further exacerbate the hypoxemia and acidosis.

Hence, care must be taken to keep the newborn warm, maintaining normal arterial oxygen and carbon dioxide tension, and minimizing anesthetic-induced myocardial depression.

## RETINOPATHY OF PREMATURITY

Oxygen toxicity and prematurity are the two main factors in the multifactorial development of retinopathy of prematurity. The retinal blood vessels grow outward from the center of the optic disc from 16- to 40-weeks' gestation. The vessels develop normally in the hypoxic intrauterine environment. As the infant is born prematurely and is exposed to high oxygen concentrations, it can lead to inhibition of growth of retinal vessels and overgrowth of abnormal vessels, including fibrous bands, which can lead to retinal detachment. The molecular mechanism is still unknown.[2] It is recommended to reduce oxygen exposure for premature infants less than 44 weeks old and maintain $PO_2$ between 60 and 80 mm Hg whenever possible.

## METABOLISM, FLUID DISTRIBUTION, AND RENAL FUNCTION

Renal function is diminished in neonates due to low perfusion pressure and immature glomerular and tubular function. Complete maturation of glomerular filtration and tubular function occurs by approximately 20 weeks after birth, and complete maturation of renal function takes place by about 2 years of age. Similarly, hepatic metabolism is underdeveloped, and the cytochrome P450 system is approximately 50% of adult values at birth. Thus, caution is required while administering medications excreted renally.

A neonate has minimal glycogen stores and is prone to hypoglycemia. Plasma levels of albumin and other proteins necessary for binding drugs are lower; therefore, the decreased protein binding of some drugs can result in greater levels of unbound drug.

The total body water is higher in neonates, and fat and muscle content is less as compared to adults. The clinical implications for those are that (a) water-soluble drugs with a large volume of distribution require a larger initial dose; and (b) drugs that depend on redistribution into fat or muscle for termination of action will have a longer clinical effect.

## THERMAL REGULATION

Newborns are vulnerable to hypothermia owing to the following:

1. High ratio of surface area to body weight.
2. Reduced subcutaneous fat.
3. There is an underdeveloped shivering response due to the neonate's smaller muscle mass. As a result, nonshivering thermogenesis is the major compensatory mechanism for cold stress. Norepinephrine and thyroid hormone stimulate the metabolism of brown fat, which is stored between the scapulae and around major abdominal organs.

A neutral thermal environment is the temperature associated with minimal oxygen consumption, and that normally corresponds to a skin temperature of 36°C and an environmental temperature of 32°C–34°C.[2]

## FETAL HEMOGLOBIN

At birth, the neonate has 70%–80% fetal hemoglobin (Hb) and it continues to decrease thereafter, reducing to less than 5% at 6 months. Fetal $Hb(\alpha_2\gamma_2)$ differs from adult $Hb(\alpha_2\beta_2)$ in that it has higher affinity for oxygen and hence a lower P50, that is, the oxygen tension at which the hemoglobin is 50% saturated. The oxyhemoglobin dissociation curve shifts to the left.

## APNEA OF PREMATURITY

Apnea is common in preterm infants and may be related to an immature respiratory control mechanism. Central apnea of infancy is defined as cessation of breathing for 15 seconds or longer or a shorter respiratory pause associated with bradycardia (<100 beat/min). These patients are prone to postoperative apnea, which led to a general consensus among pediatric anesthesiologists that infants younger than 44 weeks postconception be admitted overnight after surgeries.[2]

## BRONCHOPULMONARY DYSPLASIA

Bronchopulmonary dysplasia (BPD) is a form of chronic lung disease that occurs in patients who have survived neonatal lung disease. It is usually seen in premature infants who required prolonged and aggressive respiratory support with high pressures and high oxygen concentrations.

Key components of BPD are decreased dynamic compliance, increased airway resistance, increased physiological dead space, and increased work of breathing.

The clinical picture shows patients with intercostal retractions, nasal flaring, and wheezing. A chest x-ray shows large lung volumes, fibrosis, as well as atelectasis. Hypercapnia and hypoxia are present.

Therapy includes diuretics, bronchodilators, and respiratory support (mechanical ventilation, continuous positive airway pressure).

## REFERENCES

1. Jacob R, Thirlwell J. *Understanding Paediatric Anesthesia*. 3rd ed. Wolters Kluwer; 2015.
2. Davis PJ, Cladis Franklyn P. *Smith's Anesthesia for Infants and Children*. 9th ed. Elsevier; 2017.
3. Miller RD, et al., eds. *Miller's Anesthesia*. 7th ed. Churchill Livingstone Elsevier; 2010.

# 234.

# CARDIOVASCULAR SYSTEM

*Bilga Iana and Chike Gwam*

## INTRODUCTION

The fetal circulation transitions to the neonatal circulation, providing adaptation to extrauterine life. Changes in cardiovascular physiology continue throughout infancy and childhood toward ultimately attaining the adult functional status.

## EMBRYONAL DEVELOPMENT AND PHYSIOLOGICAL CHANGES AT BIRTH

The heart is the first functional organ of the embryo and forms between the second and eighth weeks of life. The mesoderm differentiates from the ectoderm and gives rise to the straight heart tube. The straight heart tube begins to indent to form the four initial heart structures: the truncus arteriosus, bulbus cordis, ventricle, and atrium. On day 23 occurs cardiac looping, and heart tissue begins to beat. At the end of the first month, the major structures have moved into place, and the heart circulation begins.[1-4]

Fetal circulation is relatively hypoxic compared to maternal circulation. Only a very small amount of blood is directed through the right and left pulmonary arteries to the lungs. Fetal shunts are in place to handle the limited oxygen ($O_2$) available to the developing tissues. The three shunts are the foramen ovale (right atrium to left atrium), ductus arteriosus (pulmonary artery to the aorta), and ductus venosus (umbilical vein to inferior vena cava).

At birth, transitional circulation begins when the umbilical cord is clamped, and lungs are inflated. Increased circulating oxygen leads to a decrease in pulmonary vascular resistance (PVR) and an increase in systemic vascular resistance, which eventually causes shunts to close. The patent foramen ovale (PFO) closes when left atrial pressure becomes higher than right atrial pressure. Functional closure of the PFO occurs quickly, but anatomic closure usually requires weeks. The ductus arteriosus remains patent in utero due to hypoxia, mild acidosis, and placental prostaglandins. Removal of these factors after delivery causes functional closure, with anatomic closure occurring weeks later. The ductus venosus closes after birth when portal pressure decreases, but complete closure occurs at around a week after birth. Certain conditions, such as hypothermia, hypercarbia, acidosis, hypoxia, or sepsis, can increase pulmonary pressures and lead to reverting to fetal circulation. This condition can be life threatening, and treatment is focused on decreasing PVR.[1,2,4]

## NEONATAL MYOCARDIUM

The newborn heart is qualitatively similar from embryonic stages through childhood, yet several pertinent differences exist that impact overall cardiac function. The immature neonatal myocardium has less contractile elements, poor compliance, fixed stroke volume, cardiac output that is dependent on heart rate. The myocardium comprises less contractile elements and more connective tissue than adults. Neonatal sarcoplasmic reticulum is immature with disorganized T tubules. Heart contractility mainly depends on the concentration of free calcium. It is important to know that a neonatal blood transfusion can decrease the concentration of free calcium and affect contractility.[1]

Neonatal hearts do respond to alterations in preload and afterload, but the effect is not as developed as in adults. Besides, neonates have high metabolic demand, and oxygen consumption is greatly increased (6 mL/kg vs. 3 mL/kg in adults). With high metabolic demands of the heart and other developing tissues, the neonatal heart operates at near-maximal capacity at most times. Despite the fact that anesthetics reduce myocardial $O_2$ consumption and volatile anesthetics may dilate coronary arteries, many anesthetics cause an overall reduction in the heart rate and cardiac output, risking myocardial hypoperfusion. In the setting of hypoxia and acidosis, the myocardium is significantly more sensitive to the depressant effects of anesthesia.[2]

## AUTONOMIC NERVOUS SYSTEM

Early in life, the parasympathetic system plays a major role in heart innervation as the sympathetic nervous system is still developing. Parasympathetic domination exaggerates the vagus response and plays a role in bradycardia or even asystole during induction of anesthesia, laryngoscopy, suctioning of an endotracheal tube or orogastric/nasogastric tube placement. Many clinicians pretreat with atropine or glycopyrrolate before manipulation.[1]

## HEMODYNAMIC VARIABLES FOR AGE GROUP

Oxygen saturation in the early neonatal period reflects the transition to extrauterine life. Oxygen saturation ($O_2$) in term newborns increases gradually over the first 10 minutes as follows: 1 minute of life 68%, 2 minutes 76%, 5 minutes 92%, and 10 minutes 97%. The heart rate of a neonate (<30 days of age) is 120–160 beats/min, and systolic blood pressure (SBP) is 60–75 mm Hg; the 1- to 6-month heart rate range is from 110 to 140 beats/min, and SBP is 65–85 mm Hg. At 6–12 months, heart rate is 100–140 beats/min, and SBP is 70–90 mm Hg; at 1–2 years the heart rate range is 80–130 beats/min, and SBP is 75–95 mm Hg; at 3–5 years, heart rate is 80–120 beats/min, and SBP is 80–100 mm Hg. The 6- to 12-year heart rate range is 70–115 beats/min, and SBP is 85–115 mm Hg; above 13 years, the heart rate is 60–110 beats/min, and SBP is 95–125 mm Hg.[1]

## CARDIOVASCULAR ASSESSMENT AND DRUGS

In addition to a general consideration of age-appropriate hemodynamic variables, including heart rate, blood pressure, and oxygen saturation, it is important to include other parts of assessment: capillary refill, peripheral pulses (some instances in all four extremities), respiratory status, and any heart auscultation abnormality (murmur, additional sounds). If any suspicion for inadequate oxygenation and acidosis, laboratory studies should be performed, such as venous blood gases, arterial blood gases, or capillary (mixed) blood gases. Furthermore, if assessment favors suspicion of any underlying heart pathology (congenital heart disease), chest radiography, an electrocardiogram, an echocardiogram, or a magnetic resonance tomogram may be warranted.[1]

There is controversy regarding the need for routine premedication with anticholinergics in neonates and infants to prevent vagal stimulation, which potentially can lead to severe bradycardia or asystole. Anesthesia induction, intubation, and suctioning as well as succinylcholine administration all can trigger the vagal response. Anticholinergics such as atropine and glycopyrrolate are used to prevent this response.[2]

Hypotension is a late and ominous sign in pediatric patients as children may maintain a normal blood pressure until 35% of blood volume is lost.

## REFERENCES

1. Pardo M, Miller RD. *Basics of Anesthesia*. 7th ed. Philadelphia, PA: Elsevier—Health Sciences Division; 2017.
2. Barash PG, et al, eds. *Clinical Anesthesia*. 6th ed. Philadelphia, PA: Lippincott, Williams and Wilkins; 2009.
3. Openanesthesia.org. Neonatal vs. adult cardiac physiology. Accessed August 26, 2020. https://www.openanesthesia.org/neonatal_vs-_adult_cardiac_physiology/
4. Openanesthesia.org. Pediatric anesthesia (anesthesia text). Accessed August 28, 2020. https://www.openanesthesia.org/pediatric_anesthesia_anesthesia_text/

# 235.

# METABOLISM, FLUID DISTRIBUTION, AND RENAL FUNCTION

*Elizabeth Kremen and Sahel Keshavarzi*

## METABOLISM

Glucose homeostasis is a delicate balance in neonates. At term, the fetus forms 100 kcal/d of glycogen stores, and in a healthy neonate, these glycogen stores may form 5% of the infant's total weight. Within 2 days postbirth, that store is depleted, and the infant switches to gluconeogenesis, providing glucose at 4 mg/kg/min.[1]

In terms of daily feeding, children require 0.5–3 mg/kg protein, 6–9 mg/kg glucose, and 0.5–3 g/kg fat. In the hospital and perioperative setting, critically ill children are often in a hypermetabolic state requiring hyperalimentation, often with two solutions, a fatty infusion and a glucose/protein infusion. Intraoperatively, the fat solution is often paused to avoid risks of contamination, but the glucose/protein solution should be continued at the same rate or at two-thirds to one-half the rate. Due to periods of intense stress, the child will likely have elevated insulin levels. Continuing the protein/glucose infusion, along with performing regular glucose checks, is recommended to avoid potentially severe hypoglycemia. In healthy children, intraoperatively, many physicians avoid giving dextrose as hyperglycemia may exacerbate neurological injury in the setting of an ischemic or hypoxic event.[1]

In terms of drug metabolism, the main routes of excretion are the hepatobiliary system, the kidneys, and the lungs. Due to lower organ mass compared to adults and fewer functional enzymes, decreased clearance, and increased relative volume of distribution, most drug metabolism is prolonged in neonates. For hepatically cleared drugs, half-lives are prolonged in neonates, decreased in children 4 to 10 years of age, and reach adult values in adolescents.[2]

## FLUID DISTRIBUTION

Fluid is distributed in different spaces, primarily intracellular versus extracellular (interstitial and intravascular). In utero, total body water (TBW) is approximately one-third intracellular and two-thirds extracellular initially and switches to approximately 50–50 at birth, and then two-thirds intracellular and one-third extracellular as an adult. The balance of fluid between these compartments is highly regulated (Figure 235.1). TBW content also changes with age, where it is approximately 75%–80% in neonates and progressively drops as children grow to reach adult levels, approximately 55%–60%, by adolescence, with some variation between gender as adipose tissue carries less water.[1]

During surgery, intravascular fluid loss or relative fluid loss may occur through (1) anesthetic-induced vascular relaxation resulting in a relative or "virtual" loss; (2) direct whole-blood loss; and (3) extravasation due to surgical trauma, with accompanying capillary leakage and loss of oncotic pressure. In smaller infants, direct evaporation from the surgical field is also an issue. Generally, the smaller the patient, the less the tolerance for dehydration is. The blood volume of preterm and critically ill neonates is approximately 100 mL/kg. In a healthy neonate, the blood volume is approximately 80 mL/kg. Blood volume by weight increases in the first 2 months of age, then starts to drop again, getting to 70 mL/kg at 12 months.[3]

Intraoperatively, blood loss may be replaced 1:1 with colloid (blood or albumin) or 1:1.5 with isotonic crystalloid. With procedures involving minor trauma, third-spacing repletion should be 3–4 mL/kg/h, whereas moderate trauma may require 5–7 mL/kg/h. Large traumatic cases may require 10 mL/kg/h, and severe cases in neonates (e.g., emergent necrotizing enterocolitis) may be 50 mL/kg/h. Underrepletion with crystalloid may lead to hypotension, but overrepletion may lead to hemodilution, third spacing, pulmonary edema, bowel swelling, heart failure, laryngotracheal edema, and anasarca.[1]

Water follows salt. Under normal circumstances, if there is increased retention of salt, there will be an increased retention of water and increased intravascular volume. Factors influencing fluid retention are thirst, arginine vasopressin (AVP), and renal concentrating ability. Normal serum osmolality is between 280 and 300 mOsm/L, where

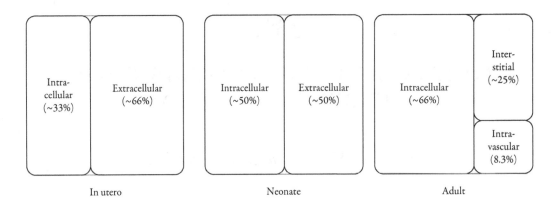

**Figure 235.1** Total body water (TBW) broken into compartments with variations by age. In adults, TBW is two-thirds intracellular, one-third extracellular. The extracellular compartment comprises approximately three-fourths interstitial fluid (or one-fourth of the TBW in adults) and one-fourth intravascular fluid (or 8.3% TBW).

even a 1% change can trigger a response. Baroreceptors, such as those in the aortic arch and carotid sinus, may override osmotic signals; thus, a hypotensive patient will be triggered to retain fluid even with low plasma osmolality.[1]

Albumin and other large soluble proteins contribute significantly to colloid oncotic pressure, as they are more likely, due to size, to stay in the intravascular space. When there is a disruption of vascular membranes, as after a major trauma, there may be an increased leak from the intravascular space.

## RENAL FUNCTION

Renal development starts at 5 weeks' gestation, and nephrons continue to develop through the 38th week.[4] The outermost cortex may continue to develop for several months. From early gestation, when renal blood flow is approximately one-fifth of normal, to the end of gestation, when it rises to one-third, renal vascular resistance slowly decreases. At birth, the vascular resistance drops further, and kidney filtration function, or the glomerular filtration rate (GFR), increases. GFR and renal plasma flow in neonates are 30% of those in adults. At 6 months, they increase to 60%, and at 1 year they become 90% of adult values.[1]

Despite having a low GFR in utero, fetal urine formation is brisk because there is poor resorption of sodium and water. In neonates, intrarenal sodium and urea gradients are much less than they are in adults; therefore, the neonate's urine-concentrating ability is much weaker than the adult kidney, with the maximum urine osmolality approximately half that of an adult. Neonates may more easily become hyponatremic due to poor renal concentrating ability. Furthermore, neonates must secrete more urine to be able to eliminate similar amounts of solutes, which may easily

lead to dehydration.[1] Similarly, renally excreted drugs have a prolonged elimination half-life in neonates.

In an acutely hypertensive child, the renal function and pressure gradient work together to move the blood pressure back to equilibrium, with both pressure diuresis and natriuresis (from decreased AVP). Additionally, atrial fibers may stretch in a fluid-overloaded patient, stimulating the release of atrial natriuretic peptide, which may lead to vasodilation, the increase of the GFR, and further diuresis.[1]

In an acutely hypotensive child, the renin-angiotensin system is activated, wherein decreased renal perfusion leads to the release of renin from the juxtaglomerular apparatus. Renin converts angiotensinogen to angiotensin I, which goes through the bloodstream to the lung epithelium and is converted to angiotensin II. Angiotensin II then stimulates the secretion of aldosterone, increases salt and water retention, and causes vasoconstriction. These homeostasis-regulating mechanisms allow the patient to maintain a narrow range of blood pressures and intravascular volume status even with a wider range of salt and water levels.[1]

## REFERENCES

1. McClain CD, McManus ML. Fluid Management. In: Coté CJ, et al., eds. *Coté and Lerman's a Practice of Anesthesia for Infants and Children*. 6th ed. Elsevier; 2019: Chap. 9.
2. Anderson BJ, et al. Pharmacokinetics and pharmacology of drugs used in children. In: Coté CJ, et al., eds. *Coté and Lerman's a Practice of Anesthesia for Infants and Children*. 6th ed. Elsevier; 2019: Chap. 7.
3. Coté CJ, et al. Strategies for blood product management, reducing transfusions, and massive blood transfusion. In: Coté CJ, et al., eds. *Coté and Lerman's a Practice of Anesthesia for Infants and Children*. 6th ed. Elsevier; 2019: Chap. 12.
4. Marciniak B. Growth and development. In: Coté CJ, et al., eds. *Coté and Lerman's a Practice of Anesthesia for Infants and Children*. 6th ed. Elsevier; 2019: Chap. 2.

# 236.

# THERMAL REGULATION

*David Bennett and Shelley Ohliger*

## INTRODUCTION

Neonates are particularly susceptible to temperature variability from environmental factors. Undergoing anesthesia and surgery can promote further temperature instability. Abnormal temperatures in pediatric patients can have significant consequences in the perioperative period.

## NEONATAL ANATOMY AND PHYSIOLOGY

Neonatal patients have up to three times the ratio of total body surface area to volume as compared to adults, allowing proportionally greater heat loss. The head of a neonate can account for up to 20% of total body surface area and can contribute to significant heat loss in the pediatric patient. The head is highly vascularized and poorly insulated due to thin cranial bones and scant hair. Other factors predisposing to hypothermia include thin skin, relatively low subcutaneous fat stores for insulation, inability to shiver, and an immature autonomic nervous system.[1]

## THERMOREGULATION

Neonatal thermoregulation is accomplished primarily by nonshivering thermogenesis, vasoconstriction and environmental control. Voluntary muscle movement, involuntary muscle movement (shivering), and dietary thermogenesis also generate heat, but are less significant in this population.[1] Infants do not develop the ability to shiver until approximately 6 months of age and rely on nonshivering thermogenesis for heat production. Nonshivering thermogenesis occurs due to the metabolism of brown fat.

Accounting for up to 5% of body mass in the neonate, brown fat has high levels of mitochondria containing thermogenin. When hypothermia occurs, noradrenergic stimulation at β-adrenergic receptors cause thermogenin to uncouple the process of oxidative phosphorylation to generate heat. Brown fat is found between the scapulae,

above the clavicles, throughout the mediastinum, and surrounding the kidneys and trachea (Figure 236.1). When fully active, brown fat may receive up to 25% of cardiac output and can double metabolic heat production. Premature and sick infants may have diminished stores of brown fat and a subsequently poor ability to generate heat. Pediatric patients anesthetized with both propofol and fentanyl demonstrate inhibition of brown adipose tissue activation in a dose-dependent fashion (Sessler, 2016). Volatile anesthetics at clinically relevant concentrations also inhibit norepinephrine-induced brown fat metabolism.[2] Anesthetics also reduce basal metabolic heat generation by about 30%.[1]

A neutral thermal environment refers to the ambient temperature at which a neonate is able to maintain a normal temperature with minimal oxygen demand. The most significant method of thermoregulation outside of a neutral thermal environment is behavioral or environmental modification by the subject, which are not significant factors in the neonate. The first autonomic response to hypothermia is peripheral vasoconstriction, which allows for up to a 25% reduction in heat loss.[1] However, most commonly used anesthetics, including volatile anesthetics, nitrous oxide, propofol, and opioids, decrease vasoconstriction temperature thresholds, thereby suppressing the ability of the patient to retain heat.[3]

## HEAT LOSS

Conditions in the perioperative period can produce clinically significant hypothermia. Humans have a range of internal temperatures at which no thermoregulatory responses are initiated, known as the interthreshold range. This range is approximately 0.4° in the awake patient; this range broadens to roughly 0.8° with regional anesthesia and 3.5° with general anesthesia, which increases the risk of hypothermia.[1]

Heat loss during anesthesia occurs through several stages. The first stage is heat redistribution caused by the profound vasodilation accompanying induction and anesthetic

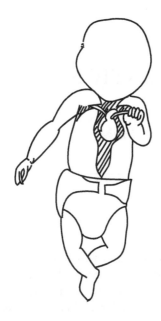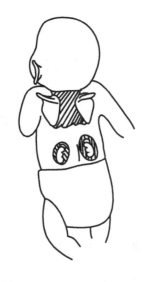

Figure 236.1 Distribution of brown fat in the neonate.

maintenance. Heat transfers from the central compartment to the periphery, such as the limbs, accounting for some 80% of the drop in central temperature in the first hour of anesthesia. The second stage is heat transferring from the skin to the environment via conduction, convection, evaporation, and radiation. The major conduit of heat loss in the newborn is radiation (39% of total heat loss), followed by convection (34%), evaporation (24%), and finally conduction (3%).[1]

With decreased temperature (below the interthreshold range), the body conserves temperature by first vasoconstriction, then nonshivering thermogenesis, and then shivering (in order). With increased temperature (above the interthreshold range), the body loses temperature by first sweating and then vasodilation (in order).

It is important to note that factors that increase heat loss in pediatric patients, such as increased surface area to volume, also increase the ease and speed of rewarming the patient.

## CONSEQUENCES OF HYPOTHERMIA

Regarding infants and children, the World Health Organization has defined mild hypothermia as a core temperature ranging from 36.0°C to 36.4°C, moderate hypothermia as 32.0°C to 35.9°C, and severe hypothermia as below 32°C. Some studies indicated that up to 50% of pediatric patients experience at least moderate intraoperative hypothermia.[4]

Hypothermia can increase metabolic oxygen demand and compensatory norepinephrine release, which can lead to pulmonary and peripheral vasoconstriction, hypoglycemia, and metabolic acidosis.[1] Vasoconstriction decreases oxygen delivery to the wound site, suppressing both wound healing and immune system activation against infection.

With a core temperature of less than 36°, anesthetized patients may experience slow intracardiac conduction, cardiac dysrhythmias (most commonly bradycardia), decreased myocardial contractility, decreased cardiac output, myocardial ischemia, respiratory depression, coagulopathy, and prolonged effect of various anesthetics. With reductions of core temperature of even 1°, blood loss can increase by 20% due to reduced release of thromboxane $A_3$ and other cold-induced coagulopathies.[5] Hypothermia decreases the minimum alveolar concentration of inhalation agents.

## CONSEQUENCES OF HYPERTHERMIA

Intraoperatively, hyperthermia occurs most commonly as a result of iatrogenic overheating. Noniatrogenic fever is rare given that both volatile anesthetics and opioids suppress the fever response. However, fever can be caused by infection, medication reactions, blood transfusion reactions, or rarely, malignant hyperthermia. Hyperthermia can result in tachycardia, dehydration, and lethargy.

## ANESTHETIC CONSIDERATIONS

- Neonates are more prone to perioperative hypothermia than adult patients due to an increased ratio of surface area to volume and also respond more readily to rewarming.
- Neonates primarily rely on brown fat for heat production, with shivering developing at around 6 months of life.
- Most anesthetics inhibit thermoregulatory responses, thereby predisposing to hypothermia.

## REFERENCES

1. Luginbuehl I, et al. Thermoregulation: physiology and perioperative disturbances. In: Davis P, Cladis F, ed. *Smith's Anesthesia for Infants and Children*. 9th ed. Philadelphia, PA: Elsevier; 2017.
2. Ohlson KBE, et al. Thermogenesis inhibition in brown adipocytes is a specific property of volatile anesthetics. *Anesthesiology*. 2003;98:437–448.
3. Kurz A. Physiology of thermoregulation. *Best Pract Res Clin Anaesthesiol*. 2008;22(4):627–644.
4. Pearce B, et al. Perioperative hypothermia in the pediatric population: prevalence, risk factors, and outcomes. *J Anesth Clin Res*. 2010;1:102.
5. Sessler D. Perioperative thermoregulation and heat balance. *Lancet*. 2016;387:2655–2664.

# 237.

# FETAL HEMOGLOBIN

*Alex Y. Chung and Dominic S. Carollo*

## INTRODUCTION

Fetal hemoglobin (HbF) is a physiologic variant of the adult hemoglobin (HbA) protein. It is primarily present in the fetus. HbA has a lower oxygen affinity than HbF. As a newborn's predominant hemoglobin transitions from HbF to HbA, the degree of oxygen saturation of hemoglobin can differ for a given partial pressure of oxygen. Transfusion with HbA blood or premature birth can affect when this transition occurs.

## PHYSIOLOGY

Maternal erythropoietin does not cross the placenta; therefore, red blood cell (RBC) production in the fetus is controlled only by fetal growth factors. HbF is not the first form of hemoglobin present in the embryo. For the first 6 weeks of the embryo, RBCs consist of embryonic hemoglobin (Hbε or hemoglobin epsilon).

Fetal hemoglobin is produced by the liver starting at 6 weeks gestational age (wGA) and becomes the dominant form after 3 months (Figure 237.1). It is composed of two α (alpha) subunits and two γ (gamma) subunits. Beginning at approximately 32 wGA, HbF begins to be replaced by HbA, which is composed of two α-subunits and two β (beta) subunits.[1] At 40 wGA, HbF accounts for 70% of fetal hemoglobin.[2] This switchover rate is consistent in infants delivered prematurely, as it is dependent on postconceptual age, not postnatal age.[1] This observation may be due to stimulation of erythropoiesis of HbF by conditions such as anemia of prematurity or history of intrauterine growth restriction due to placental insufficiency. HbF is selected for in hemoglobinopathies such as sickle cell disease and thalassemia. It is also seen in adults with chronic lung disease and anemia.[1] Hereditary presence of fetal hemoglobin is a rare, a benign condition in which the body continues to produce HbF into adulthood. About 10% of the population has an HbF level of more than 1%. Typically, HbF wanes to negligible levels 6 months after birth.[3]

Fetal hemoglobin has higher oxygen affinity than HbA. This correlates to a left shift from HbA on the oxygen-hemoglobin dissociation curve (Figure 237.2). The minimum partial pressure of oxygen needed for 50% of hemoglobin to be bound to oxygen (P50) is 19 mm Hg for HbF and 26.8 mm Hg for HbA. This allows for oxygen transfer from maternal circulation to fetal circulation across the placenta.

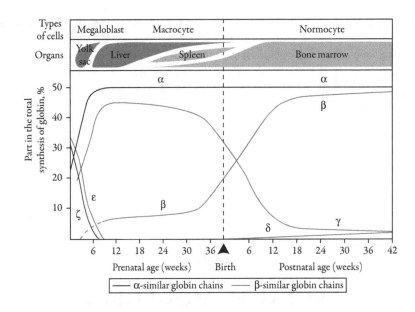

**Figure 237.1** Proportions of different hemoglobin variants over age of the fetus and infant. Different hemoglobin variants are produced in different organs. From Wood WG. Haemoglobin synthesis during human fetal development. *British Medical Journal*. 1976;32(3):282–287.

## ANESTHETIC CONSIDERATIONS

### PREOPERATIVE

A patient with history of hematologic disorders such as sickle cell anemia may need preoperative optimization, including admission and consultation with a hematologist.

Hydroxyurea is a myelosuppressive agent that increases the level of HbF and reduces sickling in sickle cell patients, as HbF does not contain the subunits affected by sickle cell anemia. Perioperatively, sickle cell children taking hydroxyurea had fewer transfusions than those not taking hydroxyurea.[4]

History of an infant should always include history of prematurity and current postconceptual age. Infants born

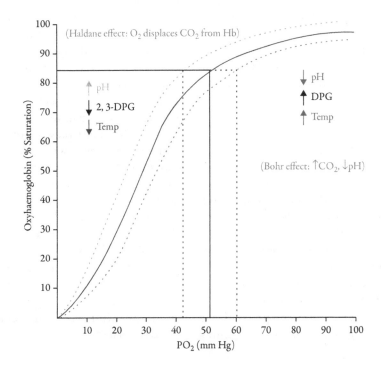

**Figure 237.2** The oxygen-hemoglobin dissociation curve for adult hemoglobin, fetal hemoglobin, and myoglobin. 2,3-DPG, 2,3-Diphosphoglycerate. From the public domain. Accessed July 1, 2020. https://en.wikipedia.org/wiki/Oxygen%E2%80%93hemoglobin_dissociation_curve

prematurely will maintain a substantial level of HbF, which affects intraoperative monitoring and management.

Review of pertinent laboratory studies such as the complete blood count is essential. The starting hematocrit is a vital part of calculating the maximum allowable blood loss to determine the transfusion threshold and adequately preparing packed RBCs before an operation with high risk of blood loss. The mean corpuscular volume (MCV) can provide a reliable estimate of the proportion of hemoglobin that is composed of HbF. HbF has a higher MCV than HbA. Therefore, a higher MCV would reflect a higher proportion of HbF. This relationship is linear and can be represented by the equation HbF (%) = (2.6 × MCV) - 215.[5]

Last, it is important to note the transfusion history of the patient. In addition to inherent risks and effects on hematocrit and volume status in the short term, transfusions can lead to antibody formation and affect HbF levels.

## INTRAOPERATIVE

When a neonate with HbF requires a transfusion, the donor packed RBCs contain HbA. This will move the oxygen-hemoglobin dissociation curve to the right of HbF, the degree depending on the percentage of circulating blood volume replaced with transfused packed RBCs. In very low-birth-weight infants, two 15-mL/kg packed RBC transfusions within the first month of life will cause HbA to be the predominant hemoglobin.[5] The change in the oxygen-hemoglobin dissociation curve creates an increase in the partial pressure of oxygen ($PO_2$) required to achieve a certain oxygen saturation ($SO_2$). For example, a neonate with 90% HbF at a certain $PO_2$ will have an $SO_2$ of 94%. After transfusion that reduces the amount of HbF to 30%, that same $PO_2$ will correlate to an $SO_2$ of 85%.[5] $PO_2$ in a patient with tenuous respiratory status may need to be improved if the patient is HbF

dominant and about to be transfused with a significant amount of HbA blood.

A blood gas analyzer has presets for HbF: 0% and 80%. A term newborn would give most accurate results using the 80% HbF preset. A newborn who has received transfusion of HbA packed RBCs would need to be analyzed using the 0% HbF preset for the most accurate results.[2] A sample of 80% HbF blood with a $PO_2$ corresponding to an $SO_2$ of 92% to 97% would be reported by a blood gas analyzer to have an $SO_2$ of 86%–95% if the blood gas analyzer was not corrected for fetal hemoglobin.[2]

The $SO_2$ is the most significant component of intravascular oxygen content and tissue delivery of oxygen. Oxygenation is one of the standards for basic anesthetic monitoring by the American Society of Anesthesiologists, and optimal oxygenation is a principal clinical goal of intraoperative management. For example, $SO_2$ is a crucial parameter in pediatric cardiac anesthesia with single-ventricle physiology, as oxygenation will affect the proportion of pulmonary blood flow and systemic blood flow. A systemic oxygen saturation of 80% is recognized as optimal for equal pulmonary and systemic blood flows.

## REFERENCES

1. Bard H, et al. The reactivation of fetal hemoglobin synthesis during anemia of prematurity. *Pediatr Res.* 1994;36(2):253–256.
2. Rabi Y, et al. Blood gases: technical aspects and interpretation. In: Goldsmith JP, et al., eds. *Assisted Ventilation of the Neonate.* Philadelphia: Elsevier; 2017:80–96.
3. Edoh D, et al. Fetal hemoglobin during infancy and in sickle cell adults. *Afr Health Sci.* 2006;6(1):51–54.
4. Hayashi M, et al. Impact of hydroxyurea on perioperative management and outcomes in children with sickle cell anemia. *J Pediatr Hematol Oncol.* 2011;33(7):487–490.
5. Barkemeyer BM, Hempe JM. Effect of transfusion on hemoglobin variants in preterm infants. *J Perinatol.* 2000;20(6):355–358.

# 238.

# PREMATURITY

*Michael J. Gyorfi and Alaa Abd-Elsayed*

## INTRODUCTION

Prematurity is defined as an infant born before 37 weeks of gestation. Preterm infants are often classified by birthweight. For example, very low birthweight is below 1500 g. Preterm birth is associated with 30% of infant mortality, 45% of cerebral palsy, and numerous other complications. The risk of mortality and morbidity are inversely related to gestational age. Extremely preterm infants are delivered before 25 weeks' gestation and are at the greatest risk.[1]

Premature infants are subject to complications in the short term and/or chronic conditions. The most prevalent complications include respiratory, retinal, gastrointestinal, cardiovascular, infectious, and neurodevelopmental disabilities.

## COMPLICATIONS OF PREMATURITY

Respiratory distress syndrome (RDS) is the earliest complication associated with prematurity. RDS is a result of decreased surfactant production in premature lungs. Surfactant increases lung compliance and helps increase gas exchange. The severity of RDS is inversely related to the gestational age. Symptoms of RDS include hypoxemia, tachypnea, hypercarbia, and acidosis. Antenatal corticosteroid therapy should be administered to all pregnant women at 23 to 34 weeks' gestation with an increased risk of preterm delivery.[1,2]

There are also long-term pulmonary complications associated with prematurity. Bronchopulmonary dysplasia (BPD), which is defined as the need for supplemental oxygen at 36 weeks' postmenstrual age. BPD affects approximately 30% of extremely low birthweight infants.[1,2] Preterm infants who required ventilatory support along with those with infections are at an increased risk of developing BPD due to the potential mechanical injury, oxidative stress, and inflammation.[1-3).

Bacterial infections leading to sepsis is seen in approximately 25% of very low birthweight infants. Preterm infants are immunocompromised due to both their innate and adaptive immune systems being underdeveloped. Premature infants often require invasive tests, such as central lines, blood draws, and intubations, which increase the risk of infection.[1-3]

Necrotizing enterocolitis (NEC) is a serious gastrointestinal complication seen in premature infants. Immature gastrointestinal mucosa has a decreased immune defense, motility, and protective barrier. Immature intestines are also susceptible to ischemic insults and are easily colonized with bacteria. The disease onset is often insidious, with symptoms such as feeding intolerance and distention. NEC may also present with intestinal perforation, hypotension, and disseminated intravascular coagulopathy.[1,2] Standard management is with urgent bowel rest and antibiotic therapy, with severe cases needing surgical intervention. Intestinal strictures, short-bowel syndrome, and feeding intolerance are potential sequelae of NEC.[2,3]

Periventricular leukomalacia (PVL) and intraventricular hemorrhage (IVH) are the most significant perinatal brain injuries seen primarily in premature infants. PVL is defined as a cerebral white matter injury. This often leads to the development of cerebral palsy. Systemic inflammation following a neonatal infection paired with an ischemic attack predisposes a premature infant to PVL. Magnetic resonance imaging is used to diagnose PVL in neonates. Parenchymal cysts and reduced white and gray matter volumes are often seen with PVL.[1-3]

Intraventricular hemorrhage is defined as bleeding within the ventricles that may extend into the surrounding parenchyma. The hemorrhage begins at the site of neuronal proliferation, termed the subependymal germinal matrix. Blood vessels supplying the matrix are fragile and are at an increased risk of rupturing with changes in pressure and cerebral blood flow. Posthemorrhagic hydrocephalus is a severe complication from IVH. IVH has a 28% to 37%

mortality in premature infants. Long-term complications include cognitive impairment, seizures, and cerebral palsy.[1-3]

Retinopathy of prematurity (ROP) affects approximately 50,000 infants worldwide each year. ROP can result in severe visual impairments and potentially blindness in infants. ROP is described as abnormal vascular proliferation within the retina. This abnormal vasculature is related to the increased local reactive oxygen species leading to angiogenic growth factors. Decreased oxygen administration has resulted in a drastic decrease in the incidence of ROP in developed countries.[1-3]

## VENTILATION AND ANESTHETIC CONSIDERATIONS

Premature infants born with an inadequate surfactant supply are surviving longer with prompt steroid administration paired with surfactant therapy. This has reduced mortality from acute RDS but has increased that of BPD due to an increased survival rate for immature infants. Limiting exposure to high oxygen concentration and tidal volumes serves to reduce mechanical and oxidative lung injury along with decreasing ROP.[1,4]

Sedatives are not routinely utilized in premature infants or young children. Distraction techniques with toys, videos, and glucose suffice for the majority of kids. Sedatives are associated with increased respiratory complications, apnea, and bradycardia, in addition to a prolonged duration of action in children due to hepatic immaturity.[4] A meta-analysis comparing randomized controlled trials of infants who received general anesthesia versus spinal anesthesia for inguinal hernia repairs demonstrated a similar incidence in apnea. However, they isolated spinal anesthesia without sedatives, which demonstrated a vastly reduced rate of apnea.[5] The downside to regional anesthesia in infants is the high technical failure rate. General anesthesia is typically performed with short-acting anesthetic medications with attempts to limit opioids and neuromuscular-blocking agents when possible.[4,5]

Postoperative pain management in infants follows a multimodal approach that utilizes local anesthetics and neuraxial and peripheral nerve block techniques. Systemic nonsteroidal anti-inflammatory drugs and acetaminophen are preferred over the use of opioids. If opioids are necessary, extended respiratory support and intensive monitoring may be required.[4]

Temperature regulation is a challenge in premature infants due to their relatively thin epidermis and increased fluid loss through the skin. The ratio of body surface area to weight increases thermal conductance and heat loss.[1,4]

## REFERENCES

1. Eichenwald EC, Stark AR. Management and outcomes of very low birth weight. *N Engl J Med*. 2008;358(16):1700–1711.
2. Natarajan G, Shankaran S. Short- and long-term outcomes of moderate and late preterm infants. *Am J Perinatol*. 2016;33(3):305–317.
3. Perlman JM, et al.; Neonatal Resuscitation Chapter Collaborators. Part 7: neonatal resuscitation: 2015 international consensus on cardiopulmonary resuscitation and emergency cardiovascular care science with treatment recommendations. *Circulation*. 2015;132(16 suppl 1):S204–S241.
4. Taneja B, et al. Physiological and anaesthetic considerations for the preterm neonate undergoing surgery. *J Neonatal Surg*. 2012;1(1):14.
5. Jones LJ, et al. Regional (spinal, epidural, caudal) versus general anaesthesia in preterm infants undergoing inguinal herniorrhaphy in early infancy. *Cochrane Database Syst Rev*. 2015;2015(6):CD003669.

# 239.

# BRONCHOPULMONARY DYSPLASIA

*Jonathan W. Klein*

## INTRODUCTION

Bronchopulmonary dysplasia (BPD), also known as arrest of lung development or evolving chronic lung disease, is a serious lung condition affecting approximately 10,000 premature infants per year. There are various criteria regarding the classification of this disease process. One of the established criteria for BPD diagnosis is the time period these infants require prolonged supplemental oxygen and/or mechanical ventilation greater than or equal to 28 postnatal days. The most widely used current classifications divides BPD into mild, moderate, and severe based on the degree of support required at critical junctures. Mild BPD is defined as any supplemental oxygen requirement at 28 days of life, moderate BPD is defined as any supplemental oxygen requirement less than 0.3 $FiO_2$ (fraction of inspired oxygen) at 36 weeks, while severe BPD is defined as a supplemental oxygen requirement with an $FiO_2$ greater than 0.3 and/or the need for positive pressure respiratory support at 36 weeks of corrected gestational age (CGA).[1] Another diagnostic feature of BPD is the chest radiograph. The chest X-ray displays a distorted parenchymal pattern with small radiolucent cysts and hyper-expanded lung fields.[2]

Bronchopulmonary dysplasia displays a pattern of arrested development of the airways with dilation of the alveolar ducts. A consistent factor regarding these patients is prematurity. Additional factors include infection, inflammation, genetics, prolonged mechanical ventilation, and greater oxygen requirements, leading to oxygen toxicity as well as chorioamnionitis and the presence of a patent ductus arteriosus.[2] Mechanical ventilation–induced trauma may be a result of volutrauma or barotrauma. However, it has been noted that some infants have developed BPD with minimal exposure to oxygen, minimal ventilation settings, and mild infective processes.[1] These numerous factors lead to an inflammatory cascade resulting in oxidative stress via increased cytokines and subsequent inflammation to the patient's lung fields.[2]

Ventilation strategies have evolved throughout the history of this profound respiratory condition. Abman et al. published ventilator strategies not only to manage severe BPD but also to aid in its prevention. These recommendations include lower tidal volumes with short inspiratory times in the first days of life for those premature infants requiring mechanical ventilation to optimize gas exchange.[3] Along with increased positive end-expiratory pressure (PEEP), $FiO_2$ to target SpO2 88%–93% and permissive hypercapnia, these strategies combine to aid in the prevention of acute lung disease.[3] However, researchers have established larger tidal volumes (10–12 mL/kg), longer inspiratory time ($\geq$0.6 seconds), $FiO_2$ to target increased $SpO_2$ (92%–96%), permissive hypercapnia, and a lower respiratory rate to prevent air stacking, especially for larger tidal volumes, aid in the treatment and management of cases of severe BPD.[3] Additionally, researchers noted that changes in rate, tidal volume, inspiratory and expiratory time, and pressure support are highly independent and may need to be altered on an individual basis. In addition to these ventilator strategies, the uses of antenatal steroids and exogenous surfactant treatments have helped to decrease the incidence of BPD.[2]

## ANESTHETIC CONSIDERATIONS

### PREOPERATIVE

Comorbidities and commonly related diagnoses of the premature patient population must be evaluated prior to the operating room. These include but are not limited to any congenital heart defects, neurological issues (i.e., intraventricular hemorrhage and/or hydrocephalus), any renal insufficiencies or impairment, and current pulmonary status and ventilation strategies.[2] An echocardiogram should be performed to establish cardiac function; also a cranial ultrasound can aid in the diagnosis of any neurological issues. Current laboratory values must be reviewed for the possibility of any anemia and any other hematologic issues or electrolyte imbalances, which must be corrected prior to the operating room. Current renal function should also be evaluated with a renal function panel. In addition to these diagnostic modalities, a focused and thorough review and plan for ventilator settings and airway evaluation must be performed due to the potential for difficult airway and ventilation. Preoperative care is aimed at optimizing an already fragile patient for the operating room.

## INTRAOPERATIVE

Ventilation aimed at the prevention of BPD and ventilation for the management of BPD require different methods of treatment and therefore require varying ventilator goals and strategies as described above. The anesthesia provider should aim to maintain these specific ventilator goals and strategies during the intraoperative period. In addition, the type of procedure performed will guide the setup and anesthetic management for each patient. Adequate warming strategies are imperative for all premature infants in the operating room due to the physiologic derangement that couples hypothermia. Also, adequate intravenous access must be established in order to provide fluid resuscitation as well as any glucose-containing fluid to prevent hypoglycemia. Analgesia may be supplied with standard narcotics; however, this patient population has a high susceptibility to postoperative respiratory depression and should be taken into consideration.

## POSTOPERATIVE

Given the fragility of this patient population and their ventilation requirements, these patients will most likely remain intubated postoperatively in the neonatal intensive care unit. Focused intraoperative fluid resuscitation and blood product replacement are vital to maintaining hemodynamics postoperatively and should be carefully evaluated. Moreover, attempting to maintain the previously prescribed ventilator strategies is key to preserving the current pulmonary function.

## REFERENCES

1. Shepherd EG, et al. Mechanical ventilation of the infant with severe bronchopulmonary dysplasia, respiratory management of newborns. IntechOpen. August 2016.
2. Roberts JD, et al. Neonatal emergencies. In: Cote CJ, et al., eds. *A Practice of Anesthesia for Infants and Children.* 6th ed. Elsevier; 2019:864–865.
3. Abman SH, et al. Interdisciplinary care of children with severe bronchopulmonary dysplasia. J Pediatr. 2017;181:12–28.

# 240.

# CONGENITAL HEART AND MAJOR VASCULAR DISEASE

*Jamie W. Sinton*

## INTRODUCTION

The global burden of congenital heart disease (CHD) remains high: approximately 6/1000 live births.[1] While there is no mechanism for decreasing the prevalence of infants born with CHD, mortality from CHD has declined in countries with a higher sociodemographic index.

Perioperative risk in children with heart disease undergoing surgery can be impacted by type of surgery,[2] stage of heart defect palliation,[3] and case volume at a given center.[4]

## CLASSIFICATION OF CONGENITAL HEART DISEASE

Congenital heart disease can be broadly classified into acyanotic, cyanotic, major vascular disease, and pulmonary hypertension (PH).

### ACYANOTIC DEFECTS

Acyanotic defects include left-to-right shunting lesions as well as obstructive and valvular lesions. See Figure 240.1

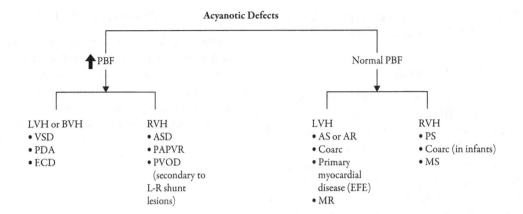

**Figure 240.1** A classification scheme for acyanotic congenital heart diseases. AR, aortic regurgitation; AS, aortic stenosis; ASD, atrial septal defect; BVH, biventricular hypertrophy; Coarc, coarctation of the aorta; ECD, endocardial cushion defect; EFE, endocardial fibroelastosis; LVH, left ventricular hypertrophy; MR, mitral regurgitation; MS, mitral stenosis; PAPVR, partially anomalous pulmonary venous return; PBF, pulmonary blood flow; PDA, patent ductus arteriosus; PS, pulmonic stenosis; PVOD, pulmonary vascular occlusive disease; RBBB, right bundle-branch block; RVH, right ventricular hypertrophy; VSD, ventricular septal defect.

for further classification of acyanotic lesions by magnitude of pulmonary blood flow.

## CYANOTIC DEFECTS

Cyanotic defects represent a wide range of pathology. Figure 240.2 further classifies cyanotic heart disease based on pulmonary blood flow. Cyanotic CHD has quite variable and often single-ventricular physiology. Lesions are discussed separately other chapters in this book.

## MAJOR VASCULAR DISEASE

The etiology of major vascular disease often occurs in the embryonic period as the primitive heart tube begins to develop. Pathology in embryonic aortic arches 4 and 6 are the major sources of major vascular diseases, such as coarctation of the aorta and vascular rings. The term *vascular ring* includes malformations such as double aortic arch, right aortic arch with ligamentum, pulmonary artery sling, and left aortic arch with aberrant right subclavian artery.

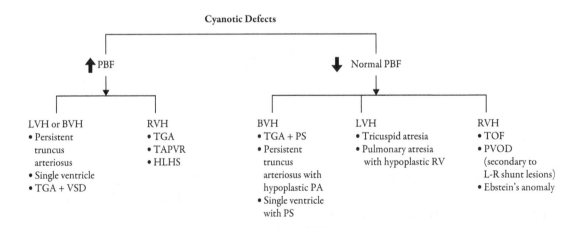

**Figure 240.2** A classification of cyanotic CHDs based on relative amount of pulmonary blood flow. Figure 240.1 shows a classification scheme for acyanotic congenital heart diseases. BVH, biventricular hypertrophy; HLHS, hypoplastic left heart syndrome; LVH, left ventricular hypertrophy; PA, pulmonary artery; PBF, pulmonary blood flow; PS, pulmonic stenosis; PVOD, pulmonary vascular occlusive disease; RBBB, right bundle-branch block; RV, right ventricle; TAPVR, totally anomalous pulmonary venous return; TGA + VSD, d-transposition of great arteries + ventricular septal defect; TOF, tetralogy of Fallot.

## Coarctation of the Aorta

Coarctation of the aorta can be classified in relation to the ductus arteriosus: preductal, ductal, postductal. Preductal coarctation obstructs aortic flow distal to the coarctation, and systemic perfusion depends on the patent ductus arteriosus (PDA). Ductal coarctations are normally not detected until around 2 weeks of life when the PDA closes. Infants present in extremis with elevated lactate levels as systemic perfusion distal to the PDA is compromised. Postductal coarctations occur in older children and adults. Patients present with upper extremity hypertension. The classic chest roentgenogram finding is rib notching due to collateral circulation.

## Vascular Rings

Congenital anomalies of the aortic arch complex can result in compression of the trachea and esophagus. Rings may be complete, incomplete, or involve the pulmonary artery. The anatomically complete ring is a double aortic arch. The incomplete ring is a right aortic arch with a left ligamentum arteriosum. Finally, a pulmonary sling occurs when the left pulmonary artery arises from the right pulmonary artery and crosses to the left side between the trachea and esophagus.

## PULMONARY HYPERTENSION

Pulmonary hypertension is classified by the World Health Organization (WHO) into groups based on etiology.[5] The five groups are as follows: (1) pulmonary arterial hypertension; (2) PH due to left heart disease; (3) PH due to lung disease and/or hypoxia; (4) chronic thromboembolic PH; and (5) PH with unclear multifactorial mechanisms. The Panama Classification of PH is very useful in pediatrics and includes a more granular cataloguing of etiologies of PH.

Pulmonary hypertension due to lung disease is commonly related to bronchopulmonary dysplasia (and prematurity). The outcome of PH in this group is directly related to respiratory robustness. Notably, children with Down syndrome have a high incidence of PH even with a structurally normal heart; PH in this population is of heterogenous origin but usually falls into WHO groups 1 and 3.

## ANESTHETIC CONSIDERATIONS

It is important to know factors that increase peripheral vascular resistance (PVR); they include hypoxia, hypercarbia, acidosis, hyperinflation, atelectasis, sympathetic stimulation, high hematocrit levels, and surgical constriction. Factors that decrease PVR include oxygen, hypocarbia, alkalosis, normal functional residual capacity, blocking sympathetic stimulation, and low hematocrit level.

## REFERENCES

1. Hoffman JIE, Kaplan S. The incidence of congenital heart disease. *J Am Coll Cardiol*. 2002;39(12):1890–1900.
2. Watkins SC, et al. Risks of noncardiac operations and other procedures in children with complex congenital heart disease. *Ann Thorac Surg*. 2013;95(1):204–211.
3. Carlo WF, et al. Interstage attrition between bidirectional Glenn and Fontan palliation in children with hypoplastic left heart syndrome. *J Thorac Cardiovasc Surg*.2011;142(3):511–516.
4. Kansy A, et al. Association of center volume with outcomes: analysis of verified data of European Association for CardioThoracic Surgery Congenital Database. *Ann Thorac Surg*. 2014;98(6):2159–2164.
5. Pulmonary Hypertension Association. About hypertension. The five groups. https://phassociation.org/types-pulmonary-hypertension-groups/.

# 241.

# CYANOTIC DEFECTS

*Jamie W. Sinton*

## CYANOTIC DEFECTS

### INTRODUCTION

Cyanotic congenital heart disease (CCHD) accounts for 1300 per million live births with congenital heart disease.[1] This review focuses on systemic complications of cyanosis and adaptations as well as hypoplastic left heart syndrome (HLHS), d-transposition of great arteries (d-TGA) and tetralogy of Fallot (TOF).

### CYANOSIS

Hypoxemia is a $PaO_2$ value below the normal 80–100 mm Hg. Cyanosis is the appearance of blue skin and mucous membranes due to at least 5 g of desaturated hemoglobin. During long-standing cyanosis, physiologic adaptations occur to preserve oxygen delivery. See Box 241.1 for details.

The three side effects of cyanosis are increased blood viscosity, coagulopathy, and urate metabolism. Bleeding tendency is attributed to inappropriate platelet activation and decreased plasma volume. Complications of chronic cyanosis include hyperviscosity and stroke, brain abscess, hypervolemia, gout, and microcytic anemia.

### HYPOPLASTIC LEFT HEART SYNDROME

Hypoplastic left heart syndrome is a CCHD in which systemic venous blood enters the right heart and the lungs,

---

**Box 241.1** PHYSIOLOGIC ADAPTATIONS TO CHRONIC CYANOSIS

---

Postnatal fetal hemoglobin production[2]

Lack of physiologic anemia of infancy[3]

Right shift of the Hb-$O_2$ dissociation curve

Increased erythropoietin production

---

followed by the pulmonary veins into the left atrium. Blood flow is obstructed at the mitral (and aortic) valve, so it crosses the atrial septal defect (ASD) and ejects into the pulmonary artery (PA), where it may cross the patent ductus arteriosus (PDA) to perfuse the body or reenter the lungs. Coronary perfusion is retrograde. An ASD and a PDA are required for survival and are maintained by balloon atrial septostomy if needed and prostaglandin $E_1$, respectively. Within the first few weeks of life, patients undergo stage 1 palliation with a Norwood or hybrid operation. The Norwood refers to the aortic arch reconstruction, while the source of pulmonary blood flow is variable.[4] The operation is performed with cardiopulmonary bypass (CPB) under regional low-flow perfusion with momentary deep hypothermic circulatory arrest. See the chapter on corrective and palliative cardiac surgery for details regarding CPB in children. Postoperatively, physiology is tenuous.

Around age 3 months, infants undergo superior cavopulmonary anastomosis (Glenn) in which the superior vena cava (SVC) is anastomosed to the PA. The prior source of pulmonary blood flow is removed. The Glenn circuit partially volume unloads the single ventricle. Postbypass ventilation favors hypercarbia as it increases oxygenation and decreases lactate.[5]

Preschool-aged children become candidates for the total cavopulmonary connection (Fontan). In the modern Fontan operation, the inferior vena cava is anastomosed to a tube that connects it to the PA. Cyanosis is relieved, ventricular volume overload decreases, and pulmonary blood flow is passive. Oxygen saturation is then normal, and the function of the single ventricle is often mildly depressed. Preload and cardiac output depend on low pulmonary vascular resistance (PVR) and adequate intravascular volume. The transpulmonary gradient (TPG) drives blood to the lungs. TPG is the difference between the mean (PA) pressure and the mean left atrial pressure or mean pulmonary capillary wedge pressure. Optimal hemodynamics incorporate sinus rhythm, low PVR, spontaneous ventilation, zero aortic arch obstruction, and minimal atrioventricular valve regurgitation.

## D-TRANSPOSITION OF THE GREAT ARTERIES

d-Transposition of the great arteries is a CCHD in which the great arteries arise from the opposite ventricles, and circulation proceeds in parallel. Systemic venous blood enters the right ventricle (RV) and then the aorta to perfuse the body with desaturated blood. Similarly, the pulmonary veins empty into the side only to be pumped back to the lungs. Clearly, a source of mixing is required for adequate oxygen delivery to the body.

Reverse differential cyanosis is pathognomonic for d-TGA physiology; the RV ejects desaturated blood into the aorta to perfuse the head and arms. At the PDA, this blood mixes with fully saturated blood from the subpulmonic ventricle to perfuse the lower body, giving the lower body a higher oxygen saturation than the upper body. Enlargement of the ASD via balloon atrial septostomy (BAS) enhances mixing. This lesion is ductal dependent. The arterial switch operation is the cure for d-TGA. The aorta and PA are transected, and the coronary arteries are translocated. ST segment change during following CPB indicates coronary obstruction.

## TETRALOGY OF FALLOT WITH PULMONARY STENOSIS

Tetralogy of Fallot is the most common CCHD. Its four classic lesions are pulmonic stenosis, ventricular septal defect (VSD), overriding aorta, and RV hypertrophy.

Newborns with TOF have a clinical course related to the severity of their right ventricular outflow tract obstruction (RVOTO). During agitation, paroxysms of RV infundibular muscle spasm trigger increased RVOTO, reduced Qp, hypotension, and ischemia: a hypercyanotic or "Tet" spell. Treatment includes oxygen, volume, afterload, and β-blockade. Prebypass management aims to preserve pulmonary blood flow.

Following CPB, the left ventricle is volume loaded, and junctional ectopic tachycardia (JET) sometimes occurs (see Figure 241.1). The ventricular rate exceeds the sinus. Treat by reducing sympathetic stimulation, preventing hyperthermia and deepening the anesthetic.

Post TOF repair, expect a dyskinetic ventricular septum due to the iatrogenic right bundle-branch block and the inability of the VSD patch to contract.

## ANESTHETIC CONSIDERATIONS

### PREOPERATIVE

Preoperatively, note the baseline oxygen saturation. Assess exercise tolerance based on weight gain and feeding. Consider cardiac anatomy, hemodynamic effect of the planned anesthetic, and the effects of cyanosis.[2]

### INTRAOPERATIVE

Intraoperatively, thoughtfully place and interpret monitors (e.g., avoid placing an arterial line on the side of a modified Blalock-Taussig shunt [MBTS] shunt or on the side of an aberrant subclavian artery if a transesophageal endotracheal

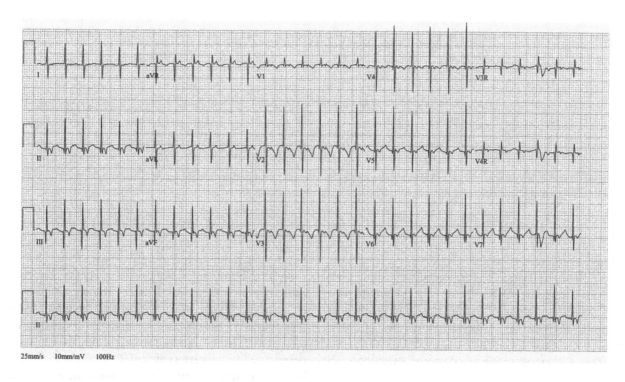

25mm/s   10mm/mV   100Hz

**Figure 241.1** An ECG of an infant in JET. Note retrograde p waves.

[TEE] is to be used). As the TEE probe enters the esophagus, it compresses the aberrant vessel, and the arterial line tracing is blunted and is of very limited utility. For patients with TOF, maintain systemic vascular resistance in order to maintain coronary perfusion and pulmonary blood flow even before a hypercyanotic spell occurs. Some would advocate for initiation of low-dose vasopressin as soon as the central line is in place. For those with HLHS, volume expansion with packed red blood cells and fresh frozen plasma is reasonable to ensure adequate hemoglobin and response to heparin. Ventilation with room air also maintains PVR and prevents overcirculation. In addition to standard and invasive monitors, give volume slowly and observe for cardiac enlargement on the surgical field. Postbypass hemostasis is challenging due to bleeding diathesis and perils of transfusion that can volume overload tenuous circulations.

## POSTOPERATIVE

Ventilation en route to the intensive care unit is exceedingly important, especially for those who are status post-Norwood with MBTS. Hyperventilation during this short transport will result in decreased PVR (avoid supplemental oxygen) and coronary steal, potentially with myocardial ischemia. Neonatal myocardium that has just undergone significant ischemic time on bypass will not tolerate it. Conversely, hypoventilation will worsen blood pH in the setting of (nearly certain) metabolic acidosis and impair myocardial function. Postoperative stroke and subclinical seizure are gaining attention. These events will be difficult to attribute to either a cannulation/bypass misadventure versus long-standing erythrocytosis.

## REFERENCES

1. Hoffman JI, Kaplan S. The incidence of congenital heart disease. *J Am Coll Cardiol.* 2002;39(12):1890–1900.
2. Zabala LM, Guzzetta NA. Cyanotic congenital heart disease (CCHD): focus on hypoxemia, secondary erythrocytosis, and coagulation alterations. *Pediatr Anesth.* 2015;25:981–989.
3. Rudolph A, et al. Hematologic adjustments to cyanotic congenital heart disease. 1953;11(5):454–465.
4. Newburger JW, et al. Transplant-free survival and interventions at 6 years in the SVR trial. *Circulation.* 2018;137(21):2246–2253.
5. Li J, et al. Effect of carbon dioxide on systemic oxygenation, oxygen consumption, and blood lactate levels after bidirectional superior cavopulmonary anastomosis. *Crit Care Med.* 2005;33(5):984–989.

# 242.

# ACYANOTIC DEFECTS

*Jamie W. Sinton*

## INTRODUCTION

Acyanotic cardiac defects include left-to-right shunting lesions, obstructive lesions, cardiomyopathy, and atrioventricular valvular (AVV) disease. Patent ductus arteriosus (PDA), tetralogy of Fallot, hypoplastic left heart syndrome, coarctation, cardiomyopathy, and pulmonic stenosis are discussed elsewhere. Isolated AVV disease are often seen following repair of complete atrioventricular canals (CAVC).

## SEPTAL DEFECTS

For categorization of left-to-right shunts see the chapter on congenital heart and major vascular disease. Left-to-right shunts are often due to septal defects. The magnitude of shunt depends on the size of the defect and the blood viscosity (determined by hematocrit). See Figure 242.1 for details.

For atrial-level shunts, the magnitude of shunt is also determined by relative ventricular compliance. In normal hearts, the right ventricle (RV) is much more elastic than

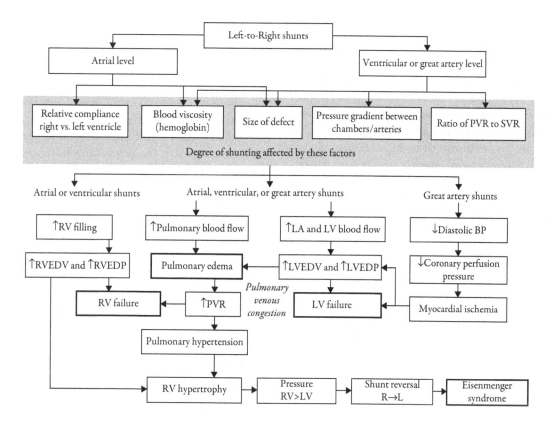

**Figure 242.1** The determinants of the degree of left-to-right shunting based on location of septal defect. BP, blood pressure; L, left; LA, left atrium; LV, left ventricle; LVEDP, left ventricle end-diastolic pressure; LVEDV, left ventricular end-diastolic volume; PVR, peripheral vascular resistance; R, right; RA, right atrium; RV, right ventricle; RVEDP, right ventricle end-diastolic pressure; RVEDV, right ventricular end-diastolic volume; SVR, systemic vascular resistance; LV, left ventricle.

the thicker left ventricle. Therefore, blood flows left to right across the atrial septum. Repair of an ASD is indicated if right heart dilation is present. Preschool age is a common time for repair of a secundum ASD. ASD repairs may be catheter-based or open surgical repairs. Figure 242.2A shows types of ASDs.

For shunts at the ventricular and great vessel level, the magnitude of shunting depends on the pressure gradient between the chambers and the ratio of pulmonary to systemic vascular resistance. Qualitatively, VSD size is compared to the aortic valve annulus size of that patient. Indications for repair of VSDs include aortic valve insufficiency and

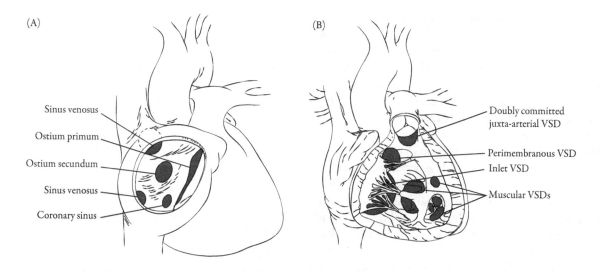

**Figure 242.2** Types of septal defects: (A) atrial septal defects and (B) ventricular septal defects (VSDs).

left-sided heart dilation. See Figure 242.2B for types of VSDs. An atrioventricular septal defect or atrioventricular canal defect is due to absence of the atrioventricular septum, an endocardial cushion defect. The atrioventricular canal forms from the endocardial cushion, and the atrioventricular septum separates the tricuspid from the mitral valve. In CAVC, the atrioventricular septum is absent, and the AVVs share an annulus. Left-to-right shunting in this defect is often torrential, and operative repair is undertaken in infancy. Davey et al. explained that repair of atrioventricular canal lesions never results in completely normal atrioventricular valves.[1]

## OBSTRUCTIVE LESIONS

Acyanotic lesions with normal pulmonary blood flow are largely obstructive lesions. Left ventricular outflow tract obstruction promotes development of left ventricular hypertrophy (LVH), increasing its myocardial oxygen consumption and reducing the ability to increase coronary perfusion pressure. Consequently, there is increased risk of demand-related myocardial ischemia. Aortic stenosis is discussed in the chapter on valvular heart disease. Critical neonatal aortic stenosis occurs when so little blood is ejected across the native aortic valve that systemic and coronary perfusion must be retrograde via the PDA. Neonates with adequate left-sided structures and isolated critical aortic stenosis undergo dilation of the aortic valve. Options for aortic valve replacement are limited in the growing child who will not tolerate anticoagulation well. The Ross procedure involves using the native pulmonary valve to replace the diseased aortic valve and placement of a conduit from the RV to pulmonary artery.

### WILLIAMS-BEUREN SYNDROME

Deletion of the elastin gene on chromosome 7 produces Williams syndrome (WS). Classically, children with WS have elfin facies and a cocktail personality. Lack of quantity and function of elastin leads to thickening and reduced compliance of arterial media. Consequently, supravalvar aortic and pulmonic stenosis often develop. Coronary ostia may be hooded or otherwise abnormal. The aorta is poorly distensible during systole and has poor diastolic recoil, leading to limited coronary perfusion (Windkessel effect). Noncardiac manifestations include generalized anxiety disorder (or other psychiatric condition), endocrine problems such as hypercalcemia, abdominal pain, subclinical hypothyroidism, and glucose intolerance. Children with WS have among the highest rates of cardiac arrest and death under anesthesia. Prolonged QT has been implicated in sudden cardiac death.[2] Surgical treatment of supravalvar aortic stenosis occurs prior to the onset of severe LVH.

### SHONE COMPLEX

The Shone complex consists of left-sided obstructive lesions with variable severity. Classic Shone complex comprises a supravalvar mitral ring (mitral stenosis), parachute mitral valve, subaortic stenosis, and coarctation of the aorta. Surgical repair of a distal lesion may unmask the hemodynamic significance of a more proximal lesion. Patients are at risk for developing postcapillary pulmonary hypertension.

## ANESTHETIC CONSIDERATIONS

### PREOPERATIVE

In left-to-right shunts, the affected heart chamber(s) are volume loaded and dilated. Cardiac dilation is often the indication for intervention. Preanesthetic management includes evaluation for difficult airway due to mandibular hypoplasia, extracorporeal membrane oxygenation (ECMO) standby for WS, and midazolam to reduce anxiety-induced tachycardia. Unrepaired adolescents with WS probably have milder disease and probably do not need ECMO backup.

### INTRAOPERATIVE

Goals of anesthetic induction intraoperatively for a WS patient include maintaining preload, afterload, and coronary perfusion pressure (CPP). Adequate CPP is a diastolic blood pressure that is 20 mm Hg above left ventricular end-diastolic pressure.

Cardiac arrest in children with cardiomyopathy was often preceded by hypotension and bradycardia, and arrest was more common following induction by agent other than an inhaled agent.[3]

### POSTOPERATIVE

Fluid resuscitation in the operating room may necessitate postoperative diuresis to minimize pulmonary congestion, especially if the mitral or left AVV is involved, such as in Shone complex or AVV disease.

## REFERENCES

1. Davey BT, Rychik J. The natural history of atrioventricular valve regurgitation throughout fetal life in patients with atrioventricular canal defects. *Pediatr Cardiol*. 2016;37:50–54.
2. Staudt GE, Eagle SS. Anesthetic considerations for patients with Williams syndrome. J Cardiothorac Vasc Anesth. 2021;35:176–186.
3. Lynch J, et al. Cardiac arrest upon induction of anesthesia in children with cardiomyopathy: an analysis of incidence and risk factors. *Pediatr Anesth*. 2011;21:951–957.

# 243.

# PULMONARY HYPERTENSION

*Benjamin Kloesel and Balazs Horvath*

## INTRODUCTION

Pulmonary hypertension (PH) in children is associated with significant morbidity and mortality. In the perioperative setting, children diagnosed with PH are at 20-fold higher risk for cardiac arrest and death, which highlights the need for careful planning and conduct of an anesthetic.[1] In contrast to adults, most cases are idiopathic or associated with congenital heart disease. Persistent pulmonary hypertension of the newborn belongs to a subcategory of PH and has a distinct underlying anatomic and pathophysiologic mechanism.

## CLASSIFICATION

The classification of pediatric PH emerged from its adult counterpart but has undergone modifications over time. Currently, two main classification schemes exist: The World Health Organization (WHO) Nice classification (updated in 2013) divides pediatric PH into 5 groups, while the Panama classification system established in 2011 by the Pulmonary Vascular Research Institute distinguishes between 10 categories (Table 243.1).[2,3]

*Table 243.1* CLASSIFICATION SYSTEMS FOR PEDIATRIC PULMONARY HYPERTENSION

| WHO NICE CLASSIFICATION | | THE PULMONARY VASCULAR RESEARCH INSTITUTE PANAMA CLASSIFICATION | |
| --- | --- | --- | --- |
| GROUP | DESCRIPTION | CATEGORY | DESCRIPTION |
| 1 | Pulmonary arterial hypertension | 1 | Prenatal or developmental pulmonary hypertensive vascular disease |
| 2 | Pulmonary hypertension due to left heart disease | 2 | Perinatal pulmonary vascular maladaptation |
| 3 | Pulmonary hypertension due to lung disease and/or hypoxia | 3 | Pediatric cardiovascular disease |
| 4 | Chronic thromboembolic pulmonary hypertension | 4 | Bronchopulmonary dysplasia |
| 5 | Pulmonary hypertension with unclear multifactorial mechanisms | 5 | Isolated pediatric pulmonary hypertensive vascular disease |
| | | 6 | Multifactorial pulmonary hypertensive vascular disease in congenital malformation syndromes |
| | | 7 | Pediatric lung disease |
| | | 8 | Pediatric thromboembolic disease |
| | | 9 | Pediatric hypobaric hypoxic exposure |
| | | 10 | Pediatric pulmonary vascular disease associated with other system disorders |

Adapted from Chau et al. The post-anesthetic care of pediatric patients with pulmonary hypertension. *Semin Cardiothorac Vasc Anesth.* 2016 Mar;20(1):63–73.

## DIAGNOSIS

Pulmonary hypertension is usually diagnosed by right heart catheterization and is defined as a resting mean pulmonary artery pressure (mPAP) equal to or greater than 25 mm Hg (normal $14 \pm 3.3$ mm Hg).[1] It is noteworthy that pulmonary vascular resistance (PVR) is not included in this definition, and that the term PH refers to increased mPAP of any cause. In cases where mPAP and PVR are increased in combination with a pulmonary artery wedge pressure (PAWP) equal to or less than 15 mm Hg, the term pulmonary arterial hypertension (PAH) is used. In PAH, the restriction to blood flow is situated in the pulmonary precapillary bed. The WHO classification system categorizes PAH as group 1, which includes idiopathic PAH (group 1.1), heritable PAH (group 1.2), and PAH associated with congenital heart disease (group 1.4.4) (Table 243.2).[3]

In children, the distinction of precapillary PH from postcapillary PH is key; in the former condition, the restriction of blood flow is located in the pulmonary precapillary bed, which has been subjected to progressive structural vascular changes, while the latter is based on left heart disease leading to left atrial or pulmonary venous hypertension.

It becomes apparent that a correct diagnosis has significant implications on treatment as the use of pulmonary vasodilators can prove detrimental in cases of postcapillary PH (e.g., pulmonary vein stenosis, aortic valve stenosis, mitral valve stenosis, cor triatriatum).[1,2]

## ANESTHETIC CONSIDERATIONS

### PREOPERATIVE

A thorough evaluation of the patient's current status with a focus on airway and cardiopulmonary system is paramount preoperatively. A review of recent cardiac studies, such as cardiac catheterization and echocardiographic data, can provide information about the severity of PH, pulmonary artery pressure, right ventricular pressure, presence of valvular abnormalities, presence of intracardiac shunts, and right/left ventricular function.[4] Presence of atrial or ventricular shunts should prompt the use of air bubble filters. In older children, the functional status serves as an important indicator of disease severity (ability of the child to participate in sports or play with peers, history of syncope, dyspnea).[2]

*Table 243.2* PULMONARY HYPERTENSION OVERVIEW

---

Pulmonary Hypertension

*Definition*: Resting mean pulmonary artery pressure equal to or greater than 25 mm Hg diagnosed by right heart catheterization

Pulmonary Vascular Resistance (PVR)

*Calculated as* $80 \times (\text{mPAP} - \text{mLAP})/\text{PBF}$
mPAP = mean pulmonary arterial pressure (mm Hg)
mLAP = mean left atrial pressure (mm Hg)
PBF = pulmonary blood flow (L/min)
During cardiac catheterization, the following values are frequently used:
PAWP for mLAP
CO for PBF
Vascular resistance is measured in dynes/s/cm$^5$, but can also be expressed in mm Hg-min/L (Wood units) by using a conversion factor of 80.

*Normal Value*: 20–130 dynes/s/cm$^5$
0.25–1.6 mm Hg/L/min (Wood units)

| Factors that ⇑ PVR | Factors that ⇓ PVR |
| --- | --- |
| Hypoxemia | Supplemental oxygen (⇑ FiO$_2$) |
| Hypercapnia | Hypocapnia |
| Acidemia | Inhaled nitric oxide |
| Hypothermia | Prostacyclin analogues (epoprostenol [intravenous], treprostinil [intravenous], iloprost [inhaled]) |
| Pain | Inodilators (milrinone, levosimendan) |
| Parasympathetic stimuli (tracheal suctioning) | Inotropes (dobutamine) |

---

CO, cardiac output; mLAP, mean left atrial pressure; mPAP, mean pulmonary artery pressure; PAWP, pulmonary artery wedge pressure; PBF, pulmonary blood flow; PVR, pulmonary vascular resistance.

If the patient is treated with a continuous infusion of prostacyclin analogues, care should be taken to avoid any interruptions. Delivery of the infusion should continue perioperatively via a reliable intravenous access site (preferably via central venous access line).

## INTRAOPERATIVE

Fluid balance needs to be optimized intraoperatively to support right ventricular function. This can be challenging as both fluid depletion and overload are detrimental. Due to required preoperative fasting times, a judicious fluid bolus prior to induction may be beneficial.[4]

Intravenous induction is largely viewed as the safer induction alternative because an existing intravenous catheter allows immediate and effective management of problems that may arise, such as bradycardia, hypotension, or laryngospasm. On the other hand, inhalation induction should not be viewed as contraindicated and may, in certain situations, be a better choice to avoid repeated, stressful, and potentially unsuccessful peripheral venous catheterization attempts.[5] Premedication can significantly aid in patient co-operation and reduce stress and anxiety. Commonly used options include midazolam (oral, nasal, intramuscular); ketamine (oral, intramuscular); and dexmedetomidine (intranasal).[4] All intravenous induction agents (propofol, ketamine, etomidate, midazolam/fentanyl) have been successfully used; it is not the agent itself but its use that determines the outcome of the induction.[1] Propofol, for example, can result in acute decompensation when given as a large bolus dose, whereas titration to the desired level of loss of consciousness with correction of its hypotensive effect can be well tolerated in selected patients.

Patient monitoring should include a five-lead electrocardiogram, and resuscitation equipment needs to be readily available.[4] The need for an invasive blood pressure monitoring cannula is dependent on the overall status of the patient and the invasiveness of the procedure. Anesthetic maintenance can be accomplished with a variety of agents, including volatile anesthetics, propofol, dexmedetomidine, ketamine, benzodiazepines, and opioids. Some combinations and dosing regimens have a larger impact on blood pressure, and care should be taken to maintain hemodynamic stability. Inotropic agents and vasopressors may be used to support blood pressure. Vasopressin plays a unique role as it does not cause pulmonary vasoconstriction, in contrast to other agents such as phenylephrine.

## POSTOPERATIVE

Postoperative care of a patient with primary PH focuses on breathing (avoidance of airway obstruction, hypoventilation, and hypercarbia); analgesia (adequate control of pain); and body temperature (avoidance of shivering). Patients with PH remain at higher risk for complications in the postoperative period, and a large portion of cardiac arrests stem from respiratory events, which highlights the need for close monitoring and judicious use of respiratory depressants. Disposition of the patient also requires careful consideration. Procedures based in the office and surgery centers should be avoided in patients with severe primary PH. Direct discharge to home from the postanesthesia care unit also needs careful consideration. For patients who will be admitted to the hospital, the decision between intensive care unit, monitored "step-down" unit, or floor should be guided by severity of the condition and magnitude/invasiveness of the procedure.[2]

## PULMONARY HYPERTENSIVE CRISIS

Pulmonary hypertensive crisis is a complication not limited to the intraoperative period. Any triggering factor that precipitates an acute rise in PVR may cause a PH crisis, and prompt intervention is necessary to avoid a vicious cycle as described below that has the potential to result in cardiopulmonary arrest. A multitude of stimuli can serve as triggering factors: hypoxia, hypercapnia, acidemia, noxious stimuli, hypothermia, vagal stimuli (airway suctioning, endotracheal intubation), and interruption of a continuous prostacyclin analogue infusion.[5] Acute increase in PVR causes an increase in right ventricular afterload, which in turn reduces right ventricular cardiac output and leads to an increase in right ventricular end-diastolic volume. Reduced cardiac output impedes left ventricular filling (preload) due to ventricular interdependence and also decreases left ventricular cardiac output. The combination of reduced left ventricular cardiac output, hypotension, and increased right ventricular wall tension decreases right ventricular coronary perfusion. Untreated, this may progressively compromise right ventricular coronary perfusion, causing myocardial ischemia that further impairs right ventricular function and cardiac output.

If a patient experiences a PH crisis, multiple steps should be taken expeditiously to restore the baseline physiologic state. Provision of 100% $FiO_2$ (fraction of inspired oxygen) and hyperventilation, either controlled or assisted via an unobstructed airway, helps to decrease PVR. Deepening the anesthetic plane and adequate analgesia can remove triggering factors. A vasoconstrictor such as phenylephrine may be helpful if low blood pressure compromises right ventricular coronary perfusion, but significant bradycardia should be avoided. If the situation is not improved with those measures, consideration should be given to inhaled nitric oxide (direct pulmonary vasodilator), sodium bicarbonate (to correct acidosis), or inhaled or intravenous prostacyclin analogues (another pulmonary vasodilator) and milrinone (systemic inodilator and pulmonary vasodilator).[1,5] If the patient suffers from severe systemic hypotension, administration of inotropes and vasopressors, including epinephrine, norepinephrine, and vasopressin should be initiated. Last, for refractory cases, extracorporeal membrane oxygenation may be a rescue therapy.[1]

## REFERENCES

1. Latham GJ, Yung D. Current understanding and perioperative management of pediatric pulmonary hypertension. *Paediatr Anaesth.* 2019;29(5):441–456.

2. Chau DF, et al. The post-anesthetic care of pediatric patients with pulmonary hypertension. *Semin Cardiothorac Vasc Anesth.* 2016;20(1):63–73.
3. Ivy DD, et al. Pediatric pulmonary hypertension. *J Am Coll Cardiol.* 2013;62(25 suppl):D117–D126.
4. Shukla AC, Almodovar MC. Anesthesia considerations for children with pulmonary hypertension. *Pediatr Crit Care Med.* 2010;11(2 suppl):S70–S73.
5. Friesen RH, Williams GD. Anesthetic management of children with pulmonary arterial hypertension. *Paediatr Anaesth.* 2008;18(3):208–216.

# 244.

# MAJOR VASCULAR MALFORMATIONS

*Benjamin Kloesel and Balazs Horvath*

## INTRODUCTION

The topic of major vascular malformations is broad and includes conditions affecting the central as well as peripheral vasculature. For the scope of this chapter, we focus on three distinct entities: coarctation of the aorta, patent ductus arteriosus (PDA), and vascular rings (Table 244.1). While the majority of patients with those conditions are diagnosed in the neonatal period, less severe forms may initially remain asymptomatic and are discovered later in life. In the neonatal period, most cases are corrected surgically. One exception is PDA, which is increasingly addressed by percutaneous closure in the cardiac catheterization laboratory.

## COARCTATION OF THE AORTA

Coarctation of the aorta is a condition in which part of the aorta is narrowed and causes obstruction to blood flow into the descending aorta. The anatomy of the proximal aorta is divided into aortic root, ascending aorta, aortic arch, aortic isthmus, and descending aorta. The aortic isthmus is located at the distal part of the aortic arch, proximal to the transition to the descending aorta and just distal to the origin of the left subclavian artery. It marks the insertion

point of the DA, which connects the aorta with the pulmonary trunk. Coarctation of the aorta typically occurs at the isthmus close to the insertion of the DA (juxtaductal). Most cases are congenital, but some may be acquired secondary to inflammatory conditions. Obstruction to forward blood flow results in left ventricular pressure overload and left ventricular hypertrophy. The effect on lower body perfusion depends on the severity of the lesion: High-grade obstruction presents in the neonatal period with poor perfusion, acidosis, progressive heart failure, and shock as the DA closes (in utero, perfusion of the lower body is maintained by the DA), while low-grade obstruction may initially go undetected. Patients later develop collaterals that supply the lower body. Depending on the age, presenting symptoms can include lower extremity claudication, right upper extremity hypertension, weak or absent femoral pulses, headaches, and fatigue.

## ANESTHETIC CONSIDERATIONS
### Preoperative

Neonates presenting with high-grade obstruction preoperatively are scheduled for operative repair via left lateral thoracotomy. The DA is kept open by a continuous infusion of

*Table 244.1*  MAJOR VASCULAR MALFORMATIONS—OVERVIEW

| | COARCTATION OF THE AORTA | PATENT DUCTUS ARTERIOSUS | VASCULAR RING |
|---|---|---|---|
| Incidence | 1.7 to 4 in 10,000 live births | 1 in 1600 term live births | Variable, depending on lesion |
| Pathophysiology | Left-sided obstruction → left ventricular pressure overload and hypertrophy | Left-to-right shunt | Compression of neighboring structures (tracheobronchial tree, esophagus) |
| Presenting symptoms | *Neonatal period:* <br>• Congestive heart failure <br>• Shock (when ductus arteriosus closes) <br>*Older child:* <br>• Hypertension <br>• Fatigue <br>• Headache <br>• Lower extremity claudication | *Large shunt:* <br>• Congestive heart failure <br>• Pulmonary overcirculation <br>• Poor feeding <br>*Moderate shunt:* <br>• Failure to thrive <br>• Recurrent upper respiratory tract infections <br>• Fatigue with exertion <br>*Small shunt:* <br>• Asymptomatic <br>• Continuous "machinery" murmur (often detected on routine preschool physical examination) | Dependent on type, location and severity of compression <br>• May be asymptomatic <br>• Respiratory distress <br>• Stridor <br>• Barky cough <br>• Recurrent upper respiratory tract infections <br>• Apnea episodes <br>• Dysphagia |
| Management | *Surgical:* <br>• Surgical repair (left lateral thoracotomy) <br>*Interventional:* <br>• Balloon dilation ± stenting | *Medical:* <br>• NSAIDs (indomethacin, ibuprofen) <br>• Acetaminophen <br>*Interventional:* <br>• Percutaneous device closure <br>*Surgical:* <br>• PDA ligation (thoracotomy) <br>• Video-assisted thoracoscopic clip closure | *Surgical:* <br>• Surgical repair/ ligation (left lateral thoracotomy; select cases via right lateral thoracotomy or median sternotomy) |

prostaglandin E$_1$, and, depending on the overall condition, the patient may require inotropic agents such as dopamine or epinephrine.[1]

## Intraoperative

Cardiopulmonary bypass is not necessary intraoperatively. The surgeon exposes the narrowed area, applies a cross clamp and removes the obstruction. There are different anastomotic techniques, with end-to-end or end-to-side anastomoses being used most frequently. From an anesthetic standpoint, the patient requires general endotracheal anesthesia. A right upper extremity arterial cannula should be placed, which provides perioperative blood pressure monitoring and allows continued blood pressure monitoring during the clamp period (aortic clamping will result in the loss of left upper extremity and lower extremity blood pressures). Some surgeons also request the placement of a femoral arterial cannula to allow assessment of the gradient across the repaired aortic segment. Aortic cross clamping has significant effects on spinal cord perfusion and the cross-clamp time should be minimized (goal less than 20 minutes). Many institutions allow the patient's body temperature to passively drift down (around 34°C-35°C) to reduce the metabolic requirements of the spinal cord. Hyperthermia should be strictly avoided. Since the

surgical approach uses a left lateral thoracotomy, regional anesthesia techniques such as paravertebral block, erector spinae block, or intercostal nerve block should be considered. Older children/adults often undergo balloon dilation and stent placement in the cardiac catheterization laboratory. Re-coarctation after surgical repair is also treated in the cardiac catheterization laboratory. Surgical exposure for older children can be improved by single-lung ventilation.[1]

## Postoperative

Postoperatively, blood pressure should be controlled with antihypertensives (sodium nitroprusside, nicardipine, esmolol) to avoid complications at the high-pressure system anastomosis site. Complications of aortic coarctation repair include perioperative hemorrhage, spinal cord injury from hypoperfusion, rebound hypertension, recurrent laryngeal nerve injury, phrenic nerve injury, thoracic duct injury, and re-coarctation.[1]

## PATENT DUCTUS ARTERIOSUS

The DA is a connection between the aorta and the pulmonary arteries. It originates from the pulmonary trunk and inserts into the upper descending thoracic aorta just distal to the origin of the left subclavian artery.[2] In the fetal period, the DA allows blood ejected by the right ventricle to bypass the pulmonary circulation as the lungs are not engaged in gas exchange. After birth, the DA closes within 2–3 days in the full-term neonate.[3] The first part of ductal closure is caused by smooth muscle contraction triggered by an increase in $PaO_2$ and a decrease in circulating prostaglandins. Over the ensuing 2 to 3 weeks, the DA becomes fibrotic and closes permanently. Failure to close results in persistent or PDA that facilitates left-to-right shunting. A PDA belongs to the group of acyanotic defects with increased pulmonary blood flow. Depending on the size of the shunt, patients may be asymptomatic (small, restrictive shunt) or develop pulmonary overcirculation and congestive heart failure (large shunt). In addition, large shunts through the PDA can cause diastolic flow reversal (retrograde flow from the descending aorta into the pulmonary arteries during diastole), which decreases systemic blood flow and raises the risk for end-organ damage, such as necrotizing enterocolitis or acute kidney injury.[2,3] Size of the PDA and shunt magnitude are monitored by transthoracic echocardiography.[3]

In certain congenital malformations, infants receive pulmonary blood through the DA, and closure of the DA can cause cyanosis. Prostaglandin $E_2$ can be infused in those infants to maintain the patency of the DA until a more permanent shunt is placed. One of the common shunts performed is the Blalock-Taussig shunt, which involves anastomosis of either the right or left subclavian artery to the respective pulmonary artery.

## ANESTHETIC CONSIDERATIONS

### Preoperative

The first attempt at closing a PDA in the neonatal period utilizes nonsteroidal anti-inflammatory drugs (NSAIDs) such as indomethacin, ibuprofen, or acetaminophen. If the medical approach fails, the PDA can be closed by surgical ligation (via either left lateral thoracotomy or video-assisted thoracoscopy) or in the cardiac catheterization laboratory via percutaneous intervention using closure devices.[3] The final decision about the closure modality is often dictated by patient condition and center preference. Surgical closure can be performed at the bedside in the neonatal intensive care unit (ICU) and critically ill neonates on high-frequency oscillatory or jet ventilation often benefit from avoidance of transport to a different procedure location preoperatively.

### Intraoperative

Surgical and catheter-based closure of the PDA is generally performed under general endotracheal anesthesia. Adequate vascular access should be present intraoperatively, and blood products need to be readily available. Ventilation goals include avoidance of increased left-to-right shunting. Avoid factors that increase pulmonary vascular resistance (hypoxia, acidosis, hypercarbia, hypothermia, sympathetic stimulation, atelectasis, high airway pressure). During surgical ligation, pulse oximetry monitoring of the right upper extremity and one lower extremity is beneficial to detect accidental ligation of the descending aorta (the surgeon typically performs a "test clamp" to exclude this). Blood pressure monitoring of the right upper extremity is beneficial if a clamp is applied to the aorta to control bleeding; this maneuver renders lower extremity blood pressure monitoring useless.[2]

### Postoperative

Postoperatively, neonates mostly remain intubated after successful PDA closure due to comorbid pulmonary conditions and are cared for in the ICU.

## VASCULAR RINGS

The term *vascular ring* includes malformations such as double aortic arch, right aortic arch with ligamentum, pulmonary artery sling, and left aortic arch with aberrant right subclavian artery. The basis of those conditions is an abnormal development of the embryonic aortic arch system. Initial formation of the aortic arch systems yields a ventral and a dorsal aorta that are connected by six primitive aortic arches. Establishment of a normal left aortic arch requires the timed involution of the first, second, right fourth, and fifth arches.[4]

Vascular rings can cause compression of neighboring vascular structures, trachea, and esophagus. In the neonatal period or early infancy, vascular rings most frequently present with respiratory symptoms (noisy breathing, barky cough, stridor, recurrent upper respiratory tract infections). Later, when solid food is introduced into the child's diet, dysphagia may occur. A computed tomography angiogram (CTA) is the diagnostic test of choice as it clearly delineates the anatomy and facilitates surgical planning. Rigid bronchoscopy can visualize the degree of airway compression and dynamic airway collapse before and after surgical repair of the vascular ring.[2,4]

## ANESTHETIC CONSIDERATIONS

### Preoperative

A review of imaging modalities, specifically CTA, is important preoperatively to gain a better understanding of the anatomy and the planned surgical approach. This also assists in planning of invasive monitoring line location.

### Intraoperative

The majority of vascular rings are repaired surgically via the left lateral thoracotomy approach. Intraoperative procedures can be as simple as a division of an atretic vessel segment or more challenging when, for example, an aberrant subclavian artery needs to be disconnected and reanastomosed to a different location on the aortic arch or the carotid artery.[2] The surgery is done under general endotracheal anesthesia. Regional anesthesia should be considered to address pain from the thoracotomy incision. Surgical exposure in older patients may be improved by single-lung ventilation.

## Postoperative

Most patients can be extubated in the operating room and are monitored in the ICU.

## REFERENCES

1. Fox EB, et al. Perioperative and anesthetic management of coarctation of the aorta. *Semin Cardiothorac Vasc Anesth.* 2019;23(2):212–224.
2. Russell HM, Backer CL. Pediatric thoracic problems: patent ductus arteriosus, vascular rings, congenital tracheal stenosis, and pectus deformities. *Surg Clin North Am.* 2010;90(5):1091–1113.
3. Conrad C, Newberry D. Understanding the pathophysiology, implications, and treatment options of patent ductus arteriosus in the neonatal population. *Adv Neonatal Care.* 2019;19(3):179–87.
4. Backer CL, et al. Vascular rings. *Semin Pediatr Surg.* 2016;25(3): 165–175.

# 245.

# ALTERED UPTAKE/DISTRIBUTION OF INTRAVENOUS AND INHALATION ANESTHETICS

*Jamie W. Sinton*

## INTRODUCTION

Developmental pharmacology challenges the anesthesiologist as there is no linear relationship between body mass and drug kinetics. Therefore, the field of allometry, the nonlinear relationship of size and function (e.g., kilograms and drug clearance) provides an improved description for drug clearance. Drug clearance more closely mirrors glomerular filtration rate and body surface area rather than kilograms. This chapter describes issues surrounding developmental pharmacology with a focus on development (e.g., organ maturity and respiratory physiology); however, in mainstream practice, most intravenous drugs are dosed in milligrams per kilogram.

## DEVELOPMENT

Developmental impact on drug kinetics depends on body composition, plasma proteins, organ maturity, and respiratory physiology. Neonates have a high percentage of total body water, especially extracellular fluid volume.[1] Total body water decreases with age.[2] Premature infants, infants, and children have much more total body water than adults. Neonates also have minimal fat and muscle.

With age concentrations of albumin and $\alpha_1$-acid glycoprotein increase. In the neonatal period, albumin is very important for binding bilirubin and preventing neonatal jaundice. Bilirubin displacement from albumin should be avoided (e.g., ceftriaxone).

Organ maturity proceeds with postmenstrual age rather than chronological age. In neonates, this is a large determinant of drug clearance. Adult hepatic and renal function is different for different drugs; however, it is generally achieved by age 2 years.[2]

Infants and children have a similar functional residual capacity (FRC) as adults: 30 mL/kg/min. Alveolar ventilation is much higher in an infant (100–150 mL/kg/min) versus an adult (60 mL/kg/min) to account for greater oxygen consumption of the infant. Therefore, a 3-kg newborn has a ratio of alveolar ventilation to FRC of 5 to 1. In contrast, an adult's ratio is closer to 2 to 1.

## INTRAVENOUS ANESTHETICS

Infants have adult levels of nonspecific plasma esterases and therefore metabolize remifentanil and cisatracurium well. For other intravenous agents, the kinetics of intravenous anesthetics largely depend on body composition, organ maturity, and plasma protein concentrations; therefore, allometric models are used to predict their clearance. Figure 245.1 shows clearance profiles for common intravenous anesthetics.

Clearance of intravenous anesthetics is complex and not linearly related to body mass; therefore, probably neither should be drug doses related to body mass. In neonates, organ maturity defines clearance kinetics. In toddlers, the relationship of age and clearance is nonlinear and is better predicted by body surface area or glomerular filtration rate.[2]

Local anesthetics are intravenous, epidural, or perineural agents whose clinical effect depends largely on albumin and $\alpha_1$-acid glycoprotein binding. Plasma protein level changes with development are complex. However, albumin reaches adult levels after 1 week of life, peaks in childhood to about 4.5–5.5 g/dL, then plateaus to around 4 mg/dL in adulthood.[4]

## INHALATIONAL ANESTHETICS

The uptake of inhaled anesthetic agents depends on drug solubility in blood, alveolar blood flow, and the difference in partial pressure between alveolar and venous blood. Clinical effect and minimum alveolar concentration (MAC) also depends on age, with infants having higher MAC for sevoflurane than neonates, children, or adults.[5]

Presently available inhalation anesthetics largely are nonionized, minimally differ from ideal gas behavior, and have low molecular weights. These properties allow for rapid diffusion and facilitation of induction and emergence.

Modern inhalation anesthetics exert their effect by obtaining an adequate brain tissue concentration. Brain tissue concentration is directly proportional to partial pressure of anesthetic in the brain. Alveolar partial pressure determines partial pressure in the brain. Inhalational agents undergo uptake, biotransformation, and elimination as in any patient.

As volatile anesthetic is inhaled and alveolar partial pressure rises, tissues and organs in the body take up small amounts of drug. In order from greatest to least uptake, these are the ones affected: vessel-rich group (brain, heart, liver); muscle group (skin and muscle); fat group; and vessel-poor group (which has insignificant uptake).

The MAC for neonates is lower than for infants. Infants have the highest MAC for sevoflurane, even higher than for older children, adolescents, and teenagers.

## FACTORS AFFECTING RATE OF INHALATION INDUCTION

Three factors affect anesthetic uptake: solubility in the blood, alveolar blood flow, and the difference in partial pressure between alveolar gas and venous blood.

As in adults, increasing the difference between inhaled and exhaled volatile agent concentration will speed inhalation induction. The greater the uptake of anesthetic agent, the greater the difference between inspired and alveolar concentrations and the slower the rate of induction.

For insoluble agents like sevoflurane, alveolar ventilation impacts rate of induction less than for soluble agents

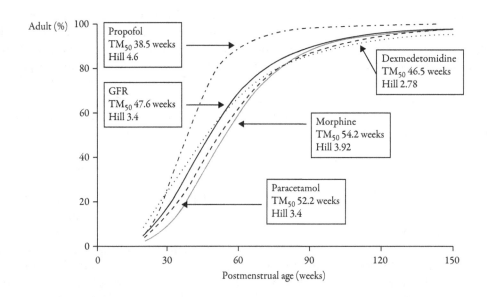

**Figure 245.1** Clearance maturation of percentage adult rate versus postmenstrual age for propofol, dexmedetomidine, and paracetamol (acetaminophen).[3] Note that clearance parallels glomerular filtration rate increases well. GFR, glomerular filtration rate.

like isoflurane. Faster inhalation induction in children can be attributed to increased minute ventilation and increased ratio of minute ventilation to FRC.[2] Other factors affecting Fi include circuit volume, fresh gas flow, and circuit absorption. The rate of rise of blood tissue concentration is also affected by tissue solubility, which may be decreased in young infants as they have relatively little fat and a high proportion of total body water.

Many of the factors that speed induction also speed recovery: elimination of rebreathing, high fresh gas flows, low anesthetic circuit volume, low absorption by the anesthetic circuit, decreased solubility, high cerebral blood flow, and increased ventilation.

The rate of rise of the alveolar concentration of inhaled anesthetic depends on inspired concentration, alveolar ventilation, and uptake. Consequently, the time constant of the inhaled anesthetic equilibrium is much shorter for infants.

## INHALATIONAL AGENTS AND THE MYOCARDIUM

The neonatal myocardium has disorganized, reduced density of muscle fibers. Neonatal myocardium also has rapid myocardial uptake of inhalation anesthetics. Due to a high ratio of minute ventilation to FRC, insoluble inhalation agents undergo faster equilibration. Consequently, infants have a higher incidence of cardiac arrest during induction.[6] In children, sevoflurane depresses myocardial function less than halothane.

## CONSIDERATIONS FOR CHILDREN WITH HEART DISEASE

The same inhalational and intravenous anesthetics used for healthy patients can be used in patients with congenital heart disease (CHD) as long as hemodynamic effects are considered. Children with an extensive history of anesthetics and intensive care unit stays may have developed significant physical dependence and tachyphylaxis to intravenous agents.

Inhalation anesthetics distribute in the body according to tissue partial pressure and solubility (partition coefficient) and, in the case of patients with CHD, pulmonary blood flow. Right-to-left intracardiac (or intrapulmonary) shunting slows the rate of inhalation induction.

Therefore, uptake of inhalational anesthetic would markedly slow in a patient with relatively little pulmonary blood flow (e.g., Qp/Qs < 1) undergoing induction with a very soluble agent (e.g., halothane).

Nitrous oxide should be used with caution in patients with CHD due to a potential impact on pulmonary vascular resistance (PVR). In infants, there is no increase in PVR when nitrous oxide is used. At the same time, inhalation induction with a potent (and more pungent) agent such as sevoflurane may precipitate crying and significant increases in PVR. In this case, the choice of use of nitrous oxide is multifactorial. However, in adults, nitrous oxide does increase PVR. Low cardiac output states predispose patients to overdose with soluble agents as the rate of rise in alveolar concentrations will be markedly increased.

## ANESTHETIC CONSIDERATIONS

### PREOPERATIVE

Preoperatively, account for postmenstrual age in order to predict anesthetic requirements.

### INTRAOPERATIVE

Intraoperatively, neonates, due to a large total body water content, require large initial doses of water-soluble medications such as succinylcholine. Given a neonate's lack of muscle, drugs that depend on redistribution into fat or muscle (e.g., fentanyl or propofol) for the termination of action will have a long clinical effect.[2] Neonates have reduced plasma protein levels, so drugs that are highly protein bound, like local anesthetics, will have a high free fraction. However, the risk of local anesthetic toxicity in this group also receives contributions from a high hepatic extraction ratio and narrow therapeutic index.[2]

### POSTOPERATIVE

In preparation for extubation in the operating room, the $FiO_2$ (fraction of inspired oxygen) is usually increased to 100%. There is controversy surrounding absorption atelectasis. Postoperatively, expect infants to emerge from inhaled anesthetics more quickly than adults. However, intravenous agents may have a prolonged duration of clinical action due to an immature clearance ability in young patients.

## REFERENCES

1. Friis-Hansen L. Body composition during growth. In vivo measurements and biochemical data correlated to differential anatomic growth. *Pediatrics*. 1971;47:264–274.
2. Vutskits L. Pediatric anesthesia. In: Gropper MA, ed. *Miller's Anesthesia*. Philadelphia, PA: Elsevier; 2020:2427–2428.
3. Sumpter A, Anderson BJ. Pediatric pharmacology in the first year of life. *Curr Opin Anaesthesiol*. 2009;22(4):469–475.
4. Ignjatovic V, et al. Age-related differences in plasma proteins: how plasma proteins change from neonates to adults. *PLoS One*. 2011;6(2):e17213.
5. Katoh T. Minimum alveolar concentration of sevoflurane in children. *Br J Anesth*. 1992. **68**: p. 139–141.
6. Anesthesia for general surgery in the neonate. In: *Smith's Anesthesia for Infants and Children*. p. 555.

# 246.

# CARDIAC SURGERY
## CORRECTIVE AND PALLIATIVE

*Jamie W. Sinton*

## INTRODUCTION

Our discussion of cardiac surgery is limited to those operations performed on cardiopulmonary bypass (CPB). Nonpump cases such as vascular ring divisions and coarctation repairs are discussed elsewhere in this book. Single-ventricle palliation is discussed in the chapter on cyanotic defects.

## ANESTHETIC CONSIDERATIONS

### PREOPERATIVE

Children presenting for elective cardiac surgery undergo extensive preoperative planning including basic laboratory tests, chest roentgenogram, echocardiogram (echo), and rarely cardiac catheterization. When major vascular disease is suspected, cardiac computed tomography or three-dimensional printed models define anatomy. Additionally, children with heart disease have a higher than average incidence of difficult airway.[1] Many children have had extensive hospital stays, and venous access may be challenging.

Preoperative anxiolysis is often administered to young infants to prevent physiologic perturbations on induction rather than for anxiety. For example, crying has a more dramatic impact on pulmonary vascular resistance than mild hypoventilation following oral midazolam.

### INTRAOPERATIVE
### Pump Circuits and Prime

Cardiopulmonary bypass pump volumes may double the blood volume of the patient and are based on body surface area. A 3-kkg neonate may have a blood volume of 225–240 mL and a pump prime volume of 215 mL. Blood primes are commonly used for children under 15 kg, although centers with very small pump primes may use crystalloid. An example of a cardiopulmonary bypass setup is shown in Figure 246.1.

### Induction

Mask or intravenous induction may be appropriate. Oxygen should be used judiciously depending on the lesion; however, brief exposure to 100% oxygen during airway management is preferable to abject hypoxia when the baseline saturation is 80%. Depending on the perceived risk of induction of anesthesia, the surgical team and perfusionist may be in attendance in case of emergent need for mechanical circulatory support. A classic example is an infant with Williams syndrome in whom coronary insufficiency and myocardial ischemia accompany induction. Cardiopulmonary resuscitation followed by neck cannulation for extracorporeal membrane oxygenation ensue. Carotid and internal jugular veins are preferred in infants as femoral vessels are too small to accommodate cannulas for adequate flow. Following sternotomy, the patient can be converted to a CPB circuit or the operation can be aborted.

### Intubation

Placement of a nasal endotracheal tube (vs. oral) may prevent dislodgement during transesophageal echocardiography (TEE).[2] Nosebleed may occur despite heparinization as infants do not have well vascularized nasal turbinates. Sometimes, oral intubation provides an excellent method of preoxygenation during nasal tube placement.

### Monitoring

In addition to American Society of Anesthesiologists monitoring and a five-lead electrocardiogram, the heart is monitored with TEE and the brain with near-infrared spectroscopy (NIRS). Temperature is measured in three locations: nasal, rectal, and skin; this helps monitor for uniform cooling and rewarming. Choose invasive monitoring line locations carefully based on the occlusions and planned anatomic connections that will be made during surgery.

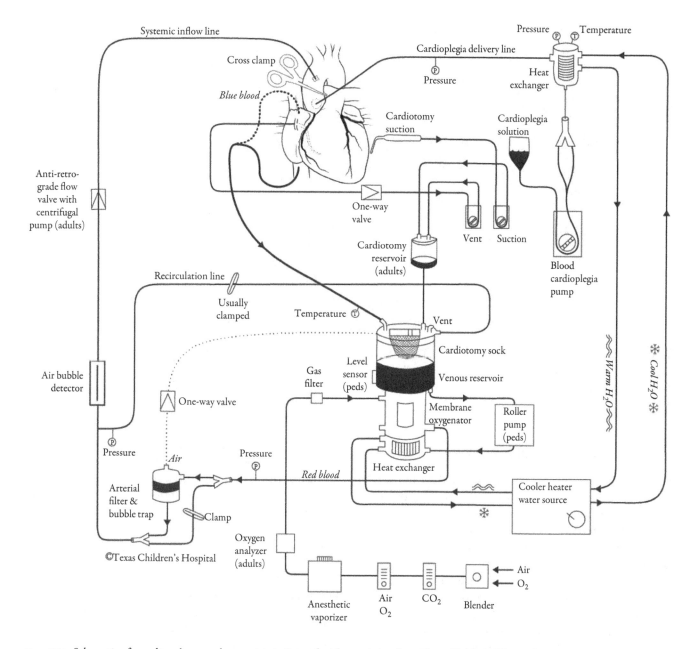

**Figure 246.1** Schematic of a cardiopulmonary bypass circuit. Printed with permission from Texas Children's Hospital.

## Incision

Antifibrinolytics are initiated prior to incision. Incision and electrocautery are quite stimulating. A deep plane of anesthesia without myocardial depression is classically achieved with fentanyl. Prior to (primary) sternotomy, ventilation should be suspended with the lungs in exhalation in order to avoid damage to the lungs or pleura.

## Cannulation

Heparin is still the most commonly used anticoagulant in children for CPB. Prior to cannulation, if antegrade cerebral perfusion (also called regional low-flow perfusion) will be used in order to minimize the time of deep hypothermic circulatory arrest, the surgeon tests the patency of the circle of Willis by sequentially clamping the carotid arteries and watching for a change in NIRS values.[3] Changes will be more easily detected if the patient is ventilated with room air.

Cannulation proceeds as in adults with arterial and then venous cannulation and is shown in Figure 246.2. However, in children, the arterial cannula may not be placed in the aorta in cases of hypoplastic left heart syndrome and interrupted aortic arch. Venous cannulation is almost universally bicaval (instead of via the right atrium) as operations require access to the right side of the heart via right atriotomy.

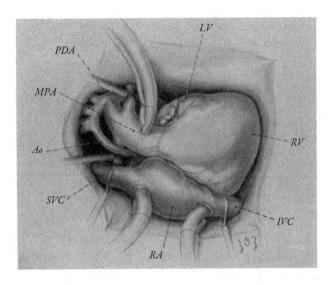

**Figure 246.2** Cannulation in hypoplastic left heart syndrome and the venous cannula are bicaval as would be common for a heart transplant. If this patient were undergoing the Norwood operation, then a right atrial venous cannula would be used instead. Ao, aorta; IVC, inferior vena cava; LV, left ventricle; PDA, patent ductus arteriosus; RA, right atrium; RV, right ventricle; SVC, superior vena cava. Printed with permission from Texas Children's Hospital.

## Initiation of Cardiopulmonary Bypass

Cardiopulmonary bypass is initiated by draining venous blood into the reservoir and the heart empties. At this time, exchange transfusion can be employed for those with sickle cell disease whose sickle cell fraction is greater than 30% or for other blood dyscrasias. Neonatal jaundice is cured. Simultaneously, the arterial cannula begins systemic perfusion. Once on full flow, check mean arterial pressure, anterior fontanelle, NIRS, and redose antibiotics, intravenous anesthetic, and muscle relaxants. Oxygenation is confirmed with venous saturation and perfusion with lactate. Cyanotic infants may have a prebypass partial pressure of oxygen ($PO_2$) of 40 mm Hg; following initiation of bypass, they may have a $PO_2$ of 500 mm Hg. The effects of hyperoxia and oxidative stress are under investigation. Cooling begins.

## Management of CPB

Children undergoing CPB are often cooled further than adults. Impressively, they maintain sinus bradycardia at very low temperatures and heart rates, whereas adults commonly fibrillate under such conditions. Expect a decreased cerebral metabolic rate of oxygen consumption (increased NIRS values), increased blood viscosity, and alterations of coagulation. Children do not have atherosclerotic vascular disease, so cerebral vasodilation and luxury perfusion are sought. Blood gas management is via pH-stat as this trends toward association with improved neurodevelopmental outcomes,[4] as does maintenance of NIRS values throughout CPB.[5] Carbon dioxide solubility in blood increases during hypothermia and may be added to the circuit to provide vasodilation. Phentolamine causes vasoplegia and also facilitates uniform cooling. Deep hypothermic circulatory arrest is employed for aortic arch operations.

## Aortic Cross Clamping and Cardioplegia

If arrest of the heart is planned, cardioplegia can be administered antegrade via the aortic root. The CPB pump will be stopped or at very low flows momentarily for clamp application. Expect asystole within 1 minute. For operations like the arterial switch operation or in the case of aortic insufficiency, cardioplegia can be given directly through each coronary.

## Rewarming and Unclamping

Establish full-flow CPB for at least 5 minutes before rewarming from deep hypothermia. During this time, maintain pH-stat management. Redose amnestics and muscle relaxant as anesthetic requirements sharply increase on rewarming. To prepare for aortic unclamping, assess for air on TEE (difficult as the heart is still and empty), vent the aortic root in Trendelenburg position, and give lidocaine 1–2 mg/kg. After unclamping, achieve sinus rhythm; defibrillate as needed. Epicardial pacing may be used in the case of heart block or to maintain a higher heart rate cardiac output. Warm slowly to prevent formation of gaseous emboli in the arterial circuit.

## Preparation for Separation From Bypass

Preparing to separate from CPB begins with returning the patient to a physiologic state. Anticipate how the operation will alter physiology to guide choice of inotropes. For example, an infant status after tetralogy of Fallot repair may have some residual right ventricular outflow tract obstruction and will separate on esmolol and dexmedetomidine. Inotropes are infused, and visual inspection and TEE confirm function and rule out residual defects. The heart is filled gradually (e.g., a neonate with an untrained left ventricle after d-transposition of great arteries) or generously (e.g., after Fontan completion).

## Postbypass

Assuming hemodynamic stability, attention postbypass turns to medical and surgical hemostasis. Protamine is slowly administered. Often, whole blood must be removed from the infant (out of the central line) in order to accommodate transfusion of platelets and cryoprecipitate. In toddlers and older children, coagulation management can be guided by point-of-care viscoelastic testing. Synthetic coagulation factors may be economical in older children.

## Emergence

Following the Collaborative Learning Initiative, children are extubated immediately postoperatively or within 6 hours of arrival to the intensive care unit. Judicious opioid use is required to accomplish this. Some advocate for fewer than 20 μg/kg of fentanyl, with most given before CPB.

## POSTOPERATIVE

Minimize distraction during transfer of care to the intensive care unit. Prevent hypoventilation, which reduces blood pH and cardiac function. Hyperventilation in a patient with a systemic-to-pulmonary shunt may be equally perilous. Chest tubes should be monitored postoperatively for function and blood loss that may be notable with position changes.

Operative mortality of congenital heart surgery is lowest from large-volume centers. Neurodevelopmental outcomes are prioritized.

## REFERENCES

1. Akpek EA, et al. Difficult intubation in pediatric cardiac anesthesia. *J Cardiothorac Vasc Anesth.* 2004;18(5):610–612.
2. Nathaniel H, et al. A study of practice behavior for endotracheal intubation site for children with congenital heart disease undergoing surgery: impact of endotracheal intubation site on perioperative outcomes—an analysis of the Society of Thoracic Surgeons Congenital Cardiac Anesthesia Society Database. *Anesth Analg.* 2019;129(4):1061–1068.
3. Pigula FA, et al. Regional low-flow perfusion provides cerebral circulatory support during neonatal aortic arch reconstruction. *J Thorac Cardiovasc Surg.* 2000;119(2):331–339.
4. Plessis AJd, et al. Perioperative effects of alpha-stat versus pH stat strategies for deep hypothermic cardiopulmonary bypass in infants. *J Thorac Cardiovasc Surg.* 1997;114:991–1001.
5. Barry D, et al. Relationship of intraoperative cerebral oxygen saturation to neurodevelopmental outcome and brain magnetic resonance imaging at 1 year of age in infants undergoing biventricular repair. *Circulation.* 2010;2010(122):245–254.

# 247.

# NONCARDIAC SURGERY

*Jamie W. Sinton*

## INTRODUCTION

The incidence of congenital heart disease (CHD) has been estimated at 6/1000.[1] The overall mortality in patients with CHD undergoing noncardiac surgery was 2.8% compared to 1.2% in patients without CHD.[2] Patients with single-ventricle heart disease, pulmonary hypertension, restrictive and dilated cardiomyopathies, hypertrophic cardiomyopathy, and ventricular-assist patients are at highest risk.[3]

## ANESTHETIC CONSIDERATIONS

### PREOPERATIVE

The child's heart disease may influence the timing of surgery. It appeals to logic that scoliosis surgery in Duchenne muscular dystrophy should occur prior to the onset of significant cardiac disease. On preoperative examination, if the patient's clinical status or objective data vary substantially from what is expected, further workup is reasonable. Additionally, children require dental clearance (and often anesthesia) prior to cardiac operations or interventions to reduce endocarditis risk.

## Upper Respiratory Infection

Elective surgery is often postponed for 4–8 weeks following an upper respiratory infection (URI) to allow airway reactivity, and therefore anesthetic risk, to decrease. In children with CHD, also consider the effects of treatment of laryngospasm or bronchospasm. While the Larson maneuver (upward pressure on the mastoid process) is benign, other treatments can cause circulatory instability. Positive pressure ventilation reduces venous return, and in a Fontan patient, cardiac output falls quickly. Succinylcholine could be used in a small dose with rapid return of spontaneous ventilation and negative intrathoracic pressure. Propofol given to reinduce anesthesia for laryngospasm has profound venodilation (and vasodilation) effects, reducing preload. This is perilous for those with poor systolic function, single-ventricle physiology, and left ventricular outflow tract obstruction. Bronchospasm treatment with albuterol or intravenous epinephrine causes tachycardia and worsens the physiology of those with obstructive cardiac lesions. Although the aforementioned considerations would imply a conservative approach to the child with CHD and a URI, data from children undergoing catheterization laboratory procedures suggested no long-term harm from perioperative consequences of URI despite the need for acute resuscitation.[4]

## Premedication

Sedative premedication may benefit those with extensive medicalization or those in whom crying would disturb physiology. Distress increases heart rate, blood pressure, and pulmonary vascular resistance. Defer premedication for those in extremis who are relying on sympathetic tone for survival preoperatively.

## INTRAOPERATIVE

Provide anticipatory guidance to operating room staff. For example, for a child at risk of ventricular arrhythmias, set the defibrillator's energy select to 2 J/kg.

Induction and maintenance of anesthesia should preserve the cardiac index. Andropoulos et al. found that in children with CHD, the cardiac index was preserved at 1 MAC (minimum alveolar concentration) and at 1.5 MAC (or equivalent) with various anesthetics. The results are shown in Figure 247.1.

Laparoscopic surgical technique tends to decrease systolic function on transesophageal echocardiography and reduced preload due to pneumoperitoneum; however; children with single-ventricle physiology tend tolerate it.

During an intraoperative emergency, use crisis resource management. Use directed, closed-loop communication, and following 6 minutes of cardiopulmonary resuscitation, activate extracorporeal membrane oxygenation. Details

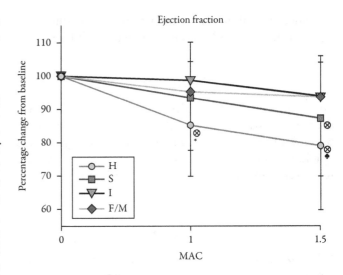

⊗ Change from baseline, $p < .05$
∗ H vs I, $p < .05$
♦ H vs I, F/M $p < .05$

**Figure 247.1** Percentage change of cardiac index from baseline in children with CHD versus minimum alveolar concentration (MAC) for various anesthetics.[5] Isoflurane preserves cardiac index well.

vary based on candidacy and feasibility of cannulation sites according to cardiac anatomy and somatic size.

## POSTOPERATIVE

Postoperatively, fluid shifts present a significant source of morbidity. Even appropriate intraoperative fluid administration may lead to pulmonary edema and dyspnea, dependent edema, and lymphatic failure with chylous pleural effusions in single-ventricle patients.

For outpatient procedures, attention should be given to the return of activities of daily living without dyspnea or hypoxia. In practice, this may include asking the patient to walk while monitoring oxygen saturation and work of breathing prior to discharge from the postanesthesia care unit.

## REFERENCES

1. Hoffman JI, Kaplan S. The incidence of congenital heart disease. *J Am Coll Cardiol.* 2002;39(12):1890–1900.
2. Faraoni D., et al. Development and validation of a risk stratification score for children with congenital heart disease undergoing noncardiac surgery. *Anesth Analg.* 2016;123(4):824–830.
3. Brown ML, et al. Anesthesia in pediatric patients with congenital heart disease undergoing noncardiac surgery: defining the risk. *J Cardiothorac Vasc Anesth.* 2020;34(2):470–478.
4. Zhang S., et al. Impact of upper respiratory tract infections on perioperative outcomes of children undergoing therapeutic cardiac catheterisation. *Acta Anaesthesiol Scand.* 2018;62(7):915–923.
5. Rivenes SM, et al. Cardiovascular effects of sevoflurane, isoflurane, halothane, and fentanyl-midazolam in children with congenital heart disease: an echocardiographic study of myocardial contractility and hemodynamics. *Anesthesiology.* 2001;94(2):223–229.

# 248.

# CHRONIC CONGENITAL HEART DISEASE

*Jamie W. Sinton*

## INTRODUCTION

By adulthood, most patients with congenital heart disease (CHD) will have undergone some type of cardiac repair. Many will have a complication, increased risk of sudden death, and eventually transition to adult care.

## CHRONIC DISEASE

Congestive heart failure encompasses cardiac dysfunction and its neurohormonal effects. It is due to pressure overload in a single ventricle or volume overload (e.g., Ebstein anomaly). Noncardiac contributors include hypertension and obstructive sleep apnea. Late complications such as pulmonary arterial hypertension are not compatible with passive pulmonary blood flow as in the Fontan. Cancer risk is elevated due to radiation exposure. Long-term cyanosis can lead to brain abscess and stroke.

## ARRHYTHMIAS AND EPICARDIAL PACEMAKER SYSTEMS

Congenital heart defects or their treatments can result in arrhythmia burden. Scar-related reentrant atrial tachycardia and atrial flutter are the most common.[1] Fontan patients would have epicardial implanted electrical systems are shown in Figure 248.1.

Epicardial systems do not obviate subacute bacterial endocarditis prophylaxis and are more prone to complications than transvenous systems.

## SPECIFIC LESIONS

### D-TRANSPOSITION OF GREAT ARTERIES

Newborns with d-transposition of the great arteries (d-TGA) can be quite sick, and undergo balloon atrial septostomy early, then an arterial switch operation as a neonate. Surgery includes great vessel suture lines and coronary reimplantation, as shown in Figure 248.2. However, long-term, these children do well.[2]

### TETRALOGY OF FALLOT

Figure 248.3 depicts anatomy in tetralogy of Fallot (TOF) both at birth and following two common types of repair. Patients with repaired TOF can be expected to have a right bundle-branch block (RBBB) on electrocardiogram. On echocardiogram (echo), dyskinesis of the ventricular septum is expected as the ventricular septal defect patch does not contract and the RBBB impairs ventricular synchrony.

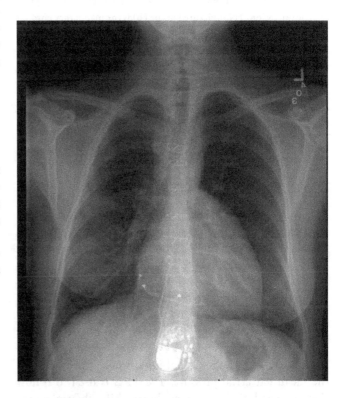

Figure 248.1 A chest roentgenogram of a patient with an epicardial pacing system. Note the subxiphoid generator location and atrial and ventricular leads external to the heart.

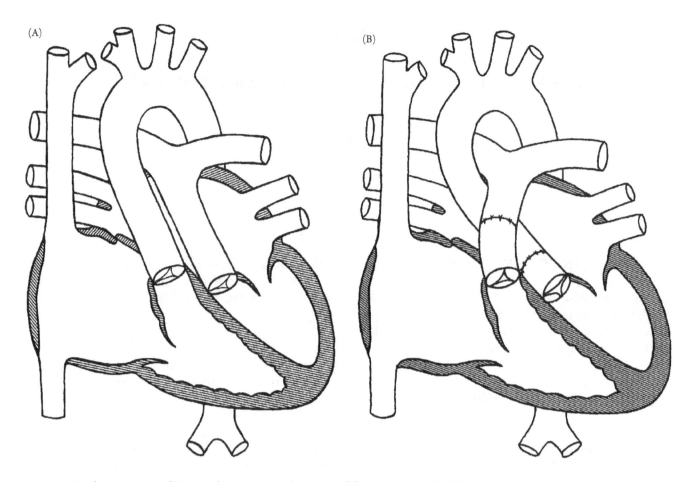

**Figure 248.2** Cardiac anatomy in d-TGA with intact ventricular septum. (A) Anatomy at birth. (B) Following the arterial switch operation (Jatene operation).[5] Not pictured in the (B) is the mandatory coronary artery reimplantation into the neoaortic root.

Pulmonic regurgitation is well tolerated even long term.[4] However, residual free pulmonary insufficiency volume loads the heart. Right ventricular volume is followed by magnetic resonance imaging to determine timing for pulmonary valve replacement.

## SINGLE-VENTRICLE DISEASE

Fontan palliation is the most common final stage for patients with many types of univentricular heart disease. See Figure 248.4 for anatomic depiction of hypoplastic left heart syndrome at birth, following Norwood, Glenn, and Fontan operations.

Total cavopulmonary anastomosis is often accomplished with an extracardiac conduit. The hemodynamic force that drives blood to the lungs is called the transpulmonary gradient (TPG). The (TPG) is the difference between the mean pulmonary artery pressure and the mean left atrial pressure. The TPG is used to follow Fontan circulation dynamics. Meanwhile, the right ventricle is pressure overloaded while pumping the systemic circulation; it is prone to failure.

### Protein-Losing Enteropathy, Plastic Bronchitis, and Liver Disease

Protein-losing enteropathy is the abnormal loss of serum proteins into the lumen of the gastrointestinal tract via diarrhea and portends a poor prognosis. Thrombosis occurs due to loss of coagulation proteins; edema, effusions, and ascites result.

Plastic bronchitis is the production of branching casts filling the airways due to aberrant lymphatic vessels. Obstructive lung disease presents with expectoration of casts. No definitive treatment exists.

Liver disease is characterized by centrilobular fibrosis. Hepatic injury may occur even before the Fontan operation.[5]

## ANESTHETIC CONSIDERATIONS

### PREOPERATIVE

Optimization prior to elective surgery involves routine preoperative cardiology care. Ensure that the patient's clinical trajectory is consistent with the natural history of palliation for that lesion. Seek subtle signs of clinical decompensation, including failure to thrive, hyperviscosity symptoms, or

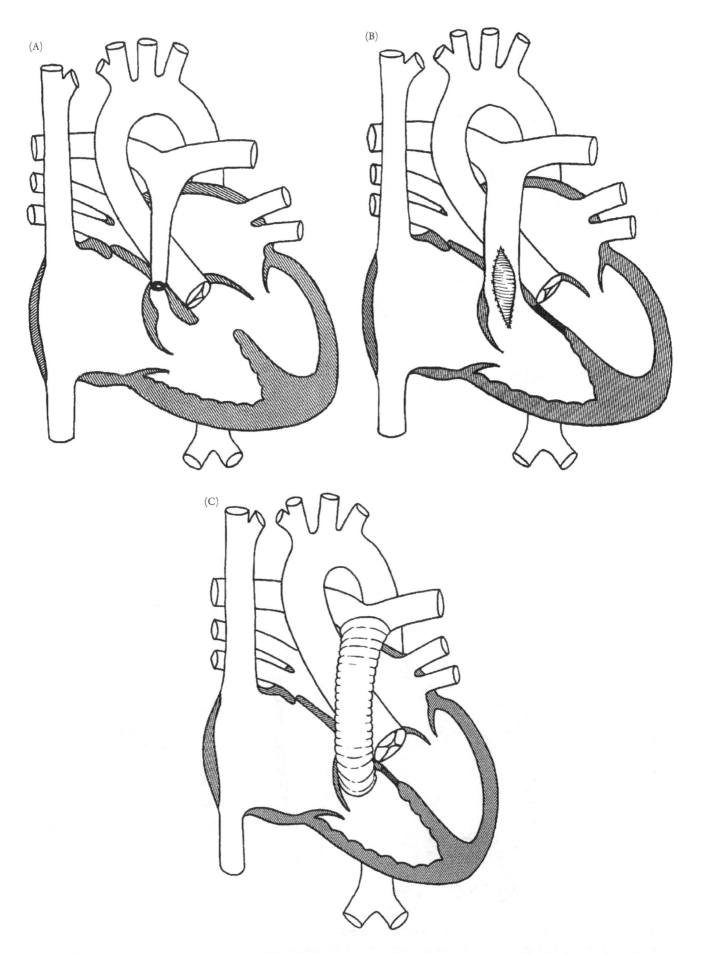

**Figure 248.3** (A) Common TOF anatomy prior to repair. (B) and (C) Common types of repairs: transannular patch (B) and right ventricle–pulmonary artery conduit (C).[3]

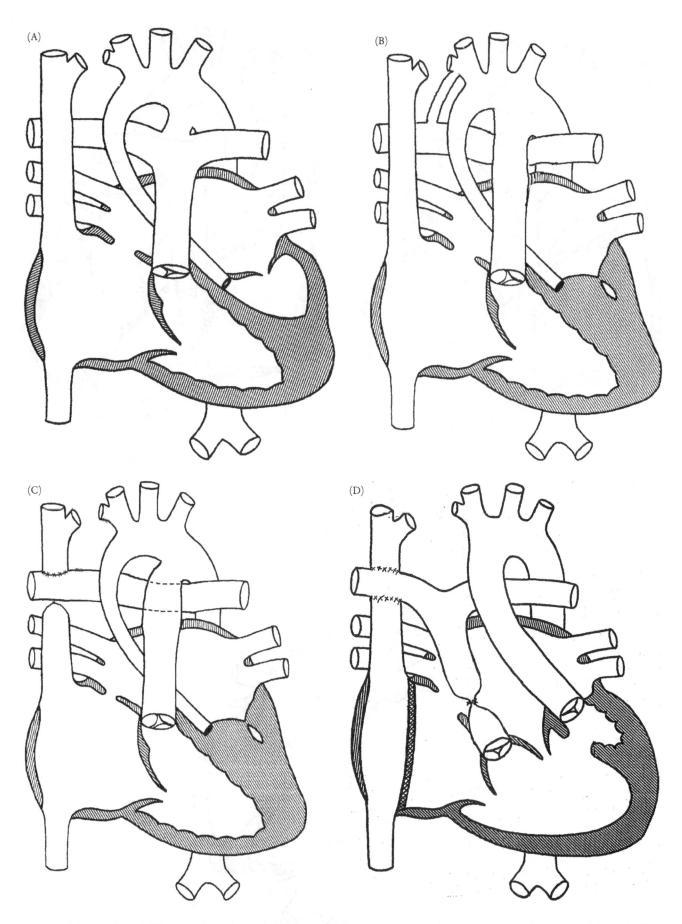

**Figure 248.4** (A) Hypoplastic left heart syndrome (HLHS). (B) Anatomy following Norwood arch reconstruction with a right modified Blalock-Taussig shunt for pulmonary blood supply. (C) Anatomy following Glenn. Note the superior cavopulmonary anastomosis. (D) Anatomy following Fontan connection with extracardiac conduit (nonfenestrated). Note that Glenn and Fontan circulations are extracardiac connections. Variable intracardiac anatomy is given for example.[3]

signs of endocarditis. Anticipate long-term effects of that patient's circulation and prior procedures.

In polycythemic patients, the amount of citrate in the tubes for coagulation studies must be adjusted in order to obtain accurate results.

## INTRAOPERATIVE

Common cardiac surgeries include Fontan conversion, arrhythmia surgery and pulmonary valve replacement. Endocarditis risk is discussed in the chapter on subacute bacterial endocarditis prophylaxis. Also, defibrillator and pacemaker generators may be subxiphoid and interfere with surgical electrocautery. In this case, disabling of the antitachycardia function is indicated intraoperatively.

## POSTOPERATIVE

Postoperatively, active pursuit of symptoms related to the cardiac system should be sought. For outpatient surgery, require some level of activity in the postanesthesia care unit that could emulate home activities.

## REFERENCES

1. Hernandez-Madrid A, et al. Arrhythmias in congenital heart disease: a position paper of the European Heart Rhythm Association (EHRA), Association for European Paediatric and Congenital Cardiology (AEPC), and the European Society of Cardiology (ESC) Working Group on Grown-up Congenital Heart Disease, endorsed by HRS, PACES, APHRS, and SOLAECE. *Europace.* 2018;20(11):1719–1753.
2. Lee J, et al. Pulmonary artery interventions after the arterial switch operation: unique and significant risks. *Congenit Heart Dis.* 2019;14(2):288–296.
3. Mullins CE. Congenital heart disease: a diagrammatic atlas. 1988;Liss;352.
4. Kendsersky P, Ward C. Right ventricular failure and congenital heart disease. *Cardiol Clin.* 2020;38(2):239–242.
5. Wu FM, et al. Portal and centrilobular hepatic fibrosis in Fontan circulation and clinical outcomes. *J Heart Lung Transplant.* 2015;34(7):883–891.

# 249.

# CONGENITAL DIAPHRAGMATIC HERNIA

*Cassandra Wasson and Christina D. Diaz*

## INTRODUCTION

Congenital diaphragmatic hernias (CDHs) are characterized by herniation of abdominal contents into the chest cavity due to a developmental defect of the diaphragm.[1-3] This herniation inhibits the normal growth of the lungs, which causes structural and functional changes to the heart, pulmonary circulation, lung parenchyma, and airways, resulting in pulmonary hypoplasia and subsequent pulmonary hypertension.[1,3] Pulmonary hypertension leads to a right-to-left shunting of blood through the patent ductus arteriosus and persistence of fetal circulation.[4]

Congenital diaphragmatic hernia is rare with a prevalence of 1 in 3000 births.[2-4] Posterolateral (or Bochdalek) hernias are the most common (70%–75%). Anterior (or Morgagni) hernias occur in 23%–28%, and the remaining 2%–7% are central hernias[1-3] (Figure 249.1). Left-sided hernias are about five times more common than right-sided ones. The etiology is unknown, but likely multifactorial.[1,3] It has been associated with vitamin A deficiency, as well as maternal mycophenolate, allopurinol, and lithium use.[3] In 50%–70% of cases, CDH is an isolated finding. The remaining 30%–50% are associated with other major structural abnormalities, chromosomal defects, or single-gene disorders.[1]

Concurrent structural abnormalities may occur in a number of organ systems. Cardiovascular anomalies occur in 25%–40% of cases and include, but are not limited to,

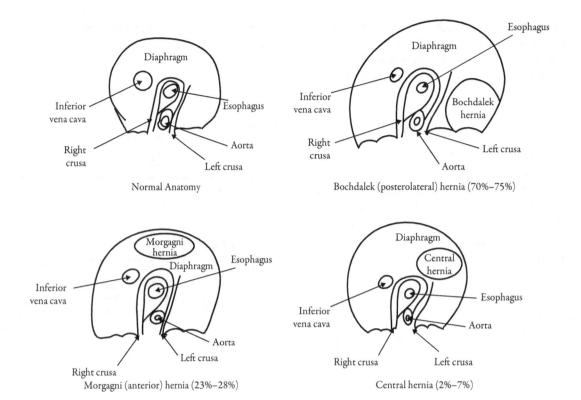

**Figure 249.1** Congenital diaphragmatic hernia types.

ventricular septal defects, atrial septal defects, tetralogy of Fallot, and aortic coarctation.[1,2] Central nervous system defects occur in 5%–10% of cases and include neural tube defects and hydrocephalus.[1,3] Musculoskeletal (e.g., polydactyly, syndactyly, limb reduction defects, club foot, vertebral anomalies, and abdominal wall defects); gastrointestinal (e.g., malrotation or imperforate anus); and urogenital (e.g., renal agenesis) abnormalities also may occur.[1,3]

Chromosomal defects are found in 10%–35% of cases.[1,3] These include aneuploidies, chromosomal deletions/duplications, and complex chromosomal rearrangements. The most common aneuploidies associated with CDH are trisomy 13, 18, and 21 and monosomy X,[1,3] but other deletion and duplication syndromes are also seen. Underlying genetic syndromes are seen in 10% of cases, with Fryns syndrome the most common. Other genetic syndromes include, but are not limited to, Apert, Beckwith-Wiedemann syndrome, and CHARGE (coloboma, heart defects, atresia of the choanae, retardation [intellectual], genital anomalies, and ear anomalies) syndrome.[1,3]

## DIAGNOSIS

Congenital diaphragmatic hernia occurs in the 4th to 12th week of gestation, and over 60% are diagnosed prenatally with routine ultrasound.[1] Herniation of the liver into the chest is a poor prognostic factor and is highly predictive

of the need for extracorporeal membrane oxygenation (ECMO) (80% with liver herniation vs. 25% in those without) and increased mortality (65% vs. 7%).[1,2] Observed-to-expected (O/E) lung area–to–head circumference ratio (LHR) has become one of the standard prenatal metrics to help predict outcomes.[1-3] It classifies severity of hypoplasia and is linked to survival (Table 249.1).

Although the majority of CDHs are diagnosed prenatally, 40% present postnatally with tachypnea, chest retractions, tachycardia, and cyanosis after birth.[1] Their physical examination is significant for barrel-shaped chest, scaphoid abdomen, and absence of breath sounds on the

*Table 249.1* OBSERVED-TO-EXPECTED LUNG AREA IN RELATION TO HEAD CIRCUMFERENCE (O/E LHR), SEVERITY SCORE, AND PERCENTAGE SURVIVAL

| O/E LHR, % | SEVERITY OF HYPOPLASIA | PERCENTAGE SURVIVAL |
|---|---|---|
| >45 | | |
| 36–45 | Mild | >75 |
| 26–35 | Moderate | 30–60 |
| 15–25 | Severe | 20 |
| <15 | Extreme | 0 |

From Reference 2.

ipsilateral side. Chest and abdominal radiographs are diagnostic and show mediastinal shift with stomach and gas-filled loops of bowel in the chest.[1,4] The primary cause of death is progressive hypoxemia and acidosis.

## MANAGEMENT

If diagnosed prenatally, fetoscopic endoluminal tracheal occlusion is an experimental option for severe cases (O/E LHR < 25% and liver herniation).[1,3] At 27–29 weeks' gestational age, a balloon is placed into the fetal trachea, causing an obstruction, which prevents fluid from leaving the lungs, increasing pulmonary pressure and subsequently increasing lung size.[1–3] The balloon is removed at 34 weeks' gestational age to allow development of type II pneumocytes and surfactant expression.[3] This intervention has led to increased survival rates but is not without risk of spontaneous preterm labor and rupture of membranes in 47% of cases, with an average delivery at 35 weeks' gestation.[1,3]

For fetuses with CDH diagnosed prenatally, delivery is planned after 39 weeks' gestation at a tertiary center.[1] The neonate is intubated immediately after delivery to avoid insufflation of the stomach and bowel with the neonate's respiratory effort.[1,2,4] An orogastric tube is inserted and placed on suction to decompress the stomach.[1–3] Both pre- and postductal saturations are monitored, with $FiO_2$ (fraction of inspired oxygen) titrated to maintain preductal saturations 80%–95% and postductal greater than 70%.[1] Surfactant is associated with lower survival rates in CDH, so it is not recommended.[1]

Ventilation management of these neonates can be challenging. Permissive hypercapnia ($PaCO_2$ 50–70 mm Hg) with gentle ventilation has been shown to increase survival.[1,2] Recommendations for ventilation include limiting peak inspiratory pressure to less than 25 cm $H_2O$, positive end-expiratory pressure of 3 to 5, and a rate of 40–60 breaths per minute.[1] If traditional ventilatory management does not provide adequate ventilation, high-frequency oscillatory ventilation (HFOV) is utilized.[1] In severe cases where HFOV is not adequate, the discussion of ECMO is warrented.[1]

The use of ECMO is contraindicated with gestational age less than 35 weeks, weight less than 2000 g, preexisting intracranial hemorrhage, congenital or neurological anomalies incompatible with good outcomes, more than a week of aggressive ventilatory therapy, and congenital heart disease.

## ANESTHETIC CONSIDERATIONS

### PREOPERATIVE

Preoperatively, timing of surgical repair of CDH is controversial.[1] Survival rates improved from 20% to 55% with delayed CDH repair and medical stabilization, which has led most centers to delay repair until lactate is less than 3 mmol/L, urine output is greater than 1 mL/kg/h, preductal saturations are 85%–95%, and mean arterial pressures are normal for gestational age.[1,2] Thus, CDH is considered a physiologic emergency, not a surgical emergency, unless herniated bowel is showing signs of ischemia.[2]

### INTRAOPERATIVE

Adequate venous access is necessary, with preference for the upper extremities because of the risk of inferior vena cava (IVC) compression after hernia reduction.[4] Nitrous oxide should be avoided.[4] Increased abdominal pressure, cephalad displacement of the diaphragm, decreased functional residual capacity, and compression of the IVC after hernia reduction should be anticipated.[4] Creation of a ventral hernia and placement of a silo is an option if the hernia requires slower reduction due to the underdeveloped abdominal cavity.[4] Aggressive positive pressure ventilation may cause a contralateral pneumothorax intraoperatively and presents as hypotension and hypoxemia.[1,4] Any deterioration of heart rate and blood pressure suggests contralateral pneumothorax, which should be treated by placing a chest tube. Some may consider prophylactic insertion of a chest tube on the contralateral side before surgery. Positive pressure ventilation with bag and mask may cause distention of the gut and should be avoided.

### POSTOPERATIVE

The overall survival rate is 70%–90% in non-ECMO neonates and up to 50% of those that require ECMO.[1,2] However, neonates that survive CDH repair continue to have long-term morbidity. Recurrent respiratory infections and respiratory insufficiency occur in 34% of patients. Patients will have gastrointestinal issues, including gastroesophageal reflux disease (30%) and failure to thrive or feeding issues (20%). Musculoskeletal deformities, such as scoliosis, pectus excavatum, or pectus carinatum, are common in 40% of adolescent CDH survivors. Cognitive impairment or developmental delay is the most common morbidity and affects up to 70% of patients.

## REFERENCES

1. Chatterjee D, et al. Update on congenital diaphragmatic hernia. *Anesth Analg.* 2020;131(3):808–821.
2. Dingeldein M. Congenital diaphragmatic hernia: management & outcomes. *Adv Pediatr.* 2018;65:241–247.
3. Kosiński P, Wielgoś M. Congenital diaphragmatic hernia: pathogenesis, prenatal diagnosis and management—literature review. *Ginekol Pol.* 2017;88(1):24–30.
4. Hines RL, Marschall KE. Pediatric diseases. In: Stoelting RK, eds. *Stoelting's Anesthesia and Co-existing Disease.* 7th ed. Philadelphia, PA: Saunders/Elsevier; 2012:635–670.

# 250.

# TRACHEOESOPHAGEAL FISTULA

*Cassandra Wasson and Christina D. Diaz*

## INTRODUCTION

Tracheoesophageal fistula (TEF), as the name suggests, is an unwanted congenital fistula between the trachea and esophagus that results in numerous aerogastric complications and occurs in 1/2500–3000 births.[1,2] The pathogenesis is not completely known but is thought to be due to incomplete separation of the tracheal bud and primitive foregut during the fourth or fifth week of embryogenesis.[1]

Prenatal ultrasound can suggest a diagnosis of TEF by the findings of polyhydramnios and a small or absent fetal stomach bubble, but it only has a positive predictive value of 44%.[1,2] The prenatal ultrasound may raise suspicions of TEF, especially if after birth the neonate is exhibiting clinical symptoms, including excessive salivation, choking with feeds, and the inability to pass a suction catheter into the stomach.[2] It is then diagnosed by radiography, which will demonstrate the presence of gas below the diaphragm.[2] Historically, contrast studies were used, such as a barium swallow or computed tomography, but these studies have a high risk of resulting aspiration and lung injury and are rarely used today.[1]

There are five subtypes of TEF that are determined by the location of the fistula and presence or absence of esophageal atresia (EA)[1] (Figure 250.1). Type C is the most common (86%) and is EA with a distal TEF.[2] Type A is isolated EA without a fistula (7%); type B is EA with a proximal TEF (2%); type D is the rarest form and is EA with proximal and distal TEF (<1%); and type E (also called type H) is a TEF without EA (4%).[2] E or H type TEF is the most difficult to diagnose, and its diagnosis may be delayed past the first month of life in 31% of patients and even up to adolescence or adulthood in some patients.[1]

Treatment for TEF can result in open surgical repair or endoscopic procedures. Endoscopic procedures, such as fibrin occlusion, sclerotherapy, electrocautery, or laser coagulation, have lower morbidity and mortality, but high recurrence rates.[1,2] Therefore, surgical repair remains the standard treatment for TEF.[1] Determining the subtype of TEF will help guide the best surgical approach. Type A is managed with a gastrostomy tube and repair of the fistula in 2–3 months.[1] The other fistulas are surgically repaired by cervical dissection, thoracotomy, or thoracoscopic surgery. If the fistula is above T2, a cervical approach is usually taken.[1] Fistulas below T2 are repaired by thoracotomy or thoracoscopic surgery.[1] Thoracoscopic approaches have lower morbidity, better surgical exposure, less surgical

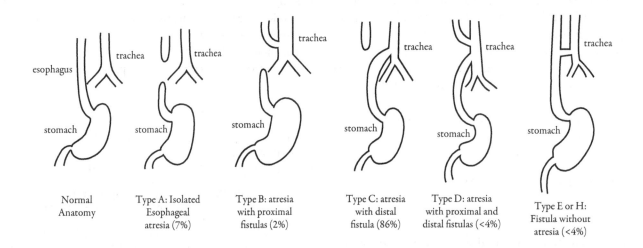

Normal Anatomy

Type A: Isolated Esophageal atresia (7%)

Type B: atresia with proximal fistulas (2%)

Type C: atresia with distal fistula (86%)

Type D: atresia with proximal and distal fistulas (<4%)

Type E or H: Fistula without atresia (<4%)

**Figure 250.1** Tracheoesophageal fistula subtypes.

trauma to the lung, faster extubation, and faster recovery. However, with thoracoscopy comes additional challenges for the anesthesia provider, as discussed below.

## ANESTHETIC CONSIDERATIONS

### PREOPERATIVE

Tracheoesophageal fistula repair is generally an urgent operation to minimize aspiration pneumonia and begin enteral nutrition.[1] Additional congenital anomalies occur in 50% of patients with TEF, and it is more common in isolated EA (65%) than isolated TEF (10%).[2] Many of these congenital anomalies are part of the VACTERL (vertebral defects, anal atresia, cardiac anomalies, TEF, renal agenesis and dysplasia, and limb anomalies) sequence.[3] Therefore, preoperative evaluation should address these organ systems.

A 12-lead electrocardiogram and echocardiogram should be obtained to diagnose associated congenital heart disease (CHD).[1,2] Cardiac anomalies are the most frequently associated abnormality at 29% and include but are not limited to ventricular septal defect, patent ductus arteriosus (PDA), atrial septal defect, and right-sided aortic arch.[2] If a neonate is found to have ductal-dependent CHD, the options include proceeding with TEF repair while maintaining prostaglandin infusion to keep the ductus arteriosus patent or proceeding with a palliating cardiac surgery first.[2]

Gastrointestinal and genitourinary anomalies are the next most common at 14% each.[2] Gastrointestinal anomalies include duodenal atresia, imperforate anus, pyloric stenosis, and malrotation.[2] Genitourinary anomalies include renal agenesis, hypospadias, and horseshoe/polycystic kidney disease.[2]

Musculoskeletal anomalies occur in 10% of TEF patients and include radial limb abnormalities, polydactyly, hemivertebrae, and scoliosis.[2] A lumbar ultrasound to evaluate for a tethered chord or other abnormalities is required for neonates with TEF and a sacral dimple, especially if a caudal catheter is being considered.[1,2]

Respiratory anomalies such as tracheobronchomalacia, pulmonary hypoplasia, and tracheal agenesis or stenosis occur in 6% of patients with TEF.[2] Last, genetic anomalies are the least prevalent occurrence at 4% of TEF patients, with trisomy 21 and trisomy 18 being the most common.

The preoperative evaluation is useful for detecting TEF patients who are at a higher risk of complications. These include patients with coexisting complex CHD, weight less than 2 kg, poor pulmonary compliance, large pericarinal fistulas, and those scheduled for thoracoscopic repairs.[2] Studies have shown that neonates less than 2 kg with CHD have a survival rate of 27%, whereas those more than 2 kg without CHD have survival rates approaching 100%.[2]

### INTRAOPERATIVE

Standard American Society of Anesthesiologists monitors and an arterial line are used for TEF repair.[1,2] Two pulse oximeters, one pre- and one postductal, are useful in neonatal surgeries to help detect excessive pulmonary arterial pressure and shunting in the presence of a PDA.[3] Vigilance is paramount in this case as the endotracheal tube (ETT) can dislodge from the trachea into the fistula and result in death.[3] Therefore, a left-sided precordial stethoscope is recommended.

Traditionally, it was taught to avoid positive pressure ventilation (PPV), including mask ventilation, until the fistula was ligated to prevent gastric distension, which would restrict ventilation and increase the risk of gastric perforation.[1] However, recent experience and studies have shown that PPV is safe in fistulas less than 3 mm in diameter.[1,2]

The preferred ETT for intubation is a microcuff ETT.[1,3] The cuff is relatively distal on the ETT,[3] and it does not have a Murphy eye.[1-3] This allows the ETT to be positioned in a way that avoids ventilation of the fistula and subsequent gastric distention.[1,3] Traditionally, the ETT is placed distal to the carina into the right mainstem bronchus and withdrawn until breath sounds become bilateral.[1,3] This works well in 67% of fistulas that are greater than 1 cm above the carina.[2,3] However, in the remaining 33% that are pericarinal, this is a poor choice. In those cases, the ETT may be placed proximal to the fistula or in the left mainstem bronchus, or a catheter can be placed into the fistula to seal it off.[3] Placing the ETT proximal to the fistula risks insufflation of the stomach, which can lead to gastric distention and rupture. Therefore, in patients at risk of requiring higher airway pressures, such as neonates with noncompliant lungs, an already distended abdomen, or a large fistula, this is not an optimal choice.[3] Placing the ETT into the left mainstem bronchus isolates ventilation from the fistula and from the right lung, which facilitates surgical exposure for thoracoscopic cases.[2,3] There are case reports of successful use of left mainstem intubation in both term and preterm infants as young as 34 weeks' postconceptual age and 1.5 kg.[2] It is important to monitor carbon dioxide ($CO_2$) via blood gases as the end-tidal $CO_2$ is falsely low in one-lung ventilation.[2]

Placing a catheter, typically a 3-French Fogarty balloon-tipped catheter, into the fistula to block it is yet another option. This allows the ETT to be placed into the midtrachea and use of PPV.[3] It is a good option for patients with a large distal fistula and poor lung compliance[2] but has the risk of dislodgement during the procedure. Furthermore, the catheter in the fistula may help the surgeons identify the TEF and distinguish it from the bronchus or aorta. However, it is important to withdraw the catheter prior to ligation of the fistula.[3] Another option is to maintain spontaneous ventilation until the fistula is ligated. Avoid nitrous oxide.

## POSTOPERATIVE

Historically, TEF malformation was 100% fatal. However, survival rates are now as high as 95% due to advancements in neonatal intensive care, anesthesia, ventilators, nutritional support, and surgical tools and techniques.[1] Postoperative mortality continues to fall, but complications are still common.[1] Postoperative vocal cord dysfunction may occur due to recurrent laryngeal nerve injury and is most common with H-type TEF.[1,2] Other complications include tracheomalacia, dysphagia, and gastroesophageal reflux disease (GERD). GERD occurs in 35%58% of patients and often persists into adulthood.[2]

Postoperatively, all TEF patients are admitted to intensive care.[1,2] Early extubation is an option for full-term neonates with no associated anomalies or respiratory impairment.[1,3] This decreases abrasion to the anastomosis from an indwelling ETT.[1] However, reintubation after repair may cause trauma to the fistula site and traction on the esophageal anastomosis.[1,3] Therefore, the risk of failing extubation is strongly evaluated prior to extubation.[1,3]

Enteral nutrition is delivered via a feeding tube beginning 48 hours after repair.[1] Oral feeding typically begins between 5 and 7 days after repair, once the neonate demonstrates adequate swallowing of saliva and after a contrast swallow study has confirmed the absence of both stenosis and leak at the anastomosis site.[1] Mark the suction catheter to make sure it will not extend past the anastomosis, which can potentially cause damage.

Analgesia options for postoperative pain include an intravenous opioid infusion, epidural catheter, caudal catheter, subcutaneous wound catheters, and local infiltration.[1,2] Regional anesthesia can facilitate earlier extubation by reducing the risk of apnea with opioid analgesia.[1,2] However, regional anesthesia is contraindicated in infants with coexisting CHD due to its tendency to decrease systemic vascular resistance.[1,2]

## REFERENCES

1. Edelman B, et al. Anesthesia practice: review of perioperative management of H-type tracheoesophageal fistula. *Anesthesiol Res Pract.* 2019;2019:8621801.
2. Broemling N, Campbell F. Anesthetic management of congenital tracheoesophageal fistula. *Pediatr Anesth.* 2010;21(11):1092–1099.
3. Ho AM-H, et al. Airway and ventilatory management options in congenital tracheoesophageal fistula repair. *J Cardiothorac Vasc Anesth.* 2016;30(2):515–520.

# 251.

# NEONATAL LOBAR EMPHYSEMA

*Jamie W. Sinton*

## INTRODUCTION

Neonatal lobar emphysema (NLE), also called congenital lobar emphysema or congenital lobar hyperinflation, is a relatively rare congenital pulmonary malformation. It represents fewer than 10% of congenital lung masses.[1] The etiology is often idiopathic but sometimes can be attributed to intrinsic disruption of bronchial morphogenesis or extrinsic (e.g., vessel) compression.[2] The lung, often the left upper lobe, has progressive air trapping and enlargement, leading to respiratory distress.

Following birth, the differential diagnosis of respiratory distress is broad and includes tension pneumothorax, congenital bronchopulmonary sequestration (intralobar or extralobar), congenital cystic adenomatoid malformation, bronchial cyst, bronchial stenosis, tracheoesophageal fistula, congenital diaphragmatic hernia, congenital pneumonia, airway malformation or malacia, respiratory distress syndrome, aberrant blood vessel, or cardiac causes such as absent pulmonary valve syndrome.

## PATHOPHYSIOLOGY

Respiratory distress in the neonatal or infant period is common. Neonatal lobar emphysema may mimic tension pneumothorax on chest roentgenogram (chest x-ray, CXR) as the lung is hyperinflated and the appearance of parenchyma is diminished. Progressive air trapping causes sudden respiratory distress. Hyperinflation leads to compression of other lung tissue, mediastinal shifting, and impaired venous return. See Figure 251.1 for an example of left lung hyperexpansion with mediastinal shifting.

## NATURAL HISTORY AND TREATMENT

The natural history of lung malformations varies from causing nonimmune hydrops fetalis and intrauterine demise, to neonatal respiratory distress, and to incidental finding on CXR in childhood. Prenatal detection of NLE is poor compared with other lung malformations.[3] Additionally, some lung lesions regress with time, causing variable respiratory distress at birth[4]; however, lung masses with cystic components are less likely to regress and more likely to be NLE. Prenatal ultrasound findings include increased echogenicity in the thorax and contralateral lung hypoplasia or polyhydramnios due to compression of the lung or esophagus, respectively.[5]

In severe cases of NLE (and other lung malformations), ex utero intrapartum therapy may facilitate resection with either placental bypass or extracorporeal membrane oxygenation. This requires complex multidisciplinary teamwork and is not discussed further.

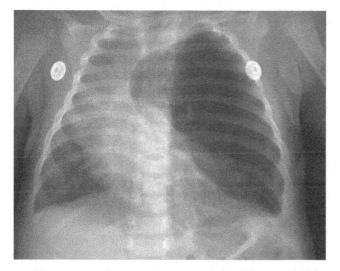

**Figure 251.1** Anteroposterior projection of a chest roentgenogram of a neonate with NLE. Note left-sided hyperexpansion and mediastinal shift.

At the other end of the spectrum, management of asymptomatic lesions is controversial, although malignization is possible, and resection may be warranted.

## ANESTHETIC CONSIDERATIONS

### PREOPERATIVE

Preoperatively, physical examination findings include asymmetric chest expansion, retractions, wheezing, diminished breath sounds, or tachycardia. Crying is poorly tolerated as it increases the amount of trapped gas in the affected lung and may precipitate respiratory distress.

Lung imaging with CXR and computed tomography are used for surgical planning and to risk stratify the lesion based on the cystic adenomatoid volume ratio. This ratio compares lesion diameter to head circumference. These patients should also undergo cardiac evaluation with echocardiography as mediastinal shift may lead to great vessel or cardiac compression. As NLE is only rarely associated with other major congenital anomalies, further workup is dictated by history and physical examination.

### INTRAOPERATIVE

Most neonates and infants with NLE undergo lung lobectomy. Operative technique of open thoracotomy or thoracoscopic resection is controversial and probably depends on the preference of the surgeon. Induction of anesthesia has been variably accomplished with focus around maintenance of spontaneous ventilation. Positive pressure ventilation can also increase the amount of trapped gas in the lung. Muscle relaxation may be deferred in order to preserve spontaneous (or assisted ventilation).

In order to facilitate surgical hemithoracic visualization, lung separation is useful. As airway equipment is limited in children younger than 6 months old, endobronchial intubation is a rational choice. Right and left bronchial diameters differ and are much smaller than tracheal diameter, so one-half size smaller endotracheal tube for age should be considered. Exact measurements of airway diameters can be made from preoperative imaging and used to plan endobronchial tube size. Lung separation can also be achieved with extraluminal bronchial blocker. The advantage of lung separation as opposed to surgical retraction is surgical visualization and improved preservation of hypoxic pulmonary vasoconstriction.

### POSTOPERATIVE

Following lobectomy, the surrounding lung tissue expands as compression by the enlarged lobe is relieved. A thoracostomy tube is placed. The infant may be extubated postoperatively, with attention to minimizing airway pressures. Some advocate for deep extubation to minimize coughing and disruption of the surgical site. Presurgical diagnosis of NLE is often confirmed on pathology but has been mistaken for adenomatoid malformation of the pulmonary airway.[1]

Pain management has been described with opioids or regional techniques. Thoracostomy tube drainage may add an element of safety in the performance of paravertebral blockade.

Outcomes are generally favorable. Children may have a residual reduction in forced vital capacity throughout childhood. Neurodevelopmental outcomes do not appear to differ among those infants with either fetal intervention or neonatal resection.

## REFERENCES

1. Rodríguez-Velasco A, et al. Cystic and pseudocystic pulmonary malformations in children: clinico-pathological correlation. *Ann Diagn Pathol*. 2019;39:78–85.
2. Durell J, Lakhoo K. Congenital cystic lesions of the lung. *Early Hum Dev*. 2014;90:935–939.
3. Kunisaki SM, et al. Current operative management of congenital lobar emphysema in children: a report from the Midwest Pediatric Surgery Consortium. *J Pediatr Surg*. 2019;54:1138–1142.
4. Kunisaki SM, et al. Vanishing fetal lung malformations: prenatal sonographic characteristics and postnatal outcomes. *J Pediatr Surg*. 2015;50:978–982.
5. Palla J, Sockrider MM. Congenital lung malformations. *Pediatr Ann*. 2019;48(4):e169–e174.

# 252.

# PYLORIC STENOSIS

*Mariam Batakji and Christina D. Diaz*

## INTRODUCTION

Pyloric stenosis presents in early infancy and is considered a medical emergency, but not a surgical emergency. It involves idiopathic thickening of the pyloric musculature, leading to gastric outlet obstruction syndrome. The patient requires medical stabilization, rehydration, correction of electrolyte abnormalities, and eventual surgical intervention. Pyloric stenosis has an incidence of 2 to 4 per 1000 live births in Western populations,[1] with a female-to-male ratio of 1:4. The etiology remains unknown, with the incidence occurring less commonly in Black or Asian ethnic groups than in Caucasians within the United States.

## CLINICAL PRESENTATION AND DIAGNOSIS

Infants present within the first 2 to 12 weeks of life with projectile, nonbilious vomiting, leading to dehydration, impaired nutritional intake, and lethargy.[2] An important clinical feature is that the infant remains hungry. Depending on the duration of the symptoms, infants can present with simple dehydration up to frank hypovolemic shock.[3,4] Clinical diagnosis is made by history and physical examination, where palpation of an "olive-like" mass in the right upper quadrant is highly suggestive of the diagnosis (Figure 252.1). Diagnosis can be confirmed by a barium swallow study or gastric ultrasonography. The classic "string sign" of the barium study due to an elongated pylorus with a narrow lumen[3] has been replaced with gastric ultrasound because it provides direct visualization of the pylorus and removes radiation exposure.[5]

## ELECTROLYTE DISTURBANCES AND RESUSCITATION

The classic presentation of pyloric stenosis is vomiting that leads to *hypochloremia hypokalemic metabolic alkalosis* because of the depletion of gastric contents, which contain sodium, potassium, and hydrochloric acid. The kidneys normally balance pH by excreting bicarbonate. This process is impaired due to a lack of chloride, leading to further

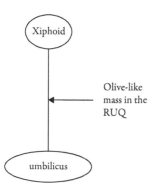

**Figure 252.1** Palpation of olive mass in right upper quadrant: The infant's lower limbs are flexed with gentle palpation of the space midway between the xiphoid and umbilicus.

alkalosis. The kidneys compensate for the gastric loss by retaining sodium/potassium at the expense of secreting hydrogen ions, leading to paradoxical aciduria[3] (Figure 252.2). As the disease progresses, the kidneys will release potassium in preference for keeping sodium, attempting to maintain the patient's fluid balance. The degree of dehydration can be determined by physical examination, urine output, and electrolyte levels. If left untreated, severe metabolic alkalosis leads to life-threatening cardiac arrhythmias, vascular collapse, and seizures.[5] Resuscitation in hemodynamically stable infants is achieved with 5% dextrose and 0.45% or 0.5% normal saline at 1.5 times maintenance fluid. Potassium is added to the resuscitative fluid once adequate urine output is achieved.[4,5] In cases of hypovolemic shock, isotonic saline boluses are given until hemodynamic stability is achieved.[3] Most infants respond to therapy within 12 to 48 hours, after which surgical correction can be performed in a nonemergent manner. Resuscitation

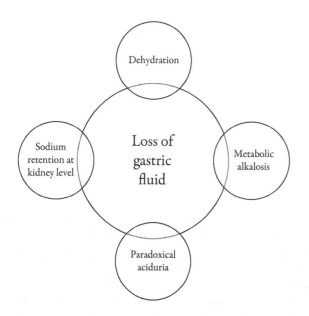

**Figure 252.2** Metabolic derangements in pyloric stenosis.

should be continued until signs of dehydration are resolved and serum electrolytes are normalized.[4] It was proposed that urine chloride concentration greater than 20 mEq/L indicates that the volume status has been corrected.

## TREATMENT

Pyloromyotomy, surgical division of the hypertrophied muscles of the pylorus, is the definitive surgical treatment for pyloric stenosis. This can be done via an open or laparoscopic approach.

## ANESTHETIC CONSIDERATIONS

### PREOPERATIVELY

Prior to proceeding to the operating room, the infant's electrolyte derangements are corrected. There is no consensus on what values can predict readiness for anesthesia, but a serum chloride concentration greater than 100 mEq/L and a serum bicarbonate concentration of less than 30 mEq/L have been suggested to be safe to proceed with the surgery.[2,3,5] It is important to note preoperatively that in infants the primary stimulus for ventilation remains $PaCO_2$. Pyloric stenosis and the resulting alkalosis depress minute ventilation by altering the pH in the cerebral spinal fluid (CSF). The infant is also at risk of aspiration as a result of the gastric outlet obstruction, independent of fasting status.[5] If the patient underwent a barium study, the patient remains at risk of barium aspiration.

### INTRAOPERATIVELY

#### Induction

Current anesthesia practice intraoperatively is to suction the infant in the right and left decubitus position to remove most of the gastric contents prior to induction.[4,5] Some clinicians will premedicate with an anticholinergic medication, such as atropine, prior to insertion of the gastric tube to counteract the parasympathetic response to oropharyngeal stimulation.[5] The high risk of aspiration warrants a rapid sequence or modified rapid sequence induction (RSI). After induction, a nasogastric tube is placed and left in place; this will allow testing the integrity of the pyloric wall after pyloromyotomy by the surgeon. An awake intubation technique has significantly decreased as a preference due to oral mucosal trauma, bradycardia, laryngospasm, longer intubation times compared to an RSI, hypoxia, and aspiration.[4,5] Infants are prone to rapid desaturations as a result of the high ratio of closing capacity to functional residual capacity and desaturate easily during brief episodes of apnea even with proper preoxygenation. As such, many clinicians use a modified RSI instead of the conventional "no ventilation" RSI in these babies. This is achieved using a gentle bag-mask ventilation (peak inflating pressure less than 10–12 cm $H_2O$) until the onset of neuromuscular paralysis.[5] Regarding cricoid pressure, its use is controversial in preventing gastric aspiration and may cause intubation difficulties due to distortion of the airway.

## Maintenance

Although the serum pH was corrected prior to proceeding to the operating room, the CSF pH is slower to correct and continues to play a role in central control of ventilation and results in an increased risk of postoperative apnea. Therefore, the use of short-duration inhalation anesthetics is warranted. Nitrous oxide is avoided, especially in laparoscopic procedures, to avoid expansion of bowel gas. The CSF alkalosis increases respiratory sensitivity to opioids in these neonates. Therefore, the use of opioids should be avoided because it delays awakening and increases risk of apnea.[2,4] Acetaminophen can be used as primary postoperative pain medication in addition to tissue infiltration with local anesthetic at the incision site.[5] Nonsteroidal anti-inflammatory drugs should be used with caution as the infant has immature kidneys.

Regional anesthesia including spinal, caudal, or thoracic epidural, have been used for open and laparoscopic pyloromyotomy.[5]

## Emergence/Postoperative Period

Extubation of these babies occurs at the end of the procedure when they are awake, breathing spontaneously, and with intact airway reflexes. Premature neonates less than 44–60 weeks of gestation should receive appropriate monitoring for postoperative apnea due to increased risk of apnea due to gestational age. Oral feeds are resumed 4 to 6 hours after surgery.[2,4,5] If respiratory depression and apnea occur after surgery, typically the cause is hyperventilation and change in CSF pH.

## REFERENCES

1. To T, et al. Population demographic indicators associated with incidence of pyloric stenosis. *Arch Pediatr Adolesc Med.* 2005;159: 520–525.
2. Sun LS, Saraiya N, Houck P. Anesthesia for abdominal surgery. In: George A. Gregory, Dean B. Andropoulos, eds. *Gregory's Pediatric Anesthesia.* Fifth Edition. Blackwell Publishing Ltd: Blackwell Publishing; 2012:Chapter 28, 720–740.
3. Aspelund G, Langer JC. Current management of hypertrophic pyloric stenosis. *Semin Pediatr Surg.* 2007;16:27–33.
4. Robert K. Williams, Helen Victoria Lauro and Peter J. Davis. *Anesthesia for General Abdominal and Urologic Surgery. Smith's Anesthesia for Infants and Children.* Ninth Edition. Elsevier Inc. 30, 2017:789–816.e4.
5. Kamata M, et al. Perioperative care of infants with pyloric stenosis. *Pediatr Anesth.* 2015;25:1193–1206.

# 253.

# NECROTIZING ENTEROCOLITIS

*Cassandra Wasson and Christina D. Diaz*

## INTRODUCTION

Necrotizing enterocolitis (NEC) is one of the most common diseases in neonates, occurring in 7% of live preterm births.[1,2] It occurs primarily in preterm infants, especially those under 32 weeks' gestational age.[3] The incidence has remained unchanged in recent years due to improved survival of premature infants.[1] In many tertiary care neonatal intensive care units caring for micropreemies, the rate has even increased.[1] NEC is an important cause of morbidity and mortality in these infants, with a rate of mortality up to 30%.[1–3] Infants who require surgery have the highest mortality rate.[1]

The pathophysiology of NEC is incompletely understood but is known to be multifactorial. Prematurity is a significant risk factor, as NEC primarily affects infants younger than 32 weeks' gestation who weigh less than 1500 g.[1,3] Other risk factors include hypoxemia, early enteral feeding with hyperosmolar solutions, cyanotic heart disease, and patent ductus arteriosus causing decreased blood supply to the gut.[2,3] These risk factors lead to increased mucosal permeability, intestinal ischemia, and sepsis, predisposing these infants to NEC.[1,3]

Necrotizing enterocolitis has many long-term effects. The most common severe complication is the need for bowel resection. In fact, NEC is the major cause of short-bowel syndrome in pediatric patients.[1] The effects of NEC are not limited to the gastrointestinal system but extend systemically. Infants recovering from NEC have a 25% chance of microcephaly and serious neurodevelopmental delays[1] as a result of the inflammatory process associated with NEC.

## DIAGNOSIS

Necrotizing enterocolitis typically presents after 8 to 10 days of life.[1] However, the more premature an infant is, the later NEC occurs after birth.[1] The initial signs and symptoms include feeding intolerance, abdominal distention, and bloody stools.[1-4] Additional signs include bilious vomiting,[2-4] temperature instability,[3,4] hyperglycemia,[4] toxic appearance,[4] hypotension, disseminated intravascular coagulation, and metabolic acidosis in severe cases. In the case of perforation, pneumoperitoneum (free air in the abdomen) may be seen on an abdominal x-ray (Figure 253.1) and is an indication for urgent surgical intervention.[2,4] Other findings on abdominal x-ray include portal venous gas and pneumatosis intestinalis (gas within the bowel wall) and are pathognomonic for NEC.[1,2]

## MANAGEMENT

Necrotizing enterocolitis is managed either medically or surgically based on the clinical presentation and severity of illness.[1] Less severe cases are managed medically with abdominal decompression, bowel rest, intravenous hyperalimentation, and broad-spectrum intravenous antibiotics.[1,3,4] Transfusions with packed red blood cells and platelets are given if necessary.[4] Medical management avoids surgery in 85% of cases.[4]

Surgery is indicated in cases of perforation, obstruction, peritonitis, and worsening acidosis.[4] Pneumoperitoneum on abdominal x-ray is an absolute indication for surgery.[3] Surgical treatment may involve a drain placement, exploratory laparotomy with resection of diseased bowel, and enterostomy with creation of a stoma.[1]

## ANESTHETIC CONSIDERATIONS

### PREOPERATIVE

Prior to surgical intervention, the neonate should be optimized as the patient's condition allows. Hypovolemia, metabolic acidosis, coagulopathy, hypocalcemia, and thrombocytopenia should be corrected as much as possible preoperatively.[4] Bleeding derangements require special attention in this particular patient population and disease process. Vitamin K, platelet transfusions, and fresh frozen plasma transfusions may be necessary prior to surgical intervention.[2]

### INTRAOPERATIVE

Intraoperative management requires anesthetic considerations for premature neonates and special considerations for

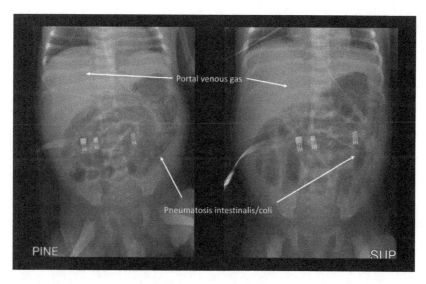

Figure 253.1 Pneumoperitoneum (free air in the abdomen) on an abdominal x-ray.

the disease process itself. Due to the risk of retinopathy of prematurity, a mixture of air and $O_2$ is recommended for ventilation with a goal $SpO_2$ of 88%–95%.[2–4] Other goals of ventilation include avoiding hyperventilation, high peak inspiratory pressures, and barotrauma.[2]

Temperature monitoring is also important for premature neonates, as they are prone to hypothermia. Intraoperative hypothermia can have multiple consequences, including hypoglycemia, apnea, and metabolic acidosis.[2] Prevention of hypothermia is achieved by increasing the room temperature, utilizing radiant heat lamps, using warm blankets, warming and humidifying inhalational gases, and wrapping the extremities and head in plastic.[4] Hypoglycemia is common in premature neonates and those with sepsis and thus may not be due to hypothermia. Therefore, intraoperative blood glucose monitoring is necessary. and dextrose-containing solutions are infused.[2,3]

Additional monitors required for NEC surgery include standard American Society of Anesthesiologist monitors and ideally a peripheral arterial line.[2–4] Umbilical arterial catheters should be removed if possible to improve mesenteric blood flow.[4] Adequate venous access is needed due to high fluid requirements, especially once the abdomen is open.[3,4] A volume of 100 mL/kg/h of crystalloids should be expected due to extreme third-space losses, preexisting hypovolemia, bleeding from coagulopathy, and metabolic acidosis.[2,4] Central venous access is helpful due to expected large fluid shifts and the possibility of needing inotropic support.[2,3]

The majority of these infants are already intubated.[4] If they are not, an awake intubation or modified rapid sequence is indicated.[4] Anesthesia is maintained with opioids, neuromuscular-blocking agents, and minimal volatile anesthetics.[3,4] Inhalational agents are minimized as they can aggravate a hypovolemic shock situation.[3] Nitrous oxide is avoided due to the already distended bowels.[3,4]

Hemodynamic collapse is common in these neonates.[3] Therefore, inotropic agents are often necessary to protect cardiovascular stability and adequate perfusion.[3,4] Blood products are often required intraoperatively as well.[3] Warmed red blood cells, fresh frozen plasma, and platelets should be immediately available.[3,4]

## POSTOPERATIVE

These neonates often require mechanical ventilatory and cardiovascular support postoperatively.[3] They will be transferred to the neonatal intensive care unit in a warmed incubator with full monitoring.[4] Parenteral nutrition is necessary postoperatively until the ileus has resolved, sepsis is controlled, and metabolic stability is maintained.[3,4]

## REFERENCES

1. Neu J, Walker WA. Necrotizing enterocolitis. *N Engl J Med.* 2011;364(3):255–264.
2. Williams A, et al. Anesthetic considerations in a preterm: extremely low birth weight neonate posted for exploratory laparotomy. *Anesth Essays Res.* 2012;6(1):81–83.
3. Caliskan E. Anesthetic management of neonatal emergency abdominal surgery. In: Garbuzenko DV, ed. *Actual Problems of Emergency Abdominal Surgery.* 2016. IntechOpen, doi:10.5772/63567. Available from: https://www.intechopen.com/chapters/51227
4. Houck PJ. Necrotizing enterocolitis. In: Atchabahian A, Gupta R, eds. *The Anesthesia Guide.* McGraw Hill; 2013:Chapter 175. https://accessanesthesiology.mhmedical.com/content.aspx?bookid=572&sectionid=42543766

# 254.

# OMPHALOCELE AND GASTROSCHISIS

*Rami Edward Karroum*

## INTRODUCTION

Omphalocele and gastroschisis represent two distinct congenital anatomical defects of the abdominal wall. However, they are often discussed together because their anesthetic management has a lot of similarities. Both are considered neonatal surgical emergencies and need to have surgical repair soon after birth (Table 254.1).

## DIAGNOSIS

Diagnosis of omphalocele and gastroschisis is usually made in the antenatal period by fetal ultrasound.

## TREATMENT

Surgical repair of the defect is the only available treatment. A primary repair is the goal of surgery as failure to replace all of the intestinal contents back into the abdominal cavity increases morbidity and mortality.

Sometimes, primary abdominal closure may not be possible due to marked increase in the intra-abdominal pressure. A partial replacement may be performed instead, and the remaining herniated abdominal contents are covered with a Silastic pouch. The size of the pouch is subsequently reduced in stages, thus allowing the abdominal cavity gradually to accommodate the increased mass without severely compromising ventilation or organ perfusion.[4]

## ANESTHETIC CONSIDERATIONS

### PREOPERATIVE

Preoperatively, immediately after delivery, the neonate is examined to ensure a patent airway and adequate ventilation and oxygenation, followed by admission to the neonatal intensive care unit.

Preoperative care is directed at

- Maintaining perfusion to the herniated viscera.
- Fluid resuscitation and correction of electrolytes and acid-base abnormalities.
- Reducing evaporative fluid loss.
- Preventing hypothermia and sepsis.

The incidence of hypothermia and dehydration is higher in gastroschisis due to the absence of a covering sac to the herniated viscera.[2] Therefore, as soon as possible after delivery, exposed viscera should be covered with sterile, saline-soaked dressings and a plastic wrap to decrease heat and evaporative fluid losses. Fluid resuscitation should be initiated with 20 mL/kg of isotonic crystalloid.

Dextrose-containing solution should be given at a maintenance rate to avoid hypoglycemia. Acid-base and electrolyte abnormalities should be corrected, and heat loss should be prevented by actively warming the newborn with a radiant heater or a heated incubator. Bowel should be decompressed with a nasogastric tube. A urinary catheter is placed to measure urine output and assess the adequacy of fluid resuscitation. Broad-spectrum antibiotics should be initiated for those with exposed bowel. Resuscitation should continue throughout the entire perioperative period. For those who are unstable or are expected to have a prolonged intensive care unit course and/or otherwise, two peripheral intravenous catheters, with at least one in the upper extremity, in the distribution of the superior vena cava, are recommended. This is due to the fact that bowel reduction into the abdominal cavity during surgery can result in compression of the inferior vena cava and impair venous return from the lower extremities.

Anesthesiologist preoperative assessment should ensure that the patient received adequate fluid resuscitation and that electrolytes and acid-base abnormalities have been corrected.

Assessment for other associated anomalies is crucial in the preoperative period, particularly in a patient with

*Table 254.1*  THE DIFFERENCE BETWEEN OMPHALOCELE AND GASTROSCHISIS

| | GASTROSCHISIS | OMPHALOCELE |
|---|---|---|
| Etiology | Occlusion of the omphalomesentric artery during gestation, resulting in ischemia and atrophy of the structures that form the paraumbilical abdominal wall. | Failure of the gut to migrate from the yolk sac into the abdomen early in gestation. |
| Location of the defect | Paramedian, usually to the right of the umbilicus. | Midline, at the site of the umbilicus. |
| Incidence | 1/2000 | 1/5000 |
| Herniated viscera | Herniated bowel is not covered by a peritoneal membrane and is therefore exposed to the irritative effects of amniotic fluid during gestation and to the air after delivery. As a result, the bowel is usually inflamed, dilated, edematous, and functionally abnormal. Has a normally situated umbilical cord.<br>Herniation of other organs is uncommon. | Herniated bowel is covered with a peritoneal membranous sac and hence not exposed to the amniotic fluid during gestation or air after delivery. Therefore, herniated bowel is usually morphologically and functionally normal, unless the ompahalocele is ruptured.<br>Large omphalocele may contain other viscera, such as liver and spleen, resulting in poorly developed abdominal and thoracic cavities and lung hypoplasia. |
| Evaporative fluid losses, dehydration, hypothermia, acidosis, electrolyte disturbances, and sepsis | More pronounced due to the lack of peritoneal membranous coverage of the herniated bowel. | Less pronounced due to the presence of peritoneal membranous sac covering the herniated viscera. If the omphalocele membranous peritoneal covering is ruptured, the extent of hypothermia and evaporative fluid loss is similar to gastroschisis. |
| Associated congenital abnormalities | Usually not associated with other congenital abnormalities.<br>Higher incidence of prematurity and low birth weight. | Common and include congenital heart disease, chromosomal defects, urological defects (e.g., bladder exstrophy and metabolic disorder such as Beckwith-Wiedemann syndrome [macroglossia, organomegaly, hypoglycemia, and polycythemia]).<br>Epigastric omphaloceles are associated with cardiac and lung anomalies, while hypogastric omphaloceles are associated with bladder and other genitourinary anomalies. |

omphalocele. Transthoracic echocardiography may be ordered if a congenital heart defect is suspected.

Patients with *Beckwith-Wiedemann syndrome* (macroglossia, organomegaly, hypoglycemia, and polycythemia) may be difficult to intubate due to macroglossia. Also, those patients can develop hypoglycemia due to pancreatic enlargement, resulting in hyperinsulinemia. Therefore, blood glucose should be monitored regularly in those patients.[1]

## INTRAOPERATIVE

The neonate should be kept warm by prewarming the ambient operating room temperature and using a radiant heater and a forced air warming device. Nasogastric suctioning should be performed before rapid sequence induction and tracheal intubation are performed. Nitrous oxide is avoided to prevent bowel distention. Fluid resuscitation should continue during the intraoperative period. Analgesia can be achieved with fentanyl or a regional technique. Adequate muscle relaxation is essential to facilitate primary closure.

Feasibility of primary closure needs to be assessed by monitoring the intra-abdominal pressure to ensure that closure will not compromise ventilation or cause abdominal compartment syndrome.

Intra-abdominal pressure may be assessed by measuring intragastric, intrabladder, peak airway, or central venous pressures. A gastric pressure that exceeds 20 mm Hg can decrease organ perfusion and ventilatory reserve, including perfusion of the intestines, liver, and kidney. This may lead to markedly altered drug metabolism and prolonged drug effects. Venous return from the lower body also may be reduced, resulting in lower extremity congestion and cyanosis.[3]

Blood pressure and pulse oximetry determinations from a lower extremity may be different from those in the upper extremity. The bowel may become edematous, and urine output may be reduced as a result of renal congestion. There are several intraoperative adverse physiologic derangements that may occur when the surgeon attempts to place a large volume of abdominal contents back into a small, restrictive abdominal cavity. Cephalad displacement of the diaphragm due to the increase in abdominal contents may significantly decrease functional residual capacity and tidal volume, which can lead to difficult ventilation, development of atelectasis, and hypoxemia. During the repair, the anesthetist may frequently need to use manual ventilation to maintain adequate tidal volumes in response to rapid changes in lung compliance. The presence of hypoxemia despite maximal ventilation may preclude completion of a primary repair.

## POSTOPERATIVE

All infants, except those with the most trivial repairs, remain intubated and mechanically ventilated in the postoperative period. Abdominal compartment syndrome and respiratory compromise may continue postoperatively; therefore, paralysis and adequate sedation with an opioid infusion are essential for optimal management. Monitoring of intra-abdominal pressure for intra-abdominal compartment syndrome could also continue in the postoperative

period. A gastric pressure that exceeds 20 mm Hg after primary closure is likely to cause abdominal ischemia and necessitate an urgent reoperation.

## REFERENCES

1. Spaeth JP, Lam JE. The extremely premature infant and common neonatal emergencies. In: Cote CJ, et al., eds. *A Practice of Anesthesia for Infants and Children.* 6th ed. Elsevier; 2019:864–865.
2. Moore TC. Gastroschisis and omphalocele: clinical differences. *Surgery.* 1977;82(5):561–568.
3. Yaster M, et al. Hemodynamic effects of primary closure of omphalocele/gastroschisis in human newborns. *Anesthesiology.* 1988;69(1):84–88.
4. Risby K, et al. Congenital abdominal wall defects: staged closure by dual mesh. *J Neonatal Surg.* 2016;5(1):2.

# 255.

# MECONIUM ASPIRATION SYNDROME

*Harsh Nathani and Chike Gwam*

## INTRODUCTION

Meconium aspiration syndrome (MAS) is a diagnosis of exclusion in a neonate with respiratory distress born through meconium-stained amniotic fluid. The syndrome can vary from mild respiratory distress to life-threatening respiratory failure and is a result of the presence of meconium in the tracheobronchial airway.[1] The aspiration of meconium can occur in the antepartum or intrapartum period. Meconium-stained amniotic fluid is noted in 10%–15% of childbirths; however only 4%–10% of these infants proceed to develop MAS. Of the infants who develop MAS, up to one-third require ventilatory support, and a fatal outcome has been noted in up to 5%–10% of cases.[2]

## RISK FACTORS

Uteroplacental insufficiency, post-term pregnancies, maternal hypertension, placenta previa, maternal pulmonary

disease, placental abruptions, cord prolapse, and cord compression are risk factors.

## PATHOPHYSIOLOGY

Meconium is the substance found within the intestines of a fetus from the 10th week of life and consists of gastrointestinal, hepatic, and pancreatic secretions; cellular debris; swallowed amniotic fluid; lanugo; vernix caseosa; and blood. Normally good anal sphincter tone and poor peristalsis keep the meconium within the rectum; however, strong vagal responses in a mature parasympathetic system triggered by fetal hypoxia or acidosis can lead to the premature passage of meconium into the amniotic fluid. Furthermore, fetal hypoxia and acidosis cause reflexive gasping, which can lead to the aspiration of meconium into the airways.[1]

Aspirated meconium causes respiratory distress through V/Q mismatch, leading to fetal/neonatal hypoxia and acidosis, pulmonary hypertension, and umbilical vessel damage through several mechanisms:

1. Airway obstruction—Meconium can become lodged in the distal airways, leading to either complete or partial obstruction. This can cause distal atelectasis and air trapping and air leak secondary to a ball-valve effect in partial obstruction. Radiographically, this process leads to the characteristic findings of areas of atelectasis and consolidation interspersed with hyperexpanded zones and along with air leaks.[1]
2. Inflammatory cytokines—Meconium is a chemical irritant to the lung and can lead to an inflammatory process that presents at 24-48 hours after inhalation. These processes can lead to pneumonitis with epithelial disruption, exudative deposits, alveolar collapse and stiffening, and cellular necrosis.[1]
3. Surfactant deficiency—Meconium is known to have deleterious effects on surfactant. Meconium leads to inactivation of surfactant, leading to decreased surface tension within alveoli, promoting atelectasis and collapse. Furthermore, surfactant is known to damage type 2 pneumocytes, leading to decreased production of surfactant.[1]
4. Pulmonary hypertension—Hypoxia from V/Q mismatch and decreased alveolar ventilation lead to acidosis and, in conjunction with vasoactive cytokines released from meconium in the airway, promotes pulmonary hypertension. Increased pulmonary arterial pressures further exacerbate hypoxia and acidosis, which in turn can worsen pulmonary hypertension, leading to a vicious cycle associated with persistent pulmonary hypertension.[1]

Last, presence of meconium in the amniotic fluid can promote an inflammatory response within the umbilical cord that can cause vasospasm and fibrosis, leading to pervasive fetal ischemia, which can contribute to neonatal mortality.[3]

## DIAGNOSIS

Meconium aspiration syndrome is diagnosed clinically based on the findings of MSAF, presence of respiratory distress, characteristic radiographic features, and presence of meconium within the airway during intubation if required. MAS should be differentiated from other causes of neonatal respiratory distress. In contrast to MAS, transient tachypnea of the newborn has a much more rapid improvement of respiratory distress and tends to occur in the late preterm infant. Respiratory distress syndrome is seen generally in preterm infants, whereas MAS is seen in postmature infants. Pneumonia can be difficult to distinguish from MAS and should be treated for aggressively while awaiting culture results. Congenital heart disease and isolated pulmonary air leaks should also be sought to exclude prior to diagnosing MAS.[4]

## PREVENTION AND MANAGEMENT

Coordination of care between obstetric and neonatology services is important in reducing the incidence of MAS and providing timely emergent therapy to reduce morbidity and mortality.

## OBSTETRIC CARE

Prevention of fetal hypoxia and postmature delivery can help reduce the incidence of MAS. The role of amnioinfusion in obstetric care is controversial and is not routinely recommended for mothers with MSAF unless there are also coincident variable decelerations. Furthermore, previously recommended routine intrapartum suctioning of the oropharynx has been abandoned due to concern for increased rates of bradycardia, laryngospasm, and stridor without significant evidence for prevention of aspiration and improved morbidity or mortality.[1]

## NEONATAL CARE

Airway clearing is not routinely recommended as part of neonatal care for infants born through MSAF or for infants suspected of having MAS with respiratory distress. Endotracheal suctioning does not provide improvements in mortality or morbidity, and as with intrapartum suctioning, the risk of bradycardia and laryngospasm are increased.[5] The goals of management for MAS remain supportive by ensuring adequate oxygenation and ventilation, maintaining blood pressure and perfusion, correcting metabolic abnormalities, and temperature management.[1] Respiratory management with supplemental oxygen therapy, assisted ventilation, and extracorporeal membrane oxygenation (ECMO) therapy should be considered. The use of surfactant has been shown to reduce the severity of respiratory distress and reduce the need for ECMO. Management of pulmonary hypertension with inhaled nitric oxide and phosphodiesterase inhibitors is associated with improved oxygenation. Circulatory support should be provided as needed with either volume or vasopressors. The role for antibiotics remains unclear as there is sparse evidence of its benefit in MAS. However, distinguishing MAS from infectious causes of neonatal respiratory distress can be challenging, and empiric anti-bacterial therapy is recommended while awaiting culture results.[1] Furthermore, there is no role for corticosteroids in the management of MAS.[1]

## REFERENCES

1. Raju U, et al. Meconium aspiration syndrome: an insight. *Med J Armed Forces India*. 2010;66(2):152–157.
2. Whitfield J, et al. Prevention of meconium aspiration syndrome: an update and the Baylor experience. *Baylor Univ Med Center Proc.* 2009;22(2):128–131.
3. Hutton E, Thorpe J. Consequences of meconium stained amniotic fluid: what does the evidence tell us? *Early Hum Dev.* 2014;90(7):333–339.
4. Wiswell T, et al. Delivery room management of the apparently vigorous meconium-stained neonate: results of the multicenter, international collaborative trial. *Pediatrics*. 2000;105(1):1–7.
5. Wyckoff M, et al. Part 13: neonatal resuscitation: 2015 American Heart Association guidelines update for cardiopulmonary resuscitation and emergency cardiovascular care (Reprint). *Pediatrics.* 2015;136(Suppl):S199–S200.

# 256.

# RESPIRATORY DISTRESS SYNDROME

*Jamie W. Sinton*

## INTRODUCTION

Infants have the highest intraoperative and postoperative anesthetic morbidity compared to older children. Respiratory (and cardiac) events are the leading cause of anesthetic adverse events in this population.[1]

Respiratory distress syndrome (RDS) is a condition of the newborn in which there is inadequate surfactant production to prevent atelectasis during tidal breathing. As surfactant is manufactured only after about 32–34 weeks' gestation, RDS and prematurity are closely linked.[2]

## PATHOPHYSIOLOGY

Respiratory distress syndrome in newborns is due to lack of pulmonary surfactant.

### SURFACTANT

Surfactant maintains alveolar patency during tidal breathing. It is normally produced following an increase in fetal cortisol between 32- and 34-weeks' gestation. Surfactant production sufficient for newborn breathing can be anticipated when the ratio of amniotic fluid lecithin to sphingomyelin (L/S) is at least 2 to 1. Maternal diabetes is a common cause of reduced lung maturity even in term infants. Maternal betamethasone administration daily for 48 hours prior to delivery improves the L/S ratio and lung maturity if delivery cannot be postponed. Surfactant synthesis may also be supported by avoiding hypovolemia, hypothermia, and acidosis—the same factors that contribute to pulmonary artery vasospasm and pulmonary hypertension. Exogenous administration of surfactant improves ventilation parameters of very premature infants as well. Surfactant is classically administered via endotracheal tube (ETT); however, less invasive delivery methods appear to be promising.[3]

## CLINICAL PRESENTATION

Respiratory distress in the newborn or young infant has many causes and is exacerbated by their relatively small number of alveoli: Newborns have approximately 1/10 that of adults: 50 million versus 500 million.[4] Newborns with RDS have cyanosis, nasal flaring, suprasternal or subcostal retractions, and accessory muscle use, including head bobbing if an infant is using his or her sternocleidomastoid muscles during breathing. Chest roentgenogram may have air bronchograms or complete whiteout relating to heterogenous distribution of ventilation. Hypoxemia and cyanosis in surfactant-deficient lungs may lead to alveolar perfusion in the absence of ventilation: intrapulmonary shunt.

Many respiratory conditions can mimic RDS. The differential diagnosis of respiratory embarrassment in this population includes abnormalities of the airway, gastrointestinal tract, and heart. Airway conditions include meconium aspiration, airway malacia, complete tracheal rings, congenital pneumonia, bronchopulmonary sequestration, congenital cystic adenomatoid malformation, neonatal lobar emphysema, persistent pulmonary hypertension, congenital diaphragmatic hernia, and tracheoesophageal fistula. Other conditions that may present with respiratory distress include newborn sepsis, osteogenesis imperfecta, thoracic insufficiency in Jeune syndrome, and others. Cardiac causes of respiratory distress include absent pulmonary valve syndrome and left-to-right shunting lesions. As the pulmonary vascular resistance of the newborn is high, left-to-right intracardiac shunts often have little clinical effect on respiration at this age.

## NATURAL HISTORY

Bronchopulmonary dysplasia (BPD) is defined as oxygen requirement at 36 weeks' postconceptual age. Patients with BPD often have coexistent patent ductus arteriosus, early pulmonary vascular disease, and pulmonary hypertension. BPD is discussed elsewhere in this book. Lung function following RDS remains reduced at age 8 years.[5]

## ANESTHETIC CONSIDERATIONS

### PREOPERATIVE

Preoperatively, these patients will usually reside in the neonatal intensive care unit (NICU), and their history often includes prematurity with coexistent, multisystem comorbidities.

Nasal continuous positive airway pressure (CPAP) reduces the severity of RDS and is a common method of respiratory support as well as intubation. Figure 256.1 provides schematic details of the setup of a bubble CPAP machine for an infant. Salient features include a

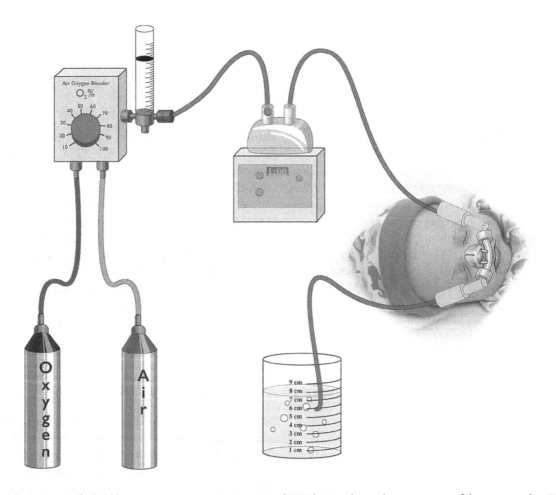

Figure 256.1 Schematic setup for bubble continuous positive airway pressure (CPAP). Note the cumbersome nature of the oxygen and air E-cylinders, tubing, and so on. This type of circuit can be used for ventilation in the intensive care unit or for transport; however, the heater and humidifier are only functional while plugged in to alternating current power.

requirement for alternating current power in order to provide heated, humidified gas.

Provision of CPAP can be maintained simply by keeping the expiratory limb of the breathing circuit submerged to the desired depth of water (e.g., 6 cm $H_2O$). Note that oxygen and air tanks are not pictured but would be required to provide fresh gas flow. Safely transporting a NICU patient to the operating room requires adjustment of preexisting respiratory support to a suitable portable modality. Inhalation of cold, dry air reduces lung compliance in infants; therefore, efforts should be made to maintain humidification even during transport. Temperature maintenance reduces cold stress which oxygen consumption and metabolic acidosis and therefore reduces the risk of development or worsening of RDS.

## INTRAOPERATIVE

In preparation for airway management, attention should focus on maintaining oxygen saturation ($SaO_2$) without contributing to pulmonary toxicity. Target partial pressure of oxygen ($PaO_2$) to 60–70 or an $SaO_2$ of 90%. However, this target has been challenged[6] and may not be a precise estimate of the newborn's needs. Greater than 40% inspired oxygen concentration is toxic to developing lungs, and consideration should be given to avoiding it if possible. If circuit disconnection or reintubation with a cuffed ETT is required intraoperatively, consider clamping the ETT during the exchange to maintain positive pressure and prevent atelectasis.

## POSTOPERATIVE

Postoperatively, arrangements should be made for the transport of this NICU patient with attention to his or her new respiratory physiology or morbidity. Often, if newborns require a procedure, there is impact on respiratory function either consciously or inadvertently.

## REFERENCES

1. Cohen MM, et al. Pediatric anesthesia morbidity and mortality in the perioperative period. *Anesth Analg.* 1990;70:160–167.
2. Glass H. Outcomes for extremely premature infants. *Anesth Analg.* 2015;120(6):1337–1351.
3. Hartel C, et al. Less invasive surfactant administration and complications of preterm birth. *Sci Rep.* 2018;8(1):8333.
4. Sapru A, et al. Pathobiology of acute respiratory distress syndrome. *Pediatr Crit Care Med.* 2015;16(5 suppl 1):S6–S22.
5. Thunqvist P, et al. Lung function at 8 and 16 years after moderate-to-late preterm birth: a prospective cohort study. *Pediatrics.* 2016;137(4):2015–2056.
6. Manja V, et al. Oxygen saturation targets in preterm infants and outcomes at 18-24 months: a systematic review. *Pediatrics.* 2017;139(1):e20161609.

# 257.

# MYELOMENINGOCELE

*Rami Edward Karroum*

## INTRODUCTION

Myelodysplasia or spinal dysraphism, or frequently referred to as spina bifida, is a group of congenital malformations involving defects in the midline structures of the back. It can involve skin, the vertebral column bones, and/or neural elements. It usually occurs at the lumbar level but can occur at any level along the vertebral column. According to the presence or absence of intact skin covering the lesion, they are further classified as follows:

1. **Spina bifida cystic:** Defect lacking skin covering and apparent at birth.
2. **Spina bifida occulta:** The defect is covered with intact skin. Neural tissue may be tethered to surrounding structures. Due to the presence of

intact skin, there may be delay of detection of the underlying deformity. Frequently, the overlying skin may show abnormalities such as midline hairy patch, fat pads, or skin dimple.

*Spina bifida cystic* is further divided based on the presence or absence of neural tissue in the meningeal sac herniating through the defect into

1. **Meningocele:** The herniating meningeal sac protruding through the defect in the back does not contain neural tissue.
2. **Myelomeningocele:** The herniated meningeal sac contains neural tissue. It is the most common congenital defect of the central nervous system, with a prevalence rate of approximately 4 per 10,000 live births. It usually occurs at the lumbar level.

## DIAGNOSIS

The defect is usually diagnosed in the prenatal period using ultrasonography.

## ANESTHETIC CONSIDERATIONS

### PREOPERATIVE

Preoperatively, myelomeningocele is a *surgical urgency*, and surgery needs to be performed within 24 hours of birth. This is due to exposure of the neural elements and the risk of infection and development of progressive neural damage.

*Hydrocephalus* is usually present and is due to type *II Chiari malformation*. Type II Chiari malformation consists of caudal displacement of the cerebellar vermis, *fourth* ventricle, and lower brainstem below the plane of the foramen magnum. Most patients will need to have a Ventriculoperitoneal *shunt* placed for hydrocephalus either at the time of the initial surgery for myelomeningocele subsequent time or before discharge home.

Neonates with myelodysplasia are at high risk for developing *latex allergy* and possibly anaphylaxis later in life. This is due to repeated exposure to latex products encountered during frequent bladder catheterizations and multiple surgical procedures, during which latex gloves are used. Avoidance of latex-containing products is begun at birth to prevent eventual development of sensitization.

Careful documentation of all neurologic deficits and review of other organ systems should be done to rule out additional congenital malformations.

Assessment of the size of the defect and the size of the dural sac is important to plan for proper positioning during induction of anesthesia and the possible need for blood transfusion.

Preoperative blood work should include at least a hemoglobin and type and screen. Packed red blood cells (PRBCs) should be available for large defects as they can be associated with significant blood loss.

Premedication is not indicated.

### INTRAOPERATIVE

*Hypothermia* risk intraoperatively is significant due to the large exposed surface area. The operating room should be prewarmed prior to patient arrival. A radiant heater can be used during induction of the anesthesia and intubation. A forced warm-air blanket should be placed underneath the infant with care to avoid contact thermal injury to the exposed dural sac. All infused fluids should be warmed.

*Positioning* for induction and airway management can be a major anesthesia challenge. In most cases with a small defect, tracheal intubation can be performed with the infant in the supine position and the uninvolved portion of the child's back supported with towels or a cushioned ring to protect the dural sac from contact injury. Alternatively, a left lateral decubitus position may be needed for induction and intubation in case of a large myelomeningocele. Standard American Society of Anesthesiologists monitors are required.

All standard intravenous and inhaled anesthetic agents are acceptable for use during induction and maintenance of general anesthesia. Succinylcholine is rarely needed for tracheal intubation, although it is not associated with hyperkalemia because the defect develops early in gestation and is not associated with muscle denervation. If succinylcholine is used, a dose of atropine should precede it due to the high incidence of bradycardia in neonates. Muscle relaxation during maintenance is relatively contraindicated because nerve stimulation may be required to identify neural structures. Alternatively, nondepolarizing muscle relaxant can be used for intubation, but the effect should be completely reversed before surgery to allow for neurophysiological monitoring.

*Airway management* can be very challenging with large hydrocephalus or very large dural sac. This can results in difficult mask fit, difficult ventilation, and / or difficult intubation. Difficult airway should be anticipated and planned for, including the need for awake/ sedated intubation.

Extreme head flexion may cause brainstem compression. Neonates born with myelomeningocele have an increased incidence of an abnormally short trachea. Therefore, the endotracheal tube position should be confirmed to ensure that the distal end of the endotracheal tube is not in the mainstem bronchus. Tube position should be rechecked again after the patient is placed in the prone position. The surgical repair is performed in the *prone position* with appropriate cushioning that provides for optimum abdominal excursion during ventilation.

Insensible loss from the skin defect can be substantial, particularly with a large defect; blood loss is usually minimal in small defects. In the case of a large defect, blood loss can be significant; therefore, packed red blood cells should be available. Two intravenous catheters are usually needed. Glucose-containing solution should be run at a maintenance rate to prevent hypoglycemia as neonates lack glycogen storage. Insensible fluid loss should be replaced with warmed crystalloids (normal saline or lactated Ringer solution). If allowable blood loss is exceeded, transfusion of PRBCs should be considered. Neonates with myelomeningocele are automatically considered latex sensitive from birth; and a latex-free operating room environment is required. Plan for tracheal extubation at the completion of the procedure.

## POSTOPERATIVE

Respiratory status needs to be carefully monitored in the postoperative period. Breathing difficulties may occur after a tight skin closure, and ventilatory responses to hypoxia and hypercarbia may be impaired due to coexisting Arnold-Chiari malformation. This is due to cranial nerve and brainstem dysfunction. VP shunt may need to be scheduled at another day prior to discharge to treat associated hydrocephalus.

## LONG-TERM OUTCOMES AND OTHER CONSIDERATIONS

Macrocephaly, vocal cord paralysis causing inspiratory stridor and respiratory distress, apnea, dysphagia, and pulmonary aspiration and cranial nerve palsy may be associated with the Arnold-Chiari malformation and usually manifests during infancy.

Children with vocal cord paralysis or an impaired gag reflex may require tracheostomy and gastrostomy to secure the airway and to minimize chronic aspiration.

Children of any age may have abnormal responses to hypoxia and hypercarbia because of cranial nerve and brainstem dysfunction.

Extreme head flexion may cause brainstem compression in otherwise asymptomatic children.

Residual neurological deficits can persist and include neurogenic bowel, bladder dysfunction, and trophic lower extremity changes. Lower extremity function depends on the levels of the lesion. Paraplegia is common with lesions above L4 level. Lower extremity functions are severely affected with L4 to S1. Patients with lesions below the S1 level are usually able to ambulate.

Children who develop latex allergy exhibit cross-reactivity with some antibiotics and fruits, such as kiwi, avocados, and bananas.

Intrauterine surgery during pregnancy has been advocated as a way of diminishing the degree of damage caused by myelodysplasia and has been practiced in some centers in the United States.

## REFERENCES

1. McClain CD, Soriano SG. Pediatric neurosurgical anesthesia. In: Cote CJ, et al, eds. *A Practice of Anesthesia for Infants and Children*. 6th ed. Elsevier; 2019:625.
2. Oren J, et al. Respiratory complications in patients with myelodysplasia and Arnold-Chiari malformation. *Am J Dis Child*. 1986;140(3):221–224.
3. Ward SL, et al. Absent hypoxic and hypercapneic arousal responses in children with myelomeningocele and apnea. *Pediatrics*. 1986;78(1):44–50.
4. Putnam PE, et al. Cricopharyngeal dysfunction associated with Chiari malformations. *Pediatrics*. 1992; 89(5 pt 1):871–876.

# 258.

# PNEUMO-, HEMO-, AND CHYLOTHORACES

*Michael J. Gyorfi and Alaa Abd-Elsayed*

## INTRODUCTION

This chapter focuses on the definitions, treatments, and anesthetic considerations of pneumo-, hemo-, and chylothoraces. Simply, a pneumothorax is the presence of air in the pleural space. Pneumothoraces can be further divided into spontaneous, traumatic, iatrogenic, and tension pneumothoraces. A hemothorax is defined as a bloody pleural effusion with a pleural fluid hematocrit of at least 50%. Last, a chylothorax is a result of thoracic duct damage causing chyle leakage into the pleural space.

## PNEUMOTHORAX OVERVIEW

The pathophysiology of a pneumothorax results from a change in pleural pressure due to the introduction of air. The pressure in the pleural space is negative relative to both the alveolar pressure throughout the respiratory cycle and the atmospheric pressure. If a communication connects to the pleural space, air will enter until the pressure gradient is eliminated or the communication is closed. After a pneumothorax occurs, there will be a decrease in the vital capacity, which is defined as the volume of air that the lungs can expel. This can be tolerated in a healthy lung; however, in abnormal lungs alveolar hypoventilation and respiratory acidosis will occur. Another consequence of a pneumothorax will be a reduced arterial $PO_2$ with an increased alveolar arterial oxygen difference due to right-left shunting.[1,2]

A spontaneous pneumothorax may occur in healthy lungs, most commonly from a ruptured subpleural bleb. This occurs most often in smokers and taller, thinner persons. You can also get a spontaneous pneumothorax secondary to underlying lung disease, such as chronic obstructive pulmonary disease and cystic fibrosis. The most common cause of pneumothorax is via iatrogenic insults, such as transthoracic needle aspirations, mechanical ventilation, and various nerve blocks.[1,2,3]

A tension pneumothorax is the result of the intrapleural pressure exceeding the atmospheric pressure. A one-way valve mechanism allows air to enter the pleural space during inspiration. Tension pneumothoraces typically occur with mechanical ventilation and cardiopulmonary resuscitation but can result from any primary pneumothorax etiology. A tension pneumothorax can lead to rapid cardiopulmonary deterioration. The increased pleural pressure results in decreased cardiac output, and in severe cases can cause a shift in mediastinal structures.[1,2,4]

A pneumothorax can present with very minimal symptoms depending on the size and pressure gradient. Shortness of breath and tachycardia are the most common symptoms. More severe pressure gradients and tension pneumothoraces will have hypotension, tactile fremitus, electrocardiographic changes, and cyanosis. An upright chest x-ray is the imaging of choice to show pathologic pleural lines indicating free air. Unlike other types of pneumothorax, a tension pneumothorax diagnosis should not rely on radiographic imaging. A clinical history and physical examination will yield a diagnosis and prompt urgent intervention.[1,2,4]

Treatment of pneumothoraces include simple modalities such as observation and supplemental oxygen, but more invasive measures such as aspiration, tube thoracostomy, and video-assisted thoracic surgery (VATS) with oversewing of blebs may be necessary for more severe cases. An emergent decompression for a tension pneumothorax should be done by placing a 14- to 16-gauge intravenous catheter into the second rib space along the midclavicular line.[1,2,3]

## HEMOTHORAX OVERVIEW

A bloody pleural effusion with a hematocrit of at least 50% of the peripheral blood is termed a hemothorax. A hemothorax can be divided into spontaneous and traumatic causes, with the latter the most common. Rib fractures are not necessary to have a traumatic hemothorax and are found in slightly over half of traumatic cases. A hemothorax may not be seen on an initial chest radiograph, and an ultrasound may demonstrate the diagnosis up to 3–6 hours after the accident. A concomitant occurrence of a pneumothorax and a hemothorax is common after blunt trauma.

Prompt chest tube drainage with a large bore is the most effective treatment. VATS may be necessary in severe cases. A spontaneous hemothorax is most commonly associated with anticoagulation (e.g., heparin for a pulmonary embolism).[4,5]

## CHYLOTHORAX OVERVIEW

Approximately 2.4 L of chyle is transported through the body every day. A large portion of this chyle passes through the thoracic, which is responsible for carrying 60%–70% of ingested fat, resulting in high amounts of cholesterol and triglycerides.[1,4,5] When there is leakage of chyle into the pleura, it is termed a chylothorax. A chylothorax is broken down into traumatic versus nontraumatic. Thoracic surgery has replaced physical injury as the leading cause of chylothoraces. Nontraumatic etiologies are vast but most commonly occur from malignancy and sarcoidosis.[5]

The clinical manifestations of a chylothorax are identical to those of a similar size pleural effusion. Chylothorax may present in neonates with respiratory distress in the first few days of life. A chylothorax is often a white, milky, odorless fluid but may appear cloudy, yellow, or even bloody. Treatment is similar to that for both a pneumothorax and hemothorax.[4,5]

## ANESTHETIC CONSIDERATIONS

General anesthesia is a rare cause of a pneumothorax, with an incidence as low as 0.5%. A pneumothorax may occur from surgical or anesthetic procedures or barotrauma. A diagnosis during surgery is often difficult because the signs are nonspecific and can be neglected with ventilatory changes until it becomes severe. Underlying lung disease, laparoscopic surgery, and barotrauma are all predisposing factors. The first signs may be tachycardia, increased oxygen needs, and signs of airway obstruction.[3]

The diagnosis is often made clinically after decompensation and with chest auscultation. An intraoperative chest tube should be placed. A chest radiograph may confirm the diagnosis if available and there is an unclear diagnosis. After stabilization and completion of the surgery, if deemed appropriate, the patient should be observed in a surgical ward and obtain postoperative computed tomography.[3]

## REFERENCES

1. Pawloski DR, Broaddus KD. Pneumothorax: a review. *J Am Anim Hosp Assoc.* 2010;46(6):385–397.
2. Sahn SA, Heffner JE. Spontaneous pneumothorax. *N Engl J Med.* 2000;342(12):868–874.
3. Heyba M, et al. Detection and management of intraoperative pneumothorax during laparoscopic cholecystectomy. *Case Rep Anesthesiol.* 2020;*2020*:9273903. https://doi.org/10.1155/2020/9273903
4. Broderick SR. Hemothorax: etiology, diagnosis, and management. *Thorac Surg Clin.* 2013;23(1):89–96, vi–vii.
5. Yeam I, Sassoon C. Hemothorax and chylothorax. *Curr Opin Pulm Med.* 1997;3(4):310–314.

# 259.

# UPPER RESPIRATORY INFECTIONS (COLDS, EPIGLOTTITIS, LARYNGOTRACHEOBRONCHITIS), BRONCHOPULMONARY DYSPLASIA, CYSTIC FIBROSIS

*Irim Salik and Ashley Kelley*

## INTRODUCTION

Upper respiratory tract infections (URIs) represent the most common infections of childhood and significantly increase a child's risk of perioperative respiratory adverse events (PRAE).

## UPPER RESPIRATORY INFECTIONS: THE COMMON COLD

Upper respiratory tract infections are a frequent problem encountered when administering anesthesia to pediatric patients. Most URIs are viral, with causative agents including rhinoviruses, coronaviruses, and adenoviruses. URIs have the potential to increase airway reactivity and the risk of PRAE, including upper airway obstruction, laryngospasm, bronchospasm, cough, stridor, apnea, and oxygen desaturation. This risk may be increased for several weeks after the resolution of URI symptoms.[1]

Anesthetic considerations:

- Children that are afebrile with clear, nonpurulent secretions and who are without serious comorbidities can generally proceed to surgery.
- Children with underlying reactive airway disease are at greater risk for developing PRAEs after a recent URI; the anesthesiologist should have a lower threshold for postponing surgery in this patient population.
- Children who present for elective surgery with more serious signs or symptoms (fever, productive cough, lethargy, dyspnea, yellow or green secretions, wheezing, and decreased oral intake) should have surgery postponed for 2–4 weeks to allow for URI resolution.
- The anesthesiologist must use their discretion when evaluating children that fall into a "gray area" or intermediate risk category

- If feasible, in children with a URI, a face mask or laryngeal mask airway should be selected instead of an endotracheal tube (ETT).
- If airway manipulation is required, children should be deeply anesthetized.
- No clear data exist to support awake versus deep removal of airway devices in pediatric patients with URIs.
- Experience of the anesthesiologist plays a large role in the reduction of PRAEs.
- In children with URIs undergoing elective surgery,
  1. Preoperative administration of $\beta_2$-agonists before surgery may reduce bronchoconstriction and PRAEs.
  2. In high-risk children, intravenous induction with propofol is preferred over inhalation induction.
  3. Following adequate suctioning, awake extubation in addition to immediate oxygen supplementation and continuous positive airway pressure (CPAP) are recommended.

## EPIGLOTTITIS

Epiglottitis is an acute onset bacterial infection of the epiglottis and aryepiglottic folds, potentially leading to cyanosis, drooling, dyspnea, dysphonia, and hoarseness in children. The most common offending pathogen is *Haemophilus influenzae* type b (Hib) (75% of cases), although group A β-hemolytic *Streptococcus pneumoniae*, *Staphylococcus aureus*, and *Klebsiella pneumoniae* are also indicated.[2] Vaccination for Hib has greatly reduced incidence in the pediatric population. Patients present with generalized toxemia, including high fevers, dysphagia, and inspiratory stridor, commonly while leaning forward in the sniffing position, known as the "tripod position." Epiglottitis constitutes an airway emergency that requires immediate intervention by the anesthesiologist and otolaryngologist, as airway loss and death can occur. Nasopharyngoscopy or laryngoscopy is the gold

**Table 259.1** COMPARISON BETWEEN CROUP AND EPIGLOTTITIS

| | CROUP | EPIGLOTTITIS |
|---|---|---|
| Age at presentation | 6 months–3 years old | 3–7 years old |
| Family history | Yes | No |
| Prodrome | Usually URI | Usually none/sore throat |
| Clinical presentation | Gradual onset (days), nontoxic appearance, barking cough, hoarseness of voice, inspiratory stridor, low-grade fever | Abrupt onset (6–24 hours), toxic appearance, acute onset of high fever, drooling, dyspnea, dysphonia, dysphagia, tripod position (one sits or stands leaning forward and supporting the upper body with hands on the knees or on another surface). Epiglottis: Cherry red, edematous |
| Etiology | Viral etiology, parainfluenza virus, influenza A and B, respiratory syncytial virus | *Haemophilus influenzae* type b, Group A β-hemolytic *Streptococcus pneumoniae, Staphylococcus aureus, Klebsiella pneumoniae* |
| X-ray findings | Subglottic narrowing (Steeple sign) on anteroposterior view | Thumbprint sign on lateral view Tracheal narrowing |
| Diagnosis | Clinical | Bronchoscopy |
| Management | Racemic epinephrine, steroids, humidification of air, fever control, hydration, antiviral agents may be helpful | Urgent airway management, antibiotics |

standard for diagnosis, and a lateral neck radiograph will reveal the "thumbprint sign" due to a "cherry-red" edematous epiglottis.[2] In severe cases, patients may become hypoxic, acidotic, and hypercapnic, predisposing them to arrhythmias and hemodynamic instability (Table 259.1).

Anesthetic considerations:

- Setup should include video laryngoscopy, a difficult airway cart, needle cricothyrotomy kit, tracheostomy setup, and an experienced anesthesiologist and otolaryngologist.
- Avoid manipulation or examination of the mouth or pharynx unless in a controlled setting, such as the operating room (OR).
- Maintain the child in a sitting position, with parental presence if necessary; transport to the OR as soon as possible; apply monitors; and provide general inhalational anesthesia with oxygen and sevoflurane. Once anesthesia is achieved, lay the child down gently.
- Intravenous line placement should be deferred until anesthetic induction and paralytics avoided until the airway is secured.
- Once a deep plane of anesthesia is achieved, nasotracheal intubation is prudent as the tube is less likely to become dislodged.
- Due to airway edema, an ETT one to two sizes smaller than would be appropriate for the age and size of the patient is appropriate.
- If spontaneous ventilation ceases or airway obstruction occurs, an emergent direct laryngoscopy or rigid bronchoscopy should be attempted.

- The surgeon must be prepared for an emergent cricothyrotomy or tracheostomy in case of a lost airway.
- Once the airway is secured, admission to the intensive care unit is mandatory as antibiotic and steroid administration is the mainstay of treatment.
- Patients remain intubated and sedated for 24–72 hours as toxemia resolves. Extubation should be attempted after resolution of pyrexia and presence of an air leak at 20 cm H$_2$O.

## CROUP

Croup, or laryngotracheobronchitis, is a viral-mediated inflammatory process involving the subglottic tracheal mucosa and tracheobronchial tree, most commonly seen in children ages 6 months to 3 years old.[3] Presentation is insidious and includes low-grade fever, cough, sore throat, and rhinorrhea prior to upper airway obstruction, characterized by a "barking cough" and inspiratory stridor. Etiology is most commonly parainfluenza type 1, but can also include types 2 and 3, influenza A and B, respiratory syncytial virus, *Mycoplasma pneumonia*, herpes simplex virus, and adenovirus.[3] Management of croup includes humidified air, nebulized racemic epinephrine to reduce airway edema, steroid administration, heliox to lower resistance to airway gas flow, and potential tracheal intubation if the patient's condition does not improve. Postintubation croup is caused by subglottic injury and edema associated with traumatic intubation, an oversize ETT, or an overinflated ETT cuff. An anteroposterior neck radiograph will reveal subglottic tracheal narrowing resembling a "steeple sign"[3] (Table 259.1).

Anesthetic considerations:

- Maintain spontaneous respirations during anesthetic induction if an intravenous line is absent
- Symptomatic patients with croup should be intubated with an ETT 0.5–1.0 mm smaller in diameter than for a child without croup.
- Following treatment with racemic epinephrine, observe patients for up to 4 hours due to risk for recurrence of symptoms.

## BRONCHOPULMONARY DYSPLASIA

Bronchopulmonary dysplasia (BPD) is defined as the continued oxygen requirement at 28 days of life in a neonate with a history of respiratory distress syndrome (RDS). It is the most common cause of chronic lung disease in infants, common in premature infants on supplementation oxygen, or in those requiring prolonged mechanical ventilation, characterized by abnormal pulmonary vascular growth and alveolar dilation.[4] Risk factors for BPD include low birth weight, nutritional deficiencies, adrenal insufficiency, meconium aspiration, and congestive heart disease. Neonates with RDS eventually develop increased airway resistance, lung hyperinflation, and airway obstruction, leading to ventilation-perfusion mismatch, compromised pulmonary compliance, and increased work of breathing. In severe cases, infants exhibiting hypoxia, hypercarbia, acidosis, and tachypnea can develop right heart failure, pulmonary hypertension, and cor pulmonale. Fluid restriction and diuretic administration may be appropriate in patients with cor pulmonale to optimize gas exchange. Mortality in patients with BPD can be reduced with more conservative ventilation strategies, including avoidance of endotracheal intubation, utilizing CPAP or noninvasive positive pressure ventilation (PPV), and timely surfactant administration. If intubation is required, lung-sparing strategies should be utilized, including small tidal volumes, permissive hypercapnia, and aggressive weaning of ventilator support.[4]

Anesthetic considerations:

- In patients with pulmonary hypertension, hypoxia, hypercarbia, and acidosis should be avoided.
- Inhalation induction with sevoflurane in infants with BPD may lead to acute desaturation due to loss of hypoxic pulmonary vasoconstriction under general anesthesia.
- Avoidance of nitrous oxide may be prudent due to elevated pulmonary vascular resistance and exacerbation of air trapping.

- Patients with prolonged intubation and mechanical ventilation may manifest subglottic stenosis, tracheomalacia, and bronchomalacia
- Patients with BPD are at higher risk of rapid desaturation, atelectasis, laryngospasm, and bronchospasm due to airway hyperactivity
- Intraoperatively, increased peak inspiratory pressures (PIP), positive end-expiratory pressure, and increased $FiO_2$ (fraction of inspired air) may be required.
- Patients with obstructive lung disease should be afforded adequate expiratory times when mechanically ventilated.
- Elevated PIP may lead to pneumothorax, pneumomediastinum, or interstitial emphysema in patients with BPD.
- Patients may require postoperative mechanical ventilation in a monitored setting.

## CYSTIC FIBROSIS

Cystic fibrosis (CF) is an autosomal recessive multisystemic syndrome that causes chronic suppurative lung disease. CF is caused by mutations on the long arm of chromosome 7, which encodes a chloride channel lining exocrine glands. The sweat test used to diagnose CF is based on abnormal sodium and chloride levels in exocrine secretions. Decreased mucociliary clearance leads to patchy atelectasis, airway inflammation, and chronic hypoxia, while bronchiectasis and air trapping lead to airway obstruction. Some patients develop a steady decline in lung function, leading to cor pulmonale, respiratory failure, and eventual death.[5] Respiratory function is maintained with physiotherapy, inhaled bronchodilators, and mucolytics. Oscillatory devices, positive expiratory pressure devices, and high-frequency chest compression devices are useful for mucous clearance. Lung and liver transplantation are increasingly common in children with CF.[5]

Anesthetic considerations:

- Prior to elective surgery, patients should be optimized with daily physiotherapy and targeted medication regimens.
- Preoperative evaluation should include chest radiography, baseline arterial blood gas analysis, and spirometric studies.
- PRAEs are increased secondary to prolonged duration of anesthesia, upper abdominal or thoracic incisions, nasogastric tube insertion, or emergency surgery.
- Glycemic control is important in patients with CF.
- Consideration for a pulmonary artery catheter or cardiac output monitoring should be utilized in patients with cor pulmonale or those undergoing major surgery.

- Placement of an ETT as opposed to supraglottic airway facilitates tracheal suctioning of secretions and allows for controlled ventilation.
- Nasal intubation should be avoided in CF patients because of the potential for nasal polyposis.
- Airway pressures should be kept low when utilizing PPV techniques, and gases should be humidified.
- Patients that are malnourished and/or cachectic must be positioned and padded to avoid nerve injury.
- Regional anesthesia can be utilized to avoid airway manipulation and facilitate analgesia for early mobilization.

## REFERENCES

1. Coté CJ, et al. *A Practice of Anesthesia for Infants and Children.* 6th ed. Elsevier Saunders; 2019.
2. Lichtor L, et al. Epiglottitis: it hasn't gone away. *Anesthesiology.* 2016;124(6):1404–1407.
3. Almeida-Chen GM. Croup. In: Houck PJ, et al., eds. *Handbook of Pediatric Anesthesia.* New York, NY: McGraw-Hill; 2015.
4. Hayes D Jr, et al. Pathogenesis of bronchopulmonary dysplasia. *Respiration.* 2010;79(5):425–436.
5. Newton TJ. Respiratory care of the hospitalized patient with cystic fibrosis. *Respir Care.* 2009;54:769–775; discussion 775–776.

# 260.

# MUSCULOSKELETAL DISEASE

*Jamie W. Sinton*

## INTRODUCTION

The particularly wide spectrum of musculoskeletal disease in children poses significant challenges in the perioperative period (e.g., method of neuromuscular blockade).[1] Although patients with muscular disease often have extreme motor challenges, they are cognitively appropriate and understand age-appropriate prognosis and expected disease course. This chapter focuses on Duchenne muscular dystrophy (DMD), spinal muscular atrophy (SMA), and osteogenesis imperfecta (OI). Disorders discussed elsewhere include cerebral palsy, malignant hyperthermia and related disorders, and achondroplasia. Other musculoskeletal diseases that are worth mentioning but are not discussed further include polymyositis, dermatomyositis, other muscular dystrophies, myotonic dystrophies, periodic paralysis, myasthenia gravis, myasthenic syndrome (Lambert-Eaton), mitochondrial myopathies, multicore myopathy, centronuclear myopathy.

## DUCHENNE MUSCULAR DYSTROPHY

Duchenne muscular dystrophy (and to a lesser extent, Becker muscular dystrophy) is a progressive muscle disorder due to dystrophin protein deficiency in skeletal muscle and myocardial and brain cells. Muscles are gradually replaced by fat and connective tissue, but the body habitus may not change. Its incidence is approximately 1/3500 live-born males.[2] DMD has an X-linked recessive genetic inheritance. The diagnosis is often suspected when children fail to meet gross motor milestones (e.g., not walking until age 18 months).[3] Cardiac manifestations are usually an acquired, progressive decline in systolic function characterized by hypertrophy and fibrosis.[4] Symptoms of heart failure include weight loss, vomiting, decreased urine output, or failure to tolerate daily activities. Resting sinus tachycardia is common on electrocardiography (ECG). Older, nonambulatory patients commonly have hypotension and risk of significant hypotension during large fluid shifts. Difficult laryngoscopy occurs in about 3.4% with masseter muscle fibrosis.[4] Muscle weakness may not be noted until the child is several years old, that is why it is recommended not to use succinylcholine in children unless it is an airway emergency.

Duchenne muscular dystrophy is not associated with malignant hyperthermia risk; however, some anesthesiologists choose to deliver a nontriggering anesthetic as fragile muscle membranes are susceptible to breakdown followed by rhabdomyolysis and hyperkalemic cardiac arrest in the presence of volatile anesthetics and succinylcholine. The children at highest risk are the younger children as they have more muscle mass (i.e., less of their muscle has already been replaced by fibrosis).

## SPINAL MUSCULAR ATROPHY

Spinal muscular atrophy is an autosomal recessive disorder of reduced production of the survival motor neuron 1 (SMN1) gene leading to α-motor neuron degeneration. Survival motor neuron 2 (SMN2) genes are ubiquitously expressed and function as motor neurons for these patients. Variation in copy number of SMN2 determines disease severity. SMA1 is also called Werdnig-Hoffmann disease, and ECG abnormalities are common, including bradycardia and intraventricular conduction delay. Milder forms of SMA are associated with acquired heart disease.[5]

An intrathecal therapy called nusinersen may improve strength in children with SMA. Due to a high incidence of scoliosis, administration is performed in interventional radiology with the child under general inhalational anesthesia.

## OSTEOGENESIS IMPERFECTA

Skeletal diseases are as diverse as muscular diseases; however, only OI is discussed here. Achondroplasia, scoliosis, and craniosynostosis are discussed elsewhere.

Osteogenesis imperfecta is an autosomal dominant disorder of deficient synthesis of type 1 collagen and results in low bone mineral density. It has four subtypes in which types 1 and 4 have mild-to-moderate severity, while types 2 and 3 are severe, and type 2 often ends in stillbirth. Table 260.1 lists anesthetic considerations for children with OI.

## ANESTHETIC CONSIDERATIONS FOR MUSCLE DISORDERS

### PREOPERATIVE

Many patients arrive to the operating room for muscle biopsy with a presumed diagnosis based on electromyographic or genetic testing. The diagnosis of myopathy is frequently unchanged following muscle biopsy; therefore, anesthetic risk could be discussed with the ordering physician.

Preoperatively, functional status and exercise tolerance will be largely unavailable by history. ECG baseline may contain artifact due to skeletal muscle tremor. The use of herbal medications, especially in the DMD population, affects coagulation. In adolescents, advanced directives and attitudes toward prolonged mechanical ventilation should be discussed.

*Table 260.1* ANESTHETIC CONSIDERATIONS IN OI

| | |
|---|---|
| Airway | Fracture risk of maxilla, mandible, cervical spine, exophthalmos (prone positioning pressure risk) |
| Cardiovascular | Cystic degeneration of aortic root and valves (regurgitant lesions), intraventricular conduction delay, congenital heart disease |
| Pulmonary | Restrictive lung disease with or without pulmonary hypertension, kyphoscoliosis |
| Monitoring | Decreased frequency of noninvasive cuff cycling or invasive blood pressure measurement |
| Positioning | Exophthalmos, fracture risk; have parent assist with positioning if possible |
| Hemorrhage | Platelet defect; may benefit from desmopressin |
| Pain control | Regional anesthesia can be accomplished safely with use of ultrasound to avoid intraosseus injection or fracture |
| Postoperative | Actively seek and treat iatrogenic trauma or fever |

### INTRAOPERATIVE

Patients often present for posterior spinal instrumentation and fusion for neuromuscular scoliosis. The timing of this repair should be prior to the onset of significant cardiac dysfunction. The Food and Drug Administration placed a black box warning on succinylcholine use in children under 8 years of age. Nondepolarizing muscle relaxants may have a prolonged effect.

Intraoperatively, surgical exposure may be preserved due to baseline muscle weakness, and muscle relaxants are often not needed. Open biopsies are often favored as a large amount of tissue is required for some metabolic studies. The surgical technique often requires a muscle tissue sample from the vastus lateralis. This site may not be densely blocked using a lateral femoral cutaneous nerve block; therefore, spinal, caudal, or femoral blocks may be considered. Further, there is some concern that infiltration with local anesthetic near the surgical site may impact biopsy results.

Nontriggering techniques and regional anesthetics should be considered when suspicion for malignant hyperthermia or AIR is present. Use caution in concluding that special safeguards were overly careful when muscle biopsy is uneventful. Regional analgesics should be considered to reduce opioid consumption.

### POSTOPERATIVE

Maintain a high index of suspicion for postoperative rhabdomyolysis if a triggering anesthetic was used. The disposition of these patients depends on respiratory reserve. Postoperative use of home continuous positive airway pressure machines is warranted.

## REFERENCES

1. Vanlinthout LE, et al. Neuromuscular-blocking agents for tracheal intubation in pediatric patients (0–12 years): a systematic review and meta-analysis. *Paediatr Anaesth*. 2020;30(4):401–414.
2. Dubowitz V. Muscle Disorders in Childhood. Philadelphia, PA: Saunders; 1995.
3. Jie Zhou AN, et al. Neuromuscular disorders including malignant hyperthermia and other genetic disorders. In: Gropper MA, eds. *Miller's Anesthesia*. Philadelphia, PA: Elsevier; 2020:1129–1130.
4. Cripe LH, Tobias JD. Cardiac considerations in the operative management of the patient with Duchenne or Becker muscular dystrophy. *Paediatr Anaesth*. 2013;23(9):777–784.
5. Wijngaarde CA, et al. Cardiac pathology in spinal muscular atrophy: a systematic review. *Orphanet J Rare Dis*. 2017;12(1):67.

# 261.

# HYDROCEPHALUS

*Jamie W. Sinton*

## INTRODUCTION

Hydrocephalus may exist with a syndrome (e.g., Arnold-Chiari malformation or myelomeningocele) or be an isolated congenital finding (i.e., neonatal intraventricular hemorrhage with compression of the aqueduct of Sylvius). It may be acquired due to (usually posterior fossa) tumor compression of cerebrospinal fluid (CSF) flow or an inflammatory mechanism or overproduction of CSF as in choroid plexus papilloma. Hydrocephalus may be noncommunicating or communicating. Noncommunicating hydrocephalus is obstructive, and communicating hydrocephalus occurs when CSF absorption is inadequate.

## PATHOPHYSIOLOGY

The Monroe-Kellie doctrine posits that intracranial volume is fixed (except in the case of infants with open fontanelles). Therefore, any obstruction to flow of CSF will increase CSF volume in the skull. Without any compensation, intracranial pressure (ICP) will rise. In order to prevent dangerous increases in ICP when CSF has no egress, venous blood can shift to accommodate. In order to maintain cerebral perfusion, mean arterial pressure (MAP) must mirror the rise in ICP. Cerebral perfusion pressure (CPP) equals MAP minus central venous pressure or ICP (whichever is greater).

In children, the most common cause of hydrocephalus is stenosis of the aqueduct of Sylvius. The delicate germinal matrix of premature infants predisposes them to germinal matrix hemorrhage, causing external compression and stenosis of the aqueduct. In this situation, CSF cannot traverse the aqueduct, and CSF accumulates in the lateral and third ventricles.

Arnold-Chiari malformation is a congenital hindbrain malformation resulting in cerebellar descent through the foramen magnum. The danger is compression of the brainstem and superior portion of the cervical spinal cord. There are four types, of which type IV is the most severe and often lethal in infancy. This cause of hydrocephalus is treated by decompression rather than CSF diversion and occipital craniectomy and laminectomy of the posterior arch of C1 and any other levels involved.

Dandy-Walker malformation is cystic of the fourth ventricle and incomplete formation of cerebellar vermis and is a common indication for CSF diversion.

Communicating hydrocephalus, more commonly seen in adults, can be treated with a shunt as well. This shunt may be placed into lumbar CSF with diversion to the peritoneal cavity.

## PRESENTATION OF HYDROCEPHALUS

In the preverbal or nonverbal child, symptoms of headache, nausea, and the like will be impossible to elicit. Refractory intracranial hypertension and impending herniation present with the Cushing triad of systolic hypertension, bradycardia, and agonal breathing. In children with open fontanelles, ICP may be quiet high; however, children are protected from herniation due to expansion of the cranial vault. Well-child checks at the pediatrician may reveal a fronto-occipital circumference that is enlarging more quickly than somatic growth. A head ultrasound can be obtained to confirm the diagnosis. On physical examination, "sun-setting" eyes appear with white sclera superior to the iris (see Figure 261.1). This is also consistent with increased ICP (often due to hydrocephalus).

## CSF DIVERSION SURGERY

Relief of obstruction to CSF flow restores intracranial volume and pressure. The ventriculoperitoneal shunt (VPS) is the most common operation. When intra-abdominal infection or peritonitis exists, CSF may be diverted elsewhere (i.e., ventriculoatrial or ventriculopleural). Shunt placement and revision are often necessary due to somatic growth of the child, malfunction (proximally at the reservoir or distally), or infection. Most VPSs are either anterior or posterior. External ventricular drains are placed for temporary relief of hydrocephalus (i.e., VPS infection or critically ill trauma patients). Third ventriculostomy, choroid plexus cauterization, or subcutaneous drain are usually considered in the case of patient prematurity, in extremis, or in a limited-resource setting.

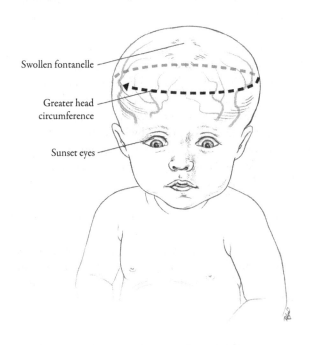

Swollen fontanelle

Greater head circumference

Sunset eyes

**Figure 261.1** An infant with an enlarged head circumference and the sclera showing superior to his irises bilaterally is shown.

## CEREBRAL HEMODYNAMICS DURING RESUSCITATION

Regardless of etiology of cardiac arrest (increased ICP or not), cerebral blood flow is reduced, and cerebral venous pressure increases. Consistent with the Monroe-Kellie hypothesis, an increased volume venous of blood in the brain due to sluggish passage through the cardiovascular system should increase ICP. To that end, if a patient with a VPS arrests, removal of CSF from an indwelling VPS may improve ICP and intracerebral hemodynamics.

## ANESTHETIC CONSIDERATIONS

### PREOPERATIVE

Normal ICP and CPP vary with age and position. An ICP less than 5 mm Hg would be acceptable for an intubated, supine infant; however, a normal alert, teenager in the sitting position could have an ICP of 10 mm Hg.[1] Preoperatively, sedative premedication should be avoided in the context of a stuporous patient and risk of herniation. Neurologic assessment may be hindered by lack of cooperation or altered mental status.

### INTRAOPERATIVE

Intraoperatively, place the operating room table in reverse Trendelenburg to allow for gravity-aided drainage of venous blood and maybe some ICP reduction. Optimal CPP likely correlates with age in pediatric neurotrauma patients.[2] Inhalation induction with early mask-assisted ventilation is acceptable in most patients when an intravenous line is not preexisting. Normocarbic ventilation is preferred unless the child is bradycardic and imminently herniating; then, momentary hyperventilation maybe of value. Goals of intubation include maintenance of CPP with minimal rise in ICP.

### POSTOPERATIVE

Postoperatively from an uncomplicated VPS (re)placement, the patient can be extubated safely. Awake extubation and coughing should be permitted as CSF is now diverted, and any increase in ICP produced by coughing should be easily abated with CSF distribution through the shunt.

### REFERENCES

1. Lovett ME, et al. Children with severe traumatic brain injury, intracranial pressure, cerebral perfusion pressure, what does it mean? A review of the literature. *Pediatr Neurol.* 2019;94:3–20.
2. Lewis PM, et al. Cerebrovascular pressure reactivity in children with traumatic brain injury. *Pediatr Crit Care Med.* 2015;16(8):739–749.

# 262.

# DEVELOPMENTAL DELAY, AUTISM, AND CEREBRAL PALSY

*Maura C. Berkelhamer*

## DEVELOPMENTAL MILESTONES

From birth to age 5 children progress from babbling to fluent speech, acquire the foundational skills for literacy, and advance from helpless immobility to running and independently performing activities of daily life. This period of rapid learning and growth follows a typical timetable from birth. Parents and pediatricians anticipate a child's progress acquiring these milestones over time using validated screening tools such as the Denver Developmental Screening Test II. There are five domains of development for a child (Table 262.1).

- Cognitive: memory, reasoning, and problem-solving
- Motor—gross and fine: tone, balance, ambulation, manipulating objects
- Social-emotional and behavioral: attachment, play, self-care
- Language: expressive, receptive, verbal comprehension

- Adaptive: hand-eye coordination, object permanence, symbolic thought

## DEVELOPMENTAL DELAYS AND DISABILITIES

Premature birth, early illness, head trauma, anoxia, or genetic abnormalities can significantly delay or interrupt a child's developmental progress. Developmental delays can be limited to one domain or global with disabilities in all domains. Delays in one domain can affect skills in another. There are comorbidities that affect people with developmental delays and disabilities (DD&D), such as seizures, hearing and visual impairment, dysmorphic facial features, somatic growth abnormalities, chronic constipation, respiratory insufficiency, gastroesophageal reflux, obstructive sleep apnea, hypothalamic dysfunction, and growth failure.

*Table 262.1* AN ABBREVIATED CHART OF DEVELOPMENTAL MILESTONES WITH IMPLICATIONS FOR ANESTHESIA

| AGE (MONTHS) | MILESTONE DESCRIPTION | ANESTHETIC IMPLICATIONS |
| --- | --- | --- |
| 0.5 | Fixes gaze on a face<br>Arms and legs flexed and tucked near body | Awake state baseline<br>Assessment of baseline strength & recovery from muscle relaxants |
| 2 | Smiles in response to a face<br>Lifts hips when supine | Awake state baseline<br>Recovery from muscle relaxants |
| 4 | Rolls (front to back first, later back to front)<br>Head control | Safety on an OR table & recovery from muscle relaxants |
| 9 | Stranger anxiety and separation anxiety<br>Babbles, dada, mama, recognizes their name<br>Places pacifier in their mouth<br>Pulls up on crib rail to stand | Consider Preoperative Sedation medication,<br>Self-soothing with pacifier & Safety in a cart |
| 24 | Can follow two-step commands<br>Imitates actions | Participation in an Inhaled Induction |

Berkelhamer MC. 2020.

Treatment is supportive and aimed at optimizing the patient's mobility and interactions with the environment as well as treating any underlying etiologies and comorbidities. Children with DD&D receive physical, speech, and occupational therapy services at home and as they progress through school. Individuals with developmental delays are often dependent on technology aides to be fed, breathe, move, or travel from home.

The neurological abnormalities causing DD&D can also be associated with behavior disturbances, which can result in injury to the patient, caregivers, and hospital staff unless they are anticipated and managed. Subsequently, individuals with developmental disabilities and their caregivers face additional challenges on the day of surgery.

## AUTISM SPECTRUM DISORDER

Autism is a term that describes DD&D originating early in childhood and impairing everyday functioning across a variety of situations, such as home, play, and school. For most patients with autism spectrum disorder (ASD), delays and disabilities exist in the domains of language and social-emotional behavior. Limitations in verbal and nonverbal communication, the ability to socialize in a typical manner, and the presence of persistent restrictive or repetitive behaviors characterize ASD. The *Diagnostic and Statistical Manual of Mental Disorders, Fifth Edition,* has combined autism, Asperger syndrome, and pervasive developmental disorder into one diagnosis: autism spectrum disorder. The etiology of ASD is varied. Genetically heterogenous abnormalities can be found on microarray analysis in some ASD patients. There are comorbidities that affect people with ASD, including sleep disorders, attention deficit hyperactivity disorder, anxiety, hearing impairment, constipation, and seizure disorders. Treatment is supportive and aimed at optimizing an individual's language abilities, social behaviors, and interactions, as well as treating any underlying comorbidities. Children with ASD have Individualized Education Plans (IEPs) throughout their schooling to provide supplemental support for learning, organization, and testing as needed. There is a spectrum of cognitive abilities among patients with the diagnosis of autism. It can be difficult for people with ASD to make the situational transitions from home through the perioperative environments that require interacting with new people and participating in unfamiliar tasks.

## CEREBRAL PALSY: MOTOR TONE ABNORMALITIES WITH OR WITHOUT STATIC ENCEPHALOPATHY

Cerebral palsy (CP) is a group of disorders characterized by abnormal motor tone, posture, and movement due to an insult to the developing brain. The disorder is not progressive or degenerative. However, an individual's clinical manifestations can change over time, and their ability to perform activities of daily life can deteriorate as they age. The diagnosis of spastic, dyskinetic, or ataxic is given to describe developmental disabilities in the motor domain that can also effect expressive language and other bulbar muscle function, such as swallowing and airway muscle tone. Static encephalopathy refers to delays and disabilities in the cognitive, adaptive, language (receptive), and social-emotional and behavior domains. Intellectual disability is associated with at least 50% of patients with CP (Table 262.2).[1]

There are many causes of brain injury that result in CP, including, anoxia, prenatal and perinatal hypoxic ischemic injury or stroke, head trauma, and brain malformations from genetic abnormalities, teratogens, or infections. Premature birth causes periventricular leukomalacia and intraventricular hemorrhage associated with CP in former premature infants. The most common risk factor for CP in premature infants is perinatal infection.[1] Comorbidities that affect individuals with CP include seizure disorders, chronic constipation, gastroesophageal reflux, dysphagia and aspiration, airway muscle tone abnormalities causing upper airway obstruction, scoliosis, and poor cough and airway clearance with subsequent respiratory insufficiency and recurrent pneumonia. For people with CP, Autonomic Nervous System dysfunction, manifested as an abnormal response in heart rate or vasomotor tone to hypovolemia, hypotension, and orthostatic stresses, or impaired thermoregulation, is exaggerated by anesthetic agents. Autonomic Storms can be seen with pain and temperature stresses during the perioperative period as sympathetic outflow is not modulated normally by parasympathetic output in patients with CP.

Treatment is supportive, such as soft tissue and bony orthopedic procedures, aimed at optimizing the patient's mobility and upright posture. Spasticity can be reduced with botulinum toxin injections, baclofen given orally or through intrathecal pumps, or dorsal rhizotomy surgery. Dental restorations, gastrostomy tube placement,

*Table 262.2* TYPES OF CEREBRAL PALSY

| | |
|---|---|
| Spastic<br>• Hemiplegia: one side of the body<br>• Diplegia: bilateral legs > arms<br>• Quadriplegia: all limbs | Upper motor neuron signs<br>Motor tone imbalances<br>  across joints<br>Contractures |
| Dyskinetic<br>• Chorea: dance-like movements<br>• Athetotic: writhing movements<br>• Dystonic: abnormal posturing | Basal ganglia signs |
| Ataxic | |

Berkelhamer MC. 2020.

fundoplication, procedures to reduce drooling, and scoliosis surgeries are often necessary.

## ANESTHETIC CONSIDERATIONS FOR PATIENTS WITH DD &D, ASD, AND CP

Preoperative evaluation and planning must consider optimizing the patients with chronic lung disease, continuing a patient's routine of anticonvulsant and psychotropic medications on the day of surgery, and continuing their use of supportive technologies. Medications can be given with small volumes of clear liquids orally or via G-tube 2 hours prior to their operating room (OR) time when necessary to maintain the patient's medication schedule of anticonvulsant and psychotropic drugs throughout their perioperative course. Caregivers must bring the technology aides necessary to support the patient in the postoperative unit; G-tube feeding extensions and specialized formulas can be necessary to ensure discharge on the day of surgery. Individuals using home bilevel positive airway pressure/continuous positive airway pressure therapy or mechanical ventilation through a tracheostomy need their equipment to have a charged battery.

Premedication with benzodiazepines or ketamine may be necessary to smooth separation from the caregiver. Assess the patient's ability to cooperate with oral sedative premedication, intravenous catheter placement, or an inhalational induction via mask or tracheostomy tube. For patients with combative behavior and those unable to cooperate with oral premedication, fast-acting intramuscular medications such as ketamine should be considered to facilitate intravenous placement or inhalational induction. Monitor patients with static encephalopathy immediately after receiving premedication as they may exhibit airway obstruction or respiratory depression. Implanted magnetic equipment such as vagal nerve stimulators and baclofen pumps may need to be inactivated during procedures using electrocautery.

Intravenous access may be difficult. Muscle tone abnormalities in the upper airway may cause airway obstruction during mask ventilation. Some patients with CP may be resistant to nondepolarizing muscle relaxants whether or not they receive seizure medication, but patients with hypotonia and reduced muscle mass are more sensitive to muscle relaxants depressing chest excursions and airway muscle tone. Train-of-four monitoring may be inaccurate if used in areas of severe muscle atrophy. CP does not cause an upregulation of acetylcholine receptors around the neuromuscular junction. In patients with CP, muscles fail to develop or atrophy but are not denervated. Succinylcholine has not been associated with exaggerated potassium release in children with CP. Patients with CP have reduced minimal alveolar concentration requirements for inhalational agents. In children with spastic quadriplegia, bispectral index values are lower when awake and at different sevoflurane concentrations compared to controls. Active warming measures are necessary to maintain body temperature because thermoregulation is impaired by hypothalamic dysfunction. Positioning patients with contracted limbs is challenging. Patients with neuromuscular scoliosis have greater blood loss during scoliosis surgery than those with idiopathic scoliosis.[2]

Patients with DD&D are more sensitive to the sedating and respiratory-depressing effects of anesthetic agents delaying emergence. After extubation, contractures and spasticity can make it difficult to maintain a head position that creates an optimally patent airway. Regional techniques can aid in reducing the need for opioid medications. Acetaminophen, ketorolac, and other nonopioid pain medications should be employed. Nonopioid pain management modalities are beneficial in reducing sedation; airway obstruction and respiratory, cough, and clearance depression; and constipation with abdominal distension, which all negatively impact respiratory parameters.

## REFERENCES

1. Gottlieb-Smith R. Weakness and ataxia. In: Dean T Jr, Bell LM, eds. *Nelson Pediatrics Board Review: Certification and Recertification.* Philadelphia, PA: Elsevier; 2019:422–423.
2. Jacobsen BL, et al. The patient with coexisting diseases. In: Bissonnette B, ed. *Pediatric Anesthesia: Basic Principals—The State of the Art-Future.* Shelton, CT: People's Medical Publishing House–USA; 2011:950.

# 263.

# CHILDHOOD OBESITY

*Irim Salik*

## INTRODUCTION

The term *obesity* refers to an excessive amount of fat. Body mass index (BMI) derived from body weight (kilograms) divided by height (meters squared) has emerged as the accepted standard to quantify obesity in children greater than 2 years of age.[1] An obese child is classified as having a BMI at or greater than the 95th percentile for age and sex. A severely obese child has a BMI at or greater than 120% of the 95th percentile.[1]

## ETIOLOGY

Obesity is the consequence of a complicated set of factors, although emotional distress, psychosocial conflicts, sugar-sweetened beverages, high-calorie "fast food" products, large portion sizes, and high glycemic index foods in addition to decreased caloric expenditure have played a pivotal role in the rise of childhood obesity. Sedentary activities and shortened sleep duration have also worsened this epidemic.

## GENETIC FACTORS

Mutation in the melanocortin 4 receptor is the most common single-gene defect currently identified in children with obesity.[2] Children with genetic syndromes predisposed to obesity generally present with characteristic physical features, including short stature, developmental delay, intellectual disability, deafness, dysmorphic facies, and deafness. Prader-Willi syndrome is most commonly associated with obesity, although trisomy 21, Albright hereditary osteodystrophy, Cohen syndrome, Bardet-Biedl syndrome, Alström syndrome, and WAGR (Wilms tumor, aniridia, genitourinary anomaly, mental retardation) are also implicated. Endocrine disorders, including hypothyroidism, growth hormone deficiency, Cushing syndrome, hypothalamic obesity, polycystic ovary syndrome (PCOS), and hyperprolactinemia are also commonly implicated.[2]

## PARENTAL FACTORS

Family-related risk factors for childhood obesity include minority ethnic and cultural background, lower maternal education, single-parent household, familial obesity history, poverty associated with supplemental food assistance, television viewing during meals, and restrictive feeding practices.

Excessive maternal gestational weight gain has been directly associated with obesity due to increased risk of macrosomia and neonatal adiposity. Cesarean delivery and maternal exposure to tobacco and alcohol have also been associated with obesity in offspring. Breastfeeding may be protective against childhood obesity.

## COMORBIDITIES OF CHILDHOOD OBESITY

### CARDIOVASCULAR

Obese children are at increased risk of hyperinsulinemia, insulin resistance, prediabetes, and type 2 diabetes mellitus (T2DM). Obese children can exhibit elevated systolic and diastolic blood pressure, low levels of high-density lipoprotein cholesterol, elevated levels of triglycerides, and elevated glycated hemoglobin levels. Echocardiographic findings include left ventricular hypertrophy, systolic and diastolic dysfunction, and increased left ventricular and left atrial diameter.

### ENDOCRINE

Childhood obesity is associated with early onset of sexual maturation in girls and higher risk for the development of PCOS, characterized by menstrual irregularities, including oligo-ovulation or anovulation, hyperandrogenism, infertility, acne, and hirsutism.

### PULMONARY

Obese children have a higher prevalence of obstructive sleep apnea (OSA), obesity hypoventilation syndrome, chronic oxygen desaturation, and asthma. Sequelae of untreated OSA include right ventricular hypertrophy and pulmonary hypertension.

## GASTROINTESTINAL

Nonalcoholic steatohepatitis is strongly associated with obesity, ranging from simple steatosis to cirrhosis and end-stage liver disease, with elevations in liver transaminases, alkaline phosphatase, and γ-glutamyl transpeptidase. Obese children have a higher incidence of gastroesophageal reflux disease (GERD) and constipation.

## MUSCULOSKELETAL

Childhood obesity increases the risk of fractures, impaired mobility, lower extremity malalignment, slipped capital femoral epiphysis, and Blount disease.

## PSYCHOSOCIAL

Childhood obesity can lead to poor self-esteem, anxiety, depression, increased risk of eating disorders, substance abuse, and social withdrawal. Adolescents are more likely to exhibit poor academic performance, missed school days, and difficulty with concentration.

## DERMATOLOGIC

Acanthosis nigracans, intertrigo, hidradenitis suppurativa, furunculosis, and stretch marks are common dermatologic manifestations of obesity.[3]

## NEUROLOGIC

Obese children may manifest pseudotumor cerebri, with headache, vomiting, retro-ocular eye pain, and vision loss due to blurred optic discs on funduscopic examination.[3]

## ONCOLOGIC

Childhood obesity is associated with malignancy in predominantly 12 cancer sites, including the pharynx and larynx, esophagus, stomach, bowel, liver, gall bladder, pancreas, postmenopausal breast, ovary, kidney, prostate, and uterus.[3]

## PHARMACOLOGICAL THERAPY

Orlistat, a lipase inhibitor, is the only medication currently approved in adolescents. Metformin is an alternative drug utilized for treatment of T2DM in children ages 10 and older. Other medications utilized for off-label treatment include topiramate and glucagon-like peptide 1 analogues such as exenatide.[4]

## BARIATRIC SURGERY

The most commonly performed bariatric procedures include the laparoscopic sleeve gastrectomy (LSG), the Roux-en-Y gastric bypass (RYGB), and the adjustable gastric band (AGB). LSG involves resection of the majority of the greater curvature of the stomach. The RYBG involves creation of a small proximal gastric pouch that is anastomosed to a Roux limb of small bowel. This procedure enables restriction of caloric intake, but leads to malabsorption of food, vitamins, and minerals. The AGB is a snug prosthetic band placed around the stomach, although it is not approved by the Food and Drug Administration for children under 18 years of age. Short-term complications of bariatric surgery include anastomotic site leakage, pulmonary embolism, wound infection, gastric ulceration, incisional hernias, postprandial hypoglycemia, small-bowel obstruction, gastrojejunal strictures or fistulas, and dumping syndrome.[5]

## ANESTHETIC CONSIDERATIONS

### PREOPERATIVE

- Obese children should be worked up for preexisting comorbid conditions, including hypertension, T2DM, asthma, GERD, and OSA.
- Children with a poor attention span, daytime somnolence, frequent snoring, and/or apnea or hypopnea episodes should be evaluated for OSA with polysomnography.
- Pulmonary function tests and arterial blood gas analyses may be indicated in children afflicted with OSA.
- Assessment for GERD is needed with appropriate preoperative prophylaxis.

### INTRAOPERATIVE

- There is a greater incidence of difficult mask ventilation (2.2% vs. 7.4%), postoperative airway obstruction (0.07% vs. 1.6%), and difficult laryngoscopy (0.4% vs. 1.3%) in obese children versus normal weight controls.
- There is a significant increase in the incidence of desaturation, difficult mask ventilation, airway obstruction, laryngospasm, and bronchospasm in obese patients.
- Intravenous induction may be preferred to avoid respiratory complications and to reduce aspiration risk.
- Intravenous access may be more challenging in obese patients due to increased subcutaneous fat deposits.

- Obese children desaturate faster than normal weight counterparts, and it may be more difficult to maintain a patent airway.
- Premedication with a sedative prior to anesthetic induction should be carefully considered as it can increase the risk of postoperative respiratory obstruction.
- Laryngeal mask airway use should be carefully considered in obese children as it may result in hypoventilation.
- Morbidly obese patients may require optimal head and neck positioning utilizing several pillows and a sniffing position to optimize visualization of the airway during laryngoscopy.
- Positive pressure ventilation with higher ventilatory pressures in addition to positive pressure end-expiratory ventilation is utilized to prevent basal collapse and manage reduced lung compliance in obese children.
- Proper positioning of obese patients during prolonged surgical procedures is essential to avoid pressure necrosis over bony prominences.
- Medication dosing based on total body weight may lead to overdose; dosing based on ideal or lean body weight may be preferred.

### POSTOPERATIVE

- Obese children have an increased risk of perioperative airway obstruction and may require a longer duration of stay in the postanesthesia care unit (PACU).

- Obese patients should be extubated fully awake after the return of airway reflexes to minimize the risk of airway obstruction.
- Multimodal analgesia is recommended in obese patients as large doses of opioids may increase the risk of delayed airway obstruction.
- The use of regional anesthesia should be encouraged in obese patients, although it may be technically difficult to achieve.
- Obese patients are at higher risk for development of deep vein thrombosis, so early postoperative mobilization and intraoperative compression stockings are recommended.
- Patients with severe OSA may require overnight hospital admission with pulse oximetry monitoring.

### REFERENCES

1. Lo JC, et al. Prevalence of obesity and extreme obesity in children aged 3–5 years. *Pediatr Obes*. 2013;9(3):167–175.
2. Dubern B, et al. Homozygous null mutation of the melanocortin-4 receptor and severe early-onset obesity. *J Pediatr*. 2007;150(6):613-617.e1.
3. Spear BA, et al. Recommendations for treatment of child and adolescent overweight and obesity. *Pediatrics*. 2007;120(suppl 4):S254–S288.
4. Kelly AS, et al. The effect of glucagonlike peptide-1 receptor agonist therapy on body mass index in adolescents with severe obesity: a randomized, placebo controlled, clinical trial. *JAMA Pediatr*. 2013;167(4):355–360.
5. Sugerman HJ, et al. Bariatric surgery for severely obese adolescents. *J Gastrointest Surg*. 2003;7(1):102–107; discussion 107–108.

# 264.

# SKELETAL ABNORMALITIES IN CHILDREN

*Gina Montone and Jonathan Adams*

### INTRODUCTION

Skeletal dysplasia is defined as abnormal development of bone and cartilage. With over 400 distinct syndromes and subtypes, it is notable that per 100,000 live births there is an incidence of 15.7 disproportionate shortening of limbs or trunks.[1] There are many physiologic implications of skeletal dysplasia. Children with skeletal abnormalities can develop respiratory failure due to developmental abnormalities of the airway and chest wall, leading to an increase in morbidity and mortality.[1] Some of the more significant disorders of skeletal dysplasia leading to respiratory depression include but, are not limited to, Down syndrome, Klippel-Feil syndrome, achondroplasia, Marfan syndrome, Morquio syndrome, and osteogenesis imperfecta. Scoliosis is common in children with these disorders and can have significant anesthetic implications, including difficulty with intubation and proper positioning.

## COMMON SKELETAL DYSPLASIA DISORDERS IN CHILDREN

### DOWN SYNDROME (TRISOMY 21)

Down syndrome, or trisomy 21, is the most prevalent genetic disorder worldwide, affecting more than 1 in 800 live births.[2] This syndrome includes features such as mental retardation and craniofacial, upper airway, cardiovascular, and gastrointestinal abnormalities.[2] Many of these anatomic abnormalities can pose challenges when administering anesthesia to a patient with Down syndrome. In some individuals with Down syndrome, there is instability involving occiput-C1 (atlanto-occipital instability) or the C1-C2 level (atlantoaxial instability). These abnormalities may be due to ligamentous laxity, which allows the C1 vertebra to sublux anteriorly on C2, compressing the spinal cord. If a general anesthetic is required, it is important to minimize head and neck movement during laryngoscopy.

### ACHONDROPLASIA

Achondroplasia is an autosomal dominant disease with an incidence of 0.36–0.60 per 10,000 live births in the United States.[3] It is caused by a fibroblast growth factor receptor 3 mutation, which leads to a disruption in cartilage proliferation and defective endochondral ossification.[3] Features of achondroplasia include a larger head diameter and atlantoaxial dislocation, which can make positioning for endotracheal intubation more challenging and necessitate axial stabilization during the procedure.[3] Other airway abnormalities include narrowed nasal passages, tracheal narrowing, sternal prominence, pharyngeal hypoplasia, and pharyngeal and laryngeal thickening. Laryngomalacia may also occur, leading to stridor. Other structural abnormalities include large tongue, tonsils, and adenoids. It has been found that roughly 40% of individuals affected by achondroplasia also have obstructive sleep apnea.[3] Additional associated abnormalities include severe scoliosis, rib hypoplasia, flattened rib cage, and pectus excavatum, which may lead to restrictive lung disease, pulmonary hypertension, cor pulmonale, and heart problems.[3]

### KLIPPEL-FEIL SYNDROME

Klippel-Feil syndrome is an autosomal disorder that is associated with features including the triad of a short neck, complete fusion of the cervical spine, and severe restriction of neck movements.[4] These spinal deformities can often lead to difficulty with patient positioning, tracheal intubation, and neuraxial anesthesia.[4]

### MARFAN SYNDROME

Marfan syndrome is an autosomal dominant connective tissue disorder with an incidence of roughly 1 in 5000 people worldwide.[5] Because the gene that controls the synthesis of fibrillin 1 (a connective tissue protein) is affected, this causes weakness in the intimal layer of vascular structures and changes in lung structure, including distal acinar emphysema. Airway management may be difficult because of a high-arched palate, potential cervical (C1 and C2) ligamentous instability, and temperomandibular joint (TMJ) laxity, which could lead to TMJ dislocation with laryngoscopy.[5] Respiratory dysfunction can occur due to associated scoliosis, pectus excavatum, restrictive lung disease, and possible spontaneous pneumothorax due to bullous lung disease.[5] Cardiovascular problems may arise from underlying valvular disease (MR, MVP, AI), aortic arch aneurysm, and aortic root dilation due to vascular weakness.[5]

### OSTEOGENESIS IMPERFECTA

Osteogenesis imperfecta consists of a group of genetic disorders characterized by brittle bones. Blue discoloration of the sclera, short stature, scoliosis, joint deformities/contractures, hearing loss, respiratory problems, and dental problems are common in osteogenesis.[1] Bone fractures are more common in pediatric patients and occur less frequently in adulthood. Laryngoscopy may be challenging in patients due to the risk of mandibular fracture, along with decreased neck mobility and kyphoscoliosis, making intubation more difficult. The use of succinylcholine and associated fasciculations can be a cause of fractures. Additional anesthetic concerns include rib fractures from minimal pressure/trauma, potentially leading to pneumothorax.[1] The use of noninvasive blood pressure cuffs causing fractures has been reported to cause fractures in severe cases, in which case one may elect to place an arterial line for monitoring blood pressure.

### MORQUIO SYNDROME

Morquio syndrome is a mucopolysaccharidoses disorder in which there is intracellular accumulation of keratin sulfate. Anesthetic implications of this disorder are related to infiltration of tissues with keratin sulfate, leading to distortion of upper airway abnormalities and subsequent difficulty with intubation. Direct laryngoscopy and intubation are often more challenging as children age, and the size of the endotracheal tube may need to be downsized. Other anatomic abnormalities include keratin sulfate infiltration of the cervical spine, leading to atlantoaxial subluxation and quadriparesis.[6]

## SCOLIOSIS

Scoliosis occurs when there is a deformity of the spine resulting in lateral curvature and rotation of the vertebrae, as well as rib cage deformities. Scoliosis can be present at birth or develop at any age, but most commonly becomes evident during rapid periods of growth. In severe cases, scoliosis can lead to cardiopulmonary abnormalities, including restrictive lung disease, ventilation-perfusion mismatch, hypoxemia, and elevated right heart pressures. Proper patient positioning can be challenging depending on the surgery being performed and the degree of scoliosis.

## REFERENCES

1. Alapati D, Shaffer TH. Skeletal dysplasia: respiratory management during infancy. *Respir Med.* 2017;131:18–26.
2. Hata T, Todd MiM. Cervical Spine considerations when anesthetizing patients with Down syndrome. *Anesthesiology.* 2005;102(3): 680–685.
3. Stokes DC, et al. Respiratory complications of achondroplasia. *J Pediatr.* 1983;102:534–541.
4. Hase Y, et al. Repeated anesthetic management for a patient with Klippel-Feil syndrome. *Anesth Prog.* 2014;61(3):103–106.
5. Ghatak T, et al. Anesthetic management of a patient with Marfan syndrome and severe aortic root dilatation undergoing cholecystectomy and partial hepatic resection. *Saudi J Anaesth.* 2013;7(4):461–463.

# 265.

# TRISOMY 21 (DOWN SYNDROME) AND VATER ASSOCIATION

*Mariam Batakji and Christina D. Diaz*

## DOWN SYNDROME

Trisomy 21 is the most common chromosomal disorder in live-born infants[1,2] and occurs in one in 700–800 infants.[1-3] It results from abnormal segregation of chromosomes 21 during gamete formation, where 95% of children with Down syndrome (DS) have an extra chromosome 21. Advanced maternal age is by far the most significant risk factor for DS.[1]

Clinical Manifestations: All DS patients have characteristic facial features of up-slanting palpebral fissures; a flat facial profile (flat occiput, short neck, epicanthal folds, Brushfield spots, and small low-set ears); and a relatively large tongue. They also have mental retardation and hypotonia.[1,3]

a- **Craniofacial/Airway Manifestations:** Down syndrome children have a narrow nasopharynx in the anterior-posterior dimension, and the craniofacial and airway proportions are smaller than non-DS children. Laryngotracheal stenosis and subglottic stenosis are often present.[3] Other airway features include macroglossia, microdontia with fused teeth, midfacial and mild mandibular hypoplasia, and a small nose with flat bridge.[3] Atlanto-occipital instability occurs in 15% of kids with DS[1,2] (refer to Figure 265.1) and can be diagnosed by obtaining lateral cervical x-rays. DS kids are at increased risk for upper airway obstruction during induction and emergence from anesthesia due to the hypotonia and described airway anatomy.[1,3] As many as 65% of children with DS screen positive for sleep-disordered breathing, including obstructive sleep apnea.[4]

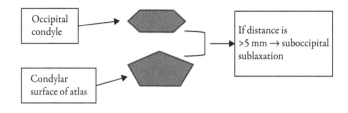

Figure 265.1 Suboccipital subluxation definition.

b- **Cardiovascular/Pulmonary Manifestations:**
Almost 40% to 50% of DS kids have associated
congenital heart disease.[2,3] Endocardial cushion defects,
patent ductus arteriosus, ventricular septal defect,
and tetralogy of Fallot are common heart defects
found in DS.[3] It is important to inquire about the
cardiac history of these kids prior to proceeding with
any surgery. Bradycardia due to high vagal tone and
sensitivity to anesthesia during induction is common
in children with DS; therefore, it is important to have
anticholinergic medications like atropine available
and to remain vigilant.[2] Pulmonary hypertension is
another disease that can be associated with Down kids.
It can result from either an underlying cardiac lesion or
chronic hypoxemia due to upper airway obstruction.[3]

c- **Gastrointestinal/Endocrinology/Hematology
Manifestations:** Gastrointestinal problems occur
in about 10% of patients with DS, with duodenal
atresia and annular pancreas being the most
common.[1] Esophageal atresia/tracheoesophageal
fistula, imperforate anus, Hirschprung disease,
gastroesophageal reflux, and congenital diaphragmatic
hernia can also be present.[1] DS patients frequently
have abnormal thyroid function, with about 2%
having congenital hypothyroidism; therefore, it
is important to ask about the history of thyroid
dysfunction and review test results before proceeding
with surgeries.[1] Down kids may have neutropenia,
thrombocytopenia, and polycythemia. In addition,
they are predisposed to certain malignancies,
including acute leukemias (Acute myeloid leukemia,
Acute lymphocytic leukemia).[1,2] Finally, these
children may be challenging for intravenous access
due to increased adipose tissue, and cannulation of
the internal jugular is difficult because of the short,
webbed neck and increased adipose tissue. Down
kids also have small radial arteries, which sometimes
makes it difficult to cannulate.[1]

## ANESTHETIC CONSIDERATIONS

### Preoperative

Even though DS kids have varying degrees of mental retardation, most are cheerful and cooperative. The dose of the
premedication should be reduced if the anesthesia provider
is concerned about airway obstruction or the presence of
congenital cardiac disease and pulmonary hypertension.[4]
A careful preoperative history and physical examination
should evaluate for undiagnosed cardiac disease, as well
as pulmonary, thyroid, and neurological problems, before
proceeding. A recent evaluation by cardiology with an echocardiogram should be considered in all patients to assess
for undiagnosed or residual heart disease and the presence
of pulmonary hypertension.[2] A recent blood test should be
reviewed to check for anemia and a platelet count, as well as
thyroid function.

### Intraoperative

Intraoperatively, peripheral intravenous access might
prove challenging and may require adjuncts such as ultrasound guidance or use of a "vein finder." Airway obstruction during mask induction may require continuous
positive airway pressure as well as airway adjuncts (oral
and nasal airways, laryngeal mask airway) and the anticipation of a difficult airway.[4] The frequent presence of
subglottic stenosis warrants the use of a smaller size endotracheal tube (ETT). The calculated age-determined ETT
size is generally decreased by half a size to accommodate
DS patients and avoid postoperative croup. Intubation
should limit neck extension as these kids are prone to
atlanto-occipital subluxation. Bradycardia during induction can be treated with decreasing the concentration of
inhalation anesthesia or atropine/glycopyrrolate.[4]

### Postoperative

DS kids are predisposed to postintubation croup. It has an
average onset of 20 to 30 minutes after ETT removal and
may be treated with intravenous dexamethasone or inhaled
racemic epinephrine.[4] When present, vigilance and rapid
intervention for desaturations are required.

## VATER ASSOCIATION

VATER association indicates congenital defects that are
not related closely enough to compose a syndrome:

- **V**ertebral defects (hemivertebrae most commonly)
- **A**nal malformation
- **T**racheoesophageal fistula with esophageal atresia
- **R**adial (radial dysplasia, absent digits, and duplication
  of the thumb) and **r**enal dysplasia (commonly unilateral
  renal agenesis)

The condition can be accompanied by cardiac malformations, especially ventricular septal defect and can be

called VACTER. Death related to this condition is commonly due to cardiac arrest.[5]

## REFERENCES

1. Mann D, et al. Anesthesia for the patient with a genetic syndrome. In: *Gregory's Pediatric Anesthesia*. 5th ed. Chapter 28. http://ebook central.proquest.com/lib/mcwlibraries ebooks/detail.action?docID= 822637

2. Lewanda AF, et al. Preoperative evaluation and comprehensive risk assessment for children with Down syndrome. *Paediatr Anaesth*. 2016;26:356–362.
3. Borland LM, et al. The frequency of anesthesia-related complications in children with Down syndrome under general anesthesia for non-cardiac procedures. *Pediatr Anesth*. 2004;14:733–738.
4. Eric P. Wittkugel and Nancy Bard Samol. Special pediatric disorders. *Smith's Anesthesia for Infants and Children*. Ninth edition. Copyright © 2017 by Elsevier Inc. Volume 52. Chapter 52, pp. 1210–1219.e3.
5. Victor C, et al. *Anesthesia for Genetic, Metabolic, & Dysmorphic Syndromes of Childhood*. 3rd ed. Lippincott, Williams & Wilkins; 2015.

# 266.

# CHROMOSOMAL ABNORMALITIES AND OTHER COMMON PEDIATRIC SYNDROMES

*Mariam Batakji and Christina D. Diaz*

## TRISOMY 18 (EDWARDS SYNDROME)

Clinical Manifestations: Trisomy 18 is a relatively common genetic syndrome that increases with maternal age and is the second most common autosomal trisomy after trisomy 21.[1] Most infants die in utero, and 90% to 95% die within the first year of life.[1] Common characteristics of this syndrome include clenched hands (characteristic), severe intellectual disability, short sternum, prominent occiput, narrow cranium, cleft lip or palate, micrognathia, small mouth opening, horseshoe kidney, and hydronephrosis, and inguinal and umbilical hernias may be present. More than 95% of these patients have a cardiac malformation. There may also be an aberrant subclavian artery present.

Anesthetic Considerations: Regarding anesthesia, difficult intubation and aberrant subclavian artery should be considered, and some patients will have congenital heart disease.[1]

## TRISOMY 13 (PATAU SYNDROME)

Clinical Manifestations: Patients affected with trisomy 13 (Patau syndrome) have multiple craniofacial, cardiac, neurologic, and renal anomalies and a limited life expectancy (95% die within the first 6 months of life). Important manifestations include an occipital scalp defect (which is characteristic), microcephaly, various neural tube defects, and severe intellectual disability.[1] The Patau patients' airway may also prove challenging as a result of cleft lip, cleft palate, cleft tongue, and micrognathia.[1] Over 80% of these children have congenital heart disease. A specific finding in trisomy 13 is the presence of microscopic pancreatic dysplasia.[1]

Anesthetic Considerations: The anesthetic considerations are similar to those for trisomy 18.

## MICROGNATHIA SYNDROMES: PIERRE ROBIN, TREACHER COLLINS, AND GOLDENHAR SYNDROME

### PIERRE ROBIN SYNDROME OR SEQUENCE

Clinical Manifestations: Pierre Robin syndrome or sequence consists of micrognathia, glossoptosis, and a soft tissue cleft palate. Pierre Robin syndrome does not have a known genetic cause, and the defect is probably due to early

*Table 266.1* CHROMOSOMAL ABNORMALITIES

| SYNDROME | CLINICAL MANIFESTATIONS | ANESTHETIC CONSIDERATIONS |
| --- | --- | --- |
| VACTREL | • Vertebral anomalies, Anal atresia, Cardiac malformations, Tracheoesophageal fistula (TEF), Esophageal atresia, Renal anomalies, and Limb anomalies[1,2]<br>• Presence of TEF is essential for the diagnosis, along with another major anomaly[1,2] | • Infants born with TEF should undergo investigation to rule out VACTREL association (echocardiography, renal ultrasound, skeletal and limb survey)[1,2]<br>• Potentially difficult intravenous access and radial artery cannulation[1] |
| CHARGE | • Coloboma, Heart defect, Atresia choanae, Retarded growth and development, Genital hypoplasia, and Ear anomalies/deafness (at least 4 criteria must be present for the diagnosis)<br>• Micrognathia, short neck, laryngomalacia, and subglottic stenosis can be present[1] | • Difficult laryngoscopy<br>• Possible airway obstruction due to laryngomalacia during mask ventilation[1]<br>• Impaired gag reflex predisposes to aspiration.<br>• Hearing loss requires an interpreter to help with communication[1]<br>• Mental retardation may make cooperation difficult[2] |
| Cri du chat (5p syndrome) one of the most common chromosomal deletion syndromes | • Microcephaly, intellectual disability<br>• Downward-slanting palpebral fissures<br>• Distinctive cat-like cry in infancy (due to laryngeal deformity) and epiglottal abnormalities (long, curved, floppy, hypoplastic, and hypotonic epiglottis)<br>• Congenital heart disease in one-third<br>• Most die in early childhood[1,2] | • Potential airway obstruction due to hypotonia of the laryngeal and pharyngeal muscles<br>• Some patients have chronic aspiration with chronic lung disease<br>• Potential difficult laryngoscopy and intubation due to airway anomalies<br>• Cardiac disease requires a tailored anesthetic plan[1,2] |
| Hurler syndrome (deficiency in α-L-iduronidase) | • Dysmorphic facial features (leads to obstructive sleep apnea), macroglossia, high larynx, TMJ (temporal mandibular joint) stiffness, short stiff neck, cervical instability, progressive joint stiffness with decreased mobility[1]<br>• Corneal clouding, glaucoma<br>• Hepatosplenomegaly<br>• Coronary artery narrowing (results in cardiac disease and arrhythmia)[5] | • Difficult mask ventilation, laryngoscopy, and intubation (suggestion that turning the mask upside down is a better fit)<br>• At risk for atlantoaxial subluxation due to presence of odontoid hypoplasia[1,2] |
| Hunter (mucopolysaccharidosis type II) (absence of the lysosomal enzyme iduronate sulfatase) | • Macrocephaly, macroglossia, adenotonsillar hypertrophy, TMJ stiffness, anterior larynx, limited neck mobility, unstable cervical spine, tracheal stenosis, obstructive sleep apnea<br>• Coronary artery narrowing<br>• Intellectual disability<br>• Hepatosplenomegaly<br>• Similar to Hurler syndrome with less severe features[1,2] | • Difficult ventilation, laryngoscopy, and intubation.<br>• Careful positioning and padding due to joint stiffness[1] |
| Becker muscular dystrophy (MD) (mutation in dystrophin gene: dystrophin of altered size or reduced abundance) | • More benign than Duchenne MD<br>• Onset of muscular dystrophy is later in life and progression is slower than in Duchenne<br>• Generalized myopathies, pseudohypertrophied calves, dilated cardiomyopathy, and in late disease stages, respiratory muscle weakness, and difficulties swallowing[1] | • Neuromuscular blockade used with caution due to preexisting muscle weakness<br>• Succinylcholine leads to fatal hyperkalemia<br>• No association with malignant hyperthermia<br>• Potential aspiration risk when swallowing difficulties present[1] |
| Duchenne muscular dystrophy (mutation in dystrophin gene resulting in absent dystrophin) | • Severe respiratory and myocardial disease is seen by mid to late teens<br>• Generalized myopathies (abnormal gait, Gower's sequence), pseudohypertrophy of the calves (classic finding); macroglossia can be observed in 33% of patients.[2] | • Respiratory complications due to restrictive lung disease<br>• Potential difficult airway management secondary to a large tongue and joint contractures<br>• Challenging positioning<br>• At risk for aspiration due to delayed gastric emptying<br>• Cautious use of neuromuscular blockade<br>• Succinylcholine leads to fatal hyperkalemia<br>• No association with malignant hyperthermia<br>• Similar to Becker MD[1,2] |

*(continued)*

*Table 266.1* CONTINUED

| SYNDROME | CLINICAL MANIFESTATIONS | ANESTHETIC CONSIDERATIONS |
|---|---|---|
| Crouzon (craniofacial dysmorphic syndrome) | • Anomalies in the craniofacial region (craniosynostosis, hypertelorism, shallow orbits with ocular proptosis, maxillary hypoplasia, and a parrot-like beaked nose)[1] | • Possible difficult mask ventilation and tracheal intubation<br>• Ocular proptosis warrants careful eye care[1] |
| Mitochondrial diseases<br>These are a group of diseases caused by mitochondrial dysfunction; patients present with various symptoms depending on the disease (muscle weakness, failure to thrive, hearing, visual problems, neurologic problems, respiratory problems, autonomic dysfunction, and dementia. | • Myopathies can result in respiratory failure, cardiac depression, conduction defects, and dysphagia<br>• Avoid circumstances that place a metabolic burden on these patients (prolonged fasting, hypoglycemia, postoperative nausea and vomiting, hypothermia [with resulting shivering], etc.)[3,4] | • Cautious use of muscle relaxants and cardiac depressant medications<br>• Avoid prolonged fasting and hypoglycemia<br>• Avoid propofol<br>• Families may request avoiding lactated Ringers[3,4] |

mandibular hypoplasia in utero, placing the tongue posteriorly, preventing the palatal shelves (which normally must grow over the tongue) from closing in the midline and thus causing a cleft.[1] Neonates generally develop obstructive sleep apnea, which in turn requires various interventions early in life (prone positioning, suturing of the tongue to the lip/jaw, nasal continuous positive airway pressure, endotracheal intubation, or tracheostomy.[1,2] In addition, these children may have feeding difficulties that warrant the insertion of a gastrostomy tube or nasogastric tube. With corrective surgeries and/or growth of the mandible, the difficulty of intubation *improves* with time.

Anesthetic Considerations: Difficult intubation must be considered. It is important to mention that prone positioning improves spontaneous ventilation by preventing the tongue from falling backward posteriorly into the pharynx[1] and can relieve obstruction. These patients require postoperative intensive care unit monitoring for airway complications after surgery.[1]

## TREACHER COLLINS SYNDROME

Clinical Manifestations: Treacher Collins syndrome is an autosomal dominant disorder of bilateral facial development, including hypoplasia of the maxilla, zygoma, and mandible. Also present is lateral downward sloping of the palpebral fissures, colobomata (notches) of the lower eyelids, defects of the external and middle ears, and sensorineural deafness.[1] These patients may require multiple facial procedures and interventions throughout their lives.

Anesthetic Considerations: Difficult intubation must be considered. Unlike Pierre Robin sequence, *laryngoscopy often becomes more difficult with aging.*[1] Like Pierre Robin syndrome, these patients may develop obstructive sleep

apnea and other respiratory complications. Prone positioning may help improve spontaneous ventilation.[1]

## GOLDENHAR SYNDROME

Clinical Manifestations: Goldenhar syndrome is due to a developmental disorder of the first and second branchial arches, resulting in ocular anomalies, vertebral anomalies, and cardiac defects. The craniofacial anomalies are usually unilateral, or at least asymmetric, hence the term *hemifacial microsomia*, which is often used to describe this syndrome.[1,2] Clinical manifestations include malformations/hypoplasia of the external and middle ear often, with sensorineural hearing loss; mandibular hypoplasia; and vertebral anomalies, including cervical spine malformations and scoliosis.[2]

Anesthetic Considerations: Prepare for difficult mask ventilation and intubation. It has been suggested that preoperative radiographs of the mandible are predictive of the degree of difficulty for laryngoscopy.[1]

Refer to Table 266.1 for other chromosomal abnormalities.

## REFERENCES

1. Victor C, et al. *Anesthesia for Genetic, Metabolic, & Dysmorphic Syndromes of Childhood.* 3rd ed. Lippincott, Williams & Wilkins; 2015.
2. Mann D, et al. Anesthesia for the patient with a genetic syndrome. In: Gregory GA, Andropoulos DB, eds. *Gregory's Pediatric Anesthesia.* 5th ed. Wiley; 2011: Chap. 28. http://ebookcentral.proquest.com/lib/mcwlibrariesebooks/detail.action?docID=822637
3. Niezgoda et al. Anesthetic considerations in patients with mitochondrial defects. *Paediatr Anaesth.* 2013;23(9):785–793.
4. Muravchick S, Levy RJ. Clinical implications of mitochondrial dysfunction. *Anesthesiology.* 2006;105:819–837.
5. Eric P. Wittkugel, Nancy Bard Samol. Special pediatric disorders. *Smith's Anesthesia for Infants and Children.* Ninth edition. Copyright © 2017 by Elsevier Inc. Volume 52. Chapter 52, pp. 1210–1219.

# 267.

# JUVENILE IDIOPATHIC ARTHRITIS

*Anthony Fritzler*

## INTRODUCTION

Juvenile idiopathic arthritis (JIA) is a wide-ranging term that includes all forms of arthritis that begin before 16 years of age, persist for more than 6 weeks, and are of unknown origin.[1] JIA is the most prevalent chronic rheumatic disease of childhood.[1] Multiple categories fall under the umbrella of JIA, including systemic JIA, enthesitis-related JIA, oligoarthritis, rheumatoid factor–positive polyarthritis, rheumatoid factor–negative polyarthritis, psoriatic arthritis, and undifferentiated JIA.[1,2] Systemic JIA is the most encompassing in terms of anesthesia-related concerns.

## ETIOLOGY

It is hypothesized that the inciting factor for the development of JIA is an autoreactive immune response initiated by T cells or B cells reacting against a self-antigen producing autoantibodies.[1] Like other autoimmune diseases, JIA likely results from genetic susceptibility and unknown environmental factors inciting an autoimmune response.[1]

Systemic JIA is unique in relation to other forms of JIA in that there is an absence of autoantibodies and no relation with human leukocyte antigen (HLA) alleles.[1] It is considered to be a polygenic autoinflammatory syndrome and not an autoimmune disease.[1] The core process in disease development appears to be an exaggerated release of pro-inflammatory cytokines. The primary cytokines in this process appear to be interleukin 1 (IL-1), IL-6, and IL-18.[1] IL-18 is the most abundant in plasma and synovial fluid; however, it is IL-1 that is key in terms of both the classification and treatment of systemic JIA.[1]

## DIAGNOSIS

Based on criteria from the American College of Rheumatology, a child must have inflammation in one or more joints lasting at least 6 weeks, be under 16 years of age, and have all other conditions ruled out before being diagnosed with JIA.[2] A comprehensive medical history and physical examination should be the first step in approaching any child suspected of having JIA. Standard laboratory tests include erythrocyte sedimentation rate (ESR), C-reactive protein (CRP), antinuclear antibody (ANA), rheumatoid factor (RF), human leukocyte antigen (HLA-B27) gene typing, and a complete blood count (CBC).[2] Typically, all types of JIA will be associated with elevated ESR and CRP levels, as well as elevated white blood cell and red blood cell counts. ANA and RF tests may be positive or negative. Most patients with enthesitis-related JIA are HLA-B27 positive.[1] Conventional x-ray imaging, ultrasonography, magnetic resonance imaging, and computed tomographic scanning are useful in determining the degree of joint damage and/or ascertaining the type of JIA.[1,2]

The usual initial presentation of systemic JIA occurs between 1 and 6 years of age, and there are equal incidences between the sexes.[3] Systemic symptoms such as fever, rash, and lymphadenopathy occur weeks or years prior to the development of arthritis.[3] Reoccurring disease exacerbations are characteristic of systemic JIA. There is an absence of autoantibodies on laboratory studies.

## TREATMENT

The treatment of JIA includes pharmacological interventions, physical and occupational therapy, and psychosocial support.[1] There is no cure for JIA, and early, aggressive treatment should be the goal. Treatment is aimed at reducing or stopping the progression of the disease and improving quality of life.[2] Pharmacological treatment involves the use of nonsteroidal anti-inflammatory drugs (NSAIDs) plus or minus corticosteroids; disease-modifying antirheumatic drugs (DMARDs); both conventional (e.g., methotrexate, leflunomide, sulfasalazine) and biologics, which include anti–tumor necrosis factor (TNF) drugs, T-cell inhibitors, B-cell inhibitors, and IL inhibitors.[2,4] The standard of care is to first attempt methotrexate, but many clinicians begin with a biologic/DMARD combination to more aggressively treat inflammation.[2] Anti-TNF drugs are not as effective for systemic JIA as for other forms of JIA.[1] The IL-1 and IL-6 inhibitors (anakinra and tocilizumab, respectively) are at the cornerstone of systemic JIA treatment.[1,4]

## ANESTHETIC CONSIDERATIONS

### PREOPERATIVE

Elective procedures should be performed only when the patient is in a stable remission period. Preoperatively, a thorough history and physical examination should be performed. Assessment of medication usage in relation to potential anesthetic implications is essential. Most commonly, patients recently or currently taking corticosteroids may need stress dosing in the perioperative period. Airway management can be very challenging, as cervical ankylosis and atlantoaxial subluxation are common.[5,6] Temporomandibular joint (TMJ) dysfunction can produce limited mouth opening and is more common in JIA and frequently associated with hypoplastic mandible.[6] Cricoarytenoid dysfunction also occurs frequently. Cardiovascular disease is the most common cause of mortality.[6] Pericarditis, pericardial effusion, myocarditis, endocarditis, and systemic vasculitis are potential complications with systemic JIA.[3] Additional extra-articular manifestations include restrictive lung defects, pleural effusions, anemia, hypoalbuminemia, chronic renal failure from drug treatment, peripheral neuropathy, and autonomic dysfunction.[5] A CBC, electrolytes, urea, electrocardiogram, and chest x-ray are the most commonly indicated studies.[5] Cervical spine x-rays are typically performed on patients who are symptomatic or have concerning findings on physical examination.[5]

### INTRAOPERATIVE

Intraoperatively, the chosen anesthetic technique should be tailored to the needs of the individual. Careful attention is essential when positioning the patient. The priority should be to limit cervical spine mobility and to utilize devices such as the laryngeal mask airway, video laryngoscope, and flexible fiber-optic scope when necessary. Coagulation status and accessibility may be deterrents to performing regional or neuraxial techniques. It is imperative to be cognizant about the possibility of systemic JIA exacerbations and the development of macrophage activation syndrome (MAS). MAS is a life-threatening complication of systemic JIA and is triggered by viral infections, drugs (NSAIDs, DMARDs), and external stresses such as cold temperature.[3] There is evidence of histamine release from mast cells during MAS.[3] Manifestations of MAS include persistent fever, generalized lymphadenopathy, disseminated intravascular coagulation, pancytopenia, hypofibrinogenemia, elevated liver enzymes, sudden fall in ESR, and central nervous system dysfunction.[3] A high index of suspicion is necessary, and high-dose corticosteroids are the treatment.[3] Avoiding NSAIDs and histamine-releasing drugs (e.g., morphine, succinylcholine, atracurium) in the operating room is reasonable. Consideration needs to be given to any preexisting hepatic or renal dysfunction when dosing medications as well.

### POSTOPERATIVE

Disease-specific goals postoperatively should include optimal positioning, maintenance of normothermia, providing effective analgesia, minimizing the risk of respiratory depression, and early mobilization.[6] Patients with rheumatoid arthritis are more sensitive to drugs and more prone to developing respiratory depression.[6] Cautious titration of opioid analgesics is essential, and a multimodal analgesic approach is optimal. A high index of suspicion should be maintained for the possibility of a systemic JIA exacerbation or MAS, with avoidance of potential triggers.

## REFERENCES

1. Prakken B, et al. Juvenile idiopathic arthritis. *Lancet.* 2011;377:2138–2149.
2. Arthritis Foundation. Juvenile idiopathic arthritis (JIA). Accessed April 21, 2020. https://www.arthritis.org/diseases/juvenile-idiopathic-arthritis
3. Garg R, et al. Perioperative anesthetic concerns in a child with systemic onset juvenile idiopathic arthritis syndrome. *Pediatr Anesth.* 2010;20:773–775.
4. Prince FHM, et al. Diagnosis and management of juvenile idiopathic arthritis. *BMJ.* 2010;341:c6434.
5. Fombon FN, Thompson JP. Anesthesia for the adult patient with rheumatoid arthritis. *Contin Educ Anaesth Crit Care Pain.* 2006;6(6):235–239.
6. Vieira EM, Goodman S, Tanaka PP. Anesthesia and rheumatoid arthritis. *Rev Bras Anestesiol.* 2011;61(3):367–375.

# 268.

# MALIGNANT HYPERTHERMIA IN CHILDREN

*Narbeh Edjiu and Howard B. Gutstein*

## INTRODUCTION

Malignant hyperthermia (MH) is a rare inherited skeletal muscle disorder resulting in exaggerated intracellular calcium release after exposure to succinylcholine and volatile anesthetics ("triggering agents"), resulting in a hypermetabolic state.[1] MH is inherited in an autosomal dominant pattern with variable penetrance. Most cases involve mutations in the ryanodine receptor (RYR1) gene, which controls calcium release from the sarcoplasmic reticulum. Pediatric patients account for approximately 50% of documented MH reactions.[2] The incidence of MH is 1:15,000 in the pediatric population and approximately 1:100,000 in adults. Males are twice as likely to develop MH as females. Also, nearly 50% of patients who suffer an episode of MH have previously been exposed to known triggering agents without incident.[1] The gold standard for diagnosis remains the caffeine-halothane contracture test (CHCT). Genetic testing is available but lacks the sensitivity and specificity of the CHCT.[3]

## CLINICAL PRESENTATION

Signs of MH can present any time from induction through an hour after emergence.[1] Early signs of MH include hypercarbia, muscle rigidity, and tachycardia. Masseter muscle rigidity (MMR) occurs in 1% of pediatric patients given succinylcholine.[3] Rapid temperature elevation (1°C every 5 minutes) presents later, and the sustained hypermetabolism can lead to markedly increased oxygen consumption, carbon dioxide production, severe metabolic acidosis, organ dysfunction, heart failure, and disseminated intravascular coagulation (DIC). Sustained rhabdomyolysis can result in severe hyperkalemia, arrhythmia, compartment syndrome due to muscle swelling, and myoglobinuria, which causes renal failure. Age-related changes in body composition may contribute to differences in clinical presentation seen in different age groups. Adolescents (13–18 years old) have greater muscle mass and develop more rhabdomyolysis and higher maximum temperatures

and creatinine phosphokinase and potassium levels than younger children, who became more acidotic and have higher lactic acid levels.[4]

## DISORDERS LINKED TO MALIGNANT HYPERTHERMIA

Malignant hyperthermia occurs after MMR about 15% of the time, but 50% of children with severe MMR have positive CHCTs. Rare genetic myopathies such as King-Denborough syndrome, central core disease, centronuclear myopathy, and multiminicore disease are strongly associated with MH. All patients suffering from these conditions should be treated as MH susceptible. Muscular dystrophies are not directly associated with MH, but can cause hyperkalemic cardiac arrest after succinylcholine administration (see further discussion).[5]

## DIFFERENTIAL DIAGNOSIS

Metabolic disorders that can mimic features of MH under anesthesia include sepsis, thyroid storm, pheochromocytoma, acute porphyria, and cocaine or MDMA ("ecstasy") abuse. Neuroleptic malignant syndrome (NMS) is caused by dopamine antagonists used to treat mental illness. Symptoms include muscle rigidity, acidosis, rhabdomyolysis, and high fevers. NMS is treated with the dopamine agonist bromocriptine and benzodiazepines. Serotonin syndrome is associated with the use of serotonin reuptake inhibitors or drugs enhancing serotonin receptor activity to treat depression. Muscle rigidity, rhabdomyolysis, and high fevers can also be observed. Treatment includes benzodiazepines and cyproheptadine, an inhibitor of serotonin synthesis. Dantrolene can be also be used to treat both of these conditions, and symptoms may respond. However, this response is nonspecific and does not indicate susceptibility to MH.[3] Patients with diagnosed or occult myopathies are at risk for hyperkalemic cardiac arrest after exposure to succinylcholine and possibly volatile anesthetics. The most common example of such a syndrome is Duchenne muscular dystrophy. Patients do develop rhabdomyolysis, but not muscle rigidity or hyperthermia.[5] If a child has an unexpected cardiac arrest, evaluate for hyperkalemia and treat this normally (calcium, bicarbonate, glucose, insulin, hyperventilation). Clinical signs will not respond to dantrolene treatment.[3] Patients with hypokalemic periodic paralysis can also present with a similar picture. Since symptoms of myopathies can present in late childhood or early adolescence, succinylcholine should not be used in children except for rapid sequence induction and in acute airway emergencies. Scoliosis and strabismus have not been formally associated with MH.[5]

## ANESTHETIC CONSIDERATIONS

### PREOPERATIVE

Patients susceptible to MH must not be exposed to any volatile anesthetics or succinylcholine preoperatively. MH-susceptible patients should be scheduled as the first case of the day, vaporizers should be removed from the anesthesia machine, and the $CO_2$ absorbent changed. The machine should be flushed with 10 L/min oxygen for at least 10 minutes or per manufacturers recommendations.[2] An activated charcoal filter should also be added to the circuit.

### INTRAOPERATIVE

Volatile anesthetics and succinylcholine must be avoided intraoperatively. Nitrous oxide and other anesthetic and analgesic agents can be used. Regional and local anesthesia may also be used, either as an adjunct or as the primary anesthetic in select older children.[3]

### MANAGEMENT OF ACUTE MH CRISIS

To manage an acute MH crisis, triggering agents must be discontinued immediately and the patient hyperventilated with 100% oxygen. An oxygen tank and ambu bag can be used until a volatile anesthetic–free machine is available. The procedure must be aborted if nonemergent; otherwise, it must proceed with nontriggering agents.[1,3] Dantrolene 2.5 mg/kg should be administered as soon as practical. The standard formulation comes in 20-mg vials, which requires additional personnel and substantial effort to solubilize. Ryanodex is a new dantrolene formulation that is easily solubilized and comes in 250-mg vials. Dantrolene is a ryanodine receptor antagonist. It inhibits calcium release from the sarcoplasmic reticulum, interfering with muscle contraction. Side effects include generalized muscle weakness due to the inhibition of calcium release, respiratory compromise, phlebitis, and gastrointestinal upset. MH signs can recur in 25% of patients; therefore dantrolene must be given every 4–8 hours for 72 hours.[3] Table 268.1 summarizes the steps for management of acute crises. More detailed explanations can be found elsewhere in this book.

*Table 268.1* PROTOCOL FOR THE MANAGEMENT OF MH CRISIS

| STEP | ACTION | ADDITIONAL DETAILS |
|---|---|---|
| 1 | Immediately discontinue volatile anesthetic | Turn vaporizer off/remove<br>Hyperventilate with 100% oxygen |
| 2 | Call for help | Notify surgeon, abort procedure |
| 3 | Administer dantrolene or Ryanodex | Initial dose: 2.5 mg/kg<br>Repeat every 10–15 minutes until MH signs resolve<br>1 mg/kg every 4–8 hours for 48–72 hours |
| 4 | Obtain access and invasive monitoring | Arterial line, Foley catheter, consider central line |
| 5 | Bicarbonate for metabolic acidosis | 1–2 mEq/kg if blood gases not available |
| 6 | Initiate cooling measures | Maintain temperature between 38°C and 39°C<br>Ice packs, chilled intravenous solutions, cooling blankets<br>Gastric lavage NOT recommended |
| 7 | Treat hyperkalemia | Hyperventilation, glucose/insulin, bicarbonate, calcium |
| 8 | Treat dysrhythmias | Amiodarone as first line; avoid calcium channel blockers—can cause cardiac arrest with dantrolene |
| 9 | Continued monitoring | Monitor (a) end-tidal $CO_2$, (b) hemodynamics, (c) electrolytes, (d) blood gases, (e) serum creatinine kinase/myoglobin, (f) coagulation status, (g) temperature, (h) urine output |

From References 1 and 3.

## POSTOPERATIVE

Patients susceptible to MH who undergo uneventful procedures with nontriggering agents can be monitored routinely postoperatively in the postanesthesia care unit. If an MH episode is suspected or confirmed, the patient should be monitored for the development of cardiac failure, DIC, and renal failure in the pediatrics intensive care unit.[2] Hemodynamic support may be required. Temperature, blood gases, serum creatine kinase/myoglobin, electrolytes, coagulation studies, and urinary output and quality need to be monitored frequently. Recrudescence can occur up to 72 hours after the procedure. Families and the patient must be educated about MH and further follow-up and testing arranged.[3]

## REFERENCES

1. Butterworth JF, et al. Thermoregulation, hypothermia, & malignant hyperthermia. In: Butterworth JF, et al., eds. *Morgan & Mikhail's Clinical Anesthesiology.* 5th ed. McGraw-Hill; 2013:1185–1191.
2. Lerman J. Perioperative management of the paediatric patient with coexisting neuromuscluar disease. *Br J Anaesth.* 2011;107(S1):i79–i89.
3. Rosenberg H, et al. Malignant hyperthermia: a review. *Orphanet J Rare Dis.* 2015;10(93): 1–19.
4. Nelson P, Litman RS. Malignant hyperthermia in children: an analysis of the North American malignant hyperthermia registry. *Anesth Analg.* 2014;118:369–374.
5. Litman RS, et al. Malignant hyperthermia susceptibility and related diseases. *Anesthesiology.* 2018;128:159–167.

# Part 20

# ANESTHETIC IMPLICATIONS FOR COMMON NONNEONATAL PEDIATRIC SUBSPECIALTY SURGERY

# 269.

# OTOLARYNGOLOGY

*Timothy Ford and Alaa Abd-Elsayed*

## CLEFT LIP AND PALATE

### INTRODUCTION

Cleft lip and palate are the most common congenital orofacial deformities. They arise from failure of the five facial prominences to fuse properly during embryogenesis. The development of cleft lip and palate is dependent on the interaction of environmental factors and genetic predisposition. As such, they can be isolated, familial, or associated with chromosomal abnormality syndromes (including but not limited to Pierre Robin sequence, Down syndrome, Treacher Collins, Klippel-Feil). Cheiloplasty typically occurs at 2–3 months of age as there is a decreased risk of complications associated with the rule of 10: age > 10 weeks of age, weight > 10 lb, and hemoglobin > 10 g/dL. Palatoplasty typically occurs at approximately 9–18 months of age to optimize speech without interfering with maxillofacial growth.

### ANESTHETIC MANAGEMENT

**Preoperative:** Preoperative airway assessment is imperative: presence of mandibular hypoplasia as seen in Pierre Robin sequence, restricted neck movement in Klippel-Feil syndrome, and presence of bilateral clefts. Difficult laryngoscopy has an incidence of 4%–7%. Palatoplasty patients are at risk of bleeding, and a type and screen is recommended.

**Intraoperative:** Induction typically occurs via standard inhalational induction in order to maintain a spontaneously ventilating patient. The airway is secured via endotracheal tube intubation. Cuffed endotracheal tubes provide benefits, including preventing aspiration risk, ensuring proper ventilation, and reducing airway fire risk. To reduce bleeding intraoperatively, the surgeon may request for permissive hypotension and/or infiltrate epinephrine at the surgical site. Precautions must be taken before extubation. The location nature of the surgery results in increased risk for postextubation airway obstruction due to reduction of the pharyngeal space, edema associated with surgical inflammation, presence of blood and secretions, and residual anesthesia. A nasopharyngeal airway is placed by the surgeon before emergence to mitigate the risk of airway obstruction and allow for suction without disrupting the repair.

**Postoperative:** Postoperatively the child is observed for 24–28 hours for airway obstruction. Postoperative analgesia is best achieved with a multimodal approach. Rectal acetaminophen in conjunction with bilateral infraorbital and external nasal nerve blocks provide analgesia and are opioid sparing.[1,2]

## TONSILLECTOMY AND ADENOIDECTOMY

### INTRODUCTION

Tonsillectomy and adenoidectomy are among the most common pediatric surgical procedures performed in the United States. Most common indications for tonsillectomy include recurrent pharyngotonsillitis, chronic tonsilitis, and peritonsillar abscess, with less common indications including unilateral tonsil enlargement concerning for malignancy and pediatric autoimmune neuropsychiatric disorders associated with streptococcus. Adenotonsillectomy is indicated in patients with adenotonsillar hyperplasia causing nocturnal upper airway obstruction with or without obstructive sleep apnea syndrome (OSAS). Tonsillectomy can be performed utilizing a variety of techniques, ranging from guillotine, cold or hot knife, monopolar or bipolar electrocautery, harmonic scalpel, bipolar radio-frequency ablation, or carbon dioxide laser.

### ANESTHETIC MANAGEMENT

**Preoperative:** Evaluate for coagulation state given the risk of bleeding after tonsillectomy. A patient history significant for easy bruising, frequent epistaxis, or positive family history warrants further coagulative evaluation. Patients with coagulopathy should be admitted early for correction of coagulopathy. Patients with hemophilia A and von Willebrand disease, more common coagulopathies in pediatric populations, can receive desmopressin (DDAVP) before induction of anesthesia. Additionally, nasal and oral patency should be carefully examined to evaluate the degree of nasal and oral airway obstruction. Finally, the teeth should also be inspected, and loose teeth noted as this patient population often loses their primary dentition, and the risk for tooth dislodgement may require a tooth to be pulled while under anesthesia.

**Intraoperative:** Anxiety can be treated with oral midazolam while bearing in mind it may be associated with emergence delirium or airway obstruction postoperatively. Anesthesia is induced most commonly with an admixture of oxygen, nitrous oxide, and sevoflurane. Airway obstruction is common following induction and likely requires jaw thrust, continuous positive airway pressure, and/or insertion of an oral airway once the gag reflex is abolished, indicating adequate anesthetic depth. Subsequently, the airway should be secured with cuffed oral endotracheal tube to reduce risk of airway fire and protect the airway from secretions. Flexible laryngeal mask airways are an alternative; however, their use is associated with higher risk of malfunction and oxygen desaturation. Fractional inspired $O_2$ should be reduced to 21%–30% to reduce the risk of airway fire. Mild hypotension can help to reduce bleeding. Children with moderate or severe OSAS should receive less opioids due to their increased risk for prolonged apnea during emergence as well as postoperative airway obstruction. Extubation should be performed in a gentle manner, in a nearly awake patient, under positive pressure to ensure the lungs are well expanded, to facilitate expulsion of secretions, and to attenuate excitation of the superior laryngeal nerve, which may diminish the risk for laryngospasm. Laryngospasm and negative pressure pulmonary edema are significant complications during emergence and the immediate postoperative period.

**Postoperative:** Postoperative analgesia should utilize a multimodal approach. Opioids should be used cautiously, especially in patients with moderate-to-severe OSAS who are at increased risk of postoperative apnea and postoperative airway obstruction. Nonsteroidal anti-inflammatory drugs (NSAIDs) have a theoretical risk of bleeding perioperatively; however, a Cochrane review demonstrated no significant correlation between NSAID use and post-tonsillectomy bleeding. Patients should be monitored closely for perioperative hypoxemia, poor oral intake, bleeding, and infection. Post-tonsillectomy bleeding is a true surgical emergency and requires expeditious intervention utilizing a team approach between the surgeon and anesthesiologist. Peritonsillar abscess is an additional complication post-tonsillectomy that is discussed in more detail further in this chapter.[1,2]

# MYRINGOTOMY AND TYMPANOSTOMY TUBE INSERTION

## INTRODUCTION

Recurrent otitis media, chronic otitis media, and chronic upper respiratory infections with the accompaniment of middle ear effusion are common childhood maladies. When medical management fails, surgical drainage is indicated because if left untreated cholesteatoma and conductive hearing loss can occur. Patients with congenital anomalies, especially craniofacial malformations and associated syndromes, are often candidates for myringotomy and tympanostomy tube insertion.

## ANESTHETIC MANAGEMENT

Myringotomy and tympanostomy tube insertion require minimal operating time and can usually be carried out using inhalational anesthesia via face mask and spontaneous ventilation. Intravenous access is rarely needed. Inhalational anesthesia typically consists of an admixture of oxygen, sevoflurane, and nitrous oxide. Because children undergoing myringotomy also have adenoidal hypertrophy, continuous positive airway pressure and oral airway insertion may be utilized to maintain airway patency once a surgical plan of anesthesia is achieved. Postoperative analgesia is facilitated by preoperative oral acetaminophen and intramuscular ketorolac intraoperatively. Intramuscular ketorolac is associated with less vomiting and minimal sedation compared to intranasal fentanyl or dexmedetomidine, the latter of which also can provide additional analgesia.[3]

## COMMON EAR PROCEDURES

### INTRODUCTION

A variety of ear procedures are performed for a diverse array of pathologies:

**Outer ear:** Otoplasty is a cosmetic procedure to reconstruct or restructure the auricle in the setting of congenital or acquired ear malformation.

**Middle ear:** Tympanoplasty is performed in the setting of tympanic membrane perforation; mastoidectomy is performed in the setting of persistent otitis media complicated by mastoiditis and cholesteatoma formation; stapedectomy is performed to treat otosclerosis.

**Inner ear procedures:** These include cochlear implant, surgery to the endolymphatic sac, and surgery to the labyrinth.

## ANESTHETIC CONSIDERATIONS

The operating room table is typically rotated 90° to 180°; thus, these procedures are mostly performed with general anesthesia with endotracheal tube placement. Neuromuscular blockade utilizing succinylcholine is preferred for facial nerve monitoring during the case. Nitrous oxide is best avoided as it easily diffuses into the middle ear and can affect the tympanic graft in the case of tympanoplasty. Deep extubation can be considered in cases where coughing and bucking on emergence can lead to displacement of graft and bone prosthesis. Postoperative nausea and vomiting (PONV) risk is increased in these procedures given their proximity to and likely stimulation of the vestibular labyrinth. PONV risk can be mitigated with intravenous dexamethasone and total intravenous anesthesia with propofol instead of maintenance with an inhalational anesthetic.[1,2]

## PERITONSILLAR ABSCESS

### INTRODUCTION

Peritonsillar abscess most frequently occurs in older children and adults. Most infections originate in the tonsils and spread to the peritonsillar space. Presenting symptoms include high fever, dysphagia, and odynophagia. It can occur as a complication following tonsillectomy. Treatment includes fluid resuscitation, antibiotics, and incision and drainage of the abscess. Peritonsillar abscess represents a significant risk for upper airway obstruction and should be treated expediently by incision and drainage. In older children, it is possible for incision and drainage of the abscess to be performed under intravenous sedation and use of local anesthetic. However, if this is not possible, general anesthesia is necessary.

### ANESTHETIC CONSIDERATIONS

General anesthesia can be induced by inhalational agents or intravenously. Neuromuscular blockade with a short-acting or rapidly reversible agent should be administered after establishing the airway, which can be maintained by mask and bag alone. Endotracheal intubation carries a risk of rupturing the abscess, and video laryngoscopy may aid in avoiding inadvertent rupture compared to direct laryngoscopy. Awake fiber-optic intubation should also be considered. Given the potential for a difficult airway and risk for upper airway obstruction, the operating room should be prepared for possible surgical airway if intubation proves difficult.[2,4]

### AIRWAY FOREIGN BODIES

### INTRODUCTION

Foreign body aspiration occurs predominantly in children 1 to 3 years of age. Commonly aspirated objections include peanuts, seeds, or other food particles, with aspiration of plastic and metal particles being less frequent. Symptoms range from coughing, wheezing, and dyspnea to bidirectional stridor and complete airway obstruction. Physical examination may reveal decreased air entry in the affected side. Due to its acute angle, the right main bronchus is the most frequent site that an object becomes lodged, with the left bronchus, larynx, and trachea less commonly involved sites. Chest radiography is helpful in determining the site of obstruction, with a lateral view helping to differentiate respiratory the foreign body from an esophageal foreign body, which may confound the diagnosis, especially since compression of the laryngeal inlet or trachea can occur in this case. Removal of the foreign body typically involves bronchoscopy. The urgency of removal depends on the severity of symptoms. Patients in respiratory distress require emergent foreign body removal and incur increased risk for aspiration depending on their fasting status.

### ANESTHETIC CONSIDERATIONS

Anesthesia is typically induced with inhalational anesthesia via mask ventilation in a spontaneously ventilating patient. Following induction, intravenous access is established and total intravenous anesthesia with propofol with or without opioids is utilized for the remainder of the procedure. Topicalization of the vocal cords is applied prior to rigid bronchoscope insertion once it is determined that there is no foreign body present at the level of the vocal cords. Short-acting muscle relaxant may be necessary to facilitate bronchoscopy. Controlled ventilation can be performed through the rigid bronchoscope utilizing either the anesthesia machine or jet ventilation. For tracheal obstruction, the foreign body is pushed distally to allow ventilation of at least one lung. Fogarty embolectomy balloon catheters may be utilized if the foreign body is impacted. Following extraction, the child is usually intubated, which allows for tracheobronchial suction, lung expansion, oxygenation, and ventilation until adequate reversal of neuromuscular blockade and return of spontaneous ventilation. Dexamethasone is given prophylactically to prevent laryngeal edema. Postoperatively, there is risk for airway swelling and the need for humidified oxygen and nebulized racemic epinephrine.[5]

### REFERENCES

1. Hammer G, et al. Anesthesia for general abdominal, thoracic, urologic, and bariatric surgery. In: Davis PJ, et al., eds. *Smith's Anesthesia for Infants and Children*. Philadelphia, PA: Mosby; 2011:786–820.
2. Motoyama EK, et al. In: Davis PJ, et al., eds. *Smith's Anesthesia for Infants and Children*. Philadelphia, PA: Mosby; 2011:831–834.
3. Robinson H, Engelhardt T. Ambulatory anesthetic care in children undergoing myringotomy and tube placement: current perspectives. *Local Reg Anesth*. 2017;10:41–49.
4. Beriault M, et al. Innovative airway management for peritonsillar abscess. *Can J Anaesth*. 2006;53(1):92–95.
5. Kendigelen P. The anaesthetic consideration of tracheobronchial foreign body aspiration in children. *J Thorac Dis*. 2016;8:3803–3807.

# 270.

# NEUROSURGERY

*Itamar Latin and Kasia Rubin*

## PEDIATRIC CRANIOTOMY AND HYDROCEPHALUS

The preoperative evaluation for a craniotomy must bear in mind why the cranial vault needs entering.[1] Potentially more so than other neurosurgical procedures, the acuity of symptom onset and extent of symptoms is of primary concern. If the craniotomy is for an acute process such as a worsening hemorrhage, evaluation of the patient's increased intracranial pressure (ICP) needs careful consideration, with increased urgency associated with symptoms such as hypertension, bradycardia, somnolence, and vomiting.[2] If the craniotomy is for a more chronic condition, such as a tumor, preoperative evaluation shifts to focus on the type of tumor and the specifics of the mass effect. Certain tumor types, due to location and/or effects on pathophysiology, lead to certain challenges intraoperatively and so require more preoperative workup.[2]

Hydrocephalus evaluation, like craniotomy procedures, focuses on how the increase in ICP affects the patient globally. In some cases, the chronic increase in ICP due to hydrocephalus will create anatomic changes unseen in other disease states.[1] On physical examination, the shape of the child's cranium warrants more attention due to how the increase in occiput may make for a more challenging intubation. Somnolence and level of arousal are also important to note preoperatively, if possible, in order to measure a baseline of the patient's mental status.

In all cases, whether craniotomy for acute or chronic mass effects, the treatment goals focus on management of the ICP. During cases of known elevated ICP, it is imperative to maintain an elevated blood pressure to maintain cerebral perfusion pressure until the ICP is normalized.[2] A discussion should be held with the neurosurgical team preoperatively to ensure clear parameters are agreed on.

An increase of ICP may lead to different airway concerns depending on the acuity of the rise. For acute rises, there may be severe emesis, leading to aspiration pneumonitis or an obstructed view when intubating. Airway management concerns are similar to those of any patient with a full stomach presenting for emergency airway management.

## PEDIATRIC CRANIOFACIAL SURGERY

From a neurosurgical perspective, craniofacial procedures tend to be mostly craniosynostosis repairs. The neurosurgery team aids in safely removing the cranial vault from the dura mater in order for the plastic surgery team to reconstruct the shape.[3] In addition to cosmetic reasons, craniosynostosis repairs are implemented within a certain age range (3–12 months) to facilitate brain growth after the constraint of prematurely fused skull plates are separated.[3] Profound blood loss can occur in these procedures.

## PERIOPERATIVE BLOOD LOSS

Many neurosurgical procedures, notably craniotomies and craniofacial procedures, can be expected to have major blood loss. There are myriad techniques and medications intraoperatively to help reduce the overall volume of blood lost. A large-bore peripheral intravenous line and an arterial line are indicated for transfusion management. Medications such as tranexamic acid (TXA) have been shown to greatly reduce intraoperative bleeding, leading to a reduced need for blood transfusions.[3] While routine use of TXA is not advisable due to seizure risk, in neurosurgical procedures with potential for significant blood loss the benefits of use far outweigh all risks in children.[3]

If possible, intraoperative blood cell salvage should be used during the procedure to transfuse back any available blood lost. Preventing hypothermia with forced air heating blankets, fluid warmers, and a warm room can prevent coagulopathy leading to blood loss.[1] If coagulopathy is suspected, tools to measure clotting such as rotational thromboelastometry or thromboelastography can help dictate which blood products to transfuse for specific clotting factors.

## NEUROINTERVENTIONAL PROCEDURES

The continued reapplication of adult interventional radiology in pediatric neurosurgical cases has offered better outcomes for patients but increased challenges for the anesthesiologist. The environment is often foreign to the anesthesiologist, and patient risk is increased. The intracranial lesions that require radiological intervention are usually vascular in origin.[2] This may be an aneurysm, arteriovenous malformation, or highly vascularized tumor. Besides the mass affect from the tumor, it is important to evaluate cardiac function in the setting of high cardiac output failure from an arteriovenous malformation.

One major challenge for pediatric patients following a neurointerventional procedure is the need for flat bed rest for 2 to 6 hours after removal of a femoral sheath to avoid postprocedural bleeding complications. Deep extubation and liberal use of $\alpha_2$-agonists may be advisable.[2]

## POSTOPERATIVE MANAGEMENT

Postoperative pain management, most notably for craniotomy and craniofacial procedures, needs forethought in order to prevent postoperative rises in blood pressure that lead to continued blood loss. While narcotics are able to reduce pain, the increased somnolence may cause confounding results in a postoperative neurological examination or an obtunded patient with a challenging postoperative airway. Dexmedetomidine may be a useful adjunct to allow for analgesia without losing respiratory drive. Short-acting oral analgesic medications are often effective.

## ANESTHETIC CONSIDERATIONS

### PREOPERATIVE

Preoperative investigations rely on integrating the patient's individualized presentation with the known expectations of the disease pathology into a comprehensive plan.

### INTRAOPERATIVE

Intraoperative importance shifts to maintaining stabilization of the dynamic elements that are required for best outcomes (blood pressure, bleeding, pH status, etc.).

### POSTOPERATIVE

Plan on providing the appropriate sedation for continued hemodynamic stabilization in the postoperative period.

## REFERENCES

1. Lamsal R, Rath GP. Pediatric neuroanesthesia. *Curr Opin Anaesthesiol.* 2018;31(5):539–543.
2. McClaine C, Landrigan-Ossar M. Challenges in pediatric neuroanesthesia. *Anesthesiol Clin.* 2014;32(1):83–100.
3. Clebone A. Pediatric neuroanesthesia. *Curr Opin Anaesthesiol.* 2015;28(5):494–497.

# 271.

# THORACIC SURGERY

*Alina Lazar*

## LUNG ISOLATION TECHNIQUES

In pediatric thoracic surgery, lung exposure can be facilitated by pushing the inflated exposed lung with surgical instruments (thoracotomy), insufflating carbon dioxide into the chest cavity (thoracoscopy), or single-lung ventilation (SLV). SLV improves surgical access, prevents expansion of cystic lesions, decreases bleeding, and reduces spillage of pus and blood into the nondiseased lung.

As opposed to adults and older children, in infants optimal oxygenation and ventilation are achieved when the diseased lung is in a dependent position. This is because the chest is floppier, and in a lateral decubitus position the dependent lung is compressed. There is less hydrostatic gradient between lungs. Children are more prone to hypoxia because they have a higher oxygen consumption and lower lung functional residual capacity.

In children younger than 2 years, SLV can be achieved by advancing the endotracheal tube (ETT) in the nonoperative lung mainstem bronchus or by placing a bronchial blocker outside the ETT (with its tip at midtrachea) into the operative lung mainstem bronchus. Advancing the ETT or bronchial blocker into the left mainstem bronchus is more challenging than into the right one because this bronchus is more steeply angled. In addition to fiber-optic or fluoroscopic guidance, bending the tip of the bronchial blocker toward the side of intended placement and orienting the bevel of the ETT and tilting the head of the child away from the bronchus to be cannulated (for mainstem intubation) facilitate the placement of the airway devices. The bronchial blocker can also be inserted through an ETT initially mainstemed into the desired bronchus and subsequently removed. Because of the short length of the right mainstem bronchus, it is very easy for airway devices to advance into the bronchus and occlude the takeoff of the right upper lobe bronchus or to slip out of the bronchus into the trachea.[1] In children older than 2 years, bronchial blockers can be placed coaxial with the ETT. Double-lumen tubes are available only for children 8 years or older. Other devices used for lung isolation in children are the bilumen (Marraro)

tube (children younger than 3 years) and the Univent tube (children older than 6 years).[2]

Incomplete deflation of the operative lung is common and can be addressed by suctioning the BB lumen and extrinsically compressing the lung with the bronchial blocker cuff deflated and the ETT disconnected. Complications of SLV are migration of bronchial blocker or double-lumen tube, ETT occlusion with blood clots or mucus, atelectasis, hypoxia, and hypercarbia.

| Indications for Single-Lung Ventilation in Children |
|---|
| Congenital pulmonary airway malformation |
| Bronchopulmonary sequestrations |
| Congenital lobar emphysema |
| Tracheoesophageal fistula |
| Bronchopleural fistula |
| Unilateral lung hemorrhage |
| Anterior spinal fusion |
| Chest neoplasms |

Pectus excavatum is a congenital chest wall disorder characterized by defective growth of the sternum and surrounding costal cartilages, resulting in posterior depression of the chest wall. Surgical correction is done usually in adolescence or young adulthood via the Nuss procedure, a minimally invasive technique in which a rigid convex bar is placed under the sternum and costal cartilages, with thoracoscopic guidance, resulting in anterior displacement of the sternum. The bar is then left in place until permanent chest wall remodeling has occurred. Pain following the Nuss procedure is severe and difficult to control. It has multiple etiologies, including outward pressure from the Nuss bar, incisional pain, muscle spasms, and release of inflammatory mediators from the primary surgical insult. Moderate-to-severe postoperative pain is expected for the first 4 postoperative days. Patients have an increased risk of chronic postoperative pain. Various management strategies have been proposed, including epidural analgesia, nerve blocks, patient-controlled analgesia, and multimodal analgesia.[3]

## ANTERIOR MEDIASTINAL MASSES

In children, the most common anterior mediastinal masses are hematological malignancies and teratomas. Of these, rapidly growing hematological malignancies (Hodgkin or non-Hodgkin lymphoma) are most likely to cause anesthetic problems. The most important diagnostic modality is computed tomographic scan. Echocardiography further assesses the degree of great vessel and myocardial compression. The usefulness of pulmonary function tests is debatable.

The following imaging findings suggest a high risk for complications: tracheal diameter 70% or less than normal and/or carinal or bronchial compression, superior vena caval obstruction, pericardial effusion, pulmonary artery outflow obstruction, and ventricular dysfunction. The presence of a cough when supine, orthopnea, stridor, or wheeze may predict respiratory complications. Syncope, upper body edema, and dysphagia are signs of superior caval obstruction and indicate an increased cardiovascular risk.

Patients at very high risk benefit from preoperative irradiation, empiric chemotherapy, and/or corticosteroid therapy; however, these may reduce the accuracy of tissue diagnosis from a subsequent biopsy. An alternative to mediastinal surgery is to biopsy a distant site, such as a pleural effusion, peripheral lymph node, or a bone marrow aspirate under local anesthesia. Sedation with dexmedetomidine, ketamine, and midazolam can facilitate the procedure, but airway compromise can be severe even under sedation.[4]

Anesthesia management should involve careful preparation and contingency planning. Muscle relaxation and general anesthetics reduce the tone of major airway and vascular structures and can lead to airway obstruction and/or cardiovascular collapse. Inhalational or intravenous induction should be carefully titrated, optimally with the child in the sitting position, and spontaneous ventilation maintained until the airway is secured. If severe airway compromise occurs, rigid bronchoscopy, a long endotracheal or double-lumen endobronchial tube, and repositioning the child in lateral decubitus or prone can be life-saving. Hemodynamic collapse not responsive to reducing anesthetic depth, vasopressors, repositioning, or rigid bronchoscopy should be managed by lifting the mass via sternotomy. Standby cardiopulmonary bypass is not a reliable strategy if severe cardiopulmonary disturbances are anticipated. Initiation of cardiopulmonary bypass under local anesthesia prior to induction is possible but difficult in children. Other anesthesia considerations include difficult intubation in patients with neck and oral masses or mucositis and tumor lysis syndrome in patients who have received chemoradiotherapy. If the tumor invades the superior vena cava, intravenous access in the lower extremity, preferably femoral vein, should be established.[5] Postoperatively, patients should be closely monitored until fully conscious and able to maintain their airways.

## REFERENCES

1. Golianu B, Hammer GB. Pediatric thoracic anesthesia. *Curr Opin Anaesthesiol.* 2005;18(1):5–11.
2. Letal M, Theam M. Paediatric lung isolation. *BJA Educ.* 2017;17:57–62.
3. Muhly WT, et al. Perioperative management and in-hospital outcomes after minimally invasive repair of pectus excavatum: a multicenter registry report from the Society for Pediatric Anesthesia Improvement Network. *Anesth Analg.* 2019;128(2):315–327.
4. McLeod M, Dobbie M. Anterior mediastinal masses in children. *BJA Educ.* 2019;19(1): 21–26.
5. Gothard JW. Anesthetic considerations for patients with anterior mediastinal masses. *Anesthesiol Clin.* 2008;26(2):305–314.

# 272.

# GENERAL AND UROLOGIC SURGERY

*Arif Valliani and Nimesh Patel*

## INTRODUCTION

In nonneonatal pediatric age groups, abdominal and urologic surgeries are more common interventions than any other surgeries for a pediatric anesthesiologist. Many of these procedures are frequently done through minimally invasive techniques, with the use of laparoscopy-assisted procedures. Most anesthesia considerations are similar to those in adults.[1]

For better perioperative care, a comprehensive preoperative evaluation is essential. Choice of anesthesia in a younger age group, due to their lack of cooperation, is mostly general anesthesia (GA). However, with the larger success of regional techniques recently and its use in postoperative analgesia, many anesthesiologists prefer these techniques along with GA.[2]

## BASIC PRINCIPLES OF ABDOMINAL SURGERY

Children coming for emergency abdominal surgeries, from either any pathologic event or trauma, are consider to have a full stomach. These patients are at risk of aspiration during induction of anesthesia. To minimize this risk and immediately secure the airway, rapid sequence induction (RSI) is recommended. For RSI, the approach is to prepare and keep ready to use all the induction anesthetic drugs and the airway according to the age and weight of the child. If appropriate, after preoxygenation, drugs are administered in a rapid sequence while applying cricoid pressure, and the trachea is rapidly intubated along with inflation of the cuff. It is still unclear whether cricoid pressure during RSI helps prevent regurgitation.[2,3]

There is significant fluid shift in most of acute abdominal surgeries due to dehydration, electrolyte imbalance, and third spacing. In such a circumstance, correction is required before proceeding to surgery. However, in some elective surgeries, electrolytes and fluid replacement depend on the particular situation, like visceral anastomosis or risk of pulmonary edema.

If the child is presenting with an ischemic bowel or sepsis, then the surgery becomes emergent, and anesthesia needs to be induced even before the patient is fully optimized. The maintenance of anesthesia is simultaneously managed by correction of fluid and electrolyte imbalance, preservation of hemodynamic stability, and in many instances the use of inotropes and vasoactive drugs.

Recently, many elective abdominal surgeries, which traditionally used to be done via open approach, are being performed laparoscopically. This is a video-assisted, minimally invasive approach, creating a pneumoperitoneum and using smaller instruments to gain clinical access.[1,2] Some common abdominal surgeries done via the laparoscopic approach are hernia repairs, Ladd procedure, ostomy, resections, abdominal exploration for bowel obstruction, mass, trauma, infection; liver surgeries like cholecystectomy, Kasai procedure, cysts, abscess; and genitourinary surgeries like nephrectomy, oophorectomy, orchidectomy, and more.

## ADVANTAGES AND DISADVANTAGES OF LAPAROSCOPIC SURGERIES

### ADVANTAGES

- Reduced bleeding
- Minimized operative wound
- Early recovery ~~and return to work~~
- Minimal postoperative pain
- Enhanced cosmesis
- Decreased adhesion formation
- Used of a three-dimensional visualization technique
- Video can be saved for references
- Diagnostic and therapeutic

### DISADVANTAGES

- Pneumoperitoneum
- Hypercapnia
- Prolong surgical time

- Technically demanding
- Low body temperature
- Insufficient ventilation
- Risk of bronchial intubation
- Mostly requires definite airway

## ANESTHESIA CONSIDERATIONS

### PREOPERATIVE

The American Society of Anesthesiology (ASA) recommendation for preoperative fasting includes 2 hours for clear liquids, 4 hours for breast milk, and 6 hours for infant formula, nonhuman milk, and solid food. Additionally, 8 hours or more required if the solid food contains high fat content and/or meat.

Most minor elective surgeries do not require preoperative laboratory investigations outside a basic history and physical examination. Some institutional policies require a pregnancy test for girls who have attained menarche. Many major cases and children with comorbidities require additional testing on a case-to-case basis. Premedication with anxiolytics is commonly used depending on the state of the patient.[4]

### INTRAOPERATIVE

Generally, intraoperatively only ASA standard monitoring is required for routine elective cases. Major intra-abdominal cases necessitate invasive or semi-invasive monitoring like arterial and central venous pressure monitoring, transesophageal echo, and/or cardiac output evaluation. As an ASA standard, temperature regulation is important, particularly in younger children. Balanced salt solutions should be used for maintenance of fluid therapy. Additionally, younger children require a sugar solution to avoid intraoperative hypoglycemia. Studies for the use of crystalloid fluids versus colloids in the resuscitation therapy are equipoise.

Choice of anesthesia depends on many factors, including anesthesiologist preference, age of the child, and type and nature of the surgery. GA with definitive airway is routinely used for many emergency intra-abdominal surgeries and cases that require pneumoperitoneum. Induction of anesthesia with either intravenous or inhalation depends on the patient's physiology and cooperation. GA with a laryngeal mask airway (LMA) can be used in elective cases for which there is minimal to no risk of aspiration (e.g., open nonobstructed hernia repairs). Regional anesthesia can be used with either supplementation of GA or sedation or as a sole anesthetic technique in awake patients.[2]

Most anesthesiologists use anesthetic adjuncts intraoperatively to reduce the risk of postoperative pain, nausea, vomiting and delirium.

### POSTOPERATIVE

Depending on the surgical and pathological course and the extent of monitoring that the child requires postoperatively, care can be done in either a recovery room or an intensive care unit. If the patient does not require ventilatory support, at the end of the surgery, spontaneous ventilation should be ensured, given appropriate anesthetic adjuvants for postoperative analgesia, nausea and vomiting, neuromuscular blocking agent reversal, and airway device (endotracheal tube or LMA) removed. Keeping the airway clear from secretions is important to the avoid risk of laryngospasm. Continuous vital signs and temperature monitoring are required until the child is fully awake for further management of care.[4]

## BASIC PRINCIPLES OF UROLOGIC SURGERY

There is a diverse assortment of pediatric urologic surgeries, ranging from ambulatory procedures to complex surgical intervention. However, most are elective, besides surgeries for acute urinary obstruction and testicular torsion. As many patients undergo multiple surgical interventions, emotional support and anxiolysis are significant measures to consider. Some common pediatric urologic procedures include hypospadias, cystoscopy, bladder exstrophy, circumcision, orchidopexy, urolithiasis, vesicoureteral reflux, testicular torsion, Eagle-Barrett syndrome, and more.

## ANESTHESIA CONSIDERATIONS

### PREOPERATIVE

Many patients coming for genitourinary surgical interventions have good renal function and a stable medical condition and do not require any investigation other than a good history and physical examination. Children with reduced renal function need to be further evaluated for the extent of their medical condition and involvement of other systems. Optimization of such conditions (e.g., dialysis, electrolyte correction) is required before proceeding for elective surgery.[1,2]

### SYSTEMIC INVOLVEMENT IN PATIENTS WITH REDUCED RENAL FUNCTION

- Anemia
- Decrease platelet function
- Acid-base imbalance
- Fluid-electrolyte abnormalities
- Congestive heart failure
- Hypertension

- Pulmonary congestion
- Gastrointestinal disturbance
- Chronic steroid dependence

## INTRAOPERATIVE

The ASA standard intraoperative monitoring is acceptable for the majority of procedures. More invasive monitors may be required depending of the extent of the surgery and in cases with associated medical problems. Urine output monitoring is also important in major cases.

As discussed for in abdominal surgery, choice of anesthesia depends on many factors and can either be GA with endotracheal intubation or LMA or a regional technique with sedation. For children with impaired renal functions, medication doses needed to be adjusted. Succinylcholine should be used with caution as there is risk of elevated potassium in the setting of poor renal function. Muscle relaxant should be reversed at the end of the surgery and extubation should only be done when full muscle strength is back and the child is fully awake.[4,5]

## POSTOPERATIVE

Children with a successful regional block require little additional analgesia in the postoperative period. Patients with impaired renal functions require careful titration of opioids. Ensure adequate ventilation and oxygenation. Correct and repeat any abnormalities in blood count, electrolytes, and acid-base balance. Finally, ensure the patient has proper follow-up with a nephrologist for continuity of care.[4]

## REFERENCES

1. Davis PJ, Cladis FP, eds. *Smith's Anesthesia for Infants and Children.* 9th ed. Elsevier; 2016.
2. Cote C, et al. *A Practice of Anesthesia for Infants and Children.* 6th Ed. Elsevier; 2018.
3. Morris J, Cook TM. Rapid sequence induction: a national survey of practice. *Anesthesia.* 2001;56:1090–1097.
4. Lerman J, et al. *Manual of Pediatric Anesthesia.* 7th ed. Springer; 2016.
5. Cote CJ, et al. Continuous noninvasive cardiac output in children: is this the next generation of operating room monitor? Initial experience in 402 pediatric patients. *Paediatr Anaesth.* 2015;25:150–159.

# 273.

# ORTHOPEDIC SURGERY

*Alina Lazar*

## INTRODUCTION

Pediatric orthopedic surgery ranges from simple ambulatory procedures to complex interventions. Common anesthetic concerns are blood loss, management of concomitant diseases, and perioperative pain. Postoperative analgesia is multimodal and includes opioids, acetaminophen, nonsteroidal anti-inflammatory drugs (NSAIDs), local anesthetics (LAs) and adjuvants for regional anesthesia (RA), and in select circumstances gabapentinoids and ketamine. Although animal studies suggest altered bone healing after fractures and bone surgery, NSAIDs have been safely used.[1] RA, either single shot or continuous infusion, has been increasingly used.[2] Caudal block is the most widely used technique for hip, leg, knee, and foot procedures, and it is usually done in children younger than 5 years. Epidural catheters can be placed for procedures with severe pain expected to last longer than 24 hours, especially if both lower extremities are involved. Single-shot peripheral nerve blocks provide analgesia for 12–16 hours. This duration may be prolonged up to a maximum of 20 hours by increasing the concentration of LA and using a combination of LA and additives.[2] Common indications and complications of RA for orthopedic procedures in children are presented in Table 273.1. Performing pediatric RA under general anesthesia/deep sedation is associated with

| BLOCK TYPE | SURGERY LOCATION | INDICATIONS FOR CONTINUOUS TECHNIQUES | COMPLICATIONS |
|---|---|---|---|
| Interscalene | Shoulder, upper arm | Shoulder arthroscopy with rotator cuff repair, proximal humerus surgery | Phrenic nerve blockade, pneumothorax, Horner syndrome, spinal cord injury, intrathecal and intravascular injection |
| Supraclavicular | Arm below shoulder | Not commonly done | Pneumothorax, phrenic nerve blockade, intravascular injection |
| Infraclavicular | Elbow, forearm, hand | Open reduction and internal fixation of distal humerus, radius, ulna, ligament repair, major polydactyly repair | Pneumothorax, intravascular injection |
| Axillary | Elbow, forearm, hand | Not commonly done | Intravascular injection |
| Lumbar plexus | Hip, femur, knee | Hip repairs, femoral head, anterior thigh tumor resections | Retroperitoneal hematoma, epidural spread |
| Fascia iliaca | Hip, femur | Not commonly done | Intravascular injection |
| Lateral femoral cutaneous | Femoral neck, hip | Not commonly done | Intravascular injection |
| Femoral | Thigh, femur, knee | Knee (ligament reconstruction, open meniscal repair), femur osteotomy | Intravascular injection |
| Adductor canal/saphenous | Medial lower leg and knee | Arthroscopic knee procedures, procedures below the knee | Motor weakness with large volume, proximal placement |
| Sciatic | Knee, leg, ankle, foot | Calcaneal, midfoot osteotomy, leg lengthening | Intravascular injection |
| Caudal/epidural | Lower extremity, hip | Complex procedures of the hip and lower extremity | Intravascular injection, infection, epidural hematoma |

acceptable safety and is the standard of care.[3] Ultrasound guidance is strongly recommended. The LAs most commonly used are bupivacaine and ropivacaine, the latter being associated with a more favorable safety profile and less motor blockade.

The most common *fractures* requiring anesthetic care in children are femur, tibia/fibula, humerus, and radius/ulna fractures. The anesthetic plan for children with fractures should take into consideration the risk of bleeding and hypovolemia, aspiration in patients with a full stomach, and coexistent intracranial, cervical, chest, and abdominal injuries. RA should be carefully considered in patients with associated nerve injury as it may interfere with postoperative neurologic evaluation.[4,5] There is no evidence that RA delays or prevents the diagnosis of compartment syndrome. In fact, increasing pain in a patient with a previously working block may indicate the development of this rare complication.[2] Avoiding dense blocks, careful postoperative monitoring, and triage of high-risk patients, such as those with tibial compartment surgery, is paramount to ensure safety.

A *slipped capital femoral epiphysis* consists of gradual or acute displacement of the femoral head from the femoral neck through the growth plate; it typically occurs in obese teenagers. Patients present with limping and pain in the groin, anterior thigh, and knee. Surgical management consists of in situ screw fixation to prevent further slippage. Any general anesthesia can be used.

*Club foot* is a common congenital anomaly that is usually treated in infancy with a series of foot stretching and casting and percutaneous Achilles tenotomy. The latter can be performed in an office with LA or in the operating room under sedation, general anesthesia, or caudal or spinal anesthesia. More severe deformities require extensive surgery. Because the postoperative pain is intense, epidural or sciatic catheters are recommended.

Developmental dysplasia of the hip is a common condition ranging from shallowness of the acetabulum, to the capsular instability, to hip dislocation. It may progress to degenerative hip osteoarthritis. More common in children born by breech delivery, it is diagnosed at birth by provocative tests or later in childhood with the Ortolani test. Surgical treatment is to relocate and stabilize the femoral head in the acetabulum with body casting within the first weeks of life. General anesthesia and caudal epidural blockade are used for the procedure.

*Cerebral palsy* (CP) is the most common neurologic disability of childhood that affects the child's ability to move and maintain balance and posture. Patients with CP require multiple orthopedic procedures to reduce spasticity in a lower extremity and around the hip girdle and progressive scoliosis. Almost any anesthesia technique can be used. Succinylcholine does not cause hyperkalemia and can be used safely. Mental retardation or limited ability to communicate make pain assessment particularly difficult. Common procedures are multilevel surgery involving tenotomies and/or osteotomies at different levels on one or both limbs and spinal fusion. Children with spastic CP develop hip dislocation over time, which makes sitting and getting dressed challenging. This condition is treated with varus derotational osteotomy, which consists of reshaping the proximal femur and hip socket, followed by spica casting. Because the orthopedic procedures intended for relieving spasm are extremely painful, continuous RA techniques are recommended in the postoperative period.

Surgery for scoliosis is done either for cosmetic reasons (idiopathic scoliosis) or to improve sitting, decrease pain, or even to prolong life if the deformity is severe and affects cardiopulmonary function (neuromuscular disorders). In the posterior approach, a growing rod system is inserted in prepubertal children or spinal fixation is performed in older children. When an anterior approach is also needed, lung isolation may be required to improve access to the spine. Anesthesia concerns are blood loss, spinal cord injury, and postoperative pain. Blood conservation techniques commonly used are blood salvage and antifibrinolytics. Because

volatile anesthetics interfere with spinal cord monitoring, intravenous anesthetic infusions (propofol, short acting opioids, ketamine, and dexmedetomidine) are used, alone or in combination with volatile anesthetic at less than 0.5 minimum alveolar concentration (MAC). Postoperative pain control can be achieved with a multimodal approach, including opioids via patient- or nurse-controlled analgesia, methadone, acetaminophen, ketamine, epidural analgesia, or intrathecal morphine. Ketorolac is controversial because it may inhibit spinal fusion.

## REFERENCES

1. Bosenberg A. Regional anaesthesia in children: an update. *South Afr J Anaesth Analg*. 2013;19:282–288.
2. Antony S, et al. Pediatric ambulatory continuous peripheral nerve blocks. *Anesthesiol Clin*. 2018;36(3):455–465.
3. Walker BJ, et al. Peripheral nerve catheters in children: an analysis of safety and practice patterns from the Pediatric Regional Anesthesia Network (PRAN). *Br J Anaesth*. 2015;115:457–462.
4. Tsui B, Suresh S. Ultrasound imaging for regional anesthesia in infants, children, and adolescents: a review of current literature and its application in the practice of extremity and trunk blocks. *Anesthesiology*. 2010;112(2):473–492.
5. Marhofer P. Upper extremity peripheral blocks. *Tech Reg Anesth Pain Manag*. 2007;11:215–221.

# 274.

# ANESTHESIA FOR PEDIATRIC OPHTHALMOLOGIC SURGERIES

*Nupur Dua and Wendy Nguyen*

## INTRODUCTION

Typically performed in an ambulatory setting, commonly performed pediatric ophthalmologic procedures include eye examination, cryotherapy or laser therapy for retinopathy of prematurity or retinoblastoma, strabismus repair, lens extraction in cataracts, and enucleation.

## ANATOMY

The orbit is formed by a complex arrangement of seven cranial bones: frontal, zygomatic, sphenoid, maxilla, palatine, lacrimal, and ethmoid. The optic foramen transmits the optic nerve, the ophthalmic artery and vein, and the sympathetic contributions from the carotid plexus (Figure 274.1).

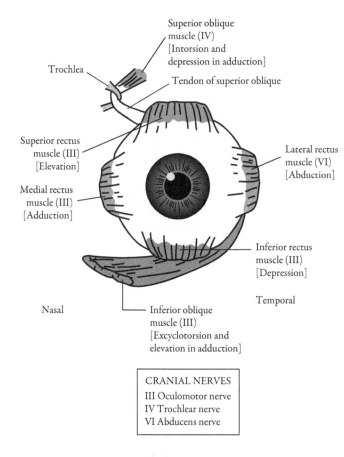

Figure 274.1 Anatomy and innervation of the eye. Reprinted with permission from Zitelli, BJ, McIntire, SC, Nowalk, AJ. *Atlas of Pediatric Physical Diagnosis.* 6th ed. Saunders; 2012:55.

The superior orbital fissure transmits branches from four other cranial nerves (oculomotor, trigeminal, trochlear, and abducens) and superior and inferior ophthalmic veins. The temporal and zygomatic branches of the facial nerve (CN VII) innervate the orbicularis oculi.

## PHYSIOLOGY

### INTRAOCULAR PRESSURE

Normal intraocular pressure (IOP) is 10–20 mm Hg. Normal pressures are slightly lower in newborns (average 9.5 mm Hg) but reach adult pressures by approximately 5 years of age. There are three primary determinants of IOP: external pressure, venous congestion, and intraocular volume.

The aqueous humor is formed primarily by the ciliary bodies, where secretion is facilitated by the carbonic anhydrase and cytochrome oxidase systems. Production is augmented by sympathetic stimulation and suppressed by parasympathetic control. Variations in the osmotic pressure of the aqueous humor and plasma

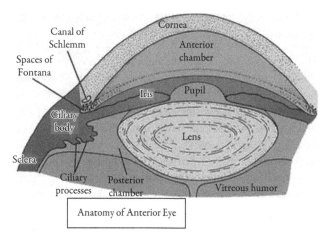

Figure 274.2 Anatomy of the anterior eye. Reprinted with permission from Motoyama ES, Davis PJ. Smith's Anesthesia for Infants and Children (6th Edition). 1996. Mosby: 872.

influence aqueous humor formation, as depicted by the following equation:

where

$k$ = coefficient of outflow

$OP_{aq}$ = osmotic pressure of aqueous humor

$OP_{pl}$ = osmotic pressure of plasma

$P_c$ = capillary perfusion pressure

The aqueous humor produced in the posterior chamber flows through the pupil into the anterior chamber, exiting the eye through the Schlem canal and into the orbital venous system (Figure 274.2). Mydriasis causes Fontana spaces to narrow, causing outflow resistance. Fluctuations in the aqueous humor outflow alter IOP based on the Hagen-Poiseuille law:

where

$A$ = volume of aqueous humor outflow per unit of time

$r$ = radius of Fontana spaces

$P_{iop}$ = IOP

$P_v$ = venous pressure

$\eta$ = viscosity

$l$ = length of Fontana spaces[1]

The following are anesthesia-related factors that impact IOP:

1. Coughing, vomiting, Valsalva maneuver ↑ due to increase in venous pressure
2. Respiratory acidosis, metabolic alkalosis ↑
3. Hypoxia ↑ by dilating intraocular vessels
4. Inadequate depth of anesthesia

## OCULOCARDIAC REFLEX

The oculocardiac reflex (OCR; also known as the Ascher reflex) is most often elicited by not only traction on the extraocular muscles but also pressure on the globe and after intraorbital or retrobulbar injections (described in more detail in the chapter on adult ophthalmology). OCR is mediated by the afferent ophthalmic division of CN V and the efferent vagal nerve (Figure 274.3). The pathway is initiated by the activation of stretch receptors in the ocular and periorbital tissues. The short and long ciliary nerves conduct impulses that carry the sensory message to the ciliary ganglion. From there the impulses are transported by way of the ophthalmic division of CN V to the Gasserian ganglion, followed by the trigeminal nucleus, where the afferent limb will terminate in the central nervous system (CNS). The CNS stimulates the efferent limb, causing impulses to exit the brainstem and transmit to the myocardium to synapse on the sinoatrial node and activate the vagal motor, causing negative chronotropy. More ominous manifestations, including atrioventricular block, ventricular bigeminy, ventricular tachycardia, and asystole, have been described. Treatment of OCR includes release of the stimulus and administration of atropine (10 to 20 µg/kg IV) or glycopyrrolate (10 µg/kg IV).

There is no consensus regarding the value of prophylaxis with vagolytics. Retrobulbar blocks are effective in preventing OCR; however, regional blocks are not commonly used during pediatric procedures, and they have triggered the reflex during placement. Sub-Tenon blocks have also been shown to decrease the incidence and severity of OCR. A sub-Tenon block is less invasive and has a lower complication rate than a retrobulbar block. With the use of local anesthetic, the afferent limb of the OCR reflex can be blocked to prevent the reflex.[2]

## OCULORESPIRATORY REFLEX AND THE OCULOEMETIC REFLEX

The oculorespiratory reflex (ORR) and oculoemetic reflex (OER) are also elicited by pressure or torsion on the extraocular muscles transmitting afferent impulses through the ophthalmic division of CN V. The ORR results in tachypnea or respiratory arrest through a connection between the trigeminal nerve, the pneumotaxic center of the pons, and the medullary respiratory centers. This reflex is not inhibited by atropine or glycopyrrolate. The exact mechanism of the OER is unknown; however, an association between the OCR and the OER has been demonstrated such that patients who exhibit the OCR intraoperatively are 2.6 times more likely to experience postoperative nausea and vomiting (PONV) than those without OCR manifestations. There is no response to anticholinergic therapy.[1]

## ANESTHETIC MANAGEMENT FOR SPECIFIC SURGERIES

### STRABISMUS

Strabismus has a prevalence of 3% to 5% in the pediatric population. Surgical correction involves isolation of one or more of the extraocular muscles with subsequent recession or resection of the muscle. Contemporary techniques

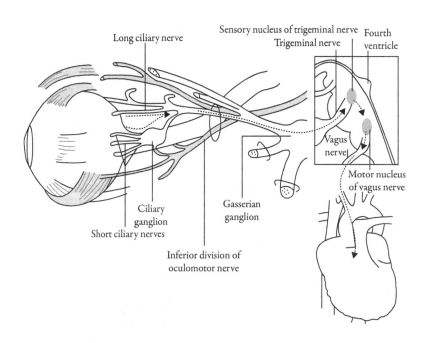

**Figure 274.3** Oculocardiac reflex arc. Reprinted with permission from Tumul Chowdhury, T, Schlaller, BJ. Trigeminocardiac Reflex. 2015. Academic Press: 91.

involving botulinum toxin injection and postoperative adjustable sutures are not commonly used in the pediatric population.

**Premedication:** As for most pediatric procedures, premedication is extremely useful to ease separation from parents and to provide for a smooth induction in children between 1 and 6 years of age. Oral midazolam (0.25 to 0.75 mg/kg) is commonly used and is effective 10 to 20 minutes after administration.

**Anesthetic Management:** Mask induction with sevoflurane for general anesthesia is common. It is common to use a laryngeal mask airway (LMA). Some ophthalmologists request the use of paralytic agents for performance of the forced duction test to more clearly differentiate paretic and restrictive disorders before surgical correction. Prolonged contractions of the extraocular muscles associated with succinylcholine administration interfere with interpretation of the forced duction test for at least 15 minutes. Problems commonly associated with strabismus surgery are OCR and PONV.[3]

**Prevention of PONV:** It is usual practice to use dual antiemetics. Methods that have demonstrated benefit include dexamethasone (0.15–0.5 mg/kg IV up to 5 mg) and ondansetron (0.1–0.15 mg/kg up to 4 mg). Adequate intravenous hydration (about 20–30 mL/kg) is also recommended. Other 5-HT$_3$ (5-hydroxytryptamine, serotonin) receptor antagonists such as granisetron and tropisetron (approved for chemotherapy-induced nausea and vomiting) may be beneficial. Avoiding opioids, when possible, will also decrease PONV.[4]

**Analgesia:** Strabismus is associated with moderate postoperative pain. Fentanyl 1–2 μg/kg supplemented with ketorolac (0.5 mg/kg IV) yields consistent analgesia. Rectal acetaminophen (30 to 40 mg/kg) may be administered to supplement.

**Emergence:** Deep extubation or removal of the LMA helps with emergence delirium. Dexmedetomidine 0.5 μg/kg just before the end of surgery is helpful in preventing delirium.[5]

## CATARACT SURGERY

The prevalence of cataracts among the pediatric population is 1.2–6 per 10,000 live births. Bilateral cataracts are most commonly associated with systemic diseases (Apert syndrome, Crouzon disease, Down syndrome, myotonic dystrophy, rubella, Turner syndrome, Stickler syndrome), whereas unilateral cataracts are typically idiopathic. Surgery for bilateral congenital cataracts must be performed within the first several weeks of life to allow for normal retinal development. Unilateral congenital disease requires surgical attention within the first 4 months of life to prohibit the development of irreversible amblyopia. Lens extraction is performed after maximal mydriasis with one or more of the topical agents. Vitrectomy instrumentation is the preferred method of extraction in young children.

**Anesthetic Management:** Akinesia and control of IOP assist in creating favorable surgical conditions. As most of these patients are infants, controlled ventilation with muscle relaxation under general anesthesia is the preferred method. The anesthesiologist should be aware of associated systemic disease and the potential systemic effects of the topical preparations used by the ophthalmologist. Analgesic requirements are usually minimal and may be met with rectal acetaminophen under normal circumstances.

Though not common, *postoperative apnea* has been reported in otherwise healthy full-term infants after cataract surgery. There is no clear mechanism. To minimize respiratory depression, a sub-Tenon block is an effective technique for postoperative analgesia compared to intravenous fentanyl in infants undergoing cataract surgery.[1] Surgical postoperative complications include formation of secondary membranes, glaucoma, and endophthalmitis. Treating nasolacrimal duct obstruction before cataract surgery and postponing cataract surgery in children with evidence of upper respiratory tract infections may avoid endophthalmitis.

## GLAUCOMA

Pediatric glaucoma is most often a congenital abnormality. Infantile glaucoma develops before 3 years of age and is a primary disorder in half of all cases. Juvenile glaucoma refers to disease that develops after 3 years of age and is most often associated with other ocular or systemic disorders (Apert syndrome, Crouzon disease, Down syndrome, Goldenhar syndrome, Marfan syndrome, Sturge-Weber syndrome). Corrective procedures include goniotomy, trabeculotomy, and cyclocryotherapy. Patients often require repeated evaluations because surgical correction is typically incremental and performed in carefully monitored stages.

**Anesthetic Management:** The management is similar for all procedures of general anesthesia with an LMA. Goals are to maintain stable IOP and complete akinesia. Short-acting opioids, in conjunction with prophylaxis for PONV, should be incorporated into the anesthetic plan.

## RETINOBLASTOMA

Treatment modalities may include combinations of enucleation, external beam radiation, localized radiotherapy, laser ablation, thermotherapy, cryotherapy, and chemotherapy.

**Anesthetic Management:** Enucleation requires similar management to those for other moderately complex ophthalmic procedures. The incidence of OCR-mediated dysrhythmias is high, and appropriate prophylaxis with atropine or glycopyrrolate may be warranted. Postoperative pain is often significant and warrants the use of opioids. External beam radiotherapy lasts only a few minutes but requires the patient to remain motionless. Brief inhalation anesthetics by insufflation methods, LMA, and endotracheal intubation can be used.[3]

## REFERENCES

1. Justice LT, et al. Anesthesia for ophthalmic surgery. In: Davis PJ, Cladis FP, eds. *Smith's Anesthesia for Infants and Children*. 9th edition. Elsevier; 2015:870–888.
2. Talebnejad MR, et al. The effect of sub-Tenon's bupivacaine on oculocardiac reflex during strabismus surgery and postoperative pain: a randomized clinical trial. *J Ophthalmic Vis Res.* 2017;12(3):296–300.
3. Waldschmidt B, Gordon N. Anesthesia for pediatric ophthalmologic surgery. *JAAPOS.* 2019;23(3):127–131.
4. Ames WA, Machovec K. An update on the management of PONV in a pediatric patient. *Best Pract Res Clin Anaesthesiol.* 2020;34(4):749–758.
5. Tan D, et al. Effect of ancillary drugs on sevoflurane related emergence agitation in children undergoing ophthalmic surgery: a Bayesian network meta-analysis. *BMC Anesthesiol.* 2019;19:138.

# 275.

# PEDIATRIC AMBULATORY SURGERY

*Megan Rodgers McCormick*

## INDICATIONS AND CONTRAINDICATIONS

Children are often excellent candidates for outpatient surgery since they are generally healthy individuals undergoing brief surgeries with few complications. These patients are usually 6 months to 18 years of age and American Society of Anesthesiologists (ASA) Physical Status Classification System I (normal and healthy patient) or II (mild, systemic disease). Common pediatric procedures for outpatient surgery include those involving otolaryngology, ophthalmology, general pediatric surgery, urology, endoscopies, plastic surgery, orthopedics, radiology, and dentistry.

There are a few firm contraindications for pediatric patients in an outpatient facility. Preterm infants should not undergo outpatient surgery until at least 60 weeks' postconceptional age (PCA) to reduce the chance of apnea. Full-term infants, those over 37 weeks' PCA, should not have outpatient procedures until they reach at least 54 weeks' PCA. Patients with higher ASA status, complex congenital heart disease, craniofacial abnormalities, moderate-to-severe obstructive sleep apnea, obesity with sleep apnea, and tonsillectomy under the age of 3 are not candidates. Patients with poorly controlled cardiopulmonary disorders are at higher risk for intraoperative and postoperative complications and are not suitable for outpatient procedures. Any patients who may require postoperative monitoring because of anesthetic-related risks or the risks related to the operative procedure should be admitted overnight. This may include surgeries with large fluid shifts and large blood loss, long duration, or pain that may be difficult to manage postoperatively with oral medications or regional blocks.

Malignant hyperthermia is not a contraindication, but individuals at risk may require prolonged postoperative stay and should be scheduled as the first case of the day with proper preparation and treatments available. Sickle cell anemia can be managed if risk factors of dehydration, hypoxia, diminished perfusion, and acidosis are avoided. Children with diseases like asthma, diabetes, and seizures can be safely managed as outpatients if these issues are controlled and medications are continued appropriately for their condition. Common causes for cancellation on day of surgery or postponement for pediatric patients are upper respiratory tract infections; undisclosed, poorly managed, or nonoptimized medical conditions; fasting violations; or no-show by patient.

## ANESTHETIC CONSIDERATIONS

### PREOPERATIVE

Instructions for nothing by mouth (nil per os, NPO) preoperatively are to abstain from clear liquids for 2 hours; breast milk for 4 hours; formula, cow's milk, or light meal (toast and clear fluids) for 6 hours; and full heavy, meat, or fatty meal for at least 8 hours.

Premedication is often used for uncooperative children or those that may exhibit anxiety. Preoperative anxiety is associated with a higher incidence of postoperative pain, disruption of sleep, and other behavioral problems postoperatively.[1] Children under 6 months do not appear to suffer anxiety when separated from parents, but children ages 1 to 5 are at greater risk. The needs of each patient must be assessed individually. Considerations for premedication are the time it takes to set in, the route of administration, possible longer postoperative recovery, and side effects. Commonly used medications include midazolam, dexmedetomidine, ketamine, and clonidine.

### INTRAOPERATIVE

Use standard ASA monitors including capnography, pulse oximeter, temperature, electrocardiogram (usually three lead), and noninvasive blood pressure.

Inhalation induction is the most common technique in children under the age of 10 who do not have intravenous access already established. A combination of nitrous, oxygen, and sevoflurane is used. Whether the child is cooperative or not will determine the time and rate at which the volatile agent is introduced. If an intravenous line is needed for surgery, it is placed after the patient reaches stage III anesthesia. Age 10 is an appropriate time to start introducing intravenous line placement in the preoperative holding area. EMLA (eutectic mixture of local anesthesia) cream may be applied for an atraumatic placement of an intravenous catheter but requires at least 15 minutes to numb and an hour to provide pain relief. Newer agents, such as the jet injection lidocaine (J-Tip) work immediately to facilitate quicker intravenous placement. Intravenous induction is usually completed with a combination of midazolam, lidocaine, propofol, and fentanyl. Neuromuscular blockade is only given when needed and is often not used in outpatient pediatric anesthesia.

Volatile anesthetics, particularly sevoflurane, is the most used maintenance technique. It titrates to effect quickly and has rapid elimination. Sevoflurane is also beneficial for reactive airways, but like all volatiles, it can cause postoperative nausea and vomiting (PONV) and emergence delirium. Patients at high risk for PONV may benefit from a propofol infusion with or without sevoflurane. Propofol allows for rapid titration of depth and prompt emergence, has antiemetic properties, and decreases the incidence of delirium and agitation compared to volatile anesthetics. Throughout the case a combination of propofol, acetaminophen, dexamethasone, ondansetron, dexmedetomidine, ketorolac, and opioids given as necessary. Since sevoflurane and propofol both do not possess analgesic properties, other pain medications need to be administered. Agents such as ketorolac and acetaminophen are used in multimodal analgesia to help minimize the use and side effects of opioids. When needed, fentanyl can be given intraoperatively and postoperatively for fast-acting analgesia. Morphine and hydromorphone can be given for longer acting analgesia.

### POSTOPERATIVE

Postoperative monitoring includes pulse oximetry, blood pressure, temperature, pain, and evaluating the surgical site at set intervals, depending on the stage of recovery. In healthy children, routine cardiac monitoring in the postanesthesia care unit (PACU) is not necessary.

Postanesthetic care is divided into three phases. The first phase overlaps the end of intraoperative care and is completed when the patient's protective reflexes and motor function have returned. This time frame has a higher risk of postoperative complications, such as laryngospasm, stridor, and emergence delirium, which require closer monitoring. Phase II is the transition of the patient to prepare for discharge from the recovery room to be cared for at home. During phases I and II, nausea, vomiting, and pain are constantly monitored and treated if necessary. PONV remains one of the most common side effects of anesthesia in children and is a cause of delayed discharge or unplanned admission. The incidence is rare under age 2 but is much higher than in adults. Since children have a higher incidence, prophylaxis should be considered. If during the recovery period a patient develops PONV, a rescue treatment should be an antiemetic from a different class than the prophylactic medications already given. A pain management strategy should include a multimodal pain regimen as well as regional anesthesia when appropriate. In most instances, acetaminophen and ketorolac have already been given in the intraoperative period and will not be able to be administered within 6 hours of the initial dose. Rescue therapy usually requires opioid administration followed by monitoring for a minimum of 30 minutes after each dose.

Phase III occurs from discharge from the PACU until full recovery. This may take days and, in outpatient practice, occurs at the patient's home. To discharge a patient from each phase, the patient must meet certain criteria. The Modified Aldrete scoring system is commonly used to determine when a patient has recovered from phase I and is ready to be transferred to phase II recovery; the Post-Anesthetic Discharge Scoring System (PADSS) and Ped-PADSS scores indicate whether the patient has recovered sufficiently and may be discharged from phase II to III, as seen in Table 275.1.[2] Both assign scores of 0, 1, or 2 to

**Table 275.1** PACU DISCHARGE CRITERIA

| ALDRETE SCORING SYSTEM | POST ANESTHETIC DISCHARGE SCORING SYSTEM (PADSS) |
|---|---|
| *Respiration*<br>Able to take deep breath and cough = 2<br>Dyspnea/shallow breath = 1<br>Apnea = 0 | *Vital Signs*<br>BP and pulse within 20% preoperative = 2<br>BP and pulse within 20%-40% preoperative = 1<br>BP and pulse within > 40% preoperative = 0 |
| $O_2$ *Saturation*<br>Maintains > 92% on room air = 2<br>Needs $O_2$ inhalation to maintain $O_2$<br>    saturation > 90% = 1<br>$O_2$ saturation < 90% even on supplemental<br>    oxygen = 0 | *Activity*<br>Steady gait, no dizziness, or meets preoperative level = 2<br>Requires assistance = 1<br>Unable to ambulate = 0 |
| *Consciousness*<br>Fully awake = 2<br>Arousable on calling = 1<br>Not responding = 0 | *Nausea and Vomiting*<br>Minimal/treated with oral medication = 2<br>Moderate/treated with parental medication = 1<br>Severe/continues despite treatment = 0 |
| *Circulation*<br>BP ± 20 mm Hg preoperative = 2<br>BP ± 20–50 mm Hg preoperative = 1<br>BP ± 50 mm Hg preoperative = 0 | *Pain*<br>Controlled with oral analgesics and acceptable to patient<br>Yes = 2<br>No = 1 |
| *Activity*<br>Able to move 4 extremities = 2<br>Able to move 2 extremities = 1<br>Able to move 0 extremities = 0 | *Surgical Bleeding*<br>Minimal/no dressing changes = 2<br>Moderate/up to two dressing changes required = 1<br>Severe/more than three dressing changes required = 0 |

BP, blood pressure.

the five categories, with 10 as the max score. A score of 8 or higher for Aldrete and 9 or higher for PADSS must be met to move on to the next phase. The PACU discharge criteria can vary greatly from facility to facility, with best practice remaining unclear. The overall picture is that a patient should be returned to their baseline with stable vital signs as well as pain, nausea, and vomiting all under control. Oral challenge and urination are no longer a requisite.[2]

A postoperative assessment is required within 48 hours of discharge to identify any adverse events related to the surgery or anesthesia as well as answer questions and guide follow-up care for patients after returning home. Follow-up phone calls are usually done by nursing staff the next business day and consist of questions regarding recovery, neuro status, pain, nausea, and vomiting.

## REFERENCES

1. Cote CJ, et al. *A Practice of Anesthesia for Infants and Children.* 5th ed. Elsevier; 2013;3:22–28.
2. Ead H. From Aldrete to PADSS: reviewing discharge criteria after ambulatory surgery. *J Perianesth Nurs.* 2006;21(4):259–267.

# 276.

# SYSTEMIC MEDICATIONS AND ROUTES OF ADMINISTRATION
## MULTIMODAL ANALGESIA

*Samiya L. Saklayen and Thomas Graul*

## INTRODUCTION

A comprehensive approach to pediatric pain management aims to address the multidimensional, biopsychosocial components of pain. Nonpharmacological measures such as caregiver contact, warm or cold compresses, and careful positioning are very low risk and may reduce the perception of pain in a child.[1] Pharmacological measures to treat postoperative pain are often combined in a multimodal approach and may include regional anesthesia, opioids, as well as nonopioid analgesics.

## NONOPIOID ANALGESICS

Concerns regarding opioid side effects and toxicities have led to the emergence of opioid-sparing techniques as an integral component of pediatric postoperative pain management. Nonopioid adjuncts to pain control include acetaminophen, nonsteroidal anti-inflammatory drugs, $\alpha_2$-agonists, *N*-methyl-D-aspartate (NMDA) receptor antagonists, steroids, and gabapentinoids.

## ACETAMINOPHEN

Several studies have found that even a single dose of acetaminophen administered preoperatively or intraoperatively, regardless of the route of administration, may reduce postoperative pain or opioid requirements for both major and minor surgeries.[2] Acetaminophen may be administered orally, intravenously, or rectally. While oral administration is most commonly preferred due to its low cost and patient comfort, intravenous injection and rectal suppository may be preferred for patients who are sedated or nauseated. The bioavailability of rectal acetaminophen is variable, partially based on the site of absorption; medication absorbed in the distal portion of the rectum bypasses the liver, whereas uptake in the proximal portion of the rectum is subject to hepatic first-pass metabolism.

## NONSTEROIDAL ANTI-INFLAMMATORY DRUGS

Multiple studies suggest perioperative nonsteroidal anti-inflammatory drug (NSAID) use decreases postoperative pain and opioid requirements for a variety of surgeries in children.[2] NSAIDs may be administered orally, intravenously, or intramuscularly. Parenteral NSAIDs approved by the Food and Drug Administration (FDA) include ibuprofen for children older than 6 months and ketorolac for children older than 2 years. Although NSAIDs have proven to be very useful and often sufficient for alleviating mild-to-moderate pain, they should be used with caution and avoided in children at risk for renal dysfunction, gastrointestinal bleeding, and coagulopathy and those at high risk of surgical bleeding.

## A$_2$-AGONISTS

Despite a lack of FDA approval for use in children, dexmedetomidine's favorable sedative and analgesic properties have led to increasing off-label use in this population. Data from randomized controlled trials revealed a lower risk of postoperative pain and opioid requirement in children who received intraoperative dexmedetomidine.[3] Although various routes of administration have been reported, dexmedetomidine is most commonly given intravenously or intranasally. Intranasal administration is fast and has no reduction in the bioavailability of the drug, making it advantageous in procedures where intravenous access is unavailable, such as myringotomy. Potential adverse events with dexmedetomidine include bradycardia, hypotension, and hypertension. Clonidine is another useful α-2 agonist that is sometimes used off label as part of a multimodal pain regimen for children. While most commonly administered orally, intravenous, epidural, and transdermal formulations are available and have been described.

## NMDA RECEPTOR ANTAGONIST

Ketamine is a potent analgesic and lacks the respiratory depressing effects of opioids, making it very useful in postoperative pain management. There is some evidence to suggest that its use may decrease postoperative nausea and vomiting due to opioid-sparing effects.[2] There is also some evidence to show that small doses of ketamine may help prevent opioid-induced hyperalgesia.[4] Ketamine is most commonly administered intravenously but can also be given intranasally or intramuscularly if intravenous access is unavailable.

## STEROIDS

Often provided for postoperative nausea and vomiting prophylaxis, the steroid dexamethasone may also be beneficial as part of a multimodal pain regimen. A meta-analysis of the perioperative use of dexamethasone in children undergoing tonsillectomy revealed lower pain scores on postoperative day 1 compared to placebo.[2] Dexamethasone is frequently administered intravenously, but oral and intramuscular routes are also available.

## GABAPENTINOIDS

Selective use of oral gabapentin or pregabalin is sometimes used as part of a multimodal pain regimen in surgeries associated with severe pain postoperatively. Although many adult studies have demonstrated gabapentin to be a useful adjunct to opioids in pain relief, pediatric data are insufficient and inconclusive.[5]

## OPIOID ANALGESICS

Open abdominal, thoracic, and orthopedic surgeries are all associated with significant pain, and inadequate analgesia affects postoperative recovery. Due to their potent analgesic effects, opioids—in addition to regional and neuraxial anesthesia—remain the mainstay of treatment for severe postoperative pain in children.

## NATURAL OPIOIDS

Morphine is one of the most commonly employed natural opioid agents used for postoperative analgesia. While most commonly administered intravenously, other routes of administration include intramuscular, subcutaneous, epidural (preservative free), as well as oral formulations. With the appropriate level of monitoring, patient-controlled analgesia is safe and efficacious even in young children.

Although codeine was once widely used for pain control in children, pharmacogenomic variability has made this drug highly problematic. Codeine is a prodrug and must be converted to morphine by cytochrome P450 2D6 (CYP2D6). Individuals who lack this enzyme have inadequate pain relief, whereas individuals with duplicated CYP2D6 genes may experience ultrarapid conversion of codeine to morphine, leading to respiratory failure and death. For this reason, the FDA has contraindicated the use of codeine in children less than 12 years and in the treatment of tonsillectomy pain in children less than 18 years old. The FDA has also warned against codeine use in children who are obese, have obstructive sleep apnea, or have severe lung disease. Tramadol, which is also a prodrug that undergoes CYP2D6 metabolism, carries similar contraindications and warnings.

## SEMISYNTHETIC OPIOIDS

Hydromorphone is a semisynthetic opioid and has a slightly more rapid onset of action compared to morphine. Routes of administration are similar to morphine.

Oxycodone is available for oral administration either alone or in combination with an adjunct such as acetaminophen.

## SYNTHETIC OPIOIDS

Fentanyl is one of the most commonly used synthetic opioids during the perioperative period due to its high potency and rapid onset of action. In addition to intravenous routes, intranasal administration may be helpful in selected procedures, such as bilateral myringotomy. Intramuscular and epidural administration may also be helpful in certain settings.

Methadone, due to its long-acting pharmacokinetic profile and NMDA receptor antagonism, may be helpful in alleviating severe postoperative pain. Methadone is available in both oral and intravenous formulations. Methadone should be avoided in patients at risk for QT prolongation.

## REFERENCES

1. Schechter W. Approach to the management of acute perioperative pain in infants and children. In: Post T, ed. *UpToDate*. Waltham, MA: UpToDate; 2020.
2. Schechter W. Pharmacological management of acute perioperative pain in infants and children. In: Post T, ed. *UpToDate*. Waltham, MA: UpToDate; 2020.
3. Zhu A, et al. Evidence for the efficacy of systemic opioid-sparing analgesics in pediatric surgical populations. *Anesth Analg.* 2017;125(5):1569–1587.
4. Schnabel A, et al. Efficacy and safety of intraoperative dexmedetomidine for acute postoperative pain in children: a meta-analysis of randomized controlled trials. *Pediatr Anesth.* 2012;23(2):170–179.
5. Hemmings HC, Egan TD. *Pharmacology and Physiology for Anesthesia: Foundations and Clinical Application*. Philadelphia, PA: Elsevier; 2019.

# 277.

# REGIONAL TECHNIQUES

*Alina Lazar*

## INTRODUCTION

Regional anesthesia (RA) provides excellent analgesia while decreasing exposure to opioids and general anesthetic agents and their associated side effects, suppresses the stress response, provides better hemodynamic stability compared to general anesthesia, and can prevent long-term behavioral responses to pain. Pediatric RA has proved to be safe despite being done under general anesthesia or deep sedation.[1] Systemic local anesthetic (LA) toxicity is more likely to occur in infants than in adults because of low protein binding and decreased intrinsic clearance. LA should be based on the patient's age, ideal body weight, surgical procedure, and desired duration of analgesia and should not exceed recommended dosage (Table 277.1).[2] Adjuvants (epinephrine, clonidine or dexmedetomidine, and intravenous dexamethasone) prolong the duration of RA. The use of clonidine in infants younger than 3 months is controversial because of a hypothesized risk of apnea in this age group.

## CENTRAL NEURAXIAL TECHNIQUES

A *caudal block* is performed in children, usually 5 years and younger, who undergo surgery in the lower extremities and infraumbilical area. A styletted needle with a blunt tip is advanced through the sacrococcygeal ligament into the caudal space. A "pop" is felt as the needle penetrates the ligament. Contraindications to caudal anesthesia in children include local site infection and spinal dysraphism. The duration of the caudal block depends on the volume of LA and is typically 4 to 6 hours. Depending on the volume of LA (bupivacaine and ropivacaine with epinephrine 1:200,000), the block can extend from the sacral area (0.5 mL/kg) to the lumbar and low thoracic area (1–1.5 mL/kg, maximum of 30 mL). Clonidine prolongs the block duration by 4 hours, while dexmedetomidine extends it by a factor of 2.5–3. Morphine not only prolongs the block duration but also causes ileus, postoperative nausea/vomiting, pruritus, and delayed-onset respiratory depression.

*Table 277.1* MAXIMUM AND USUAL DOSES OF LOCAL ANESTHETIC RECOMMENDED BY THE AMERICAN SOCIETY OF REGIONAL ANESTHESIA AND PAIN MEDICINE (ASRA)/EUROPEAN SOCIETY OF REGIONAL ANESTHESIA (ESRA) FOR PEDIATRIC REGIONAL ANESTHESIA

| | BUPIVACAINE ROPIVACAINE | CHLOROPROCAINE |
|---|---|---|
| Epidural single injection (mg/kg) | 1.7 | 30–45 |
| Epidural continuous infusion (mg/kg/h) | 0.2 (<3 months old) 0.3 (3 months–1 year) 0.4 (>1 year old) | 0.2 (<3 months old) 0.3 (3 months–1 year) 0.5 (>1 year old) |
| Upper and lower extremity nerve blocks, single injection (mg/kg) | 0.5–1.5 | Not used |
| Upper and lower extremity nerve blocks, continuous infusion (mg/kg/h) | 0.1–0.3 | Not used |
| Fascial plane blocks, single injection (mg/kg) | 0.25–0.75 | Not used |
| Fascial plane blocks, continuous infusion (mg/kg/h) | 0.1–0.3 | Not used |

From Reference 2.

**Table 277.2** RECOMMENDED DOSES OF ADJUVANTS FOR PEDIATRIC EPIDURAL ANALGESIA

| MEDICATION | INITIAL BOLUS | INFUSION SOLUTION | INFUSION LIMITS |
|---|---|---|---|
| Fentanyl | 1–2 mg/kg | 2–5 mg/mL | 0.5–2 mg/kg/h |
| Morphine | 10–30 mg/kg | 5–10 mg/mL | 1–5 mg/kg/h |
| Hydromorphone | 2–6 mg/kg | 2–5 mg/mL | 1–2.5 mg/kg/h |
| Clonidine | 1–2 mg/kg | 0.5–1 mg/mL | 0.5–1 mg/kg/h |

*Epidural catheters* can be placed directly or, in infants, inserted in the caudal space and threaded cephalad to the desired dermatome. In infants, the tip of the conus medullaris and dural sac is lower than in adults (L3 and S4, respectively), thus increasing the risk of dural puncture or spinal cord injury. There is a more subtle "give" as the ligamentum flavum is pierced. Generally, the epidural space is found at 1 mm/kg of body weight, but variations exist. Loss of resistance to saline is recommended to avoid massive air embolism. Epidural anesthesia is contraindicated in children with coagulopathy, skin infection at the insertion site, bacteremia, and lack of consent. A ventriculoperitoneal shunt is a relative contraindication. Because of LA age and weight limitations, the precise placement of the catheter at the surgical dermatome should be verified in infants by radiologic, ultrasound, or nerve-stimulating techniques. Epidural analgesic and adjuvant doses are listed in Tables 277.1 and 277.2. Possible complications of epidural analgesia are bleeding, infection, and spinal cord injury. Hypotension is infrequent in children younger than 8 years.

Spinal anesthesia is mostly indicated in the sick neonate or preterm babies to avoid postoperative apnea and hypotension associated with general anesthesia.[3] Hyperbaric or isobaric bupivacaine (0.5 mg/kg) is the most common choice. Compared to adults, spinal blockade in infants is less dense and has a shorter duration and a higher failure rate. It is associated with remarkable hemodynamic stability.

A *paravertebral block* is used for thoracic and abdominal surgery. It is less likely to cause hypotension from sympathectomy when placed unilaterally and has an efficacy comparable to epidural anesthesia without the risk of spinal cord injury.

Truncal blocks are easier to place and safer than epidural and paravertebral blocks, but less potent. They are particularly useful in patients with spinal abnormalities or abnormal coagulation and as a component to multimodal analgesia. They provide somatic analgesia to the thoracic and abdominal wall and possibly visceral analgesia (erector spinae plane and quadratus lumborum blocks).[4]

The *erector spinae plane* block can be placed in the plane between the erector spinae muscles and spinal transverse process. It targets the dorsal and lateral branches of the spinal nerves, but paravertebral, and even epidural, spread has been reported. It has been used for a variety of thoracoabdominal procedures, as either a single-shot or continuous technique.

Depending on the site of placement (lateral, posterior, subcostal), the transversus abdominus plane (TAP) block provides analgesia to the anterior infraumbilical, anterior and lateral infraumbilical, and anterior supraumbilical areas of the upper abdomen, respectively. The quadratus lumborum block, placed at the lateral, posterior, or anterior border of the quadratus lumborum muscle, provides superior and longer duration analgesia compared to the TAP block, in the T8–L1 dermatomes depending on the location of the block.

The rectus sheath blocks are effective for midline abdominal incisions in umbilical hernia, laparoscopic appendectomy, and cholecystectomy.

The ilioinguinal/iliohypogastric block provides equivalent quality but longer duration of analgesia compared to caudal block to the inguinal area and anterior scrotum.

The pudendal nerve innervates the penis, scrotum, and perineum. In circumcision and hypospadias repair, the pudendal nerve block provides better analgesia of longer duration than caudal analgesia and without urinary retention or leg weakness.

As for peripheral nerve blocks of the upper and lower extremities, in children brachial plexus blockade can be done via axillary, infraclavicular, interscalene, and supraclavicular approaches, the latter being the most frequently used. Lower extremity blocks include lumbar plexus, fascia iliaca, femoral, sciatic, and saphenous or adductor canal blocks.[5]

## REFERENCES

1. Polaner DM, et al. Pediatric Regional Anesthesia Network (PRAN): a multi-institutional study of the use and incidence of complications of pediatric regional anesthesia. *Anesth Analg.* 2012;1156:1353–1364.
2. Suresh S, et al. The European Society of Regional Anaesthesia and Pain Therapy/American Society of Regional Anesthesia and Pain Medicine recommendations on local anesthetics and adjuvants dosage in pediatric regional anesthesia. *Reg Anesth Pain Med.* 2018;43(2):211–216.
3. Boretsky KR. A review of regional anesthesia in infants. *Paediatr Drugs.* 2019;21(6):439–449.
4. Visoiu M. Paediatric regional anaesthesia: a current perspective. *Curr Opin Anaesthesiol.* 2015;28(5):577–582.
5. Shah RD, Suresh S. Applications of regional anaesthesia in paediatrics. *Br J Anaesth.* 2013;111(suppl 1):i114–i124.

# 278.

# PEDIATRIC MANAGEMENT OF POSTOPERATIVE NAUSEA AND VOMITING

*Lisgelia Santana*

## INTRODUCTION

The incidence of postoperative nausea and vomiting (PONV) in children is high, as it is estimated to be between 33.2% and 82% depending on patient risk factors.[1] PONV typically describes nausea, vomiting, or retching that can occur starting in the postanesthesia care unit (PACU) and continuing up to 24 hours after surgery. Postdischarge nausea and vomiting includes symptoms that persist for up to 7 days after anesthesia. PONV occurs twice as often in children than in adults and can lead to delays in hospital discharge, readmission, longer PACU stays, and a significant financial burden. The syndrome of nausea, vomiting, and dehydration is one of the leading causes of pediatric readmissions, accounting for 51.2% of such cases.[2]

A wide range of antiemetic regimens is recommended for the prevention and treatment of PONV in children, including pharmacotherapy with corticosteroids, 5-HT$_3$ (5-hydroxytryptamine, serotonin) antagonists, prokinetics, butyrophenones, antihistamines, and anticholinergics.

## RISK FACTORS

Various independent risk factors have been implicated in the development of pediatric PONV. In a multicenter study of 1257 children, the following major risk factors were identified: history of PONV in the child or immediate relatives (parents or siblings), age 3 years or older, duration of surgery more than 30 minutes, and strabismus surgery. It is estimated that the risk of developing PONV is 9%, 10%, 30%, 55%, and 70% depending on the presence of 0, 1, 2, 3, or 4 risk factors, respectively[3] (Table 278.1).

Various surgeries are associated with a higher risk of developing PONV, including tonsillectomy, adenoidectomy, and strabismus surgery. One study found that PONV rates were as high as 82% in pediatric patients undergoing tonsillectomy, and another reported PONV rates of 54% in children undergoing strabismus surgery.[3] Several agents are used for the treatment of PONV (Table 278.2)

To guide pediatric PONV prophylaxis, Bourdaud et al.[4] created a risk-predictive scoring model for vomiting in the postoperative period (Table 278.3).

## ANESTHETIC CONSIDERATIONS

### PREOPERATIVE

A major factor that may influence the incidence of PONV is preoperative fasting. The purpose of fasting is to reduce the volume of gastric contents and thus lower risk of aspiration.

*Table 278.1* RISK FACTORS FOR PONV IN PEDIATRIC PATIENTS

| Surgical factors | Strabismus surgery |
| | Duration greater than 30 minutes |
| | Ear, nose, and throat surgery |
| Anesthetic management | Use of opioids |
| | Increased postoperative pain |
| | Use of volatile anesthetic |
| Patient risk factors | Dehydration |
| | 3 years old or older |
| | Immediate family history of PONV |
| | Prolonged preoperative fast |

*Table 278.2* PHARMACOLOGICAL MANAGEMENT

| DRUG CLASS | MECHANISM OF ACTION | ADVERSE EFFECTS | DOSE AND TIME OF ADMINISTRATION |
|---|---|---|---|
| Corticosteroid<br>1. Dexamethasone | Thought to act on glucocorticoid receptors; ability to reduce local inflammatory reactions after surgery | Tumor lysis syndrome, hyperglycemia, increased postoperative infection risk, and cancer recurrence | 150 µg/kg up to 8 mg IV; drug administered immediately before or after induction of anesthesia instead of after surgery |
| 5-HT$_3$ Antagonist<br>1. Ondansetron<br>2. Granisetron<br>3. Dolasetron | Antagonizing the action of serotonin in the 5-HT$_3$ receptor-rich areas of the brain | Headache, dizziness, elevated liver enzymes, constipation, diarrhea, arrhythmias, and QT prolongation | Ondansetron:<br>a. 100 µg/kg or maximum 4 mg IV<br>b. 8 mg oral<br>c. Administer at the end of surgery<br>Granisetron:<br>a. 0.35 to 3 mg IV (5–20 µg/kg)<br>b. Administer at the end of surgery<br>Dolasetron:<br>a. 12.5 mg IV at the end of surgery or at the time of induction |
| Butyrophenone<br>1. Droperidol | Potent centrally acting D$_2$ receptor antagonist | Drowsiness, sedation, headaches; rare extrapyramidal symptoms; black box warning of sudden cardiac death | 50 µg/kg IV 30 minutes before the end of surgery |
| Prokinetics<br>1. Metoclopramide | Peripheral and central (basal ganglia) dopamine receptor antagonist | Extrapyramidal symptoms, sedation, diarrhea; rare apnea, anaphylaxis, respiratory distress or arrest, galactorrhea, gynecomastia, urinary retention, and priapism | 0.1 to 0.5 mg/kg IV |
| Anticholinergics<br>1. Scopolamine | Competitive smooth muscle muscarinic antagonist; percutaneous absorption; detected in plasma within 4 hours of patch application | Sedation, dry mouth, vision changes, decreased gastric motility, and delayed gastric emptying; caution with other anticholinergics (antihistamine, tricyclic, muscle relaxant) | 0.25–0.75 mg via a transdermal patch |
| Antihistamines<br>1. Dimenhydrinate<br>2. Hydroxyzine<br>3. Diphenhydramine | Reversible H$_1$ receptor inhibition; more commonly used for motion sickness | Sedation, CYP450 inhibitor, dry mouth, constipation, confusion, blurry vision, urine retention | 0.5 mg/kg, up to 25 mg IV<br>2 mg/kg/d orally<br>1.1 mg/kg IM |

The preoperative intake of a carbohydrate-rich fluid or carbohydrate loading has also been suggested as a method to reduce PONV.

## INTRAOPERATIVE

It is important for clinicians to try to use different techniques to minimize the risk of PONV in their patients. One such strategy is to avoid the use of volatile anesthetics in favor of total intravenous anesthesia (TIVA) with propofol during the intraoperative period. This change alone can reduce the rate of PONV by as much as 25%. Nonopioid, multimodal pain management for postoperative pain control is also important to prevent PONV. It has been shown that using caudal blocks for regional anesthesia in patients undergoing renal, bladder, or ureteral procedures reduced PONV and was associated with lower use of opioids and rescue antiemetics.[5] Nitrous oxide has also been associated with PONV and is recommended to be avoided in patients at an increased risk for developing PONV. A combination of most 5-HT$_3$ antagonists with dexamethasone offers effective emesis risk reduction and is supported for use in children. One article proposed the use of monotherapy for small surgeries or minimal PONV predictive risk and multimodal prophylaxis in patients with moderate-to-high risk.[5]

## POSTOPERATIVE

Acetaminophen and nonsteroidal anti-inflammatory drugs are used to manage postoperative pain in the pediatric population. Consider prokinetics and antihistamine for rescue management of PONV.

*Table 278.3* VOMITING IN THE POSTOPERATIVE PERIOD SCORING SYSTEM

| | |
|---|---|
| Age | 0 point < or equal to 3 years<br>1 point > 3 years and < 6 years<br>2 points > or equal to 6 years and less than or equal to 13 years |
| Duration of anesthesia | 0 point < 45 minutes<br>1 point > 45 minutes |
| Surgery at risk | 1 point for tonsillectomy, tympanoplasty, strabismus surgery<br>0 point other surgeries |
| Predisposition to PONV | 0 point no<br>1 point yes |
| Multiple opioid doses | 0 point no<br>1 point yes |
| Scoring and percentage incidence | 0 = 5% for 0–1 low risk<br>1 = 6%<br>2 = 13% for 2–3 moderate risk<br>3 = 21%<br>4= 36% > 4 high risk<br>5 = 48%<br>6 = 52% |

## REFERENCES

1. Eberhart LHJ, et al. Applicability of risk scores for postoperative nausea and vomiting in adults to paediatric patients. *Br J Anaesth.* 2004;93:386–392.
2. Edler AA, et al. An analysis of factors influencing postanesthesia recovery after pediatric ambulatory tonsillectomy and adenoidectomy. *Anesth Analg.* 2007;104:784–789.
3. Eberhart LHJ, et al. The development and validation of a risk score to predict the probability of postoperative vomiting in pediatric patients. *Anesth Analg.* 2004;99:1630–1637.
4. Bourdaud N, et al. Development and validation of a risk score to predict the probability of postoperative vomiting in pediatric patients: the VPOP score. *Paediatr Anaesth.* 2014;24:945–952.
5. Gan TJJ, et al. Consensus guidelines for the management of postoperative nausea and vomiting. *Anesth Analg.* 2014;118:85–113.

# 279.

# PEDIATRIC SEDATION

*Kasia Rubin*

## PATIENT SELECTION

Careful patient selection is critical to maintaining excellent outcomes for pediatric sedation. A careful presedation assessment is needed to determine whether the patient has specific risk factors that may increase the chance of adverse events. In addition to a standard preoperative assessment, focusing on abnormalities of cardiac, pulmonary, renal, and hepatic systems, particular attention to current or recent upper respiratory tract infections must be emphasized. The presence of an upper respiratory tract infection within the past 2 weeks significantly increased the risk of airway events in large-scale studies of pediatric procedural sedations. Airway concerns, especially those suggestive of difficult mask ventilation such as snoring, may indicate that sedation without airway protection would be unacceptable as respiratory-related adverse events are the most significant risks in pediatric sedation.[1–3]

## PREOPERATIVE SEDATION

Preoperative anxiolysis often requires preoperative sedation in the pediatric patient, despite the best attempts of the staff to address fears and provide reassurance. Given that children come to the preoperative holding area without a preoperative consultation and without intravenous access, such premedication often needs to be administered via nonintravenous routes. The ideal anxiolytic will provide effective and reliable anxiolysis with minimal discomfort on administration, a rapid onset of action without prolongation of recovery time, and no respiratory depression. Midazolam is the most commonly administered premedication and is considered the gold standard via oral administration when intravenous access is unavailable. In healthy children, no cardiac or respiratory depression occurs. Nasal administration via an atomizer also provides effective anxiolysis but is very irritating to the nasal mucosa, producing discomfort and a crying child. Ketamine may be administered orally or via the intramuscular route, although it prolongs recovery from anesthesia, and there is a high incidence of minor adverse effects, including nystagmus, random limb movements, and tongue fasciculation.[4] Dexmedetomidine also provides an excellent level of sedation with nasal administration, providing a sedation that mimics natural sleep patterns with minimal respiratory depression effects.[1]

## LEVEL OF SEDATION

Sedation level may be divided into categories ranging from minimal sedation, or anxiolysis, to deep sedation and general anesthesia. The principle differences are described in terms of level of consciousness, ability to maintain a patent airway, ability to maintain spontaneous ventilation, and the effects of the sedation medications on cardiovascular function. It is recognized that sedation exists along a continuum, rather than in separate categories, and the potential for inducing general anesthesia always exists, as described in Table 279.1.[2]

The end goal of sedation may be achieved with a variety of medications, many of which are familiar to the anesthesiologist as part of a general anesthesia armamentarium.

## RISKS OF SEDATION

Both oversedation and inadequate sedation may occur. Inadequate sedation may not allow the procedure to be completed and cause injury to self or caregivers. Concerns associated with oversedation include respiratory depression, cardiovascular depression, aspiration, loss of protective airway reflexes, and hemodynamic instability. A plan for increased intensity of care is necessary in any place where sedation is provided. Adequate monitoring aids in early detection of adverse events and immediate action can be taken. Monitoring pulmonary function via observation and auscultation is sufficient in a patient who maintains purposeful responses to gentle stimulation, but monitoring of exhaled carbon dioxide is critical in deeper levels of sedation as it can provide early detection of respiratory depression, loss of airway, and aspiration.[2] End-tidal $CO_2$ monitoring allows for immediate escalation of care. Blood oxygen saturation is appropriate with pulse oximetry, and early detection of changes of heart rate and blood pressure allow the anesthesiologist to detect problems in a timely fashion.

## POSTSEDATION RECOVERY

Following moderate or deeper levels of sedation, the patient must be observed in an environment with adequate suction apparatus, oxygen, and positive pressure ventilation. Vital signs and level of consciousness must be monitored. Recovery is considered complete when the patient is awake and oriented. Simple evaluation tools should provide observation-based evaluation of level of sedation and ensure appropriate discharge criteria. Regardless of which discharge tool is utilized, the patient should have stable vital signs, adequate analgesia, and minimal nausea/vomiting.[5]

*Table 279.1* DIFFERENT LEVELS OF SEDATION

| | MINIMAL SEDATION ANXIOLYSIS | MODERATE SEDATION/ANALGESIA ("CONSCIOUS SEDATION") | DEEP SEDATION/ANALGESIA | GENERAL ANESTHESIA |
|---|---|---|---|---|
| Responsiveness | Normal response to verbal stimulation | Purposeful** response to verbal or tactile stimulation | Purposeful** response following repeated or painful stimulation | Unarousable even with painful stimulus |
| Airway | Unaffected | No intervention required | Intervention may be required | Intervention often required |
| Spontaneous ventilation | Unaffected | Adequate | May be inadequate | Frequently inadequate |
| Cardiovascular function | Unaffected | Usually maintained | Usually maintained | May be impaired |

## REFERENCES

1. Mason KP, Seth N. The pearls of pediatric sedation: polish the old and embrace the new. *Minerva Anestesiol.* 2019;85(10):1105–1117.
2. Cote CJ, Wilson S. Guidelines for monitoring and management of pediatric patients before, during, and after sedation for diagnostic and therapeutic procedures. *Pediatrics.* 2019;143(6):e20191000.
3. ASAHQ continuum of depth of sedation. Last amended October 23, 2019.
4. Tripi P. Preoperative anxiolysis and sedation. In: Kaye AD, et al., eds. *Essentials of Pediatric Anesthesiology.* Cambridge University Press, Cambridge, UK; 2015.
5. Ead H. From Aldrete to PADSS: reviewing discharge criteria after ambulatory surgery. J Perianesth Nurs. 2006;21(4):259–267.

# 280.

# PEDIATRIC ANESTHESIA OUTSIDE THE OPERATING ROOM

*Hannah Masters and Christina D. Diaz*

## INTRODUCTION

Over the last several decades, the number of diagnostic and therapeutic procedures has significantly increased, necessitating a higher volume of anesthetics performed in environments outside of the operating room (OOR). Advancements in technology enable greater diagnostic capabilities with computed tomography (CT), magnetic resonance imaging (MRI), and nuclear medicine, as well as therapeutic interventions with interventional radiology (IR) and radiation therapy. Procedural sites are utilized for endoscopies, lumbar punctures or bone marrow aspirates, and burn dressing changes.[1,2]

## COMPUTED TOMOGRAPHY

Computed tomographic images are useful for fractures and head trauma to assess for mass effect and acute bleeding. Compared to plain radiographs, CT is associated with higher radiation exposure, and safety measures should be taken for the patient and all providers. The goal is to maximize distance between the provider and scanner as appropriate and shield the patient as appropriate. Regulations recently changed with new CT scanners limiting the radiation exposure; therefore, not all patients require shielding. Older children and recently fed and swaddled infants can often remain still long enough with minimal-to-no sedation. Toddlers and preschool-aged children often require sedation.[3,4]

Intravenous contrast is often used for CT imaging. Low osmolar agents (Omnipaque) exhibit lower rates of adverse reactions and allergy (about 1–2 in 10,000) compared to high osmolar agents (1 in 1000) such as Hypaque and Conray. Potential complications include extravasation, mild allergic reactions with vomiting and hives, or more severe reactions resulting in anaphylaxis with bronchospasm, facial or airway swelling, hypotension, seizures, or cardiac arrest. Observation and administration of an antihistamine are indicated for mild reactions, with the addition of steroids and bronchodilators for moderate reactions. Providers should have appropriate medications and equipment to provide pediatric advanced life support for severe reactions as indicated. Additional precautions should be taken in patients with renal insufficiency, such as additional intravenous fluids or a lower total dose of contrast. Pregnancy tests should be obtained for all postmenarchal female patients. Oral contrast is used for gastrointestinal imaging of the stomach and small intestines and can negate fasting status.

## MAGNETIC RESONANCE IMAGING

Magnetic resonance imaging utilizes magnetic fields and radio-frequency pulses to orient hydrogen protons to generate images; therefore, there is no radiation exposure. MRI is employed for detailed assessments of soft tissues or vasculature, and the scan duration is often significantly longer than CT. All providers working with MRI technology need to understand magnetic safety concerns and take the necessary precautions. MRI contraindications include ferromagnetic vascular clips, metallic foreign bodies, and ventricular assist devices. It is important to note the magnet is *always on*, even when the scanner is not actively being used. There are four MRI safety zones defined by proximity to the MRI scanner magnet. Screening for ferromagnetic objects occurs when interfacing in zone 2, with restricted access to zones 3 and 4. For patient emergencies, the priority is to remove the patient from the scanner to zone 1 or 2 to allow for appropriate resuscitation (Table 280.1).[5]

All equipment must be MRI safe or "conditional," including electrocardiography leads, anesthesia machines, pulse oximetry probes, and intravenous pumps. The distance between the scanner and control room may require intravenous extensions. Monitors must be easily visible, as direct visualization of the patient is typically difficult. During MRI scanning, loud noises are generated, and patients should have ear protection. Claustrophobia can hinder image acquisition without sedation or general anesthesia. The patient must remain motionless for a prolonged period of time, which can impact one's anesthetic choice depending on patient age, developmental stage, and comorbidities.

## INTERVENTIONAL RADIOLOGY

Interventional radiology procedures include vascular interventions such as angiograms, sclerotherapy, coiling procedures, or central venous line (CVL) placement, as well as lumbar punctures, drain placement, and tumor or solid-organ biopsies. Unique considerations include the proceduralist's needs for immobility, prone positioning, or breath holds, which often necessitate general endotracheal

*Table 280.1* MRI ZONES

| | |
|---|---|
| Zone 1 | Public access. No precautions. |
| Zone 2 | Semirestricted. Patients and staff can interact (e.g., reception area, dressing room). |
| Zone 3 | Completely and physically restricted from non-MRI personnel and the general public (e.g., control room, computer room). |
| Zone 4 | The magnet room. Always contained within zone 3. |

anesthesia. These procedures may also be stimulating or painful and require treatment by the anesthesiologist. Cerebral angiograms in particular warrant minimization of extreme hemodynamic changes due to the risk of stroke or hemorrhage. Due to significant radiation exposure, the use of shields and maximization of distance from the radiation source should be utilized by the patient and all providers.

## NUCLEAR MEDICINE

Nuclear medicine helps determine the extent of neoplasms, infections, and epileptic foci in refractory seizures. Positron electron tomography (PET) involves the injection of radionuclide tracers of glucose metabolism, requiring peripheral intravenous access prior to the procedure for tracer administration. The tracer's half-life is about 110 minutes, requiring the scan within an hour of administration. For single-photon emission computed tomography (SPECT) to map an epileptic focus, radio-labeled technetium 99m with a half-life of 6.5 hours is injected during a seizure. Therefore, the scan must occur within 1–6 hours from time of injection. Neither PET nor SPECT are painful procedures.

## RADIATION THERAPY

Pediatric patients with cancers including Wilms tumor, retinoblastoma, and acute leukemias and lymphomas may undergo radiation therapy using an external beam of ionizing photons or brachytherapy. Anesthesia is often required for this patient population to tolerate the use of immobilizers/masks and enable them to remain motionless. No one other than the patient may remain in the room during a treatment.

## OTHER OOR ENVIRONMENTS

Procedure rooms are sometimes utilized by gastroenterologists for endoscopies. Unique considerations include abnormal gastric motility, aspiration risk following insufflation of the stomach, as well as the risk of tracheal compression in infants by the endoscope. Oncologists utilize procedure rooms for lumbar punctures and bone marrow aspirates. Oncology patients are often severely immunocompromised, requiring heightened infection precautions, particularly if accessing a CVL. Procedure rooms can also be used for burn dressing changes; an increased room temperature is imperative to diminish increased evaporative losses. A paucity of intact skin surface area can make placing standard monitors difficult. Auditory brainstem response testing is often performed OOR and requires anesthesia for older infants and children to remain still for the duration of the procedure (Table 280.2).

*Table 280.2* SUMMARY OF OOR PROCEDURES AND KEY POINTS

| PROCEDURE | LENGTH | MAJOR ANESTHETIC CONSIDERATIONS | COMPLICATIONS |
|---|---|---|---|
| CT | 15–30 minutes | Significant radiation exposure<br>Oral contrast can negate fasting status; consider rapid sequence induction followed by nasogastric tube placement. | Oral contrast: aspiration, pneumonitis, pulmonary edema<br>Intravenous contrast: allergic reaction, avoid in hyperthyroidism |
| MRI | 30–90 minutes | The magnet is always on.<br>Use MRI safe/conditional devices and equipment. | Projectile ferromagnetic objects in zone 4<br>Potential burns from looped wires left on the patient |
| IR | Variable | Significant radiation exposure. Avoid major hemodynamic swings with cerebral angiograms.<br>Possible breath holds for imaging.<br>May need to treat pain. | Migration of glue/coils<br>Tissue necrosis or agitation/delirium from 99% ethanol |
| Nuclear medicine | 30–60 minutes | Intravenous for tracer preprocedure.<br>Radioactive tracer expelled in urine. | |
| Gastroenterology | 30–90 minutes | Upper endoscopy can compress airway if < 1 year or < 10 kg.<br>ERCP lazy lateral or prone position. | Hypotension from bowel prep<br>Methemoglobinemia can occur with topical benzocaine |
| Radiation therapy | Variable | Pain free; may notice unpleasant smell.<br>Shielded room and use of stereotactic head frame/positioning devices. | Patient monitored via camera can delay interventions<br>Only patient present in a sealed room during treatment |

ERCP—Endoscopic retrograde cholangiopancreatography.

# REFERENCES

1. Coté CJ, Wilson S; American Academy of Pediatrics et al. Guidelines for monitoring and management of pediatric patients before, during, and after sedation for diagnostic and therapeutic procedures: update 2016. *Pediatrics*. 2016;138(1): e20161212

2. Kaplan RF, Yang CI. Sedation and analgesia in pediatric patients for procedures outside the operating room. *Anesthesiol Clin North Am*. 2002;20(1):181–194, vii

3. Gregory GA, Andropoulos DB. *Gregory's Pediatric Anesthesia*. 5th ed. Chichester, UK: Wiley-Blackwell; 2012. https://ebookcentral.proquest.com/lib/mcwlibraries-ebooks/reader.action?docID=822637

4. Allison DJ, Grainger RG. *Grainger & Allison's Diagnostic Radiology: A Textbook of Medical Imaging*. 6th ed. (Adam A, et al., eds.). Edinburgh, Scotland: Churchill Livingstone/Elsevier; 2015. https://www-clinicalkey-com.proxy.lib.mcw.edu/#!/browse/book/3-s2.0-C20091628458

5. Kanal E, et al. ACR guidance document on MR safe practices: 2013. *J Magn Reson Imaging*. 2013;37: 501–530.

# Part 21
# OBSTETRIC ANESTHESIA

# 281.

# MATERNAL PHYSIOLOGY

*Nimit K. Shah and Piotr Al-Jindi*

## INTRODUCTION

There are various anatomical and physiological changes in pregnancy to meet the increased metabolic needs of a growing fetus.[1]

## PHYSIOLOGIC CHANGES DURING PREGNANCY

### CARDIOVASCULAR SYSTEM

Cardiac output (CO) begins to increase by 35%–40% by the end of the first trimester and 50% by the end of the second trimester.[2] It remains unchanged in the third trimester. The initial increase is from an increase in heart rate (HR), which increases by 15%–25% (stroke volume [SV] increases by 20%) by the end of the first trimester and then remains relatively unchanged during the remaining pregnancy. SV increases by 25%–30% above baseline during the second trimester. CO further increases during labor: 10%–25% during the first stage, 40% in the second stage, and 80%–100% after delivery.[2] Normal pregnant patients can sustain this enormous increase in the CO, but pregnant patients with heart disease may decompensate.

Plasma volume (PV) increases by 50% by 34 weeks and then either stabilizes or decreases slightly. This is due to the stimulation of the renin-angiotensin system (RAS) by progesterone, leading to sodium and water reabsorption.[2] Red blood cell (RBC) count increases by 30% at term. The relative increase of PV over RBC volume typically causes the *physiological anemia of pregnancy*[3] with hemoglobin around 11.6.

Systolic, diastolic, and mean arterial pressure (MAP) decrease by 5%–20% by 20 weeks, then gradually increase toward prepregnancy values by term.[2] This is due to the vasodilatory effects of progesterone and low-resistance uteroplacental vascular bed. Peripheral vascular resistance decreases by 35%. Central venous pressure and pulmonary capillary wedge pressure remain unchanged despite an increase in intravascular PV because of venous capacitance increases.

## SUPINE HYPOTENSION SYNDROME

The gravid uterus compresses both the inferior vena cava (IVC) and aorta significantly from the 20th week, which can lead to supine hypotension syndrome SHS in about 10% of patients when they lie supine. SHS is defined as a decrease in MAP greater than 15 mm hg and an increase in HR greater than 20 beats/min when supine[2] and is often accompanied by sweating, nausea, vomiting, and changes in mentation. IVC compression decreases venous return and therefore CO and blood pressure. This can decrease fetal blood supply and lead to fetal acidosis, which is further worsened by aortal compression (placental perfusion is dependent on perfusion pressure). Most patients have compensatory mechanisms, such as increased sympathetic activity, which leads to an increase in HR and SVR and maintaining adequate CO. Patients who receive neuraxial or general anesthesia (GA) may have impaired sympathetic response and may develop SHS.

## RESPIRATORY SYSTEM CHANGES

Minute ventilation increases by 45%–50% in the first trimester and remains elevated throughout the pregnancy.[2] This is due to increased tidal volumes due to the progesterone sensitization of central chemoreceptors, increasing the ventilatory response to $CO_2$. Maternal $PaCO_2$ decreases from 40 mm Hg to approximately 30 mm Hg during the first trimester.

| Arterial Blood Gas Values | Pregnancy | Nonpregnancy |
|---|---|---|
| $PaO_2$ | 103 | 100 |
| $PaCO_2$ | 30 | 40 |
| $HCO_3$ | 20 | 24 |
| pH | 7.44 | 7.4 |
| P50 | 30 | 27 |

Oxygen consumption increases from 40% to 60%. The gravid uterus pushes the diaphragm cephalad, which decreases the functional residual capacity (FRC) by 20% in the standing position and 30% in the supine position at term (expiratory reserve volume and residual volume are equally reduced).

## GASTROINTESTINAL SYSTEM

In the gastrointestinal system, the stomach is pushed cephalad by the gravid uterus, which pushes the intra-abdominal portion of the esophagus into the chest and decreases the competence of the LES. The LES tone is reduced by progesterone, and estrogen and intragastric pressures are elevated due to pressure from the gravid uterus, which further reduces the lower esophageal barrier pressure. Gastric volume is increased and gastric pH is decreased due to gastrin secreted from the placenta.[2]

## HEPATIC SYSTEM

In the hepatic system, the albumin concentration decreases, and this can result in elevated free levels of highly protein-bound drugs. The globulin level increases to 10% at term, and the total protein and albumin/globulin ratio (A/G) ratio decreases from 1.4 to 0.9. Plasma cholinesterase activity is decreased by approximately 25%–30% beginning from the 10th week of gestation to 6 weeks' postpartum but is not commonly associated with the prolongation of a neuromuscular block by succinylcholine.

## RENAL SYSTEM

Renal blood flow increases by 60%–80% due to an increase in CO. The glomerular filtration rate increases by 50%. This increases clearance of creatinine, urea, and uric acid, and their levels are reduced by 40%.

## HEMATOLOGY SYSTEM

For the hematology system, pregnancy is a hypercoagulable state. The risk of venous thromboembolism is 10-fold during pregnancy and 25-fold during the postpartum period. The concentrations of factors I, VII, VIII, IX, X, XII, and von Willebrand factor increase. Factors II and V remain unchanged; factors XI and XIII decrease. Fibrinogen levels increase and, at term, are more than 400 mg/dL. Normal D-dimer in pregnancy can be as high as 500–1700 ng/mL compared to less than 500 ng/mL in nonpregnant patients. The levels of antithrombin III and protein S are decreased, whereas the levels of protein C remain unchanged.

## CENTRAL NERVOUS SYSTEM

In the central nervous system, the MAC 50 (minimum alveolar concentration in 50% of subjects) is reduced by about 30%–40% in pregnant patients. Inhalational induction is faster because of increased minute ventilation (MV) and decreased FRC.

## ANESTHETIC CONSIDERATIONS

### PREOPERATIVE

Preoperatively, all patients are considered at risk of aspiration and hence should receive sodium citrate 15–30 minutes before induction. An H$_2$ blocker and a prokinetic agent are also given. There is a higher incidence of difficult mask ventilation and difficult intubation in pregnant patients (1 in 250–300). The time of the last dose of thromboprophylaxis should be checked before commencing a neuraxial block.

### INTRAOPERATIVE

Intraoperatively, neuraxial blocks should be preferred to GA for the risk of aspiration and difficult intubation. The dose of local anesthetic for neuraxial blocks should be reduced by 25%–40% as there is a contraction of epidural space and cerebrospinal fluid volume due to IVC compression[2]; for the same reason, there is an increased incidence of bloody taps with epidurals.

Maternal hypotension should be immediately corrected. Several studies have shown phenylephrine ($\alpha$-adrenergic agonist) is effective in preventing hypotension; it also is associated with less fetal acidosis than ephedrine.[4] With GA, these patients desaturate faster on induction, so they should be adequately preoxygenated.[1] Rapid sequence induction with cricoid pressure should be employed for induction. Patients should be tilted 15°–30° to the left to prevent aortocaval compression. The MAC requirement is reduced by 30%–40%.

### POSTOPERATIVE

Postoperatively, patients should be extubated awake. Thromboprophylaxis is routinely prescribed and should be appropriately timed if neuraxial block is used.

## REFERENCES

1. Bedson R, Riccoboni A. Physiology of pregnancy: clinical anaesthetic implications. *Contin Educ Anaesth Crit Care Pain.* 2014;14(2):69–72.
2. Sharpe EE, Arendt KW. Anesthesia for obstetrics,—In: Miller RD, ed. *Anesthesia.* 9 ed. Elsevier; 2020:2006–2040.
3. Gaiser R. Physiologic changes of pregnancy. In: Chestnut DH, et al., eds. *Chestnut's Obstetric Anesthesia: Principles and Practice.* 5th ed. Philadelphia, PA: Elsevier Science, Mosby; 2014:15–36.
4. Cooper DW, et al. Fetal and maternal effects of phenylephrine and ephedrine during spinal anesthesia for cesarean delivery. *Anesthesiology.* 2002;97:1582–1590.

# 282.

# PLACENTA

*Roneisha McLendon*

## INTRODUCTION

The placenta is a very important organ integral to fetal development and primarily responsible for providing oxygen and nutrition. In return, the placenta allows for transfer of deoxygenated blood and fetal waste elimination through the maternal circulation. Deficiencies in placental development and alterations to uteroplacental blood flow can have acute implications affecting fetal viability, as well as far-reaching implications related to cardiovascular health as an adult.[1]

## ANATOMY AND STRUCTURE

Following blastocyst implantation, the placenta begins to develop secondary to blastocyst and trophoblast fusion, which creates the syncytiotrophoblast. The syncytiotrophoblast functions as the metabolically active layer of the placenta with endocrine function as well. The syncytiotrophoblast proliferates via fusion of the cytotrophoblast cells, leading to lacunae formation and trophoblast invasion. Trophoblast invasion is important for decreasing resistance and increasing blood flow through loss of smooth muscle in the spiral arteries. Next, the spiral arteries begin to undergo remodeling in the maternal uterine wall, with resulting arteriovenous connections forming in the lacunae and trophoblast branching to form a network of villous trees filled with maternal blood flow.[2] The ultimate purpose of this chain of events is to develop a low-resistance uterine blood flow system to increase blood flow to the placenta. Any deviation or abnormalities in the placental development of the syncytium or villous maturation and growth can contribute to fetal morbidity or fetal demise.[3] In regard to maternal effects, abnormal trophoblast invasion into the spiral arteries is a severe misstep contributing to preeclampsia.[1]

## CHANGES AND FUNCTION

The placenta evolves as the pregnancy advances, changing to meet the needs of the growing fetus. There are three primary layers in the villous circulation of the placenta, separating maternal and fetal blood circulation[4]:

- Trophoblast layer, composed of the cytotrophoblast and syncytiotrophoblast, which are metabolically active and perform endocrine functions of the placenta
- Basal lamina and fetal connective tissue, which are primarily supportive in function
- Endothelium of fetal capillaries

## UTEROPLACENTAL CIRCULATION

### UTERINE BLOOD FLOW

Uterine blood flow is very important in regulating gas exchange between maternal and fetal circulations and providing nutrients to the placenta and developing fetus. The spiral arteries initiate oxygenated maternal blood flow into the intervillous space, where very important gas exchange occurs as well as exchange of nutrients and waste between the maternal-fetal interface. This oxygenated maternal blood originates from the uterine arteries. The return of blood flow to the maternal circulation is facilitated through the drainage of multiple collecting veins. Within the placenta, the umbilical arteries are what provides the oxygenated, nutrient-rich blood, and after exchange, the blood return occurs via the umbilical vein.[1,5]

## ANESTHETIC DRUG CONSIDERATIONS FOR THE PLACENTA

### NEURAXIAL ANESTHESIA

There are several factors contributing to how neuraxial anesthesia affects uteroplacental blood flow and ultimately fetal perfusion. Pain relief with epidural analgesia decreases the catecholamine release that is associated with the pain of labor and also reduces hyperventilation, which contributes to maintenance of uteroplacental blood flow. Conversely, decreases in uterine blood flow have been attributed to maternal hypotension from sympathectomy associated with epidural or spinal anesthesia, as well as maternal respiratory depression from inadvertent intravenous or intrathecal injection of local anesthetic. The overall observation is that in the absence of hypotension, epidural analgesia either increases or does not change uteroplacental blood flow.[1]

- Hypotension—Neuraxial analgesia–induced hypotension can decrease uteroplacental blood flow due to reduction in perfusion pressure and reflexive release of catecholamines (vasoconstrictors).
- Vasopressors—Many studies showed uteroplacental blood flow is better maintained with ephedrine; however, clinical studies favored the use of phenylephrine for maintaining maternal blood pressure without negatively affecting fetal pH or base excess.
- Local anesthetics—Uteroplacental blood flow is maintained at clinically appropriate doses. However, high concentrations of local anesthetic from inadvertent intravascular injection or paracervical block may decrease uteroplacental flow via vasoconstriction and increased myometrial contractility.
- Opioids—Research studies have observed no significant effect of opioids on uteroplacental blood flow; however, intrathecal opioids have been identified as contributing to fetal bradycardia secondary to an increase in resting uterine tone and a subsequent decrease in uteroplacental blood flow.

## GENERAL ANESTHESIA

- Intravenous induction agents—Many studies exist; the overall finding was that there is minimal effect on uteroplacental blood flow.
- Inhalational anesthetics—For all commonly used inhalational agents, there has been minimal or no effect on uteroplacental blood flow in standard clinical doses.

- Mechanical ventilation—Significant hypoxemia or hypercapnia can reduce uteroplacental blood flow. The overall recommendation is to avoid hyper- and hypoventilation in parturients in an effort to maintain uteroplacental blood flow.[5]

## EFFECTS OF OTHER DRUGS

- Magnesium—This increases uteroplacental blood flow.
- Antihypertensives—Studies have shown varying results, but overall no significant change has been observed.
- Calcium channel blockers—Verapamil decreased uteroplacental blood flow, while nifedipine has shown controversial results.
- Vasodilators—Nitroglycerin studies have shown an increase in uterine artery blood flow that did not necessarily translate to an improvement in uteroplacental blood flow; more studies are needed.
- Inotropes—Dopamine and epinephrine decrease uteroplacental blood flow; milrinone and amrinone can increase uteroplacental blood flow. These drugs are not commonly used in obstetric patients, but when needed for emergency situations of maternal resuscitation or cardiac arrest, effects on uteroplacental blood flow are not the primary concern.[5]

## REFERENCES

1. Chestnut DH, Ngan Kee WD. Uteroplacental blood flow. In: *Chestnut's Obstetric Anesthesia: Principles and Practice*. 6th ed. Philadephia, PA: Elsevier; 2020:38–55.
2. Al-Enazy S, et al. Placental control of drug delivery. *Adv Drug Deliv Rev*. 2017;116:63–72.
3. Resnik R, et al. Normal early development. In: *Creasy and Resnik's Maternal-Fetal Medicine: Principles and Practice*. 7th ed. Philadelphia, PA: Elsevier; 2019:37–46.
4. Kliman HJ. Uteroplacental blood flow: the story of decidualization, menstruation, and trophoblast invasion. *Am J Pathol*. 2000;157(6):1759–1768.
5. Rosen MA, et al. Uteroplacental circulation and respiratory gas exchange. In: *Shnider and Levinson's Anesthesia for Obstetrics*. 4th ed. Lippincott, Williams and Wilkins; 2013:19–40.

# 283.

# DRUGS AND ADJUVANTS

*M. Anthony Cometa and Jordan Thompson*

## VAGINAL DELIVERY: SYSTEMIC MEDICATIONS

Physiologic changes in pregnancy alter the maternal volume of distribution, plasma protein concentrations, and the elimination half-life of intravenous medications (Box 283.1).

### INTRAVENOUS ANALGESIA

Intravenous opioids are commonly used for analgesia during labor. All opioids cross the placenta and can affect fetal heart rate variability.

- **Meperidine:** One of the most common opioids worldwide for the first stage of labor; it has an active

---

**Box 283.1** TAKE-HOME POINTS

1. All intravenous opioids cross the placenta.
2. Meperidine should be used with caution due to its active metabolite, normeperidine.
3. Remifentanil crosses the placenta, but it is rapidly metabolized by the fetus.
4. Neuraxial opioids act at the dorsal horn of the spinal cord and work synergistically with LAs for analgesia to facilitate a decreased LA concentration.
5. The most common LAs for labor analgesia are the amide-linked bupivacaine and ropivacaine.
6. The rapid onset of 3% 2-chloroprocaine is due to its high delivered concentration rather than its pKa.
7. Neuraxial clonidine, a partial $\alpha_2$-agonist, acts on the dorsal horn of the spinal cord to decrease nociceptive transmission.
8. Sodium bicarbonate increases the nonionized proportion of the LA to speed up onset.
9. Volatile agent concentration should be minimized to avoid uterine atony.
10. The relative risk of mortality for the parturient is 1.7 for general anesthesia compared to neuraxial anesthesia.

---

metabolite, normeperidine, that can cause maternal seizures and cross the placenta to negatively affect the neonate.[1]

- **Nalbuphine:** An opioid agonist-antagonist with a pharmacokinetic profile similar to morphine, it may partially reverse opioid induced respiratory depression. It may induce opioid withdrawal in opioid-dependent parturients.
- **Fentanyl:** A synthetic, lipophilic opioid agonist with a rapid onset and short half-life and duration of action. It has a minimal effect on neonatal Apgar scores if given in small intravenous doses of 50 to 100 μg/h.
- **Remifentanil:** Administered via patient-controlled analgesia, it may be an alternative in parturients with contraindications for a neuraxial technique. Although it crosses the placenta freely, it is metabolized via nonspecific esterases and eliminated in the neonate by metabolism and redistribution.[1]

### INHALATIONAL ANALGESIA

- **Nitrous oxide:** Although it may be given alone, it acts synergistically when coadministered with opioids. It is indicated in women who want to avoid intravenous analgesia and/or who have contraindications to neuraxial interventions. Studies show that it is inferior to neuraxial analgesia, but maternal satisfaction is adequate.[2]

## VAGINAL DELIVERY: NEURAXIAL MEDICATIONS

Labor analgesia is best achieved by the neuraxial route. Local anesthetics (LAs) with opioid adjuvants are the mainstay, delivered via epidural, combined spinal-epidural, or single-shot spinal techniques.

### LOCAL ANESTHETICS

- **Bupivacaine/ropivacaine:** The most common amide LAs for labor epidural analgesia, they are typically administered via epidural infusion to provide excellent analgesia with minimal motor block. They are highly protein bound and exhibit minimal placental transfer. Relative to other LAs, bupivacaine has a high cardiotoxic profile due to its avid affinity for cardiac voltage-gated sodium channels.

- **Lidocaine:** Compared to bupivacaine/ropivacaine, it has a quicker onset but shorter duration of action and is less protein bound, resulting in more placental transfer. It is rarely used for labor analgesia due to increased motor block.
- **2-Chloroprocaine:** It has minimal placental transfer due to hydrolysis by nonspecific esterases. The quick onset of action of 3% 2-chloroprocaine is due to its high delivered concentration rather than its pKa. This is particularly useful during conversion of labor epidural analgesia for emergent cesarean delivery.

## DRUG ADJUVANTS

- **Opioids:** Neuraxial opioids act synergistically with LAs for analgesia, enabling a reduced LA concentration.[3] Opioids bind to presynaptic and postsynaptic receptor sites in the dorsal horn of the spinal cord.
- **Fentanyl/sufentanil:** This lipid-soluble adjuvant produces rapid analgesic effects (5–10 minutes) with a short duration of action (60–90 minutes). Side effects include nausea, pruritus, and respiratory depression.
- **Epinephrine:** It results in constriction of epidural veins to decrease systemic LA and opioid uptake and is typically administered in a 1:200,000 dilution with lidocaine.

## CESAREAN DELIVERY: NEURAXIAL MEDICATIONS

Epidural, combined spinal-epidural, or single-shot spinal anesthesia are common techniques for cesarean delivery. The medications include an LA and typically an opioid adjunct.

### LOCAL ANESTHETICS

Choice of neuraxial medication matches the pharmacokinetic profile to demands of the obstetric scenario (e.g., urgent cesarean delivery). If spinal anesthesia is utilized, a hyperbaric LA must be used to ensure appropriate rostral spread. Baricity describes the density of an LA relative to cerebrospinal fluid, with hyperbaric efficacy following the direction of gravity. Hyperbaric bupivacaine is typically administered for single-shot spinal and combined

spinal-epidural routes to ensure appropriate surgical anesthesia coverage during cesarean delivery. Preservative-free 2% lidocaine with 1:200,000 epinephrine is typically administered if an epidural technique is used; intrathecal administration of lidocaine is avoided due to increased risk of transient neurologic syndrome when compared to bupivacaine. In more urgent cases, pH-adjusted 3% 2-chloroprocaine is administered via epidural.

### ADJUVANTS

- **Opioids:** A lipid-soluble opioid (fentanyl/sufentanil) can be administered to enhance neuraxial blockade. Preservative-free morphine, the mainstay additive for postcesarean analgesia, can be administered via epidural or spinal anesthesia; however, it is hydrophilic, and patients must be monitored for delayed respiratory depression. Morphine has rostral spread in the cerebrospinal fluid and can activate the μ-opioid receptors in the ventral medulla, potentially causing respiratory depression.[4] Caution should be exercised if supplemental opioids are administered.
- **Epinephrine:** When administered intrathecally, it can improve the quality and duration of the spinal anesthetic. Activation of $\alpha_2$-adrenergic receptors can provide additional analgesia.
- **Clonidine:** A centrally acting partial $\alpha_2$-adrenoreceptor agonist acting on the dorsal horn of the spinal cord to decrease nociceptive transmission, its benefits include increased spinal duration of action and decreased epidural LA requirement.
- **Sodium bicarbonate (NaHCO$_3$):** This is coadministered with epidural lidocaine to reduce the time required for onset of action. By altering the pH of the solution, lidocaine is more readily available in the nonionized form, allowing for faster diffusion and onset of action in urgent cesarean delivery. Use with bupivacaine should be avoided because it causes precipitation.

## REFERENCES

1. Evron S, Ezri T. Options for systemic labor analgesia. *Curr Opin Anaesthesiol.* 2007;20:181–185.
2. Richardson MG, et al. Nitrous oxide during labor: maternal satisfaction does not depend exclusively on analgesic effectiveness. *Anesth Analg.* 2017;124:548–553.
3. Chestnut DH, et al. Continuous infusion epidural analgesia during labor: a randomized, double-blind comparison of 0.0625% bupivacaine/0.0002% fentanyl versus 0.125% bupivacaine. *Anesthesiology.* 1988;68:754–759.
4. Sultan P, et al. Neuraxial morphine and respiratory depression: finding the right balance. *Drugs.* 2011;71:1807–1819.

# 284.

## OXYTOCIC DRUGS

*Piotr Al-Jindi and Nimit K. Shah*

## INTRODUCTION

Postpartum hemorrhage has been defined as blood loss of more than 500 mL within 24 hours of delivery.[1] It is estimated that it affects 10% of deliveries. The most common cause of postpartum hemorrhage is uterine atony. Oxytocic drugs are agents used to increase uterine tone.

## OXYTOCIC AGENTS

### OXYTOCIN

Oxytocin is considered as the first-line drug in uterine atony. It does decrease the risk of postpartum hemorrhage by 60%. Other uses are induction and augmentation of labor. The number of oxytocin receptors increases during pregnancy. Oxytocin binds to the G protein–coupled receptor closely related to the vasopressin receptor and stimulates the contractions by increasing the concentration of free calcium.[2] The synthetic derivative Pitocin is used to limit the antidiuretic and cardiovascular side effects of vasopressin that may contaminate oxytocin in vivo because of its proximity of production.

It is used for the prevention of hemorrhage as 10 IU IM or 5–10 IU IV bolus, but no benefit was demonstrated for bolus compared to infusion. For the treatment of uterine atony and postpartum bleeding, the dose of 30 IU of oxytocin in 500 L normal saline infused as 300 mL/h in a patient with no previous exposure to oxytocin, the rate can be increased to 600 and 900 mL/h if uterine atony develops. However, if the patient had exposure to oxytocin, then a rate of 600 mL/h should be given and increased to 900 mL/h if needed.[1] The onset of action is 30 seconds if given intravenously and 3–5 min if given intramuscularly. This should be started immediately after the clamping of the umbilical cord or placenta delivery for a vaginal birth.[2]

Common side effects include hypotension (direct vasodilatory effect on vessels' musculature); fetal distress (it causes the upper segment of the myometrium to contract rhythmically, constricting spiral arteries and decreasing blood flow through the uterus); uterine atony (when used for prolonged labor); uterine rupture; water retention; and hyponatremia (due to its structure, which is similar to vasopressin). Myocardial ischemia was reported.[1] When used in large doses over a long duration, antidiuretics may produce water intoxication and hyponatremia.

## PROSTAGLANDINS

Prostaglandin (Carboprost, Misoprostol) levels increase during pregnancy with a peak at placenta separation. The failure of an increase in the levels of prostaglandins might contribute to uterine atony.[1] These medications can be used in uterine atony when oxytocin infusion fails to contract the uterus. It has been reported that there is a decreased response to prostaglandins in chorioamnionitis.[3]

### CARBOPROST (HEMABATE)

Carboprost (Hemabate), a synthetic analogue of F2-α prostaglandin considered as a second-line agent for uterine atony, can be given intramuscularly or into the myometrium and repeated every 15 minutes, with a total dose of 2 mg (8 doses). The onset of action is within minutes. It increases myometrial free calcium concentration.[3] It is contraindicated in asthma, active hepatic disease, and cardiac disease. It may be less effective in chorioamnionitis, as with other uterotonic agents. Common side effects include diarrhea, nausea and vomiting, fever and chills, and bronchospasm.

### MISOPROSTOL (CYTOTEC)

Misoprostol (Cytotec) is a prostaglandin $E_1$ analogue. Off-label, it is used for uterine atony and obstetrical hemorrhage. It can be given sublingually or rectally. It is metabolized to prostaglandin F. So, it is unlikely that it would work if the patient failed to respond to Carboprost. The dose range is

800–1000 µg, with action onset in minutes. The only contraindication is hypersensitivity to the drug. Side effects include diarrhea, shivering, and headache. It does not cause bronchospasm, so it can be used in asthmatic patients. If the patient is on a high dose of oxytocin, misoprostol does not provide any benefit.[1]

## METHYLERGONOVINE (METHERGINE)

An ergot alkaloid, methylergonovine (Methergine), stimulates uterine contraction by acting directly on uterine smooth muscle tissue to increase tone. The onset of action is 2–5 minutes. The plasma half-life is 3.4 hours. It should not be given intravascularly.[1] The dose is 0.2 mg IM; repeat every 2–4 hours. The most common side effects are nausea and vomiting. It is not recommended to be given intravenously due to its potential cardiovascular side effects. In the case of toxicity, chest pain and myocardial infarctions have been reported. It is relatively contraindicated in the setting of hypertension and preeclampsia. It can be used only in the postpartum period.[1]

Methylergonovine is a substrate of cytochrome P450 (CYP) 3A4. Therefore, if given concurrently with strong CYP3A4 inhibitors, vasospasm, cerebral ischemia, and/or ischemia of the lower extremities can occur. Avoid use with CYP3A4 inhibitors such as macrolide antibiotics, ketoconazole, and other azole antifungals or protease inhibitors.[3]

## ANESTHETIC CONSIDERATIONS

### PREOPERATIVE

The anesthesiologist should be able to access the risk for uterine atony and hemorrhage preoperatively. Uterine atony is the most common cause of postpartum hemorrhage. Risk factors for postpartum uterine atony include retained products, long labor, high parity, macrosomia, polyhydramnios, excessive oxytocin augmentation, chorioamnionitis, precipitous labor, and use of volatile anesthetics, magnesium sulfate, or terbutaline.[1] If the patient is at high risk for uterine atony, then it is recommended

to have two large-bore intravenous lines. Uterotonics and blood products should be readily available.

### INTRAOPERATIVE

Intraoperatively, during cesarean section, after clamping the umbilical cord oxytocin should be started. Oxytocin should be started as an infusion. Oxytocin can cause hypotension, and this can be treated with phenylephrine if needed.[1] High doses of oxytocin and free water can lead to hyponatremia and seizure. The half-life of oxytocin is 6 minutes, so prolonged infusion is needed.

If first-line treatment fails, then second-line drugs based on the patient's comorbidity should be used.

High concentrations of halogenated agents exacerbate uterine atony, so nitrous oxide can be used to decrease the minimum alveolar concentration of halogenated agents. If hemorrhage persists despite uterotonics and bimanual uterine massage, then balloon tamponade of the uterus, uterine compression suture, embolization, or ligation of the uterine arteries is considered. The last option is a hysterectomy. Avoidance of hypothermia is important as it can exacerbate coagulopathy. Fibrinogen levels greater than 150–200 mg/dL should be maintained. Results from the WOMAN trial showed that tranexamic acid given within 3 hours of diagnosis of hemorrhage had fewer deaths than the placebo group. Tranexamic acid is likely to decrease blood loss and transfusion rates. The dose is 1 g IV given over 10 minutes. Side effects of tranexamic acid include thromboembolism and seizure.[1]

### POSTOPERATIVE

Postoperative care should concentrate on reversing coagulopathy and maintaining hemodynamic stability and normothermia.

## REFERENCES

1. Chestnut D, et al. *Chestnut's Obstetric Anesthesia: Principles and Practice*. 6th ed. Elsevier; 2020.
2. Payton RG, Brucker MC. Drugs and uterine motility. *J Obstet Gynecol Neonatal Nurs*. 1999;28:628–638.
3. Drugs@FDA. US Food and Drug Administration. Accessed August 2020. http://www.accessdata.fda.gov/scripts/cder/drugsatfda/index.cfm?fuseaction=Search.Label_ApprovalHistory

# 285.

# TOCOLYTIC DRUGS

*Piotr Al-Jindi and Bethany Potere*

## INTRODUCTION

Preterm labor is the labor that occurs after the 20th week and before the 37th week of pregnancy. It is one of the leading causes of mortality and neurodevelopment impairment worldwide. In the United States, preterm labor accounts for 11.4% of labor, and it accounts for 70% of neonatal death.

Tocolytic drugs are considered between 22 and 34 weeks of gestational age. The purpose of tocolytic drugs is to delay labor and allow enough time for the administration of corticosteroids, which will facilitate lung maturity. Additionally, evidence suggests that magnesium sulfate reduces the severity of cerebral palsy in surviving infants if administered when the birth is anticipated before 32 weeks of gestation.[1]

## CONTRAINDICATIONS TO TOCOLYTIC THERAPY

Contraindications to tocolytic therapy are intrauterine fetal demise, lethal fetal anomaly, nonreasoning fetal status, severe preeclampsia or eclampsia, maternal bleeding with hemodynamic instability, chorioamnionitis, preterm premature rupture of membranes (when maternal infection is present), and maternal contraindications to specific agents.

## TOCOLYTICS CLASSES

### BETAMIMETICS (RITODRINE, TERBUTALINE)

$\beta_2$-Receptor agonists (betamimetics ritodrine and terbutaline) work by increasing cyclic adenosine monophosphate. They deplete intracellular calcium levels, which diminish uterine contractility due to its action on $\beta_2$-receptors. Tachyphylaxis has been reported with these drugs, and that is the reason for the short duration of action. Terbutaline is used subcutaneously, and a typical dose is 0.25 mg, which

can be repeated every 4 hours.[2] It is rarely used intravenously as an infusion, and the oral route is contraindicated in the treatment of preterm labor. In 2011, the Food and Drug Administration issued a warning about the use of terbutaline and stated that injectable terbutaline should not be used for prolonged treatment (beyond 48 hours) due to potential maternal side effects and death.[1]

Cardiac (maternal tachycardia, hypotension, arrhythmias, myocardial infarction, pulmonary edema) and metabolic (hypokalemia and hyperglycemia) side effects are due to its action on $\beta_1$-receptors. Tremors and palpitations are also reported. It can cause neonatal hypoglycemia, hypocalcemia, and ileus. Terbutaline is contraindicated in heart disease, patients with cardiac arrhythmias, hemorrhage, and uncontrolled diabetes mellitus.[2]

## CALCIUM CHANNEL BLOCKING AGENTS (NIFEDIPINE)

Calcium channel blocking agents (nifedipine) are considered to be the first-line agents for the treatment of preterm labor.[3] A meta-analysis suggested that calcium channel blockers are more beneficial than $\beta$-adrenergic agents with respect to prolongation of pregnancy, neonatal morbidity, and maternal side effects. They work through blocking voltage-gated calcium channels and preventing the release of calcium from the sarcoplasmic reticulum. This will result in the relaxation of smooth muscles.

Nifedipine has much fewer side effects than terbutaline. The most common side effects are headache, flushing, dizziness, nausea, and palpitation.

A contraindications is maternal hypotension.

## MAGNESIUM SULFATE

Magnesium sulfate, as a tocolytic agent, works through a competitive antagonism to calcium for entry into myocytes. It also decreases the release of acetylcholine. A Cochrane review in 2014 concluded that magnesium sulfate is not effective in delaying labor, and it does not have an advantage over other tocolytic agents when it comes to neonatal and maternal outcomes.[5]

Individual titration to uterine relaxation and maternal side effects is recommended. Most physicians titrate the dosing of $MgSO_4$ once the serum level exceeds 8 mg/dL.

Contraindications are myasthenia gravis and heart failure. Caution should be exerted in patients with renal failure.

As for maternal side effects, magnesium sulfate is generally well tolerated. Side effects include flushing, headache, lethargy, muscle weakness, diplopia, chest tightness, shortness of breath, and pulmonary edema. Side effects can be minimized by monitoring urinary output, deep tendon reflexes, respiratory rate, and pulse. Loss of patellar reflexes is seen at serum levels of 8–12 mg/dL, respiratory depression at serum level 15–17 mg/dL, and cardiac arrest at levels 30–35 mg/dL. Calcium gluconate 1 g IV bolus can be used to reverse magnesium side effects. Magnesium sulfate does cross the placenta, and fetal lethargy, hypotonia, and decrease in fetal bone density might be observed.

## PROSTAGLANDIN SYNTHETASE INHIBITORS (INDOMETHACIN, SULINDAC, KETOROLAC)

Prostaglandins E and F are mediators of uterine contraction. They work by inhibiting the cyclooxygenase that decreases prostaglandin synthetase and blocks the conversion of arachidonic acid to prostaglandins.

Nausea and heartburn are the two most common side effects. Adverse effects on neonates are unlikely (closure of the ductus arteriosus) if indomethacin is used for less than 48 hours. Indomethacin is also associated with oligohydramnios secondary to decreased fetal urinary output. So, cyclooxygenase inhibitors are not used beyond 32 weeks of gestation as potential side effects outweigh the benefits of their use.

## ANESTHETIC CONSIDERATIONS

### PREOPERATIVE

Preoperatively, it is accepted to stop magnesium during transportation to the operating room for an emergent cesarean section to minimize the risk of an unintentional bolus. If it is given for fetal neuroprotection, it can be discontinued at the time of delivery.

### INTRAOPERATIVE

Patients on terbutaline therapy are at risk for the development of pulmonary edema, so aggressive hydration is to be avoided intraoperatively. Also, drugs that increase maternal tachycardia are to be avoided. Due to the tachycardia, assessing the depth of anesthesia and volume status is more difficult. If general anesthesia is induced, hyperventilation should be avoided because it will exacerbate hypokalemia.

Calcium channel blockers can potentiate the hypotension of inhaled anesthetics. Concomitant use of magnesium sulfate and nifedipine is not advised due to the risk of neuromuscular blockade.[4]

Hypermagnesemia can potentiate the hypotension associated with neuraxial epidural administration. Magnesium overdose can carry severe consequences for the mother and the fetus.

Magnesium sulfate potentiates the action of depolarizing and nondepolarizing muscle relaxants (it decreases the release of acetylcholine at the neuromuscular junction and decreases the sensitivity of the motor end plate to acetylcholine). Defasciculating doses of nondepolarizing muscle relaxants should be avoided. However, it is recommended to use a standard dose of muscle relaxants for intubation because the effect of potentiation is variable. It is also recommended to avoid or reduce any subsequent dose of muscle relaxants. Magnesium sulfate also decreases the minimum alveolar concentration.

The American Society for Reginal Anesthesia recommends caution when the patient is on nonsteroidal anti-inflammatory drugs and there is the concurrent use of other medications affecting clotting.

### POSTOPERATIVE

For patients on magnesium sulfate, postoperative monitoring for weakness is warranted.

### REFERENCES

1. American College of Obstetricians and Gynecologists' Committee on Practice Bulletins—Obstetrics. Practice bulletin no. 171: management of preterm labor. *Obstet Gynecol.* 2016;128(4):e155–e164.
2. Creasy RK, et al. *Creasy and Resnik's Maternal Fetal Medicine: Principles and Practice.* 6th ed. Philadelphia, PA: Saunders; 2009.
3. Chestnut D, et al. *Chestnut's Obstetric Anesthesia: Principles and Practice.* 6th ed. Elsevier; 2020.
4. Flenady V, et al. Calcium channel blockers for inhibiting preterm labour and birth. *Cochrane Database Syst Rev.* 2014;2014(6): CD002255.
5. Crowther CA, et al. Magnesium sulphate for preventing preterm birth in threatened preterm labour. *Cochrane Database Syst Rev.* 2014;(8):CD001060.

# 286.

# MECHANISMS OF PLACENTAL TRANSFER AND PLACENTAL TRANSFER OF SPECIFIC DRUGS

*Muhammad Fayyaz Ahmed and Ihab Kamel*

## INTRODUCTION

The placenta is closely involved in exchange of fetal and maternal blood for transfer of waste, nutrients, gases, and drugs.[1,2]

## MECHANISM OF PLACENTAL TRANSFER

The placenta allows bidirectional transfer of various substances through an imperfect barrier involving a complex transport mechanism. The permeability of the membrane and availability of certain processes limit free movement. Transfer of substances between the maternal and fetal system occurs through the processes outlined next.

**Passive Transport:** Passive transport or simple diffusion occurs primarily across a concentration gradient. It takes place across the lipid membrane, where water and lipophilic molecules move, or through the protein channel, where charged substances move. Substances with less than 600 Da can only move by passive diffusion. Factors impacting the passive movement of molecules are lipid solubility, molecular weight, concentration gradient, thickness of the membrane, exchange surface area, and extent of ionization. Oxygen and carbon dioxide utilize this process to cross the placenta.[1,2]

**Facilitated Transport:** Facilitated transport is defined as passive transport of substances that use an adenosine triphosphate (ATP) independent carrier to transport comparatively lipid insoluble molecules down the concentration gradient. The rate of transfer depends on the amount of carrier protein complexes across the membrane and the extent of interaction between the channel and the substance for transport. Glucose moves through facilitated diffusion. Fatty acid movement primarily occurs through simple diffusion; fatty acid binding proteins may facilitate transport. Amino acid is transported through secondary active transport or cotransport, which functions by uphill transport of a substance linked to another molecule moving down its own concentration gradient without using energy.[1,2]

**Active Transport:** Active transport is defined as movement of a substance through the membrane, usually against the concentration gradient, utilizing energy in the form of ATP. It operates with a protein membrane carrier. The classic example is of the Na+/K+ ATPase (adenosine phosphatase) pump. Active transport protein is vital in protecting the fetus from teratogenic and foreign substances. It transports many antibiotics and lipophilic drugs, removes waste material from the fetus, and prevents certain drugs, such as methadone, from entering the fetal circulation. Drugs with similar characteristics may competitively compete with endogenous compounds for active transport.[1,2]

**Pinocytosis:** Pinocytosis is an energy-requiring process of enveloping large molecules with cell membrane and moving contents across the membrane that cannot be transported through diffusion. Immunoglobulin G uses this mode of transport.[1,2]

The following characteristics influence the exchange of maternal and fetal substances: gestational age, pH gradient, concentration of plasma protein, diffusion capacity, placental metabolism, fetal and maternal blood flow, and placental metabolism.

## PLACENTAL TRANSFER OF DRUGS

The ratio of fetus/maternal (F/M) is a quantitative number demonstrating the exposure of fetus to drugs in relation to the mother. The pharmacokinetics and membrane permeability determine the exposure the fetus gets to maternal drugs. Factors affecting drug transfer across the placental membrane are protein binding, pKa, lipid solubility, tissue binding, blood flow, and pH. It is also to note that fetal

**Table 286.1** FACTORS AFFECTING DRUG TRANSFER ACROSS THE PLACENTAL MEMBRANE

|  | INCREASED TRANSFER | DECREASED TRANSFER |
|---|---|---|
| Size | <1000 Da | >1000 Da |
| Lipid solubility | Lipophilic | Hydrophobic |
| Charge of molecule | Uncharged | Charge |
| Free unbound drug | High | Low |
| Binding protein | Albumin | $\alpha_1$-Acid glycoprotein |

acidemia increases maternal fetal transfer of basic drugs such as local anesthetics and opioids. In general, highly ionized molecules and large molecules are less likely to cross the placenta. Factors determining placental transfer of drugs are summarized in Table 286.1.

A summary of placental transfer of drugs commonly used during pregnancy and delivery is in Table 286.2.

## ANESTHETIC CONSIDERATIONS

Prolonged exposure (>10 minutes) to high doses of inhaled anesthetics (>1 minimum alveolar concentration) can cause neonatal depression. An induction dose of propofol may have sedative effects on the neonate. Opioids can lead to neonatal respiratory and central nervous system depression if administered prior to delivery. Thus, the administration of intravenous opioids after delivery is preferred. Atropine and scopolamine cross the placenta easily, while glycopyrolate poorly moves through the membrane.

**Table 286.2** DRUGS THAT CROSS THE PLACENTA READILY AND DRUGS THAT DO NOT CROSS THE PLACENTA EASILY PLUS IMPORTANT CLINICAL CONSIDERATIONS

| DRUGS THAT CROSS THE PLACENTA | DRUGS THAT DO NOT CROSS THE PLACENTA |
|---|---|
| **Induction agents**<br>Propofol, etomidate, ketamine, and dexmedetomidine<br><br>**Inhalational agents**<br><br>**Opioids**<br>*Morphine* can cause significant reduction in fetal breathing and fetal heart rate acceleration within 20 minutes of administration. *Fentanyl* readily crosses the placenta and can be found in the fetal brain and placenta. *Nalbuphine* causes less neonatal, maternal, and fetal side effects.<br><br>**Benzodiazepines**<br>Midazolam, lorazepam, and diazepam<br><br>**Anticholinergic agents**<br>Atropine and scopolamine<br><br>**Anticoagulants**<br>Warfarin (risk of congenital anomalies), apixaban, and rivaroxaban<br><br>**Vasopressors**<br>Ephedrine<br>Phenylephrine<br><br>**Antihypertensives**<br>β-Adrenergic antagonist (labetalol and esmolol)<br>Nitroprusside (can lead to cyanide toxicity)<br>Nitroglycerin<br>Hydralazine (Can cause umbilical artery vasodilation)<br><br>**Local anesthetics**<br>Chlorprocaine has the least transfer. Bupivacaine and ropivacaine have lower fetal blood levels than lidocaine.<br><br>**Angiotensin-converting enzyme inhibitors**<br>Affect fetus renal activity<br><br>**Steroids**<br>Dexamethasone been associated with a 3- to 4-fold increase in cleft lip incidence when used during first trimester.[2]<br><br>**Antiemetics**<br>Ondansetron and metoclopramide can be used safely during pregnancy.<br><br>**Acetaminophen**<br>Concern for liver toxicity of the fetus. Possible increased incidence of developing asthma and attention deficit hyperactivity disorder with long-term use.[3] | **Muscle relaxants and reversal agents**<br>Depolarizing agents (succinylcholine)<br>Nondepolarizing agents<br>Neostigmine (limited transfer across placenta)<br>Sugammadex<br><br>**Anticoagulants**<br>Heparin<br>Enoxaparin<br>Low-molecular-weight heparin (limited transfer)<br><br>**Anticholinergic agent**<br>Glycopyrolate<br><br>Insulin |

From References 1, 2, and 4.

Although neostigmine does not cross the placental membrane easily, it crosses the placenta relatively more than glycopyrolate. Thus, atropine should be used during reversal of neuromuscular blockade in pregnant patients presenting for nonobstetric surgery to avoid fetal bradycardia.

## REFERENCES

1. Zakowski MI, Geller A. The placenta: anatomy, physiology, and transfer of drugs. In: Chestnut DH, et al., eds. *Chestnut's Obstetric Anesthesia: Principles and Practice.* 6th ed. Philadelphia, PA: Elsevier Health Sciences; 2020:56–76.
2. Campbell DC, Vincente MS. Placental transfer of drugs and perinatal pharmacology. In: Suresh MS, et al., eds. *Shnider and Levinson's Anesthesia for Obstetrics.* 5th ed. Philadelphia, PA: Lippincott, Williams & Wilkins; 2013:46–55.
3. Tumukunde J, et al. Effects of propofol versus thiopental on Apgar scores in newborns and peri-operative outcomes of women undergoing emergency cesarean section: a randomized clinical trial. BMC Anesthesiol. 2015;15:63.
4. Thiele K et al. Acetaminophen and pregnancy: short- and long-term consequences for mother and child. J Reprod Immunol. 2013;97(1):128–139.

# 287.

# FETAL DISPOSITION OF DRUGS

*Afshin Heidari and Ben Aquino*

## INTRODUCTION

Due to immature metabolism and potentially teratogenic consequences during organogenesis, fetal disposition of medications is critically important. Surveys of drug use in pregnancy demonstrated that a significant proportion of human fetuses are exposed to prescription and nonprescription drugs antenatally or during labor. Anesthetic medications are no exception and can be transferred to the fetus after maternal administration.

Placental exchange can occur by one of five mechanisms:

- Bulk flow (water)
- Active transport (amino acids, vitamins, ions, calcium, iron)
- Pinocytosis (large molecules, e.g., immunoglobulins)
- Breaks (direct mixing of blood; responsible for Rh sensitization)
- Diffusion (respiratory gases and most drugs used in anesthesia)[1]

## ANESTHETIC DRUGS

All inhalational agents and most intravenous agents freely cross the placenta; however, inhalational agents cause little fetal depression provided they are given in limited doses (<1 minimum alveolar concentration) and delivery occurs within 10 minutes of the induction of anesthesia.

Intravenous agents readily cross the placenta into the fetal circulation. Except for benzodiazepines, fetal effects are limited by drug distribution, metabolism, and possibly placental uptake.[2]

Corticosteroids, commonly used for postoperative and chemotherapy-induced nausea and vomiting, are associated with cleft lip with or without cleft palate when used before 10 weeks' gestation.

Opiates readily cross the placenta, but neonatal effects vary considerably. In terms of respiratory depression, morphine produces the most, fentanyl the least. Remifentanil readily crosses the placenta and has the potential to produce respiratory depression. The umbilical artery to umbilical vein ratio (UA/UV ratio) is about 30%, suggesting fairly rapid metabolism of remifentanil in the neonate. Epidural or intrathecal opiates to a lesser extent generally produce minimal neonatal effects.

Intrathecal lipophilic opioids may contribute to fetal bradycardia, possibly from decreased circulating maternal catecholamines accompanying rapid onset of analgesia. Decreasing epinephrine (tocolytic via $\beta_2$-receptor agonism) may increase uterine tone, leading to decreased uteroplacental perfusion and fetal hypoxia, since uteroplacental perfusion occurs during uterine relaxation.

Muscle relaxants are highly ionized, which impedes placental transfer, resulting in minimal effects on the fetus.

Local anesthetics are weakly basic drugs that are principally bound to 1-acid glycoprotein. Placental transfer depends on (1) pKa, (2) maternal and fetal pH, and (3) degree of protein binding. Except for chloroprocaine, fetal acidosis produces higher fetal-to-maternal drug ratios because binding of hydrogen ions to the nonionized form causes trapping of the local anesthetic in the fetal circulation. Highly protein-bound agents diffuse poorly across the placenta; thus, greater protein binding of bupivacaine and ropivacaine, compared with that of lidocaine, likely accounts for their lower fetal blood levels. Chloroprocaine has the least placental transfer because it is rapidly broken down by maternal plasma cholinesterases.

Anesthetic adjuncts like maternally administered ephedrine, β-adrenergic blockers, vasodilators, phenothiazines, antihistamines ($H_1$ and $H_2$), and metoclopramide are transferred to the fetus. Atropine and scopolamine cross the placenta; glycopyrrolate has a quaternary ammonium (ionized) structure, resulting in only limited transfer.

## OTHER MEDICATIONS

Some commonly used medications can have adverse effects on fetal development during the pregnancy due to fetal disposition. Examples include the following[3]: antidepressants, warfarin, hypothyroid medications, and angiotensin-converting enzyme (ACE) inhibitors.

### ANTIDEPRESSANTS

Tricyclic antidepressants (e.g., amitriptyline, imipramine) are associated with congenital malformations and should be replaced by selective serotonin reuptake inhibitors for first-line therapy for depression in pregnancy. Most have no major risk for malformations and abnormalities. Paroxetine may be associated with increased risk for right ventricular outflow tract obstruction, so it should be avoided, and women who used paroxetine during early pregnancy need fetal echocardiography. Lithium during pregnancy remains controversial. Discontinuation is associated with higher chance of relapse of the affective disorder in 1 year, but it can cause hypotonia, lethargy, and poor feeding in newborns.

### WARFARIN

Warfarin can cause fetal warfarin syndrome: nasal hypoplasia, depressed nasal bridge (often with a deep groove between the alae and nasal tip), stippled epiphyses, nail hypoplasia, mental retardation, and growth restriction. Second and third trimester exposure can cause microcephaly, blindness, deafness, and growth restriction.

### HYPERTHYROIDISM MEDICATIONS

Propylthiouracil can cause fetal and neonatal hypothyroidism and, rarely, goiter. Methimazole causes aplasia cutis of the scalp in newborns.

### ACE INHIBITORS

The ACE inhibitors may increase cardiac and central nervous system defects. They can cause fetal renal failure and oligohydramnios, which may result in fetal limb contractures, craniofacial deformities, and pulmonary hypoplasia.[3]

See Table 287.1 for common anesthetic drugs that have limited placental transfer.

## FETAL PHYSIOLOGY

Some special features of fetal physiology and pharmacology make this issue even more significant.

Fetal tissue uptake of local anesthetics is influenced by

- Fetal plasma protein binding
- Lipid solubility
- Degree of ionization of the drug
- Hemodynamic changes that affect the distribution of fetal cardiac output
- Increased blood flow to vital organs (e.g., heart, brain, adrenal glands) during asphyxia

*Table 287.1* LIST OF DRUGS WITH LIMITED PLACENTAL TRANSFER

| DRUG | RATIONALE FOR LIMITED PLACENTAL TRANSFER |
|---|---|
| Nondepolarizing muscle relaxants | Highly ionized and large molecular weight |
| Succinylcholine | Highly ionized |
| Glycopyrrolate | Highly ionized due to quaternary ammonium structure |
| Heparin | Large molecular weight |
| Protamine | Large molecular weight |
| Chloroprocaine | Metabolized by plasma esterases in maternal circulation |
| Insulin | Large molecular weight |

The fetal liver may be less important to drug elimination than in the adult, but conjugated drug metabolites in the fetus may persist because of limited placental transfer. Accumulation of intact drugs in amniotic fluid also occurs via fetal renal excretion and perhaps via fetal membranes. A number of basic amine drugs are also concentrated in fetal tracheal fluid, probably due to pulmonary uptake, which also takes place in the adult. However, this could result in high levels of agents in the fetal lung, such as $\beta_2$-adrenergic agonists, which have potent effects on pulmonary function and maturation.

## REFERENCES

1. Zakowski MI, Geller A. The placenta: anatomy, physiology, and transfer of drugs. In: Chestnut D, et al., eds. *Chestnut's Obstetric Anesthesia: Principles and Practice.* 5th ed. Philadelphia, PA: Elsevier Saunders; 2014: Chap 4.
2. Isoherranen N, Thummel KE. Drug metabolism and transport during pregnancy: how does drug disposition change during pregnancy and what are the mechanisms that cause such changes? *Drug Metab Dispos.* 2013;41(2):256–262.
3. Wasson C, et al. Fetal disposition of drugs. In: *Absolute Obstetric Anesthesia Review.* New York, NY: Springer, 2019.

# 288.

# DRUG EFFECTS ON THE NEWBORN

*Ben Aquino*

## INTRODUCTION

Important factors in maternal-fetal drug transmission are the mode of transmission, fetal physiology affecting drug effects, and salient points of a few commonly used peripartum maternal drugs and their effects on the fetus and neonate.

## PLACENTAL TRANSFER

Though several transport systems act as means for substances to cross the placenta, most maternal-fetal drug transmission occurs via simple diffusion. Molecules 1000 Da or less generally cross the placenta, driven by the drug maternal-fetal concentration gradients. Other factors affecting drug transfer include drug charge, lipophilicity, and degree of ionization, which relates to the drug's pKa in relation to physiologic pH.[1] Plasma protein binding is also a factor—albumin binds drugs with great affinity, but α-acid-glycoprotein (AAG) does not.[2] Gestational age also affects placental transfer; the placenta is more permeable early in pregnancy (Table 288.1).

## FETAL/NEONATAL PHYSIOLOGY

The fetal liver, though immature, has enzymatic metabolic and synthetic capabilities (clotting factors, albumin, and AAG). Because umbilical vein input goes through the portal circulation before entering the heart, many drugs undergo first-pass metabolism in the liver, which decreases fetal drug levels. Fetal protein binding is approximately 50% of an adult, meaning with any drug at a given plasma concentration, there will be more free drug in fetal blood than in maternal blood.

Fetal blood pH also influences drug effects. In contrast to the maternal compensated respiratory alkalosis and blood pH of around 7.45, fetal pH values as low as 7.25 can be normal. In the immediate peripartum period, this can influence movement of drugs with pKa values close to physiologic pH. Local anesthetics, being weak bases, are largely nonionized in maternal circulation, but when they enter fetal circulation, lower fetal pH makes the local anesthetic more ionized and less lipid soluble, hindering transport back into maternal circulation. This can raise fetal drug levels, especially in situations of fetal distress and acidosis.

**Table 288.1** FACTORS INCREASING FETAL/NEONATAL PLASMA DRUG CONCENTRATIONS

| FACTOR | RATIONALE | EXAMPLES |
|---|---|---|
| Lipophilicity | Diffuses easily through placental and cell membranes | Induction agents<br>Fentanyl |
| Low molecular weight < 1000 Da | Diffuses easily through placental and cell membranes | Atropine<br>Volatile anesthetics |
| Low degree of maternal ionization | Decreases relative polarity of molecule and increases its lipid solubility | Local anesthetics (weak bases) |
| Fetal acidosis | Ion trapping: in more acidic fetal blood, greater percentage of drug is ionized and does not recross placenta from fetal to maternal circulation | Local anesthetics |
| High (albumin) maternal protein binding | Protein binding prevents drug metabolism (only free drug is metabolized) | Diazepam |
| High fetal-maternal concentration gradient | Fick's first law of diffusion | Drugs in maternal plasma with any of the previous characteristics |

## SPECIFIC DRUGS

### LOCAL ANESTHETICS

Local anesthetic effects, such as seizures and cardiovascular collapse, can occur in the fetus and neonate as well as the adult. Animal studies have shown that fetuses can tolerate higher doses of local anesthetic (in mg/kg), possibly because of fetal drug excretion back across the placenta to the mother. By contrast, the higher dose tolerated by neonates is likely due to a larger volume of distribution.[2] Local anesthetics, metabolized by neonatal liver enzymes, have longer elimination half-lives in the neonate. In contrast, fetal and maternal elimination half-lives of these drugs are similar, again likely from transplacental fetal excretion of drug back to the mother.

### OPIOIDS AND BENZODIAZEPINES

All commonly used opioids readily cross the placenta. Maternal meperidine administration is associated with neonatal central nervous system depression; fetal/maternal levels rise quickly, neonatal metabolism is slower, and neonates are more susceptible to the active metabolite normeperidine. Morphine also has an active metabolite metabolized more slowly in neonates. Remifentanil has the advantage of being metabolized by plasma esterases (fully mature in the term fetus and neonate). Of the benzodiazepines, diazepam (lipid soluble, unionized) reaches high fetal levels quickly. Midazolam, less polar, takes longer (20 minutes) to reach similar fetal levels, but fetal/neonatal levels decrease rapidly within 3 hours.

### INDUCTION AGENTS

Propofol—the most commonly used induction agent—is lipophilic, crosses the placenta, and when given in standard induction doses for cesarean section has been associated with lower neonatal Apgar scores than equivalent induction doses of thiopental.[2] The neonatal plasma levels, and subsequent clinical effect, are less if the delivery is within 10 minutes of induction of anesthesia.

Thiopental crosses the placenta easily, but because of significant variation between individuals, both maternal and fetal, concentrations of the drug are strongly dependent on maternal and fetal protein concentrations.

### INHALATION ANESTHETICS

Inhalational agents (lipid soluble, low molecular weight) cross the placenta readily. All cause neonatal depression and lower Apgar scores if incision-to-delivery times are prolonged during cesarean section.

Nitrous oxide ($N_2O$) has rapid placental transfer and is associated with neonatal depression, possibly because it decreases fetal central vascular resistance by 30%. Diffusion hypoxia is possible during rapid elimination of $N_2O$, and any exposed neonate needs supplemental oxygen as soon as possible.[2]

### MUSCLE RELAXANTS

The muscle relaxant succinylcholine is low molecular weight but highly charged and does not readily cross the placenta unless given in supraclinical doses. Maternal administration rarely causes neonatal weakness unless both mother and baby are homozygous for pseudocholinesterase deficiency.[3]

Nondepolarizing relaxants, fully ionized with high molecular weight, do not easily cross the placenta.

## PRESSORS

The pressor ephedrine is no longer the first-choice drug for maternal hypotension, partially due to fetal/neonatal effects. It crosses the placenta easily (10 times more lipid soluble than phenylephrine). It is associated with fetal acidosis; drug levels are much higher, and it stimulates fetal β-adrenergic activity, raising plasma lactate, glucose, and norepinephrine to a greater extent than phenylephrine.[4]

## SPECIAL EXCEPTIONS

For special exceptions, the muscarinic antagonist glycopyrrolate (highly charged) is poorly transferred across the placenta. Scopolamine crosses the placenta, as does atropine; atropine is associated with lower fetal heart rate variability and fetal tachycardia.

Heparin is highly charged and does not readily cross the placenta.

## REFERENCES

1. Flood P, Rollins MD. Obstetric anesthesia. In: Miller RD, et al., eds. *Miller's Anesthesia*. Philadelphia, PA: Elsevier Saunders; 2015: Chap. 77.
2. Zakowski MI, Geller A. The placenta: anatomy, physiology, and transfer of drugs. In: Chestnut DH, et al. *Chestnut's Obstetric Anesthesia: Principles and Practice*. 5th ed. Philadelphia, PA: Elsevier Saunders; 2014: Chap. 4.
3. Baraka A, et al. Response of the newborn to succinylcholine injection in homozygotic atypical mothers. *Anesthesiology*. 1975;43(1):115–116.
4. Ngan Kee WD, et al. Placental transfer and fetal metabolic effects of phenylephrine and ephedrine during spinal anesthesia for cesarean delivery. *Anesthesiology*. 2009;111(3):506–512.

# 289.

# AMNIOTIC FLUID

*James Urness and Ami Attali*

## INTRODUCTION

The developing fetus is surrounded by free-flowing, complex fluid that changes in function, composition, and volume as the pregnancy progresses to term. This medium supports the developing fetus in a multitude of ways, from forming a protective environment to preventing injury from the outside, allowing free movements, a means of nutrient and signaling transfer, and a defense system against foreign microbes. The production and maintenance of amniotic fluid balance relies on a number of sources depending on the stage of fetal development, maternal hydration, hormonal status, and placental perfusion.[1]

## FLUID CHARACTERISTICS

Amniotic fluid originates from numerous sources throughout gestation; during embryogenesis fluid is principally derived from maternal plasma by the passage of water through aquaporin channels expressed on the fetal maternal membranes and secretions from amniotic epithelium of the chorionic plate. Initially, the composition of amniotic fluid is like that of fetal extracellular fluid, as there is an absence of keratin in the fetal skin, allowing flow of nutrients and signaling molecules to developing cells. After keratinization is completed by 25 weeks, the developing gut has decreased permeability, and the volume of amniotic fluid becomes a function of fetal urine production and lung secretions. As the fetal kidneys produce urine, the composition of amniotic fluid steadily increases in concentrations of urea and creatinine and a decrease in concentrations of sodium and chloride.[2] Amniotic fluid volume relies on aquaporin channels and follows a predictable linear increase between 10 and 20 weeks' gestation, from 25 mL at 10 weeks to 400 mL at 20 weeks, then over 700 mL by 28 weeks, where it stays until term, after which it decreases to 400 mL.

Another important role of amniotic fluid is antimicrobial defense within the fluid, primarily composed of maternal humoral and cellular mediators, which all have significant activity against bacteria, viruses, and fungi. Neutrophils are usually absent from the amniotic fluid; however, if present can signify an inflammatory or infectious process such as chorioamnionitis.[1] Cellular mediators are poorly characterized in amniotic fluid, and it remains unclear if the immune cells that are present serve a scavenging or antimicrobial role.[1]

## CLINICAL CORRELATIONS

During routine antenatal visits, the amniotic fluid volume is measured and expressed as an amniotic fluid index to compare to expected volumes. If there is less than expected amniotic fluid, it is termed oligohydramnios, and if there is more than expected, it is deemed polyhydramnios. Oligohydramnios in the second or third trimester is usually the result of lack of urine production or an obstructive process of the lower urinary tract. The major concern with oligohydramnios before 20 weeks' gestation is increased risk of pulmonary hypoplasia and neonatal morbidity. On the other hand, excessive amniotic fluid is generally caused by overproduction of fluid via polyuria or there could be a gastrointestinal obstruction or functional swallowing impairment.[2]

During delivery, an amniotic fluid embolism (AFE) is one of the most feared and devastating obstetric complications for maternal prognosis. Fortunately, AFEs are very rare, but are associated with extremely high mortality, accounting for almost 10% of all maternal deaths in developed countries, most commonly occurring during labor and cesarean sections.[3] Historically, it was thought that emboli of amniotic fluid obstructed the maternal pulmonary circulation; however, a more contemporary etiology is that of abnormal immunologic reaction to fetal antigen(s). The hypothesized pathway is that the antigen(s) trigger a hypersensitivity immunologic response that activated the complement system, leading to platelet and mast cell degranulation, subsequently releasing thromboxane and serotonin, which further amplify the immunologic systems, leading to shock. With the amplified immune response, paired with procoagulants from the amniotic fluid, the activated coagulation cascade leads to disseminated intravascular coagulation (DIC) and hypofibrinogenemia, causing massive hemorrhaging.[3,4]

## ANESTHETIC MANAGEMENT

Clinical sequela of AFE can be divided into three stages that evolve sequentially: respiratory distress, cardiovascular collapse, and coagulopathy. More likely diagnoses need to be considered first, such as high spinal, anaphylaxis, pulmonary embolism or venous air embolism, local anesthetic toxicity, aspiration, or any obstetrical possibilities such as eclampsia, massive hemorrhage.[4] Once AFE enters as a possible diagnosis, rapid recognition and supportive aggressive resuscitation are key for favorable fetal and maternal outcomes. The following discussion is guidance to take into consideration in the event of a possible diagnosis of AFE.

### PREOPERATIVE

The preoperative key for a robust response to the unpredictable is to be prepared and vigilant. Before a parturient starts active labor or beginning a cesarean section, it is imperative that consent is obtained for potential blood products, type and screen has been performed, and two large-bore intravenous lines are present and working. Fetal monitoring is recommended for identifying distress as an early sign of AFE is fetal bradycardia. The patient should be positioned with left uterine displacement to relieve inferior vena cava compression maintaining preload.

### INTRAOPERATIVE

All patients should have standard American Society of Anesthesiologists monitors (pulse oximeter, electrocardiography, blood pressure monitor, end-tidal $CO_2$, and temperature monitor) once in the operating room. Intraoperatively, an initial heralding symptom of AFE is maternal loss of consciousness, likely a result of acute pulmonary hypertension and dramatic decrease in cardiac output. At the first sign of cardiopulmonary decompensation, a protected airway needs to be immediately established with endotracheal intubation to ensure proper ventilation and reduced risk of aspiration.[4,5] Hemodynamics can rapidly deteriorate from biventricular failure, first with right heart failure, then cardiovascular collapse and arrest, requiring initiation of cardiopulmonary resuscitation and consideration of a stat cesarean delivery if return of circulation has not been established within 4 minutes.[3,5] Immediate establishment of invasive, large-bore, and central venous access needs to be obtained with an available rapid infuser for fluid and vasopressor resuscitation. Also consider a pulmonary artery catheter and transthoracic or transesophageal ultrasound for guided hemodynamic therapies for persistent shock.[5] If the patient survives this hemodynamic collapse, there will likely be evidence of acute hemorrhage or laboratory findings of abnormal coagulopathy. The use of viscoelastic testing for coagulation information is ideal to properly monitor coagulopathy status in real time; commonly, there is DIC with significant hyperfibrinolysis seen in AFE that can be revealed by viscoelastic testing, and it should be corrected with antifibrinolytic therapy.[4,5] Using these data and considering the patient's clinical status, blood products and/or massive transfusion protocol should be utilized in a 1:1:1 ratio to correct ongoing coagulopathies. Normothermia should be a priority with forced air warmers to prevent any further coagulopathy from hypothermia. Uterine atony in the setting of potential AFE should be treated with standard pharmacological interventions, including necessary surgical interventions.[3]

## POSTOPERATIVE

The patient should be admitted to the intensive care unit for close observation postoperatively. If the patient had a cardiac arrest, it is recommended to have therapeutic hypothermia in an attempt to preserve neurologic function as up to 60% of patients who survive AFE have long-term neurologic impairment. There should be continued serial blood draws to monitor for additional blood losses and coagulopathies, especially fibrinogen level as it is frequently low in obstetric hemorrhages.[3] In patients who are

unresponsive to continued resuscitative efforts for their cardiopulmonary shock, advanced life support devices and invasive hemodynamic support (extracorporeal membrane oxygenation) may be beneficial.[5] Once AFE is identified, using a multidisciplinary approach to management of this complex pathology is highly recommended.

## REFERENCES

1. Soens M, et al. Fetal development. In: *Chestnut's Obstetric Anesthesia*. 6th ed. Elsevier; 2020:77–95.
2. Standring, S. Implantation and placentation. In: *Gray's Anatomy: The Anatomical Basis of Clinical Practice*. 42nd ed. Elsevier Health Sciences; 2020:178–187.
3. Sultan P, et al. Amniotic fluid embolism. *Curr Opin Anaesthesiol*. 2016;29(3):288–296.
4. Chestnut DH, Toledo P. Embolic disorders. In: *Chestnut's Obstetric Anesthesia*. 6th ed. Elsevier; 2020:937–955.
5. Pacheco LD, et al. Amniotic fluid embolism: principles of early clinical management. *Am J Obstet Gynecol*. 2020;222(1):48–52.

# 290.

# LABOR ANALGESIA

*Ifomachukwu Uzodinma and Piotr Al-Jindi*

## INTRODUCTION

Labor pain has complex contributions from visceral, sympathetic, and somatic inputs that result in maternal discomfort.[1] Neuraxial anesthesia is the most reliable and effective method to control labor pain. The most common methods of neuraxial anesthesia implemented in the treatment of labor pain include epidurals, combined spinal-epidural (CSE), or spinals for labor pain. In the setting that neuraxial is contraindicated, other regional blocks, such as the paracervical, lumbar sympathetic, and pudendal nerve blocks, may also be used to control labor pain.

## LABOR PAIN

During the first stage of labor, the effacement and dilation of the cervix lead to stimulation of visceral afferent nerves. The visceral nerve impulses travel with sympathetic nerve fibers from the cervix and uterus until they ultimately enter the dorsal root ganglia at levels T10 through L1.[1] During the second stage of labor, it is the intense stretching of the vagina and perineum that contributes to the somatic component of labor pain. These somatic contributions of the second stage of labor pain are conducted along the pudendal nerves to the dorsal nerve roots of S2 through S4[1] (Figure 290.1).

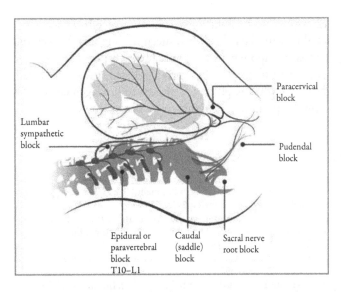

**Figure 290.1** Labor related nerve blocks

## PREPROCEDURAL ASSESSMENT

Prior to any neuraxial placement, an appropriate history and physical should be completed. The provider should pay special attention to maternal history, surgical history, previous anesthetics, and a focused physical examination.[1,2] Detailed examination of the anatomy of the spine is important prior to placing any neuraxial block. Maternal vital signs and fetal heart monitoring should occur during neuraxial placement.[1,2] The provider should be prepared with resuscitative medications and airway devices in the event of complications such as subdural placement, high spinal, or total spinal. Adequate hydration with isotonic fluids is necessary as neuraxial procedures can result in significant sympathectomy.[1] Additional potential side effects that may occur with neuraxial procedures include shivering, fever, delayed gastric emptying, and urinary retention[1] (Table 290.1).

## EPIDURAL ANALGESIA

Epidural analgesia provides excellent pain relief throughout labor. Lumbar epidurals are often inserted at the L2-L4 levels. Typically, a low concentration of an amide local anesthetic such as bupivacaine 0.0625%–0.125% or ropivacaine 0.1%–0.2% is used in the continuous epidural infusions (CEIs). The local anesthetic is combined with a low concentration of a lipid-soluble opioid (fentanyl 2 μg/mL or sufentanil 0.2 μg/mL), which typically provides satisfactory analgesia, improves latency, and limits extensive motor blockade. Amides are highly protein bound and therefore have the added benefit of limiting transplacental transfer. A test dose of 3 mL of lidocaine 1.5% with 1:200,000 epinephrine can be administered to rule out intrathecal or intravascular placement. If the catheter happens to be intrathecal, a dense motor block will result. In the event of a rapid sensory block, concern for subdural placement should be considered. In the setting that the test dose is intravascular, the epinephrine at 1:200,000 will contribute toward a 20%–30% increase in heart rate and blood pressure.[1] Particular caution should be taken as the gravid uterus often leads to inferior vena cava compression, resulting in engorgement of the epidural veins, increasing the risk of potential intravascular placement of the epidural catheter.[1] If a denser block is required due to instrumented delivery or episiotomy tears, lidocaine 2% with 1:200,000 epinephrine or 2-chloroprocaine (3%) are the medications often used.

## CAUDAL ANALGESIA

Caudal analgesia can be beneficial when used within the active phase of the first stage of labor and the early second stage of labor. The Tuohy needle will pass through the sacrococcygeal ligament and then into the caudal space. It may be used in a parturient who has a history of spinal surgery with hardware, making interlaminar access to the epidural space difficult. Caudal placement in a parturient may be technically challenging due to the increased sacral edema that occurs during labor.[1] Caudal epidurals carry increased risk of injury to the fetal head, potential risk of injury to the rectum, and increased volumes of local anesthetic to achieve adequate sensory blockage.[1]

## SPINAL ANALGESIA

A single-shot spinal can be used for rapidly progressing labor or for analgesia immediately prior to vaginal delivery requiring a dense sacral block. The benefit in spinal analgesia is its rapid onset. Typical intrathecal medications include a local anesthetic, opioids, or the combination of both a local anesthetic and a lipid-soluble opioid (e.g., fentanyl 12.5–25 μg and bupivacaine 6 mg).[2] The combination of the local anesthetic and the opioid work to ensure better sensory blockade and analgesia. Prolonged labor may surpass the duration of the spinal medication, which would lead to patient dissatisfaction and the potential requirement for readministering the neuraxial analgesia.[1,2] Intrathecal opioids carry an elevated risk of pruritis when compared to epidural administration; this also may lead to patient discontent.[1]

## COMBINED SPINAL-EPIDURAL ANALGESIA

The CSE technique has the benefit of administering intrathecal medication for rapid onset of analgesia while continuing maintenance through the epidural catheter infusion.[1–3] The epidural space is identified, then a spinal needle is introduced through the Tuohy needle. After puncture of the dura,

*Table 290.1* RELATIVE INFANT DOSE (RID) OF ANESTHESIA MEDICATIONS AND RECOMMENDATIONS

| MEDICATION CLASS (DRUG) | MEAN RID (%)[a] |
|---|---|
| Anticholinergics (atropine, glycopyrrolate) | Unknown: generally considered safe with single systemic or ophthalmic dosing |
| Anticholinesterases (neostigmine, pyridostigmine) | 0.1 |
| Antiemetics (metoclopramide, ondansetron) | Unknown: considered safe due to lack of sedating side effects |
| Benzodiazepines (diazepam, lorazepam, midazolam) | 0.3 |
| Intravenous Anesthetics | |
| Etomidate | 0.1 |
| Ketamine | Unknown: recommended only if medically necessary |
| Propofol | 0.1 |
| Local Anesthetics (bupivacaine, lidocaine, ropivacaine) | 0.1 |
| Narcotics | |
| Fentanyl | 1 |
| Hydrocodone | 3 |
| Hydromorphone | 3 |
| Morphine | 9 |
| Oxycodone | 3 (maximum daily dose 30 mg[b]) |
| Remifentanil | Unknown: considered safe secondary to short half-life |
| Codeine/Tramadol | Avoid: Food and Drug Administration warning against use in women with a cytochrome P450 2D6 mutation |
| Nonnarcotic Analgesics | |
| Acetaminophen | 4 (maximum daily dose < 3g[c]) |
| Ibuprofen | 0.5 |
| Ketorolac | 0.3 |
| Miscellaneous | |
| Gabapentin | 3 |
| Dexamethasone | Unknown: considered safe (may cause temporary loss of milk secondary to ↓ prolactin levels) |
| Diphenhydramine | Unknown: generally considered safe |
| Volatile Gases | Unknown: considered safe secondary to rapid excretion, poor bioavailability, and/or scavenging of gases |

[a] Mean RID is an estimated average from multiple sources reviewed.

[b] LactMed. Toxicology Data Network. US National Library of Medicine. NIH. HMS. Bethesda, MD. https://toxnet.nlm.nih.gov/cgi-bin/sis/search2

[c] FDA acetaminophen dosage announcement 468. 2012. https://www.medicaid.nv.gov/Downloads/provider/web_announcement_468_20120425.pdf

aspiration should result in the return of cerebrospinal fluid. The intrathecal medication is administered, and the spinal needle is removed. The catheter is then inserted into the epidural space. CSE delivers a faster onset of analgesia, particularly in the sacral region, when compared to the traditional epidural.[1] The onset of analgesia for CSE is 2–5 minutes, compared to the epidural alone, which takes approximately 15–20 minutes.[1]

## PROGRAMMED INTERMITTENT EPIDURAL BOLUS

A variety of different methods for administering epidural solutions exist; most recently, programmed intermittent epidural boluses (PIEBs) have been shown to provide superior analgesia for the laboring patient.[4] The popular use of the combined delivery modes that include patient-controlled epidural analgesia (PCEA) and CEIs have been shown to be beneficial in the parturient; however, they do not prevent requests for additional top-off dosing.[4,5] The introduction of the PIEB relies on the concept of providing consistently timed boluses to the laboring patient at fixed intervals. Regularly spaced intermittent boluses result in improved spread of the local anesthetic within the epidural space and thus better sensory block.[3–5] Evidence shows that laboring patients who receive the PIEB have better pain control, better sensory blockage, less motor blockade, and fewer requirements for vaginal delivery with instrumentation.[1,5] Caution should be maintained when implementing CEI plus PCEA and PIEB. Limitations may include pressure alarms with epidural pumps due to frequent boluses.[4] Providers should maintain vigilance when first using the PIEB system in conjunction with PCEA and CEI delivery systems and diligence to maternal hypotension, fetal heart rate changes, and sensory and motor blockade.[3–5]

## REFERENCES

1. Wong CA. Epidural and spinal analgesia: anesthesia for labor and vaginal delivery. In: Chestnut DH, et al., eds. *Chestnut's Obstetric Anesthesia: Principles and Practice*. 6th ed. Philadelphia, PA: Elsevier; 2020:474–539.
2. Practice guidelines for obstetric anesthesia: an updated report by the American Society of Anesthesiologists Task Force on Obstetric Anesthesia and the Society for Obstetric Anesthesia and Perinatology. *Anesthesiology*. 2016; 124: 270–300.
3. Fettes PDW, et al. Intermittent vs continuous administration of epidural ropivacaine with fentanyl for analgesia during labour. *Br J Anaesth*. 2006; 97(3):359–364.
4. Carvalho B, et al. Implementation of programmed intermittent epidural bolus for maintenance of labor analgesia. *Anesth Analg*. 2016;123(4):965–971.
5. Onuoha O. Epidural analgesia for labor. *Anesthesiol Clin*. 2017;35(1):1–14.

# 291.

# SYSTEMIC MEDICATIONS

*Ifomachukwu Uzodinma and Piotr Al-Jindi*

## INTRODUCTION

Early use of systemic analgesia in labor pain was surrounded with controversies based on religion, women's rights, and the unknown potential effects that the agents may have on the mother and neonate. Early methods often included ether or chloroform; such agents have since been abandoned as they resulted in poor fetal effects.[1,2] Systemic medications are a good alternative for the laboring patient who refuses neuraxial analgesia or prefers an alternative method to treat labor pain.[1]

## MORPHINE

Morphine is a potent analgesic with a prolonged duration of action of 3–4 hours when administered intravenously.

Morphine may be beneficial during the latent phase of labor; however, it is generally avoided during the active phase of labor due to its prolonged duration of action and potent metabolite morphine-6-glucoronide. Morphine can cause decreased fetal heart rate variability, respiratory depression, and low Apgar scores with increased use.[1,2] Maternal side effects include pruritis from the histamine release, sedation, and dysphoria.[1]

## MEPERIDINE

Meperidine acts as an agonist at μ- and κ-receptors, undergoes metabolism in the liver, and has an active metabolite, normeperidine.[1] The maternal half-life for meperidine is 4.5 hours, compared to that of normeperidine, which has a half-life of 14–21 hours.[1,3] Due to the prolonged half-life of normeperidine combined with the reduced clearance in the neonate, the respiratory depressant effects of normeperidine may last up to 3–5 days.[3]

## FENTANYL

Common delivery methods for administering opioids to the laboring patient are via patient-controlled analgesia (PCA) systems. Fentanyl PCAs are often used to treat labor pain. Fentanyl is a lipid-soluble synthetic opioid. It is particularly advantageous to the laboring patient due to its lack of active metabolites.[1] A fentanyl PCA is typically ordered as 25 μg every 10–15 minutes, with a lockout of 100 μg per hour.[1,2] The onset is within 2–4 minutes, and the duration is 30–60 minutes. The risks associated with a fentanyl PCA for labor analgesia include maternal sedation and dizziness.[1,2] Fentanyl does have transplacental transfer; however, typical maternal and fetal vein transfer is low, as fentanyl is easily redistributed.[1]

## REMIFENTANIL

In the past decade, remifentanil PCAs have been introduced in labor analgesia.[2,3] Remifentanil is known for its ultrarapid onset, at approximately 30 seconds, with a peak analgesic effect at 90 seconds.[1] Some limitation with remifentanil is the difficulty that arises when trying to match the exact timing of the bolus with the peak of uterine contractions.[2] Remifentanil undergoes metabolism via rapid hydrolysis by nonspecific plasma and tissue esterases; it has a short context-sensitive half-time of 3 minutes.[3] Adverse effects of remifentanil are not often seen in the neonate due to redistribution and rapid metabolism.[1–3] When compared with fentanyl, remifentanil does lead to increased maternal sedation and the potential for respiratory depression. When ordering a remifentanil PCA, optimal monitoring with 1-to-1 provider observation, and continuous pulse oximetry helps to ensure maternal safety.[1]

## ALFENTANIL

Alfentanil is a fentanyl derivative; it is highly selective to the μ-opioid receptor. If considered as an agent for labor analgesia, it is primarily administered with a PCA. Compared to fentanyl, alfentanil has a shorter context-sensitive half-time when administered for a prolonged duration.[3] Comparative studies between fentanyl and alfentanil noted that the two are similarly effective until cervical dilation reaches 6 cm. After the active phase of labor, fentanyl is superior; this may be related to alfentanil's shorter duration of action and rapid clearance.[1]

## KETAMINE

Ketamine is a phencyclidine derivative known for its effects as a N-methyl-D-aspartic acid (NMDA) and glutamate receptor antagonist. Ketamine acts by providing dissociative analgesia and works synergistically with systemic opioids. Typical onset occurs within 30 seconds of intravenous administration.[1] If neuraxial analgesia is suboptimal, small doses of ketamine at 0.2 mg/kg may be used as an adjunct during labor.[1] Ketamine has sympathomimetic properties; it should be avoided in the parturient with preeclampsia or gestational hypertension.

## NITROUS OXIDE

Nitrous oxide is an inhalational agent used worldwide for labor analgesia; it is colorless, odorless, and fairly inexpensive.[1,2,4] Despite its variable effectiveness at treating labor pain, it has been shown to increase maternal satisfaction due to its ability to allow the mother the option to have control in the birthing process.[2] Optimal analgesic effects are experienced at concentrations of approximately 50% nitrous oxide and 50% oxygen.[5] Concentrations higher than 60% nitrous oxide potentiate adverse effects, such as nausea and vomiting. Nitrous oxide works fairly rapidly due to its low blood/gas solubility at 0.42; peak concentrations occur within 1 minute.[4] The exact mechanism of action of nitrous oxide is not fully understood, but it is postulated that it works through multiple different neuromodulators in the spinal cord. It is specifically thought to act via modulation of opioid receptors within the periaqueductal gray, descending pain pathways within the spinal cord, and NMDA receptor antagonism.[1,4] Despite the capability of nitrous oxide to cross the placenta, there is no evidence that it leads to neonatal respiratory depression, altered neurobehavioral scores, decreased Apgar scores, or changes in fetal umbilical blood gases.[1,5] Potential adverse effects of nitrous oxide are increased maternal dizziness, nausea, emesis, and detachment.[5] Continuous exposure of anesthesia providers to nitrous oxide without proper scavenging systems may lead to potential neurotoxicity, reproductive toxicity, and DNA mutations as nitrous oxide inactivates methionine synthetase.[2,5]

## REFERENCES

1. Setty T, Fernando R. Systemic analgesia: parenteral and inhalational agents. In: Chestnut DH, et al., eds. *Chestnut's Obstetric Anesthesia: Principles and Practice*. 6th ed. Philadelphia, PA: Elsevier; 2020:453–473.
2. Lim G, et al. A review of the impact of obstetric anesthesia on maternal and neonatal outcomes. *Anesthesiology*. 2018;129(1):192–215.
3. Evron S, Ezri T. Options for systemic labor analgesia. *Curr Opin Anaesthesiol*. 2007;20(3):181–185.
4. Becker DE, Rosenberg M. Nitrous oxide and the inhalation anesthetics. *Anesth Prog*. 2008;55(4):124–132.
5. Vallejo MC, Zakowski MI. Pro-con debate: nitrous oxide for labor analgesia. *Biomed Research Int*. 2019;2019(4618798):1–12.

# 292.

# OTHER BLOCKS

*Mark L. Stram*

## INTRODUCTION

Epidural and spinal anesthesia/analgesia are the cornerstone of labor pain management for obstetric patients. These techniques are the most widely used for obstetric analgesia; however, there are circumstances where they may not be employed due to either patient factors (coagulopathy, thrombocytopenia, hemorrhage, prior lumbar spine surgery, or patient refusal) or lack of availability and expertise.

The paracervical block and lumbar sympathetic block are effective in managing pain during the first stage of labor, where the pain impulses result from dilation and thinning of the cervix and distention of the lower uterine segment and upper vagina. These impulses travel through the L2-3 sympathetic chain fibers via inferior hypogastric plexus and enter the spinal cord at T10-L1. The paracervical block stops impulses through the paracervical ganglion, which lies lateral and posterior to the cervicouterine junction, and is typically placed by an obstetrician during active labor with the cervix dilated between 4 and 8 cm. Paracervical block beyond 8 cm increases risk of fetal bradycardia; additionally, scalp injury or injection may occur due to

cervical thinning. Lumbar sympathetic (also known as paravertebral lumbar sympathetic) blocks are used to impede visceral pain impulses at the L2-3 sympathetic chain ganglion. This technique is useful for patients who have had previous lumbar spine surgery that precludes epidural catheter placement. Pudendal nerve blockade provides analgesia to the perineum, vulva, and lower vagina. It is performed by the obstetrician during the second stage of labor. The nerve arises from the S2-4 level of the sacral plexus and passes beneath the sacrospinous ligament and medial to the ischial spine, which is the target area for this block.

## TECHNIQUE

### PARACERVICAL BLOCK

For a paracervical block (Figure 292.1), position the patient in modified lithotomy position with left uterine displacement. Two injections will be made, at the 4 and 8 o'clock positions with reference to the cervix. For the 4 o'clock (left side) injection, insert the gloved left hand into the vagina with the needle guide ("Iowa trumpet") containing

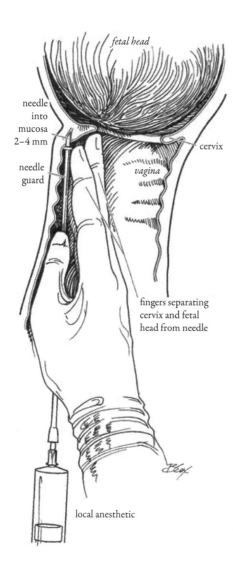

needle into mucosa 2–4 mm

fetal head

needle guard

cervix

vagina

fingers separating cervix and fetal head from needle

local anesthetic

Figure 292.1  To come

*Table 292.1* MATERNAL AND FETAL COMPLICATIONS

| MATERNAL COMPLICATIONS | FETAL COMPLICATIONS |
| --- | --- |
| Bleeding: hematoma and/or mucosal laceration | Fetal bradycardia |
| Infection/abscess formation | Scalp injection[3] |
| Vasovagal syncope | LAST |
| Local anesthetic systemic toxicity (LAST) | |
| Sacral neuropathy due to needle trauma or hematoma | |

of analgesia is relatively short. Repeated injections can be made, however, this was not without additional risk, primarily to the fetus (bradycardia, fetal scalp injection causing local anesthetic toxicity and death[3]). Although considered off-label use in the United States, 0.125% bupivacaine has been safely used, especially in Europe, and provides longer duration of analgesia. The most common complication is fetal bradycardia, felt to be about 15% (Table 292.1).[4]

## LUMBAR SYMPATHETIC BLOCK

For the lumbar sympathetic block (Figure 292.2), the patient should be sitting. The usual sterile technique should be used. The L2 transverse process is identified. Skin and soft tissue are infiltrated with 1% lidocaine at the needle insertion point, located approximately 7–8 cm from the midline. A 10-cm spinal needle is introduced with the tip angled medially toward the lateral surface of the L2 vertebral body, then "walked off" anterolaterally until the tip is located just anterior to the psoas muscle attachment. The syringe should

a 20-gauge, 6-inch (15.2 cm) needle between index and middle fingers and directed as far laterally as possible into the fornix. The needle is advanced no more than 3 mm beyond the end of the needle guide. The risk of fetal bradycardia and scalp injection is reduced by keeping the injection depth less than 4 mm. Maternal local anesthetic systemic absorption is also reduced with shallower injection depth of 2–3 mm.[1] The physician should aspirate prior to injection in an effort to avoid intravascular injection. Use 5–10 mL of local without epinephrine. Before proceeding to the other side, the clinician should monitor fetal heart tones for 10 minutes, watching for fetal bradycardia. Repeat the same process for injecting at the 8 o'clock position using the right index and middle fingers to direct the needle guide. Extreme care should be taken to avoid needlestick injury to the physician. The needle guide does not consistently protect the physician from needle injury[2] and risk of HIV or hepatitis.

The choice of local anesthetic is controversial. Traditionally, 1% lidocaine has been used; however, the duration

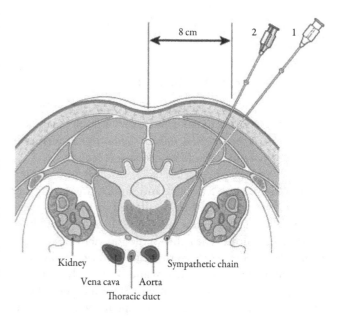

8 cm

2    1

Kidney

Sympathetic chain

Vena cava    Aorta

Thoracic duct

Figure 292.2  To come

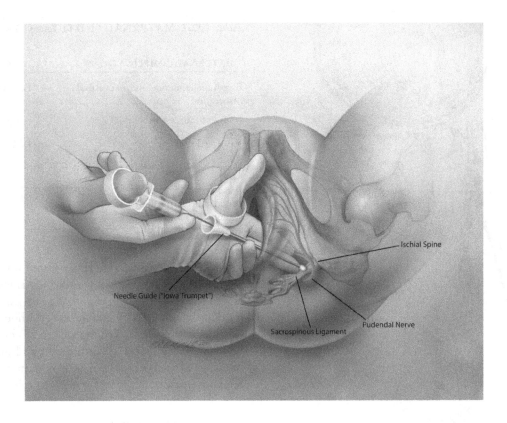

Figure 292.3 To come

be aspirated to avoid intravascular injection. Inject 10 mL of 0.5%–0.375% bupivacaine with epinephrine 2.5 μg/mL in several incremental doses. If inadequate analgesia is achieved, a second injection may be performed on the opposite side. Maternal hypotension is the most common complication and may be mitigated by administration of 500–1000 mL of intravenous crystalloid prior to placing the block. The main risk to the fetus would stem from any prolonged maternal hypotension. Other complications include local anesthetic systemic toxicity (LAST), retroperitoneal hematoma, inadvertent dural puncture,[5] and total spinal block.

## PUDENDAL BLOCK

The pudendal block (Figure 292.3) may be performed with either a transvaginal or transperineal approach. The transvaginal technique is most commonly done in the United States and is described in the next section.

Similar to the paracervical block, a needle guide is positioned between the left index and middle fingers to place the left pudendal nerve block, followed by the right index and middle fingers to place the right side block. The obstetrician then palpates the ischial spine and sacrospinous ligament. The needle is placed into the mucosa and through the sacrospinous ligament medially and posteriorly to the ischial spine. The needle is advanced 1–1.5 cm beyond the tip of the guide. The physician should aspirate before injecting

to avoid intravascular injection into the pudendal artery, which lies in close proximity to the nerve. Concentrated local anesthetic should not be used and is not necessary. Typically, 1% lidocaine or mepivacaine is preferred over 2-chloroprocaine due to the longer duration. Like the paracervical block, this technique requires blind needle insertion and has similar risk for needlestick injury to the operator.[2] Complications include LAST; hematoma formation (retroperitoneal, ischiorectal, or vaginal); vaginal mucosal laceration; fetal needle trauma; and direct injection of local into the fetus.

## REFERENCES

1. Jägerhorn M. Paracervical block in obstetrics. An improved injection method. A clinical and radiological study. *Acta Obstet Gynecol Scand*. 1975;54:9–27.
2. Chestnut DH. Alternative regional anesthetic techniques: paracervical block, lumbar sympathetic block, pudendal nerve block, and perineal infiltration. In: Chestnut DH, et al., eds. *Chestnut's Obstetric Anesthesia Principles and Practice*. 4th ed. Philadelphia, PA: Mosby Elsevier; 2009:493–503.
3. Shnider SM, et al. Regional anesthesia for labor and delivery. In: Shnider SM, Levinson G, eds. *Anesthesia for Obstetrics*. 3rd ed. Baltimore, MD: Williams & Wilkins; 1993:135–153.
4. Rosen MA. Paracervical block for labor analgesia: a brief historic review. *Am J Obstet Gynecol*. 2002;186(5 suppl):S127–S130.
5. Artuso JD, et al. Postdural puncture headache after lumbar sympathetic block: a report of two cases. *Reg Anesth*. 1991;16:288–291

# 293.

# COMPLICATIONS OF OBSTETRIC ANESTHESIA

*Peter Lampert and Kristopher M. Schroeder*

## POSTDURAL PUNCTURE HEADACHE

### INTRODUCTION

Postdural puncture headache (PDPH) is one of the most commonly encountered postpartum complications of neuraxial anesthesia. However, it is just one of many potential etiologies that contribute to the diagnosis of postpartum headaches. PDPH can occur following unintentional dural puncture with an epidural needle or after intentional dural puncture with a spinal needle. The rate at which an unintentional puncture of the dura is encountered is roughly 1 in 100 epidural attempts. Following the incidental dural puncture, the risk of headache is approximately 50%; however, it has been reported as up to 75% in some populations with other associated risk factors. This is compared to the headache rate following intentional dural puncture, which carries a 1.5% to 11.2% risk of the individual developing a headache. The pathophysiology behind PDPH remains heavily debated, but it is theorized to be a result of cerebrospinal fluid (CSF) leakage through the dural puncture causing sagging of intracranial structures, thereby stretching the cerebral pain fibers. This occurs in conjunction with CSF hypotension, leading to a compensatory increase in cerebral blood flow secondary to cerebral venodilation, which causes further traction on intracranial structures.[1]

### SYMPTOMS

Symptoms of a PDPH include a headache that usually occurs within 5 days of a dural puncture. The headache is always symmetric, with pain localized to the frontal, occipital, or, most commonly, a combination of the frontal and occipital regions. Classically, there is a positional nature directly associated with the headache, wherein the symptoms are exacerbated when assuming the upright position and relieved with recumbency. Associated symptoms include ocular disturbances (photophobia, diplopia); auditory manifestations (phonophobia, hearing loss, and tinnitus);

neck stiffness; and nausea. Cranial nerve palsies can also be encountered with PDPH and are thought to be a consequence of low CSF volumes causing traction on cranial nerves. Most susceptible to this traction is cranial nerve VI (abducens) due to its long and tortuous path, manifesting itself clinically as diplopia and failure of the involved eye to abduct. Onset of symptoms is delayed, usually within 12 to 48 hours, and can rarely present 5 days following a dural puncture. Development of headache symptoms within 12 to 24 hours raises the concern for pneumocephalus rather than PDPH.[1,2]

### RISK FACTORS

- Age—This is very unlikely in patients older than 60 and younger than 10 years of age, with peak incidence occurring in the late teens and early 20s (Table 293.1).
- Gender—The incidence is 11.1% for nonpregnant females compared to 3.6% for age-matched males.
- Vaginal delivery—The mechanical consequences of Valsalva during the expulsive efforts in the second stage of labor may promote increased CSF leakage.

*Table 293.1* RISK FACTORS FOR THE DEVELOPMENT OF PDPH

| RISK FACTORS FOR PDPH | |
| --- | --- |
| **Modifiable** | Beveled (Quincke), cutting needle<br>Larger needle (decreased gauge)<br>Spinal needle bevel orientation<br>Vaginal delivery, specifically prolonged second stage of labor<br>Multiple dural punctures |
| **Nonmodifiable** | Female gender<br>Pregnancy<br>Younger age<br>Lower BMI (controversial)<br>History of prior dural puncture headache or chronic headaches |

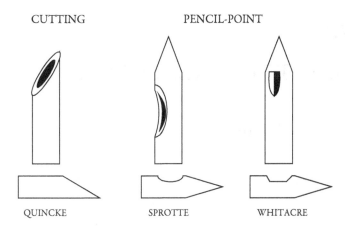

CUTTING          PENCIL-POINT

QUINCKE          SPROTTE          WHITACRE

**Figure 293.1** Common types of spinal needles

- Obesity—Patients with a higher body mass index (BMI) were associated with lower rates of PDPH. This finding is fraught with conflicting data due to the added procedural complexity inherent to patients with larger BMIs and difficulty locating surface landmarks, often requiring multiple attempts.
- Neuraxial technique.
  - Spinal needle design—Beveled cutting needles such as the Quincke increase the risk of PDPH. As a result, pencil-point needles like the Whitacre or Sprotte needles are preferred (Figure 293.1).
  - Spinal needle size—Larger needle diameter is associated with an elevated risk of PDPH.
  - Direction of needle bevel when using a cutting needle (Quincke needle) for spinal anesthesia—Accessing the intrathecal space with a Quincke needle parallel to the long axis of the spine reduces the risk of PDPH.
- Multiple dural punctures.
- History of previous PDPH.

## TREATMENT

In the setting of unintentional dural punctures, no interventions have reliably demonstrated efficacy in preventing PDPH. Initial treatment is generally supportive through scheduled analgesics, hydration, and encouraging horizontal positioning. Even though the evidence fails to show improvement in symptoms with increased hydration, dehydration should be avoided.

The gold standard therapy is considered to be the autologous epidural blood patch (EBP). Typically, 15–30 mL of the patient's own blood is injected into the epidural space via an epidural needle. Prophylactic EBP was historically advocated in the setting of known unintentional dural puncture, but recent evidence does not support this practice. Consistent with this, observational studies have demonstrated an increased risk of treatment failure if the EBP is performed within 24–48 hours of dural puncture. The

ideal timing of EBP has not definitively been elucidated; however, severity of symptoms often influences the timing of administration, especially in the setting of a presumed cranial nerve palsy. Performing an EBP has been shown to prevent the progression of ocular symptoms if they are associated with cranial nerve palsies. If symptoms fail to improve with a second EBP attempt or additional neurologic deficits develop, further patient evaluation is warranted, and other etiologies of postpartum headache must be considered.[2]

Alternatively, several regional techniques, including sphenopalantine ganglion and greater occipital nerve blocks, have been shown to improve the symptoms of PDPH. Bilateral transnasal sphenopalantine ganglion blocks using topical local anesthetic is emerging as a promising alternative to EBP as it abates symptoms via blockade of autonomic and sensory nerves that contribute to symptomology.[1]

## PERIPHERAL NEUROPATHIES

### INTRODUCTION

Postpartum neuropathies are frequently encountered and mistakenly attributed to neuraxial analgesia; however, it is important to emphasize that obstetric causes are more likely to result in peripheral neuropathies than anesthetic-related injury. Neuraxial anesthesia is more likely to cause central compared to peripheral nerve injuries, which generally occur as a result of direct nerve trauma. Intrapartum nerve compression may be more frequently undetected if neuraxial anesthesia is utilized secondary to a decreased ability to perceive the sensation of positional extremes. (Table 293.2) summarizes the frequently encountered postpartum nerve palsies.[3,4]

### RISK FACTORS

Certain obstetric factors contribute to an increased incidence of postpartum nerve palsies during the delivery process. These include compression by the fetal head, prolonged second stage of labor, nerve injury as the fetus traverses the birth canal, difficult instrumented delivery, nulliparity, and maternal positioning to facilitate delivery, including prolonged use of the lithotomy position. To reduce peripartum nerve injuries, mindful patient positioning and frequent position changes should be performed, particularly after administration of neuraxial blockade. Additionally, the use of low-dose local anesthetic and neuraxial opioids should be administered to allow for maximal mobility. Perhaps most importantly, the anesthetic provider should have a keen understanding that not all numbness and tingling can be attributed to neuraxial anesthesia but rather can represent more insidious nerve compression or injury.[4]

*Table 293.2* COMMON POSTPARTUM NEUROPATHIES

| PERIPHERAL NERVE | CAUSE | MOTOR/SENSORY DISTURBANCE |
|---|---|---|
| Lumbosacral trunk (L4-5) | Compression by the fetal head at the level of the pelvic brim, often related to cephalopelvic disproportion and difficult vaginal deliveries | Commonly affects medial fibers that comprise the peroneal nerve, thereby sparing the tibial nerve<br>*Motor*—reduced ankle dorsiflexion and toe extension (foot-drop)<br>*Sensory*—disturbances to the L5 dermatome (lateral leg and dorsum of the foot) |
| Obturator (L2-4) | Susceptible as it crosses the pelvic brim or within the obturator canal<br>Compression of the nerve between the pelvis and fetal head/forceps | *Motor*—weakness of hip adduction and internal rotation, leading to gait disturbances<br>*Sensory*—disturbances to medial thigh |
| Femoral (L2-4) | Vulnerable to stretch as it traverses beneath the inguinal ligament, anterior to the iliopsoas<br>Results from prolonged hip flexion, abduction, and external rotation consistent with extreme lithotomy | *Motor*—proximal injury at the level of the inguinal ligament leads to weakness in hip flexion; however, more distal injuries spare the iliopsoas motor supply<br>*Sensory*—disturbances of the anteromedial thigh and medial leg/foot |
| Meralgia Paresthetica (L2-3) | Nerve entrapment as the lateral femoral cutaneous nerve passes around the anterior superior iliac spine (ASIS) through the inguinal ligament<br>Associated with increased intra-abdominal pressure and the downward force applied by the gravid uterus<br>Compressive forces from retractors during cesarean delivery | *Sensory*—paresthesias and numbness over the anterolateral aspect of the thigh |
| Peroneal (L4—S2) | Susceptible to compression as the common peroneal nerve passes around the lateral head of the fibula<br>Prolonged compression of the lateral knee against a hard surface (lithotomy stirrups, patient's hand, side of the bed) | *Motor*—reduced ankle dorsiflexion and toe extension (foot-drop), decreased strength with ankle eversion<br>*Sensory*—deficits in the anterolateral calf and dorsum of the foot |

# REFERENCES

1. Peralta F, McArthur A. Postpartum headaches. In: *Chestnut's Obstetric Anesthesia: Principles and Practice*. Elsevier; 2020;30:724–751.
2. Maronge L, Bogod D. Complications in obstetric anesthesia. *Anesthesia*. 2018;73:61–66.
3. Duncan A, Patel S. Neurological complications in obstetric regional anesthetic practice. *J Obstet Anesth Crit Care*. 2016;6:3–10.
4. Sviggum H, Reynolds F. Neurologic complications of pregnancy and neuraxial anesthesia. In: *Chestnut's Obstetric Anesthesia: Principles and Practice*. Elsevier. 2020;30:752–776.

# 294.

# PHYSIOLOGY OF LABOR

*Nwadiogo Ejiogu and Barbara Orlando*

## INTRODUCTION

As detailed in a separate chapter, pregnancy is marked by several profound anatomic, physiologic, and pharmacological changes that affect every organ system.

## STAGES OF LABOR

Labor is a complex physiologic event that involves multiple different organ systems, all collaborating to reach an end of parturition. This process has been categorized in stages.

The first stage of labor is defined as the beginning of uterine contractions, causing effacement and dilation of the cervix; it ends with complete cervical dilation of 10 cm. This stage of labor includes a latent phase with slow cervical dilation (with a lack of consensus regarding absolute diagnostic criteria on when it starts and when it ends), and an active phase, which generally occurs when at least 6 cm dilation is reached. Pain during stage 1 is mediated by T10-L1 sympathetic nerve fibers that travel via the inferior hypogastric plexus to the sympathetic chain.

Complete cervical dilation of 10 cm marks the beginning of the second stage of labor, with completion being the delivery of the neonate. Second-stage pain is transmitted via the pudendal nerve (S2-4).

Finally, the third stage of labor begins with the delivery of the newborn and ends with the delivery of the placenta. While labor analgesia is covered in another chapter in this book, the stages of labor are critical to understanding the physiologic changes associated with parturition.

## HEMODYNAMIC CHANGES DURING LABOR

Cardiac output increases throughout pregnancy.[1] Labor is associated with further increases in cardiac output, from 10% in the early first stage of labor to 25% in the late first stage of labor, compared to prelabor values. During the second stage of labor, those numbers in cardiac output go up to 40% compared to prelabor values.[2] This phenomenon is thought to be a result of three things:

1. Increased venous return during contractions: With each uterine contraction there is approximately 300 to 500 mL of blood from the uterus that is "autotransfused" into the circulating blood volume. This leads to increased venous return and a concomitant increase in stroke volume and cardiac output.
2. Increase in sympathetic tone secondary to heightened pain and/or anxiety in the parturient: Pain (in the unmedicated parturient) and/or excitement/anxiety cause heart rate and blood pressure elevation by 10%–25%.
3. The parturient's process of pushing results in the sympathetically mediated increase in heart rate contributing to alterations in cardiac output during labor.

Cardiac output peaks in the immediate postpartum period and can increase by as much as 150% above prepregnancy values. The postpartum peak of cardiac output is again caused by both myometrial contraction and the elimination of vena cava compression. Cardiac output begins to decrease 1 hour postpartum and returns to prelabor and prepregnancy values at 24 hours and 3 to 6 months postpartum, respectively.[3]

Knowledge of these profound changes in cardiac output in the parturient are especially critical in caring for patients with cardiovascular comorbidities such as heart failure, pulmonary hypertension, and stenotic valvular lesions. Those diseases can be severely affected by the labor period and lead to dangerous decompensation that can put the parturient's life in jeopardy.

## CHANGES IN VENTILATION AND AIRWAY ANATOMY DURING LABOR

Hormonal changes in pregnancy lead to increases in minute ventilation that continue during labor.[1] The unmedicated parturient experiences an increase in minute ventilation by 70% to 140% during the first stage and up to 200% in the second stage of labor, compared with prepregnancy values.[2] An outcome of this change in minute ventilation is a further decreased $PaCO_2$, with values as low as 10 mm Hg. These changes in ventilation are thought to be primarily due to pain, anxiety, and an up to 75% increase in oxygen consumption. Neuraxial analgesia can mitigate changes in ventilation by reducing pain and, by extension, reducing the increased metabolic demands of hyperventilation.

After delivery, it takes approximately 6 to 8 weeks for minute ventilation, tidal volume, and oxygen consumption to return to prepregnancy values, while functional residual capacity and $PaCO_2$ both increase postpartum but remain below nonpregnant values at 2 weeks and 8 weeks, respectively.[2]

Airway edema can also worsen with labor.[4] Specifically, during the second stage of labor, airway edema is more pronounced due to the increase in venous pressure with active pushing. This is a major physiologic alteration that is important to consider when attempting laryngoscopy and choosing endotracheal tube size (preference given to 6.0–6.5 mm).

## GASTROINTESTINAL PHYSIOLOGIC CHANGES DURING LABOR

The pregnant population is at an increased risk of gastric aspiration, likely from both mechanical factors, which lead to an increase in intra-abdominal pressure, and the progesterone hormone, which relaxes the lower esophageal sphincter. The highest risk of aspiration is during labor or immediately postpartum. This increased risk of aspiration immediately before and after delivery is thought to be secondary to two factors: sedation and the parturient's recumbent position. Other gastrointestinal changes during labor include new onset of delayed gastric emptying (worsened during labor because of the pain) and an increased prevalence of patients with gastric volumes greater than 25 mL. This prolonged gastric emptying occurs if the parturient is given a sedative or opiate drug. It is, however, unclear whether gastric acid secretion is changed in laboring people.[2]

## OTHER PHYSIOLOGIC CHANGES WITH LABOR

Pregnancy has been associated with leukocytosis.[5] A normal white blood cell (WBC) count is greater than 10,000 cells/μL during pregnancy. This leukocytosis increases both at term and during labor, with an upper level as high as 29,000 cells/μL. These elevated WBC values return to normal 4 to 5 days postpartum.

There are neurologic changes also experienced during labor. For instance, cerebral spinal fluid pressure and intracranial pressure (ICP) are both increased with contractions and pushing during the second stage of labor (especially during the Valsalva maneuver used by the parturient during the pushing period). This change in ICP during labor can make vaginal delivery a contraindication in some patients with a baseline elevated ICP.

## REFERENCES

1. Gaiser R. Physiologic changes of pregnancy." In: Chestnut D, et al., eds. *Chestnut's Obstetric Anesthesia: Principles and Practice.* 5th ed. 2014:15–38.
2. Ouzounian JG, Elkayam U. Physiologic changes during normal pregnancy and delivery. *Cardiol Clin.* 2012;30(3):317–329.
3. Capeless EL, Clapp JF. When do cardiovascular parameters return to their preconception values? *Am J Obstet Gynecol.* 1991;165(4 pt 1):883–886.
4. Bhavani-Shankar K, et al. Airway changes during labor and delivery. *Anesthesiology.* 2018;108(3):357–353.
5. Molberg P, et al. Leukocytosis in labor: what are its implications? *Fam Pract Res J.* 1994;14:229.

# 295.

# INFLUENCE OF ANESTHETIC TECHNIQUE ON LABOR

*Mary J. Im and Ihab Kamel*

## INTRODUCTION

Epidural analgesia does not impact the risk of cesarean section. Nevertheless, epidural analgesia was found to be associated with a prolongation of the second stage of labor and increased risk of assisted vaginal birth.

## EFFECT OF LABOR PROGRESS AND CESAREAN SECTION RATE

### LABOR PROGRESS

#### First Stage of Labor

The duration of the first stage of labor and the epidural effect is difficult to assess. Most of the randomized controlled studies and meta-analyses evaluated the duration of the first stage of labor as a secondary outcome, and there were mixed findings among the studies. The duration of the first stage is defined as the time from the beginning of regular uterine contraction to the complete cervical dilation of 10 cm. Because of the effect of epidural analgesia, women who received and epidural may not feel the rectal pressure with complete cervical dilation, which may artificially prolong the duration of the first stage of labor by delaying cervical examination.[1]

#### Second Stage of Labor

Epidural analgesia is associated with the prolongation of the second stage of labor. In nulliparous women, the 95th percentile of the second stage of labor was 3.6 hours with epidural analgesia and 2.8 hours without epidural analgesia.[2] The Society of Maternal-Fetal Medicine and the American College of Obstetricians and Gynecologists (ACOG) reflected the epidural analgesia effect on the prolongation of the second stage of labor (Table 295.1) by using different definitions of prolonged labor in women who received neuraxial analgesia or not.[3]

The association of epidural analgesia with the prolongation of the second stage of labor was not significant when a low concentration of local anesthetics (LCLA; <0.15% of ropivacaine or < 0.1% of bupivacaine) was used. A recent meta-analysis did not show a significant difference in duration of the second stage of labor between the group of epidural analgesia with LCLA and the group of nonepidural analgesia.[2]

There have been concerns about maternal and neonatal outcomes associated with the duration of the second stage of labor or active pushing. The risks of postpartum hemorrhage, advanced degree of perineal lacerations, chorioamnionitis, as well as neonatal complications, were observed to be higher with the prolongation of the second stage of labor.[2]

### ASSISTED VAGINAL DELIVERY RATE

Epidural analgesia has been associated with high assisted vaginal delivery (AVD) rate. A recent meta-analysis found that women who received epidural analgesia were more likely to experience instrumental vaginal delivery.[4] However, when the authors reanalyzed the trials only after 2005, the higher rate of AVD was no longer present, which suggests that modern epidural medication with LCLA is not associated an increase in instrumental vaginal delivery rate. The higher rate of AVD observed in women who

*Table 295.1* DEFINITION OF SECOND-STAGE ARREST DISORDER

| | NULLIPAROUS WOMEN | MULTIPAROUS WOMEN |
|---|---|---|
| With epidural analgesia | No progress for ≥ 4 hours | No progress for ≥ 3 hours |
| Without epidural analgesia | No progress for ≥ 3 hours | No progress for ≥ 2 hours |

received epidural analgesia may result from a prolonged second stage of labor with a high concentration of local anesthetics in the epidural infusion. Although it is not clearly defined, motor impairment induced by the dense epidural block may result in prolongation of the second stage and higher incidence of AVD.

## CESAREAN SECTION RATE

About 32% of pregnant women deliver by cesarean section in the United States.[1] Multiple randomized controlled trials have been conducted to assess the effect of epidural analgesia on the cesarean delivery rate, which did not show significant findings compared with nonepidural analgesia or no analgesia.[4] In one population-based, retrospective cohort study from the Netherlands, there was no significant association between epidural analgesia and cesarean delivery rate. A meta-analysis of the impact of epidural analgesia before and after the availability of epidural analgesia did not show any significant change in the cesarean delivery rate with an increase in epidural analgesia. Overall, epidural analgesia has no significant effect on the cesarean delivery rate.[1]

## TIMING OF NEURAXIAL ANALGESIA AND DELIVERY OUTCOMES

Multiple randomized controlled trials investigated the effect of early epidural analgesia, and obstetrical outcomes on the mode of delivery did not show any evidence of the risk of cesarean delivery or instrumental vaginal delivery rate. Overall, there was no difference in the rate of cesarean section or AVD among women given epidural analgesia at less than 4 cm of cervical dilation compared to women who received epidural analgesia later in labor.

## ANESTHETIC CONSIDERATIONS

### PREOPERATIVE

Women should receive epidural analgesia for the labor pain preoperatively, when requested, regardless of the stage of labor. According to a practice bulletin in 2017, ACOG stated that "In the absence of a medical contraindication, maternal request is a sufficient medical indication for pain relief during labor."[5]

### INTRAOPERATIVE

An LCLA such as of ropivacaine less than 0.15% or bupivacaine less than 0.1% should be used for labor epidural analgesia to avoid a motor block and minimize the likelihood of prolongation of the second stage of labor. Supplementing the epidural local anesthetic solution with a low-dose opioid medication (e.g., fentanyl 2 µg/mL) will improve the quality of analgesia while avoiding a motor block.

## REFERENCES

1. Wong CA. Epidural and spinal analgesia: anesthesia for labor and vaginal delivery. In: Chestnut DH, et al., eds. *Chestnut's Obstetric Anesthesia: Principles and Practice.* 6th ed. Philadelphia, PA: Elsevier Health Sciences; 2020:474–539.
2. Lim G, et al. A review of the impact of obstetric anesthesia on maternal and neonatal outcomes. *Anesthesiology.* 2018;129(1):192–215.
3. Spong CY, et al. Preventing the first cesarean delivery: summary of a joint Eunice Kennedy Shriver National Institute of Child Health and Human Development, Society for Maternal-Fetal Medicine, and American College of Obstetricians and Gynecologists Workshop. *Obstet Gynecol.* 2012;120(5):1181–1193.
4. Anim-Somuah M, et al. Epidural versus non-epidural or no analgesia for pain management in labour. *Cochrane Database Syst Rev.* 2018;5:CD000331.
5. Committee on Practice Bulletins—Obstetrics. Practice bulletin no. 177. Obstetric analgesia and anesthesia. *Obstet Gynecol.* 2017;129(4):e73.

# 296.

# CESAREAN SECTION

*Piotr Al-Jindi and Ami Attali*

## INTRODUCTION

Cesarean delivery is the most common surgical procedure performed worldwide. It is defined as the birth of an infant through an abdominal and uterine incision.

A clear designation of urgency is vital for the best maternal and fetal outcome.[1] Cases may be categorized as stat/emergent when there is an immediate threat to the life of mother or fetus. An urgent designation is when a maternal or fetal compromise is not immediately life threatening. A scheduled case is when early delivery without any maternal or fetal compromise is performed electively.

## INDICATIONS

Indications for cesarean section can be classified into one of three groups: maternal, fetal, and uterine or placental.

Maternal indications include antepartum/intrapartum hemorrhage, labor arrest, genital herpes, failed induction, deteriorating maternal conditions, multiple gestation, or maternal request.

Fetal indications include malpresentation, intolerance of labor, suspected macrosomia, dystocia, and nonreassuring fetal status.

Uterine or placental indications include uterine rupture, placental rupture, placenta previa, prolapsed fetal cord, previous myomectomy, and chorioamnionitis.

## TECHNIQUE

The low transverse uterine incision is associated with reduced risk of infection, blood loss, and abdominal adhesions. Other commonly used surgical approaches include midline vertical abdomen incision, which allows greater surgical exposure, and horizontal suprapubic incision, which offers better wound healing.

## COMPLICATIONS

Some complications associated with a cesarean section include hemorrhage, uterine atony, uterine laceration, broad ligament hematoma, endometritis, wound infection, venous thromboembolism, ileus, adhesions, and bladder/ureteral injury.

## ANESTHETIC CONSIDERATIONS

### PREOPERATIVE

Preoperative evaluation should occur early in the admission process and should include a review of the past medical and obstetric history, including a physical examination of the patient's airway, heart, and lungs. A blood type and cross-match and large-bore intravenous line should be obtained for these patients due to an increased risk of hemorrhage.

Aspiration prophylaxis with a nonparticulate antacid, $H_2$ receptor antagonist, proton pump inhibitor, and metoclopramide in select patients should be given within 30 minutes prior to cesarean section.[2] The anesthesia provider should use multimodal pharmacological therapies to help prevent postoperative nausea and vomiting. Preventing intraoperative or sympathetically mediated maternal hypotension may be the most effective means of preventing nausea and vomiting. Administration of prophylactic antibiotics within 1 hour of surgical incision reduces the risk of infectious complications after cesarean section.[3]

### INTRAOPERATIVE

Intraoperative preparation for cesarean section involves ensuring communication with the obstetric team about anticipated surgical complications and risk factors for hemorrhage and ensuring medication availability, including uterotonic agents and vasopressors, and having airway equipment at hand.

Neuraxial anesthesia is the preferred method of anesthesia for cesarean section unless there is an absolute contraindication. Even in some cases of obstetrical emergencies, such as umbilical cord prolapse, neuraxial anesthesia may be useful if the prolapse can be decompressed and if the fetal status remains reassuring. Neuraxial anesthesia is used for most elective cases and in certain emergent cesarean sections in the United States. Advantages of neuraxial anesthesia include decreasing maternal mortality, limited neonatal drug transfer, ability of the parents to be awake and take part in the delivery during the birth of their child, and avoiding airway manipulation in patients who have both a potentially difficult airway and an aspiration risk.

There are different neuraxial techniques that can be used:

- An epidural can be used for early labor analgesia and, in the event of a cesarean section, activated to provide surgical anesthesia.
- A single-shot spinal has a limited duration of anesthesia and cannot be redosed if needed for longer than anticipated.
- A combined spinal-epidural has the benefit of deep spinal anesthesia with the ability to titrate and extend intraoperative anesthesia via the epidural catheter for postoperative analgesia.
- A continuous spinal catheter can be used for rapid onset of dense anesthesia but has an increased risk of postdural puncture headache. It can also be mistaken as an epidural catheter, and if dosed as an epidural catheter can lead to high spinal anesthesia and cardiovascular collapse.

When general anesthesia is indicated, a multidisciplinary team discussion should ensure that all equipment is readily available for the patient. Adequate intravenous access should be obtained, the patient should be placed supine with left uterine displacement, and a nonparticulate antacid and $H_2$ receptor antagonist should be given. Standard American Society of Anesthesiologist monitoring, including pulse oximetry, electrocardiography, capnography, and noninvasive blood pressure should be started. A proper team time out is essential even in emergent scenarios. If general anesthesia is planned, patients should be preoxygenated with 100% $FiO_2$ (fraction of inspired oxygen) to prevent hypoxemia during apnea. Rapid sequence induction and intubation with cricoid pressure should follow as the patient is at an increased risk for aspiration. If a patient has a potentially difficult airway, then awake intubation should be considered. Maintenance during the anesthetic should ensure adequate fetal and maternal oxygenation, appropriate depth of anesthesia, and minimal effects on uterine tone and the neonate. The patient should be placed in a semirecumbent position prior to extubation.

Regardless of which anesthesia technique was used, it is crucial that there is communication between the obstetric and anesthesia team during the cesarean section to see if additional uterotonic agents are required.

Anesthetic complications include intraoperative awareness and recall, dyspnea following neuraxial anesthesia, hypotension, failure of neuraxial blockade, high neuraxial blockade, difficult airway/trauma to the airway, and nausea and vomiting.

## POSTOPERATIVE

There are multiple important postoperative aspects to consider following a cesarean section. Some of these include postoperative pain, pruritus, hypothermia, hemorrhage, and thromboembolic events. A combination of different agents and techniques can be considered for postoperative pain management, including opioids, epidural catheter, and transversus abdominal plane blocks. Pruritus is a common side effect of intrathecal and epidural opioids. Opioid receptor antagonists and partial antagonists/agonists are currently the most effective treatment of choice.[4] Neuraxial anesthesia is also associated with perioperative hypothermia and shivering, which can be managed with warming devices and pharmacological agents.

Peripartum hemorrhage is the leading cause of maternal mortality worldwide.[5] Postpartum uterine atony is the most common cause of blood transfusion and postpartum hysterectomy. Management includes uterine massage, uterotonic agents, operative maneuvers, and hysterectomy. Pregnancy and cesarean section also have an increased risk of thromboembolic events. Recommended measures include hydration, early mobilization, and pneumatic compression devices.

## REFERENCES

1. Lucas DN, et al. Urgency of caesarean section: a new classification. *J R Soc Med.* 2000;93:346–350.
2. American Society of Anesthesiologists, Society for Obstetric Anesthesia and Perinatology. Practice guidelines for obstetric anesthesia: an updated report by the American Society of Anesthesiologists Task Force on Obstetric Anesthesia and the Society for Obstetric Anesthesia and Perinatology. *Anesthesiology.* 2016;124:270–300.
3. American College of Obstetricians and Gynecologists. Practice bulletin no. 199: use of prophylactic antibiotics in labor and delivery. *Obstet Gynecol.* 2018;132:e103–e119.
4. Szarvas S, et al. Neuraxial opioid-induced pruritus: a review. *J Clin Anesth.* 2003;15:234–239.
5. GBD 2015 Maternal Mortality Collaborators. Global, regional, and national levels of maternal mortality, 1990–2015: a systematic analysis for the Global Burden of Disease Study 2015. *Lancet.* 2016;388:1775–1812.

# 297.

# ANESTHESIA FOR CERCLAGE OR NONOBSTETRIC SURGERY

*Rowaa Ibrahim and Ami Attali*

## INTRODUCTION

Procedures during pregnancy may be pregnancy related or non–pregnancy related. Procedures unrelated to delivery occur between 0.3% and 2.2% of cases, with parturient women often presenting emergently. A thorough anesthetic plan should be in place to ensure the safety of both the mother and the baby. The choice of anesthetic is guided by the physiological changes associated with pregnancy, the effects on the fetus, as well as the nature of the procedures.

Studies analyzing information from the National Surgical Quality Improvement Program database showed similar rates of major complications in pregnant and nonpregnant women (7%). Fetal risks of antenatal surgery include the effects of the disease process itself, teratogenicity of the drugs used, uteroplacental insufficiency, preterm labor, or fetal demise. American College of Obstetricians and Gynecologists/American Society of Anesthesiologists (ACOG/ASA) guidelines on nonobstetric surgery during pregnancy recommend delaying elective surgery until after delivery. However, if surgery should be deemed necessary, the second trimester is preferred because of its association with the lowest risk for spontaneous abortion and preterm labor (Figure 297.1).

## ANESTHETIC CONSIDERATIONS

### PREOPERATIVE

Preoperative assessment of pregnant patients undergoing nonobstetric surgery is essential. Given the increased risk of aspiration following 18 weeks' gestation, premedication with a histamine antagonist, metoclopramide, or nonparticulate antacid is used. Caution must be taken with the use of premedication for anxiety.

Fetal heart rate monitoring is feasible at 18 weeks but may be technically difficult prior to 22 weeks. ACOG and ASA have published guidelines for fetal monitoring during nonobstetric surgery. For a pre-viable fetus, fetal heart rate (FHR) is measured by Doppler before and after the procedure. With a viable fetus, simultaneous electronic FHR and tocometric monitoring should be performed before and after the procedure.

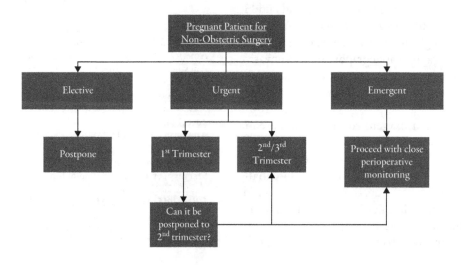

Figure 297.1 To come

## INTRAOPERATIVE

Changes in physiology during pregnancy can lead to the rapid development of hypoxemia and acidosis during periods of hypoventilation or apnea. By 8 weeks, most of the cardiovascular changes seen, such as the increase in cardiac output and stroke volume and decrease in systemic vascular resistance, have occurred, reaching a peak at 24 weeks. Compression of the inferior vena cava by the gravid uterus can occur. Intraoperative management should focus on avoiding hypoxemia, hypotension, acidosis, and hyperventilation, which are the most critical elements of anesthetic management.

Monitoring can be achieved by noninvasive or invasive blood pressure measurement, electrocardiography, pulse oximetry, capnography, temperature monitoring, and peripheral nerve stimulator. Hypotension in the pregnant patient undergoing surgery can be caused by deep levels of general anesthesia, sympathectomy due to spinal or epidural blockade, aortocaval compression or hypovolemia. Intraoperative electronic FHR monitoring may be done when feasible. Transabdominal monitoring can be challenging, and the use of transvaginal Doppler may be necessary. FHR and uterine activity should be monitored and documented prior to the procedure.

Studies have shown an association between general anesthesia and a significantly low birth weight. Maternal airway and pulmonary complications can complicate the general anesthesia picture. Depending on the nature of the procedure, the use of local, regional, neuraxial, or total intravenous anesthesia option may be preferred. No studies have conclusively determined superiority of any of these techniques.

Given the physiological changes that occur with pregnancy, general anesthesia requires endotracheal intubation. Adequate preoxygenation should be done prior to attempts. Several studies have indicated the safety of laryngeal mask airway (LMA), but the LMA cohort had normal body mass index and the devices were placed following fasting with the use of aspiration precautions.

Medications that are known to be safe include thiopental, propofol, morphine, fentanyl, succinylcholine, and the nondepolarizing muscle relaxants. Changes in volume of distribution, metabolic activity, and hepatic or renal elimination may contribute to changes in drug effects and metabolism. Although halogenated volatile anesthetics can cross the placenta and affect the fetus, moderate levels have been found to be safe with adequate compensation in uterine artery tone up to 1.5 MAC (minimum alveolar concentration). There is a 30%–40% decrease in volatile anesthetic MAC requirements during pregnancy. Nitrous oxide causes methionine synthase inhibition, which could lead to a decrease in DNA synthesis. Evidence does not support the avoidance of nitrous oxide in pregnancy, especially after the first 6 weeks of gestation. The risk of awareness under anesthesia has been noted to be higher during cesarean sections, and a similar increased risk is seen with nonobstetric surgery during pregnancy.

## POSTOPERATIVE

Postoperative pain control can be achieved by opioids, neuraxial procedures, nerve blocks, and the use of multimodal pain control. Nonsteroidal anti-inflammatory drugs should be avoided due to concerns for risk of premature closure of the fetal ductus arteriosus and oligohydramnios, while opioid use should be kept at a minimum. Given the hypercoagulable state, thromboprophylaxis is necessary unless contraindicated.

In the event of cardiac arrest or resuscitation, left uterine placement should be maintained, oxygen should be administered, and hypotension should be treated with vasopressors. Surgical manipulation or insufflation should stop, and the use of medications to promote uterine relaxation should be considered. Maternal hemoglobin and acid-base status should be checked. Cesarean delivery may be necessary, with a focus on maternal survival, and should be considered, with the goal of delivery within 5 minutes of arrest. Causes of arrest specific to pregnancy include amniotic fluid embolism, eclampsia, placental abruption, and hemorrhage.

## ANESTHETIC MANAGEMENT OF CERCLAGE

Preoperative and postoperative management of patients presenting for cerclage is similar to nonobstetric procedures. The greatest risk during cerclage procedures is rupture of the membranes, leading to emergent delivery. It is performed most commonly under spinal anesthesia with a saddle block but can be done with epidural or general anesthesia, which will depend on the degree of cervical dilation. Spinal anesthesia allows for rapid and reliable anesthesia, while general anesthesia carries the same risks previously described for parturient patients. Sensory blockade is needed from sacral to T10 dermatome to cover the cervix (L1 to T10) and vagina and perineum (S2 to S4). General anesthesia may be preferred if the cervix is dilated with bulging membranes. Uterine smooth muscles can be relaxed by volatile anesthetics or nitroglycerin and decreases intrauterine pressure, which facilitates re-placement of the bulging membranes and placement of the cerclage. There is limited evidence comparing general and neuraxial anesthesia for cerclage.

## REFERENCES

1. American College of Obstetricians and Gynecologists and American Society of Anesthesiologists. ACOG committee opinion no. 696: nonobstetric surgery during pregnancy. *Obstet Gynecol.* 2017;129:777–778.
2. Moore HB, et al. Effect of pregnancy on adverse outcomes after general surgery. *JAMA Surg.* 2015;150:637–643.
3. Chestnut D, et al. In: *Chestnut's Obstetric Anesthesia.* 17, 350–367, 368–391.

# 298.

# ECTOPIC PREGNANCY

*Edward Noguera*

## INTRODUCTION

Ectopic pregnancy is the leading cause of obstetric hemorrhage in the United States. Obstetric hemorrhage is the leading cause of maternal death. Ectopic pregnancy is the leading cause of maternal deaths (10%–15%). During ectopic pregnancy, the fertilized egg grows in an abnormal place, outside the uterus, commonly the fallopian tubes. As the sac grows, it could eventually rupture (15%–20% of cases), causing hemorrhage. Tubal rupture is a surgical emergency. The prevalence of ectopic pregnancy is 6%–16%. The implantation sites are the fallopian tubes (95%), ovary (3%), and abdomen (2%).

## CLINICAL MANAGEMENT

In addition to the general considerations for obstetric patients, the management of ectopic pregnancy is based on three main pillars: (1) early recognition, (2) prompt resuscitation, and (3) definitive treatment.

### RISK FACTORS

Risk factors for ectopic pregnancy include history of previous ectopic pregnancy; tubal damage (sexually transmitted disease, pelvic inflammatory disease, previous tubal surgery); smoking history; multiple partners; oral contraceptives or intrauterine devices; and history of longer than 2 years of infertility.

### CLINICAL PRESENTATION

The typical presentation for ectopic pregnancy is a woman of childbirth age who has missed a period presenting with acute abdominal pain, vaginal bleeding, lightheadedness, dizziness, fever, vomiting, and hypotension. Some patients with late presentation can have signs of circulatory shock: tachycardia, tachypnea, pallor, oliguria, and respiratory distress.[1,2]

## DIAGNOSIS

The diagnosis is based on a positive test for pregnancy (β-hCG [human chorionic gonadotrophin], pregnancy hormone) and ultrasound (vaginal and abdominal). The β-HCG concentration helps identify the viability of a pregnancy and expected findings for normal pregnancy during ultrasound. Typical ultrasound findings include empty uterine cavity, complex extra-adnexal cyst or mass, tubal ring, free pelvic fluid, or hemoperitoneum in the pouch of Douglas.[3]

## THERAPEUTIC OPTIONS

Medical management is considered in patients who are hemodynamically stable and have no contraindications to methotrexate (MTX) (Table 298.1).

There are several dose regimens for administration of MTX: single-dose, two-dose, and fixed multiple-dose

*Table 298.1* CONTRAINDICATIONS TO USING METHOTREXATE

| ABSOLUTE CONTRAINDICATIONS TO MTX | RELATIVE CONTRAINDICATIONS TO MTX |
|---|---|
| Intrauterine pregnancy, ruptured ectopic | Embryonic cardiac activity by transvaginal ultrasound |
| Evidence of immunodeficiency | High initial hGC concentration |
| Moderate-to-severe pancytopenia | Ectopic pregnancy > 4 cm in size |
| Sensitivity to MTX | Refusal to accept blood transfusion |
| Active pulmonary disease | |
| Active peptic ulcer disease | |
| Hepatic or severe renal dysfunction | |

protocols. Most protocols include follow-up with β-hCG concentrations to assess efficiency and results.[4]

## RUPTURED ECTOPIC PREGNANCY

Ruptured ectopic pregnancy is a surgical emergency. Laparoscopic techniques are preferred. Occasionally, laparotomy is indicated in very unstable patients or failed laparoscopy. Patients with ruptured ectopic pregnancy can become hemodynamically unstable at any time. This could happen preoperatively, intraoperatively, or postoperatively. Thus, appropriate preparation is of paramount importance.

## ANESTHETIC CONSIDERATIONS

### PREOPERATIVE

The preoperative general anesthetic considerations of pregnant patients include risk of aspiration, friable airway, potentially difficult airway, increased oral secretions, and hemodynamic changes related to hormonal changes of pregnancy.

A review of systems and physical examination to assess a potentially difficult airway are important. Hemodynamically unstable patients need fluid resuscitation before induction of anesthesia. Level of anemia and possible coagulopathies should be assessed. Blood products should be available for surgery, and large-bore peripheral intravenous access should be established.

### INTRAOPERATIVE

Aspiration risk is increased in pregnant woman; thus, full-stomach precautions are warranted. Consider rapid sequence induction technique. If nausea and vomiting are severe, gastric decompression via nasogastric tube can be considered. Oral antacids and antisialagogues should be given ahead of time before induction of anesthesia. Maintenance of anesthesia can be based on volatile agents or intravenous techniques. There is no evidence supporting one or another in this scenario. Neuraxial techniques have very limited use in the setting of laparoscopy and high probability of hypotension intraoperatively.

Plans for management of a potentially difficult airway should be contemplated, and equipment should be ready for use. Gentle management of the airway tissues can avoid bleeding in the pregnant patient.

Surgery for ectopic pregnancy can be lengthy. There is a possibility for potential intraoperative deterioration and unforeseen technical difficulties. Intravenous access with large-bore intravenous lines is of paramount importance during ruptured ectopic pregnancy procedures. Hypothermia during bleeding is associated with poor patient outcomes. Thus, hypothermia avoidance techniques should be considered: intravenous fluid warmers, covering the patient appropriately, increasing the room temperature, and effective fluid resuscitation.

Hypotension during surgery for ruptured ectopic pregnancy is usually related to hemorrhagic complications. Circulatory shock requires a proactive management approach. Avoiding prolonged episodes of hypotension can help prevent further end-organ damage. Triggers for blood product transfusion should be planned and rapidly implemented.

### POSTOPERATIVE

The postoperative management of ruptured ectopic pregnancy patients depends on the intraoperative findings and course. If the patient is no longer hypotensive, hypothermic, acidotic, or severely coagulopathic, extubation in the operating room can be safely accomplished. The usual criteria are followed, bearing in mind that there is always a potential for both aspiration and difficult airway in the pregnant patient. Thus, preferably, the patient should be extubated fully awake, following commands while extubation parameters are reassuring. In this scenario, anesthesia recovery in the postanesthesia recovery unit is indicated.

However, if the patient has developed organ failure intraoperatively, recovery in the intensive care unit is the next step to follow. Continuation of intraoperative hemodynamic goals, assessment of volume status, and assessment of possible ongoing bleeding or unresolved coagulopathy will guide postoperative management goals.

## REFERENCES

1. Problems of early pregnancy. In: *Chestnut's Obstetric Anesthesia*. 6th ed. 2020:351–355.
2. Physiologic changes of pregnancy. In: Barash PG, et al., eds. *Clinical Anesthesia*. 8th ed. Lippincott, Williams & Wilkins; 2017:1145–1147.
3. Ectopic pregnancy. In: *Stoelting's Anesthesia and Coexisting Disease*. 3rd South Asia ed. Elsevier; 2019:699.
4. Transvaginal sonography of ectopic pregnancy. *Fleischer's Sonography in Obstetrics and Gynecology*. 8th ed. McGraw-Hill Education; 2018:81–108.

# 299.

# SPONTANEOUS ABORTION

*Joshua D. Younger and Monica Prasad*

## INTRODUCTION

The medical definition of abortion is a pregnancy that is lost or terminated before 20 weeks' gestation. This is not to be confused with the definition used in the vernacular. Abortion can occur both spontaneously and electively. An abortion can be performed either medically or surgically. Medical abortions are usually managed with medications, such as methotrexate, mifepristone, and misoprostol. Surgical abortions are performed with a manual vacuum aspirator (MVA), metal curette, a suction device, or any combination of these.[1]

Spontaneous abortion occurs in 10%–15% of pregnancies,[1] of which 50%–80% are due to fetal chromosomal abnormalities.[2] These spontaneous abortions most usually occur before 8 weeks of gestation. Of note, 5% of all pregnancy-related deaths are associated with either an elective or a spontaneous abortion.[3] These maternal deaths are usually linked to sepsis and/or hemorrhage.

## MEDICAL AND SURGICAL CONSIDERATIONS

The choice of abortion management is often dictated by the presentation. An abortion can present in many ways, and this gives way to a classification system used to describe the presentation. Spontaneous abortions are classified as threatened, inevitable, complete, incomplete, and missed. There is also the dreaded septic abortion. Table 299.1 displays this classification system in depth.[4] These terms and classifications are not mutually exclusive. For example, an incomplete abortion can also be a septic abortion.

One of the major complications of a medically induced abortion is the potential for hemorrhage. This may even require the patient to subsequently undergo a surgical abortion. Depending on the degree of the hemorrhage, it can be life threatening and may even require the use of a massive transfusion protocol. If blood was needed before an active blood type and screen was available, O-negative blood should be given. Another serious risk can be procedure failure, leading to retained products of conception and subsequent bleeding and/or infection.

There are myriad complications associated with surgical abortions. Most of these complications are similarly associated with bleeding and infection. In terms of bleeding risks, there is the risk of uterine perforation, cervical laceration, and retained products of conception leading to hemorrhage. The infection risk, as mentioned, can also stem from retained product of conception and/or an unsterile procedure.

It is important to remember that a mother who is Rh negative and has significant bleeding from an abortion is at risk for Rh isoimmunization.[5] It is imperative to consider Rh immunoglobulin, RhoGAM, to mitigate this risk. If a patient were to become isoimmunized, it could have ever-lasting deleterious effects on her subsequent pregnancies.

*Table 299.1* MISCARRIAGE TYPES AND PHYSICAL EXAMINATION FINDINGS

| TYPE | CERVICAL OS | DESCRIPTION |
| --- | --- | --- |
| Threatened | Closed | Vaginal bleeding with viable IUP (intrauterine pregnancy) |
| Complete | Closed | All products of conception (POC) expelled from uterus |
| Missed | Closed | Nonviable IUP (without fetal heart activity) still present in uterus |
| Inevitable | Open | Nonviable IUP with fetal heart activity present in the uterus but an open cervical os |
| Incomplete | Open | Partial expulsion of POC from the uterus in a nonviable IUP |
| Septic | Either | An abortion that causes an infective process that leads to sepsis |

## ANESTHETIC CONSIDERATIONS

The anesthetic considerations are dependent on the active issues that present when the patient enters the operating suite. The most concerning of them is the rapid management of hemorrhage and infection. Hemorrhage will require large-bore intravenous access and possibly an arterial line, with a central line if there is hemodynamic instability. Infection may also come with hemodynamic instability (i.e., sepsis), also requiring central access and an arterial line for monitoring. Infections should be treated with source control (i.e., evacuation of the uterus) and broad-spectrum antibiotics.

1. *Anesthetic Type*: A regional anesthetic such as a paracervical block can be used for office-based and minor procedures such as those using an MVA. However, if the procedure was to be more invasive and there was no imminent danger, a neuraxial procedure could be utilized. If there was sepsis or hemorrhage, a general anesthetic with an endotracheal tube would be preferred. Consideration of induction agent should be based on the patient's preoperative state. In periods of hemodynamic instability, ketamine is often favorably considered given its desirable hemodynamic effects and its ability to serve as a uterotonic.[6]
2. *Intravenous Access*: Hemorrhage is a real possibility during these cases, and large-bore intravenous access

should be employed. An active type and screen should be available, so expedited transfusion can be employed as needed. Uterotonic medications should be readily available, though their efficacy is questionable at early gestational ages.
3. *Invasive Monitoring*: This would be situationally dependent on the present existing comorbidities. If the patient is hemodynamically unstable in the setting of sepsis and/or hemorrhage, this would warrant placement.
4. *Postoperative*: Intensive care should not be routinely required unless there were significant comorbidities preoperatively or during an intraoperative event.

## REFERENCES

1. Wilcox AJ, et al. Incidence of early loss of pregnancy. *N Engl J Med*. 1988;319:189–194.
2. Strom CM, et al. Analyses of 95 first-trimester spontaneous abortions by chorionic villus sampling and karyotype. *J Assist Reprod Genet*. 1992;9:458–461.
3. Berg CJ, et al. Pregnancy-related mortality in the United States 1991–1997. *Obstet Gynecol*. 2003;101:289–296.
4. Pedigo R. First trimester pregnancy emergencies: recognition and management. *Emerg Med Pract*. 2019;21(1):1–20.
5. American College of Obstetricians and Gynecologists Committee on Practice Bulletins-Obstetrics. Practice bulletin no. 181: prevention of Rh D alloimmunization. *Obstet Gynecol*. 2017;130:e57–e70.
6. Oats JN, et al. Effects of ketamine on the pregnant uterus. *Br J Anaesth*. 1979;51:1163–1166.

# 300.

# GESTATIONAL TROPHOBLASTIC DISEASE

*Joshua D. Younger*

## INTRODUCTION

Trophoblastic tissue develops as early as 4 days after fertilization. The tissue serves to feed and nourish the developing embryo. The trophoblastic tissue ultimately becomes a major component of the placenta.

Maldevelopment of this can occur and ultimately leads to a spectrum of diseases called gestational trophoblastic disease (GTD). This disease spectrum can range from benign to lethal. Albeit rare, there can be multiple medical and specific anesthetic considerations that need to be appreciated.

## GESTATIONAL TROPHOBLASTIC DISEASE SPECTRUM

Included in the GTD disease spectrum is a partial hydatiform molar pregnancy, complete molar pregnancy, invasive molar pregnancy, placental site trophoblastic tumor, and last gestational choriocarcinoma. This list is ordered from most benign to most lethal and mirrors the classification system that is used by the Society of Gynecologic Oncology (SGO) and the American College of Obstetrics and Gynecology (ACOG).[1]

### HYDATIFORM MOLE

1. Complete
2. Partial

### MALIGNANT GTD

1. Invasive mole
2. Gestational choriocarcinoma
3. Placental site trophoplastic tumor

As implied in the listed names, there is a carcinogenic component of this disease spectrum, and treatment for the most lethal forms is accompanied by chemotherapies and radiation. Even the "benign" forms of partial and complete molar pregnancies will have sequelae that require chemotherapy. Partial moles will have persistent disease after termination of pregnancy, requiring chemotherapy in up to 5% of cases and for complete moles up to 20%.[2]

As this disease is a product of an abnormal pregnancy, it produces human chorionic gonadotropin (hCG). An overproduction of hCG is a characteristic component of this disease spectrum. The abnormal laboratory values are followed to indicate disease progression and recession. Of note, overproduction of hCG can lead to anesthetic challenges, discussed further in this chapter.

## MEDICAL AND SURGICAL CONSIDERATIONS

There are a slew of medical conditions and derangements linked to this spectrum of diseases. While specific pathology may differ, generalizations are employed here. In over a quarter of cases, the uterus will be excessive in size due to the abnormal proliferation of this trophoblastic tissue. Other common pathology includes bilateral ovarian cysts, hyperemesis gravidarum, and gestational hypertension. Anemia may also be present in these patients, as bleeding may be either vaginal or intratumor.

The overproduction of this trophoblastic tissue generates an excessive amount of hCG. This leads to the development and excessive growth of intrauterine tissue, with ovarian theca-lutein cysts causing the above conditions. The cysts may lead to emergency intra-abdominal processes such as ovarian torsion or ruptured cysts. While nausea and vomiting are well-known phenomena of pregnancy, the excess hCG often leads to incessant vomiting, causing hyperemesis gravidarum. Hyperemesis is not a benign pathology and is accompanied with multiple electrolyte derangements. In extreme cases, patients may even require total parenteral nutrition treatment.[3]

While it is rare, hyperthyroidism may be present in these cases. As hCG and thyroid-stimulating hormone (thyrotropin) are very close in structure, the body can mistakenly overproduce thyroxine and triiodothyronine. This overproduction can lead to a thyroid storm, which has a host of medical and anesthetic concerns.[4]

Acute cardiopulmonary distress following evacuation of these aberrant pregnancies was noted in past. This presented with chest pain, tachycardia, tachypnea, hypoxemia, diffuse rales, and chest imaging demonstrating pulmonary infiltrates. The etiology of this distress was not well understood, and varying hypotheses presented. However, this is a rare findings in current medical practice as earlier diagnosis and treatment methods have been discovered and employed and mitigated this distress.[5]

## ANESTHETIC CONSIDERATIONS

The most important anesthetic considerations include the significant bleeding risk that accompanies these uterine evacuations and the potential for acute cardiopulmonary distress.

### PREOPERATIVE

Given the concern for incessant vomiting, uterine/abdominal distention, potential postprocedure respiratory compromise, and known decrease in esophageal tone during pregnancy, it would seem that a general anesthetic with an endotracheal tube using a rapid sequence induction would be preferred. Consideration of induction agent would be based on the patient's preoperative state. This being said, molar pregnancies have been described under neuraxial anesthesia, and the anesthetic should be individualized.

### INTRAOPERATIVE

*Intravenous Access*: Hemorrhage is a real possibility during these cases, and large-bore intravenous access should be employed intraoperatively. An active blood type and screen should be available so expedited transfusion can be employed as needed. Uterotonic medications should be readily available.

*Invasive Monitoring*: This would be situationally dependent on the comorbidities that were present with the GTD. If the patient had pathologic metabolic and/or physiologic derangements, arterial line placement should be highly considered. Severe anemia and hemodynamic instability would also warrant this.

## POSTOPERATIVE

Intensive care would should not be routinely required unless there were significant metabolic derangements preoperatively or an intraoperative event.

## REFERENCES

1. Soper JT et al.; American College of Obstetricians and Gynecologists. Diagnosis and treatment of gestational trophoblastic disease: ACOG practice bulletin no. 53. *Gynecol Oncol*. 2004;93(3):575–585.
2. Kohorn EI. Gestational trophoblastic neoplasia and evidence-based medicine. *J Reprod Med*. 2002;47:427–432.
3. Lurain JR. Gestational trophoblastic disease. I. Epidemiology, pathology, clinical presentation and diagnosis of gestational trophoblastic disease, and management of hydatidiform mole. *Am J Obstet Gynecol*. 2010;203:531–539.
4. Amir SM, et al: Human chorionic gonadotropin and thyroid function in patients with hydatidiform mole. *Am J Obstet Gynecol*. 1984;150:723–728.
5. Orr JW, et al. Acute pulmonary edema associated with molar pregnancies: a high-risk factor for development of persistent trophoblastic disease. *Am J Obstet Gynecol*. 1980;136:412–415.

# 301.

# AUTOIMMUNE DISORDERS

*Anuschka Bhatia and Kevin W. Chung*

## SYSTEMIC LUPUS ERYTHEMATOSUS

### INTRODUCTION

Systemic lupus erythematosus (SLE) is an autoimmune disorder characterized by autoantibody formation, multisystem immune complex deposition, and organ inflammation.[1] Patients with SLE experience higher rates of maternal and fetal complications during pregnancy.[2] Clinical manifestations are diverse, and diagnosis requires the presence of four or more criteria (Table 301.1).

### EFFECTS ON PREGNANCY AND MANAGEMENT PRIOR TO DELIVERY

Parturients with SLE experience more lupus flares during pregnancy and experience a higher incidence of obstetrical complications like preterm labor, unplanned cesarean delivery, and preeclampsia/eclampsia.[2] Management during pregnancy should involve a multidisciplinary approach between the rheumatologist, obstetrician, and anesthesiologist.

Risk factors that predispose to lupus exacerbation during pregnancy include active disease within 6 months of conception, lupus nephritis history, discontinuation of hydroxychloroquine, and primigravida. These, in addition to preexisting hypertension, presence of antiphospholipid antibodies (aPL), and decreasing complement levels, are significantly associated with adverse pregnancy outcomes.[3]

A preconception evaluation (Table 301.2) should be completed to stratify risk, optimize disease activity, and transition to pregnancy-compatible medications.[2] If possible, high-risk patients should wait for 6 months of disease quiescence prior to conception. SLE activity should be monitored at least each trimester, with active disease requiring more frequent monitoring.

Both normal and aberrant physiologic changes of pregnancy can overlap with features of active lupus. Mild anemia of pregnancy may mask worsening anemia of chronic disease or autoimmune hemolytic anemia in the setting of lupus flare. Thrombocytopenia may be physiologic or a pathologic sign of lupus nephritis, preeclampsia, or antiphospholipid syndrome (APS). Proteinuria during pregnancy does not normally exceed 300 mg daily and

**Table 301.1** LUPUS INTERNATIONAL COLLABORATING CLINIC CRITERIA FOR CLASSIFICATION OF SYSTEMIC LUPUS ERYTHEMATOSUS

| CLINICAL MANIFESTATIONS | IMMUNOLOGIC MANIFESTATIONS |
|---|---|
| Skin | Antinuclear antibody > reference negative value |
|   Acute, subacute cutaneous LE (photosensitive, malar, maculopapular, bullous) | Anti–double-stranded DNA > reference, if by enzyme-linked immunosorbent assay 2× reference |
|   Chronic cutaneous LE (discoid lupus, panniculitis, lichen planus-like, hypertrophic verrucous, chilblains) | Anti-Sm |
| Oral or nasal ulcers | Antiphospholipid (any of lupus anticoagulant, false-positive rapid plasma reagin, anticardiolipin, anti-β-glycoprotein I |
| Nonscarring alopecia | Low serum complement (C3, C4, or CH50) |
| Synovitis involving ≥ 2 joints | Positive direct Coombs test in absence of hemolytic anemia |
| Serositis (pleurisy, pericarditis) | |
| Renal | |
|   Protein/creatinine (Cr) ≥ 0.5 | |
|   Red blood cell casts | |
|   Biopsy | |
| Neurologic | |
|   Seizures, psychosis, mononeuritis, myelitis, peripheral or cranial neuropathies, acute confusional state | |
| Hemolytic anemia | |
| Leukopenia (<4000/μL) or lymphopenia (<1000/μL) | |
| Thrombocytopenia (<100,000/μL) | |

Taken from Reference 1.

should not be accompanied by worsening renal function, as is seen in lupus nephritis and preeclampsia. Clinical context and active monitoring of high-risk SLE patients will aid subsequent diagnosis and treatment.

Effects of SLE on the fetus include fetal loss, intrauterine growth restriction (IUGR), premature birth, and neonatal lupus. Neonatal lupus is the result of passive transplacental transfer of anti-Ro/SSA or anti-LA/SSB antibodies and is classically associated with complete congenital heart block, though it can also have cutaneous, hematologic, and hepatic manifestations. A positive antibody test warrants more frequent fetal surveillance.[1]

**Table 301.2** PRECONCEPTION EVALUATION IN THE PARTURIENT WITH SYSTEMIC LUPUS ERYTHEMATOSUS

| COMPONENTS OF INITIAL EVALUATION |
|---|
| Physical examination (including blood pressure check) |
| Complete blood count (CBC) |
| Renal function tests (blood urea nitrogen [BUN]/Cr, spot urine protein:creatinine ratio or 24-hour urine collection, and urinalysis) |
| Liver function tests (LFTs) |
| Lupus anticoagulant (LA), anticardiolipin antibodies (aCL), and anti-β$_2$-glycoprotein (aβ$_2$-gp) |
| Anti-RO/SSA and anti-La/SSB antibodies |
| Anti–double-stranded DNA (dsDNA) antibodies |
| Complement levels (CH50, C3, and C4) |
| Serum uric acid |

## MEDICAL MANAGEMENT

Medication regimens should be reviewed and adjusted prior to conception with the acknowledgment that cessation or alteration can increase the risk of lupus flares. Disease-modifying antirheumatic drugs (DMARDs) such as hydroxychloroquine, azathioprine, cyclosporine, and tacrolimus have all been shown to be compatible with pregnancy.[2] Cyclophosphamide, mycophenolate mofetil, and methotrexate are known teratogens and are contraindicated in pregnancy. Corticosteroids are often used to treat SLE flares, and while low-dose prednisone is safe in pregnancy, regular use of dexamethasone and betamethasone are associated with IUGR. Nonsteroidal anti-inflammatory drug use for joint pain should be avoided after 30 weeks' gestation due to risk of premature closure of the ductus arteriosus. Low-dose aspirin is recommended for use in all women with SLE.[2]

## ANESTHETIC MANAGEMENT

It is critical to perform thorough review of the patient's medical history and to formulate a multidisciplinary plan for delivery. Evaluation as outlined previously can help guide further testing like electrocardiography, echocardiography, and/or chest x-ray.

Potential coagulopathy may contraindicate neuraxial techniques and should be investigated prior to delivery. SLE patients can rarely have autoantibodies against coagulation factors and are more likely to have asymptomatic or active APS; both can manifest as elevated activated partial thromboplastin time (aPTT) and warrant early hematology consultation.[1,2] Neurologic manifestations of SLE should be properly evaluated and monitored throughout the peripartum period. Any preexisting autonomic or sensorimotor neuropathies should be documented prior to administration of regional anesthetics.

During the peripartum period, preparedness for obstetrical complications in the mother, such as preterm labor and acute lupus exacerbation, and neonatal complications in the fetus, such as congenital heart block, is essential. Invasive monitoring may be warranted in patients with prior history of cardiovascular disease, such as myocarditis and valvular disease. Renal-protective strategies should be utilized, especially in those with preexisting kidney disease. Chronic steroid use is associated with hyperglycemia, adrenal suppression, and osteoporosis and may warrant blood glucose monitoring and stress-dose steroids.

Systemic lupus erythematosus is associated with cervical osteoarthritis, cricoarytenoid arthritis, vocal cord palsy, and subglottic and/or laryngeal edema, which may result in more challenging airway management.[4] Smaller endotracheal tubes, laryngeal mask airways, and difficult airway equipment such as a video laryngoscope should be readily available.

## ANTIPHOSPHOLIPID SYNDROME

### INTRODUCTION

Antiphospholipid syndrome is an autoimmune disorder characterized by recurrent venous and arterial thrombosis or fetal loss and the presence of aPLs.[1] Though it can exist as a separate disease entity, it is classically associated with SLE, as approximately 40% of SLE patients will also have aPLs.[2]

### CLINICAL FEATURES

Diagnosis is based on fulfillment of one clinical (e.g., evidence of venous or arterial thrombosis or recurrent fetal loss) and one laboratory criterion (e.g., lupus anticoagulant, anticardiolipin antibodies, anti-$\beta_2$-glycoprotein).[1] APS will also characteristically result in mild prolongation of aPTT and thrombocytopenia. Women with recurrent thrombosis or more than three unexplained pregnancy losses should be tested for aPLs.[2] Pregnant women with APS are at risk for venous and arterial thrombosis, myocardial infarction, pulmonary embolism, and fetal loss.[4] Catastrophic APS is an accelerated form of disease that occurs in 1% of APS patients; there is presence of aPLs, involvement of three or more organs, and rapid progression of disease.[2]

### MEDICAL AND OBSTETRIC MANAGEMENT

Thrombophylaxis is the mainstay of APS management. Improved maternal thrombotic risk and fetal survival are seen in women on low-dose aspirin and heparin, and prophylactic dosing during pregnancy through 6–8 weeks' postpartum should be considered.[2]

### ANESTHETIC MANAGEMENT

Despite mild prolonged aPTT and thrombocytopenia, APS patients are more likely to be hypercoagulable, and neuraxial anesthesia can be provided safely in the absence of anticoagulant therapy. Aspirin therapy does not contraindicate neuraxial anesthesia. Neuraxial anesthesia can be administered 4 hours after prophylactic unfractionated heparin, 12 hours after prophylactic low-molecular-weight heparin (LMWH), and 24 hours after therapeutic LMWH.[5] Due to high risk of thrombosis, hypothermia and dehydration should be avoided. Sequential compression devices, early ambulation, and warm intravenous fluids can be utilized to help mitigate risk.

### REFERENCES

1. Jameson J, et al. *Harrison's Principles of Internal Medicine.* 20th ed. McGraw-Hill; 2018.
2. Chestnut DH. *Chestnut's Obstetric Anesthesia: Principles and Practice.* Elsevier, 2020.
3. Buyon JP, et al. Predictors of pregnancy outcomes in patients with lupus. *Ann Intern Med.* 2015;163(3):153.
4. Teitel AD, et al. Laryngeal involvement in systemic lupus erythematosus. *Semin Arthritis Rheum.* 1992;22(no. 3):203–214.
5. Horlocker TT, et al. Regional anesthesia in the patient receiving antithrombotic or thrombolytic therapy. *Reg Anesth Pain Med.* 2018;43(no. 3):263–309.

# 302.

# ENDOCRINE DISORDERS

*Eric P. Zhou and Kevin W. Chung*

## INTRODUCTION

### DIABETES

According to the Centers for Disease Control and Prevention, approximately 1% to 2% of pregnant women have type 1 or 2 diabetes, while the prevalence of gestational diabetes is between 6% and 9%.

### CLINICAL FEATURES

Type 1 diabetes is typically secondary to destruction of islet β-cells, causing an absolute insulin deficiency, whereas type 2 diabetes is often correlated with obesity and other lifestyle factors, resulting in systemic insulin resistance.[1] Gestational diabetes is caused by the development of insulin resistance in the setting of pregnancy. Ninety percent of gestational diabetes cases resolve after delivery.

The effects of hyperglycemia are multisystemic. Diabetics have an increased risk of small- and large-vessel disease, resulting in myriad consequences, such as cerebrovascular disease, myocardial ischemia, renal parenchymal disease, and autonomic neuropathy. Patients with diabetes are at an increased risk of postoperative complications, including poor wound healing and ketoacidosis.

In the parturient, diabetes can result in fetal macrosomia, preeclampsia, stillbirth, or polyhydramnios. Fetal macrosomia is the most common complication and results in an increased risk for operative delivery, cardiomegaly, heart failure, shoulder dystocia, or brachial plexus injury.[1] All viscera except the brain can be affected by the macrosomic process. Chronic fetal hyperinsulinemia leads to neonatal hypoglycemia at delivery. In addition, maternal diabetes mellitus can lead to several fetal congenital anomalies, with the cardiac and skeletal systems most commonly affected.

### DIAGNOSIS

The American Diabetes Association defines a hemoglobin $A_{1c}$ (Hb$A_{1c}$) greater than or equal to 6.5%, a fasting plasma glucose of 126 mg/dL or higher, or an oral glucose tolerance test of 200 mg/dL or higher as diagnostic of diabetes mellitus.

### TREATMENT

Intraoperative management of glucose is crucial in order to reduce the risk of neonatal hypoglycemia. Short-acting insulin is utilized to target a blood glucose level of between 110 and 180 mg/dL.

### ANESTHETIC CONSIDERATIONS

There is an increased risk of infection, such as an epidural abscess related to the neuraxial block placement, and exaggerated sympathetic blockade may result in profound hypotension.[2] Diabetic parturients may have gastroparesis and limited atlanto-occipital joint extension, which increase the risks and difficulty of securing an airway when undergoing general anesthesia. Aspiration prophylaxis and preparation for a difficult airway should be considered.[2]

## THYROID DISORDERS

### INTRODUCTION

The most common thyroid disorders encountered during pregnancy are hyperthyroidism and hypothyroidism. Both can lead to an increased risk of perinatal morbidity and preterm delivery.

### CLINICAL FEATURES

Common symptoms of hyperthyroidism include tremor, palpitations, weight loss, anxiety, heat intolerance, and dyspnea.[3] A goiter may be present on physical examination. Patients with hypothyroidism may have symptoms such as weight gain, cold intolerance, and fatigue.

## DIAGNOSIS

Hyperthyroidism is most commonly secondary to Graves disease or human chorionic gonadotropin–mediated hyperthyroidism. Diagnosis is based on a suppressed (<0.1 mU/L) thyroid-stimulating hormone (TSH, thyrotropin) level with elevated thyroid hormone levels.[3]

Hypothyroidism is most commonly caused by chronic autoimmune thyroiditis. Diagnosis is made from an elevated TSH level (>4.0 mU/L) and decreased concentration (Table 302.1).[3]

## TREATMENT

For moderate-to-severe hyperthyroidism, women should be placed on a β-blocker. Propylthiouracil is preferred to suppress hormonal levels, while radioiodine therapy is absolutely contraindicated in the pregnant patient. Levothyroxine is used for hormonal supplementation in chronic hypothyroidism.

## ANESTHETIC CONSIDERATIONS

Thyroid disorders can affect a wide range of physiological processes. Hyperthyroid patients are more predisposed to hemodynamic instability in the form of an increased heart rate, higher myocardial oxygen consumption, and reduced systemic vascular resistance. These patients may have more pronounced hemodynamic response to neuraxial anesthesia and increased sensitivity to catecholamines.[3] Phenylephrine is recommended as a first-line treatment for hypotension rather than ephedrine. Although rare, the clinician should be cognizant of the clinical signs of thyroid storms, such as hyperthermia, altered mentation, and cardiac dysfunction. A β-blocker should be administered if not contraindicated, and an immediate endocrinology consult should be placed.

Patients with hypothyroidism may also have intraoperative hemodynamic instability in the form of bradycardia, increased systemic vascular resistance, and a decreased response to vasopressors. These patients may demonstrate a more pronounced hemodynamic response to neuraxial anesthesia and may be more sensitive to anesthetic agents and opioids. In addition, postoperative respiratory muscle weakness may occur.[3]

## PHEOCHROMOCYTOMA

### INTRODUCTION

Pheochromocytoma in pregnancy is rare, with a reported incidence of 0.2 per 10,000 pregnancies.[4]

### CLINICAL FEATURES

Pheochromocytoma arises from catecholamine-secreting tumors in the chromaffin cells of the adrenal medulla. The gravid uterus may stimulate catecholamine secretion. The classical triad associated with pheochromocytoma is headache, diaphoresis, and tachycardia. Patients may have severe hypertension prior to 20 weeks of gestation.

### DIAGNOSIS

Initial diagnosis is confirmed with a two-fold elevation of 24-hour urine fractionated metanephrines and catecholamines. Normetanephrine levels greater than 900 μg or metanephrine levels greater than 400 μg are confirmative.[4] Imaging is used to localize the tumor.

### TREATMENT

α-Adrenergic blockade agents such as phenoxybenzamine and β-blockers may be used to control hypertension. β-Blockade should never be started before starting an α-adrenergic antagonist, as doing so could result in profound unopposed α-mediated vasoconstriction that can precipitate hypertensive crisis and/or pulmonary edema. If the diagnosis is confirmed prior to 24 weeks of gestational age, surgical excision is recommended, whereas a diagnosis made after 24 weeks' gestational age should be medically managed until delivery. Elective cesarean section is the preferred method of delivery if the tumor is still present.

### ANESTHETIC CONSIDERATIONS

Undiagnosed pheochromocytoma may result in fatal episodes of hypertension that are precipitated by vaginal delivery, general anesthesia, or uterine contractions. Such a crisis can cause uteroplacental insufficiency and, ultimately, fetal hypoxia and demise. It is critical to avoid hemodynamic instability in the peripartum period.

In a patient undergoing general anesthesia for tumor excision or delivery, the patient should receive 10 to 14 days of α-adrenergic blockade.[4] Intubation, tumor manipulation, and insufflation of the peritoneum are the times of greatest risk for catecholamine release and resultant hypertensive

*Table 302.1* LABORATORY DIAGNOSIS OF THYROID DISORDERS

| HYPOTHYROIDISM | HYPERTHYROIDISM |
| --- | --- |
| TSH > 4.0 mIU/mL | TSH < 0.1 mIU/mL |
| Total T$_4$ < 4.0 mIU/mL | Total T$_4$ > 12.5 mIU/mL |
| Free T$_4$ < 0.7 mIU/mL | Free T$_4$ > 2.0 mIU/mL |
| Total T$_3$ < 80 ng/dL | Total T$_3$ > 220 ng/dL |

T$_3$, triiodothyronine; T$_4$, thyroxine.

crisis. A preinduction arterial line is recommended, as is an adequate depth of anesthesia prior to laryngoscopy.[4] Ketamine and ephedrine are contraindicated. Desflurane is relatively contraindicated due to its catecholamine-secreting properties. In a tumor excision surgery, severe hypotension may occur after the effluent vein is clamped due to a sudden drop in catecholamines, so vasopressors should be immediately available for when this occurs.[5]

## REFERENCES

1. Lazer S, et al. Complications associated with the macrosomic fetus. *J Reprod Med.* 1986;31(6):501.
2. McAnulty G, et al. Anaesthetic management of patients with diabetes mellitus. *Br J Anaesth.* 2000;85(1):80–90.
3. Wissler R. Endocrine disorders. In: Chestnut DH, ed. *Obstetric Anesthesia. Principles and Practice.* 2nd ed. New York, NY: Mosby Year Book; 1999:828–832.
4. Lau P, et al. Phaeochromocytoma in pregnancy. *Aust NZ J Obstet Gynaecol.* 1996;36:472–476.
5. Kercher K, et al. Laparoscopic curative resection of pheochromocytomas. *Ann Surg.* 2005;241:919–928.

# 303.

# HEART DISEASE

*Muhammad Fayyaz Ahmed and Ihab Kamel*

## INTRODUCTION

Cardiovascular disease affects 1%–4% of pregnancies in the United Stated annually. Risk factors for future development of cardiovascular disease include hypertensive disorders of pregnancy, preeclampsia, and gestational diabetes mellitus. In the United States, maternal mortality from hypertensive disorders and hemorrhage is declining, and mortality from cardiovascular conditions has been slowly increasing.[1,2]

The physiologic changes of pregnancy may provide favorable outcome to most patient with heart disease. In certain situations, it may exacerbate cardiovascular conditions. In rare circumstances, it is advisable to avoid pregnancy as it can increase maternal morbidity and mortality.

## CONGENITAL HEART DISEASE

Patients with uncorrected *left-to-right* shunt such as atrial septal defect (ASD), ventricular septal defect (VSD),

and patent ductus arteriosus (PDA) may become symptomatic during pregnancy due to changes in cardiovascular physiology. The most common ASD defect is the secundum-type ASD. Compared to the general obstetric population, patients with ASD will have a higher incidence of precelampsia, fetal demise, and small for gestational age. Parturients with a repaired VSD or a small VSD (without pulmonary hypertension) tolerate pregnancy well. Preeclampsia is encountered more frequently in women with an unrepaired VSD. Pregnancy is well tolerated in patients with PDA. If a patient with right-to-left shunt develops pulmonary hypertension and Eisenmenger syndrome, pregnancy is associated with high risk of mortality and is not recommended. Eisenmenger syndrome develops due to increased blood flow to the pulmonary circulation, leading to pulmonary hypertension, right ventricular failure, and shunt reversal (right-to-left shunt).

Congenital defects associated with *right-to-left shunt* include tetralogy of Fallot, tricuspid atresia, and transposition of the great vessels. Patients with right-to-left shunts that are not surgically corrected are usually cyanotic, and pregnancy is not recommended. Patients who had a surgical repair should be evaluated by a cardiologist as part of multidisciplinary management before conception and throughout pregnancy. In the United States, most women born with tetralogy of Fallot present in pregnancy after surgical repair of the defect. Unrepaired tetralogy of Fallot consists of a VSD, an aorta that overrides the VSD, right ventricular hypertrophy, and right ventricular outflow tract obstruction (pulmonary stenosis).

## PULMONARY ARTERIAL HYPERTENSION

Pulmonary arterial hypertension is defined as a mean pulmonary artery pressure greater than 25 mm Hg with a *normal* pulmonary artery occlusion pressure (≤15 mm Hg) and pulmonary vascular resistance greater than 3 Wood[*] units. Group 1 (pulmonary arterial hypertension) includes idiopathic pulmonary arterial hypertension and pulmonary hypertension due to congenital heart disease. It is associated with exceptionally high maternal mortality, ranging from 17% to 56%. Pregnancy should be discouraged in women with severe pulmonary hypertension due the possibility of acute increase in the pulmonary artery pressure leading to acute right ventricular failure and death.[2,3]

## ARRHYTHMIAS

The incidence of arrhythmias increases during pregnancy due to an increase in intravascular volume causing atrial and ventricular stretch. Increase in resting heart rate and autonomic and hormonal changes during pregnancy also contributes to the higher incidence. Supraventricular arrhythmias (most common during pregnancy) and atrial fibrillation usually resolve after delivery. Pregnancy may exacerbate underlying supraventricular tachycardia. Structural heart disease is commonly associated with ventricular arrhythmias.

## VALVULAR HEART DISEASE

Cardiovascular physiologic changes of pregnancy present a challenge to women with underlying valvular heart disease. The general management of pregnant women with valvular heart disease focuses on hemodynamic goals and anticoagulation for patients with a mechanical valve. Generally, regurgitant valvular lesions are better tolerated than stenotic lesions. Both regional and general anesthesia can be safely administered if the hemodynamic goals of anesthetic management are satisfied.

## PERIPARTUM CARDIOMYOPATHY

Peripartum cardiomyopathy occurs during the last month of pregnancy or within 5 months postpartum. The patient should not have any other identifiable cause of heart failure and no heart disease before pregnancy. Echocardiographic diagnostic criteria include left ventricular ejection fraction less than 45%, left ventricular end-diastolic ventricular dimension greater than 27 mm/m$^2$ body surface area, and fractional shortening less than 30%.[2] When a patient develops cardiomyopathy before the last month of pregnancy, it is referred to as pregnancy-associated cardiomyopathy. Incidence is 1 per 3000 to 4000 live births in the United States. Risk factors include age older than 30 years, preeclampsia, gestational hypertension, multiparity, multiple gestation, African race, use of tocolytic agents, and cocaine abuse. Patients present with signs and symptoms of systolic heart failure.[2]

## HYPERTROPHIC CARDIOMYOPATHY

Pregnant patients with hypertrophic obstructive cardiomyopathy may present with dyspnea, fatigue, angina, palpitations, and/or syncope. Patients with atrial fibrillation typically present with symptoms of congestive heart failure. The increase in blood volume during pregnancy is beneficial for patients with hypertrophic cardiomyopathy. A general anesthesia technique should be considered for the parturient since it avoids a significant decrease in preload, and the negative effect of inhalation anesthetic agents may reduce the degree of dynamic outflow obstruction. Neuraxial anesthesia can be cautiously used in these patients, carefully titrating the medications to avoid an abrupt decrease in preload, leading to an increased degree of left ventricular outflow tract, leading to dynamic obstruction.

## ANESTHETIC CONSIDERATIONS

### PREOPERATIVE

Multidisciplinary management and obtaining an echocardiogram are usually warranted for the parturient with heart disease. Patients with ventricular arrhythmias should be investigated for underlying cardiomyopathy. Patients with pulmonary hypertension on continuous intravenous prostanoids are at higher risk for bleeding due to the adverse effect of these drugs on platelet function. However, this is not a contraindication to neuraxial anesthesia. Intravenous prostanoids should not be abruptly discontinued to avoid life-threatening rebound pulmonary hypertension.

## INTRAOPERATIVE

The goals of intraoperative anesthetic management for common cardiac conditions during pregnancy are summarized in the table below.

| HEART DISEASE | GOALS OF ANESTHETIC MANAGEMENT |
|---|---|
| Aortic stenosis (AS) Mitral stenosis (MS) | (1) *Maintenance of a normal heart rate and sinus rhythm* (to maximize ventricular filling)<br>(2) *Aggressive treatment of atrial fibrillation*<br>(2) *Maintenance of SVR* (to maintain systemic and coronary perfusion beyond stenosis)<br>(3) Maintenance of preload (optimize intravascular volume and avoid aortacaval compression)<br>(4) Avoidance of myocardial depression during general anesthesia<br>(5) Avoidance of an increase in PVR (avoid pain, hypoxemia, hypercarbia, and acidosis) |
| Aortic regurgitation (AR) Mitral regurgitation (MR) | (1) *Maintenance of a normal to slightly elevated heart rate and sinus rhythm*<br>(2) *Prevention of an increase in SVR* (minimize regurgitant blood flow through the valve)<br>(3) Maintenance preload (optimize intravascular volume and avoid aortacaval compression)<br>(4) Avoidance of myocardial depression during general anesthesia<br>(5) Avoidance of an increase in PVR (avoid pain, hypoxemia, hypercarbia, and acidosis) |
| Left-to-right cardiac shunts | (1) Maintenance of preload and be careful in<br>(2) Judicial application of positive pressure ventilation as it can decrease preload and increase intrathoracic pressure, which is deleterious to venous return and RV function<br>(3) Meticulous attention in de-airing all venous access tubing and avoid using a loss of resistance to air technique to identify the epidural space to minimize the risk of paradoxical embolism |
| Right-to-left cardiac shunts | An asymptomatic patient with fully corrected congenital condition such as tetralogy of Fallot can be managed as a normal pregnant patient after consultation.<br>Patients symptomatic due to partial or unsuccessful correction should be managed with the following goals in mind:<br>(1) Optimization preload guided by preoperative systolic and diastolic function (echo)<br>(2) Avoidance of myocardial depression during general anesthesia<br>(3) *Maintenance of SVR to maximize the blood flow through the pulmonary circulation.* Neuraxial anesthesia should be used with caution due the profound and sudden vasodilation, which may lead to more systemic diversion of the deoxygenated blood rather than maximizing its flow to the pulmonary circulation.<br>(4) Avoidance of an increase in PVR (avoid pain, hypoxemia, hypercarbia, and acidosis) |
| Pulmonary hypertension | (1) Maintenance of adequate SVR<br>(2) Maintenance preload (optimize intravascular volume and avoid aortacaval compression)<br>(3) Avoidance of an increase in PVR (avoid pain, hypoxemia, hypercarbia, and acidosis)<br>(4) Avoidance of myocardial depression during general anesthesia<br>(5) Neuraxial analgesia can be administered during early labor by gently titrating local anesthetic and/or use of opioid to attenuate the surge of catecholamines with minimal effect on SVR.<br>(6) Minimizing tissue and the number of needle passes is advised if the patient is on intravenous prostanoids. Switching to inhaled prostanoids should be considered if the patient is on a *low dose* of intravenous prostanoids due to the limited systemic effects of inhaled prostanoid on platelet function. |
| Hypertrophic cardiomyopathy | The goal is to reduce the dynamic left ventricular outflow obstruction.<br>(1) Maintenance preload (optimize intravascular volume and avoid aortacaval compression)<br>(2) Maintenance of SVR (phenylephrine is drug of choice to treat hypotension)<br>(3) Avoidance of an increase in heart rate<br>(4) Avoidance of an increase in myocardial contractility<br>(5) Consider invasive blood pressure monitoring<br>(6) Use of β-blockers if necessary |

| HEART DISEASE | GOALS OF ANESTHETIC MANAGEMENT |
|---|---|
| Peripartum cardiomyopathy | Neuraxial anesthesia appears ideally suited for patients with peripartum cardiomyopathy because it results in a beneficial decrease in both preload and afterload. Avoidance of myocardial depression during induction and maintenance of general anesthesia is important. |

echo, echocardiogram; PVR, peripheral vascular resistance; RV, right ventricle; SVR, systemic vascular resistance.

## POSTOPERATIVE

Closely monitor the patient postoperatively due to the higher incidence of arrhythmia. In patients with peripartum cardiomyopathy and mitral stenosis, the patient should be closely monitored in the immediate postpartum period when auto-transfusion combined with the regression of neuraxial anesthesia (leading to an increase in SVR and PVR) may cause worsening of heart failure.

## REFERENCES

1. ACOG practice bulletin no. 212: pregnancy and heart disease. Obst Gynecol. 2019;133(5):e320–e356.
2. Vidovich MI. Cardiovascular disease. In: Chestnut DH, et al., eds. *Chestnut's Obstetric Anesthesia: Principles and Practice.* 6th ed. Philadelphia, PA: Elsevier Health Sciences; 2020:988–1023.
3. Chandrasekhar S, et al. Anesthetic management of the pregnant cardiac patient. In: Suresh MS, et al., eds. *Shnider and Levinson's Anesthesia for Obstetrics.* 5th ed. Philadelphia, PA: Lippincott, Williams & Wilkins; 2013:484–523.

# 304.

# HEMATOLOGIC DISORDERS

*Benjamin M. Hyers and Kevin W. Chung*

## INTRODUCTION

Hematologic disorders present a unique challenge in the laboring patient. While neuraxial anesthesia is commonly performed in laboring patients, the presence of hematologic disorders increases the risk of a catastrophic epidural hematoma.[1]

## SICKLE CELL ANEMIA

In sickle cell anemia, patients are homozygous for hemoglobin S, a hemoglobin variant that causes erythrocytes to "sickle" (i.e., become elongated and crescent shaped) when exposed to deoxygenated environments. Many factors, such as dehydration, acidosis, and hypothermia, increase the risk of sickling, but the most important determinant of sickling is oxygen tension, with sickling occurring at $PO_2$ levels of less than 50 mm Hg.[1]

Sickle cells can form aggregates and cause vaso-occlusive crises, leading to end-organ damage. Sickle cell complications can be exacerbated in pregnancy, and these patients have a higher incidence of placental abruption, preterm labor, fetal growth restriction, and preeclampsia/eclampsia. The primary goal of anesthetic management is to avoid sickling by ensuring excellent pain control, adequate hydration and oxygenation, and maintenance of normothermia.

## IDIOPATHIC THROMBOCYTOPENIC PURPURA

Idiopathic thrombocytopenic purpura comprises the majority of cases of thrombocytopenia in the first trimester.

Many of these patients can present later in pregnancy with profound thrombocytopenia, with the degree of thrombocytopenia directly proportional to the risk of postpartum hemorrhage. Corticosteroids are usually reserved for patients with a platelet count of less than 20,000–30,000/μL of blood during labor and less than 50,000/μL of blood during delivery, and intravenous immunoglobulin can be administered for a fast but temporary increase in platelet count.[1]

These patients generally have a stable quantitative defect; therefore, in the absence of bleeding diatheses, it is reasonable to proceed with neuraxial anesthesia with a platelet count of 50,000/μL or greater.[1,2] A low concentration of local anesthetic should be used to preserve motor function, and frequent neurologic examinations are necessary to ensure the motor blockade is not more profound than expected and is not progressing with time. Physical examination findings concerning for an epidural hematoma (see Box 304.1) warrant emergent magnetic resonance imaging and decompression to prevent permanent nerve damage and paralysis.[2,3]

## VON WILLEBRAND DISEASE

Von Willebrand disease (VWD) is the most common hemostatic disorder in the general population and is due to either a quantitative or qualitative defect in von Willebrand factor (VWF).[1,2] Symptoms, treatment, and prophylaxis for patients with VWD depend on the type of disease, timing, and presentation.[1] For example, since VWF can increase by 200%–375% during a normal pregnancy, patients with type 1 disease rarely have bleeding after the first trimester.[2] Preoperatively, it may be reasonable to test factor VIII concentrations and to perform a von Willebrand ristocetin cofactor activity assay (VWF:RCo) test to determine the functional concentration of VWF. Patients with a normal VWF:RCo, factor VIII, and VWF antigen concentrations are candidates for neuraxial anesthesia. Catheters should be removed immediately after delivery since VWF concentrations will return to the patient's baseline quickly in the postpartum period.[2]

## DISSEMINATED INTRAVASCULAR COAGULATION

In disseminated intravascular coagulation (DIC), abnormal activation of the coagulation system results in increased thrombin production, fibrinolytic system activation, and depletion of coagulation factors, thereby leading to both a hypocoagulable and hypercoagulable state with resultant hemorrhage, microvascular thrombosis, and end-organ damage. The most common causes of DIC in the parturient population are placental abruption, amniotic fluid embolism, retained dead fetus syndrome, preeclampsia, sepsis, and postpartum hemorrhage.[1]

Treating the precipitating cause of DIC is imperative as it will lead to a return to normalcy of the coagulation cascade. Treatment is largely supportive, consisting of blood product transfusions to replete coagulation factors.[1] Patients in DIC are not candidates for neuraxial anesthetics and would need general anesthesia for cesarean deliveries.[1]

## ANTICOAGULANT THERAPY

The most common anticoagulants used during pregnancy are unfractionated heparin (UFH) and low-molecular-weight heparin (LMWH).[2,3] While LMWH does not require laboratory testing and has a lower risk of causing heparin-induced thrombocytopenia and osteoporosis, LMWH is associated with a higher risk of epidural hematoma formation compared to UFH, likely due to its longer duration of action.[2]

Appropriate timing of neuraxial placement in pregnant patients taking anticoagulation therapy is important to prevent serious complications. Table 304.1 depicts specific time intervals for neuraxial placement after anticoagulant administration and the time intervals for resuming anticoagulation in the postpartum period.[3,4]

## RH AND ABO INCOMPATIBILITY

Hemolytic disease of the newborn is a deadly disease where maternal antibodies cross the placenta and target the newborn's red blood cells (RBCs). This is commonly caused by an incompatibility with the Rh blood group, usually the D antigen, between the fetus and mother. When an Rh D-negative mother gives birth to an Rh D-positive child for the first time, sensitization can occur during labor and delivery when there is a high chance of the maternal circulation being exposed to fetal blood. The mother mounts an immune response by producing immunoglobulin (Ig) M anti-D antibodies, which are not able to cross the placenta. During a subsequent pregnancy with an Rh-positive fetus and repeat exposure to the Rh D antigen, the mother mounts

**Table 304.1** RECOMMENDED TIMING INTERVALS FOR NEURAXIAL ANESTHESIA PLACEMENT, CATHETER REMOVAL, AND POSTPARTUM ANTICOAGULATION FOR COMMON ANTICOAGULANT THERAPIES

| MEDICATION AND DOSAGE | MINIMUM TIMING BETWEEN LAST DOSE OF ANTICOAGULANT AND NEURAXIAL PLACEMENT OR CATHETER REMOVAL | MINIMUM TIMING BETWEEN NEURAXIAL PLACEMENT OR CATHETER REMOVAL AND INITIATION OF POSTPARTUM ANTICOAGULATION |
|---|---|---|
| SC UFH 5000 U twice or three times daily | 4–6 hours | 1 hour |
| SC UFH 7500–10000 U twice daily | 12 hours<br>Check aPTT | 1 hour |
| SC UFH greater than 10,000 U/dose or greater than 20,000 U/d | 24 hours<br>Check aPTT | 1 hour |
| Intravenous UFH | 4–6 hours<br>Check aPTT | 1 hour |
| SC enoxaparin 40 mg daily | 12 hours | 4 hours after catheter removal but also at least 12 hours after initial neuraxial placement |
| Enoxaparin 1 mg/kg twice daily or 1.5 mg/kg daily | 24 hours | 4 hours after catheter removal but also at least 24 hours after initial neuraxial placement |

aPTT, activated partial thromboplastin time; SC, subcutaneous; UFH, unfractionated heparin.

From References 3 and 4.

a robust immune response consisting of mostly IgG anti-D antibodies, which are able to cross the placenta and bind to the Rh antigen on fetal RBCs, resulting in hemolysis.[5]

# REFERENCES

1. Mhyre JM. Hematologic and coagulation disorders. In: Chestnut DH. ed. *Chestnut's Obstetric Anesthesia Principles and Practice.* 6th ed. Philadelphia, PA: Elsevier; 2020:1088–1111.

2. Katz D, Beilin Y. Disorders of coagulation in pregnancy. *Br J Anaesth.* 2015;115(suppl 2):ii75–ii88.

3. Toledo P. Embolic disorders. In: Chestnut DH, ed. *Chestnut's Obstetric Anesthesia Principles and Practice.* 6th ed. Philadelphia, PA: Elsevier; 2020:937–955.

4. Horlocker TT, et al. Regional anesthesia in the patient receiving antithrombotic or thrombolytic therapy: American Society of Regional Anesthesia and Pain Medicine evidence-based guidelines (fourth edition). *Reg Anesth Pain Med.* 2018;43(3):263–309.

5. Dean L. *Blood Groups and Red Cell Antigens.* Bethesda, MD: National Center for Biotechnology Information; 2005. https://www.ncbi.nlm.nih.gov/books/NBK2261/

# 305.

# HYPERTENSION

*Muhammad Fayyaz Ahmed and Ihab Kamel*

## INTRODUCTION

Hypertension complicates 5% to 10% of all pregnancies and is a major cause of maternal morbidity and mortality worldwide.[1] Hypertensive disorders during pregnancy include chronic hypertension, gestational hypertension, preeclampsia superimposed on chronic hypertension preeclampsia, and eclampsia. The clinical presentation and symptoms often overlap, making it a challenge to diagnose. The updated classification by the American College of Obstetricians and Gynecologists in 2013 assisted in clarifying the different classes of hypertension during pregnancy.[2,3]

## CLASSIFICATION OF HYPERTENSION DURING PREGNANCY

### CHRONIC HYPERTENSION

Chronic hypertension is defined as either prepregnancy systolic blood pressure of 140 mm Hg or higher and/or diastolic blood pressure of 90 mm Hg on two occasions at least 4 hours apart in a previously normotensive patient *or* increased blood pressure during pregnancy that fails to resolve within 12 weeks of delivery. Chronic hypertension develops into preeclampsia in around 20% to 25% of affected patients. Chronic hypertension is associated with a higher incidence of adverse maternal and fetal pregnancy outcomes even in the absence of preeclampsia.[2]

### CHRONIC HYPERTENSION WITH SUPERIMPOSED PREECLAMPSIA

Chronic hypertension with superimposed preeclampsia is defined as having preeclampsia in a woman with chronic hypertension before pregnancy. Clinical presentation includes sudden increase in the blood pressure, new-onset proteinuria, and signs and symptoms of severe preeclampsia. Maternal and fetal morbidity is increased compared to preeclampsia alone.

## GESTATIONAL HYPERTENSION

Gestational hypertension is defined as elevated blood pressure after 20 weeks of gestation without proteinuria and the absence of diagnosis of chronic hypertension. The hypertension resolves by 12 weeks' postpartum. Gestational hypertension usually develops after 37 weeks of gestation. Approximately 25% of patients with gestational hypertension develop preeclampsia. Treatment is not usually required since most patients will have only mild hypertension. Uncomplicated gestational hypertension at term has minimal effect on maternal or perinatal morbidity or mortality. Patients with severe gestational hypertension (systolic blood pressure > 160 mm Hg and/or diastolic blood pressure > 110 mm Hg) are at increased risk for adverse maternal and perinatal outcomes and therefore should be treated with antihypertensive agents.

## PREECLAMPSIA

Preeclampsia is defined as new-onset hypertension after 20 weeks' gestation with proteinuria and/or end-organ involvement. The presence of proteinuria is defined as 0.3 g or higher in 24 hours, a protein/creatinine ratio of 0.3 or higher, or a urine dipstick protein of 1+. End-organ involvement includes cerebral symptoms (visual disturbance, hyperreflexia, headache, and coma); epigastric or right upper quadrant pain; fetal growth restriction; thrombocytopenia; and elevated serum liver enzymes.

## MANAGEMENT OF HYPERTENSION DURING PREGNANCY

Blood pressure should be controlled in patients with severe hypertension and in patients with nonsevere hypertension with evidence of end-organ damage. The ideal target blood pressure below 160/110 mm Hg remains debatable. Current treatment recommendations for severe hypertension include intravenous hydralazine (5–10 mg every 20–40 minutes, maximum 20 mg OR 0.5–10 mg/h infusion); oral immediate-release nifedipine (10–20 mg every 2–6 hours, maximum 180 mg/d); intravenous labetalol (10–20 mg → 20–80 mg every 10–30 minutes, maximum 300 mg); and intravenous labetalol (1–2 mg/min infusion). Current recommendations for treatment of nonsevere hypertension include oral extended-release nifedipine (20–120 mg/d), oral labetalol (200–2400 mg/d), and oral methyldopa (500–3000 mg/d). β-Blockers and diuretics are acceptable treatment options, while renin-angiotensin-aldosterone system inhibitors are contraindicated due to association with fetal adverse effects.

## ANESTHETIC CONSIDERATIONS

### PREOPERATIVE

Unless contraindicated, neuraxial anesthesia is the anesthetic of choice preoperatively for cesarean section in patients with hypertensive disorders. Patients with preeclampsia are *less likely* to develop hypotension associated with spinal anesthesia compared to patients who do not have preeclampsia complicating their pregnancy. Epidural anesthesia and analgesia are considered beneficial due the effect on systemic vascular resistance and the resulting improvement of uteroplacental perfusion. Furthermore, regional anesthesia allows for cesarean delivery while avoiding direct laryngoscopy and endotracheal intubation.

### INTRAOPERATIVE

Acute severe hypertension associated with endotracheal intubation in hypertensive patients can lead to fatal consequences, such as intracranial hemorrhage.

Intraoperatively, achieving adequate anesthetic depth before direct laryngoscopy and intubation, minimizing the time of direct laryngoscopy (preferably under 15 seconds) to avoid an exaggerated sympathetic response, and immediate treatment of ensuing blood pressure elevation with esmolol are among the most important considerations during induction of general anesthesia. Methergine (methylergonovine maleate) should be avoided in patients with a history of hypertension as it leads to severe hypertension and intracerebral hemorrhage. Judicious use of phenylephrine intravenous infusion during cesarean delivery to counteract the concomitant hypotension resulting from the spinal block is highly recommended. Cautious titration of adrenergic agents in patients with hypertensive disorders is recommended due to increased sensitivity to their effect.

### POSTOPERATIVE

Hypertensive patients may demonstrate signs and symptoms of hypertension in the immediate postoperative period. Careful monitoring of blood pressure and prompt treatment are recommended to avoid maternal complications.

## REFERENCES

1. Ramanathan J, et al. Hypertensive disorders of pregnancy. In: Suresh MS, et al., eds. *Shnider and Levinson's Anesthesia for Obstetrics.* 5th ed. Philadelphia, PA: Lippincott, Williams & Wilkins; 2013:437–461.
2. Dyer RA, et al. Hypertensive disorders. In: Chestnut DH, et al., eds. *Chestnut's Obstetric Anesthesia: Principles and Practice.* 6th ed. Philadelphia, PA: Elsevier Health Sciences; 2020:840–868.
3. American College of Obstetricians and Gynecologists, Task Force on Hypertension in Pregnancy. Hypertension in pregnancy. Report of the American College of Obstetricians and Gynecologists' Task Force on Hypertension in Pregnancy. *Obstet Gynecol.* 2013;122(5):1122–1131.

# 306.

# NEUROLOGIC DISORDERS

*Katrina Brakoniecki and Kevin W. Chung*

## INTRODUCTION

As the medical management of women with neurologic diseases advances, many of these women are carrying healthy babies to term. The physiologic changes of pregnancy can greatly affect these individuals' anesthetic management.

## SEIZURES

Epilepsy is one of the most common neurologic conditions, affecting about 5 per 1000 people.[1] While most women have little increase in seizure frequency or severity while continuing antiepileptic drugs (AEDs) during pregnancy, up to 33% of pregnant patients will face increased disease burden due to physiological and emotional stresses.[1,2] Seizures during pregnancy can cause fetal bradycardia, fetal hypoxia, placental abruption, and miscarriage.

For anesthetic management, uncontrolled pain during labor and delivery can cause stress and hyperventilation, which may precipitate a seizure.[1] There is no contraindication to general or neuraxial anesthesia, and the choice of technique should be based on patient preference and clinical judgment. If general anesthesia is pursued, recognize that some AEDs may antagonize neuromuscular blocking drugs (NMBDs).

If seizures occur in the peripartum or perioperative period, benzodiazepines are the first drug of choice for acute seizure management.[3] Other alternatives include phenytoin, valproate, and, if needed, general anesthesia.[3] Fetal monitoring should commence as soon as possible.

## MYASTHENIA GRAVIS

Myasthenia gravis (MG) is an autoimmune disease with an incidence of 15 in 100,000 and is most common in women of childbearing age.[1,3] The effects of pregnancy on MG are highly variable; about 30% of MG patients will deteriorate during pregnancy and require higher doses of oral steroids and respiratory intervention.[3] Pregnant patients with MG are at higher risk of preterm premature rupture of membranes, premature labor, and intrauterine growth restriction.[1]

Preoperative evaluation should focus on medication dosages and bulbar and pulmonary function. Many patients take anticholinesterase therapy, which should be continued in the peripartum period. Patients should also be given stress-dose steroids as indicated. The patient with MG and preeclampsia presents a unique challenge. Commonly used medications to treat preeclampsia, including magnesium, nifedipine, and labetalol, are contraindicated in MG due to concern for precipitation of myasthenic crisis.[1] Recommended alternatives include levetiracetam and hydralazine.[4]

There is no contraindication to neuraxial anesthetics in MG patients, though amide local anesthetics should be considered for patients on anticholinesterase medications, which may impair the hydrolysis of ester local anesthetics, resulting in prolonged neuraxial blockade.[1] If general anesthesia is pursued, these patients should be treated similarly to their nonpregnant MG counterparts: avoid neuromuscular blocking agents, give medications in minimal doses, and avoid hypothermia.

## SPINAL CORD INJURIES

Every year in the United States there are about 12,000 new spinal cord injuries (SCIs) reported.[1] Women with SCIs are more likely to deliver preterm and require either instrumental delivery or cesarean section.[1]

An SCI is not a contraindication for neuraxial anesthesia, although it may be technically difficult in patients with previous spinal surgery. Early placement of neuraxial anesthetics is ideal as poorly controlled pain despite the lack of patient perception can precipitate autonomic dysreflexia, which is most commonly associated with SCI above T6.[1]

Uncontrolled hypertension can lead to headache, sweating, cerebral hemorrhage and edema, fetal bradycardia, and/ or placental abruption.[1] For this reason, dense neuraxial blocks are often utilized, including spinal catheters if necessary, in conjunction with antihypertensives.

In the case of scheduled or urgent/emergent cesarean section, regional anesthesia is preferred. These patients may present difficult intubations if they have contracted limbs or fixed cervical injuries. Succinylcholine should be avoided due to concerns for hyperkalemia. Following induction of general anesthesia, lack of sympathetic response can lead to profound hypotension. Additionally, temperature should be monitored closely; thermoregulation is often impaired in these patients.

## MULTIPLE SCLEROSIS

Multiple sclerosis (MS) is an immune-mediated, demyelinating disease that affects an estimated 2.5 million people worldwide.[1] Most of the disease-modifying drugs, such as interferon, have few data supporting their safe use during pregnancy, and patients are advised to stop treatment during pregnancy.[1] While conflicting data exists, the general consensus is that symptoms of MS decrease during pregnancy and increase in the postpartum period. This is supported by the Pregnancy in Multiple Sclerosis (PRIMS) study, which followed 254 women and found the highest rate of relapse during the 3-month postpartum period, whereas a protective effect was seen during pregnancy.[5] Overall, pregnancy does not accelerate disease severity or progression, and MS does not affect neonatal outcomes.

Epidural anesthesia has been used safely in MS patients, while spinal anesthesia is relatively contraindicated due to concerns that it increases MS exacerbations.[3] For patients in active relapse, demyelinated neurons will be more sensitive to the effects of local anesthetics and more susceptible to toxicity. If general anesthesia is pursued for cesarean section, similar precautions as would be undertaken for a nonpregnant MS patient should be taken, such as avoiding succinylcholine, careful use of neuromuscular blockers, and prevention of hypothermia.

## SUBARACHNOID HEMORRHAGE

Subarachnoid hemorrhage (SAH) is a rare but potentially catastrophic event and is most commonly related to rupture of an intracranial aneurysm. During pregnancy, SAH is associated with a 35% risk of poor feto-maternal outcomes and a maternal mortality rate of 35%–83%.[1] Each trimester, the risk of aneurysm rupture increases, peaking during the peripartum period. Arteriovenous malformations can also cause SAH, and the risk of bleeding is greatest in the second trimester due to changes in circulating blood volume and cardiovascular status.[1] Interventions such as endovascular coiling can and should be safely pursued during pregnancy.

Intraoperative management of these patients includes careful monitoring of hemodynamics and avoidance of agents and techniques that increase intracranial pressure (ICP), which could potentiate herniation. In the intubated patient, maternal carbon dioxide tension should be kept in the low-normal range to decrease ICP while avoiding hyperventilation-induced uterine artery spasm.[3] In a laboring but otherwise stable patient during the peripartum period, an epidural is preferred over a spinal because of the avoidance of intentional dural puncture, which can result in an uncontrolled significant drop in ICP with risk of herniation.[3] While inadvertent dural puncture may occur with epidural placement, the benefits of labor analgesia and avoidance of large blood pressure swings likely outweighs these risks. General anesthesia is generally reserved for cases of emergent cesarean section and fetal distress.

## REFERENCES

1. Gunaydin B, and Ismail S, eds. *Obstetric Anesthesia for Co-morbid Conditions.* Springer International; 2017.
2. Pennell PB, Hovinga CA. Antiepileptic drug therapy in pregnancy I: gestation-induced effects on AED pharmacokinetics. *Int Rev Neurobiol.* 2007; 83:227–240.
3. Palmer CM, et al. *Obstetric Anesthesia.* Oxford University Press, 2011.
4. Waters J. Management of myasthenia gravis in pregnancy. *Neurol Clin.* 2019;37(1):113–120.
5. Vukusic S, et al. Pregnancy and multiple sclerosis (the PRIMS study): clinical predictors of post-partum relapse. *Brain J Neurol.* 2004;127(pt 6):1353–1360.

# 307.

# RESPIRATORY DISORDERS

*Devin O'Conor and Kevin W. Chung*

## EPIDEMIOLOGY OF RESPIRATORY FAILURE IN PREGNANCY

The incidence of respiratory failure during pregnancy has been estimated to be as high as 1 in 500.[1] There are a number of etiologies of respiratory failure in the pregnant patient (Table 307.1). Respiratory failure in pregnant patients has serious consequences for both the mother and the fetus as maternal hypoxemia and hypotension result in impaired fetal oxygen delivery.

*Asthma* is a disease process classified by reversible airway obstruction, airway inflammation, and airway hyperresponsiveness to certain stimuli.[2] There are two main categories of pharmacological management for asthma: bronchodilators and anti-inflammatory agents. Examples of bronchodilators include β-agonists, methylxanthines, and magnesium sulfate; examples of anti-inflammatory agents include inhaled corticosteroids, cromolyn sodium, and leukotriene receptor antagonists.[2]

Asthma is associated with an increased incidence of preeclampsia, cesarean delivery, low birth weight, preterm labor, antepartum and postpartum hemorrhage, and perinatal mortality.[3] Poorly controlled asthma leads to increased morbidity and mortality secondary to hypoxemia, hypocapnea, inflammation, and altered placental function from asthma-induced mediator release (Table 307.2).[3]

## ANESTHETIC MANAGEMENT

The overall goal is to manage predisposing conditions, limit fluid transudation, and optimize maternal oxygen delivery. These goals may vary depending on the etiology of respiratory failure. Oxygen delivery to the fetus decreases significantly at maternal $PaO_2$ levels less than 70 mm Hg or $SaO_2$ levels below 95%.[4]

The use of positive end-expiratory pressure must be balanced with maintaining cardiac output to provide adequate blood flow to the uterus.

*Table 307.1* ETIOLOGIES OF RESPIRATORY FAILURE DURING PREGNANCY

Acute respiratory distress syndrome

Infection—bacteria or viral pneumonia, endometritis, chorioamnionitis, pyelonephritis, sepsis

Preeclampsia

Hemorrhage—multiplatelet transfusions, disseminated intravascular coagulation

Gastric acid aspiration

Embolism

Drugs—salicylates, opioids

Pulmonary embolism—amniotic fluid embolism, venous air embolism, venous thromboembolism

Pulmonary edema—cardiomyopathy, transfusion-associated circulatory overload (TACO)

Cystic fibrosis

Asthma

Valvular heart disease

Pulmonary hypertension

*Table 307.2* EFFECTS OF HORMONAL CHANGES DURING PREGNANCY ON ASTHMATIC PATIENTS

- Progesterone results in relaxation of uterine, gastrointestinal, and possibly airway smooth muscle. Progesterone is also associated with increased inflammation.

- There is an increased production of both bronchoconstricting and bronchodilating prostaglandins during pregnancy.

- The elevated cortisol levels during pregnancy are associated with an improvement in asthma status.

Adapted from Reference 2.

## PREOPERATIVE

Specific preoperative questions should relate to current symptoms (e.g., cough, dyspnea, and wheezing), frequency and severity of attacks, and the most recent exacerbation.

The physical examination in the asthmatic patient focuses on chest auscultation for the presence or absence of wheezing, air movement, duration of expiration, pulsus paradoxus, and use of accessory muscles. In stable asthmatics, laboratory values usually have little value. In the setting of an acute exacerbation, arterial blood gases can show respiratory alkalemia from hyperventilation.[2] Normalization of or elevation in $PaCO_2$ is an ominous sign and may suggest impending respiratory failure due to patient fatigue. Chest x-rays can show complications of asthma (e.g., pneumonia, pneumothorax, and heart failure). Finally, spirometry can be used for measurement of exhaled gas over time, with peak expiratory flow rate used to assess for airway obstruction.[1]

For the induction of labor, prostaglandins should be administered cautiously as they can have a variable response in regard to bronchodilating or constricting the airways.[2] Asthma represents a relative contraindication to 15-methyl prostaglandin F2a (carboprost, Hemabate) for the management of uterine atony. Additionally, ergot alkaloids have been associated with episodes of acute bronchospasm. Oxytocin, which is not associated with increased airway smooth muscle/tone, is the preferred uterotonic agent for asthmatics.[2]

## INTRAOPERATIVE

### Management During Labor and Vaginal Delivery

The goals for analgesia during the peripartum period do not differ drastically from the nonasthmatic parturient. It is important to prevent hyperventilation/hyperpnea and corresponding hypocapnea in asthmatic patients as the decrease in partial pressure of arterial $CO_2$ will subsequently result in decreased uterine blood flow. Pain relief in the pregnant population can additionally help decrease the stimulus for hyperventilation. Options for pain relief to the laboring patient include systemic opioids and, most commonly, lumbar epidural placement. Of note, morphine and nonfentanyl narcotics carry a risk of histamine release, which can trigger bronchospasm.[2]

Lumbar epidurals provide pain relief and a reduction in the stimulus to hyperventilate while minimizing maternal respiratory depression and obviating the need for airway manipulation in the event that a cesarean delivery is necessary. The main respiratory concern associated with lumbar epidural placement is the risk of a high thoracic motor block with resulting respiratory insufficiency.[2] To minimize this risk, maintenance of sensation at the T10 level is desirable.[2] Additionally, the combination of an opioid and local anesthetic epidural solution allows for a lower local anesthetic

dose than would be necessary for a narcotic-sparing epidural infusion. This is all done while providing desirable analgesia with less motor blockade.[5]

### Management During Cesarean Delivery

Airway manipulation with endotracheal intubation provides a potent trigger for bronchospasm in a patient with preexisting reactive airway disease. If a neuraxial technique is used for delivery, then this risk can be avoided. However, if the patient is experiencing an acute asthma exacerbation and is using accessory muscles for respiration, she may be unable to tolerate a neuraxial anesthetic if the motor block extends too far cephalad. Additionally, there are other times where neuraxial anesthesia is contraindicated and a general anesthetic must be performed, such as in the setting of coagulopathy or patient refusal.

The pregnant patient is a higher aspiration risk than her nonlaboring counterpart. As such, a rapid sequence intubation is generally the safest option for securing the airway. Intravenous adjuvants may reduce airway reactivity. For instance, ketamine causes bronchodilation through neural mechanisms and catecholamine release, while intravenous lidocaine has been shown to result in a reduction of airway reactivity via inhibition of airway reflexes and a reduction in irritant-induced bronchoconstriction.[2]

Maintenance of general anesthesia during cesarean delivery in an asthmatic patient should consider the bronchodilating properties of volatile inhalational agents while balancing it against the dose-dependent decrease in uterine tone that accompanies them. The potent inhalational agents attenuate airway responsiveness through direct bronchodilating properties and inhibition of airway reflexes. If possible, minimization or avoidance of systemic opioids should be delayed until after delivery of the baby to avoid neonatal respiratory depression.[2]

## POSTOPERATIVE

Continue to manage the source of respiratory failure or asthma. If general anesthesia was performed in an asthmatic, one must balance the decision between a deep extubation, which minimizes tracheal tube stimulation while increasing the risk for aspiration, versus awake extubation.

## REFERENCES

1. Lapinsky SE. Management of acute respiratory failure in pregnancy. *Semin Respir Crit Care Med*. 2017;38(2):201–207.
2. Lindeman K. (2019). Respiratory diseases. In Chestnut D, Wong C, Tsen L, Ngan Kee WD, Beilin Y, Myhre J, Bateman BT, Nathan N, eds. *Chestnut's Obstetric Anesthesia: Principles and Practice*. 6th ed. Philadelphia, PA: Elsevier; 2019:1231–1247.

3. Murphy VE, et al. A meta-analysis of adverse perinatal outcomes in women with asthma. *BJOG.* 2011;118(11):1314–1323.
4. Cole DE, et al. Acute respiratory distress syndrome in pregnancy. *Crit Care Med.* 2005;33(10 suppl):S269–S278.
5. Chestnut DH, et al. Continuous infusion epidural analgesia during labor: a randomized, double-blind comparison of 0.0625% bupivacaine/0.0002% fentanyl versus 0.125% bupivacaine. *Anesthesiology.* 1988;68(5):754–759.

# 308.

# RENAL CHANGES IN PREGNANCY

*Jarna Shah*

## INTRODUCTION

Several important physiologic alterations occur during pregnancy (Table 308.1). In particular, renal function undergoes significant changes before, during, and after delivery. Physiologic renal dysfunction can adversely affect the health of the fetus and mother.

## PHYSIOLOGIC CHANGES

### GLOMERULAR FILTRATION RATE

The glomerular filtration rate (GFR) begins to rise very early during the pregnancy. It will typically increase by 50% by the second trimester.[1] This elevated GFR persists until the parturient is full term and is often sustained for some time before returning to prepregnancy levels. Oncotic pressure is decreased, and plasma volume is increased. This contributes to an elevated GFR.[2]

### SERUM CREATININE

While the GFR increases during pregnancy, serum creatinine levels decrease in the first trimester and plateau during the second trimester. Traditional creatinine calculators will not accurately reflect appropriate values in the pregnant population.[3,4] Serum creatinine levels are lowered in pregnancy due to a variety of factors, including increased GFR and a higher circulating plasma volume.[3]

The mean serum creatinine range is between 0.5 and 0.6 mg/dL. Values greater than 0.8 mg/dL may be indicative of underlying disease[1] and may alter drug metabolism and

*Table 308.1* PHYSIOLOGIC TRENDS DURING PREGNANCY

|  | FIRST TRIMESTER | SECOND TRIMESTER | THIRD TRIMESTER | IMMEDIATELY POSTPARTUM |
|---|---|---|---|---|
| Serum creatinine | ↓ | ↓↓↓ | ↓↓ | — |
| GFR | ↑↑ | ↑↑↑ | ↑↑ | ↑ |
| Renal blood flow | ↑↑↑ | ↑ | ↑ | — |
| Creatinine clearance | ↑ | ↑ | ↑ | — |

elimination. If elevated creatinine levels are noted in the parturient, the provider should pursue further evaluation. For example, one study demonstrated that 70% of pregnant women with a creatinine greater than 2.5 mg/dL experienced a preterm delivery, and more than 40% developed preeclampsia.[3]

## CREATININE CLEARANCE

Creatinine clearance rises slightly during the first trimester and remains elevated during the pregnancy.[2]

## RENAL PLASMA FLOW

Renal plasma flow increases by over 80% during the first and second trimesters. These levels decline slowly during the remainder of pregnancy, and they then begin to decline slowly in the postpartum period. Relaxin releases nitric oxide, which contributes to renal vasodilation.[1] This also contributes to glomerular hyperfiltration.

## RENIN-ANGIOTENSIN-ALDOSTERONE SYSTEM

Upregulation of the renin-angiotensin-aldosterone system is a common finding in pregnancy. The placenta produces estrogen, which leads to increased production of angiotensin II. However, in spite of this, blood pressures tend to be lower than prepregnancy values.[2] This is thought to be related to increased levels of progesterone.

## URINE GLUCOSE

Typically, glucose is filtered through the glomerulus and reabsorbed in the proximal tubule. In pregnancy, glucose is less effectively reabsorbed due to hyperfiltration and the increased GFR. Therefore, it is often common to note mild glucosuria in healthy parturients. However, elevated levels of urine glucose may also be related to gestational diabetes, which would require further workup.[2]

## URINE PROTEIN

Pregnancy is associated with elevated urinary protein and albumin excretion, and it increases with each trimester. Abnormal or increased levels of proteinuria may be associated with risk factors for preeclampsia.[2]

## ANATOMIC CHANGES

During pregnancy, the anatomic size of the kidneys increases by 1–1.5cm. They decrease in size within 6 months of the postpartum period. This change is thought to be related to the increased interstitial volume. In addition, there is a higher incidence of hydronephrosis. Physiologic hydronephrosis occurs in up to 80% of women, and prevalence increases with each trimester. Some theorize this may be due to mechanical compression of the ureters. Progesterone may also contribute to reduction of ureteral tone.[2]

## REFERENCES

1. Cunningham G, et al. Maternal physiology. In: Williams Obstetrics. McGraw-Hill Education; 2018.
2. Cheung KL, Lafayette RA. Renal physiology of pregnancy. *Adv Chronic Kidney Dis.* 2013;20(3):209–214.
3. Maynard SE, Thadhani R. Pregnancy and the kidney." *J Am Soc Nephrol.* 2009;20(1):14–22.
4. Harel Z, et al. Serum creatinine levels before, during, and after pregnancy. *JAMA.* 2019;321(2):205–207.

# 309.

# FETAL MONITORING

*Shuchi Jain and Joshua D. Younger*

## INTRODUCTION

There are a multitude of methods employed to ensure fetal well-being throughout the gestational period. Biochemical markers as well as imaging are the foundation of this testing. α-Fetoprotein, human chorionic gonadotropin, estriol, inhibin A, and pregnancy-associated plasma protein A are used antenatally to detect various syndromes and fetal malformations. Ultrasound is used in conjunction with the biomarkers to evaluate the fetal anatomy, placenta and amniotic fluid. Additionally, cell-free DNA can be extracted from maternal blood, and invasive testing can be averted. However, if needed, further invasive testing can be performed via chorionic villi sampling and/or amniocentesis. The nonstress test, NST, evaluates fetal well-being. The NST looks at the baseline fetal heart rate (FHR), accelerations, decelerations, baseline variability, and fetal movements during a 20-minutes period, it is either reassuring or not. When not, additional testing is often employed. A stress test utilizes oxytocin to cause uterine contractions and can demonstrate compromised fetal blood flow. This oxytocin challenge test is positive if persistent FHR decelerations occur repeatedly with the uterine contractions.

All the above testing is done in the antenatal period. However, intrapartum testing most frequently involves electronic fetal monitoring (EFM) and occasionally fetal scalp pH sampling and/or ultrasonography. Fetal pH is normally 7.25–7.45; if below 7.2, this indicates fetal acidosis.

The goal of fetal assessment and monitoring is to improve neonatal outcomes by reducing neonatal mortality and neurologic morbidity.[1] A knowledge of EFM allows the obstetric anesthesiologist to anticipate problems and communicate concerns with obstetricians and perinatologists.[2] Fetal monitoring allows for the detection of poor fetal oxygenation and acid-base abnormalities to allow for prompt interventions. Even though fetal monitoring technology has improved over the past 50 years, accurate fetal assessment in labor still remains challenging.[2–4] High surgical delivery rates and persistent cases of fetal/neonatal neurologic injuries demonstrate a need to further optimize fetal assessment tools.[3]

## ELECTRONIC FETAL HEART RATE MONITORING

Most assessments of fetal health during labor and delivery include assessment of the FHR. The FHR can be monitored through several inputs, typically one that records uterine contractions and one that may receive fetal or maternal electrocardiographic (ECG) input. The most common FHR monitoring is done through a noninvasive external Doppler transducer applied to the parturient's abdomen. Another option is a fetal scalp electrode (FSE) placed on the fetal scalp skin to provide direct ECG input.[4] An external tocodynamometer is typically built into these monitors to help assess uterine contraction patterns in conjunction with FHR. Another option is insertion of an intrauterine pressure catheter (IUPC), which allows quantitative assessment of uterine strength. Use of both FSE and IUPC is limited to parturients with ruptured membranes.[4]

## INTERPRETATION OF ELECTRONIC FETAL HEART RATE MONITORING

A normal baseline FHR is defined as 110–160 beats per minute (beats/min). Table 309.1 describes the characteristics of FHR tracings, and Table 309.2 describes the categories of FHR tracings as defined by the National Institute of Child Health and Human Development.[1,3] Normal baseline FHR indicates normal cardiac conduction, autonomic innervation, and fetal catecholamine levels. Generally, term fetuses have a lower baseline FHR than preterm given the former's greater parasympathetic nervous system activity. Variability indicates that the sympathetic and parasympathetic nervous systems of the fetus are intact, and thus there is adequate oxygenation of the fetal central nervous system (CNS).[3]

*Table 309.1* INTRAPARTUM FHR TRACING ASSESSMENT AND CHARACTERISTICS

CHARACTERISTICS OF FHR TRACINGS

| CHARACTERISTICS | DEFINITION | CAUSES |
|---|---|---|
| Baseline | <ul><li>*Normal*: 110–160 beats/min</li><li>*Abnormal*<ul><li>Fetal bradycardia: < 110 beats/min</li><li>Fetal tachycardia: > 160 beats/min</li></ul></li></ul> | <ul><li>Fetal bradycardia: maternal hypotension, hypoxemia, hypothermia, hypoglycemia, maternal β-blocker therapy, congenital heart block</li><li>Fetal tachycardia: maternal medications, maternal fever, chorioamniotis, thyrotoxicosis, fetal anemia, fetal tachyarrhythmia, increased fetal catecholamines</li></ul> |
| Variability | <ul><li>*Normal*: 5–25 beats/min</li><li>*Abnormal*<ul><li>Absent: 0 beats/min</li><li>Minimal: ≤5 beats/min</li><li>Moderate: 5–25 beats/min</li><li>Marked: >25 beats/min</li></ul></li></ul> | <ul><li>Absent or minimal: acidemia or hypoxia; also prematurity, sleep cycle, anesthesia, arrhythmias, neurologic injury, congenital abnormalities</li><li>Moderate: absence of fetal acidemia or hypoxia</li><li>Marked: unknown</li></ul> |
| Decelerations | <ul><li>*Normal*: early</li><li>*Abnormal*<ul><li>Variable</li><li>Late</li></ul></li></ul> | <ul><li>Early: head compression</li><li>Variable: cord compression</li><li>Late: uteroplacental insufficiency</li></ul> |

Decelerations demonstrate FHR slowing in relation to uterine contractions.[1,3] Early decelerations are typically not associated with fetal distress and often occur as a result of reflex vagal activity secondary to head compression. Variable decelerations are often secondary to cord compression, causing increased vagal tones. Late decelerations are due to uteroplacental insufficiency and often occur 10 to 30 seconds after the onset of uterine contractions.[1,3]

A variety of systems for EFM interpretation have been used worldwide. However, a three-tiered categorization system of FHR patterns is the most common (Figure 309.1).[1] The three-tiered evaluation system allows for assessment of current fetal acid-base status (Table 309.2). It is important to understand that FHR tracings may move back and forth through the three categories, depending on the clinical situation.[1]

## ANESTHETIC CONSIDERATIONS

Neuraxial anesthesia, typically used for vaginal and cesarean deliveries, can lead to decreased uteroplacental perfusion, fetal hypoxemia, and fetal decelerations. FHR decelerations can be seen even in the absence of maternal hypotension. This is thought to be due to a decrease in circulating maternal catecholamines from rapid onset of neuraxial analgesia, causing uterine hypertonus. Opioids are often added to neuraxial anesthesia as an adjunct to local anesthetics and are readily taken up by systemic maternal circulation. They appear to have no effect on EFM.[4] Epidural clonidine is found to redistribute rapidly into maternal and then fetal circulation.[4] Clonidine has been shown to lower FHR when combined with dilute bupivacaine.[4]

General anesthesia decreases maternal sympathetic output, which can cause maternal hypotension, diminished

*Table 309.2* CATEGORIES OF FHR TRACINGS

| CATEGORIES | FHR PATTERN | CAUSES |
|---|---|---|
| Category I | <ul><li>Baseline 110–160 beats/min</li><li>Moderate variability</li><li>Absence of late/variable decelerations</li></ul> | Normal fetal acid-base status, low likelihood of acidemia or fetal hypoxemia |
| Category II | All patterns that are not category I or category II | Indeterminant in terms of reliability of predicting fetal acid-base status |
| Category III | Absent baseline variability with any of the following:<ul><li>Recurrent late decelerations</li><li>Recurrent variable decelerations</li><li>Bradycardia</li><li>Sinusoidal pattern</li></ul> | Highly predictive of abnormal acid-base status |

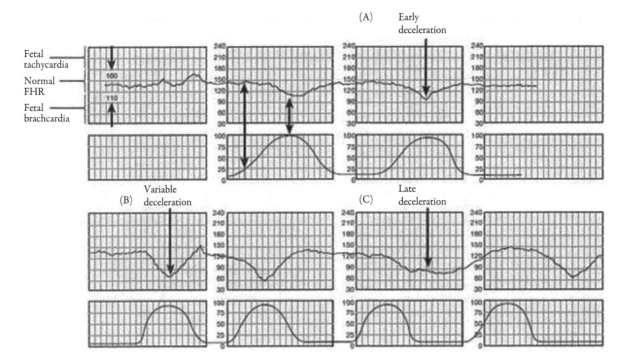

**Figure 309.1** Fetal heart rate (FHR) patterns. (A) Early deceleration. Notice how the nadir of the deceleration occurs at the same time as the peak of the uterine contraction; they are mirror images of each other. (B) Variable deceleration. These decelerations may start before, during, or after a uterine contraction starts. (C) Late deceleration. The onset, nadir, and recovery of the deceleration occur, respectively, after the beginning, peak, and end of the contraction.

fetal oxygen delivery, and EFM changes. Both general anesthetics and opioids cause CNS depression and can cross the placenta, leading to fetal CNS depression. This can cause decreased fetal movement, altering EFM patterns, particularly decreasing variability. Neostigmine, an acetylcholinesterase inhibitor used to antagonize neuromuscular blockade, is a positively charged amide that can cross the placenta. When administered, it can cause bradycardia or asystole and is typically given with glycopyrrolate to prevent muscarinic effects. However, in the case of pregnancy, atropine may be more beneficial as atropine crosses the placenta to decrease the risk of bradycardia or asystole.[4]

## LIMITATIONS OF ELECTRONIC FETAL HEART RATE MONITORING

There is limited evidence to suggest FHR monitoring accurately reflects fetal health. Nevertheless, retrospective reports demonstrated that continuous FHR monitoring is associated with lower incidence of intrauterine fetal demise, neonatal seizures, and neonatal death. As a result, FHR monitoring is utilized in about 85% of monitored deliveries and remains the standard of care of intrapartum obstetric patients.

## REFERENCES

1. ACOG Practice Bulletin No. 106: Intrapartum fetal heart rate monitoring: nomenclature, interpretation, and general management principles. *Obstet Gynecol.* 2009 Jul;114(1):192–202. doi:10.1097/AOG.0b013e3181aef106. PMID: 19546798.
2. Livingston EG. Intrapartum fetal assessment and therapy. In: *Chestnut's Obstetric Anesthesia: Principles and Practice.* 6th ed. Philadelphia, PA: Elsevier; 2020:155–170.
3. Molitor RJ. Fetal assessment and intrapartum fetal monitoring. In: *Faust's Anesthesiology Review.* 5th ed. Philadelphia, PA: Elsevier; 2020:524–526.
4. Richardson MG, et al. Fetal assessment and monitoring. In: *A Practical Approach to Obstetric Anesthesia.* 2nd ed. Philadelphia, PA: Elsevier; 2020:152–182.

# 310.

# PREECLAMPSIA AND ECLAMPSIA

*Alina Genis*

## INTRODUCTION

Up to 10% of pregnancies in the United States are affected by hypertensive disorders of pregnancy.[1] The spectrum of disorders is a dynamic continuum that ranges from gestational hypertension to preeclampsia and preeclampsia with severe features. These disorders can be superimposed on chronic hypertension when symptoms occur after 20 weeks' gestation. Preeclampsia is one of the leading causes of fetal growth restriction, intrauterine fetal demise, and preterm birth. Known risk factors can help identify patients in need of frequent reevaluation, although healthy women without any obvious risk factors are most commonly diagnosed. Symptoms can be multisystemic, and management of preeclampsia includes blood pressure control, seizure prophylaxis, and optimizing timing of delivery. Anesthetic goals include early neuraxial analgesia, avoidance of general anesthesia, management of drastic hemodynamic changes, and fluid optimization.

## DIAGNOSIS

Based on the 2013 criteria released by the American College of Obstetrics and Gynecology, preeclampsia is diagnosed when the patient has two blood pressure readings above 140/90 mm Hg at rest, at least 4 hours apart, along with proteinuria. The diagnosis becomes preeclampsia with severe features when either the systolic blood pressure readings are 160 mm Hg or more or diastolic blood pressure is 110 mm Hg or more and/or there is additional evidence of end-organ involvement. Signs of end-organ damage include renal insufficiency (creatinine 1.1 or doubling of the baseline creatinine); thrombocytopenia (platelet count < 100,000); impaired hepatic function (persistent right upper quadrant or epigastric pain, liver enzymes twice the normal value); pulmonary edema or new-onset cerebral or visual disturbances, such as headaches or scotomata. Preeclampsia can rapidly progress from mild to severe disease. Risk factors include increased maternal age, previous preeclampsia, family history of preeclampsia, chronic hypertension and renal disease, thrombophilia, multiple pregnancy, assisted reproductive techniques, types 1 and 2 diabetes, obesity, and systemic lupus erythematosus.

The HELLP syndrome comprises hemolysis, elevated liver enzymes, and low platelets.

## PATHOPHYSIOLOGY

The pathophysiology of preeclampsia is believed to originate from failure of the spiral arteries to deeply invade the myometrium. This structural change is thought to result from an imbalance of the placental production of prostacyclin and thromboxane. While these two substances are normally produced in equal amounts, in preeclampsia there can be up to seven times more thromboxane than prostacyclin.[2] The deficiency of the spiral arteries to invade the myometrium prevents them from becoming low-resistance vessels and leads to an increase in uterine arterial resistance. Placental hypoperfusion results in the release of various factors and biomarkers, leading to endothelial damage and maternal vascular remodeling.[3] Generalized arteriolar vasoconstriction leads to maternal hypertension with organ hypoperfusion and clinically the various multisystemic signs and symptoms found in preeclamptic patients.

## MANAGEMENT

Management of preeclamptic patients involves blood pressure control, seizure prophylaxis, careful fluid management, and optimizing timing of delivery. The most common agents used for antihypertensive management include labetalol, hydralazine, or nifedipine, with second-line agents including nicardipine, sodium nitroprusside, or esmolol infusions. Preeclamptic women are at higher risk for intracranial bleeding at much lower blood pressures secondary to the lack of cerebral autoregulation associated with this disease state. Blood pressure must be carefully managed to avoid overcorrection, which can compromise uteroplacental blood flow. Mortality occurs most frequently secondary to hemorrhagic stroke and the complications of seizures. The only curative treatment is delivery of the fetus and placenta; however, this often leads to a complex clinical scenario where preterm delivery of the fetus must be taken into consideration.

Eclamptic seizures are thought to occur secondary to vasogenic edema after acute severe hypertension.[4] Eclamptic seizures may be preceded by increasingly severe hypertension and neurological disturbances but can also occur in asymptomatic patients. Magnesium is the most commonly used agent for prophylaxis of seizures and is recommended for women with preeclampsia with severe features. It is typically administered as a 4-g loading dose and then continued as a 1- to 2-g/h infusion. The infusion is often continued intraoperatively during a cesarean delivery and postoperatively for 24–48 hours after delivery. Patients are monitored closely for signs of magnesium toxicity with assessment of serial deep tendon reflexes and serum magnesium levels. Acute kidney injury can increase the likelihood of magnesium toxicity due to its renal excretion, and patients with renal impairment should be monitored more closely. Common side effects of magnesium therapy include flushing, nausea, vomiting, drowsiness, and weakness. Signs of magnesium toxicity begin with electrocardiographic changes (prolonged PR interval, widened QRS) and gradually lead to decreased deep tendon reflexes, muscle weakness, and respiratory depression at levels of 10 mEq/L; respiratory arrest and SA and SV conduction defects at 15 mEq/L; and subsequently can lead to cardiac arrest at levels of 25 mEq/L.

## ANESTHETIC CONSIDERATIONS

Delivery is recommended at 34 weeks' gestation for preeclampsia with severe features and at 37 weeks' gestation in the absence of severe features, although deteriorating maternal or fetal status can change delivery status to urgent or emergent.[4] Preeclamptic patients have increased rates of cesarean delivery compared to healthy parturients. Early neuraxial anesthesia, if not contraindicated by thrombocytopenia or coagulopathy, is recommended in these patients in order to avoid general anesthesia if an emergent cesarean delivery becomes necessary. In laboring patients with hypertensive disorders of pregnancy, neuraxial labor analgesia may help avoid drastic increases in maternal blood pressure during contractions. Spinal anesthesia does not result in more severe hypotension when compared to the healthy pregnant patient, as was initially anticipated due to a rapid sympathectomy.[4] In addition, neuraxial anesthesia avoids the need for endotracheal intubation. Patients with preeclampsia tend to have greater laryngeal edema, complicating an already potentially difficult airway associated with pregnancy. The anesthesia provider should aim to attenuate the hypertensive pressor response to laryngoscopy, intubation, skin incision, and extubation. If general anesthesia is utilized, the effects of nondepolarizing muscle relaxants can be prolonged secondary to magnesium infusion. Methylergonovine is contraindicated in patients with preeclampsia in the case of postpartum hemorrhage due to the possibility of inciting severe hypertension.[3] Conservative fluid management is recommended as excessive elevation in pulmonary vascular hydrostatic pressure combined with decreased plasma oncotic pressure may produce pulmonary edema.

## REFERENCES

1. Aronow WS. Hypertensive disorders in pregnancy. *Ann Transl Med*. 2017;5(12):266.
2. Barash P, et al., eds. *Clinical Anesthesia*. Philadelphia, PA: Lippincott Williams & Wilkins; 2006.
3. Wan Po JL, Bhatia K. Pre-eclampsia and the anaesthetist. *Anaesth Intensive Care Med*. 2103;14(7):283–286.
4. Siddiqui MM, et al. Preeclampsia through the eyes of the obstetrician and anesthesiologist. *Int J Obstet Anesth*. 2019;40:140–148.
5. Russell R. Preeclampsia and the anaesthesiologist: current management. *Curr Opin Anaesthesiol*. 2020;33(3):305–310.

# 311.

# SUPINE HYPOTENSIVE SYNDROME

*Muhammad Fayyaz Ahmed and Ihab Kamel*

## INTRODUCTION

The supine hypotension syndrome (SHS) is defined as a systolic blood pressure reduction of 15 and 30 mm Hg or an increase in heart rate of 20 beats/min, with or without symptoms, when the parturient assumes the supine position. SHS is caused by compression of the aorta and inferior vena cava by the gravid uterus against the lumbar vertebral bodies in the supine positon. It begins around 18–20 weeks of gestation and typically manifests as pallor, hypotension, dizziness, nausea, tachycardia, and sweating during the third trimester.[1]

## SUPINE HYPOTENSIVE SYNDROME PHYSIOLOGY

The uteroplacental perfusion has minimal autoregulation during pregnancy. Thus, uterine blood flow is proportional to uterine arterial pressure and inversely proportional to uterine venous pressures and uterine vascular resistance. At term, SHS occurs due to partial obstruction of the inferior vena cava occurs in the lateral position, and complete obstruction in the supine position. Aortocaval compression by the gravid uterus is responsible for a 30% reduction in cardiac output (due to a decrease in venous return), an increase in uterine venous pressure, and a 20% reduction in the uteroplacental blood flow.[1] Aortacaval compression also leads to an increase in the venous pressure in the lower extremities, decreasing its blood flow by 50%. Blood flow in the upper extremities is normal.[2] Uterine artery perfusion pressure may decrease in the supine position despite normal maternal blood pressure due to an increases in uterine venous pressure or aortic compression.

## CLINICAL PRESENTATION

Despite the significant aortocaval compression that occurs in the third trimester, only 10%–15% of parturients experience SHS. This is due to the fact that most patient gradually develop adequate collateral venous flow through the intraosseous, vertebral, azygos, paravertebral, and epidural veins to increase the right atrial pressure and maintain cardiac output.[3,4] Symptoms of SHS develop over a few minutes when the cardiovascular system partially compensates for the obstruction of the inferior vena cava. Risk factors for SHS include multiple gestation, polyhydramnios, maternal obesity, and increased fetal weight. In the lateral position, venous return and ventricular filling pressures are maintained due to partial relief of the venal caval obstruction. A 15° to 30° left tilt is usually required to relieve venacaval compression and improve cardiac output. Patients with autonomic neuropathy secondary to diabetes may be more prone to SHS due to inadequate increase in heart rate, stroke volume, and cardiac output.[2] SHS symptoms are exacerbated by peripheral vasodilation induced by anesthetic agents and regional anesthesia, primarily due to a reduction in venous return.[2] Nonreassuring fetal heart rate patterns are more frequently observed in the supine position after induction of neuraxial or general anesthesia.

## ANESTHETIC CONSIDERATIONS

### PREOPERATIVE

Preoperatively, all patients beyond 20 weeks of gestation should be in left lateral tilt to mitigate SHS. Compared to the supine position, left uterine displacement has been associated with higher umbilical arterial blood pH and better neonatal outcomes. Maternal blood pressure measured at the level of the brachial artery may not always predict uteroplacental perfusion. Significant tilt, up to 30°, may be required to minimize aortic compression during the third trimester. Physical methods to mitigate SHS include use of lower limb compression bandages or pneumatic compression devices. Preparation to resuscitate patients with SHS should always be in place, such as large-bore intravenous access, fluids, and vasopressor drugs such as ephedrine or phenylephrine.[2]

## INTRAOPERATIVE

During a cesarean delivery and after neuraxial anesthesia administration, a 15° to 30° left tilt is recommended to mitigate SHS. If a patient develops SHS intraoperatively after neuraxial analgesia or anesthesia administration, the first intervention is to place the patient in a left lateral tilt position. The impact of repositioning on maternal blood pressure is quick. Occasionally, right uterine displacement or right lateral position may be the most effective intervention. Trendelenburg position without left uterine displacement should be avoided as it may lead to worsening of maternal hypotension due to shifting of the uterus back, leading to aortic and caval compression. Second-line interventions include intravenous infusion of colloids or crystalloids and use of vasopressors such as phenylephrine.

In cardiac arrest during pregnancy, it is important to perform left uterine displacement during resuscitation to alleviate aortocaval compression and improve effectiveness of cardiopulmonary resuscitation (CPR). Left uterine displacement approaches during CPR include manual two-hand displacement of the gravid uterus, using a solid wedge, application of a "human wedge" (left uterine displacement maintained by supporting the patient on the rescuer's knees to provide a stable position), and tilting the patient onto the back of an upturned chair. Application of any of the aforementioned techniques is pivotal to maintaining the effectiveness of chest compressions.

## REFERENCES

1. Kacmar RM, Gaiser R. Physiologic changes of pregnancy. In: Chestnut D., ed. *Chestnut's Obstetric Anesthesia: Principles and Practice.* 6th ed. Philadelphia, PA: Elsevier Health Sciences; 2020:13–37.
2. Bucklin BA, Fuller AJ. Physiologic changes of pregnancy. In: Suresh MS, et al., eds. *Shnider and Levinson's Anesthesia for Obstetrics.* 5th ed. Philadelphia, PA: Lippincott, Williams & Wilkins; 2013:1–17.
3. Hawkins JL. Abnormal presentation and multiple gestation. In: Chestnut DH, et al., eds. *Chestnut's Obstetric Anesthesia: Principles and Practice.* 6th ed. Philadelphia, PA: Elsevier Health Sciences; 2020:822–839.
4. Humphries A, et al. Hemodynamic changes in women with symptoms of supine hypotensive syndrome. *Acta Obstet Gynecol Scand.* 2020;99(5):631–636.

# 312.

# ASPIRATION OF GASTRIC CONTENTS

*Muhammad Fayyaz Ahmed and Ihab Kamel*

## INTRODUCTION

The incidence of aspiration in women undergoing cesarean section is estimated to be 0.15%, which is three-fold higher than the general population. Factors determining the morbidity and mortality associated with aspiration include the type and volume of aspirate, the therapy administered, the physical status of the patient, and the criteria used for making the diagnosis. The incidence of aspiration during delivery has significantly decreased in the past years, mainly due to frequent use of neuraxial anesthesia.[1]

## GASTROINTESTINAL CHANGES DURING PREGNANCY

The physiologic changes of pregnancy that increase the risk of aspiration are gastroesophageal reflux and decreases in gastric emptying.[2] Progesterone relaxes the smooth muscles, leading to a decrease in the lower esophageal sphincter tone, leading to a higher incidence of gastroesophageal reflux. Parenteral opioids and neuraxial boluses of opioids cause a significant delay in gastric emptying. Gastric emptying is not usually delayed with continuous epidural infusion of low-dose local anesthetic with fentanyl if the total dose of fentanyl is less than 100 µg.

## RISK FACTORS FOR ASPIRATION

Factors predisposing to aspiration in obstetrics include emergency surgery, difficult/failed tracheal intubation, light anesthesia, and gastroesophageal reflux. Risk of failed intubation is higher in pregnant patients compared to the nonpregnant patients. This is primarily due to airway edema, breast enlargement, obesity, and high likelihood of emergent surgery. Gastric fluid pH less than 2.5 and volume of greater than 25 mL are risk factors for aspiration pneumonitis. Volume and chemical and physical properties of the aspirate are the main factors determining the morbidity and mortality associated with aspiration pneumonitis. Clinically, the most severe lung injury is observed in patients who aspirate acidic gastric contents with particulate matter and a volume greater than 25 mL.[1,2]

## PATHOPHYSIOLOGY

Aspiration pneumonitis is a chemical injury to the alveoli and bronchial tree secondary to the inhalation of sterile gastric contents. Aspiration pneumonia describes an infectious process if the aspirate is colonized by pathogenic bacteria. Damage of the alveolar epithelium by acidic aspirate leads to the production of alveolar exudates composed of fibrin, cellular debris, edema, albumin, and red blood cells. It decreases pulmonary compliance and causes intrapulmonary shunting. Large particle aspiration leads to obstruction of large airways and atelectasis. Inflammation of the bronchioles and alveolar ducts occurs with aspiration of smaller particulate matter. Aspiration in the upright position affects lower lobes. Aspiration in the supine position affects the posterior segments of the upper lobe and the apical segments of the lower lobe. The most common anatomic location for aspiration is the right lower lobe due to its anatomic location.[1,2]

## CLINICAL PRESENTATION

Aspiration while spontaneously breathing results in a brief episode of breath holding, followed by tachypnea, tachycardia, and a respiratory acidosis. Significant aspiration results in hypoxemia and bronchospasm. Abnormalities in a chest x-ray can be seen after 12–24 hours.

## MANAGEMENT OF ASPIRATION

Initial management of aspiration includes suction of the gastric contents from the upper airway or trachea if the patient is intubated, administration of 100% $FiO_2$ (fraction of inspired oxygen), application of positive end-expiratory pressure (continuous positive airway pressure to nonintubated patient), and the use of a rigid bronchoscope to extract large solid particles. Prophylactic antibiotic has not been shown to be beneficial and can lead to infections with resistant organisms. Administration of corticosteroid has not been shown to be beneficial and is not recommended. Aspiration leading to respiratory failure presents clinically as acute respiratory distress syndrome, and its recommended management focuses on lung-protective ventilation strategies.

## PROPHYLAXIS

Aspiration is best managed by prevention and preoperative strategies to reduce the severity of aspiration. The risk is low when gastric emptying is normal and patients follow nothing by mouth (NPO, nil per os) guidelines. It has been stated by the American Society of Anesthesiologists Guidelines for Obstetric Anesthesia that uncomplicated patient undergoing elective cesarean section may have a modest amount of clear liquids up to 2 hours before induction of anesthesia. It also states that before surgical procedures (e.g., cesarean delivery and postpartum tubal ligation) consider timely administration of nonparticulate antacids, $H_2$ receptor antagonist, and/or metoclopramide for aspiration prophylaxis.[3] Pharmacological prophylaxis is summarized in Table 312.1.

## ANESTHETIC CONSIDERATIONS

### PREOPERATIVE

Preoperative strategies to decrease the risk of aspiration include enforcement of NPO guidelines, the use of neuraxial anesthesia, use of medications to reduce gastric acidity and gastric acid production, use of promotility agents, and rapid sequence induction of general anesthesia. For elective cesarean delivery, administration of $H_2$ receptor antagonists, oral sodium citrate, and intravenous metoclopramide before induction of anesthesia is recommended. For emergency cesarean delivery under general anesthesia, 30 mL of sodium citrate should be administered orally before induction, while ranitidine 50 mg (or famotidine 20 mg or omeprazole 40 mg) and metoclopramide 10 mg should be given intravenously.

### INTRAOPERATIVE

Intraoperatively, rapid sequence induction is recommended in parturients with head elevated to 30° as it increases the functional residual capacity. Application for cricoid

*Table 312.1* PHARMACOLOGICAL PROPHYLAXIS FOR ASPIRATION

| DRUG | MECHANISM OF ACTION | EFFECT ON GASTROINTESTINAL SYSTEM | DOSAGE |
|---|---|---|---|
| Bicitra, sodium citrate | Antacid: neutralizes gastric acid | A volume of 30 mL of sodium citrate neutralizes 255 mL of hydrochloric acid with a pH of 1.0 | Oral 30 mL within 20 minutes of induction |
| Cimetidine, ranitidine | Histamine 2 receptor antagonist | Reduces gastric acidity and volume by reducing gastric acid production | Cimetidine 200 to 400 mg IV or orally; ranitidine IV or IM dose of 50 to 100 mg or an oral dose of 150 mg |
| Metoclopramide | Peripheral cholinergic agonist and a central dopamine antagonist | Increases lower esophageal sphincter tone and reduces gastric emptying by increasing gastric peristalsis | Intravenous dose of 10 mg |

IM, intramuscular; IV, intravenous.

From References 1 and 3.

pressure is controversial. Thus, if cricoid pressure distorts the laryngoscopy view, the pressure should be promptly released. In addition to pharmacological prophylaxis, further protection against aspiration can be achieved by using an orogastric tube to empty the stomach contents before extubation.

## POSTOPERATIVE

After aspiration in a nonintubated patient, the severity of hypoxia and hemodynamic stability should be assessed to determine if patient needs to be intubated. If the patient requires intubation or has significant hypoxia, the patient may need to be transferred postoperatively to intensive care for close monitoring. Avoid administration of corticosteroids, routine use of prophylactic antibiotics, and

lung lavage with saline and bicarbonate as these treatments lack evidence to support their use.

## REFERENCES

1. Farber MK. Aspiration: risk, prophylaxis, and treatment. In: Chestnut DH, et al., eds. *Chestnut's Obstetric Anesthesia: Principles and Practice*. 6th ed.. Philadelphia, PA: Elsevier Health Sciences; 2020:671–691.
2. O'Sullivan G, Segal S. NPO controversies—pulmonary aspiration: risks and management. In: Suresh MS, et al., eds. *Shnider and Levinson's Anesthesia for Obstetrics*. 5th ed. Philadelphia, PA: Lippincott, Williams & Wilkins; 2013:403–411.
3. American Society of Anesthesiologists. Practice guidelines for obstetric anesthesia: an updated report by the American Society of Anesthesiologists Task Force on Obstetric Anesthesia and the Society for Obstetric Anesthesia and Perinatology. *Anesthesiology*. 2016;124:270–300.

# 313.

# EMBOLIC DISORDERS

*Muhammad Fayyaz Ahmed and Ihab Kamel*


## INTRODUCTION

Embolic disorders are a major cause of maternal mortality in the United States, accounting for around 20% of all maternal deaths. Embolic disorders include amniotic fluid embolism (AFE), venous thromboembolism, and venous air embolism. Each of the disorders has a different clinical course and management. Early recognition and management are necessary to reduce morbidity and mortality.[1,2]


## AMNIOTIC FLUID EMBOLISM

The incidence of AFE in the United States is 7.7 per 100,000 deliveries, and the reported incidence of maternal mortality is between 0.5 and 1.7 deaths per 100,000 live births. It accounts for 7.5% of pregnancy-related deaths in the United States. Although it remains unclear, the pathophysiology of AFE may involve a systemic inflammatory response; activation of a coagulation cascade, leading to pulmonary vasoconstriction; systemic vasodilation; and right heart failure. Risk factors associated with AFE are multiple gestation, multiparity, older age, placental abruption, abnormal placentation, eclampsia, cesarean section, induction of labor, and artificial or spontaneous rupture of membranes.[1]


## CLINICAL PRESENTATION OF AFE

Amniotic fluid embolism is a diagnosis of exclusion. AFE most often occurs during labor.[1,2] Signs and symptoms of AFE include cardiovascular collapse, acute respiratory distress, and coagulopathy during or after delivery. According to the United States AFE national registry, the diagnosis of AFE is confirmed based on meeting the following criteria: acute hypotension or cardiac arrest; acute hypoxia; coagulopathy (laboratory evidence or hemorrhage); onset of symptoms during labor, cesarean section, dilation and evacuation, or within 30 minutes postpartum; and absence of an alternative explanation for the observed signs/symptoms. AFE presents a biphasic cardiovascular response, with the initial phase of acute pulmonary hypertension resulting in right ventricular failure and hypoxia. It is followed with a brief episode of systemic hypertension from release of catecholamines that precedes hypotension and cardiac arrest.


## PULMONARY THROMBOEMBOLISM

The incidence of pregnancy-related deep venous thrombosis (DVT) and pulmonary thromboembolism (PTE) is 1.36 and 0.36 per 1000 pregnancies, respectively. Fifteen to twenty-four percent of untreated pregnant women with DVT develop PTE. The highest risk of DVT and PTE is in the first week postpartum. Risk factors include history of thromboembolism, prior diagnosis of thrombophilia (factor V Leiden mutation), antenatal immobilization, obesity, preeclampsia with fetal growth restriction, heart disease, sickle cell disease, postpartum hemorrhage, blood transfusion, and postpartum infection.[1,3] The pathophysiology of PTE is characterized by vascular damage, venous stasis, and hypercoagulability (Virchow triad).[1] Massive PTE occludes the pulmonary vasculature, leading to right ventricular failure and cardiopulmonary arrest.


## CLINICAL PRESENTATION OF PTE

In PTE, patients usually present with shortness of breath, tachypnea, palpitations, fever, anxiety, pleuritic chest pain, cyanosis, diaphoresis, and cough with or without hemoptysis. Invasive monitoring demonstrates normal-to-low pulmonary artery occlusion pressure, increased mean pulmonary artery pressure, and increased central venous pressure. Ventilation perfusion (V/Q) scan or computed tomography angiography should be performed to confirm the diagnosis and initiate anticoagulation. It is recommended to use low-molecular-weight heparin rather than unfractionated heparin for prophylactic and therapeutic anticoagulation for pregnant women.[1,3]

## ANESTHETIC CONSIDERATIONS

### PREOPERATIVE

High-risk patients with a history of thrombosis, acquired or inherited thrombophilias, or with a mechanical heart valve should be anticoagulated during pregnancy as well as the postpartum period. Patients clinically developing signs and symptoms of AFE or PTE should be managed by a multidisciplinary team. Patients with severe massive venous thrombosis and pulmonary emboli may need to continue anticoagulation; thus, cesarean delivery under general anesthesia may be the most prudent choice. Preoperative recommendations for management of anticoagulation prior to neuraxial anesthesia administration are summarized in Table 313.1.

### INTRAOPERATIVE

If symptoms and signs of AFE or PTE are identified intraoperatively, maternal resuscitation should focus on

*Table 313.1* ASRA RECOMMENDED GUIDELINES FOR TIME INTERVAL BETWEEN ANTICOAGULATION ADMINISTRATION AND INITIATION OF NEURAXIAL ANESTHESIA

| | |
|---|---|
| **(a) Interval between anticoagulant administration and initiation of neuraxial anesthesia** | |
| UFH | 4–6-hour delay for subcutaneous low-dose prophylactic |
| | 4–6-hour delay for intravenous dosing |
| | 12-hour delay for subcutaneous intermediate dose |
| | 24-hour delay for subcutaneous therapeutic dose |
| LMWH | 12-hour delay for prophylactic dose |
| | 24-hour delay for therapeutic dose |
| **(b) Interval between placement of neuraxial block or catheter removal and initiation of anticoagulation** | |
| UFH | 1-hour delay regardless of dose or route of administration |
| LMWH | 12-hour delay for prophylactic dose |
| | 24-hour delay for therapeutic dose |

These guidelines undergo continuous updates, so please check most recent guidelines every year.

From Reference 1.

hemodynamic support, maintenance of oxygenation, and correction of coagulopathy. Administration of 100% oxygen and maintaining left uterine displacement should be immediate first-line interventions. Intubation and assisted ventilation may be required. Establishing adequate vascular access and activation of the massive transfusion protocol is necessary if cardiovascular instability ensues. An arterial line facilitates hemodynamic monitoring and arterial blood gas sampling. A central venous catheter may be needed for vasopressor infusions and massive fluid resuscitation. Increased pulmonary artery pressure and right ventricular strain can be managed with inhaled nitric oxide, prostacyclin infusion, inodilators such milrinone or dobutamine, and a right ventricular assist device. Vasopressors such as vasopressin and epinephrine can be used to support systemic blood pressure. Fetal well-being should be monitored closely. Delivery should be expedited if nonreassuring fetal heart rate tracing ensues.[1] In the case of maternal cardiovascular collapse and cardiac arrest, delivery of the fetus within 4 minutes of initiation of resuscitation is essential to improve neonatal survival. In case of disseminated intravascular coagulation associated with AFE, recombinant factor VII should be avoided as it is associated with increased mortality due to multiorgan failure.

### POSTOPERATIVE

Patients with significant hemodynamic instability, respiratory failure, or neurologic compromise postoperatively should be transferred to the intensive care unit. PTE most commonly occurs during the first week postpartum.

### REFERENCES

1. Toledo P. Embolic disorders. In: Chestnut DH, et al., eds. *Chestnut's Obstetric Anesthesia: Principles and Practice.* 6th ed. Philadelphia, PA: Elsevier Health Sciences; 2020:937–955.
2. Palacios QT. Amniotic fluid embolism. In: Suresh MS, et al., eds. *Shnider and Levinson's Anesthesia for Obstetrics.* 5th ed. Philadelphia, PA: Lippincott, Williams & Wilkins; 2013: 333–348.
3. Palacios QT. Venous thromboembolism in pregnancy and guidelines for neuraxial anesthesia following anticoagulant and antithrombotic drugs. In: Suresh MS, et al., eds. *Shnider and Levinson's Anesthesia for Obstetrics.* 5th ed. Philadelphia, PA: Lippincott, Williams & Wilkins; 2013:349–362.

# 314.

# ANTEPARTUM HEMORRHAGE

*Mary J. Im and Ihab Kamel*

## INTRODUCTION

Antepartum vaginal bleeding may occur in as many as 25% of pregnant women. Etiologies of antepartum hemorrhage include placenta previa, placenta abruption, vasa previa, and uterine rupture.[1]

## PLACENTA PREVIA

Placenta previa is defined as placental implantation that covers the cervical os. The incidence of placenta previa ranges from 1% to 4% in the second trimester and 0.3% to 0.5% at term. Risk factors for placenta previa include advanced maternal age, multiparity, prior cesarean delivery or other uterine surgery, previous placenta previa, multifetal gestation, and smoking.[1,2] The classic clinical sign is painless vaginal bleeding during the second or third trimester. The diagnosis is based on transvaginal ultrasonography.

## PLACENTAL ABRUPTION

Placental abruption is defined as the separation of the placenta from the decidua basalis before delivery of the fetus. It occurs usually after the 20th week of pregnancy. Typical symptoms and signs of placental abruption include abdominal pain with bleeding, uterine tenderness, increased uterine tone, and nonreassuring fetal heart rate tracing. Incidence of placental abruption is 0.4% to 1.0% of pregnancies.[1] Risk factors for placental abruption include advanced maternal age, multiparity, hypertensive disorder during pregnancy, premature rupture of membranes, chorioamnionitis, substance abuse, and direct or indirect trauma. The diagnosis of placental abruption is based on clinical presentation and history primarily, but ultrasonography may be helpful. Placental abruption can cause significant adverse outcomes, including maternal hemodynamic instability, coagulopathy, and fetal demise.

## UTERINE RUPTURE

Uterine rupture or dehiscence can cause antepartum bleeding, which leads to maternal and neonatal adverse outcomes. Risk factors include prior uterine surgery, induction of labor, high-dose oxytocin induction, prostaglandin induction, grand multiparity, congenital uterine anomaly, connective tissue disorder, and trauma. The classical vertical uterine incision is associated with a higher risk of uterine rupture and greater morbidity because the incision involves the muscular uterine fundus and anterior uterine wall (highly vascular). The incidence of true uterine rupture after cesarean delivery is less than 1%. An abnormal fetal heart rate tracing can be the first sign of uterine rupture. Other symptoms and signs include abdominal pain and vaginal bleeding.

## VASA PREVIA

Vasa previa occurs when the fetal blood vessels traverse the internal cervical os. Velamentous cord insertion refers to the cord insertion into the fetal membranes, with the fetal vessels not protected by the placenta. The rupture of membranes can cause the exsanguination of the fetus. The incidence of vasa previa is approximately 1 in 2500 pregnancies.[2] Risk factors include the presence of velamentous cord insertion, placenta previa or low-lying placenta, placental accessory lobes, in vitro fertilization, and multiple gestation.

## ANESTHETIC CONSIDERATION

### PREOPERATIVE CONSIDERATIONS

The timing of delivery is recommended at 36–37 weeks of gestation for stable placenta previa patients and between 34 and 37 weeks of gestation for vasa previa patients.[2] Women presenting with active, ongoing obstetric hemorrhage require stabilization and preparation for delivery by cesarean section. Preoperative evaluation should include airway examination, intravascular volume assessment, blood product availability, adequate intravenous access, and coagulation status. Potential intraoperative bleeding risks exist without active bleeding preoperatively. If the placenta is located anteriorly, there is a risk of heavy bleeding during uterine incision. The lower uterine segment implantation site does not contract well because of the lack of uterine muscles. Also, placenta previa is associated with an increased incidence of placental accreta if the patient has a history of previous cesarean section.

## INTRAOPERATIVE CONSIDERATIONS

Intraoperatively, the choice of anesthetic technique should be determined by the urgency of the delivery, the maternal hemodynamic conditions, and the obstetric concerns, such as previous surgical history, placental location, or abnormal adhesion of the abdominal wall. General anesthesia is preferred for urgent cesarean delivery. Intravenous oxytocin infusion should be administered immediately after delivery and other uterotonic agents as well to prevent postpartum hemorrhage. If general anesthesia is indicated and the bleeding continues after delivery, intravenous anesthetics should be considered instead of inhalational anesthetics to avoid significant uterine relaxation. After delivery, if inhalational anesthetics should be used during general anesthesia, a lower dose of halogenated inhalational agents should be used while supplementing the anesthetic with nitrous oxide (50%–70%) due to the favorable effect of nitrous on uterine contractility. A bispectral index monitor should be considered in the setting of hemodynamic instability under general anesthesia using inhalation agents to strike the delicate balance between providing adequate anesthesia and minimizing the uterine relaxation induced by inhalational agents. In cases of severe hemorrhage and unstable hemodynamics, an intra-arterial catheter and invasive monitoring is indicated to assess blood pressure and hematologic status. Patients with abruption are at risk for developing coagulopathy, such as disseminated intravascular coagulation. It is recommended to replace coagulation factors, especially fibrinogen, to minimize the risk of massive hemorrhage and developing a coagulopathy.[1]

## POSTOPERATIVE CONSIDERATIONS

Postoperatively, most patients recover quickly without adverse outcomes. Patients who experienced massive hemorrhage and were resuscitated with multiple blood products should be monitored for hemodynamic instability and for the development of disseminated intravascular coagulopathy in the intensive care unit.

## REFERENCES

1. Banayan JM, et al. Antepartum and postpartum hemorrhage. In: Chestnut DH, et al., eds. *Chestnut's Obstetric Anesthesia: Principles and Practice.* 6th ed.. Philadelphia, PA: Elsevier Health Sciences; 2020:901–936.
2. Gyamfi-Bannerman C, for the Society for Maternal-Fetal Medicine (SMFM). Society for Maternal-Fetal Medicine (SMFM) consult series #44: management of bleeding in the late preterm period. Am J Obstet Gynecol. 2018; 218:B2–B8.

# 315.

# POSTPARTUM HEMORRHAGE

*Mary J. Im and Ihab Kamel*

## INTRODUCTION

Postpartum hemorrhage (PPH) is defined as blood loss greater than or equal to 1000 mL or blood loss accompanied by signs or symptoms of hypovolemia within 24 hours of birth.[1] The incidence of PPH in the United States is approximately 3%. Uterine blood flow (UBF) reaches 700 mL/min at term. This significant increase in the UBF can lead to massive life-threatening bleeding. In addition, the control of uterine bleeding depends on multiple factors, which include coagulation factors and uterine musculature tone. Etiologies of PPH include uterine atony, genital trauma, retained placenta, uterine inversion, and placenta accreta.

## UTERINE ATONY

Uterine atony is the most common cause of PPH. Risk factors for uterine atony are listed in Table 315.1.[2]

Active management of the third stage of labor can reduce the risk of PPH. Prophylactic oxytocin administration after delivery would be the first choice of uterotonics because of the increase in oxytocin receptors at term pregnancy. In the case of inadequate response to oxytocin, additional uterotonic agents should be employed.

*Table 315.1* CONDITIONS ASSOCIATED WITH UTERINE ATONY

- Advanced maternal age
- Hypertensive disorder during pregnancy
- Diabetes
- Cesarean delivery
- Induction of labor, augmentation of labor
- Multiple gestation
- Multiparity
- Macrosomia
- Polyhydramnios
- Prolonged labor
- Precipitous labor
- Chorioamnionitis
- Volatile anesthetics
- Tocolytics

## GENITAL TRAUMA

Perineal lacerations and hematomas can be associated with significant PPH. Risk factors include instrumental deliveries using forceps and vacuum extraction, nulliparity, advanced maternal age, macrosomia, prolonged second stage of labor, multiple gestation, preeclampsia, and vulvovaginal varicosities. Retroperitoneal hematomas are the most dangerous hematomas; they result from laceration of one of the branches of the hypogastric artery.

## RETAINED PLACENTA

Retained placenta occurs when the placenta fails to be delivered completely within 30 minutes of delivery of the infant. The incidence is estimated at 3% of vaginal deliveries approximately. The risk for retained placenta increases with a history of retained placenta, preterm delivery, oxytocin use during labor, preeclampsia, and nulliparity.

Management of retained placenta involves gentle cord traction, uterine massage, manual removal, or a dilation and curettage procedure to remove the retained tissue. Uterine relaxation is required to facilitate placental passage. Small boluses of intravenous nitroglycerin (50 to 100 μg) or sublingual administration of nitroglycerine spray provide reliable smooth muscle relaxation without causing prolonged uterine atony.[2]

## UTERINE INVERSION

Uterine inversion refers to the turning inside-out of all or part of the uterus. Risk factors include excessive manual umbilical cord traction, uterine atony, a short umbilical cord, uterine anomalies, use of uterine-relaxing agents, uterine overdistension, fetal macrosomia, and connective tissue disorders. Once the diagnosis has been made, immediate intervention to reposition the uterus and control hemorrhage is required. Uterine relaxation using nitroglycerine, tocolytics, or inhaled anesthetics is necessary to correct the

**Table 315.2** AN EXAMPLE OF AN OBSTETRIC HEMORRHAGE MTP

| ROUND | RED BLOOD CELLS (UNIT) | FRESH FROZEN PLASMA (UNIT) | PLATELETS (UNIT) | CRYOPRECIPITATE (UNIT) | TXA |
|---|---|---|---|---|---|
| 1 | 6 | 6 | 6 | | 1 gram IV over 10 minutes |
| 2 | 6 | 6 | 6 | | |
| 3 | 6 | 6 | 6 | 10 | |

From Reference 4.

inversion. After the replacement, oxytocin and additional uterotonic drugs may be needed.

## PLACENTA ACCRETA

Placenta accreta is defined as a pathologic adherence of the placenta to the uterine wall. The placenta accreta spectrum includes placenta increta, placenta percreta, and placenta accreta. Placenta accreta refers to adherence of chorionic villi to the myometrium in the absence of the decidua basalis. Placenta increta and percreta represent the invasion of chorionic villi into the myometrium only and invasion through the myometrium into serosa, respectively. The risk factors include previous cesarean delivery, placenta previa, advanced maternal age, multiparity, prior uterine surgeries or curettage, and Asherman syndrome.[3] The risk of placenta accreta is increased with placenta previa and history of cesarean section. The incidence of placenta accreta with placenta previa and no prior uterine surgery is approximately 3%, whereas the incidence is increased above 60% with placenta previa and a history of three or more previous cesarean sections. The American College of Obstetricians and Gynecologists advises that patients with placenta accreta should undergo planned cesarean delivery and possible hysterectomy with the placenta left in situ, with the surgery occurring with a multidisciplinary team approach.[3]

## ANESTHETIC IMPLICATIONS

### PREOPERATIVE

Preoperative assessment includes the airway examination, intravascular volume assessment, blood product availability, adequate intravenous access, and the determination of hemoglobin concentration and coagulation status. Invasive blood pressure monitoring with an arterial line will be useful for the prompt recognition of hypotension and frequent blood sampling to monitor coagulation status. The massive transfusion protocol should

be accessible, and the autologous cell saver technique can be utilized.

### INTRAOPERATIVE

Intraoperatively, the choice of anesthetic technique depends on the hemodynamic status of the patient, ongoing blood loss, and anticipation of surgical time. General anesthesia is the anesthetic technique of choice in massive PPH. Airway protection is necessary for severely hypotensive patients with massive volume resuscitation, which increases airway edema and the risk of difficult intubation.

A massive transfusion protocol (MTP) should be considered when bleeding continues after the transfusion of 2 units of red blood cells within 1–2 hours, cumulative blood loss greater than 1500 mL, unstable vital signs, or the suspicion of disseminated intravascular coagulation (DIC). An example of obstetric hemorrhage MTP is described in Table 315.2.[4] The fibrinogen level during obstetric hemorrhage has been described as a biomarker for severe PPH. Cryoprecipitate may be considered to maintain the serum fibrinogen at 150–200 mg/dL. Antifibrinolytic therapy may be useful in the setting of PPH. A recent international trial to investigate the effect of early tranexamic acid (TXA) administration showed TXA reduced death caused by PPH when it was used within 3 hours of giving birth.[5]

After the third round, if an MTP is not terminated, it will repeat from round 1. A second dose of TXA may be given 30 minutes after the first dose if bleeding persists.

### POSTOPERATIVE

Patients with massive PPH should be observed postoperatively for recurrence of hemorrhage. Bleeding may occur due incomplete management of the primary cause of bleeding or from the DIC primarily due to dilution of coagulation factor. Assessment of the coagulation profile and fibrinogen level, as well as assessment of clinical bleeding, should be included in the immediate postoperative management routine.

## REFERENCES

1. Committee on Practice Bulletins-Obstetrics. Practice bulletin no. 183. *Obstet Gynecol.* 2017;130(4):e168–e186.
2. Banayan JM, et al. Antepartum and postpartum hemorrhage. In: Chestnut DH, et al., eds. *Chestnut's Obstetric Anesthesia: Principles and Practice.* 6th ed. Philadelphia, PA: Elsevier Health Sciences; 2020:901–936.
3. Obstetric care consensus no. 7: placenta accreta spectrum. *Obstet Gynecol.* 2018;132(6):1519–1521.
4. Pacheco LD, et al. An update on the use of massive transfusion protocols in obstetrics. *Am J Obstet Gynecol.* 2016;214(3):340–344.
5. WOMAN Trial Collaborators, et al. Effect of early tranexamic acid administration on mortality, hysterectomy, and other morbidities in women with post-partum haemorrhage (WOMAN): an international, randomised, double-blind, placebo-controlled trial. *Lancet.* 2017;389(10084):2105–2116.

# 316.

# CORD PROLAPSE

*Muhammad Fayyaz Ahmed and Ihab Kamel*

## INTRODUCTION

Umbilical cord prolapse (UCP) is an obstetrical emergency that occurs when the cord slips ahead (overt UCP) or alongside (occult UCP) the presenting part of the fetus and protrudes into the cervical canal or beyond. Compression of the prolapsed cord leads to occlusion of the umbilical vein and vasospasm of the umbilical artery, which compromises fetal oxygenation.[1] The reported incidence of UCP is around 0.16% to 0.18% of live-born deliveries. Risk factors for UCP are divided into two main categories: maternal-fetal and iatrogenic risk factors.[1] Maternal-fetal risk factors include nonvertex fetal presentation (with highest frequency associated with the transverse followed by breech presentation), preterm labor, low birth weight, second twin, polyhydramnios, and pelvic deformities. Iatrogenic risk factors include artificial rupture of membrane, induction of labor, external cephalic version, and application of forceps or vacuum.

## CLINICAL PRESENTATION

Cord prolapse usually presents as an abrupt onset of severe prolonged fetal bradycardia or moderate-to-severe variable fetal heart rate decelerations. The fetal heart rate changes typically occur soon after membrane rupture or an obstetric intervention that dislodges the presenting part. Rarely, the physician might palpate a pulsating cord incidentally.[2]

## PATHOPHYSIOLOGY

Compression of the umbilical cord leads to significant or total blockage of fetal oxygenation, causing near-total or total acute asphyxia. This results in failure of the normal cerebral autoregulatory mechanisms and cell death of the brainstem—the most metabolically active area of the brain.

## MANAGEMENT OF UMBILICAL CORD PROLAPSE

Umbilical cord prolapse is an obstetrical emergency that requires attention to deliver the fetus immediately. The route of delivery taken is the one that is quicker, which typically is emergent caesarian section. It is recommended to deliver the baby within 30 minutes of the diagnosis in order to reduce perinatal mortality.[3]

It is important to call for help when the diagnosis is made and make aware the teams involved aware, including the anesthetist, operating room staff, and pediatrician. Continuous fetal monitoring and supplemental oxygen should be maintained while emergently transporting the patient to the operating room for immediate delivery. An alternative to a cesarean delivery is vaginal delivery if deemed safe and quick. It is vital to manually decompress the presenting part before and during the delivery, which involves two fingers/hand in the vagina plus elevation of the presenting part, steep Trendelenburg position or knee-chest position, insertion of a Foley catheter, and infusion of saline into the urinary bladder. Manual replacement of the umbilical cord is rarely used. Tocolytics can be considered to decrease uterine contractions to relieve pressure on the prolapsed cord.[3]

## CHOICE OF ANESTHESIA

In UCP, the best choice of anesthesia is the one that has the shortest interval between diagnosis and delivery due to the increase in neonatal mortality by delaying the delivery.[3] An existing labor epidural anesthesia that can be used in an emergency may be an acceptable approach due to the potential benefits of regional anesthesia compared to general anesthesia. However, the time to administer general anesthesia is shorter compared to regional anesthesia. It has been shown that general anesthesia has a shorter interval time compared to regional anesthesia, except for a functional epidural, which can be rapidly extended to provide surgical block.

In the circumstance of cord prolapse, it is unlikely that the asphyxiated neonate receives a significant proportion of general anesthetic drugs via the placenta. The risks associated with general anesthesia are unlikely to be any greater than a usual cesarean delivery under general anesthesia. In contrast, in the context of cord prolapse, the difficulties posed by regional anesthesia are considerably higher than usual. Expected concerns are higher failure rate due to time constraint and distressed patient, increased risk of high spinal block due to abnormal position, and challenges in maintaining a sterile field and aseptic technique. Considering these factors, general anesthesia is favored as it is a safe and quicker method with relatively fewer disadvantages.[3]

## PREVENTION

Knowing the risk factors of UCP does not significantly decrease its occurrence; however, the anticipation of the situation assists in better planning and may lead to improvement of fetal morbidity and mortality. It is also important to note that cord prolapse can occur in pregnancies without obvious risk factors, which renders this complication unpreventable.[2]

## ANESTHETIC CONSIDERATIONS

### PREOPERATIVE

Preoperatively, know that umbilical cord prolapse is an obstetrical emergency that can lead to neonatal asphyxiation and death if not managed properly. The anesthetic of choice is general anesthesia, while the delivery mode of choice is cesarean delivery. Delay of delivery due to administering a local anesthetic via a functional epidural catheter to obtain surgical block of anesthesia should be avoided. If there is a delay in achieving a surgical block and the obstetrical team is ready, quickly switching to general anesthesia to reduce neonatal mortality is the most appropriate approach.

### INTRAOPERATIVE

Manual decompression of the umbilical cord by elevating the presenting part while maintaining a steep Trendelenburg position must be maintained intraoperatively until delivery. Maintaining material physiological parameters such as hemoglobin oxygen saturation and systemic blood pressure is important to optimize fetal perfusion.

## REFERENCES

1. Bush M, et al. Umbilical cord prolapse. In: Post TW, ed. *UpToDate*. UpToDate; Updated March 18, 2019. https://www.uptodate.com/contents/umbilical-cord-prolapse
2. Ahmed S, et al. Optimal management of umbilical cord prolapse. *Int J Womens Health*. 2018;10:459–465.
3. Bythell V. Cord prolapse demands general anaesthesia. *Int J Obst Anesth*. 2003:12(4):287–289.

# 317.

# RETAINED PLACENTA

*Muhammad Fayyaz Ahmed and Ihab Kamel*

## INTRODUCTION

Retained placenta is defined as failure to deliver the placenta completely within 30 minutes (active management of labor) or 60 minutes (physiologic management of labor) after the delivery of the fetus. Reported incidence of retained placenta ranges from 0.01% to 6.3% of vaginal deliveries. Complications of placenta accreta include primary and secondary postpartum hemorrhage, uterine prolapse, and puerperal sepsis. Postpartum hemorrhage can be life threatening, requiring transfusion.[1,2] Types of retained placenta include trapped placenta (the placenta is trapped behind a partially closed cervix); placenta adherens (the placenta is adherent to the endometrial lining of the uterus, but manually separable); and placenta accreta (the placenta is abnormally adherent to the myometrium).[2]

## RISK FACTORS

Risk factors for retained placenta include history of uterine surgery, history of retained placenta, preterm delivery, older maternal age, small or low-lying placenta, preterm delivery, in vitro fertilization conception, congenital uterine anomaly, prolonged use of oxytocin during labor, diagnosis of preeclampsia, and nulliparity.[3,4]

## OBSTETRIC MANAGEMENT

The retained placenta does not allow the uterus to contract, leading to postpartum hemorrhage. Early removal of the retained placenta can reduce the risk of hemorrhage. The risk of postpartum hemorrhage increases when the duration of placenta retention exceeds 30 minutes versus 18 minutes from delivery of the infant.[2] Early management of retained placenta involves manual removal of the placenta and inspecting it. In certain circumstances, curettage may be needed for complete removal. Once the placenta is removed, it is essential to evaluate the tone of the uterus and augment it with oxytocin. The patient should be monitored for recurrent hemorrhage leading to hemodynamic compromise.

## ANESTHETIC CONSIDERATIONS

### PREOPERATIVE

In the preoperative period, evaluate the patient's airway, ensure good intravenous access (a second intravenous access), and availability of crossmatched blood. Evaluate the patient's hemodynamics and the status of ongoing bleeding. If the plan is to proceed with labor epidural for curettage, evaluate the epidural site and its functionality. If the plan is to proceed with general anesthesia, administer aspiration prophylaxis.

### INTRAOPERATIVE

#### Anesthetic Management

Intraoperatively, the process of proper examination and removal of the retained placenta through either manual extraction or use of curettage involves significant pain and requires analgesia and anxiolysis. The choice of anesthetic use depends on the severity of hemorrhage, hemodynamic stability, and patient risk factors. In some cases, monitored anesthesia care will allow the obstetrician to perform an examination and manually extract the placenta. General anesthesia is required if the patient is having significant bleeding causing hemodynamic compromise. If general anesthesia is planned, rapid sequence induction and tracheal intubation are recommended. Closely monitoring the patient's hemodynamic parameters and surgical field assessment for ongoing hemorrhage is important to determine the need for blood product administration. Neuraxial anesthesia can be considered in hemodynamically stable patients with moderate bleeding. Neuraxial anesthesia is achieved by placing spinal anesthesia or the administration of additional local anesthetic, with or without opioids, through an existing functioning labor epidural. The goal is to obtain a sensory level covering the dermatomes from T10 to S4.

## Uterine Relaxation

Manual removal of the placenta is usually facilitated by uterine relaxation. Interventions to achieve uterine relaxation include intravenous nitroglycerin administration and general endotracheal anesthesia with volatile agents.

**Nitroglycerin:** Nitroglycerin can be administered intravenously for uterine relaxation by releasing nitric oxide to cause smooth muscle relaxation. Nitroglycerin has a rapid onset of action and a short plasma half-life of 2–3 minutes. The dose used can be titrated to effect; it may be initiated with a small dose of 20 μg, increasing as needed. Studies have shown the use of intravenous nitroglycerin doses of 50 to 500 μg are usually needed achieve uterine relaxation. It can also be administered sublingually. It is important to closely monitor the patient's blood pressure and heart rate when administering nitroglycerin in the setting of ongoing hemorrhage. Brief hypotension should be treated with boluses of adrenergic agents, such as phenylephrine.

**General Endotracheal Anesthesia With Volatile Agents:** Uterine relaxation can be achieved by performing general anesthesia and administering a high dose of volatile anesthetic. Consider the risks, such as difficulty in endotracheal intubation and mask ventilation, aspiration of gastric content, and hemodynamic effects of inhaled anesthetics. Perform rapid sequence induction followed by intubation and administration of around 1.5 MAC (minimum alveolar concentration) volatile anesthetic agent. It has been shown that 1.5 MAC of volatile anesthetic agent can decrease uterine contractility by 50%.[1] The degree of uterine relaxation is similar between the different volatile agents used, provided equipotent doses are used. It is vital to have typed, screened, and crossmatched blood available. Close monitoring of hemodynamic parameters and obtaining crossmatched blood are critical.

## POSTOPERATIVE

Postoperatively, evaluate the patient's hemodynamic status with attention to uterine bleeding, heart rate, and blood pressure before discharge from the postanesthesia care unit. Sustained tachycardia is usually a concerning sign and should be investigated prior to discharge. In some cases, tachycardia is the earliest and only sign of hemodynamic compromise. Checking hemoglobin and hematocrit is recommended in cases of severe bleeding.

## REFERENCES

1. Banayan JM, et al. Antepartum and postpartum hemorrhage. In: Chestnut DH, et al., eds. *Chestnut's Obstetric Anesthesia: Principles and Practice.* 6th ed. Philadelphia, PA: Elsevier Health Sciences; 2020:901–936.
2. Wali A, Waters JH. Obstetric hemorrhage, novel pharmacologic interventions, blood conservation techniques, and hemorrhage protocols. In: Suresh MS, et al., eds. *Shnider and Levinson's Anesthesia for Obstetrics.* (5th ed. Philadelphia, PA: Lippincott, Williams & Wilkins; 2013:311–332.
3. Coviello EM, et al. Risk factors for retained placenta. *Obstet Anesth Digest.* 2016;36(4):202–203.
4. Perlman NC, Carusi DA. Retained placenta after vaginal delivery: risk factors and management. *Int J Womens Health.* 2019;11:527–534.

# 318.

# DYSTOCIA, MALPOSITION, AND MALPRESENTATION

*Diana Feinstein and Daniella Miele*

## INTRODUCTION

Spontaneous vaginal delivery most often occurs with a head-down (cephalic) and flexed fetus in the occiput anterior (OA) position.[1] This position is beneficial as it minimizes the fetal head diameter and puts the body in an optimal position to pass through the maternal pelvis. Deviation from this positioning complicates the delivery.

## MALPOSITION

Fetal malposition means the fetus is rotated, rendering the occiput posterior (OP) or occiput transverse (OT). The diagnosis is commonly made with a digital vaginal examination and confirmed with ultrasound.[2] If a malposition is noted in the second stage of labor, most often the obstetrics team waits to see if the fetus naturally rotates into the OA position. Epidural analgesia may decrease the likelihood of fetal rotation by relaxing the maternal pelvic floor muscles.[2] However, this has not been proven, and these patients frequently have increased labor pain, therefore benefiting from epidural placement.

Occiput posterior presentation is associated with longer labor, increased cesarean section and instrumental delivery rates, extreme maternal perineal tears (third and fourth degree), and elevated blood loss with delivery.[3] Furthermore, malposition adversely affects the fetus with increased 5-minute Apgar scores less than 7, umbilical cord gas acidemia, neonatal intensive care unit admissions, and longer hospitalizations.[2] Successful rotation of the fetus from OP or OT position to OA is associated with decreased second stage of labor, reduced maternal perineal trauma, and a reduction in blood loss.[3]

## MALPRESENTATION

A noncephalic or nonvertex presentation is termed malpresentation. Breech presentation is the most common malpresentation (3%–4%) and occurs when the buttocks or feet enter the pelvic inlet.[1] If the term fetus is in breech position, the obstetric team may perform an external cephalic version (ECV) in an effort to manually move the fetus to a head-down position. This maneuver is successful in 50%–65% of cases but may lead to complications.[1] Most ECVs are performed under epidural analgesia, with the anesthesia team prepared for emergency cesarean delivery if persistent fetal bradycardia ensues. Risks of ECV include cord prolapse, placental abruption, rupture of membranes, cord compression, and emergency cesarean section. If the patient declines an ECV, an elective cesarean section is considered the safest delivery option for breech position.

If a patient with a fetus in the breech position presents with rupture of membranes, there is a risk of cord prolapse and cord compression, so most often an emergency cesarean section is performed. Maternal and fetal risks are reduced when a planned cesarean section is performed for the breech position.

## SHOULDER DYSTOCIA

Shoulder dystocia is an unpredictable and unpreventable obstetrical emergency. It is associated with an increased risk of injury to the mother and fetus. Diagnosis is subjective and made at the time of delivery when excessive traction is needed to deliver the fetal trunk after delivery of the head. Use of increased traction during delivery increases the risk of injury to the fetal brachial plexus.[4]

Shoulder dystocia with a normal size fetus is most often related to two risk factors. The first risk factor is precipitous delivery that does not allow adequate rotation of the fetal body, leading to misalignment of fetal shoulders and maternal pelvis. The second risk factor is iatrogenic, and it involves the use of operative delivery instruments such as forceps to deliver a normal size fetus. Other risk factors include fetopelvic disproportion, as seen with fetal macrosomia or when the fetus's trunk grows faster and asymmetrically compared to the size of its head. To a lesser extent, shoulder dystocia may also be caused by a normal size fetus in a mother of short stature or with a small or misshapen pelvis.

Maternal risk factors for large-for-gestational-age babies associated with increased risk of shoulder dystocia include history of previous shoulder dystocia (highest risk factor and predictor), gestational diabetes, maternal obesity, excessive weight gain during pregnancy, parity, and postdate deliveries.

## ANESTHETIC CONSIDERATIONS

### PREOPERATIVE

If the parturient has preexisting risk factors, it is important preoperatively to ensure adequate intravenous access and to obtain a blood type and screen in the event of postpartum hemorrhage. Early placement of epidural analgesia to facilitate instrumental delivery or ECV should be considered in these patients.

### INTRAOPERATIVE

Intraoperatively, the goal of epidural analgesia during ECV is to treat maternal pain, which is the most common reason for terminating an ECV attempt. Epidural analgesia significantly increases the chances of ECV success by reducing maternal pain, abdominal muscle tone, and guarding. Both high-dose surgical anesthesia and low-dose epidural analgesia can be used. Epidural analgesia sensory level should be confirmed before an ECV attempt. The use of high-dose local anesthesia (T6 sensory level) has the advantage of providing optimal analgesia for ECV and adequate surgical anesthesia for an immediate cesarean delivery if necessary. However, it may be associated with a higher incidence of hypotension. Maternal blood pressure should be monitored frequently, and hypotension should be treated immediately with left uterine displacement, phenylephrine, and fluid boluses. Although epidural opioids can be added to provide analgesia, they should be avoided due to a possible systemic effect on maternal ventilation and fetal central nervous system. The anesthesia team must be prepared for an emergency cesarean section and increased risk of bleeding.

### POSTOPERATIVE

Fetal malposition and malpresentation predispose the patient to postpartum hemorrhage. Postoperatively, the patient should be closely monitored after delivery for vaginal bleeding and signs of hemodynamic instability. Persistent postpartum tachycardia should be investigated.

### REFERENCES

1. Pilliod R, Caughey A. Fetal malpresentation and malposition: diagnosis and management. *Obstet Gynecol Clin N Am.* 2017;44:631–643.
2. Caughey A, et al. Fetal malposition: impact and management. *Clin Obstet & Gynecol.* 2015;58(2):241–245.
3. Aiken A, et al. Management of fetal malposition in the second stage of labor: a propensity score analysis. *Am J Obstet Gynecol.* 2015;212:355.e1–7.
4. Allen EG, Allen RH. Management of shoulder dystocia. In: Malvasi A, et al., *Management and Therapy of Late Pregnancy Complications.* Cham, Switzerland: Springer; 2017:167–178.

# 319.

# MATERNAL CARDIOPULMONARY RESUSCITATION

*Steven Zhou and Nasir Hussain*

## INTRODUCTION

Cardiac arrest during pregnancy is a relatively rare phenomenon, as the majority of parturients tend to be younger with fewer comorbidities. Recent data from the US Nationwide Inpatient Sample suggests that cardiac arrest occurs in 1:12,000 admissions for delivery.[1] Risk factors for cardiac arrest, such as advanced maternal age; history of cardiac disease (congenital disease, valvular lesions); preeclampsia; history of seizures; and strokes need to be identified and evaluated prior to pregnancy.

## PHYSIOLOGIC CHANGES IN PREGNANCY

Numerous changes in anatomy and physiology occur in pregnancy, brought on by a change in circulating hormones, biochemical changes associated with the demands of the fetus, and mechanical displacement of internal structures by the developing fetus.[2,3] These changes affect nearly all organ systems, with the most pertinent to this chapter being the cardiovascular, pulmonary, hematologic, and renal systems. A summary of these changes is highlighted in Table 319.1.

## CARDIOPULMONARY RESUSCITATION

The basics of maternal cardiopulmonary resuscitation (CPR) follow basic life support/advanced cardiac life support (BLS/ACLS) algorithms with additions necessitated by the distinctive physiologic changes of pregnancy. Promptly obtaining large-bore intravenous access, timely request for help/code activation, and high-quality chest compressions are all essential steps in ACLS. As in nonpregnant ACLS, prompt defibrillation of ventricular fibrillation or pulseless ventricular tachycardia is critical.[4] The developing fetus is also particularly sensitive to hypotension, further necessitating a rapid emergency response.

## SPECIAL CONSIDERATIONS

During maternal CPR, care is provided for not only the mother but also the developing fetus. Maintenance of pregnancy and fetal development is paramount whenever possible. As such, code activation must involve both specialized personnel and equipment. Healthcare providers such as a neonatologists, obstetricians, anesthesiologists, and others are needed for timely recognition and treatment of instigating causal pathologies, such as hemorrhage, sepsis, pulmonary embolism, and others. Surgical supplies for a possible resuscitative hysterotomy and the preparation of an operation room for the delivery of a neonate are essential.[4] Fetal heart rate monitoring under the care of an obstetrician may be useful but should not impede resuscitation.

## DETERMINING GESTATIONAL AGE

Determining age and fetal viability is important during CPR as it can help dictate management. Different approaches are necessary for nonviable versus viable fetuses. Age can be approximated by classically accepted rule-of-thumb landmarks if no information is known: gestational age of 12 weeks if uterus is palpable at the pubic symphysis, 20 weeks if the uterus is palpable at the umbilicus.[4] Fundal height may be skewed during periods of pregnancy, so the expertise of all available team members should be utilized.

## AORTOCAVAL COMPRESSION

An important consideration of the of the gravid uterus on the cardiovascular system is aortocaval compression, which is generally seen at more than 20 weeks of gestation.[4] In the supine position, compression of the aorta and vena cava can decrease preload, cardiac output, and systemic blood pressure.[2–4] When performing chest compressions, manual left uterine displacement has been shown to be more useful than bed tilt as maintaining quality compressions may be more difficult with a tilt. The uterus should be pushed

## Table 319.1 PHYSIOLOGIC CHANGES IN PREGNANCY WITH HIGH-YIELD COMMENTS

| ORGAN SYSTEM | HIGH-YIELD COMMENTS |
| --- | --- |
| Cardiovascular | • Increased cardiac output by 30%–50% (increased stroke volume and heart rate); most pronounced immediately after delivery<br>• Increase in intravascular fluid volume (relative anemia)<br>• Decrease in systemic vascular resistance (due to endogenous hormones and vasodilators)<br>• Supine aortocaval compression (by gravid uterus → supine hypotension syndrome with nausea/vomiting, diaphoresis, neurological symptoms) |
| Pulmonary | • Decreased functional residual capacity<br>• Increased minute ventilation (increase in tidal volume)<br>• Increased $O_2$ consumption<br>• Shift in $O_2$ dissociation curve (right in mother to increase offloading to placenta/fetus) |
| Renal/gastrointestinal | • Increased regurgitation/aspiration risk → consider rapid sequence induction/high aspiration risk/cricoid pressure<br>• Decreased competence of esophageal sphincter tone, prolonged gastric transit time<br>• Increased glomerular filtration rate and renal blood flow<br>• Altered drug metabolism |
| Hematologic | • Hypercoagulable → increased factor I, VII, VIII, IX, X, and XII<br>• Decreased factors XI, XIII, antithrombin III |

Based on References 2–4.

upward and leftward to offset pressure on maternal vessels, thus promoting return of preload to the heart and improved fetal blood flow. Adequate CPR may not be possible until the compression is relieved.

## AIRWAY MANAGEMENT

Parturients have a decreased functional reserve in contrast to nonpregnant patients. As a result, rapid airway and ventilatory interventions are essential.[4] Due to increased capillary engorgement in the upper airway, tissue edema, and increased tissue friability, special care must be taken when intubating.[2,3] As such, it may be beneficial to begin with a smaller endotracheal tube (6.0 or 6.5 mm). The presence of preeclampsia, pushing during labor, or weight gain during pregnancy can further exacerbate airway tissue edema, making intubation and ventilation even more challenging.

## HEMORRHAGE

Hemorrhage is one of the leading causes of sudden cardiac arrest in women and can be precipitated by placental or uterine abnormalities. A thorough history and physical examination is critical since placental pathologies in prior pregnancies often increase the risk for subsequent complications. These can include abnormal uterine implantation of the placenta, uterine rupture, retained placenta, and uterine atony. While the specific management of each pathology is outside the scope of this chapter, prompt recognition and communication with the obstetric team is essential. In the event of a massive transfusion activation, general anesthesia may be required in some cases.

## AMNIOTIC FLUID EMBOLISM

While rare, an amniotic fluid embolism (AFE) is a potentially lethal condition of pregnancy. Clinical features of AFE include the triad of sudden onset hypotension, hypoxic respiratory failure, and coagulopathy.[5] While previous studies have suggested a link with retained fragments of amniotic debris in maternal circulation, the current theory revolves on a hypersensitivity reaction and abnormal activation of pro-inflammation mediator systems. Currently, there is no diagnostic marker, and AFE remains a clinical diagnosis of exclusion. Differentials are often difficult to distinguish, but include pulmonary embolism, sepsis, venous air embolism, hemorrhage, anaphylaxis, cardiomyopathy, and others. Treatment is supportive, involving immediate high-quality CPR, transfusions for the coagulopathy and hemorrhage, ionotropic support, and correction of hypoxemia. Assessment of the patient's coagulation profile may be useful. Intubation is almost always indicated, and extracorporeal membrane oxygenation may be necessary as a last resort.

## RESUSCITATIVE HYSTEROTOMY

Despite maneuvers to reduce aortocaval compression, CPR may not be successful at restoring spontaneous circulation without delivery of the fetus. Without restoring cardiac output, both the mother and fetus are at significant risk for hypoxia and anoxia.[4] During CPR, hysterotomy has dual effects. First, removal of the uterus relieves aortocaval obstruction/compression by the fetus and may improve resuscitation efforts with improved venous return to the heart. Second, delivery of the baby is of critical importance to relieve anoxia and reduce the risk of permanent neurological damage in the event of inadequate maternal blood supply. The exact timeline for resuscitation hysterotomy remains controversial, but the American

Heart Association recommends a "5-minute window," where efforts for delivery should begin 5 minutes after unsuccessful CPR.

## REFERENCES

1. Mhyre JM, et al. Cardiac arrest during hospitalization for delivery in the United States, 1998–2011. *Anesthesiology*. 2014;120:810–818.

2. Cheek TG, Gutsche BB. Maternal physiologic alterations. In: Huges SC, et al., eds. *Schnider and Levinson's Anesthesia for Obstetrics*. 4th ed. Philadelphia, PA: Lippincott, Williams & Wilkins; 2002:3–18.

3. Gaiser R. Physiologic changes of pregnancy. In: Chestnut DH, et al., eds. *Chestnut's Obstetric Anesthesia: Principles and Practice*. 4th ed. Philadelphia, PA: Elsevier; 2009:15–36.

4. Jeejeebhoy FM, et al. Cardiac arrest in pregnancy: a scientific statement from the American Heart Association. *Circulation*. 2015;132:1747.

5. Pacheco L, et al. Amniotic fluid embolism: diagnosis and management. *Am J Obstet Gynecol*. 2016;215(2):B16–B24.

# 320.

# FEVER AND INFECTION

*Helen Pappas and Elizabeth Lange*

## INTRODUCTION

Fever is classically defined as a temperature of 38°C (100.4°F) or greater. The incidence of maternal fever varies from 10% to as high as one-third of all deliveries. Maternal fever has been associated with severe adverse neonatal outcomes, including hypotonia, need for assisted ventilation, neonatal seizures, and cerebral palsy. The etiology of maternal fever varies and includes both infectious and noninfectious causes. Intra-amniotic infection, or chorioamnionitis, occurs in about 2%–5% of deliveries.[1,2] Independent of etiology, adverse events occur as a result of maternal fever.

## CLINICAL FEATURES

Maternal fever can present antepartum, intrapartum, and postpartum. Maternal oral temperature is the best indicator of intrauterine temperature but may underestimate by about 0.8°C. Predominant risk factors for the development of maternal fever include nulliparous state, premature rupture of membranes, prolonged labor and rupture of membranes, pregnancy-induced hypertension, and diabetes mellitus.[3]

Maternal fever may be a result of intrauterine or extrauterine causes. Frequently, maternal fever is attributed to chorioamnionitis; however, other infectious etiologies, including bacterial and viral infections, can cause women to develop a fever during labor. Infectious etiologies have the potential to progress to sepsis. Sepsis in pregnancy can be difficult to diagnose clinically due to normal maternal physiologic changes, such as alterations in blood pressure, heart rate, and leukocytosis. Noninfectious causes can include the administration of medications that raise maternal temperature such as prostaglandin $E_2$ agents and elevated ambient temperature and fever related to neuraxial labor analgesia (coined epidural fever).

Maternal fever is associated with both maternal and neonatal morbidity. Maternal complications include dysfunctional labor, uterine atony, maternal hemorrhage, and maternal sepsis.[1] Fetal core temperature in utero is approximately 0.5°C to 0.9°C higher than maternal core temperature; therefore, fetuses of febrile mothers are exposed to higher temperatures than suggested by the degree of maternal temperature elevation. Maternal fever is associated with fetal tachycardia in utero. In addition to an increased incidence of low (<7) Apgar scores, several adverse neonatal outcomes have been associated with maternal fever, such as increased need for resuscitation and assisted ventilation, hypotonia, neonatal seizures, and encephalopathy.[2] These adverse neonatal outcomes have also been associated with more conservative definitions of fever, such as 37.5°C.

## DIAGNOSIS

Intra-amniotic infection, or chorioamnionitis, an infection of the fluid, placenta, or fetal parts, is the most common cause of maternal fever in the peripartum period. While historically a diagnosis of intra-amniotic infection could be made when maternal temperature was 39°C or greater or 38°C–39°C with additional clinical indictors, including fetal tachycardia or purulent vaginal discharge, recently a more general description has been advocated. Triple I criteria describe maternal fever as a result of intrauterine inflammation, infection, or both. It requires a maternal fever of 38°C or greater and one of the following: fetal tachycardia, maternal leukocytosis in the absence of corticosteroid use, purulent cervical fluid, or microbial invasion of the amniotic cavity. It is estimated that 2%–5% of deliveries are complicated by intra-amniotic infection.[1]

## TREATMENT/MANAGEMENT

Maternal fever regardless of etiology confounds clinical decision-making. It can prompt providers to treat women with antibiotics for presumed chorioamnionitis, as well as lead to sepsis evaluation of the neonate, resulting in separation of the mother from the newborn during the first hours or days of life.

Prompt recognition of intra-amniotic infection and treatment with empiric antibiotics are the mainstay of minimizing maternal and fetal complications, with multiple studies documenting decreased incidence of neonatal bacteremia and sepsis with adequate maternal antibiotic administration. First-line antibiotics are ampicillin and gentamicin, with cefazolin and clindamycin as substitutes for penicillin-allergic patients. Antibiotic therapy is recommended during labor and continued postpartum if there are additional risk factors for postpartum endometritis.[1] Although current recommendations from the American College of Obstetricians and Gynecologists state that the presence of intra-amniotic infection is not an indication for cesarean delivery, there is a higher incidence of cesarean and assisted delivery for these patients. When maternal sepsis is suspected, it is managed with supportive, goal-directed therapy and source control as in the nonpregnant population.

For maternal fever thought to be secondary to noninfectious etiologies, management is supportive with antipyretics as indicated. There is no definitive evidence to support specific treatment or management of epidural fever.

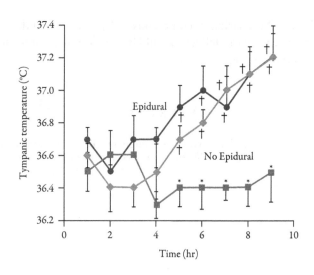

Figure 320.1 Maternal temperature regulation during labor.

## ANESTHETIC CONSIDERATIONS

Data from observational and retrospective studies reveal that roughly 20% of women who receive labor epidural analgesia will have a significant increase in temperature during labor.[4] Epidural fever was first described in 1989. While the exact mechanism is unclear, the underlying process appears to be inflammatory, not infectious, with elevations of pro-inflammatory cytokines interleukin (IL) 6 and IL-8 detected in patients who develop fever.[4] Significant differences in temperature can be seen between 4 and 6 hours after the initiation of analgesia in patients who use neuraxial labor analgesia compared to those who do not, as depicted in Figure 320.1.[5]

The leading proposed mechanisms for epidural fever involve alterations in immunomodulation and cell injury. The mechanism by which epidural analgesia induces maternal fever is currently unknown, but the prevailing theory involves a noninfectious, inflammatory pathway induced by local anesthetics or the indwelling catheter. Local anesthetics are known to inhibit neutrophil activity and immune function, which is thought to create a pro-inflammatory environment. Local anesthetics are also known to cause cell injury and death, which causes release of pro-inflammatory mediators and cytokines.[4]

## NO EPIDURAL OR EPIDURAL

Studies aimed at treating and preventing epidural fever have evaluated use of prophylactic acetaminophen and antibiotics prior to neuraxial analgesia placement. Both of these strategies yielded no significant difference in maternal temperature curves. While steroid regimens have been shown to decrease the incidence of epidural fever, they are not clinically used for this purpose due to an increased incidence of neonatal bacteremia associated with their use. Other potential prevention strategies include magnesium sulfate, which decreases inflammatory mediators associated with epidural fever. Further research is needed to determine the best approach to decreasing the incidence of and managing epidural-induced maternal fever.

Camann and associates studied the effect of epidural analgesia on maternal oral and tympanic membrane temperature measurements in laboring women who self-selected IV nalbuphine or epidural analgesia. Women who requested epidural analgesia were randomized to receive either epidural bupivacaine only or epidural bupivacaine with fentanyl. At hour 5, the mean tympanic membrane temperature was significantly higher in both epidural groups (circles and diamonds [in Figure 320.1]) when compared with the IV nalbuphine group (squares). (Reprinted with permission from Elsevier.)[5]

## REFERENCES

1. Committee on Obstetric Practice. Committee opinion no. 712: intrapartum management of intraamniotic infection. *Obstet Gynecol*. 2017;130(2):e95–e101.
2. Greenwell EA, et al. Intrapartum temperature elevation, epidural use, and adverse outcome in term infants. *Pediatrics*. 2012;129(2):e447–e454.
3. Petrova A, et al. Association of maternal fever during labor with neonatal and infant morbidity and mortality. *Obstet Gynecol*. 2001;98(1):20–27.
4. Sultan P, et al. Inflammation and epidural-related maternal fever: proposed mechanisms. *Anesth Analg*. 2016;122(5):1546–1553.
5. Camann WR, et al. Maternal temperature regulation during extradural analgesia for labour. *Br J Anaesth*. 1991;67(5):565–568.

# 321.

# PRETERM LABOR

*Erika Taco and Kevin Spencer*

## INTRODUCTION

Preterm labor is defined as regular uterine contractions accompanied by a change in cervical dilation, effacement, or both occurring at less than 37 and more than 20 weeks' gestational age. It can alternatively be defined by an initial presentation with regular contractions and cervical dilation of at least 2 cm.

## RISK FACTORS FOR PRETERM LABOR

In the United States, African American women have a prematurity rate ranging from 16% to 18% compared to 7% to 9% for white women. Low socioeconomic status is also associated with preterm labor. Extremes in maternal prenatal weight, specifically a body mass index of less than 19.5 cm²/kg and obesity carry a higher risk of preterm delivery. A history of preterm labor increases the risk from 17% to 40% in the second pregnancy, and other studies have found a 2.5-fold increased risk of spontaneous preterm labor. The earlier the preterm delivery history, the greater the risk of preterm delivery. Multiple gestations carries the greatest risk of preterm delivery as the length of gestation decreases with the number of babies, twins (36 weeks), triplets (33 weeks), and quadruplets (31 weeks).

In addition to the factors mentioned, extremes in the volume of amniotic fluid (oligohydramnios and polyhydramnios) are associated with preterm labor. Infections like asymptomatic bacteriuria, pyelonephritis, and appendicitis can cause reactive uterine contractions.[1–3]

## PATHOPHYSIOLOGY OF PRETERM LABOR

Preterm labor genesis is not well understood. Various theories have been proposed:

1. Progesterone withdrawal: Increased fetal susceptibility to adenocorticotropic hormone, increasing cortisol secretion. Fetal cortisol decreases the production of progesterone and increases the estrogen/progesterone ratio, subsequently increasing prostaglandin formation, provoking preterm labor.
2. Oxytocin initiation: It is thought that oxytocin is an initiator of labor as it increases the frequency and intensity of uterine contractions. However, this is contradictory to the physiology because the oxytocin levels do not rise before labor, and clearance is constant.
3. Premature decidual activation: This theory is the most supported. Decidual activation through the fetal-decidual paracrine system, potentially by uterine bleeding or infection, can trigger uterine contractions.[1,3]

## DIAGNOSIS

### BIOCHEMICAL, ULTRASONOGRAPHIC PREDICTORS

Fetal fibronectin is a glycoprotein produced after the 20th week of pregnancy in the extracellular matrix, apparently when there is a choriodecidual disruption. It is highly specific to rule out preterm labor; if negative, there is a less than 1% chance of delivering in the next 1 to 2 weeks.

Ultrasound (US) also produces an objective measurement to examine the cervix. Short cervical length, as assessed by transvaginal US, is associated with a greater risk for preterm delivery.[2]

### TOCOLYTICS VERSUS DELIVERY

Obstetric clinical decision-making regarding use of tocolysis versus proceeding with delivery depends on the reason for delivery. Tocolytic therapy can be considered in the absence of a compelling explanation for why labor was triggered and to allow the fetus time to receive 48 hours of steroid therapy. Neonates that received antenatal corticosteroids have significantly lower severity and frequency of respiratory distress syndrome, intracranial hemorrhage, necrotizing enterocolitis, and death in comparison with neonates whose mothers did not receive antenatal steroids. They are recommended in women between 24 and 34 weeks of gestation who are at risk of delivery within 7 days and whose prior course of antenatal corticosteroids was administered more than 14 days previously. Maintenance therapy with tocolytics is not effective for preventing preterm birth or improving the neonatal outcomes. In the absence of maternal infection with a premature rupture of membranes, tocolytics may be considered for the purposes of maternal transport, steroid administration, or both.

No evidence exists that tocolytic therapy has any direct favorable effect on neonatal outcomes or that any prolongation of pregnancy afforded by tocolytics actually translates into a statistically significant neonatal benefit.

Common contraindications to tocolysis include intrauterine fetal demise, lethal fetal anomaly, nonreassuring fetal status, severe preeclampsia or eclampsia, significant maternal bleeding, chorioamnionitis, preterm premature rupture of membranes, and maternal contraindications to a specific tocolysis agent.

## ANESTHETIC CONSIDERATIONS

### PREOPERATIVE

Preoperatively, reasons to deliver an early pregnancy are either suspected fetal acidosis or maternal conditions. Timing is important for late preterm (34, 35, and 36 weeks) versus early term (37 and 38 weeks of gestation). Neonates born between 34 and 37 weeks account for most admissions to the neonatal intensive care unit. Reddy found that infants born at 37 weeks are twice likely to die before their first birthday than those born at 40 weeks. Common causes are sudden infant death syndrome, birth defects, and intrauterine and birth hypoxemia.[1]

### INTRAOPERATIVE

Anesthetic intraoperative considerations for delivering a preterm fetus are largely the same as for a full-term fetus; however, there is a greater risk for cesarean delivery. Neuraxial anesthesia reduces maternal catecholamines, potentially improving uteroplacental perfusion if hypotension is avoided. The timing of initiation of epidural anesthesia can be problematic in preterm labor due to the uncertainty that women having contractions are in labor, prolongation of the latent phase of labor, and last, rapid progression through labor. It is therefore advisable to initiate epidural anesthesia early.[4]

When vaginal delivery is imminent, combined spinal-epidural (CSE) analgesia may be preferred in contrast to a single-shot spinal technique. Although both provide quick pain relief and perineal relaxation, if forceps or emergent cesarean delivery is required, CSE decreases the risk of undergoing emergent general anesthesia.

If cesarean delivery is warranted, it remains preferable to resort to a neuraxial technique to avoid the depressant effects of agents used with general anesthesia. However, if there is insufficient time to perform the aforementioned techniques, administration of general anesthesia for preterm cesarean delivery is largely the same as that for full-term deliveries.[4]

To date, while animal data show neuronal apoptosis following general anesthetic exposure, there is no substantial evidence that a general anesthetic administered to a human mother of a preterm fetus could have dire consequences for fetal or child brain development.[1,2]

## POSTOPERATIVE

Removal time for the catheter should be immediately after delivery, but a 24-hour postoperative follow-up should be done to assess headache, mobility, bowel and bladder control, and paresthesias or weakness.

## REFERENCES

1. Suresh M, et al. *Shnider and Levinson's Anesthesia for Obstetrics.* Lippincott Williams & Wilkins; December 10, 2012.
2. American College of Obstetricians and Gynecologists. Practice bulletin no. 171: management of preterm labor. *Obstet Gynecol.* 2016;128(4):e155.
3. Goldenberg RL. The management of preterm labor. *Obstet Gynecol.* 2002;100(5):1020–1037.
4. Chestnut DH, et al. *Chestnut's Obstetric Anesthesia: Principles and Practice.* Elsevier Saunders; 2014.

# 322.

# TRIAL OF LABOR AFTER CESAREAN DELIVERY

*Piotr Al-Jindi and Nasir Hussain*

## INTRODUCTION

(trial of labor after cesarean, TOLAC) is a trial of labor in women who have had a previous cesarean delivery regardless of the mode of delivery. This does not mean the trial ended in successful vaginal delivery.

Vaginal birth after cesarean (VBAC) is a vaginal birth after a previous cesarean delivery. The VBAC rates have been increasing, from 2% in the 1980s to 13.3% in 2018 (up 7% from 2016).

Cesarean section rates have plateaued around 32% in the United States.[1] It is a sharp increase from 5% in 1970. This was due to the introduction of fetal heart rate monitoring and a decrease in operative vaginal deliveries. In the 1990s, the number of TOLAC was going up, as were reports of uterine rupture and complications associated with TOLAC. This resulted in the drop of VBAC rates from 28.3% to 8.5% in 2006, and cesarean section rates went up to 31%. In 2010, the National Institutes of Health (NIH) had a consensus conference, during which it was found that many females undergoing repeated cesarean section were candidates for TOLAC and successful VBAC.[2]

Repeated cesarean deliveries carry the risk of increased maternal mortality, related to abnormal placentation (placenta accreta and placenta previa), uterine rupture, massive transfusion, hysterectomy, and prolonged hospital stay. These risks increase with the number of subsequent cesareansections.[2]

## MATERNAL RISKS AND OUTCOME

Use of TOLAC provides an option for the delivering mother to experience a vaginal delivery. Those who successfully achieve a VBAC have a lower maternal mortality (related to avoidance of surgery and its risks and complications), hysterectomy, maternal fever, and shorter hospital stays, but increased risk of uterine rupture, blood transfusion, and perinatal mortality. Reports showed that the chance of having a VBAC after a TOLAC is around 75%.[1]

The incidence of uterine rupture with TOLAC is 0.8%, which is higher than in the repeated cesarean section group, 0.16%,[3] and this incidence increases with subsequent cesarean sections and pregnancies. So, to summarize the risk, maternal morbidity is lower when VBAC is successful, slightly higher when elective repeat cesarean delivery (ERCD) is done, and the highest when a patient with TOLAC needs a cesarean delivery.

## NEONATAL RISKS AND OUTCOMES

The NIH panel in 2010 concluded that the neonatal mortality rate is increased with TOLAC when compared with ERCD (110 deaths/100,000 vs. 50/100,000). It also concluded that there is insufficient evidence to determine whether there is a substantial difference between neonates born via repeat cesarean section or TOLAC when it comes to respiratory complications.

## SELECTION CRITERIA

The classic uterine incision is a vertical incision in the upper uterus. This incision is associated with a high risk of uterine rupture during a subsequent pregnancy (6%–10%) and is often associated with significant mortality and morbidity for the mother and the fetus. It is rarely performed now and is reserved for cases when the fetus position or placental implantation is abnormal. Most obstetricians prefer to make a low transverse uterine incision, which carries the lowest risk during subsequent pregnancies and has the highest healing rates.

The greatest predictor for a successful VBAC is a previous successful VBAC (2, 3). It is also noted that spontaneous labor and prior vaginal delivery will increase the probability of successful VBAC. A calculator for the likelihood of VBAC is available online.[4] The America College of Obstetricians and Gynecologists (ACOG) recommends that women with at least a 60%–70% chance of successful VBAC undergo TOLAC since they have equal or fewer complications undergoing TOLAC than a repeated cesarean section.[2] The ACOG concluded that most women with one previous cesarean delivery with a low transverse incision are candidates for TOLAC. History of dystocia, the need for labor induction, and maternal obesity are associated with lower success rates for TOLAC.[2]

The ACOG states that it is reasonable to offer TOLAC for patients with two low transverse cesarean deliveries. Data regarding the risk of TOLAC in females with more than two cesarean sections is limited. Macrosomia, twin pregnancy, gestation beyond 40 weeks, previous low vertical incision, and high body mass index should not be contraindications for TOLAC if vaginal delivery is not contraindicated otherwise.[2]

Misoprostol (prostaglandins) used for induction of labor was found to increase the risk of uterine rupture during TOLAC. Other induction agents have been shown to decrease the incidence of successful VBAC after TOLAC, but this finding was not consistent in all studies.[2]

## CONTRAINDICATIONS

Previous classic or T-shape incision or extensive uterine surgery, previous uterine rupture, a medical or obstetric complication that precludes labor and vaginal delivery, and inability to perform an emergency cesarean delivery are contraindications to TOLAC.[2]

## ANESTHESIA CONSIDERATIONS

### PREOPERATIVE

Preoperatively, all females who undergo TOLAC should have early large-bore intravenous access, and blood products should be immediately available.

Continuous fetal heart tone monitoring is recommended because it is the best mode for detecting uterine rupture, with severe bradycardia the most sensitive sign of uterine rupture. Intrauterine pressure monitoring was not found to detect uterine rupture.[2] Symptoms of uterine rupture include, but are not limited to, increased abdominal pain, fetal heart rate abnormalities, especially fetal bradycardia, bleeding, loss of fetal station, and palpable uterine defects. Not all cases of uterine rupture are apparent.[4]

Epidural analgesia does not decrease the likelihood of successful VBAC, and it does not mask the signs of uterine rupture. Sudden onset of pain during successful epidural analgesia might be a sign of uterine rupture.[2] Ultrasound might be helpful in diagnosis.

### INTRAOPERATIVE

If a uterine rupture is suspected, intraoperative efforts should concentrate on saving the mother and the fetus. Oxytocin should be stopped immediately. Tocolytics can be used, but they can exacerbate the hypotension. These patients require emergency cesarean section; there is a concern that the epidural will attenuate the physiological response to hemorrhage and can worsen the hypotension. However, most lower segment dehiscence does not lead to hemorrhage.

Invasive hemodynamic monitoring may be required and should be dictated by the stability of the patient. These cases might be associated with severe blood loss and massive transfusion, and in some cases, a hysterectomy may be required.[5]

## POSTOPERATIVE

Postoperative efforts should be concentrated on hemodynamic stability and monitoring the patient for bleeding.

## REFERENCES

1. Osterman MJK. Recent trends in vaginal birth after cesarean delivery: United States, 2016–2018. NCHS Data Brief No. 359, March 2020. Accessed August 2020. https://www.cdc.gov/nchs/products/databriefs/db359.htm?fbclid=IwAR1fwYKPz0lP80mvwVA5hlannuekSwSZOzgy7NrABiUYcO8n-W1s89F2bjk

2. Practice bulletin no. 184: vaginal birth after cesarean delivery. *Obstet Gynecol.* 2017;130:e217–e233.

3. Mercer BM, et al. Labor outcomes with increasing number of prior vaginal births after cesarean delivery. *Obstet Gynecol.* 2008;111:285–291.

4. Vaginal birth after cesarean. VABC online calculator. https://mfmunetwork.bsc.gwu.edu/web/mfmunetwork/vaginal-birth-after-cesarean-calculator

5. Goynumer G, et al. Spontaneous uterine rupture during a second trimester pregnancy with a history of laparoscopic myomectomy. *J Obstet Gynaecol Res.* 2009;35(6):1132–1135.

# 323.

# MULTIPLE GESTATION

*Steven Knoblock and Joshua D. Younger*

## INTRODUCTION

The United States has roughly 3.7 million births per year according to National Center for Health Statistics. Of these births, roughly 127,000 births were the result of multiple-gestation pregnancies. Since 2005 the rate of multiple gestations has increased by 70%. It is important to become familiar with the needs and challenges a multiple-gestation pregnancy may present. An anesthesia provider in the obstetric environment is tasked with not only caring for the laboring patient, but also tailoring an anesthetic for the most desirable outcomes for the expectant multiples. This necessitates familiarity with how a multiple-gestation pregnancy physiologically differs from a single gestation. It is also essential to acknowledge the fetal effects of a multiple-gestation pregnancy. Last, anesthesia optimization in the setting of multiple gestation is critical to the success during the labor and delivery course.

A multiple-gestation pregnancy is the result of one of two scenarios. The first is when a single fertilized ovum divides into two or more ova, resulting in what is called a monozygotic twin pregnancy. The second scenario is when two or more ova are fertilized, resulting in a single pregnancy called a dizygotic twin pregnancy. When considering the type of multiple pregnancy, either monozygotic or dizygotic, a provider is often concerned with the placenta of each fetus. There are four types of placentations for a multiple-gestation pregnancy: (1) dichorionic diamniotic fused placentae; (2) dichorionic diamniotic separate placentae; (3) monochorionic diamniotic; and (4) monochorionic monoamniotic. In all dizygotic multiple-gestation pregnancies, the placenta is dichorionic diamniotic. The placenta presentation is important because it is a determinant of potential vascular complications, such as twin-to-twin transfusion reactions and cord complications.

Umbilical cord accidents resulting in higher rates of intrauterine fetal death are usually associated with monochorionic placentations. Vascular communication is extremely rare with dichorionic placentations. In all monochorionic placentations, a vascular communication takes place to some degree.

Unfortunately, multiple-gestation pregnancies are not immune to other non-vascular–related complications. There are multiple fetal complications associated with multiple gestations. As stated, intrauterine growth restriction can be related to vascular abnormalities, but it can also be a result of polyhydramnios within one fetal sac. This can limit the intrauterine size and growth of the second fetus. Independently, limited uterine size may also be a factor. Both fetuses are also subject to the risks of intrauterine growth restriction associated with single pregnancies.

Preterm labor is when a child is born prior to 37 weeks. Preterm labor is more common with a multiple-gestation pregnancy. Twin pregnancies that are a result of in vitro fertilization experience preterm labor at a rate of 52%. Only 6% of triplets reach full term. These pregnancies often receive tocolytic therapies. Anesthetic consideration is imperative during tocolytic therapy due to certain risks these agents may have on the patient. Risks associated with tocolytic agents may include a higher risk for postpartum hemorrhage and pulmonary edema.

Also, fetal presentation during multiple gestations warrants attention. In order to accommodate multiple gestations, a fetus may be found in an abnormal presentation, leading to increased risk of umbilical cord prolapse. In this case, there is an increase in fetal morbidity and mortality. In summary, fetal mortality in the setting of twin pregnancy is four times higher than for a single-gestation pregnancy. Potential concern and complications for both mother and fetuses continue to increase with the number of gestations, mostly due to preterm labor; however, other contributing factors include twin-to-twin transfusion, congenital malformations, preeclampsia, malpresentation, and/or prolapsed umbilical cord.

Emphasis should also be directed toward the female physiologic changes that occur with pregnancy. These changes are often accelerated and exaggerated with multiple gestations. Anesthetic consideration is significant not only during the labor and delivery setting but also in the surgical setting in the case of elective/emergency procedures. The cardiovascular status of a mother carrying multiples has an increased cardiac output of 20% in comparison to a single-gestation pregnancy. This is due to an increase in stroke volume of 15% and heart rate by 3.5%. Due to the increase in uterine size, aortocaval compression and supine hypotension syndrome are more likely to occur.

The increased uterine size during multiple-gestational pregnancies affects the pulmonary status to varying degrees. As the uterus increases in size, it pushes cephalad on the thoracic cavity. This leads to a decrease in lung volume and capacity. Increased total metabolic rate occurring during pregnancy coupled with a decreased functional residual capacity results in serious risk of hypoxia. This can occur more quickly during periods of apnea and hypoventilation.

When comparing a pregnant mother carrying multiples to a single gestation, there is an enhanced displacement of the stomach in the cephalad direction. This leads to an even higher risk for aspiration. Airway changes can also occur due to increase in weight, especially after 30 weeks of pregnancy. The threat of aspiration and overall airway changes necessitates the anesthesia provider to be thorough and prepared when approaching any anesthetic being administered.

Multiple gestations increase a mother's risks for mortality and morbidity. Maternal mortality and morbidity increase in proportion to the number of fetuses a woman carries. Common maternal complications associated with multiple gestations are: preterm delivery, congenital anomalies, polyhydramnios, umbilical cord prolapse, intrauterine growth restriction, twin-to-twin transfusion, and malpresentation..

The delivery method for a multiple-gestation pregnancy is usually based on fetal age and the position of the first child that is expected to be delivered (twin A). When both twins are in the vertex position, a vaginal birth is usually attempted. If twin A is in the breach or shoulder-first position, a cesarean section is usually preferred. An anesthesia provider should beware if twin A is in the breach position and twin B is in the vertex position. When this occurs, the chin of each twin may become interlocked during a vaginal delivery, leading to devastating results.

There are multiple anesthetic considerations to be accounted for when caring for a multiple-gestation delivery. An operating room is often desirable for delivery as it allows for a quick abdominal surgical approach if required. Epidural anesthesia has been found to be the ideal form of analgesia for these patients. A lumbar epidural has the advantage of providing quality analgesia for a laboring patient, with the option to quickly address a change in anesthetic plan if a cesarean section is required. If there is any doubt in the placement or quality of effectiveness of an epidural catheter, replacement of the catheter should be done prior to delivery. An anesthetic level around T8 to T6 with an increased concentration of local anesthetic solution is desirable when delivery is about to take place. This provides adequate anesthesia for an internal podalic version and breach extraction of twin B. An epidural catheter also has the ability to provide analgesia for prolonged labor, where other forms of neuraxial anesthetics may fall short. There is an increased risk for blood loss during multiple-gestation deliveries. With each additional fetus, there is an estimated increased risk of 500 mL blood loss. This is often due to increased uterine atony from advanced uterine distention and prolonged delivery times. As technology has improved to allow for advanced fetal monitoring, safe delivery times between twin delivery has increased up to 134 minutes. An anesthesia provider should ensure the laboring mother has at least two intravenous access points, a blood type and screen, and a complete blood count drawn on admission.

## REFERENCES

1. Hamilton BE, et al. Population and vital statistics report. In: *Statistical Papers—United Nations (Ser. A), Population and Vital Statistics Report*. United Nations; 2020. doi:10.18356/6412774e-en
2. Hawkins JL. Abnormal presentation and multiple gestation. In: Chestnut DH, Nathan N, eds. *Chestnut's Obstetric Anesthesia: Principles and Practice*, 6th ed. Philadelphia, PA: Elsevier; 2020:822–839.
3. Frolick MA. Obstetric anesthesia. In: Butterworth JF IV, Mackey DC, Wasnick JD, eds. *Morgan & Mikhail's Clinical Anesthesiology*, 6th ed. New York, NY: McGraw-Hill Education; 2018:861–896.
4. Braveman FR, Scavone BM, Blessing ME, Wong CA. Obstetric anesthesia. In: Barash PG, Cullen BF, Stoelting RK, et al. *Clinical Anesthesia*, 8th ed. Philadelphia, PA: Wolters Kluwer; 2017:1144–1177.

# 324.

# NEONATAL RESUSCITATION

## *Irim Salik and Tara Doherty*

## INTRODUCTION

The successful transition from intrauterine to extrauterine life is dependent on physiologic changes that occur following delivery. Most newborns are able to make this transition without assistance, but 10% of all newborns need some intervention, and 1% require extensive resuscitation measures.[1] Infants more likely to require resuscitation can be identified by risk factors, including advanced or very young maternal age, maternal diabetes mellitus, hypertension, or previous history of fetal demise. Placental anomalies, delivery complications, prematurity, postmaturity, congenital anomalies, or multiple gestations also increase risk of intervention. Evidence presented at the 2015 International Consensus on Cardiopulmonary Resuscitation and Emergency Cardiovascular Care Science with Treatment Recommendations (CoSTR) is presented in this chapter.[2]

## INITIAL STEPS

There are three important questions that can be utilized to identify whether newborns will require resuscitation: Did the baby have a term gestation? Does the neonate have good tone? Is the infant breathing or crying? If the answer to any of these questions is "no," the infant should be moved to a radiant warmer to receive one or more of the following four interventions: (1) warming, drying, stimulation, and maintenance of normothermia and positioning of the airway with clearing of secretions if they are copious or obstructing the airway; (2) ventilation and oxygenation; (3) initiation of chest compressions; and (4) administration of medication and/or volume resuscitation as appropriate. Initial steps of newborn resuscitation include normothermia maintenance, positioning of the infant's head in a "sniffing" position to open the airway, clearing secretions with a bulb syringe or suction catheter, drying, and stimulation of the infant to breathe. Approximately 60 seconds, or "the golden minute," is allocated for completion of initial steps, reevaluation, and ventilation, if required. It is imperative to avoid an unnecessary delay in the initiation of ventilation, as this is the most important step for successful neonatal resuscitation in an infant unresponsive to initial steps. Progression beyond initial steps is based on heart rate less than 100 beats/min and labored respirations, including apnea or gasping (Figure 324.1).

## TEMPERATURE REGULATION

Preterm infants are especially prone to hypothermia, associated with increased risk of intraventricular hemorrhage (IVH), respiratory depression, hypoglycemia, and late-onset sepsis.[3] Therefore, neonatal admission temperature

# Resuscitation Algorithm for Neonates

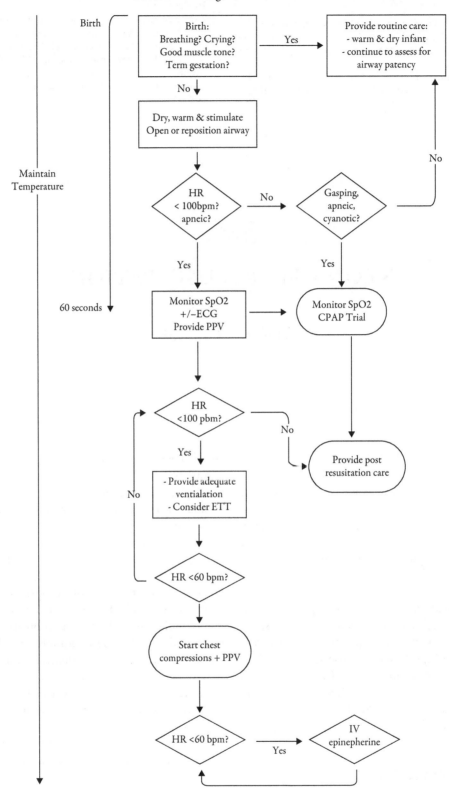

**Figure 324.1** Neonatal resuscitation.

is recorded as an outcome predictor and quality indicator. Temperature of newborns should be maintained between 36.5°C and 37.5°C after birth through admission via the utilization of radiant warmers, plastic wrap, a head cap, increased room temperature, thermal mattresses, and warmed and humidified resuscitation gases. Historically, slower rewarming was recommended to avoid complications, including apnea and arrhythmias in neonates, but there is insufficient current evidence to recommend a preference for either rapid (0.5°C/h or greater) or slow (less than 0.5°C/h) rewarming. For infants born at greater than 36 weeks of gestation with moderate-to-severe hypoxic-ischemic encephalopathy, therapeutic hypothermia should be offered.

## AIRWAY CLEARANCE

If a newborn's airway is obstructed or positive pressure ventilation (PPV) is required, suctioning with a bulb syringe or suction catheter should be considered. Unnecessary nasopharyngeal suctioning should be avoided as it can elicit reflex bradycardia. Meconium-stained amniotic fluid may indicate fetal distress in a neonate. In an infant with meconium-stained amniotic fluid who presents with poor muscle tone or inadequate respiratory effort, initial resuscitation steps should be completed under the radiant warmer. With a heart rate less than 100 beats/min or respiratory embarrassment, PPV should be initiated. Routine intubation for tracheal suctioning in infants with meconium staining is not suggested as there is insufficient evidence to continue this practice, and infants may benefit from the avoidance of an intubation attempt.[2]

## HEART RATE ASSESSMENT

Following delivery, assessment of neonatal heart rate is utilized to evaluate the effectiveness of spontaneous respiratory effort and determine the need for subsequent intervention. An increase in a newborn's heart rate is considered the most sensitive indicator of successful response to an intervention during resuscitation. The three-lead electrocardiogram (ECG) is considered to be a more reliable measure of neonatal heart rate than pulse oximetry during the first minute of life.[4] Pulse oximetry can underestimate a newborn's heart rate and lead to potentially unnecessary interventions. The use of ECG is adjunctive and does not replace the need for pulse oximetry to evaluate a newborn's oxygenation.

## OXYGENATION ASSESSMENT AND OXYGEN ADMINISTRATION

Pulse oximetry should be utilized when resuscitation is anticipated, if PPV is administered, when central cyanosis persists beyond 5 to 10 minutes of life, or when supplementary oxygen is administered.[2] In apneic infants, administration of PPV is the standard recommended treatment via a flow-inflating or self-inflating resuscitation bag or T-piece resuscitator. If PPV is administered to preterm neonates, use of 5 cm $H_2O$ positive end-expiratory pressure is suggested. Resuscitation of infants less than 35 weeks' gestational age should be initiated with low $FiO_2$ (fraction of inspired air; 21% to 30%) as the oxygen concentration is titrated to achieve preductal oxygen saturation in the interquartile range measured in healthy term infants.[3]

## UMBILICAL CORD MANAGEMENT

During the 2010 CoSTR review, it was revealed that delayed cord clamping (DCC) may be beneficial for infants who do not require immediate resuscitation at birth.[3] Although overall mortality or long-term outcomes are not affected by DCC, it may be associated with reduced incidence of IVH, less need for transfusion requirements after birth, improved initial mean arterial pressure, and a decreased incidence of necrotizing enterocolitis. Unfortunately, DCC does cause hyperbilirubinemia, associated with increased need for phototherapy. National recommendations indicate that DCC for greater than 30 seconds should be practiced in both term and preterm infants who do not require resuscitation at birth.

## AIRWAY MANAGEMENT

Laryngeal mask airways (LMAs) fit over the laryngeal inlet and facilitate ventilation in infants born at 34 weeks of gestation or weighing greater than 2000 g. An LMA is utilized as an alternative to intubation if a face mask is unsuccessful at effective ventilation or if tracheal intubation is unsuccessful or not feasible. LMA use has not been evaluated during chest compressions or for the administration of emergency medications. Endotracheal tube placement is indicated during neonatal resuscitation when bag-mask ventilation is ineffective or prolonged, if chest compressions are utilized, or for special circumstances, including an infant with congenital diaphragmatic hernia. When PPV is provided through an appropriately placed endotracheal tube, a prompt increase in heart rate is commonly seen. Exhaled end-tidal $CO_2$ ($ETCO_2$) detection remains the most reliable method of confirmation for endotracheal tube placement. $ETCO_2$ may not be detected in a neonate suffering from cardiac arrest despite appropriate tube placement.

## CONTINUOUS POSITIVE AIRWAY PRESSURE

A number of randomized controlled trials with 2358 preterm infants indicated that for infants born at less than

30 weeks of gestation, continuous positive airway pressure (CPAP) may be beneficial, as opposed to endotracheal intubation and PPV.[5] The use of CPAP resulted in decreased rate of intubation in the delivery room, reduced duration of mechanical ventilation with decreased mortality and bronchopulmonary dysplasia, and no significant increase in air leak or severe IVH. Spontaneously breathing preterm infants with respiratory distress may be supported with CPAP rather than routine intubation for administering PPV.

## CHEST COMPRESSIONS

Chest compressions are indicated in an infant with heart rate less than 60 beats/min despite adequate ventilation with an endotracheal tube. Because ventilation is of primary importance in neonatal resuscitation, rescuers should ensure that assisted ventilation is optimally delivered during initiation of chest compressions.[2] Compressions are delivered on the lower third of the sternum to a depth of approximately one-third of the anteroposterior diameter of the chest. The two techniques commonly utilized are the two-thumb technique or the two-finger technique. Compression with two thumbs involves the rescuer encircling the chest and supporting the back. This is the preferred technique as it generates higher blood pressure and coronary perfusion pressure with reduced rescuer fatigue. Although the rescuer's thumbs should not leave the chest, the newborn's chest should be allowed to reexpand fully during relaxation. The two-finger technique involves compression with two fingers with a second hand supporting the back. The compression-to-ventilation ratio should be 3:1, with 90 compressions and 30 breaths to achieve 120 events per minute to maximize ventilation.[3]

## MEDICATIONS AND VOLUME EXPANSION

Drugs are not commonly indicated in newborn resuscitation. Bradycardia is usually the result of inadequate lung inflation or profound hypoxemia, and ensuring adequate ventilation is generally the most useful means for correction. If the neonate's heart rate remains less than 60 beats/min despite adequate ventilation with 100% oxygen via an endotracheal tube and chest compressions, administration of epinephrine, or volume, or both is indicated.[2]

Hypoglycemia has been associated with an increased risk for brain injury, while hyperglycemia may be protective in neonates. There is currently no recommended target glucose concentration in infants. Intravenous administration of epinephrine should be given at a dose of 0.01 to 0.03 mg/kg of 1:10,000 epinephrine. If intravenous access is not yet established, a dose of 0.05 to 0.1 mg/kg can be given through the endotracheal tube. In a neonate with signs of hypovolemia, including pale skin, weak pulse, or poor perfusion, volume expansion can be considered if the heart rate has not responded adequately to other resuscitative measures. Blood or an isotonic crystalloid solution can be considered at a dose of 10 mL/kg, which can be repeated if necessary. Rapid volume expansion should be avoided in preterm infants as it can lead to IVH.[2]

## DISCONTINUING RESUSCITATION

An Apgar score (based on muscle tone, pulse, reflex irritability, skin color, and respirations) of 0 at 10 minutes is a strong predictor of morbidity and mortality in preterm and term infants alike. Following 10 minutes of resuscitation, if the heart rate remains undetectable, it is appropriate to cease assisted ventilation. However, the decision to discontinue resuscitation should be based on each patient's unique circumstances. Resources and factors, including availability of advanced neonatal care, including therapeutic hypothermia; timing of insult; parental wishes; and whether the resuscitation was optimal should be thoroughly assessed.

## REFERENCES

1. Wyckoff MH, et al. Part 13: neonatal resuscitation: 2015 American Heart Association guidelines update for cardiopulmonary resuscitation and emergency cardiovascular care. *Circulation*. 2015;132:S543.
2. Wyllie J, et al.; on behalf of the Neonatal Resuscitation Chapter Collaborators. Part 7: neonatal resuscitation: 2015 international consensus on cardiopulmonary resuscitation and emergency cardiovascular care science with treatment recommendations. *Resuscitation*. 2015;95:e171–e203.
3. Perlman JM, et al. Neonatal resuscitation chapter. Part 11: neonatal resuscitation: international consensus on cardiopulmonary resuscitation and emergency cardiovascular care science with treatment recommendations. *Circulation*. 2010;122:S516–538.
4. Mizumoto H, et al. Electrocardiogram shows reliable heart rates much earlier than pulse oximetry during neonatal resuscitation. *Pediatr Int*. 2012;54:205–207.
5. Dunn MS et al.; Vermont Oxford Network DRM Study Group. Randomized trial comparing 3 approaches to the initial respiratory management of preterm neonates. *Pediatrics*. 2011;128:e1069–e1076.

# 325.

# APGAR SCORING

*Muhammad Fayyaz Ahmed and Ihab Kamel*

## INTRODUCTION

The Apgar scoring system is a simple and sensitive method for neonatal assessment at 1 minute and 5 minutes after delivery. Apgar scoring is performed while care is being delivered. The Apgar scoring consists of five components that are evaluated at 1 and 5 minutes after birth and may undergo further scoring at 10 minutes if the initial scores are low.[1] The five components of the Apgar scoring system are **a**ppearance, **p**ulse, **g**rimace, **a**ctivity, and **r**espiration. A score of 0, 1, or 2 is assigned for each of these five entities (Table 325.1). A total score of 8 to 10 is normal, a score of 4 to 7 indicates moderate impairment, and a score of 0 to 3 is a sign of fetal distress requiring immediate resuscitation. The Neonatal Encephalopathy and Neurologic Outcome report defined a 5-minute Apgar score of 7 to 10 as reassuring and a score of 4 to 6 as moderately abnormal. A score of 0 to 3 is defined as low in the term infant and late-preterm infant and is considered a nonspecific sign of illness, which may be one of the first indications of encephalopathy.[2]

## IMPORTANCE OF THE APGAR SCORE

The Apgar scoring helps predict mortality and neurologic morbidity in the population of infants. An Apgar score that remains 3 or less at 10, 15, and 20 minutes is predictive of a poor neurologic outcome. An Apgar score that remains 0 beyond 10 minutes of age is useful in determining the need to continue with resuscitative efforts as very few infants with an Apgar score of 0 at 10 minutes have been reported to survive with a normal neurological outcome.[2]

The 1-minute and 5-minute Apgar scores of 0 to 3 have been shown to correlate with neonatal mortality in a large population but do not predict *individual* mortality or future neurologic dysfunction. However, based on *population* studies, a low 5-minute Apgar score clearly relates to an increased relative risk of cerebral palsy, reported to be as high as 20- to 100-fold over that of infants with a 5-minute Apgar score of 7 to 10.[2] The majority of infants with low Apgar scores will not develop cerebral palsy.

Factors affecting the Apgar score include antenatal drug exposure, gestational age, maternal sedation or anesthesia, preterm delivery, congenital anomalies, neuromuscular diseases, trauma, manipulation at delivery, and subjectivity. It is unlikely that peripartum hypoxia-ischemia is a cause of neonatal encephalopathy if the Apgar score at 5 minutes is 7 or greater.

## LIMITATIONS

The Apgar scoring system is a reporting of the neonate's physiologic condition at a point in time, and it includes

*Table 325.1* **APGAR SCORING SYSTEM**

| | PARAMETERS | 0 | 1 | 2 |
|---|---|---|---|---|
| A | Appearance (skin color) | Blue or pale | Pink body, blue extremities | Pink |
| P | Pulse (heart rate, beats/min) | Absent | <100 beats/min | >100 beats/min |
| G | Grimace (reflex irritability) | No response to stimulation | Grimace on aggressive stimulation | Cough, sneezes, or cries with stimulation |
| A | Activity (muscle tone) | Flaccid, floppy, limp | Some flexion of extremities | Active spontaneous movement |
| R | Respiration | Absent | Irregular, slow, or shallow respiration; weak cry | Normal rate and effort; good cry |

subjective components. Although it is widely used to assess neonates at birth, it does not replace a detailed physical examination and serial evaluation of the neonate after birth. Low Apgar scores alone do not provide sufficient evidence of perinatal asphyxia; rather, Apgar scores can be affected for a variety of reasons, as mentioned previously. Preterm infants also often have low Apgar scores despite the presence of normal umbilical cord blood gas and pH measurements; therefore, the assessment of umbilical cord blood may be especially helpful in the evaluation of preterm neonates.

## ANESTHESIA EFFECT ON THE APGAR SCORE

The impact of regional versus general anesthesia on the Apgar score has been studied extensively. While some studies reported no difference in Apgar scores, others have shown that general anesthesia is associated with lower Apgar scores and worse outcome. However, some studies reported an association between neonatal acidosis and regional anesthesia, which may be related to the use of ephedrine to support maternal blood pressure. In a large retrospective review, general anesthesia was associated with lower Apgar scores at 1 and 5 minutes and with greater requirements for intubation and artificial ventilation compared to regional anesthesia. There were no differences in neonatal death rates.[3] Another study comparing general anesthesia with spinal anesthesia for elective cesarean delivery at term showed no difference in Apgar scores and short-term neonatal outcomes.[4] Epidural anesthesia was associated with higher Apgar scores in a randomized study comparing general anesthesia and epidural anesthesia for cesarean delivery at term.[4] Existing data and clinical reports suggest that general anesthesia is associated with lower neonatal Apgar scores and lower resuscitation rates. However, the long-term clinical significance of these findings is unclear.

## ANESTHETIC CONSIDERATIONS

### PREOPERATIVE

Preoperatively, each patient should be evaluated clinically for the best anesthetic choice.

### INTRAOPERATIVE

Intraoperatively, if a cesarean delivery is performed under general anesthesia, rapid delivery of the fetus is recommended. Maintenance of maternal blood pressure close to baseline during cesarean delivery is helpful to optimize fetal perfusion and oxygenation. This can be achieved by maintaining left uterine displacement, using phenylephrine infusion and boluses, and administering adequate intravenous colloid and crystalloid loads during induction of anesthesia. During cesarean delivery under general anesthesia, it is prudent to avoid excessive induction doses of anesthetic agents given that the anesthetic requirements are decreased during pregnancy and minimize induction-to-delivery time.

### POSTOPERATIVE

A newborn infant with an Apgar score of 5 or less at 5 minutes, obtaining an umbilical arterial blood gas sample from a clamped section of the umbilical cord and submitting the placenta for pathologic examination should be considered postoperatively.

## REFERENCES

1. American Academy of Pediatrics Committee on Fetus and Newborn, American College of Obstetricians and Gynecologists Committee on Obstetric Practice. The Apgar score. *Pediatrics*. 2015;136(4):819–822.
2. Ong BY, et al. Anesthesia for cesarean section—effects on neonates. *Anesth Analg*. 1989;68: 270–275.
3. Kavak ZN, et al. Short-term outcome of newborn infants: spinal versus general anesthesia for elective cesarean section. A prospective randomized study. *Eur J Obstet Gynecol*. 2001;100:50–54.
4. Sener EB, et al. Comparison of neonatal effects of epidural and general anesthesia for cesarean section. *Gynecol Obstet Invest*. 2003;55:41–45.

# 326.

# UMBILICAL CORD BLOOD GAS

*Pritee Tarwade and Christine Acho*

## INTRODUCTION

Umbilical cord blood gas analysis was first described by James et al. in 1958; since then it has been widely studied and is now recommended in all high-risk deliveries by both British and American College of Obstetrics and Gynecology. Umbilical cord gas along with the Apgar score are two of the most common tools used to assess fetal well-being.

## UMBILICAL CORD ANATOMY

Oxygenated blood is carried from the mother to the fetus via a single, large umbilical vein. Deoxygenated blood is carried from the fetus to the mother via umbilical arteries. If there is difficulty in obtaining a sample from the umbilical arteries, it is common to access the umbilical vein for a cord gas sample. Usually, the umbilical cord has a single larger umbilical vein and two smaller umbilical arteries. Because of the size, the umbilical vein is easier to access than the artery. Hence, when sampling is difficult and only one sample is achieved, it is usually a venous sample. It is not always easy to differentiate between umbilical venous and arterial cord gas samples.

**Technique of Sampling:** Umbilical artery blood is more reflective of fetal metabolism compared to umbilical venous blood, which is more reflective of the placental function. Almost immediately after delivery, a 10- to 20-cm segment of umbilical cord is doubly clamped, and blood is drawn from this segment. A heparinized syringe is used to collect the sample, and blood is sent to the laboratory immediately. If delay is anticipated in sending the sample to the laboratory, it is kept on ice. The sample can also be obtained from a clamped umbilical cord segment kept at room temperature for no more than 20 minutes. If the sample is acquired more than 20 minutes later, up to 90 minutes, values can be estimated based on the multiple studies done to observe the rate of fall of pH over time. If kept at room temperature for over 60 minutes, arterial or venous pH can fall by more than 0.2 pH units.

However, if the cord is doubly clamped at birth and kept aside at room temperature, these changes are not marked at the end of 1 hour. Hence, whenever there is a delay in sampling the blood gas, it is important to know if the blood was drawn from isolated cord or cord connected to the placenta (as there is continuous metabolism occurring in the placenta).

**Effect of Delayed Cord Clamping:** All the reference values of umbilical cord arterial and venous blood gas are from samples obtained immediately after birth. However, delayed cord clamping is the preferred management. A number of studies have examined the effect of delayed cord clamping on umbilical blood gas. A systematic review was done recently by Nudelman et al. of two randomized controlled trials and three observational studies. The randomized controlled trials showed samples obtained after delayed cord clamping were slightly more academic than immediate samples, but still fell within the normal range. On the other hand, the observational studies showed that delayed clamping of just 2 minutes had an effect on gas values, but the magnitude of change was clinically insignificant in normal healthy, vaginally delivered newborns.

Do we need both arterial and venous blood gas samples? A normal umbilical vein pH is higher than the umbilical artery pH. For prognostic purposes, either sample should suffice, keeping in mind the normal differences between the two. In cases of fetal distress, both umbilical arterial and venous blood gas should be obtained. Any restriction to umbilical blood flow will widen the gap between arterial and venous values. Placental insufficiencies affect both umbilical arterial and venous blood gases, and there is no difference between the arterial and venous gas. A study done by Johnson et al. comparing infants born after cord prolapse and those after placental abruption found umbilical venoarterial differences in pH up to 0.3 units was observed in cord prolapse compared to 0.15 units in placental abruption.[1] Looking at these data, it is essential to sample both umbilical arterial and venous gas whenever an infant is depressed at birth. In case of umbilical cord obstruction, you can obtain a normal umbilical venous gas concealing severe mixed umbilical arterial acidosis.

*Table 326.1* NORMAL VALUES

| | UMBILICAL ARTERY | UMBILICAL VEIN |
|---|---|---|
| pH | $7.27 \pm 0.069$ | $7.35 \pm 0.05$ |
| $pCO_2$ | $50.5 \pm 11.1$ | $38.2 \pm 5.6$ |
| $pO_2$ | $22.0 \pm 3.6$ | $29.2 \pm 6.9$ |
| $HCO_3$ | $22.3 \pm 2.5$ | $20.4 \pm 2.1$ |

An easy way to remember this is the $PaO_2$ of the umbilical artery, vein, and $PaCO_2$ of the umbilical vein and artery are about 20, 30, 40, and 50, respectively, in that order (Table 326.1).

Umbilical cord blood gas can be a predictor of fetal mortality and morbidity. According to the 197b fetal health surveillance guideline: (1) Ideally, cord blood sampling of both umbilical arterial and umbilical venous blood is recommended for *all* births for quality assurance and improvement purposes. If only one sample is possible, it should preferably be arterial (III-B). (2) When risk factors for adverse perinatal outcome exist or when intervention for fetal indications occurs, sampling of arterial and venous cord gases is strongly recommended.[2]

Multiple studies have looked at cord blood gases as a tool to predict fetal morbidity and mortality along with other tools, like the Apgar score and fetal scalp studies. One such study looked at 7789 patients with paired umbilical cord $PaO_2$; 106 patients (1.4%) had a composite neonatal morbidity. The $PaO_2$ was significantly lower in patients with neonatal morbidity compared to those without ($p < .001$), but the $PaO_2$ was a poor predictor of morbidity.[3] Most of the studies have consistently showed a relationship between fetal morbidity and umbilical gas abnormalities but have failed to show its value, if any, as a predictor of morbidity.

## ANESTHESIA IMPLICATIONS

For a long time, efforts have been made to study if the types of labor analgesia or anesthesia make any difference in the fetal acid-base balance. A meta-analysis published in 2006 concluded that umbilical artery pH was lower in patients with spinal anesthesia compared to those who received either general or epidural anesthesia. However, a retrospective study done by Duke University, which included 1064 patients who underwent cesarean section, found the type of anesthesia was an important predictor of lower umbilical artery pH in patients undergoing emergent cesarean sections. Patients who received general anesthesia had lower umbilical artery pH when compared to those who had either a spinal or epidural anesthetic. For nonemergency cesarean sections, no differences were noted.[4] An important point to keep in mind is that general anesthesia is typically used in an emergency situation where fetal distress is already present, independent of the anesthetic employed.

Another retrospective cohort study looked at all the elective scheduled cesarean sections between 2014 and 2017 under spinal anesthesia. Stepwise linear regression was performed to identify predictors of decreasing umbilical arterial pH; the following factors were deemed predictive of decreasing umbilical arterial pH: maternal body mass index, noncephalic presentation, spinal start-to-delivery interval, uterine incision–to-delivery, and maximum reduction in blood pressure from baseline.[5]

Another area where extensive research has been done is choice of vasopressor for spinal-induced hypotension and its effect on umbilical artery acidosis. However, there is insufficient evidence to recommend one vasopressor over the other.

## REFERENCES

1. Johnson JW, Richards DS. The etiology of fetal acidosis as determined by umbilical cord acid-base studies. *Am J Obstet Gynecol.* 1997;177(2):274–282.
2. Liston R, et al. No. 197b-fetal health surveillance: intrapartum consensus guideline. *J Obstet Gynaecol Canada.* 2018;40(4):e298–e322.
3. Raghuraman N, et al. Umbilical cord oxygen content and neonatal morbidity at term. *Am J Perinatol.* 2018;35(4):331–335.
4. Strouch Z, et al. Anesthetic technique for cesarean delivery and neonatal acid–base status: a retrospective database analysis. *Int J Obstet Anesth.* 2015;24(1):22–29.
5. Rimsza RR, et al. Time from neuraxial anesthesia placement to delivery is inversely proportional to umbilical arterial cord pH at scheduled cesarean delivery. *Am J Obstet Gynecol.* 2019;220(4):389.e1–e9.

# 327.

# INTRAUTERINE SURGERY

*Jarna Shah*

## INTRODUCTION

Intrauterine surgery is fraught with many risks and challenges. Some fetal abnormalities are amenable to intervention in the antepartum period. However, often with certain underlying conditions, intervention is required prior to delivery. Techniques utilized include minimally invasive surgery, open fetal surgery, and ex utero intrapartum treatment (EXIT) procedures.[1] Concerns lie with the risks of fetal demise, maternal injury, and the potential fetal teratogenic effects of anesthetics used while performing these procedures.

## OPEN FETAL SURGERY

Open fetal surgery is considered for a few indications, which include severe myelomeningocele, cystic lung lesion, and sacrococcygeal teratoma.[2] Prior to any open fetal surgery, extensive family counseling and multidisciplinary planning is highly recommended.[1] A low transverse hysterotomy incision is made over the abdomen while under general anesthesia. Uterine relaxation is required before the fetus can be manipulated, with careful monitoring of the mother and the fetus. Risks involved with open fetal surgery include placental abruption, pulmonary edema, premature rupture of the membranes, preterm delivery, blood loss requiring transfusions, and fetal demise.

## MINIMALLY INVASIVE FETAL SURGERY

Advances in fetal surgery have allowed for more procedures to be performed either percutaneously or by endoscopic surgery. Indications include laser atrial septostomy, treatment of tracheal occlusions, intrauterine transfusion, selective feticide of a nonviable twin, and laser coagulation of connecting vessels in twin-to-twin transfusion syndrome.[1] Procedures like fetal blood sampling can be performed using ultrasound guidance and do not require general anesthesia; in these cases, a regional anesthetic can be considered.

## EX UTERO INTRAPARTUM TREATMENT PROCEDURES

Ex utero intrapartum treatment is a procedure that is used to deliver babies with airway compression due to cervical teratomas, cystic hygromas, and blockage of the airway.[1] EXIT procedures require profound uterine relaxation to prevent uterine rupture and placental separation. It is usually performed under general anesthesia. Using high-dose volatile anesthetic agents and sometimes intravenous nitroglycerin can accomplish this.[3] However, high concentrations of inhaled anesthetics can result in maternal hypotension. Vasopressors and fluids help promote maternal hemodynamic stability, maintaining uteroplacental perfusion. Risks include uterine atony and significant postoperative maternal blood loss.[1] Tocolytics, such as a magnesium sulfate infusion, can be used to help maintain uterine tone.[1,2]

## ANESTHETIC CONSIDERATIONS

### PREOPERATIVE

The anesthesiologist must complete a thorough history and physical for the mother preoperatively. Another critical component is the airway assessment since pregnancy is often associated with changes in the airway examination. This is due to an increase in body weight, nasal mucosa vascularity, and nasopharyngeal edema.[3] Advanced airway supplies such as video laryngoscopy should be readily available. Underlying respiratory and cardiovascular conditions may require changes to the anesthetic plan. In addition, functional residual capacity decreases by as much as 20% during pregnancy compared to nonpregnant patients. Oxygen consumption and alveolar ventilation are also increased. These patients are likely to desaturate with periods of prolonged apnea. The pregnant patient has a lower minimal alveolar concentration and thus a higher sensitivity to anesthetics.[2]

## INTRAOPERATIVE

During the intraoperative period, the anesthesiologist must consider how best to maintain stable maternal hemodynamics. Uterine perfusion is dependent on maternal blood pressure, and vasopressors such as phenylephrine and ephedrine should be readily available.[3] Adequate fluid resuscitation is also crucial due to expected fluid losses during longer cases. Maintaining appropriate urine output promotes adequate renal perfusion.

## POSTOPERATIVE

Postoperative blood loss due to uterine atony must be treated appropriately and in a timely manner. Resuscitation requires adequate intravenous access and careful monitoring, as patients do not outwardly show signs of decompensation until they have already lost a significant blood volume. Pregnant patients are in a hypercoagulable state, and prophylactic measures such as anticoagulation status should be considered.[2]

## REFERENCES

1. Cunningham G, et al. Fetal therapy. In: Williams Obstetrics. McGraw-Hill Education; 2018.
2. Van de Velde M, De Buck F. Fetal and maternal analgesia/anesthesia for fetal procedures. *Fetal Diagn Ther.* 2012;31(4):201–209.
3. Tran KM, et al. Anesthesia for fetal surgery: miles to go before we sleep. *Anesthesiology.* 2013;118(4):772–774.

# 328.

# ANESTHETIC CONSIDERATIONS IN BREASTFEEDING

*Lora B. Levin and Jeffrey W. Cannon*

## INTRODUCTION

The benefits of breastfeeding are well established. From reduction of pediatric illnesses such as bacteremia and diarrhea to reduction of maternal complications such as postpartum bleeding—breast feeding is unequivocally beneficial in numerous ways.[1] Breast feeding is recommended by the World Health Organization for at least the first 6 months and up to the first 2 years of the child's life.[1] For patients who are breastfeeding, undergoing anesthesia can be a stress-inducing experience. Not only are they concerned about the procedure, but also they are concerned about the implications the anesthesia may have on their ability to breastfeed. It is likely they have heard that they will need to "pump and dump," meaning they discard their breast milk for up to 24 hours after undergoing anesthesia. However, this is not the current recommendation and may cause lactating women to have undue stress regarding the effect of anesthesia on breastfeeding.

Breast milk is the product of synthesis in the mammary gland of female humans. Prolactin is an endogenous hormone that is secreted from the anterior pituitary gland and controls the synthesis of breast milk. Oxytocin is an endogenous hormone that is secreted from the posterior pituitary gland and controls the ejection of breast milk by causing the myoepithelial cells of the mammary gland to contract. Breast milk comprises nutritional components, cytokines, growth factors, antibodies, and other products of lactocytes. This milk is expressed into the lactiferous ducts and sinuses before ultimately being expelled through the areolar pores.

The process of inducing, maintaining, and emerging from anesthesia requires the administration of several different pharmacological agents by various routes: oral, intravenous, and inhalational. When a patient is or will be breastfeeding, a point of primary concern is how exposure to these agents will affect the infant. Drugs diffuse from maternal blood into the breast milk based on several factors, including protein binding, lipid solubility, molecular weight, pKa, and maternal plasma level of the drug. Anesthetic gases, propofol, and narcotics, for instance, are lipophilic and tend to accumulate in adipose tissue until fully eliminated after administration. In fact, all anesthetic and analgesic drugs administered to the mother are secreted in breast milk. The ideal drug would be one with minimal transfer into breast milk, a short elimination half-life, and no active metabolites. The amount of a drug that transfers from mother to infant via breast milk is commonly expressed as the relative infant dose (RID). RID is defined as the

*Table 328.1* RELATIVE INFANT DOSE (RID) OF ANESTHESIA MEDICATIONS AND RECOMMENDATIONS

| MEDICATION CLASS (DRUG) | MEAN RID (%)[a] |
| --- | --- |
| *Anticholinergics* (atropine, glycopyrrolate) | Unknown: generally considered safe with single systemic or ophthalmic dosing |
| *Anticholinesterases* (neostigmine, pyridostigmine) | 0.1 |
| *Antiemetics* (metoclopramide, ondansetron) | Unknown: considered safe due to lack of sedating side effects |
| *Benzodiazepines* (diazepam, lorazepam, midazolam) | 0.3 |
| *Intravenous Anesthetics* | |
| Etomidate | 0.1 |
| Ketamine | Unknown: recommended only if medically necessary |
| Propofol | 0.1 |
| *Local Anesthetics* (bupivacaine, lidocaine, ropivacaine) | 0.1 |
| *Narcotics* | |
| Fentanyl | 1 |
| Hydrocodone | 3 |
| Hydromorphone | 3 |
| Morphine | 9 |
| Oxycodone | 3 (maximum daily dose 30 mg[b]) |
| Remifentanil | Unknown: considered safe secondary to short half-life |
| Codeine/tramadol | Avoid: Food and Drug Administration warning against use in women with a cytochrome P450 2D6 mutation |
| *Nonnarcotic Analgesics* | |
| Acetaminophen | 4 (maximum daily dose < 3g[c]) |
| Ibuprofen | 0.5 |
| Ketorolac | 0.3 |
| *Miscellaneous* | |
| Gabapentin | 3 |
| Dexamethasone | Unknown: considered safe (may cause temporary loss of milk secondary to ↓ prolactin levels) |
| Diphenhydramine | Unknown: generally considered safe |
| *Volatile Gases* | Unknown: considered safe secondary to rapid excretion, poor bioavailability, and/or scavenging of gases |

[a] Mean RID is an estimated average from multiple sources reviewed.

[b] LactMed. Toxicology Data Network. US National Library of Medicine, National Institutes of Health, Harvard Medical School, Bethesda, MD. https://toxnet.nlm.nih.gov/cgi-bin/sis/search2

[c] Acetaminophen dosage announcement. FDA Announcement 468, 2012. https://www.medicaid.nv.gov/Downloads/provider/web_announ cement_468_20120425.pdf

proportion of drug in maternal blood flow that transfers to the infant via breast milk and breastfeeding. Agents with RID less than 10% are considered safe for a healthy, term breastfeeding infant. The majority of anesthetic agents pass into breast milk in small amounts, with RID much less than 10%.[2,3] Morphine has a higher RID of 9, but a long history of safe use (Table 328.1). Two common anesthetic medications that are metabolized into active metabolites, codeine and tramadol, should be avoided in breastfeeding mothers as metabolic variability between mother and infant could result in higher infant levels.[3,4]

The anesthetic goals for breastfeeding mothers should aim to prevent interruption or cessation of breastfeeding after surgery; to ensure breast feeding patients receive needed medications; and to take into account the transfer of all anesthetic and analgesic medicines into breastmilk.[4] Based on available data, including RID, anesthetic agents transfer to breast milk in very low concentrations, and breastfeeding after anesthesia is considered safe for healthy term infants once the mother is awake, alert, and stable after anesthesia. Best recommendations include the following:

1. Keep the mother well hydrated and provide good pain control since dehydration and poor pain control can interfere with breastfeeding.
2. Resume breastfeeding as soon as the mother is awake, alert, stable, and able to hold the infant.
3. Consider neuraxial anesthesia with long-acting neuraxial narcotic.
4. For general anesthesia, use short-acting agents and agents with RID less than 10.
5. Minimize benzodiazepine use.
6. Minimize narcotic use by employing multimodal analgesia, including nonsteroidal anti-inflammatory drugs, acetaminophen, and peripheral nerve blocks.
7. Avoid medications with active metabolites (i.e., codeine, meperidine, and tramadol).

8. Breastfeeding mothers, especially those who require higher doses of pain medicine or a postoperative course of narcotics or whose infants are premature or have medical issues, should be counseled to watch the infant for signs of sedation, such as difficulty to arouse or slowed breathing rate.
9. For information on specific drugs and breastfeeding, consult the Lactation Database (LactMed) from the National Library of Medicine.[5]

Breastfeeding can be a point of stress for mothers, especially when undergoing surgery and anesthesia. Having pump and dump as a recommendation after anesthesia adds another stressor to the situation. Fortunately, current recommendations indicate that breastfeeding for healthy, term infants after anesthesia is safe once the mother is awake, alert, and stable. With good patient education, anesthesiologists can help reduce a patient's stress related to anesthesia and breastfeeding and provide a safe and effective anesthetic to help maintain breastfeeding postoperatively.

## REFERENCES

1. Infant and young child feeding fact sheet. World Health Organization. Accessed July 31, 2020. https://www.who.int/news-room/fact-sheets/detail/infant-and-young-child-feeding
2. Wanderer J, Rathmell J. Anesthesia & breastfeeding: more often than not, they are compatible. *Anesthesiology.* 2017;127:A15.
3. Cobb BT, et al. Breastfeeding after anesthesia: a review for anesthesia providers regarding the transfer of medications into breast milk. *Transl Perioper Pain Med.* 2015;2(2):2–7.
4. Committee on Obstetric Anesthesia. Statement on resuming breastfeeding after anesthesia. American Society of Anesthesiologists. 2019. https://www.asahq.org/standards-and-guidelines/statement-on-resuming-breastfeeding-after-anesthesia?&ct=d38ffdbd56b81d7 3384b93597bdf0c831549d4899e03d35c4f5cbce7954091f4bf431bf ad2f09ef346e789081e89271af46f16c011367d6aefe3783085092b2c
5. Drugs and Lactation Database (LactMed). United States National Library of Medicine, National Institutes of Health, Department of Health and Human Services. https://toxnet.nlm.nih.gov/newtox net/lactmed.htm

# Part 22

# OTORHINOLARYNGOLOGY (ENT) ANESTHESIA

# 329.

# AIRWAY ENDOSCOPY, MICROLARYNGEAL SURGERY, AND LASER SURGERY

*Rotem Naftalovich and James Schiffenhaus*

## ENDOSCOPY

Endoscopy includes laryngoscopy, microlaryngoscopy (aided by use of operative microscope), esophagoscopy, and bronchoscopy. When developing anesthetic plans for these procedures, potential airway problems should be actively sought from history, physical examination, and preoperative studies. If available, preoperative imaging, flow-volume loop studies, and insight from preoperative indirect laryngoscopy performed in the ear, nose, and throat (ENT) clinic can aid in the evaluation.[1]

Preoperatively, the anesthesiologist must assess whether there could be difficulty with either positive pressure *ventilation* via face or laryngeal mask or *intubation*. If difficulty is suggested, consideration should be made to secure the airway *prior* to induction. The cooperative patient may be amenable to awake direct or fiber-optic intubation, whereas the uncooperative patient may be a better candidate for an inhalational induction prior to intubation.[1] Regardless of the scenario, equipment and experienced personnel capable of emergent surgical airway should be immediately available. If paralysis is deemed safe prior to securing the airway, succinylcholine was historically considered the paralytic of choice due to its rapid onset and relatively short duration: By enabling return of muscle function and respiration in the scenario of a failed intubation and failed ventilation, it provides a theoretical "backup" plan. The introduction of sugammadex into clinical practice is an additional option that can be used in conjunction with high-dose rocuronium on induction and also to reverse paralysis after induction for monitoring and/or nerve stimulation.

Endoscopic ENT surgeries can involve intermittent intubations as well as surgical stimulation to the airway, which is an extremely innervated anatomical area, and hemodynamic instability from sympathetic drive is therefore common. A baseline total intravenous anesthesia (TIVA) supplemented with boluses of short-acting anesthetics (e.g., propofol, remifentanil) or adrenergic antagonists (e.g., esmolol) is an anesthetic option. Regional nerve blocks (e.g., glossopharyngeal or superior laryngeal) can also help attenuate hypertensive responses to surgical stimulation.[1]

Maintenance of adequate ventilation and oxygenation is paramount yet challenging in these surgeries as the anesthesiologist attempts to minimize interference with the surgical field. One of the most common strategies involves use of the *microlaryngeal endotracheal tube* (ETT). These smaller diameter tubes are standard length (unlike similar size 4.0, 5.0, and 6.0 standard tubes, which are shorter and designed for pediatric patients) and may enable a secured airway when a larger diameter tube would be not feasible; this can have the benefit of protection against aspiration, the ability to monitor concentrations of end-tidal $CO_2$, and the ability to utilize inhaled anesthetics. These tubes, however, may still obstruct the surgical field, and their smaller diameter increases airway pressures.[1]

Another ideal technique involves connecting a manual *jet ventilator* to a laryngoscope side port. Jet ventilation involves delivering a high-pressure jet of oxygen through the glottic opening, which entrains oxygen and room air into the lungs. Delivered tidal volumes are determined by the driving pressure, inspiratory time, and lung compliance. Adequate time (~4–6 seconds) must be given for exhalation, which is passively driven by the elastic recoil of the lung. Air trapping and barotrauma are potential complications if adequate time is not given for exhalation. TIVA is required, and end-tidal $CO_2$ monitoring is compromised. An alternate approach is to use a specialized ETT (Hunsaker tube) that passes through the glottic to deliver subglottic jet ventilation. While this method may impede the surgical field, it delivers oxygen more accurately and can better allow end-tidal $CO_2$ monitoring.[2]

*Intermittent apnea* is another option when a completely unobstructed surgical field is required. Periods of positive pressure ventilation via mask or ETT are alternated with periods of apnea, during which the surgical procedure is performed. Risks with this approach include inability to ventilate, hypoventilation, and pulmonary aspiration.[1]

Paralysis during these cases may be optimal to reduce the risk of laryngospasm and optimize laryngoscopy conditions with relaxation of the masseter muscle to allow positioning of the suspension laryngoscope. If laryngospasm does occur while a scope (e.g., a fiber-optic wire) is in the bronchus, the presence of the scope prevents complete closure of the airway, and the decision of whether to remove or maintain the scope in position can be critical.

## LASER SURGERY

Endoscopic ENT procedures commonly employ lasers, which generate focused beams of electromagnetic energy and give the surgeon optimal accuracy and hemostasis with minimal postoperative edema. While many risks exist with the use of lasers, retinal injury, laser plume, and airway fire can be devastating ones.[3]

Lasers can aerosolize destructed, microscopic tissue into toxic fumes and transmit microbial diseases. Standard precautions include suction evacuation and use of properly fitted filtering respirators (i.e., N95) by operating (OR) team.[3]

Carbon dioxide, argon, YAG (yttrium, aluminum, garnet), and ruby lasers can all cause rapid, permanent *damage to the retina*. As such, all OR personnel and the patient should wear eye protection specific for the wavelength and type of laser being used.[3]

The most feared complication of laser surgery, however, is the airway fire. Surgeries of the head and neck pose the greatest risk of OR fires because of the proximity of ignition sources to oxygen. The components of a fire ("fire triad") are (1) *ignition source*, (2) *fuel*, and (3) *oxidizer*. OR oxidizers include oxygen, air, and nitrous oxide. Ignition sources include cautery and lasers. Potential fuels include drapes, ETTs, dressings, alcohol, and patient hair.[3]

Because lasers are powerful, potential ignition sources, multiple steps can and should be taken to minimize the risk of an airway fire:

- Keeping the $FiO_2$ (fraction of inspired air) as low as possible (ideally < 30%).
- Avoiding use of nitrous oxide.
- Using stainless steel, laser-resistant ETTs when possible.
- Filling the ETT cuff with saline with or without methylene blue to make cuff damage noticeable.
- Having a 60-mL syringe filled with saline prepared to flood surgical field.

Should an airway fire occur, first the oxidizer source should be removed, so the oxygen/gas flows should be turned off, and the anesthesia circuit should be disconnected. The ETT should be removed immediately. Residual flames should be extinguished with fluids. Ventilation should then be resumed via face mask or reintubation. Once an airway is secured, bronchoscopy can be performed to assess for damage.[1]

## REFERENCES

1. Butterworth JF IV, et al. Anesthesia for otolaryngology–head & neck surgery. In: *Morgan & Mikhail's Clinical Anesthesiology*. 6th ed. New York, NY: McGraw-Hill Education; 2018.
2. Evans E, et al. Jet ventilation. *Contin Educ Anaesth Crit Care Pain*. 2007;7(1):2–5.
3. Gupta B, et al. Hazards of laser surgery. *Anesthesiology*. 1984;61(3): A146–A146.

# 330.

# HAZARDS AND COMPLICATIONS

*Rotem Naftalovich and Manan Nimish Shah*

Ear, nose, and throat (ENT) surgery necessitates unique considerations for surgical complications that can jeopardize the airway, preexisting conditions with the potential to render difficulties in oxygenation and ventilation, and intraoperative field avoidance. The confluence of ways by which ENT pathology can potentially complicate the airway cannot be underestimated.

To illustrate, the American Society of Anesthesiologists practice guideline for management of the *difficult airway* highlights 11 preoperative airway physical examination features of particular concern that can predispose to difficult orotracheal intubation: length of upper incisors, relationship of maxillary and mandibular incisors during normal jaw closure and during voluntary protrusion of mandible, interincisor distance, visibility of uvula, shape of the palate, compliance of the mandibular space, thyromental distance, neck length, neck thickness, and head and neck range of motion[1]—Any of these examination components can present as nonreassuring due to ENT pathology. Poor *compliance of the mandibular space* can occur with fibrosis and ankylosis, such as from prior radiation therapy. Fibrosis can also affect the temporomandibular joint, which can reduce the *interincisor distance*. Mouth opening may also be limited secondary to pain, trismus, or mechanical etiologies (e.g., from prior facial trauma). Pain and trismus are generally overcome by anesthesia and muscle relaxation, but mechanical limitations may render orotracheal intubation impossible; nasotracheal fiber-optic intubation may be a better option in such scenarios.[2] Consideration should be given to the degree of facial trauma and the risk of an endotracheal tube (ETT) entering the cranial cavity with a nasotracheal intubation, which is contraindicated in LeFort III fractures.[2]

A large *mass* in close proximity to the airway may best be managed by securing the airway in the awake state. This is because general anesthesia and paralysis result in loss of protective muscle tone that may be maintaining airway patency during normal sleep.[3] For a mass threatening tracheal collapse, rigid bronchoscopy should be available to stent open the airway, and a reinforced ETT should be considered. The location of the hazard should be identified by imaging as the ETT may need to be advanced past it in the event of compression. If the above techniques fail, emergent proning to relieve mass compression may be life saving. Depending on the location of the hazard, awake tracheostomy with local anesthesia may be a feasible option that is commonly considered safe.[2] Interestingly, a peritonsillar abscess is usually fixed in the lateral pharynx, so mask ventilation is unlikely to be compromised with anesthesia and muscle paralysis.[2] Nonetheless, vigilance during laryngoscopy and intubation is warranted because the abscess can bleed or rupture and purulent material could be aspirated.

Foreign body aspiration is a hazard that varies in nature based on the aspirated object. Vegetables expand with moisture from the respiratory tract, which can worsen obstruction. They can also fragment into multiple pieces and hence further migrate through the respiratory tract. Oil-containing objects such as peanuts can cause chemical inflammation, which can also worsen obstruction as the airway itself swells and narrows with time. Of note, plastic is radiolucent and will not appear well on x-ray–based imaging. Maintaining spontaneous ventilation in this setting is an important consideration as positive pressure ventilation and even the ETT can push the object further downstream in the airway. Upper gastrointestinal bleeding in the airway can lead to continuous swallowing of blood and hence a "full" and irritated stomach, with subsequent higher risk for gastric content aspiration; rapid sequence induction should be considered. Aspiration of blood can also occur from an active bleed, a complication commonly seen posttonsillectomy or occasionally with massive epistaxis or a swallowed sharp object, and carries the added risk of blood pooling in the pharynx and obstructing visualization of the vocal cords during laryngoscopy. Preparation of an adequate suction device is important with a backup suction advised. If suctioning fails to clear pooling blood and visualization is compromised, an attempt should be made to visualize air bubbles emitting from the trachea. If the patient is not breathing spontaneously, pressure can be applied to the stomach externally to produce air bubbles and aid in tracheal intubation.

Edematous tissue can lead to upper airway obstruction; it is also more friable and bleeds easily, which can further compromise the airway. Edema can be seen with upper airway infections and can occur postoperatively from surgical stress itself. Prophylaxis with intraoperative dexamethasone and judicious fluid management can be important. Postoperative humidified oxygen and nebulized bronchodilators are also treatment options, but maintaining an intubated airway is a vital consideration.

Extra vigilance when securing the airway or positioning the patient is warranted to prevent accidental endobronchial intubation, tube occlusion, cuff leaks, disconnections, and even frank dislodgement. Head and neck manipulation by the surgeon could lead to airway obstruction: Good *communication* between teams is important. In the same vein, epinephrine is commonly used to decrease bleeding and improve visualization; this often leads to iatrogenic hemodynamic changes, which can easily be misdiagnosed. Decreased mean arterial pressure and reverse Trendelenburg positioning are other options to decrease venous congestion and bleeding.[3] Avoiding elevated venous pressures is a consideration in ear and graft surgeries; this can occur from disruptions such as bleeding, bucking, or coughing. Options for smoother emergence include deep extubation in a reassuring airway, remifentanil or propofol infusion on emergence, and antiemetic prophylaxis. If throat packing is used, removal is crucial prior to extubation.

Thyroid or parathyroid surgery can be complicated by an enlarging neck hematoma early in the postoperative course; protecting the airway is a priority, but evacuating the hematoma prior to induction may be life saving. Other complications include recurrent laryngeal nerve damage (with ipsilateral vocal cord paralysis), phrenic nerve damage (affecting ipsilateral hemidiaphragm), or superior laryngeal nerve damage (causing paralysis of the cricothyroid muscle). Iatrogenic hypocalcemia can occur following parathyroidectomy (or accidentally with thyroidectomy) and may present later in the postoperative period with parasthesias, muscle spasms, tetany, apnea, laryngospasm, and even bronchospasm.

*Nitrous oxide* use is generally avoided or limited in ear procedures because it can quickly diffuse into closed spaces, causing air trapping and problems such as increased middle ear pressure after placement of a tympanoplasty graft or graft dislodgement.[3]

## REFERENCES

1. Apfelbaum JL, et al. Practice guidelines for management of the difficult airway: an updated report by the American Society of Anesthesiologists Task Force on Management of the Difficult Airway. *Anesthesiology.* 2013;118(2):251–270.
2. Barash PG. Anesthesia for otolaryngologic surgery. In: *Clinical Anesthesia.* 7th ed. Philadelphia, PA: Lippincott Williams & Wilkins; 2013:1356–1372.
3. Pardo MC Jr, Miller RD. Ophthalmology and otolaryngology. In: *Basics of Anesthesia.* 7th ed. Philadelphia, PA: Elsevier; 2018:524–536.

# 331.

# INTRAOPERATIVE THYROID AND PARATHYROID FUNCTION MONITORING

*Kelsey E. Lacourrege and Alan D. Kaye*

## THYROID MONITORING

### DIAGNOSIS

In asymptomatic patients with no signs of thyroid disease, no screening is warranted. However, for those in whom a thorough history and physical raises concern for a hypo- or hypermetabolic state, preoperative evaluation should be undertaken by assessing thyrotropin (TSH, formerly thyroid-stimulating hormone) levels. In patients with known thyroid disease, TSH levels should be obtained to ensure that the patient is in a euthyroid state prior to surgery.[1]

### ANESTHETIC CONSIDERATIONS

It should be noted that hypo- or hyperthyroidism does not affect the minimum alveolar concentration (MAC) dosing of anesthesia. For patients with hyperthyroid states, elective procedures should be postponed until a euthyroid state can be achieved with the use of β-blockers, propylthiouracil, methimazole, and/or iodine. For patients requiring emergent operations, caution should be taken with high doses of β-blockers in order to avoid complications such as congestive heart failure and bronchospasm.[1,2] Thyroid crisis can be triggered by events like surgery in the hyperthyroid patient and can mimic malignant hyperthermia. Management of these patients should include magnesium sulfate to protect against arrythmias brought on by these patients' increased sensitivity to catecholamines.[2]

For patients with hypothyroidism, $T_3$ (triiodothyronine) and $T_4$ (thyroxine) should be administered preoperatively to attain a euthyroid state. On the day of the operation, the usual $T_4$ dose (levothyroxine) can be skipped as it has a half-life of about 7 days.[1,2] For patients also taking $T_3$ (liothyronine), this medication should ideally be taken on the day of surgery.[2]

## PARATHYROID MONITORING

The parathyroid glands are responsible for the secretion of parathyroid hormone (PTH), which has a significant role in regulation of calcium levels in the blood. The parathyroid glands are four small, ovoid-shaped glands weighing an average of approximately 40 mg, and two are superior and approximately 1 cm from the recurrent laryngeal nerves and two are inferior. PTH release is controlled directly by the plasma calcium concentration. Since PTH directly effects calcium, surgery to remove the parathyroid glands will alter calcium, which directly mediates muscle contraction; exocrine, endocrine, and neurocrine secretion; cell growth; and transport and secretion of fluids and electrolytes. Surgery has evolved in recent years, and the use of minimally invasive techniques in parathyroidectomy depends on accurate identification and removal of hyperfunctioning tissue. Intraoperative PTH assays provide an effective method for assessing the persistence of hypersecreting parathyroid tissue and thus the need for further dissection and excision during parathyroidectomy. This technique is an integral part of minimally invasive parathyroidectomy and is widely used by surgeons today.[3] Success rates of 97%–99% have been reported with use of intraoperative monitoring.[4]

### UTILITY

Hyperparathyroidism is classified into primary, secondary, and tertiary forms. Additionally, multiple endocrine neoplasia (MEN) syndrome and parathyroid cancer can lead to elevated parathyroid hormone levels. Intraoperative parathyroid hormone monitoring (IPM) has been evaluated in the surgical management of multiple forms of hyperparathyroidism and has achieved varying levels of accuracy depending on the etiology of the hyperparathyroidism. Currently, IPM appears most accurate and thus has the highest utility in the management of sporadic primary hyperparathyroidism. This form of hyperparathyroidism typically occurs in relation to a single hyperfunctioning gland.[3]

The exact role of IPM will vary depending on the circumstances of each case and needs of the surgeon. An appropriate decline in PTH levels, described below, throughout the case can be used to ensure complete removal of hyperfunctioning tissue and prevent unnecessary further dissection and normal tissue excision. Conversely, persistently elevated PTH levels guide further surgical exploration and excision and help prevent operative failure. Differential jugular venous sampling facilitates lateralization and localization of the hyperfunctioning gland. Finally, IPM can also be used in fine-needle aspiration samples to aid in tissue identification.[3]

Hypoparathyoidectomy includes risk of injury to the recurrent laryngeal nerve and postoperative hypocalcemia. There are several devices that are available that are effective for minimizing nerve injury, and typically they are connected through a specialized endotracheal tube and provide information as the surgeon moves closer to the recurrent laryngeal nerve. Meticulous measurement of calcium and appreciation of clinical signs and symptoms of hypocalcemia are paramount to identify and to treat patients postsurgery. The major signs and symptoms of hypocalcemia include mental status changes, tetany, positive Chvostek and Trousseau signs, laryngospasm, hypotension, and dysrhythmias.[5] Electrocardiogram study may demonstrate prolongation of the QT interval or heart block. Treatment, often in response to hypotension, involves intravenous infusion of 10% calcium chloride (1.36 mEq/mL) or calcium gluconate (0.45 mEq/mL).[3,5] Extubation should be done with careful consideration of operative site to avoid trauma and potential hematoma formation, which can compromise the airway in parathyroid surgery.[3,5]

## REFERENCES

1. Palace MR. Perioperative management of thyroid dysfunction. *Heal Serv Insights*. 2017;10. https://doi.org/10.1177/1178632916689677
2. Bacuzzi A, et al. Anaesthesia for thyroid surgery: perioperative management. *Int J Surg*. 2008;6(suppl 1):S82–S85.
3. Khan ZF, Lew JI. Intraoperative parathyroid hormone monitoring in the surgical management of sporadic primary hyperparathyroidism. *Endocrinol Metab*. 2019;34:327–339.
4. Wilhelm SM, et al. The American Association of Endocrine Surgeons Guidelines for definitive management of primary hyperparathyroidism. *JAMA Surg*. 2016;151(10):959–968.
5. Prejean R, Kaye AD. Parathyroid anatomy & physiology. In: Abd-Elsayed AA, ed. *Basic Anesthesia Review*. In press.

# 332.

# NERVE INJURY MONITORING DURING ENT SURGERY

*Garrett W. Burnett*

## INTRODUCTION

Intraoperative nerve monitoring during otolaryngologic (ENT; ear, nose, and throat) surgery allows for identification of nerves susceptible to injury during surgery. Careful and deliberate surgical technique is a vital component of reducing the risk of nerve injury, but intraoperative monitoring with electromyography (EMG) can further reduce the risk of complications associated with intraoperative injury.[1,2]

Spontaneous and evoked EMG are utilized during intraoperative monitoring. Spontaneous EMG refers to the intrinsic muscle activity and may be altered with stretch or trauma to cranial nerves during surgery. Evoked EMG involves an extrinsic stimulation that results in a larger EMG response and allows for identification of nerves during dissection.[3]

Basic components of EMG include a stimulus source, recording electrodes, and a recording device. The stimulus source may be a specialized probe or surgical instrument

## Table 332.1 COMMONLY MONITORED NERVES DURING ENT SURGERY

| NERVE | FUNCTION | SURGERY | COMPLICATION OF INJURY |
|---|---|---|---|
| Facial nerve (VII) | Motor, sensory | Middle ear, mastoid, parotid surgeries | Facial muscle paralysis |
| Recurrent laryngeal nerve (X) | Motor, sensory | Thyroidectomy, parathyroidectomy | Hoarseness, stridor, aphonia, airway obstruction, aspiration |
| Spinal accessory nerve (XI) | Motor | Neck dissection, lymph node biopsy | Pain, functional impairment |

that allows for direct stimulation of nerves. Recording electrodes may be needles in the target innervated muscle or sensors on tracheal tubes that identify vocal cord contraction. Recording devices are computers that display EMG readings.[3,4]

Cranial nerves commonly monitored include the facial nerve, vagus nerve, recurrent laryngeal nerve, and spinal accessory nerve. EMG monitoring requires nerves with motor components; therefore, only nerves with motor function can be monitored.[4] See Table 332.1 for more information regarding commonly monitored cranial nerves.

## ANESTHESIA CONSIDERATIONS

### PREOPERATIVE

Specialized sensors that may attach to or be embedded in endotracheal tubes are required for monitoring of the recurrent laryngeal nerve, while needle electrodes are needed to monitor other nerves, such as the facial nerve or spinal accessory nerve. Preoperatively, any specialized stimulating probes used by the otolaryngologists and the computer device the monitors are connected to should be available and in working order prior to induction of anesthesia.

The patient should be evaluated for any preexisting neurological deficit during the preanesthetic interview. Any deficits should be noted as these could confound intraoperative monitoring.

### INTRAOPERATIVE

Anesthetic technique may alter intraoperative nerve monitoring. Neuromuscular blockade should be avoided due to its interference with EMG signals during surgery.[1,4] If necessary, succinylcholine or a shorter acting, nondepolarizing neuromuscular blocker such as rocuronium should be used, but care must be taken to make certain the neuromuscular blockade has worn off prior to surgical dissection. If necessary, neostigmine paired with glycopyrrolate or sugammadex reversal of rocuronium-induced neuromuscular blockade may be required.

One method to reduce the need for neuromuscular blockade is the use of a potent, rapid-acting opioid such as remifentanil as an adjunct to induction and maintenance of anesthesia. Maintenance of anesthesia can be achieved using a total intravenous anesthesia technique or with inhaled drugs such as nitrous oxide or volatile gas. EMG monitoring is interfered by volatile gases in the same way somatosensory evoked potentials or motor evoked potentials are in spinal surgery and neurosurgery.

Additionally, local anesthetics should not be used near nerves being monitored. Local anesthetics will prevent EMG signals from the nerve to the target muscle and limit intraoperative monitoring capabilities.

Depending on the cranial nerves being monitored, the anesthesiologist may be required to place the sensing device, as in the case of the endotracheal tube sensor, to monitor the recurrent laryngeal nerve. These sensors typically have two horizontal lines or a blue stripe on the endotracheal tube, and the vocal cords should be positioned between these lines. Positioning of this sensor is important to allow for reliable monitoring of the recurrent laryngeal nerve, and the endotracheal tube should be fully secured to prevent tube migration. Needle electrodes are placed by otolaryngologists for monitoring of target muscles for the facial and spinal accessory nerves.

Vigilance of monitoring the EMG monitor abnormalities is important for the otolaryngologist and anesthesiologist. Spontaneous EMG is suggestive of stretch or surgical trauma to the nerves during dissection.[4] Spontaneous EMG may also be suggestive of light anesthesia, and an adequate depth of anesthesia should be confirmed.[1] When using the stimulating probe, otolaryngologists will look for evoked potentials to identify nerves and avoid injury during the surgery.

### POSTOPERATIVE

Although intraoperative cranial nerve monitoring has been shown to decrease the rate of intraoperative nerve injury during otolaryngologic surgery, nerve injury may be recognized in the postoperative period.

Recurrent laryngeal nerve injury may result in deficits of the intrinsic muscles of the larynx, except the cricothyroid muscle. Unilateral recurrent laryngeal nerve injury may result in hoarseness or stridor, while bilateral recurrent laryngeal nerve injury may result in aphonia or airway obstruction. Additionally, aspiration is a risk for patients with recurrent laryngeal nerve injury.[4]

Facial nerve injury may result in facial muscle paralysis, which may result in functional and cosmetic deficits.[2] Spinal accessory nerve injury may lead to pain or functional impairment through impaired innervation of the trapezius and sternocleidomastoid muscles.[4]

## REFERENCES

1. Dinh CT, et al. Intraoperative neurophyiological monitoring. In: Bracchmann D, et al., eds. *Otologic Surgery*. 4th ed. Philadelphia, PA: Elsevier; 2016:678–689.
2. Gidley PW, et al. Contemporary opinions on intraoperative facial nerve monitoring. *OTO Open*. 2018;2(3):1–7.
3. Dillon FX. Electromyographic (EMG) neuromonitoring in otolaryngology-head and neck surgery. *Anesthesiol Clin*. 2010;28(3):423–442.
4. Holland NR. Intraoperative electromyography. *J Clin Neurophysiol*. 2002;19(5):444–453.

# Part 23

# MISCELLANEOUS

# 333.

# LIPOSUCTION

*Alexandra N. Cole and Balram Sharma*

## INTRODUCTION

Liposuction has become a popular means of expedient weight loss. It is a cosmetic surgery procedure where metal cannulas are inserted through small incisions into the subcutaneous adipose tissue, with suctioned into a canister using negative pressure.[1] There are four techniques used: dry, wet, superwet, and tumescent. The first introduced was dry liposuction and was associated with hypovolemia and blood loss. Wet techniques followed with a 1:1 ratio of injectate to aspirate volume, but the techniques continued to have significant blood losses associated with them.[2] Klein introduced the tumescent solution, which consisted of 0.05%–0.1% lidocaine and 1:100,000 epinephrine added to normal saline, which allowed for a 2–3:1 ratio of injectate to aspirate volume.[2,3] Sodium bicarbonate was later added to decrease the burning sensation on injection. Tumescent liposuction quickly became the popular choice due to the increased volume of aspirate that can be removed during a single procedure and the relatively small amount of blood loss (<1%) associated with this technique due to the vasoconstrictive properties of epinephrine, in contrast to 20%–45% blood loss using the dry technique.[2,3] Small-volume aspiration procedures are often office based under local anesthesia or sedation, with larger volume (>4–5 L) aspiration or multiple sites typically being done under general anesthesia in the operating room.[1]

The liposuction guidelines of the American Society for Dermatologic Surgery recommends that the maximal safe milligram-per-kilogram dosage of tumescent lidocaine for liposuction totally by local anesthesia is 55 mg/kg.

## ANESTHETIC CONSIDERATIONS

### PREOPERATIVE

Appropriate selection of patients who are healthy with a body mass index of less than 30% is important in determining which patients can safely undergo office-based liposuction versus those who need liposuction to be performed at a tertiary center in the operating room. Due to the fluid shifts, dosage of lidocaine and epinephrine administered intraoperatively with large -volume tumescent liposuction requires detailed medical histories are needed to document medications, herbs, and vitamins and ensure there are no pre-existing cardiovascular, renal, pulmonary, or hepatic diseases as healthy patients should be able to tolerate increased intravascular volume.[2] Patients taking herbal or over-the-counter weight loss medications should be instructed to discontinue them as they can interfere with coagulation or pose interactions with epinephrine.[4] Baseline electrocardiogram, complete blood count, coagulation studies, chemistry panel, and pregnancy test for women of childbearing age should be obtained. Liposuction is contraindicated in pregnancy, severe cardiovascular disease, or coagulation disorder.

### INTRAOPERATIVE

There are numerous complications that can happen intraoperatively during these procedures. The most common is pulmonary thromboembolism.[5] Placement of pneumatic compression devices is required, and patients who are at high risk should be considered for thromboprophylaxis. Careful consideration should be taken in regard to fluid management due to patients receiving large volumes of subcutaneous fluid with 60%–70% of it being displaced intravascularly. The increase in intravascular volume can lead to pulmonary edema or congestive heart failure. Procedures with less than 4–5 L of aspirate should not require large amounts of intravenous fluid resuscitation or maintenance fluids, whereas, high-volume liposuction supplemental fluids should be titrated to urinary output.[2] Other complications include abdominal or pleural perforation, development of local anesthetic systemic toxicity (LAST), drug reaction, fat embolism, pulmonary edema, or hypothermia. The development of LAST during this time would not present with the more subtle symptoms of perioral numbness, tinnitus, or metallic taste in the mouth but rather cardiovascular collapse or seizures.[1] Thermoregulation with warmed fluids and a forced air warmer is important during this period as hypothermia occurs from general anesthesia and the temperature of the tumescent fluids injected, which can lead to worsening coagulopathy or cardiac dysrhythmias.

## POSTOPERATIVE

Although lidocaine toxicity can occur during the intraoperative setting, it is more likely to happen in the postoperative setting. Tissue-bound lidocaine will slowly continue to be absorbed and contribute to intravascular volume reaching peak plasma levels 10–14 hours postoperatively.[1] During this period, patients can develop LAST and should be monitored.

## REFERENCES

1. Matarasso A, Hutchinson OHZ. Liposuction. *JAMA*. 2001;285(3): 266–268.
2. Wang G, et al.. Fluid management in extensive liposuction. *Medicine*. 2018;97(41):e12655.
3. de Jong RH, Grazer FM. Perioperative management of cosmetic liposuction. *Plast Reconstr Surg*. 2001;107(4):1039–1044.
4. Granados-Tinajero S, et al. Anesthesia management for large-volume liposuction. In: Whizar-Lugo VM, ed. *Anesthesia Topics for Plastic and Reconstructive Surgery*. IntechOpen; February 4, 2019. doi:10.5772/intechopen.83630
5. Grazer FM, dc Jong RH. Fatal outcomes from liposuction: census survey of cosmetic surgeons. *Plast Reconstr Surg*. 2000;105(1): 436–448.

# 334.

# ANESTHESIA FOR LAPAROSCOPIC SURGERY

*Maria F. Ramirez and J. P. Cata*

## INTRODUCTION

Laparoscopic surgery is considered a common procedure that is performed around the world every day. Its advantages compared to conventional open abdominal surgery include the reduction of (1) postoperative pain and ileus, (2) respiratory complications, (3) blood loss, and (4) reduction of hospital stays, which allows a rapid return to normal activities. Laparoscopic surgery requires intraperitoneal insufflation of $CO_2$ to create a pneumoperitoneum, which is essential to facilitate visualization. $CO_2$ is the most commonly used gas for abdominal insufflation because it is highly soluble, not flammable, and rapidly absorbed in the peritoneal cavity (which decreases the risk of air embolism). Limiting the intra-abdominal pressure below 12–15 mm Hg during insufflation and using slow insufflation when the pneumoperitoneum is established are strategies to prevent significant cardiopulmonary compromise, particularly in patients with cardiopulmonary comorbidities.

Anesthetic concerns for patients undergoing laparoscopic surgery include cardiopulmonary effects of pneumoperitoneum, systemic absorption of $CO_2$, venous air embolism, unintentional injuries to intraperitoneal structures, and patient positioning.[1] Laparoscopic surgery is routinely performed under balanced general anesthesia with controlled ventilation. Appropriate anesthesia techniques and monitoring improve surgical conditions and allow early detection of fatal complications (Table 334.1).

## PHYSIOLOGICAL CHANGES ASSOCIATED WITH LAPAROSCOPIC SURGERY

### CARDIOVASCULAR EFFECTS

In laparoscopic surgery, hemodynamic alterations are secondary to three components: (1) the increase of the intra-abdominal pressure, (2) the increase of $CO_2$ and acidosis, and (3) the position, either Trendelenburg or reverse Trendelenburg. The increase of intra-abdominal pressure decreases venous return secondary to inferior vena cava compression and increased central venous pressure. The $CO_2$ absorption produces an increase in sympathetic stimulation with consequently increased

## Table 334.1 COMPLICATION ASSOCIATED WITH LAPAROSCOPIC SURGERY

| COMPLICATION | MECHANISM |
|---|---|
| Bradycardia and asystole | Pneumoperitoneum produces a vasovagal reflex secondary to peritoneal stretch. *Treatment*: Immediate desufflation of the abdomen, atropine administration, and cardiopulmonary resuscitation. |
| Subcutaneous emphysema | Unintentional extraperitoneal insufflation in the subcutaneous and preperitoneal tissue. *Treatment*: Observation and spontaneous resolution after the abdomen is deflated. |
| Endobronchial intubation | Elevation of diaphragm. *Treatment*: Withdrawal of endotracheal tube as needed. |
| Gas embolism | Unintentional introduction of $CO_2$ through the Veress needle into the large veins. *Treatment*: Telease of pneumoperitoneum and supportive measures; aspiration of the intracardiac gas. Patient should be turned to the left lateral decubitus with head-down position to prevent gas from entering the pulmonary circulation. |
| Trocar-associated injuries | Hemorrhage and visceral trauma. |

## Table 334.2 PHYSIOLOGIC CHANGES ASSOCIATED WITH LAPAROSCOPIC SURGERY

| PHYSIOLOGIC CHANGE | MECHANISM |
|---|---|
| **CARDIOVASCULAR** | |
| ↑SVR, peripheral vascular resistance, MAP | Increased release of catecholamines and vasopressin<br>Hypercarbia<br>Increased intra-abdominal pressure |
| ↓Brady- or tachycardia | Peritoneal stretch<br>Hypercarbia<br>Hypoxia |
| ↓Venous return | Vena cava compression |
| ↓Cardiac index | Increased afterload<br>Decreased preload |
| **PULMONARY** | |
| ↓Lung volumes | Increased intra-abdominal pressure<br>Decreased diaphragmatic excursion<br>Trendelenburg position |
| ↓Lung compliance | Increased intra-abdominal pressure<br>Increased intra-thoracic pressure |
| ↑Airway pressure | Increased intra-abdominal pressure<br>Trendelenburg position |
| ↑ETCO$_2$ and acidosis | $CO_2$ insufflation<br>Decreased alveolar ventilation |
| **NEUROLOGICAL** | |
| ↑Intracranial | Increased cerebral blood flow secondary to hypercarbia<br>Decreased venous return<br>Trendelenburg position |
| **RENAL** | |
| ↓Urinary output | Decreased blood flow<br>Increased antidiuretic hormone |

systemic vascular resistance (SVR), mean arterial pressure (MAP), pulmonary resistance, myocardial wall tension, and myocardial oxygen demand.[2] Moderate-to-severe hypercapnia has negative consequences in cardiac function due to vasodilation, myocardial depression, and sensibilization of myocardium to the arrhythmogenic effect of catecholamines. Furthermore, the negative hemodynamic effects are accentuated in patients with cardiovascular disease, such as heart failure, ischemic heart disease, valvular heart disease, and pulmonary hypertension. The pneumoperitoneum produces a vasovagal reflex secondary to peritoneal stretch, and although this reaction is usually benign and self-limited, on occasion, it can lead to profound bradycardia, asystole, and cardiovascular collapse (Table 334.2).

### RESPIRATORY EFFECTS

Laparoscopic surgery alters the pulmonary mechanics and acid-base balance but does not significantly affect oxygenation. The rise of intra-abdominal pressure impedes diaphragm excursion and induces basal lung collapse, reduces functional residual capacity, and increases the intrapulmonary shunt. The $CO_2$ insufflation increases intrathoracic pressure, decreases pulmonary compliance, and increases peak pressure, plateau pressure, and end-tidal $CO_2$.[3] Maintenance of the appropriate ventilation may be achieved by an increase in respiratory rate and/or increase of delivered tidal volume.

### NEUROLOGICAL EFFECTS

The pneumoperitoneum and subsequent increase in intra-abdominal pressure decrease the venous return and increase intracranial pressure. This increase can be accentuated by the increase in PaCO$_2$ (increased cerebral blood flow) and steep Trendelenburg position. Nevertheless, cerebral perfusion is maintained by the increase in MAP in healthy patients.

### SPLANCHNIC EFFECT

The abdominal insufflation decreases the splanchnic circulation and reduces hepatic, bowel, and renal blood flow (decreases glomerular filtration and urinary output).

However, this effect is attenuated by vasodilation caused by hypercapnia.

## ANESTHETIC CONSIDERATIONS

### PREOPERATIVE

Adherence to fundamental principles of preoperative evaluation, along with special attention to the cardiovascular and pulmonary systems, is required. The anesthetic concerns of patients undergoing laparoscopic surgery are primarily related to the use of pneumoperitoneum and steep Trendelenburg position. Relative contraindications to laparoscopic surgery should be considered, and an open procedure is advised. Close communication between the surgeon and the anesthesiologist is required in relation to positioning.

### INTRAOPERATIVE

**Patient Monitoring:** Standard American Society of Anesthesiologists monitoring includes pulse oximeter, electrocardiography, noninvasive blood pressure, and temperature. Neuromuscular block monitors are recommended to ensure adequate surgical conditions. An arterial line and arterial blood gases should be considered in patients with cardiopulmonary comorbidities.

**Anesthesia Technique:** Laparoscopic surgery is routinely performed with general anesthesia and tracheal intubation. This technique is commonly used because it allows the control of mechanical ventilation necessary to adjust airway pressures and to reduce the end-tidal $CO_2$. Optimal surgical conditions are facilitated by decompression of the gastrointestinal tract, proper neuromuscular blockage, and proper positioning (Trendelenburg or reverse Trendelenburg). Maintenance of general anesthesia can be achieved with either volatile agents or propofol-based total intravenous anesthesia. Opioids should be carefully titrated, and neuromuscular blockers should be administered to ensure proper muscle relaxation. Management of intravenous fluids must be optimized to avoid tissue hypoperfusion or fluid overload, but in general terms, laparoscopic surgery has a lower requirement for intravenous fluid compared to open procedures. In regard to mechanical ventilation, pressure-controlled ventilation rather than volume-controlled ventilation (specifically in morbidly obese patients), positive pressure at the end of the expiration (positive end-expiratory pressure 5 to 10 cm $H_2O$) and recruitment maneuvers have been shown to improve respiratory mechanics.[4]

### POSTOPERATIVE

**Pain:** Postoperative pain is significantly less severe and shorter compared to open procedures. The etiology is multifactorial and includes neuropraxia of the phrenic nerve during gas insufflation, residual intra-abdominal gas, and surgical trauma. Pain can be reduced by a combination of simple measures, including preoperative acetaminophen, injection of local anesthetic at the port site at the beginning of the operation, maintaining a pneumoperitoneum below 15 mm Hg, ensuring proper evacuation of the insufflated $CO_2$ at the end of the operation, and intraoperative medications like nonsteroidal anti-inflammatory drugs and opioids.

**Postoperative Nauseas and Vomit (PONV):** PONV is common in laparoscopic surgery and is secondary to stretching and irritation of the peritoneum (from insufflation of gas) as well as bowel manipulation. Multimodal prophylactic medications include dexamethasone after induction of anesthesia, ondasentron at the end of surgery, proper intravenous hydration, and adequate analgesia.[5]

## REFERENCES

1. Bajwa SJ, Kulshrestha A. Anaesthesia for laparoscopic surgery: general vs regional anaesthesia. *J Minim Access Surg.* 2016;12(1):4–9.
2. Buia A, et al. Laparoscopic surgery: a qualified systematic review. *World J Methodol.* 2015;5(4):238–254.
3. Cunningham AJ. Anesthetic implications of laparoscopic surgery. *Yale J Biol Med.* 1998;71(6):551–578.
4. Dec M, Andruszkiewicz P. Anaesthesia for minimally invasive surgery. *Wideochir Inne Tech Maloinwazyjne.* 2016;10(4):509–514.
5. Chatterjee S, et al. Current concepts in the management of postoperative nausea and vomiting. *Anesthesiol Res Pract.* 2011;2011:748031.

# 335.

# OPHTHALMOLOGIC ANESTHESIA

*Camila Teixeira and Steven Minear*

## INTRODUCTION

Ophthalmologic anesthesia encompasses care delivered to multiple surgical areas (intraocular, extraocular, oculoplastic), all done in a great variety of settings. Providing anesthesia for ophthalmic surgery also involves the care of a wide range of patients who may show a high incidence of comorbidities from systemic diseases with ocular manifestation. Therefore, the anesthesia technique choice should be individualized.

## RETROBULBAR AND PERIBULBAR BLOCKS

Regional anesthesia has several advantages over general and topical anesthesia, especially postoperative analgesia, intraoperative akinesia, oculocardiac reflex (OCR) prevention, and emesis reduction. A combination of bupivacaine 0.75% and lidocaine 2% without epinephrine is most commonly used. Following injection, the intraocular pressure (IOP) increases; therefore, gentle digital pressure or a Honan balloon set at 30 mm Hg should be applied to the globe. Special care must be taken in eyes with axial length greater than 25 mm due to the increased risk of ocular penetration.

- *Retrobulbar Block*: Primarily blocks ciliary ganglion; ciliary nerves; cranial nerves II, III, and VI. A 23- to 25-gauge, 31-cm long needle is placed between the inferior and lateral orbit, just above the inferior rim. Once past the globe equator, the needle is turned superiorly (Figure 335.1a). A small volume of local anesthetic (3–5 mL) is injected inside the muscular cone. All extraocular muscles are paralyzed except the superior oblique, located outside the cone. An additional eyelid block might be needed.[1] The superior and nasal sites of puncture should be avoided due to the reduced distance between the roof and the globe at this location. The main hazard of this technique is injury to the globe or intraconal elements.

- *Peribulbar Block*: This technique has largely replaced the retrobulbar block. A 23- to 25-gauge, 25-mm long needle is placed into the extraconal space. Limiting the depth of the needle insertion is safer because the rectus muscles are in contact with orbit walls, making the extraconal space virtual.[2] Classically there are two injections (Figure 335.1b), but it is advocated to use

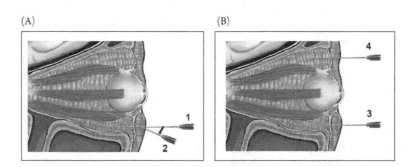

(A)   (B)

**Figure 335.1** (a) Retrobulbar block: (1) needle insertion and (2) intraconal needle placement. (b) Peribulbar block: (3) extraconal needle placement and (4) second injection.

the second injection only if the previous has failed. Disadvantages of peribulbar blocks include longer onset, higher volume of anesthetic, and lower incidence of akinesia.

Complications of needle blocks:

- *Retrobulbar Hemorrhage*: Most common complication and consequences may vary from subconjunctival chemosis to a compressive hematoma threatening retinal perfusion and vision.
- *Diplopia and Ptosis*: Extraocular muscle injury from needle insertion or hematoma.
- *Globe Damage*: Risk factors include myopia, staphyloma, and physician inexperience. Retinal detachment and vitreous loss have been reported.
- *Brainstem Anesthesia*: Accidental injection through the optic nerve sheath or via retrograde flow in the internal carotid after an intra-arterial injection.
- *Direct Optic Nerve Damage*: Rare nerve atrophy and blindness.

## OPEN EYE INJURIES

Traumatic eye injuries are either open globe (ocular wall integrity is violated by rupture or laceration) or closed globe (ocular wall is preserved). Lacerations are penetrating (entry wound only) or perforating (entry and exit wounds). The combination of open eye injury and a patient with a full stomach is an anesthesiology challenge. Patients are at risk of worsening eye injury from either induction of general anesthesia or administration of regional block. The goal is to protect the patient from aspiration and to avoid elevation of IOP.[3] Mask pressure, coughing, hypercarbia, hypoxia, and blood pressure elevation are avoided. A rapid sequence induction is used for general anesthesia, with use of medications that minimize IOP elevation. Traditionally, the use of succinylcholine is discouraged because the drug raises IOP; however, reports of vitreous extrusion are extremely rare. Regional and topical anesthesia are reserved for less serious injuries in a comorbid patient.

## INTRAOCULAR PRESSURE

The globe is a relatively noncompliant compartment. The volume of internal structures is fixed except for the aqueous fluid and choroidal blood volume. Therefore, the volume of both factors regulates IOP.[4] Normal IOP ranges from 10 to 20 mm Hg, and its elevation is a result of aqueous drainage impairment or a change in choroidal blood volume caused by hypercapnia. Coughing, vomiting, face mask pressure,

and laryngoscopy can increase IOP. IOP impacts intraocular perfusion pressure, which is mean arterial pressure less IOP. Reflexive IOP elevation can lead to catastrophic events: optic nerve ischemia, intraocular content extrusion, and permanent visual loss. Anesthetics in general decrease IOP. Ketamine, etomidate, atropine, and succinylcholine confer a modest rise in IOP when usual doses are used.

## OCULOCARDIAC REFLEX

The OCR is a decrease in heart rate greater than 20% from extraocular muscle traction or globe pressure.[5] This reflex is most notable during strabismus surgery, but orbital injections can also be a trigger. It fatigues after repeated stimulation. Pediatric patients are more susceptible and at most risk for hemodynamic changes. Stretch receptors localized in the ocular and periorbital tissues send sensory impulses via the ciliary ganglion to the ophthalmic division of the trigeminal nerve. Impulses are carried from the visceral motor nucleus of the vagus to the sinoatrial node. Complications of OCR include hypotension, dizziness, nausea and vomiting, atrioventricular block, and asystole.

## ANESTHETIC CONSIDERATIONS

### PREOPERATIVE

Most ophthalmic surgeries are done as outpatient procedures under local anesthesia. Preoperative assessment should identify patients who are not suitable for this approach. Physical examination should pay special attention to not only positioning problems but also hearing loss, cooperation, and tremor. For low-risk procedures, cardiovascular evaluation should be limited to eliciting major risk factors. Ophthalmic evaluation includes previous ophthalmic surgery, glaucoma, globe axial length, and presence of staphyloma. Anticoagulant medications can be continued for cataract surgery (least risk for hemorrhage), assuming a therapeutic international ratio.[4]

### INTRAOPERATIVE

Intraoperatively, proper sedation is crucial in the setting of relative airway inaccessibility. If IOP is elevated, mannitol may be requested. This osmotic diuretic has a risk of worsening congestive heart failure or bladder distention. In some vitreoretinal procedures with intraocular gas, nitrous oxide must be discontinued for 15 minutes prior to the insufflation and for the following 7–45 days. The OCR incidence is increased with topical anesthesia alone, and eye blocks can decrease its occurrence. Definitive treatment is to stop the triggering stimulus by immediately discontinuing eye manipulation and occasionally by intravenous anticholinergics.

## POSTOPERATIVE

Emesis leads to delayed suprachoroidal hemorrhage, and prophylaxis is required. Regional anesthesia is often associated with general anesthesia, especially in children, and its intention is to avoid postoperative pain, eye manipulation, and emesis.

## REFERENCES

1. Nouvellon E, et al. Regional anesthesia and eye surgery. *Anesthesiology.* 2010;113(5):1236–1242.
2. Jaichandran VV. Ophthalmic regional anaesthesia: a review and update. *Indian J Anaesth.* 2013;57:7–13.
3. Sinha AC, Baumann B. Anesthesia for ocular trauma. *Curr Anaesth Crit Care.* 2010;21(4):184–188.
4. Miller RD. *Miller's Anesthesia.* 8th ed. Philadelphia, PA: Churchill Livingstone/Elsevier; 2015:2512–2521.
5. Dunville LM, Kramer J. Oculocardiac reflex. In: *StatPearls.* Treasure Island, FL: Stat Pearls Publishing; January 2020.

# 336.

# ORTHOPEDIC ANESTHESIA
## TOURNIQUET MANAGEMENT, COMPLICATIONS OF ORTHOPEDIC SURGERY, REGIONAL VERSUS GENERAL ANESTHESIA

*Alberto Thomas and Jason Bang*

## INTRODUCTION

During orthopedic surgery, the tourniquet pressure and duration of the cuff may result in muscle and nerve damage. For this reason, cuff pressure is recommended to be done with the lowest amount of pressure possible. Currently, methods such as limb occlusion pressures (LOPs) are utilized to minimize the required pressure.[1-3] Every anesthesiologist should be aware of complications in orthopedic surgery such as air embolism, fat embolism, and fat embolism syndrome (FES). Other complications include compartment syndrome and coexisting diseases, such as rheumatoid arthritis, which will have disorders such as atlantoaxial subluxation and temporomandibular joint involvement.[1] Among the most important advantages of regional anesthesia versus general anesthesia are postoperative pain management and reductions in perioperative complications, such as venous thromboembolism, myocardial infarction, respiratory depression, and bleeding complications.[4]

## TOURNIQUET MANAGEMENT

Compression devices used to control bleeding have been used and documented since ancient times. The tourniquet pressure and extended duration of cuff inflation may result in muscle and nerve damage. For this reason, cuff pressure is recommended to be done with the lowest amount of pressure possible. Previously, fixed pressures were used: for upper extremities 250 mm Hg and 300 mm Hg for lower limbs. Current methods such as LOPs are utilized to minimize the required pressure. LOP is the minimum pressure required to stop the flow of arterial blood into the limb distal to the cuff. Although tourniquet time and pressure continue to be controversial, the recommended time of cuff inflation is 90–120 minutes, and if the anticipated time will be longer, the cuff should be deflated for 10 minutes every 1-hour interval. (C. Franco, regarding tourniquet in surgery of the extremities, personal communication, 2020) Table 336.1 suggests a safety margin to be added to the LOP.

Table 336.1 SAFETY MARGIN ADDED TO LIMB
OCCLUSION PRESSURE

| SAFETY MARGIN | LIMB OCCLUSION PRESSURE |
|---|---|
| 40 mm Hg | <130 |
| 60 mm Hg | 131–190 |
| 80 mm Hg | >191 |
| 50 mm Hg | Pediatric patients |

Some of the problems associated with tourniquet use include posttourniquet nerve palsy and posttourniquet syndrome. The latter is caused by a prolonged time of ischemia that will manifest as arm weakness, edema, and numbness. Both of these complications will usually resolve in a manner of weeks after surgery.[3] After the tourniquet is released, the increase in blood flow to the ischemic limb will cause an increase in lactic acidosis and increase in potassium levels. To manage the intraoperative pain due to tourniquet use, an intercostobrachial block (T2 block) was wrongly used as a tourniquet block. Because the pain associated with the tourniquet is an ischemic pain and not one due to a cutaneous pain, this block should be used only if the medial side of the arm is being worked on (C. Franco, regarding tourniquet in surgery of the extremities, personal communication, 2020).

## COMPLICATIONS

Fat embolism and FES are complications that are known in orthopedic surgery. The pathophysiology relates to fat embolization and bone marrow debris, which, when released, may produce a vascular blockage. This in itself may produce a systemic inflammatory response. A petechial rash that is commonly present in the conjunctiva and oral mucosa is suggestive of FES. Respiratory signs include hypoxemia, tachypnea, and radiologic signs of diffuse alveolar infiltrates. Drowsiness and confusion are some of the neurologic symptoms that may also be manifested. The treatment of FES is that of support and early resuscitation. Although some clinicians recommend use of steroids, there are investigators who do not support this management.[1]

Air embolism in orthopedic surgery should be considered in procedures that involve a sitting position, such as shoulder surgery in a beach chair position. Air embolism may occur when a pressure gradient is in favor of entry through a blood vessel that is open. Any procedure where the surgical field is above the level of the heart should be monitored closely. Cardiovascular collapse and cardiac dysrhythmias may occur. Pulmonary symptoms in awake patients will present acute dyspnea, tachypnea, and wheezing. The end-tidal carbon dioxide and arterial oxygen saturation will decrease. Immediate management of acute venous air embolism includes notifying the surgeon to flood or pack the field, apply jugular compression, lower the patients head to a Trendelenburg position, administer 100% oxygen, and provide circulatory support.[2]

Other important concepts to consider include bone cement during total hip replacement. The polymerization reaction that is produced may lead to embolization of fat, air, or bone marrow. Due to the reaction of the cement, vasodilation may occur, and thus hypotension, degranulation of mast cells, and histamine release may be produced.[1]

Common coexisting diseases should be taken into account when performing orthopedic surgery. Anterior atlantoaxial subluxation is seen in about 25% of patients with rheumatoid arthritis, and temporomandibular joint involvement should also be considered when manipulating the airway.

Orthopedic trauma is a major risk factor for compartment syndrome, especially if there are any tibial fractures involved. Clinicians should consider looking for a palpable pulse, pallor, paralysis, paresthesia, and pain. Treatment is a fasciotomy to relieve the pressure and is done when intracompartmental pressure is more than 30 cm $H_2O$.[1]

## REGIONAL VERSUS GENERAL ANESTHESIA

The use of regional anesthesia in orthopedic surgery has shown its advantages over general anesthesia. Among the most important advantages is the postoperative management for pain control. Orthopedic surgery can be very painful, and the use of peripheral blocks has been shown to be superior in pain control. It also gives the opportunity for placement of nerve catheters that can be used with a home infusion pump, which may deliver local anesthetics for a prolonged period of time.[1]

Incidence of major perioperative complications have been reduced when comparing regional anesthesia to general anesthesia. In a systematic review of trials using randomization to intraoperative neuroaxial block or not, 9559 patients were included. In this trial, significant reductions in perioperative complications, such as venous thromboembolism, myocardial infarction, respiratory depression, and bleeding complications were seen. It is suggested that some of the reasons for this include multiple factors, such as better capacity for breathing from pain-free management, reduction in stress response from surgery, and increased blood flow.[4]

## REFERENCES

1. Urban MK. Anesthesia for orthopedic surgery. In: *Miller's Anesthesia*. 7th ed. Philadelphia, PA: Elsevier; 2010:2241–2257.
2. Hegde RT, Avatgere RN. 'Air embolism during anaesthesia for shoulder arthroscopy'. British Journal of Anaesthesia.2000.85;6:926–927

3. Kumar K, et al. Tourniquet application during anesthesia: "What we need to know?" *J Anaesthesiol Clin Pharmacol*. 2016;2:61–70.
4. Rodgers A, et al. Reduction of postoperative mortality and morbidity with epidural or spinal anaesthesia: results from overview of randomized trials. *BMJ*. 2000;321:1493.

# 337.

# ANESTHESIA FOR THE TRAUMA PATIENT

*Alexander Rothkrug and Karim Fikry*

## INTRODUCTION

The assessment of a trauma patient begins with a brief overview of their stability and any external injury. Obtain any information from prehospital personnel/first responders. The primary survey assesses the ABCs: airway, breathing, and circulation. It may also include a targeted neurological examination, assignment of a Glasgow Coma Scale (GCS) score, and other immediate interventions such as portable films, laboratory tests, a focused assessment with sonography in trauma examination, and limited transthoracic echocardiogram to assess the patient's myocardial contractility, volume status, and presence of pericardial effusion.

The secondary survey includes a detailed assessment of the fully exposed patient while immediate resuscitation efforts are ongoing. Missed diagnoses can prove to be problematic later intraoperatively. Hypercarbia can impede an adequate neurological examination but is improved with establishment of ventilation and circulation. Also consider intoxication with alcohol or other drugs, hypoglycemia, traumatic brain injury (TBI), and spinal cord injury (SCI) when performing the neurological examination. Shock and aggressive fluid resuscitation expose the patient to risk of hypothermia; thus, close attention should be paid to maintaining normothermia with warmed fluids and forced air warming.

Intraoperative management for damage control surgery (DCS) should work under the assumption that the patient presents with a full stomach and the possibility of TBI or SCI.

The postoperative period is heavily concerned with pain control, management of complications, and disposition. The tertiary survey takes place 24 hours after injury and generally repeats both the primary and secondary surveys while assessing for any injuries that may have been missed.

## INITIAL EVALUATION AND PREOPERATIVE ASSESSMENT

### AIRWAY

In all trauma patients, one must assume the stomach is full and that a cervical spine injury is present until proven otherwise. Keep in mind the airway may be obstructed from edema, hematoma formation, bleeding, secretions, or foreign body or be displaced by bone and soft tissue. Management may begin with chin lift and jaw thrust, suctioning of the airway, placement of an oral airway, and use of a bag valve mask with supplemental oxygen. Caution should be exercised with placement of a nasopharyngeal airway in the event of facial or basilar skull fracture. If intubation is required, it should be done in a rapid sequence technique. Manual inline stabilization is the standard of care for direct laryngoscopy to avoid new or further cervical spine injury.[1] Use of video laryngoscopy may improve the glottic view but can exert the same amount of pressure on the cervical spine as direct laryngoscopy. Awake fiber-optic bronchoscopy is safe and effective, but timely and limited by the staff and equipment available.

## BREATHING

In a hypoxemic and hypotensive patient, suspicion for tension pneumothorax should be high. Assess for cyanosis, tachypnea, and jugular venous distension and listen for bilateral breath sounds as well. In addition to chest x-ray, ultrasound is highly sensitive for identifying pneumothorax, which may present with absence of lung sliding and comet tail artifact. Presence of the lung point is a diagnostic sign.[2] If already on mechanical ventilation, assess peak inspiratory pressures and tidal volume. Disconnecting from mechanical ventilation and performing needle thoracostomy via insertion of a 14-gauge angiocatheter into either the fourth or fifth intercostal space of the midaxillary line or the second intercostal space of the midclavicular line can be life saving. Later, thoracostomy tubes can be placed.

## CIRCULATION

Pulse and blood pressure provide insight into the presence of circulation and will help determine if emergent exploration, embolization by interventional radiology, or intensive care unit (ICU) level of care is required. At a minimum, two large-bore intravenous lines should be placed and blood for laboratory tests drawn for hemoglobin/hematocrit and type and screen. Arterial blood gas, venous blood gas, and coagulation studies provide additional information. Tissue hypoperfusion and the resultant severe metabolic acidosis with elevated base deficit are responsible for the development of coagulopathy in a large proportion of major traumas (see separate chapters for the mechanism of coagulopathy).[3] Severe hemorrhagic shock usually demands initiation of a massive transfusion protocol (MTP) and DCS. Imaging can aid in diagnosing internal hemorrhage.

Tension pneumothorax can compromise circulation. The ACS Committee on Trauma recommends against emergency thoracotomy following blunt trauma in patients without reassuring signs of circulation but maintains the recommendation in penetrating trauma if patients have a preserved organized cardiac rhythm. Bilateral thoracostomy tubes and fluid resuscitation should be rapidly performed following penetrating trauma even in a pulseless patient.

## INTRAOPERATIVE MANAGEMENT

In addition to standard American Society of Anesthesiologists monitors and availability of airway equipment, having adequate intravenous access is important for the trauma patient. In severe hypotension or hypovolemia, large-bore peripheral access as well as placement of invasive monitors such as an arterial line may be difficult. Subclavian access for central lines or intraosseous access may be preferred alternatives when attaining peripheral access is not feasible.

If not already intubated prior to operating room arrival, take hemodynamics into consideration when planning induction. If using propofol, pretreating with vasopressors may help with hypotension caused by its vasodilatory effects. Etomidate and ketamine are associated with more favorable hemodynamics and preservation of sympathetic tone. Ketamine maintains mean arterial pressure (MAP) without causing large increases in intraocular pressure (IOP) and intracranial pressure (ICP), thus minimizing the extent of head, eye, and major vessel injuries.[4] Etomidate can cause delayed hypotension secondary to adrenal insufficiency. Nitrous should be avoided, especially when suspicion is high for perforated viscus or pneumothorax. To achieve neuromuscular blockade for rapid sequence intubation, both rocuronium and succinylcholine may be used; however succinylcholine is relatively contraindicated in several cases (see Table 337.1).

The objective of DCS is to achieve hemostasis and prevent intra-abdominal contamination from perforated viscus injury by stapling and/or resection. Areas of bleeding are compressed and packed. The aorta may be compressed if bleeding persists. Repair of complex injuries is performed at a later time. If intraoperatively the patient becomes unstable, hypothermic, and/or hemodynamically unresponsive to transfusion, the decision should be made to stop surgery, pack any bleeding locations, and determine whether to engage interventional radiology for endovascular procedures versus transfer to the ICU for further resuscitative and stabilizing efforts.

If undiagnosed TBI or SCI (see separate chapters) is suspected, ensure adequate cerebral perfusion pressure through a reasonable MAP and by minimizing ICP with hyperventilation and use of osmotic diuretics such as mannitol. In certain cases, invasive ICP monitoring may be required.

## POSTOPERATIVE

Following major trauma and any subsequent urgent intervention, patients should be managed in the ICU. Pain control is multimodal and especially important in patients with chest and abdominal injuries that limit inspiratory effort and perpetuate atelectasis. Lung-protective ventilation is utilized in acute lung injury or acute respiratory distress syndrome.

Acute kidney injury can be a sequela of trauma, ureteral/urethral injury, retroperitoneal hematoma, septic shock, MTP, and abdominal compartment syndrome. Acute renal failure in crush syndrome is likely secondary

*Table 337.1* NEUROMUSCULAR BLOCKADE FOR RAPID SEQUENCE INTUBATION

|  | SUCCINYLCHOLINE | ROCURONIUM |
|---|---|---|
| Standard dose | 1–1.5 mg/kg | 0.6–1 mg/kg |
| RSI dose | 1–1.5 mg/kg | 1.2 mg/kg |
| Time for onset | 30 seconds to 1 minute | 1–3 minutes |
| Duration of action | 3–10 minutes | 30 minutes to 1 hour |
| Contraindications | Personal or family history of MH (unless ruled out), muscular dystrophy, severe burns, and crush injury (>24–48 hours), SCI (>1 week), allergy, severe hyperkalemia | Allergy |
| Adverse effects/complications | Hyperkalemia, increased ICP, IOP, and intragastric pressure; MH; masseter spasm; anaphylaxis | Bradycardia, possible vagolytic effect, anaphylaxis |

ICP, intracranial pressure; IDBW, ideal body weight; IOP, intraocular pressure; MH, malignant hyperthermia; RSI, rapid sequence intubation; SCI, spinal cord injury; TBW, total body weight.

to rhabdomyolysis, which may present with an increase in creatinine, creatine kinase, and presence of oliguria or myoglobinuria.

Abdominal compartment syndrome is characterized as intra-abdominal hypertension and end-organ dysfunction secondary to edema that develops through the actions of inflammatory mediators elevated in shock, massive fluid resuscitation, and surgical manipulation. Clinical signs include a distended abdomen, elevated peak airway pressures, and oliguria. Intravesical pressure measured with a Foley catheter attached to a transducer approximates the intra-abdominal pressure. Pressures consistently above 20 mm Hg may compromise organ perfusion; thus, decompression should be pursued without delay. Limiting crystalloid infusion is one of the biggest determinants in preventing end-organ failure as a result of abdominal compartment syndrome.[5]

Trauma patients are at increased risk for venous thromboembolism. Mechanical and chemoprophylaxis with sequential compression devices (SCDs) and low molecular weight heparin should be initiated as soon as clinically safe. Hypoxemia with dyspnea, tachycardia, and/or fever should raise suspicion for pulmonary embolism. Diagnosis is confirmed with spiral computed tomography (CT) or CT pulmonary angiography. Temporary placement of an inferior vena cava filter may be indicated if the risk of bleeding with anticoagulation is high.

## REFERENCES

1. Santoni BG, et al. Manual in-line stabilization increases pressures applied by the laryngoscope blade during direct laryngoscopy and orotracheal intubation. *Anesthesiology.* 2009;110(1):24–31.
2. Zhang M, et al. Rapid detection of pneumothorax by ultrasonography in patients with multiple trauma. *Crit Care.* 2006;10(4):R112.
3. Simmons JW, Powell MF. Acute traumatic coagulopathy: pathophysiology and resuscitation. *Br J Anaesth.* 2016;117(suppl 3):iii31–iii43.
4. Grathwohl KW, et al. Total intravenous anesthesia including ketamine versus volatile gas anesthesia for combat-related operative traumatic brain injury. *Anesthesiology.* 2008;109(1):44–53.
5. Vatankhah S, et al. The relationship between fluid resuscitation and intra-abdominal hypertension in patients with blunt abdominal trauma. *Int J Crit Illn Inj Sci.* 2018;8(3):149–153.

# 338.

# ANESTHESIA FOR MRI

*Adi Cosic and Soozan S. Abouhassan*

Magnetic resonance imaging (MRI) is a technology that has roots in the early 1970s, when it was first developed by Paul Lauterbur at Stony Brook University. Using strong magnetic fields, magnetic gradients, and radio waves at multiple axes, MRIs interact with individual atoms in tissue. Nuclei of atoms (particularly hydrogen atoms, which most MRI machines are tuned to interact with) possess a net spin that gives them a characteristic magnetic dipole moment. When presented with the force of a magnetic field, these nuclei can orient themselves in parallel with the formed external magnetic field or at an angle to it, antiparallel. By applying oscillating fields, the nuclei can move between the parallel and antiparallel. Both of these positions cause a strain on the nuclei, and once the magnetic field is released, they return to their resting orientation and release energy, which is detected by a receiving coil in the MRI machine. In total, MRI machines produce three magnetic fields. The static, the radio-frequency (the weakest field, which can cause burns), and the gradient field. Most modern MRI machines operate between 0.5 and 3 Tesla (T), with most operating at about 1.5 T. Compare this to Earth's relatively weak magnetic field at 0.00005 T.

It is because of the strength of the magnetic fields that the development of "safety zones" in the MRI suite arose. Zone I includes all freely accessible areas to the public where the magnet has no effect. Zone II includes the reception area, dressing rooms, and all other areas immediately past zone I. Zone III is an access-restricted area in which all approved personnel must be screened for magnetic objects on their person before entering. Of note, the MRI control room is in zone III. Zone IV is the room that houses the MRI machine and is designed in such a way that the perimeter line limit contains 0.5 mT of magnetic field.

In the event of medical emergencies in zone IV, such as a cardiopulmonary arrest, current practice advisories from the American Society of Anesthesiologists (ASA) calls for the immediate removal of the patient from zone IV while initiating cardiopulmonary resuscitation if indicated, calling for help, and transporting the patient to a designated safe area that is not in zone IV. This area should be as close to zone IV as possible so resuscitation is not delayed.

The MRI machines in the United States are generally produced as *superconducting* magnets that necessitate a very low temperature (4K, -270°C) at all times to operate effectively, and because of this inherent quality, magnets are active at all times. Although another type of magnet exists (resistive magnets), these are not generally used, and stabilization of the magnetic field can take 30–60 minutes, and therefore they are usually left on. The low temperature magnets require is attained by the use of liquid helium and a series of heat exchangers and coils, which must be maintained at a cost of tens of thousands of dollars.

"Magnet quench" is the sudden loss of the nearly absolute zero temperature of the magnetic coils, which can happen either accidently or in the event of an emergency. In this process, the superconducting magnet loses its magnetic field, and helium in the cryogen bath is released quickly. While most MRI suites have helium venting systems, some do not, and this rapid release of helium can decrease oxygen concentrations below critical levels, decreasing temperature below freezing, as well as increasing pressure in the room to a high level. If scan room doors are closed when a quench occurs, the increase in pressure can prevent the doors from opening, trapping anyone inside. Irreparable damage during a quench can cost multiple millions of dollars to replace a MRI machine.[1]

The MRI scanners produce high-resolution images of body tissues that are used for guidance in therapy as well as diagnostics. Through nearly four decades of research, and with the emergence of semiconductors, MRI became what we know it as now. With 39 million scans performed per year, it is one of the most common modalities of imaging in the United States.

The strong magnetic fields and remote locations of MRI machines pose a unique set of challenges for the practitioners. Even small ferromagnetic objects such as ID clips and stethoscopes can become lethal projectiles when exposed to the magnetic field of an MRI machine. Additionally, most modern MRIs keep the magnetic field on even between scans. To avoid unwanted events, only clinicians who have undergone a safety check should be permitted within range of the MRI machine. In addition to visible and obvious ferromagnetic objects, there are also those that do not come to mind as quickly. Patients with implantable cardiac devices are at particularly high risk if they possess an incompatible device and can experience a fault of the device, switching it to asynchronous mode or turning it off. Medical devices are often labeled in one of three categories: MRI safe, conditional, or unsafe.[2]

High levels of noise that can potentially cause hearing damage can be experienced by the patient, even under sedation. Typically, sounds over 85 dB are produced by the MRI machine, which is on par with a freight train passing by. Because of this, it is pertinent to protect the patient's hearing and place earplugs to prevent hearing loss.

Systemic and localized heating due to reactions between incompatible monitor wires and the magnetic field can occur if incompatible wiring is used. Personal jewelry that a patient wears is also prohibited in this setting for this reason. Patients are especially susceptible to burns when there is no barrier placed between the skin and the wiring, particularly when coils are formed. This is evidenced by Faraday's law of induction, which implies that the current in a wire is directly proportional to the number of coils present. To avoid this, electrocardiography (ECG) pads, as well as any other wired monitor, should be placed in close proximity at the center of the chest with no coiling, exiting with no crossing. Pulse oximeters with wireless or fiber-optic cables now exist.[2] Among the most common complications is ECG interference caused by the magnetic field produced by the MRI machine. Even MRI-compatible leads are not immune to the effects, most commonly imitating malignant arrhythmias or ST segment abnormalities.

Because of the above listed complications, as well as a claustrophobic environment, potentially developmentally disabled patients, anxious patients, or patients otherwise unable to cooperate, sedation is sometimes necessary to provide a motionless patient and therefore high-quality image. Thought should be given to the length of tubing needed to reach a patient. Typically, a practitioner will set outside of the MRI suite and remotely monitor the patient's vitals. Immediate access to the patient is limited. Extension sets on intravenous tubing as well as airways are sometimes necessary to provide adequate anesthesia without being in close proximity to the patient.[4]

Visualization of the patient can be obscured by a darkened room, interrupted line of sight, or other distractions. Due to these challenges, practice advisories have been formed in regard to patient care in the MRI suite.[2] Even though these difficulties exist, and through the often unfamiliar environments that are encountered, proper charting is always necessary.

A multitude of options for anesthesia exist when presented with a patient in the MRI suite. It is imperative the ASA standard monitors are connected to the patient and verified prior to beginning a case as it is difficult to troubleshoot after the start of the scan. Intravenous anesthesia, achieved by propofol or ketamine, titrated to maintain respiratory drive is a viable option if the patient lacks any contraindications, such as obstructive sleep apnea or other signs of difficult airway. As noted previously, extension tubing long enough to reach the patient for intravenous access is necessary to titrate medications. If presented with patients who possess contraindications for intravenous anesthesia, general anesthesia is considered the next best step. MRI-compatible anesthesia machines exist and are commonly used in these settings.

## REFERENCES

1. Ye L, et al. Magnetic field dependent stability and quench behavior and degradation limits in conduction-cooled $MgB_2$ wires and coils. *Supercond Sci Technol*. 2015;28(3):035015. Accessed November 2, 2020. https://www.ncbi.nlm.nih.gov/pmc/articles/PMC4394391/
2. Reddy U, et al. Anaesthesia for magnetic resonance imaging. *Contin Educ Anaesth Crit Care Pain*. 2012;12(Issue 3):140–144.
3. Deen J, et al. Challenges in the anesthetic management of ambulatory patients in the MRI suites. *Curr Opin Anaesthesiol*. 2017;30(6):670–675.
4. Berkow LC. Anesthetic management and human factors in the intraoperative MRI environment. *Curr Opin Anaesthesiol*. 2016;29(5):563–567.

# 339.

# HEMORRHAGIC SHOCK

*Colby B. Tanner and Elaine A. Boydston*

## INTRODUCTION

Hemorrhagic shock results in impaired organ perfusion and drastically reduced oxygen delivery to vital organs. If not corrected quickly, hemorrhagic shock results in end-organ damage and ultimately death.[1] Hemorrhagic shock accounts for more than 60,000 deaths annually in the United States and approximately 1.9 million deaths worldwide. Trauma is the cause of the vast majority of hemorrhagic shock–related deaths (1.5 million annual deaths worldwide). Of patients who die from potentially survivable traumatic injuries, 80%–90% of the deaths are from hemorrhage.[1,2] Other significant causes of hemorrhage include surgical bleeding, gastrointestinal bleeding, pregnancy and peripartum bleeding, and ruptured abdominal aortic aneurysms. No matter the cause of the hemorrhage, rapid resuscitation with blood products improves patient outcomes and decreases mortality.[1]

## PHYSIOLOGY OF HEMORRHAGIC SHOCK

Hemodynamically significant hemorrhage causes an immediate release of catecholamines and activation of the renin-angiotensin system, which acts to maintain blood pressure within the normal range. This response allows healthy individuals to lose up to 30% of their blood volume before showing signs of shock.[3] The intense vasoconstriction due to catecholamine release can cause ischemia of vital organs and tissues, resulting in anaerobic metabolism.[3,4] Anaerobic metabolites accumulate, including lactic acid, inorganic phosphates, and oxygen radicals. This combination of poor organ perfusion from vasoconstriction and decreased oxygen delivery with worsening acidosis ultimately causes cellular apoptosis and organ dysfunction.[1,3]

At the site of tissue injury, endothelial damage activates the coagulation cascade and triggers platelet aggregation, leading to thrombin clot formation and hemostasis. This response is opposed by circulating plasmin and autoheparinization from glycocalyx shedding by damaged vascular endothelium,[1,4] tending toward a state of coagulopathy and hyperfibrinolysis.[1] In patients with severe traumatic injuries, the procoagulopathic effect can be especially pronounced and has been demonstrated almost immediately following injury. Untreated, coagulopathy worsens over time, as demonstrated by laboratory tests, including thromboelastography (TEG), and hyperfibrinolysis is frequently detected within hours.[4]

## DIAGNOSIS

The initial assessment of bleeding patients should involve a detailed history, including estimated blood volume lost at the scene and en route to the hospital, extent of suspected injuries, mechanism of blood loss, and history of anticoagulant use. Physical examination, including initial vital signs, can help estimate the severity of hemorrhagic shock Table 339.1). Normal heart rate and blood pressure in a patient with significant hemorrhage indicates stage I shock. Tachycardia indicates progression to stage II, while hypotension indicates progression to stage III. Once patients become hypotensive from hemorrhage, it is probable that they have lost at least 30% of their total blood volume. Physical examination should focus on body compartments that can hold a large volume of blood, including the thoracic cavity, abdomen, pelvis, retroperitoneum, and proximal thighs. Providers should look for signs of blood extravasation as they sometimes are evident prior to changes in vital signs. Laboratory tests may help elucidate the extent of hemorrhage by indicating tissue hypoperfusion, as evidenced by acidemia and elevated blood lactate. Abnormal hemoglobin and international normalized ratio values can also help predict the need for massive transfusion.[1] Last, in situations of traumatic injury, several imaging modalities can be employed rapidly to screen for the source of bleeding, including computed tomographic scans and ultrasound (i.e., focused assessment with sonography in trauma examination).

**Table 339.1 STAGES OF HEMORRHAGIC SHOCK**

| STAGE | BLOOD LOSS, % | HEART RATE | BLOOD PRESSURE | RESPIRATORY RATE |
|-------|-----|-----|-------------|-------|
| I | <15 | <100 | Normotensive | 14–20 |
| II | 15–30 | 100–120 | Normotensive | 20–30 |
| III | 30–40 | 120–140 | Hypotensive | 30–40 |
| IV | >40 | >140 | Hypotensive | >35 |

Based on values from American College of Surgeons Committee on Trauma.[1]

## MANAGEMENT

Early diagnosis and treatment of hemorrhagic shock results in decreased organ damage and improved mortality by minimizing the accumulation of oxygen debt by organs undergoing anaerobic metabolism.[1,4] While intravascular volume expansion is critical to the restoration of adequate perfusion, the choice of fluid for volume expansion can play a significant role in determining patient outcomes.

### INITIAL MANAGEMENT

Early attempts at hemostasis after traumatic injury include placement of mechanical pressure at the site of bleeding if possible (e.g., tourniquet for extremity injuries, direct pressure at injury site, pelvic binder, etc.). Additionally, avoidance or correction of hypothermia is especially important. Diagnostic measures to determine the site of bleeding and the extent of hemorrhage should be employed as soon as possible to allow for planning of surgical, endoscopic, and/or angiographic means of obtaining hemostasis.

### RESUSCITATION

Blood products should be preferentially employed for volume expansion as they are less likely to result in dilutional coagulopathy and acidosis, as compared to crystalloid or other colloid solutions. If whole blood is not available, it is important to transfuse balanced ratios of blood products to maintain near-normal blood composition. Ratios closest to 1:1:1 red blood cells to plasma to platelets have been shown to improve mortality when administered early in the resuscitation of hemorrhagic shock.[1] While awaiting definitive treatment (i.e., repair of the injury and ultimately hemostasis), it is important to also evaluate the extent of coagulopathy via laboratory tests, including prothrombin time, activated partial thromboplastin time, and viscoelastic tests such as TEG or rotational thromboelastometry. Coagulopathy can be treated with procoagulant therapies, including recombinant factor VIIa, antifibrinolytics, prothrombin complex concentrate, and fibrinogen complex concentrate. The use of these agents to reduce hemorrhage should be weighed against the risks of thrombotic complications depending on individual patient risk factors.[1]

### BLOOD PRESSURE CONTROL

Vasopressor use remains controversial in hemorrhagic shock and is generally employed only when hypotension persists despite volume resuscitation.[3,5] Norepinephrine and vasopressin can counteract the vasodilatory components of shock, while inotropes such as epinephrine or dobutamine can be employed in the presence of myocardial dysfunction. These agents should be used judiciously as treatment of hypotension without concomitant volume expansion can worsen outcomes and increase mortality.[3] In a 2018 meta-analysis, Tran et al. evaluated studies comparing conventional resuscitation strategies (goal of maintaining mean arterial pressure [MAP] between 65 and 100 mm Hg) to permissive hypotension (goal of maintaining MAP between 50 and 70 mm Hg). The authors found that permissive hypotension was associated with decreased total blood loss and fewer blood transfusions. While this suggests a potential survival benefit to resuscitation while allowing for permissive hypotension, higher powered studies are needed to make a definitive recommendation.[5] Blood pressure management should be individualized based on the patient's risk of bleeding and underlying medical problems predisposing them to organ dysfunction due to hypoperfusion.

## REFERENCES

1. Cannon JW. Hemorrhagic shock. *N Engl J Med.* 2018;378(4): 370–379.
2. Eastridge BJ, et al. Outcomes of traumatic hemorrhagic shock and the epidemiology of preventable death from injury. *Transfusion.* 2019;59(S2):1423–1428.
3. Gupta B, et al. Vasopressors: do they have any role in hemorrhagic shock? *J Anaesthesiol Clin Pharmacol.* 2017;33(1):3–8.
4. White NJ, et al. Hemorrhagic blood failure: oxygen debt, coagulopathy, and endothelial damage. *J Trauma Acute Care Surg.* 2017;82(6S suppl 1):S41–S49.
5. Tran A, et al. Permissive hypotension versus conventional resuscitation strategies in adult trauma patients with hemorrhagic shock: a systematic review and meta-analysis of randomized controlled trials. *J Trauma Acute Care Surg.* 2018;84(5):802–808.

# 340.

# MANAGEMENT OF TRAUMATIC BRAIN INJURY

*Bharathram Vasudevan and Ned F. Nasr*

## INTRODUCTION

Traumatic brain injury (TBI) is a major cause of mortality and disability, accounting for 2.8 million emergency department visits, hospitalizations, and deaths each year in the United States.[1] Most common causes are falls and motor vehicle accidents.[1]

## PATHOPHYSIOLOGY

Pathophysiology of TBI is divided into primary and secondary brain injuries. Primary brain injury is injury to intracranial structures from external mechanical forces during initial trauma.[2] Various pathologies include contusions, hematomas, diffuse axonal injury, and cerebral edema. Secondary brain injury starts after initial trauma and continues for days, mediated by inflammation, neurotransmitter excitotoxicity, free radical injury, apoptosis, ischemia, and electrolyte imbalances, leading to neuronal death, cerebral edema, and elevated intracranial pressure (ICP).[2]

## ANESTHETIC CONSIDERATIONS

Patients with severe TBI may undergo emergent or non-emergent intracranial or extracranial surgeries. The main goal is to prevent secondary brain injury by maintenance of cerebral perfusion pressure (CPP), treating elevated ICP, avoiding hypoxia, hypotension, hyper-/hypocarbia, hyper-/hypoglycemia, hyperthermia, seizures, and coagulopathy. The 2016 Brain Trauma Foundation guidelines provide evidence-based recommendations for management.[3]

## GLASGOW COMA SCALE

### EYE-OPENING RESPONSE

Spontaneous, open with blinking at baseline, 4 points

To verbal stimuli, command, speech, 3 points

To pain only (not applied to face), 2 points

No response, 1 point

### VERBAL RESPONSE

Oriented, 5 points

Confused conversation, but able to answer questions, 4 points

Inappropriate words, 3 points

Incomprehensible speech, 2 points

No response, 1 point

### MOTOR RESPONSE

Obeys commands for movement, 6 points

Purposeful movement to painful stimulus, 5 points

Withdraws in response to pain, 4 points

Flexion in response to pain (decorticate posturing), 3 points

Extension response in response to pain (decerebrate posturing), 2 points

No response, 1 point

## PREOPERATIVE EVALUATION

A comprehensive preanesthetic evaluation should be performed, including pupillary and neurological examination. Based on the Glasgow Coma Scale (GCS), TBI is classified as mild (GCS 13–15), moderate (GCS 9–12), and severe (GCS 3–8). Patients with GCS of 8 or less need emergent intubation. Signs of impending herniation should necessitate immediate measures to lower ICP. Imaging and laboratory testing should be reviewed, including complete blood count, electrolytes, glucose, blood gases, and coagulation profile.

## INTRAOPERATIVE MANAGEMENT

### AIRWAY MANAGEMENT

Airway management is challenging due to associated cervical spine injuries, facial trauma, full stomach, and depressed respiration. The method of choice is rapid sequence induction (RSI) and intubation with manual inline stabilization and cricoid pressure.[4] Video laryngoscopy improves visualization but takes longer and does not decrease cervical movement.[4] Fiber-optic intubation ensures minimal movement but may be difficult in emergencies. Nasal intubation should be avoided in skull base fractures.

### CHOICE OF ANESTHETIC DRUGS

Intravenous induction agents decrease cerebral blood flow (CBF), cerebral metabolic rate for oxygen ($CMRO_2$), and ICP except for ketamine, which increases these.[5] Recent studies reported ketamine is safe but is best avoided. Propofol and etomidate can be safely used. Succinylcholine is used for neuromuscular blockade during RSI unless otherwise contraindicated. Though it can transiently increase ICP, administering a defasciculating dose of nondepolarizing muscle relaxant before succinylcholine may prevent that.[4] Alternatively, rocuronium (1.2 mg/kg) can be used. Short-acting opioids are administered for analgesia and blunting intubation response. Longer acting opioids are avoided to facilitate early neurological examination. Maintenance can be with intravenous or inhalational agents. All potent volatile agents decrease $CMRO_2$ but increase CBF and ICP by vasodilation. This effect is minimal under 1 minimum alveolar concentration. Nitrous oxide increases $CMRO_2$, CBF, and ICP and is avoided.[5]

## VENTILATION

Hypoxia leads to increased mortality. The oxygenation goal is partial pressure of oxygen greater than 60 mm Hg.[3] Adequate ventilation should ensure normocarbia: partial pressure of carbon dioxide ($PaCO_2$) 35–40 mm Hg. Hypercarbia can increase CBF and ICP. Mild hyperventilation can be used temporarily to decrease ICP for short periods with target $PaCO_2$ of 30–35 mm Hg.[5] Further hyperventilation to $PaCO_2$ 25–30 mm Hg can cause cerebral ischemia and is avoided. Hyperventilation is also avoided during the first 24 hours after TBI.[3]

## ICP MONITORING AND MANAGEMENT

Intracranial pressure monitoring is frequently done. Elevated ICP of more than 22 mm Hg is associated with increased mortality.[3] Management includes ensuring adequate analgesia and sedation, elevating the head more than 30°, discontinuing positive end-expiratory pressure, temporary hyperventilation, switching to intravenous anesthesia, and treating hyperthermia and seizures. When a ventriculostomy drain is present, cerebrospinal fluid can be drained in small increments. Osmotherapy with mannitol (0.25 to 1 g/kg) or hypertonic saline can be used. Therapeutic coma with barbiturate or propofol is reserved for refractory cases.[3]

## HEMODYNAMIC MANAGEMENT

The goal of hemodynamic management is to maintain adequate CPP. CPP is equal to the mean arterial pressure (MAP) minus the ICP. Invasive arterial blood pressure monitoring is performed with a transducer leveled at the level of the external auditory meatus. Normally, cerebral autoregulation preserves CBF between MAP of 60 and 160 mm Hg. TBI disrupts this, and CBF becomes dependent on systemic pressures (pressure passive). The goal systolic blood pressure is 100 mm Hg or greater in patients 50–69 years old and 110 mm Hg or greater in patients 15–49 years old or 70 years old or older.[3] The minimum CPP goal is 60–70 mm Hg.[3] When CPP is low, the first step is to decrease the ICP if elevated. The next would be to raise the MAP by vasopressors or fluid administration. Isotonic crystalloids like normal saline are used for fluid management.[5] Hypotonic solutions can cause cerebral edema and are avoided. Lactated Ringer solution is mildly hypo-osmolar and should be used with caution. Use of albumin is generally avoided in TBI as it can increase cerebral edema.[5]

## OTHER IMPORTANT CONSIDERATIONS

Traumatic brain injury can cause coagulopathy by systemic release of tissue factor and phospholipids. Fresh frozen plasma, prothrombin complex concentrate, and vitamin K may be administered to maintain a target international normalized ratio of less than 1.4. For thrombocytopenia,[4] platelets may be transfused to maintain a count greater than 75,000/mm[3]. Anemia can lead to decreased cerebral oxygen delivery. However, a liberal transfusion threshold of hemoglobin less than 10 g/dL is not associated with better outcomes compared to a threshold of 7 g/dL.[4] Hyper-/hypoglycemia should be avoided. The target glucose range is 80–180 mg/dL. Temperature monitoring is done to maintain normothermia. Hyperthermia worsens brain injury, while hypothermia has not improved outcomes. Antiseizure drugs are recommended to prevent early posttraumatic seizures.[3] Steroids can be harmful in TBI and are avoided.[3] Advanced cerebral monitoring techniques including jugular venous oximetry (normal value 55%–75%) and brain tissue oxygen monitoring (normal value 20–35 mm Hg) can be used.[3] Lower values reflect decreased CPP, anemia, or hypoxemia.

## POSTOPERATIVE CARE

Patients with severe TBI are usually not extubated and require further care in the intensive care unit (ICU). Mild-to-moderate TBI patients should be evaluated on an individual basis for neurological status, spontaneous ventilation, and airway protection before extubation. Care should be taken to prevent any increase in ICP at emergence. Further care in the ICU is directed by the same principles to avoid secondary brain injury and allow early recovery and rehabilitation.

## REFERENCES

1. Taylor CA, et al. Traumatic brain injury–related emergency department visits, hospitalizations, and deaths—United States, 2007 and 2013. *MMWR Surveill Summ*. 2017:66(no. SS-9):1–16.
2. Farrell D, Bendo AA. Perioperative management of severe traumatic brain injury: what is new? *Curr Anesthesiol Rep*. 2018;8(3):279–289.
3. Carney N, et al. Guidelines for the management of severe traumatic brain injury, fourth edition. *Neurosurgery*. 2017;80(1):6–15.
4. Qureshi H, et al. Anesthetic *Management of Traumatic Brain Injury. Clin Med Rev Case Rep*. 2017;4:159.
5. Khandelwal A, et al. Anesthetic considerations for extracranial injuries in patients with associated brain trauma. *J Anaesthesiol Clin Pharmacol*. 2019;35(3):302–311.

# 341.

# MASS CASUALTY EVENTS

*Ashok Kumar Manepalli and Stacey Watt*

## INTRODUCTION

Mass casualty events are disasters that result in casualties that overwhelm the healthcare system in which they occur. They can range from natural disasters such as forest fires to man-made disasters such as bomb explosions.

## MASS CASUALTY EVENTS

There are various types of mass casualty events[1]:

- Radiation exposure from nuclear bombs or plant accidents has the greatest impact on tissue with high regeneration rate (i.e., gastrointestinal, skin, bone marrow, lymphatics). Potassium iodide must be given within 24 hours of exposure to effectively prevent adverse thyroid effects or cancers caused by radioactive iodine I 131 ($^{131}$I).

- Chemical agents have historically been used as weapons of war, but such attacks have subsided since the Chemical Weapons Convention (1993). Still, attacks can occur from terrorist groups and countries not bound by the treaty. Chemical agents include tabun, sarin, soman, cyanides, phosgene, chlorine, and sulfur mustard. Nerve agents are classically treated with atropine, oximes, and benzodiazepines.
- Biological agents are usually weaponized forms of existing infectious agents, such as Ebola, anthrax, salmonella, or hantavirus. Most agents have a predictable symptomology and presentation, which anesthesiologists should be able to recognize once alerted to the disaster.
- In the event of an infectious disease pandemic, anesthesiologists should familiarize themselves with the pathophysiology of the offending agent and the appropriate contact/isolation precautions. Treatment should include the use of proper personal protective equipment (PPE) to ensure the safety of healthcare workers. Aerosol-generating procedures such as intubation and bag-mask ventilation require extra protection as exposure is maximized to the provider and surrounding personnel.
- Mass shootings and bombings are quick to overwhelm hospitals due to the polytrauma nature of the victims who require immediate surgical intervention. Emergency room staff, surgical staff, blood banks, operating rooms, and intensive care unit (ICU) staff are the first to be stressed by such disasters. Strong leadership and guidelines are required to appropriately triage patients and allocate appropriate resources. Additionally, leadership should work to recruit additional staffing in times of crises. As anesthesiologists, we are trained in emergency situations and can help direct emergency plans on a systemwide scale.

## DISASTER MANAGEMENT

- During a mass casualty event, the goals of disaster management[1] are to effectively minimize casualties, triage and treat victims, and facilitate recovery. This is only done through effective collaboration of hospital systems, government agencies, and local communities. The four phases of a disaster are mitigation, preparedness, response, and recovery.

- Mitigation: preventing or attenuating the effects of the disaster before it occurs (e.g., flood insurance)
- Preparedness: planning the appropriate response; notifying the appropriate personnel; establishing required resources (e.g., evacuation routes, emergency kits)
- Response: execute disaster response plan; mitigate hazardous situations created by disasters (e.g., medical care, food, water, search and rescue)
- Recovery: return to normalcy, reconstruction, data collection (e.g., temporary housing, postdisaster medical care, rebuilding communities)

### ROLE

- Anesthesiologists' breadth of knowledge in physiology, pharmacology, airway management, trauma, line placement, and resuscitation make them a vital resource to serve an important role during mass casualty events.[2] Their training provides for high adaptability and allows them to be readily deployed to a variety of hospital settings such as the operating room/postanesthesia care unit, emergency department, and ICU. Depending on the type of disaster, anesthesiologists may be called to act as first responders and/or triage leaders.

### TRIAGE

- Sorting patients into severity categories to determine who receives care first *is one of the most important steps in mass casualty event treatment*. The two most commonly used triage algorithms are SALT[3] (sort, assess, life-saving interventions, treatment/transport) and START[4] (simple triage and rapid treatment). The purpose of the triage system is to organize patients by severity of injury and likelihood of survival and subsequently allocate the appropriate resources for management (see Table 341.1).

### AIRWAY MANAGEMENT

- Airway management[5] is often the responsibility of anesthesiologists during mass casualty events. Endotracheal intubation via rapid sequence intubation (RSI) is the gold standard for securing the airway. Avoid succinylcholine during RSI in the setting of nerve agent toxicity. The use of PPE may prolong intubation time by reducing manual dexterity and impairing airway visualization. Although a supraglottic airway can be implemented faster, or required in the case of a difficult intubation, it should be replaced by an endotracheal tube as soon as feasible (only used as a bridge to intubation).

**Table 341.1** MASS CASUALTY VICTIM TRIAGE

| INJURY SEVERITY | DESCRIPTION | MANAGEMENT |
|---|---|---|
| Immediate | Survivable life-threatening injuries | Immediate intervention |
| Delayed | Hemodynamically stable | Injuries may be addressed later without adverse outcomes |
| Minimal | Minor injuries | Hospitalization not required |
| Expectant | Severe injuries, unlikely to survive | Medicate for comfort to alleviate pain and suffering |
| Dead | Unsurvivable injuries; pulseless | Should not start resuscitative efforts |

FROM *Adv Anesth*. 2018;36(1):39–66. doi: 10.1016/j.aan.2018.07.002

## PREPAREDNESS

- Mass casualty events can easily overwhelm a hospital system with a sudden increase in patients, damage to infrastructure, and responder exposure to toxins. The initial hazard vulnerability analysis is used to identify the source of the disaster, institutional impact, and response capability. Hospital emergency preparedness plans[5] provide a chain of command and establish a command center to coordinate the disaster response.

- The Joint Commission requires all accredited hospitals have a disaster plan prepared and tested at least twice a year. The Hospital Incident Command System (HICS) consists of a command-and-control framework headed by the incident commander and contains prioritized tasks for others. A single leader would quickly be overwhelmed, so responsibilities are delegated per expertise. The HICS does not address specific operating room management and triage, so an experienced anesthesiologist would be well suited for the role.

## REFERENCES

1. Kuza CM, McIsaac JH 3rd. Emergency preparedness and mass casualty considerations for anesthesiologists. *Adv Anesth*. 2018;36(1):39–66.
2. Pardo M, Miller RD. Trauma, bioterrorism and natural disasters. In: Manual C. Pardo, Ronald D. Miller, eds. *Basics of Anesthesia*. 7th ed. Philadelphia, PA: Elsevier; 2018:681–688.
3. SALT mass casualty triage: concept endorsed by the American College of Emergency Physicians, American College of Surgeons Committee on Trauma, American Trauma Society, National Association of EMS Physicians, National Disaster Life Support Education Consortium, and State and Territorial Injury Prevention Directors Association. *Disaster Med Public Health Prep*. 2008;2(4):245–246.
4. Dudaryk RA, Pretto EA. Resuscitation in a multiple casualty event. *Anesthesiol Clin*. 2013;31(1):85–106.
5. Hagberg CA, et al. Disaster preparedness, cardiopulmonary resuscitation, and airway management. In: Carin A. Hagberg, Carlos A. Artime, Mkhael F. Aziz, eds. *Hagberg and Benumofs Airway Management*. 3rd ed. Philadelphia, PA: Elsevier; 2018:692–694.

# 342.

# CHEMICAL AND BIOLOGICAL WARFARE

*Cassian Horoszczak and Stacey Watt*

## INTRODUCTION

Chemical and biological warfare agents pose as major health threats not only in modern warfare, but also for their potential use in domestic terrorism.

## CHEMICAL WARFARE AGENT CLASSES

Modern chemical warfare began during World War I with the use of pulmonary agents. Since then, chemical weapon development was expanded by governments to include the following[1]:

- *Toxic agents* are intended to cause serious injury or death; they are divided into four classes:
  - *Nerve agents* (acetylcholinesterase inhibitors): All nerve agents are organophosphorus esters. G-series agents (second generation) include tabun, sarin, soman, and cyclosarin. V-series agents (third generation) include VX. A-series agents (fourth generation) or Novichok compounds are characterized by low volatility (persist as liquids at room temperature). Toxidrome includes cholinergic hyperactivity ("dumbbells": diarrhea, urination, miosis, bradycardia, bronchoconstriction, excitation or involuntary muscle contraction, lacrimation, lethargy, salivation). Pharmacological treatment following exposure includes atropine and pralidoxime. If exposure to a nerve agent is anticipated, pretreatment with pyridostigmine should be considered.
  - *Pulmonary agents/asphyxiants*: Type 1 agents affect large airways (e.g., smoke products, sulfur mustard). Type 2 agents affect terminal and respiratory bronchioles and alveoli (e.g., phosgene). Mixed-effect agents affect both (e.g., chlorine, lewisite). Treatment of type 1 agents includes early intubation, humidified 100% $O_2$, bronchodilators, with or without corticosteroids, and antibiotics for secondary infection. Treatment of type 2 agents includes positive

pressure ventilation (continuous positive airway pressure [CPAP] or positive end-expiratory pressure [PEEP]), bronchodilators, and rarely corticosteroids.
  - *Systemic (hematologic) asphyxiants* include cyanide salts and hydrogen sulfide. Both inactivate the cytochrome oxidase needed for mitochondrial oxidative phosphorylation in the electron transport chain, leading to cellular anoxia. Central apnea is usually the mechanism of death in cyanide poisoning. First-line treatment includes airway support and specific cyanide antidotes, including the combination of sodium thiosulfate and hydroxocobalamin. Where hydroxocobalamin is not available, the cyanide antidote kit may be available in some centers (no longer manufactured); it contains amyl nitrite, sodium nitrite, and sodium thiosulfate.
  - *Vesicants (blistering agents)* include mustards (DNA alkylating agents), lewisite, and phosgene. Treatment includes decontamination, treating skin lesions similar to burns, and airway support as many vesicants are also pulmonary agents.
- *Incapacitating agents* are intended to cause temporary, nonlethal injury:
  - *Anticholinergic agents*: 3-Quinuclidinyl (NATO [North American Treaty Organization] code BZ) is a solid disseminated by heat-generating artillery rounds and can persist in the environment for 3 to 4 weeks. BZ binds to and blocks muscarinic cholinergic receptors in the central nervous system, smooth muscle, and exocrine glands to inhibit acetylcholine binding at these sites. Treatment is supportive care, including cooling. Some may benefit from physostigmine.
  - *Riot-control agents* include chloroacetophenone (CN, Mace˙), chlorobenzylidenemalononitrile (CS), dibenzoxazepine (CR), diphenylaminoarsine (DM, adamsite), and oleoresin capsicum (OC, pepper spray). Treatment is supportive.
  - *Opioids*, especially potent fentanyl derivatives. In 2002, Russian Special Forces deployed a chemical aerosol against Chechen terrorists to rescue hostages

from a Moscow theater. Mass spectrometry of clothing from survivors demonstrated a mixture of carfentanil and remifentanil. Inadequate use of naloxone resulted in significant postevacuation casualties.

- *Incendiary/burn-causing agents* are intended to create not only light and flame, but also thermal injuries. Agents include magnesium powder, chlorine trifluoride, white phosphorus, napalm, and thermite. These agents undergo high-temperature exothermic redox reactions in the presence of an oxidant (usually oxygen) and a source of ignition. Hydrogen fluoride (HF) may cause chemical burns through an acid-base reaction. HF boils at 19.5°C, forming a gas at room temperature. On contact with moisture or tissue, HF gas immediately converts to hydrofluoric acid, which is highly corrosive and systemically toxic, resulting in severe electrolyte abnormalities, including hypocalcemia and hyperkalemia.

## BIOLOGICAL WARFARE AGENT CLASSES

Rudimentary forms of biological warfare have been practiced since antiquity through to modern times, where in most cases the bioagent is either a bacterial agent, viral agent, or toxin. The Centers for Disease Control and Prevention categorizes bioagents with the potential for bioterrorism use into three categories[2]:

- Category A: High-priority agents that pose a risk to national security because they easily disseminate, result in high mortality rates, have the potential for major public health impact and might cause public panic.
- *Anthrax (Bacillus anthracis)*: Cutaneous anthrax is the most common form of the disease. Cutaneous anthrax involves papule, to vesicle, to eschar formation with painful regional lymphadenopathy and fever. Pulmonary anthrax (wool sorter's disease) involves severe pneumonia and mediastinal hemorrhagic lymphadenitis (mediastinal widening on chest x-ray). Gastrointestinal disease is rare, but edema and blockage of the gastrointestinal tract can occur.
- *Botulism (Clostridium botulinum* toxin): The toxin blocks release of acetylcholine at the neuromuscular junction of peripheral nerve synapses, resulting in flaccid paralysis. Preformed toxin in poorly canned foods infects adults. Infants may ingest spores in household dust or honey.
- *Plague (Yersinia pestis)*: Bubonic plague includes symptoms of rapidly increasing fever, regional buboes in the groin or axilla, and conjunctivitis. Pneumonic plague results from septic emboli in bubonic plague or inhalation from infected individuals.
- *Smallpox (Variola major)*: One serotype exists. There is a 5- to 17-day incubation period, starting with a flu-like prodrome for 2–4 days followed by synchronous rash (all vesicles same stage), which begins in the mouth and spreads to extremities to cover the whole body within 24 hours (Figure 432.1).
- *Tularemia (Francisella tularensis)*: This is endemic in every state of the United States. Reservoir includes wild animals, especially rabbits. Traumatic

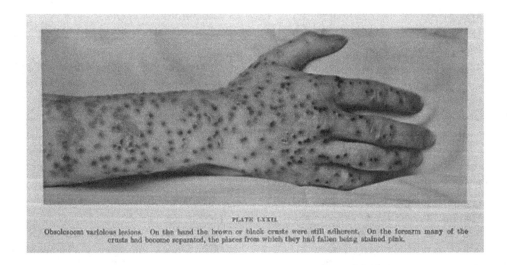

PLATE LXXII.
Obsolescent variolous lesions. On the hand the brown or black crusts were still adherent. On the forearm many of the crusts had become separated, the places from which they had fallen being stained pink.

**Figure 342.1** *Gross anatomical specimen of forearm with smallpox.* The fur trade of North America carried smallpox to Native Americans of the continental interior, and even intentional infection of Natives by British soldiers was implicated. In 1796, Edward Jenner demonstrated that inoculation with cowpox protected against smallpox. Subsequently, vaccinia virus became the basis for the smallpox vaccine, with the global eradication of the disease certified by the World Health Organization in 1980. Credit: Obsolescent variolous lesions, smallpox. Credit: Wellcome Collection. Attribution 4.0 International (CC BY 4.0).

implantation causes ulceroglandular disease. Aerosolization can cause pneumonia.

- *Viral hemorrhagic fevers*: Filoviruses (Ebola, Marburg) and arenavirus species (Lassa, Machupo) are agents with high fatality rates. Rodent hosts of arenavirus species shed the virus into the environment in urine or droppings. Lassa and Machupo are also associated with secondary person-to-person and nosocomial transmission. Airborne transmission has also been reported.
- *Category B*: These are midpriority agents that are moderately easy to disseminate, have moderate morbidity rates and low mortality rates, and require enhanced diagnostic capacity and disease surveillance.
  - Brucellosis (*Brucella* species); epsilon toxin of *Clostridium perfringens*; hemorrhagic diarrhea (*Salmonella* species, *Escherichia coli* O157:H7, *Shigella*); glanders (*Burkholderia mallei*); melioidosis (*Burkholderia pseudomallei*); psittacosis (*Chlamydia psittaci*); Q fever (*Coxiella burnetii*); ricin toxin from *Ricinus communis* (castor beans); staphylococcal enterotoxin B; typhus fever (*Rickettsia prowazekii*); viral encephalitis (alphaviruses, e.g., eastern equine encephalitis, Venezuelan equine encephalitis, as well as western equine encephalitis and water safety threats [*Vibrio cholerae, Cryptosporidium parvum*].
- *Category C*: These are lower priority, including emerging pathogens with the potential for mass dissemination because of availability, ease of production/dissemination, and potential for high morbidity/ mortality rates and major health impact.
  - Nipah virus (*Paramyxoviridae* species) and hantavirus.

## CONCLUSION

The 1972 Biological Weapons Convention supplemented the 1925 Geneva Protocol in prohibiting the use but not possession or development of chemical and biological weapons.[3] The 1993 Chemical Weapons Convention outlawed production, stockpiling, and use of chemical weapons, as well as obligated member states to destroy currently stockpiled chemical weapons.[4]

## ANESTHETIC CONSIDERATIONS

- *Preoperative*: Diagnosis of the infection or toxidrome is usually based on clinical presentation and exposure history as there may be insufficient time to wait for microbiology or pathology.
- *Intraoperative*: Decontaminate infected material. Care is often supportive.
- *Postoperative*: Administer vaccines, when available, and maintain appropriate transmission precautions.

## REFERENCES

1. Madsen J. Overview of chemical-warfare agents. *Merck Manuals Professional Edition*. Last full review/revision May 2019; content last modified May 2019. Accessed April 18, 2020. http://www.merckmanuals.com/en-ca/professional/injuries-poisoning/mass-casualty-weapons/overview-of-chemical-warfare-agents
2. Centers for Disease Control and Prevention. Bioterrorism agents and diseases. April 4, 2018. Accessed April 18, 2020. https://emergency.cdc.gov/agent/agentlist-category.asp
3. Biological Weapons—UNODA. United Nations. Accessed April 18, 2020. http://www.un.org/disarmament/wmd/bio/
4. Chemical Weapons Convention. OPCW. Accessed April 18, 2020. http://www.opcw.org/chemical-weapons-convention

# 343.

# ANESTHESIA FOR OUTPATIENT SURGERY

*M. Anthony Cometa and Christopher Giordano*

## INTRODUCTION

Ambulatory surgery originated due to resource constraints and recognition of its economic advantages.[1] It is estimated that outpatient surgery costs are approximately five times lower than inpatient.[2] The first outpatient surgery unit opened in the 1950s, and more facilities followed. In turn, initial recognition of ambulatory anesthesia as a subspecialty was augmented by the formation of the Society for Ambulatory Anesthesia. Currently, ambulatory surgery constitutes approximately 80% of elective surgeries in the United States,[1] a significant economic footprint in today's healthcare revenue.

## PREOPERATIVE MANAGEMENT: SELECTION FACTORS FOR OUTPATIENT SURGERY

Contraindications to outpatient surgery are relative based on patient risk stratification for a particular procedure rather than absolute. It is paramount that both the procedure and the patient are appropriate for an outpatient surgery setting. For example, a patient with severe aortic stenosis and pulmonary hypertension would not be appropriate for laparoscopic cholecystectomy in an outpatient surgery center, but that same patient may be able to undergo cataract surgery. The advancement of minimally invasive surgical procedures coupled with appropriate anesthetic techniques facilitating site-specific surgery (e.g., regional anesthesia) with multimodal analgesic regimens increase the feasibility. Developing policies and algorithms to minimize variation and achieve predictability is essential to optimize patient safety and economic viability.[3]

## SURGICAL FACTORS

### PROCEDURE COMPLEXITY

Selecting procedures with limited complexity helps to ensure a predictable intraoperative course. The requisite surgical instruments, technical hazards, potential for significant blood loss, and intraoperative monitoring needs must be anticipated. The most common outpatient surgical procedures are cataract surgery, orthopedic surgery, and laparoscopic cholecystectomy.

## NEED FOR COMPLEX OR SPECIALIZED POSTOPERATIVE CARE

Many surgical specialties, such as neurosurgery and orthopedic surgery, that have required complex or specialized postoperative care are embracing outpatient surgical pathways for their procedures by implementing protocols and hiring appropriate personnel (e.g., on-site physical therapy) to facilitate immediate postoperative rehabilitation.

## PATIENT FACTORS

### EXISTING COMORBIDITIES RELATIVE TO PROPOSED PROCEDURE

Consideration of the patient's age and comorbidities coupled with the proposed procedure can ensure optimization of the patient's medical status to mitigate potential adverse events that require postoperative hospital admission. Patients with an American Society of Anesthesiologists (ASA) physical status of 3 or 4 who undergo surgeries longer than 60 minutes have a substantially elevated risk of hospital transfer along with an unanticipated admission.[3] Examples of these comorbidities include morbid obesity (body mass index > 40), severe obstructive sleep apnea, oxygen-dependent chronic obstructive pulmonary disease (COPD), hemodialysis-dependent end-stage renal disease, pacemaker dependency, severe cardiomyopathy, and others. The ambulatory surgery perioperative mortality rate is less than 1 in 11,000.[1]

### SOCIAL FACTORS

Patients undergoing procedures requiring general anesthesia (GA) or sedation should have a responsible adult escort them on the day of surgery to ensure postoperative instructions are received appropriately and the patient safely returns to their home. Patients without this support system are not good candidates for outpatient surgery.

## INTRAOPERATIVE MANAGEMENT: ANESTHETIC TECHNIQUES

The anesthetic technique should appropriately balance patient safety and comfort with a timely and efficient recovery.

### MONITORED ANESTHESIA CARE

The billing terminology monitored anesthesia care can encompass various forms of sedation used to permit surgical approaches: minimal sedation, moderate sedation, and deep sedation. Each of these will impact intraoperative risk as well as postoperative recovery time.

### GENERAL ANESTHESIA

General anesthesia can be administered safely in the outpatient surgery setting, and many patients may require GA due to refusal or contraindications to regional or neuraxial techniques. Severe anxiety, intellectual disability, as well as procedural location may limit sedation techniques, making GA the appropriate and safest anesthetic technique.

### REGIONAL ANESTHESIA

Regional anesthesia, with or without sedation or in combination with GA, may be employed to facilitate site-specific surgery. Regional nerve blocks have been shown to decrease overall anesthesia and postanesthesia care unit (PACU) times.[4] When regional catheters are used, postoperative analgesia may be effective for days after surgery, improving overall patient satisfaction and facilitating rehabilitation.

### NEURAXIAL ANESTHESIA

Neuraxial anesthesia techniques, with or without sedation, may be used for lower extremity, pelvic/gynecologic, and abdominal surgeries. This technique may be particularly beneficial for patients with comorbid chronic pulmonary disease. It is important to choose local anesthetics that provide surgical anesthesia that facilitates a duration of recovery appropriate for an ambulatory setting. An example of an appropriate local anesthetic for spinal anesthesia in an outpatient surgery setting is 2-chloroprocaine.

## POSTOPERATIVE MANAGEMENT: PACU ISSUES AND DISCHARGE CRITERIA

When appropriate preoperative planning and intraoperative management are well coordinated, the patient may be safely discharged. The most common complication in the PACU is postoperative nausea and vomiting (PONV), followed by respiratory insufficiency and hypotension.[5]

### POSTOPERATIVE NAUSEA AND VOMITING

It is important that prophylaxis be provided to patients with risk factors for PONV to mitigate increased costs associated with prolonged PACU stays and prevent unanticipated hospital admission. These risk factors include female gender, nonsmoker, history of motion sickness or PONV, and use of postoperative opioids (Table 343.1).

### RESPIRATORY INSUFFICIENCY

Hypoventilation due to residual inhaled/intravenous anesthetic, opioid overdose, residual neuromuscular blockade, or splinting due to pain are common. Treatment should proceed according to etiology. Additionally, asthma/COPD exacerbations may occur in the PACU, and appropriate treatment should be initiated promptly to prevent further exacerbation and unplanned admission.

### HYPOTENSION

Factors affecting the patient's preload, afterload, contractility, or heart rate should be evaluated and treated

*Table 343.1* POSTOPERATIVE NAUSEA AND VOMITING (PONV) RISK SCORE

| FACTOR | PONV RISK SCORE |
| --- | --- |
| *Gender* | |
| Male | 0 |
| Female | 1 |
| *History of Motion Sickness or PONV* | |
| No | 0 |
| Yes | 1 |
| *Nonsmoker* | |
| No | 0 |
| Yes | 1 |
| *Use of Postoperative Opioids* | |
| No | 0 |
| Yes | 1 |

The presence of none, one, two, three, or four of these risk factors predicts the incidence of PONV at 10%, 21%, 39%, 61%, and 79%, respectively.

Adapted from Apfel CC, Läärä E, Koivuranta M, Greim CA, Roewer N. A simplified risk score for predicting postoperative nausea and vomiting. *Anesthesiology.* 1999;91:693–700.

accordingly. Discharge to home versus escalation of care is based on clinical assessment.

Patients can be safely discharged home when criteria via the Modified Aldrete Score is met. A minimum time in the PACU is not required. The patient's mental and cardiovascular status should be at baseline, and the patient should no longer be at risk for depression of ventilation. A responsible adult to accompany the patient home is strongly recommended. Finally, based on the ASA standards of care, a physician must accept responsibility for discharge of patients from the PACU.

## REFERENCES

1. Gropper MA, et al., eds. *Miller's Anesthesia*. 9th ed. Philadelphia, PA: Elsevier, 2020.
2. Mathis MR, et al. Patient selection for day case-eligible surgery: identifying those at high risk for major complications. *Anesthesiology*. 2013;119:1310–1321.
3. Pardo MC, Miller RD. *Basics of Anesthesia*. 7th ed. Philadelphia, PA: Elsevier, 2018.
4. Marioano ER, et al. Anesthesia-controlled time and turnover time for ambulatory upper extremity surgery performed with regional versus general anesthesia. *J Clin Anesth*. 2009;21:253–257.
5. Hines R, et al. Complications occurring in the postanesthesia care unit: a survey. *Anesth Analg*. 1992;74:503–509.

# 344.

# PATIENT SELECTION AND PREOPERATIVE MANAGEMENT

*Anna Moskal*

## INTRODUCTION

The development of minimally invasive surgery, improvement in surgical technique and pain control, as well as better patient selection and preoperative management contribute to significant expansion of ambulatory anesthesia. The surgical procedures suitable for same-day surgery are characterized by modest surgical trauma, no likelihood of continuing blood loss or large perioperative fluid shifts, or the need for complex postoperative care. In the outpatient setting, effective preoperative assessment and patient selection significantly influence perioperative outcome. Ambulatory surgery is very safe, with low perioperative mortality. Predictors for morbidity and mortality are obesity, prolonged operative time, prior cardiac surgical intervention, hypertension, and a history of transient ischemic attack or stroke. Preoperative assessment clinics screen patients by telephone or health history questionnaire, with clinic attendance required only if unexpected problems are uncovered or if requested by the patient. The American Society of Anesthesiologists physical status (ASA-PS) classification provides a starting point for triaging patients. ASA-PS III and IV patients may benefit from more intensive assessment and optimization before the day of surgery. Chronic conditions should be relatively stable and must be optimized.

## OBESITY

Obese patients benefit from ambulatory management with early mobilization, the use of short-acting drugs, and avoidance of opioid analgesia. Obesity does not increase the rate of unanticipated admission, postoperative complications, or readmission. Even morbid obesity (body mass index [BMI] > 40 kg/m²) is no longer considered an absolute contraindication to same-day discharge as long as comorbidities are optimized before surgery. However, super obese patients with BMI greater than 50 kg/m² are at increased risk for infectious, thromboembolic, and surgical complications.

# OBSTRUCTIVE SLEEP APNEA

The bidirectional relationship between obstructive sleep apnea (OSA) and difficult airway contributes to a high rate of adverse respiratory events. Chronic intermittent hypoxia and sleep fragmentation may cause upregulation of μ-opioid receptors, which results in increased sensitivity to pain and hyperalgesia. Compliance with continuous positive airway pressure (CPAP) therapy may potentially improve pain intensity and decrease the need for opioid analgesics. In a recent retrospective analysis, patients diagnosed with moderate-to-high risk for OSA did not have a higher hospital transfer rate, but developed more frequent respiratory complications.[1] The suitability of ambulatory surgery in patients with OSA remains controversial; therefore, the Society for Ambulatory Anesthesia (SAMBA) developed a consensus statement. The recommendations include the use of the STOP-Bang questionnaire for preoperative OSA screening and consider patients' comorbid conditions in the selection process (Table 344.1). According to SAMBA guidelines, patients with a diagnosis of OSA, compliant with CPAP, optimized comorbidities, and minimal postoperative opioid requirements can be considered for ambulatory surgery if they are able to use a CPAP device in the postoperative period. Patients with a presumed diagnosis of OSA, based on screening with the STOP-Bang questionnaire, and with optimized comorbid conditions can be considered for ambulatory surgery if postoperative pain can be managed predominantly with nonopioid analgesic techniques. On the other hand, OSA patients with nonoptimized comorbid medical conditions may not be good candidates for ambulatory surgery.[2]

*Table 344.1* STOP-BANG SCORING MODEL

| QUESTIONS | YES | NO |
|---|---|---|
| SNORING<br>Do you snore loudly (louder than talking or loud enough to be heard through closed doors) | ☐ | ☐ |
| TIRED<br>Do you often feel tired, fatigued, or sleepy during daytime? | ☐ | ☐ |
| OBSERVED<br>Has anyone observed you stop breathing during your sleep? | ☐ | ☐ |
| BLOOD PRESSURE<br>Do you have or are you being treated for high blood pressure? | ☐ | ☐ |
| BMI<br>BMI more than 35 kg/m²? | ☐ | ☐ |
| AGE<br>Age over 50 years old? | ☐ | ☐ |
| NECK CIRCUMFERENCE<br>Neck circumference greater than 40 cm? | ☐ | ☐ |
| GENDER<br>Gender male? | ☐ | ☐ |

High risk of OSA: answering yes to three or more items
Low risk of OSA: answering yes to less than three items

Reprinted with permission from Chung F, Yegneswaran B, Liao P, et al. STOP questionnaire: a tool to screen patients for obstructive sleep apnea. Anesthesiology 2008; 108: 812–21.

# AGE

Elderly patients have increased postoperative complications, including pulmonary, cardiovascular, and infectious events. Patients older than 70 years have increased hospital admissions following ambulatory surgery, with an odds ratio of 1.54 (1.29–1.84). The American Geriatrics Society recommends using the Immediate Preoperative Management Checklist for the optimal perioperative management of the geriatric patient. The checklist recommendations include confirming outcome goals, including advance directives, identifying a surrogate decision-maker, limiting fluid fasting (clear liquids up to 2 hours before anesthesia), and providing appropriate medication instruction.[3] Comorbidities unique to the elderly such as frailty, cognitive impairment, decreased functional status, and impaired nutrition are associated with postoperative morbidity and mortality. At the same time, the occurrence of early postoperative complications seems to be reduced. In particular, older patients seem to experience far less postoperative pain, dizziness, nausea, and vomiting than younger patients.[4] Age itself is an independent risk factor for venous thromboembolism, so the use of either intermittent pneumatic compression or pharmacological prophylaxis is essential. The dose adjustment may be needed for low-molecular-weight heparin because of reduced renal clearance.

# CARDIOVASCULAR DISEASE

Even though hypertension is the most common cardiovascular disease, the blood pressure value that is too high to proceed with a surgery is not well defined. The 2017 American College of Cardiology/American Heart Association Task Force for Management of High Blood Pressure (BP) in adults recommends deferring major elective surgery for patients with a systolic BP greater than 180 mm Hg or diastolic BP greater than 110 mm Hg. However, there are no recommendations for low-risk surgeries.

# CORONARY ARTERY DISEASE

Cardiac risk assessment in patients with coronary artery disease (CAD) considers patient and surgical factors to estimate the risk of major adverse cardiac events (MACEs). Exercise tolerance is a major determinant of perioperative risk in patients with elevated MACE. An inability to climb a flight of stairs (4 metabolic equivalent tasks, i.e., METs) is highly predictive (89%) of postoperative cardiopulmonary complications. The most common risk assessment tools include the National Surgical Quality Improvement Project (NSQIP), Myocardial Infarction or Cardiac Arrest (MICA), and Revised Cardiac Risk Index (RCRI). The NSQIP calculator likely best determines overall surgical risk because it considers type of planned surgery. Furthermore, the calculator was derived from populations that included ambulatory surgical patients. Cardiac testing is indicated only if expected test results impact management. However, cataract and minor plastic surgery are considered very low risk; therefore, preoperative cardiac testing is not indicated.

## DIABETES MELLITUS

SAMBA recommends delaying surgery only if there is evidence of severe dehydration, ketoacidosis, or hypo-osmolar nonketotic state, but not for a specific blood glucose level. Acceptable levels of hemoglobin $A_{1c}$ ($HbA_{1c}$) for surgery are controversial. An $HbA_{1c}$ greater than 8% is associated with significantly decreased wound healing. The target glucose range for the perioperative period should be 80–180 mg/dL (4.4–10.0 mmol/L). The morning of surgery, any oral hypoglycemic agents should be withheld. Patients should receive either half an NPH dose, full doses of a long-acting analogue, or pump basal insulin. Blood glucose should be monitored every 4–6 hours during fasting with doses of short-acting insulin as needed.

## DIALYSIS-DEPENDENT PATIENTS

Elective surgery for dialysis-dependent patients should be scheduled within 24 hours of dialysis to ensure acceptable volume status, normal electrolytes, and acid-base status. It is reasonable to proceed with ambulatory surgery with mild hyperkalemia (<5.7 mEq/L) without acidosis in a patient receiving regular dialysis. Patients with moderate (5.7–6.3 mEq/L) to severe (>6.3 mEq/L) hyperkalemia should have surgery delayed.

## PATIENTS WITH CHRONIC PAIN

Patients with anticipated difficult-to-control postoperative pain should have preoperative planning, including multimodal analgesia and regional/neuraxial anesthesia. Preoperative nonsteroidal anti-inflammatory drugs, celecoxib, acetaminophen, gabapentin, or pregabalin are beneficial.

Patients taking opioid agonist-antagonists require special management. Those taking buprenorphine require large doses of opioids for analgesia. Buprenorphine has higher affinity for opioid receptors than fentanyl or morphine with slow dissociation, but low overall agonist activity. In consultation with the patient's pain or addiction specialist, buprenorphine may be held for at least 3 days before surgery and resumed after pain has diminished.

Naloxone combined with buprenorphine or oxycodone in oral preparations has limited bioavailability due to first-pass metabolism and limited systemic opioid antagonism.

Patients with opioid dependence or alcohol abuse who take extended-release injectable suspension of naltrexone have an opioid receptor blockade for 30 days, rendering opioids ineffective for analgesia except at extremely high doses. Surgery should be timed for the fourth week of treatment, when receptor blockade can be overcome with opioids. Postoperative resumption of naltrexone should be coordinated with the patient's surgeon to avoid withdrawal symptoms.[4]

## REFERENCES

1. Wanderer JP, et al. Putting positive pressure on ambulatory surgery criteria: sleep apnea and short-term outcomes. *Anesth Analg.* 2019;129(2):322.
2. Joshi GP, et al. Society for Ambulatory Anesthesia consensus statement on preoperative selection of adult patients with obstructive sleep apnea scheduled for ambulatory surgery. *Anesth Analg.* 2012;115(5):1060–1068
3. Mohanty S, et al. Optimal perioperative management of the geriatric patient: a best practices guideline from the American College of Surgeons NSQIP and the American Geriatrics Society. *J Am Coll Surg.* 2016;222(5):930–947.
4. Okocha O, et al. Preoperative evaluation for ambulatory anesthesia: what, when, and how? *Anesthesiol Clin.* 2019;37(2):195–213.
5. American Diabetes Association. Diabetes care in the hospital. *Diabetes Care.* 2016;39(suppl 1):S99–S104.

# 345.

# DISCHARGE CRITERIA AND POSTOPERATIVE FOLLOW-UP

*Matthew T. Connolly and Alaa Abd-Elsayed*

## INTRODUCTION

The postoperative recovery process consists of three components: phase I, phase II, and discharge. Phase I begins immediately from leaving the operating room and ends when specific discharge criteria are met, with monitoring taking place in the postanesthesia care unit (PACU). Phase II places emphasis on readiness to discharge home, with the primary criteria being stable/baseline vital signs, controlled nausea/vomiting, and tolerating oral liquids. Discharge consists of receiving patient postoperative instructions and necessary medications and patient transported home with a designated, responsible caregiver.

## DISCHARGE FROM THE PACU

### GENERAL PRINCIPLES

The American Society of Anesthesiologists (ASA) developed guidelines that should be universally incorporated into the anesthesiologist's specific criteria.[1] The two most common scoring systems employed in the United States employ the following principles, which are further addressed in this chapter. Although urinary voiding is no longer a requirement for discharge, high-risk patients should be bladder scanned to assess for volume and urinary retention.

- Patients should be alert and oriented or mental status returned to baseline.
- A minimum mandatory stay is not required.
- Vital signs should be stable and within acceptable limits.
- Discharge should occur after patients have met specified criteria.
- Use of scoring systems may assist in documenting fitness for discharge.
  - Urination before discharge and drinking and retaining clear liquids should *not* be part of a routine discharge protocol, although these requirements may be appropriate for selected patients.
- Outpatients should be discharged to a responsible adult who will accompany them home

## MODIFIED ALDRETE SCORING SYSTEM

The Modified Aldrete Scoring System was modified from the original 1970 criteria developed by Aldrete and Kroulik, with pulse oximetry replacing the visual assessment of oxygenation. A score of 9 or greater is considered acceptable for discharge.[2]

- **Activity** (score 0–2)
  - Able to move four extremities on command—2 points
  - Able to move two extremities on command—1 point
    - Able to move no extremities on command—0 points
- **Breathing** (score 0–2)
  - Able to breathe deeply and cough freely—2 points
  - Dyspnea—1 point
  - Apnea—0 points
- **Circulation** (score 0–2)
  - Systemic blood pressure of 20% or less than the preanesthetic level—2 points
  - Systemic blood pressure 20% to 50% of the preanesthetic level—1 point
  - Systemic blood pressure 50% or greater of the preanesthetic level—0 points
- **Consciousness** (score 0–2)
  - Fully awake—2 points
  - Arousable—1 point
  - Not responding—0 points
- **Oxygen Saturation** (score 0–2)
  - Maintains $SpO_2$ (oxygen saturation as measured by pulse oximetry) more than 92% on room air (2 points)
  - Requires supplemental oxygen to pain $SpO_2$ greater than 90% (1 point)
  - Unable to maintain $SpO_2$ greater than 90% with supplemental oxygen (0 points)

## POST-ANESTHETIC DISCHARGE SCORING SYSTEM

The Post-Anesthetic Discharge Scoring System (PADSS) is a set of criteria that continues to evolve, with the ability to urinate having been removed as a requirement for discharge and separating pain from nausea/vomiting. As with the Modified Aldrete Scoring System, a score of 9 or greater allows for discharge.

- **Vital Signs** (score 0–2)
  - Blood pressure and pulse within 20% of preoperative baseline—2 points
  - Blood pressure and pulse within 20%–40% of preoperative baseline—1 point
  - Blood pressure and pulse more than 40% of preoperative baseline—0 points
- **Activity**
  - Steady gait, no dizziness, or meets preoperative baseline—2 points
  - Requires assistance—1 point
  - Unable to ambulate—0 points
- **Nausea and Vomiting**
  - Minimal/treated with oral medication—2 points
  - Moderate/treated with parenteral medication—1 point
  - Severe/continues despite treatment—0 points
- **Pain**
  - Controlled with oral analgesics/acceptable to patient—2 points
  - Not acceptable to patient/not controlled with oral analgesics—1 point
- **Surgical Bleeding**
  - Minimal/no dressing changes—2 points
  - Moderate/up to two dressing changes required—1 point
  - Severe/more than three dressing changes required—0 points

## DISCHARGE FROM PHASE II TO HOME AND ANESTHESIA FOLLOW-UP

As mentioned previously, numerous scoring systems exist to assist in the consistent assessment of patient readiness to discharge, with PADSS the most commonly implemented and focusing on discharge from phase II. A written postoperative evaluation must be written within 48 hours postprocedure per the Centers for Medicare and Medicaid Services and must be performed only after the patient has recovered from anesthesia to participate appropriately. The written evaluation must contain a description related to respiratory function (including respiratory rate, airway patency, and oxygen saturation); cardiovascular function (including pulse rate and blood pressure); mental status; temperature; pain; nausea and vomiting; and postoperative hydration/volume status.[3]

## SPECIAL CONSIDERATIONS

### FAST TRACKING

Many institutions are attempting to bypass the PACU to phase II for quicker discharge while preserving safety standards in select patient populations and surgical procedures, with the intent to reduce nursing workload and hospital costs. However, several studies have found the nursing workload is merely shifted to phase II with no significant reduction in either nursing care or overall costs.[4] One of the key elements of successful implementation of fast tracking is properly identifying patients who could qualify for bypassing the PACU in order to avoid additional nursing workload and preserve safety standards.

### PEDIATRIC POPULATION

The majority of pediatric procedures are same-day outpatient surgeries.[5] The pediatric population is unique in regard to the extreme variability among age groups and developmental milestones. It can be challenging for the provider to assess patients who are nonverbal and properly instructing and giving anticipatory guidance to parents for care while at home following discharge. Additionally, separation anxiety in the younger population can cloud patient assessment. It is necessary for the anesthesia provider to avoid systems criteria and evaluate readiness for home in the context of the patient's previous baseline and developmental milestones.

### REGIONAL ANESTHESIA

Patients receiving peripheral nerve blocks and neuraxial anesthesia typically require longer periods of monitoring prior to discharge to ensure resolution of local anesthetic effects and assess for any neurologic deficits or other complications, such as local anesthetic toxicity. Moreover, adequate pain control without the augmentation of regional anesthesia should be assessed with a comprehensive plan for pain control and monitoring for any residual symptoms from regional anesthesia that may require medical attention.[3]

## REFERENCES

1. Apfelbaum JL. Practice guidelines for postanesthetic care: an updated report by the American Society of Anesthesiologists Task Force on Postanesthetic Care. *Anesthesiology*. 2013:118:291–307.
2. Miller R. *Miller's Anesthesia*. 9th ed. Philadelphia, PA: Elsevier Churchill Livingstone; 2020.
3. Barash P. *Clinical Anesthesia*. 7th ed. Philadelphia, PA: Lippincott, Williams & Wilkens; 2015.
4. Abdullah HR, Chung F. Postoperative issues: discharge criteria. *Anesthesiol Clin*. 2014;32(2):487–493.
5. Ryals M, Palokas M. Pediatric post-anesthesia care unit discharge criteria: a scoping review protocol. *JBI Database Syst Rev Implement Rep*. 2017;15(8):2033–2039.

# 346.

# OFFICE-BASED ANESTHESIA (OBA)

*Afshin Heidari and Ben Aquino*

## INTRODUCTION

Ambulatory surgery has become increasingly prevalent over the last few decades, and office-based surgery (OBA) has as well. This is due to (1) newer and safer surgical and anesthetic techniques; (2) diminished overhead costs; (3) increased convenience and control for the surgeon; and (4) patient convenience. The proportion of surgeries done as outpatient has increased from less than 10% in 1979 to close to 80%,[1] 15% to 20% of which are in an office-based setting.[2] More invasive procedures—on more medically complex patients—are being done in nonhospital, office-based settings. However, justified safety concerns remain.[2] One study has shown a 10-fold increase in adverse outcomes and deaths when procedures are performed in an office setting instead of an ambulatory facility.[1] Suspected causes include inadequately trained staff, suboptimal monitoring equipment, lack of vigilance, and oversedation.

Currently, there is little to no regulation over the practice of office-based surgery. The anesthesiologist who participates in an OBA setting needs to take into consideration a lot of factors, both medical and administrative, that might be taken for granted in a larger setting. The American Society of Anesthesiologists (ASA) came out with OBA guidelines in 1999 and last amended it in 2019. OBA is a subset of ambulatory anesthesia, and all parameters and standards defined in the ASA's "Guidelines for Ambulatory Anesthesia and Surgery" apply.[3]

## GUIDELINES FOR OBA

### ADMINISTRATIVE

Because office-based anesthesia currently lacks regulation, it is up to the offices themselves, and the anesthesiologist, to maintain a standard of care that, at minimum, meets ASA standards. The offices are also responsible for all administrative components of administering anesthesia. The ASA's OBA guidelines recommend a medical director, whose role includes "establish[ing] policy and [being] responsible for

the activities of the facility and its staff."[3] The specifics of this include establishing and reviewing policies and procedures, ensuring adherence to "all applicable local, state, and federal regulations," and hiring licensed, qualified staff. The guidelines mention safety concerns, including dealing with medical waste and complying with controlled substance regulations.

## CLINICAL

### PATIENT/PROCEDURE SELECTION

Patient selection guidelines need to be more stringent and specific than in other settings. Factors to be taken into mind include the scope of practice, qualifications, and comfort level of the operative and anesthesia teams. The overall health of the patient, including significant comorbidities, need to be taken into account as well. Patients at risk must be identified and referred to appropriate facilities. Procedures must be simple enough and short enough (in planned duration) "that [they] will permit the patient to recover and be discharged from the facility."[3]

### PERIOPERATIVE CARE

The ASA standards must be upheld in the office-based practice, including those for preoperative assessment, intraoperative monitoring, and postoperative care. The anesthesiologist and trained resuscitation personnel must be present until the last patient is discharged home.[4]

### MONITORING AND EQUIPMENT

The ASA guidelines also state "all facilities should have a reliable source of oxygen, suction, resuscitation equipment, and emergency drugs."[3] ASA standard monitoring equipment, periodic maintenance, sufficient space to contain it, and backup power sources are also needed. Also, any facility caring for pediatric patients must have appropriate equipment.

## EMERGENCIES AND TRANSFERS

The guidelines emphasize equipment (including malignant hyperthermia treatment kit, when indicated) and personnel trained to handle emergencies and protocols to deal with and transfer emergencies.

## ANESTHESIA CONSIDERATIONS

### PREOPERATIVE

Preparation in the preoperative period is the most important component of safe and successful OBA. Meeting facility and practice rules and regulations, including those for safety and controlled substances, is critical. Safety standards must not be compromised just to save time or money. Staff must be trained for the level of surgery being performed and participate in quality assurance and continuing education.[1] Likewise, equipment, protocols, staffing, and contingency plans must be appropriate for the complexity of the cases and patients. See Table 346.11 for a list of these patient selection factors.

*Table 346.1* PATIENT FACTORS AFFECTING APPROPRIATENESS OF OFFICE-BASED ANESTHESIA

| PSYCHOLOGICAL/SOCIAL | MEDICAL |
| --- | --- |
| • Patient's psychological status<br>• Presence of responsible adult to take patient home<br>• Patient's home and support situation—availability of help in providing pertinent postdischarge care<br>• History of substance or alcohol abuse | • Patient's medical comorbidities and stability of these conditions<br>• Risk of postoperative thromboembolic event<br>• Prior anesthesia problems<br>• Morbid obesity<br>• Airway issues—obstructive sleep apnea, known difficult airway<br>• Complexity/duration of postoperative care and monitoring |

From Massachusetts Medical Society. Office-Based Surgery Guidelines. Accessed August 29, 2020. http://www.massmed.org/Physicians/Legal-and-Regulatory/Office-Based-Surgery-Guidelines-(pdf)/

### INTRAOPERATIVE

Office-based anesthesia *must* adhere to ASA standards, including preoperative evaluation, monitoring, and postanesthesia care. Sedation is on a continuum from (1) minimal sedation (anxiolysis), (2) moderate (conscious) sedation, (3) deep sedation, to (4) general anesthesia. The anesthesia provider must have the training and equipment available intraoperatively to safely care for a patient who reaches a deeper level of sedation than intended.[4]

### POSTOPERATIVE

In addition to upholding ASA standards, the anesthesiologist and resuscitation-trained personnel need to be present for discharge. Fast-track anesthesia is the goal, meaning the patient will be awake and alert enough to have moved themselves onto the cart after emergence. It is important to prevent not only postoperative nausea and vomiting but also postdischarge nausea and vomiting.[1]

## REFERENCES

1. Smith I, et al. Ambulatory (outpatient) anesthesia. In: Miller RD, et al., eds. *Miller's Anesthesia*. 8th ed. Philadelphia, PA: Elsevier Saunders; 2015: Chap. 89.
2. Osman BM, Shapiro FE. Office-based anesthesia: a comprehensive review and 2019 update. *Anesthesiol Clin*. 2019;37(2):317–331.
3. Ambulatory Surgical Care Committee, ASA. Guidelines for office-based anesthesia. Approved by ASA House of Delegates on October 13, 1999. Last amended October 23, 2019. https://www.asahq.org/standards-and-guidelines/guidelines-for-office-based-anesthesia
4. Practice guidelines for moderate procedural sedation and analgesia 2018: a report by the American Society of Anesthesiologists Task Force on Moderate Procedural Sedation and Analgesia, the American Association of Oral and Maxillofacial Surgeons, American College of Radiology, American Dental Association, American Society of Dental Anesthesiologists, and Society of Interventional Radiology. Approved by the ASA House of Delegates on October 25, 2017. *Anesthesiology*. 2018;128(3):437–479.

# 347.

# GERIATRICS

*Maggie W. Mechlin and Courtney R. Jones*

## INTRODUCTION

As of 2018, approximately 16% of Americans were greater than 65 years old[1]; this percentage is expected to continue to rise. As patients live longer, they are requiring and qualifying for more invasive procedures and operations than ever before. Due to the anatomic and physiologic changes of aging, anesthetic management of elderly patients can pose unique challenges. These difficulties can range from the obvious need to plan a safe, balanced anesthetic and minimize the risk of complications to the more subtle need to prepare the patient, their family, and sometimes even the surgeon/proceduralist for the expected risk of morbidity and mortality.

## CHANGES WITH AGING

As we age, our bodies progressively lose the ability to adjust to and compensate for physiologic derangements. The most prominent changes that impact anesthetic planning and management are neurocognitive decline and decreased compliance of the cardiovascular system.

Neurologically, the loss of volume of brain tissue and decrease in neurotransmitter production ultimately lead to decreased MAC (minimum alveolar concentration) requirements and increased sensitivity to sedatives and analgesics. After the age of 40, MAC decreases approximately 6% per decade of life.[2] In addition, a patient's response to medications, particularly benzodiazepines, can change. Elderly patients are at an elevated risk for confusion, agitation, and disinhibition following a dose of benzodiazepines.[3] This so-called paradoxical response and associated psychomotor agitation may be enough to preclude safely performing a procedure under sedation.

Loss of compliance throughout the heart and vasculature makes it more challenging to manage hemodynamics in elderly patients. The stiffened left ventricle, which causes diastolic dysfunction, is less able to compensate for changes in intravascular volume status. This means patients will have a narrower range of filling pressures over which they will be able to maintain normal hemodynamics. In addition, the increasing stiffness of the blood vessels leads to hypertension and more dramatic variations in vascular tone in response to medications (particularly vasopressors and vasodilators).

In addition to the neurologic and cardiovascular changes with aging, patients experience decreases in both renal and hepatic function. Patients consistently have a decline in their glomerular filtration rate with age, though their creatinine may appear to be within normal limits. Furthermore, hepatic blood flow decreases with age. These changes lead to decreased ability to metabolize and excrete medications. Taken with the decrease in MAC of the halogenated gases, one could inadvertently administer more anesthetic than required for the intended effect.

## REQUIRED DISCUSSION OF END-OF-LIFE WISHES

While not all elderly patients will have reflected on their own wishes for their code status, this cohort of patients is more likely to hold a preexisting do not attempt resuscitation (DNAR) order than their younger counterparts. The old approach of "automatically suspending" a patient's DNAR order perioperatively violates patient autonomy, as well as the recommendations of the American Society of Anesthesiologists and American College of Surgeons.[4,5] Both professional organizations recommend a specific discussion with the patient or surrogate decision-maker prior to their procedure to determine whether it is consistent with the patient's values to continue their DNAR status perioperatively or whether it is more consistent with the patient's values to temporarily rescind their DNAR order and be a full-code in the perioperative period. In the event that the patient opts to become full code, the conversation must include a discussion of when the patient wishes to return to their preoperative DNAR status.

## ANESTHETIC CONSIDERATIONS

### PREOPERATIVE

Preoperative preparation of the elderly patient is largely based on the premise of risk stratification. There is a plethora of published information regarding the risk of major adverse cardiac events based on patient history and planned procedure. With the use of the Revised Cardiac Risk Index and other prediction models, anesthesiologists are adept at identifying which patients are at elevated risk for perioperative cardiac events. This information, together with the American College of Cardiologists/American Heart Association preoperative assessment algorithm can be used to identify which patients may benefit from additional testing or medication management to decrease the likelihood of unplanned major adverse cardiac events.

Postoperative neurologic function is frequently a major concern for elderly patients. One relatively holistic approach to this assessment is the Frail Scale. This scale (Table 347.1) takes into account a patient's fatigue, resistance, ambulation, illness, and loss of weight (over the preceding year). The 11 illnesses the scale considers are hypertension, diabetes, cancer, chronic lung disease, heart attack, congestive heart failure, angina, asthma, arthritis, stroke, and kidney disease. A total FRAIL score of zero is considered "robust," with a 1 or a 2 categorized as "prefrail," and a 3, 4, or 5 qualifying as "frail." The preoperative FRAIL score has been linked to likelihood of developing postoperative delirium in elderly patients.[6] Interestingly, in this study increasing frailty was not associated with postoperative cognitive dysfunction.

### INTRAOPERATIVE

As discussed, alterations in organ function with aging lead to increased medication sensitivity. Intraoperatively, patients are able to be both induced and maintained with much smaller doses of medications.

There are myriad studies that attempted to elucidate the superiority of regional or general anesthesia in elderly patients. The bulk of the scientific evaluation of this has occurred in patients having orthopedic surgeries. There is no conclusive proof of the advantage of regional versus general on morbidity or mortality in elderly patients. Like with younger patients, the decision should be made based on the nature of the operation, patient comorbidities, any risks associated with anticoagulation and regional technique, and the surgeon and patient preferences.

### POSTOPERATIVE

The crux of postoperative care of the geriatric patient is maintaining physiologic normalcy to the extent possible. Ensure hemodynamics are such that there is adequate end-organ perfusion. Minimize the risk of postoperative delirium by assisting the patient in maintaining a normal sleep/wake cycle when possible, incorporate the patient's loved ones in their planning and care, and consider use of a physician or team expert in the care of geriatric patients when necessary.

*Table 347.1* FRAIL SCALE

|  | 0 | 1 |
|---|---|---|
| **Fatigue** | Some of the time, a little of the time, none of the time | All or most of the time |
| How much of the time during the past 4 weeks have you felt tired | | |
| **Resistance** | No | Yes |
| By yourself and not using aids, do you have difficulty walking up 10 steps without resting | | |
| **Ambulation** | No | Yes |
| By yourself and not using aids, do you have difficulty walking several hundred yards | | |
| **Illness** | 0–4/11 | ≥5/11 |
| Did a doctor ever tell you that you have [insert illness] | | |
| **Loss of Weight** | Change < 5% | Change > 5% |
| How much do you weigh with your clothes on but without shoes? One year ago, how much did you weigh with your clothes on without shoes? | | |

## REFERENCES

1. Bureau U. 2020. Tables. United States Census Bureau. Accessed August 29, 2020. https://www.census.gov/data/tables.html
2. Eger EI 2nd. Age, minimum alveolar anesthetic concentration, and minimum alveolar anesthetic concentration-awake. *Anesth Analg.* 2001;93(4):947–953.
3. Silva JM Jr, et al. Comparison of dexmedetomidine and benzodiazepine for intraoperative sedation in elderly patients: a randomized clinical trial. *Reg Anesth Pain Med.* 2019;44:319–324.
4. Mohanty S, et al. Optimal perioperative management of the geriatric patient: a best practices guideline from the American College of Surgeons NSQIP and the American Geriatrics Society. *J Am Coll Surg.* 2016;222(5):930–947.
5. Committee on Ethics. 2020. Ethical guidelines for the anesthesia care of patients with do-not-resuscitate orders or other directives that limit treatment. American Society of Anesthesiologists. Accessed August 29, 2020. https://www.asahq.org/standards-and-guidelines/ethical-guidelines-for-the-anesthesia-care-of-patients-with-do-not-resuscitate-orders-or-other-directives-that-limit-treatment
6. Mahanna-Gabrielli E, et al. Frailty is associated with postoperative delirium but not with postoperative cognitive decline in older noncardiac surgery patients. *Anesth Analg.* 2020;130(6):1516–1523.

# 348.

# PHARMACOLOGICAL IMPLICATIONS
## EFFECT OF INHALATIONAL AGENTS ON ALL ORGANS

*Dillon Tinevez and Jai Jani*

## INTRODUCTION

The common inhalational agents used today are nitrous oxide ($N_2O$) and the volatile anesthetics: sevoflurane, desflurane, and isoflurane. There have been several other volatile anesthetics used in the past but have been discontinued, mainly due to undesirable effects on various organ systems. The primary target of inhaled anesthetics is on the central nervous system to reach desirable levels of anesthesia. They also have profound effects on different body systems.

## CENTRAL NERVOUS SYSTEM

All volatile anesthetics decrease the cerebral metabolic rate of oxygen consumption ($CMRO_2$). Under normal circumstances, a decrease in $CMRO_2$ is associated with a decrease in cerebral blood flow (CBF). However, at concentrations above 0.6 minimum alveolar concentration (MAC), volatile anesthetics cause cerebral vasodilatation.[1] At concentrations greater than 1 MAC, the vasodilatory effects of the volatile anesthetics exceed the vasoconstricting effects of the reduction in $CMRO_2$.[1] This leads to an increase in CBF and increased intracranial pressure (ICP), especially if the awake blood pressure (BP) is maintained. The increase in ICP associated with all volatile anesthetics can be counteracted by hypocapnia.[1] When volatile anesthetics are given at doses less than 1 MAC, cerebral autoregulation is impaired; therefore, if the patient's BP drops, the increase in CBF will be diminished or even abolished. Isoflurane causes the least cerebral vasodilation and conserves autoregulation better than the other volatile anesthetics. Desflurane increases cerebrospinal fluid (CSF) production with no effects on CSF reabsorption. Isoflurane does not affect CSF production but decreases resistance to CSF absorption.[2] When $N_2O$ is administered alone, it causes an increase in $CMRO_2$, CBF, and ICP.[1] The increase in ICP associated with $N_2O$ can be attenuated with hypocapnia, barbiturates, and opioids. Inhaled anesthetics do not abolish the cerebral vascular responsiveness to changes in $PaCO_2$.[1]

Both volatile anesthetics and $N_2O$ decrease the amplitude and increase the latency of somatosensory evoked potentials (SSEPs) in a dose-dependent manner. SSEPs may be abolished at 1 MAC of a volatile anesthetic alone or at 0.5 MAC with 50% $N_2O$. Low concentrations of volatile anesthetics (0.2–0.3 MAC) can decrease the reliability of motor evoked potentials.[1] Multipulse stimuli may overcome this effect. Increasing the depth of anesthesia is associated with an increase of amplitude and synchrony of electroencephalographic signals. Deeper levels of anesthesia can cause periods of electrical silence known as burst suppression, and a complete isoelectric pattern can be seen at a MAC of 1.5–2 or greater. Sevoflurane may cause epileptiform activity at high concentrations or during controlled hyperventilation, but the clinical significance of this is not clear.[1]

## CIRCULATORY

Volatile anesthetics have similar circulatory effects at equipotent doses, especially during maintenance of anesthesia. These effects are typically dose dependent but are hard to predict with accuracy due to factors such as age, volume status, coexisting disease, and concurrent medications.[1]

During maintenance of anesthesia, the mean arterial pressure (MAP) decreases with increasing concentrations of all volatile anesthetics in a dose-dependent manner. The decrease in MAP is primarily a result of decreased systemic vascular resistance (SVR) with the exception of halothane, which is mainly due to a decrease in cardiac output. Partial substitution of a volatile anesthetic with $N_2O$ can attenuate the decrease in SVR. $N_2O$ may cause a mild increase in MAP, if any change at all.[1]

All of the volatile anesthetics cause a stepwise increase in heart rate (HR) at different concentrations. Isoflurane starts at 0.25 MAC, desflurane starts at 1 MAC, and sevoflurane starts at 1.5 MAC.[2] The increases in HR with isoflurane and sevoflurane are thought to be due to reflex baroreceptor activity in response to decreased MAP. Rapid increases in concentration of desflurane above 1 MAC are associated with increased levels of plasma epinephrine, norepinephrine, and activation of the sympathetic nervous system. The activation causes an increase in both HR and MAP. Increasing desflurane from 4% to 8% in less than 1 minute can double the HR and BP above baseline. This can be attenuated with the use of β-blockers (esmolol), opioids (fentanyl), clonidine, or time (10–15 minutes). This phenomenon can also be seen to a lesser degree with isoflurane and cannot be attenuated by partial substitution of the volatile anesthetic with $N_2O$. Sevoflurane can cause tachycardia in both adults and children with a single breath induction of 8% sevoflurane under controlled hyperventilation.[1] This is also thought to be caused by stimulation of the sympathetic nervous system and has been associated with epileptiform brain activity.

All volatile anesthetics diminish the baroreceptor response in a dose dependent manner. Sevoflurane can

prolong the QT interval on electrocardiogram and should be avoided in patients with known congenital long QT syndrome. All anesthetics have been proven to be safe in long QT syndrome with the use of β-blockers, which is the mainstay therapy for this condition.[1] All volatile anesthetics depress myocardial contractility due to sensitization of the myocardium to epinephrine.[2] Desflurane, sevoflurane, and isoflurane have minimal effects on cardiac index (CI), while halothane has a significant dose-dependent decrease on CI.[1] Transesophageal echocardiographic data suggest that desflurane produces minor increases in ejection fraction.[1]

Volatile anesthetics have not been shown to have different outcomes in patients with coronary artery disease undergoing coronary artery bypass grafting when compared to one another or to intravenous anesthesia.[2] Volatile anesthetics have protective benefits against myocardial ischemia due to cardiac preconditioning via opening of the mitochondrial adenosine triphosphate–sensitive potassium channels. Isoflurane has coronary vasodilating properties but has not been shown to increase the risk for intraoperative myocardial ischemia due to coronary steal syndrome compared to other anesthetics.[2]

## RESPIRATORY

Volatile anesthetics cause a decrease in tidal volume and an increase in respiratory rate. Minute ventilation is preserved; however, the decrease in tidal volume increases the dead space to alveolar ventilation fraction. Patients who are spontaneously breathing have increased atelectasis.[2] Deeper levels of anesthesia have less efficient gas exchange, and $PaCO_2$ increases proportionally with the concentration of anesthetic. Substitution with $N_2O$ may attenuate the increase in $PaCO_2$ at deeper levels of anesthesia. Volatile anesthetics blunt $CO_2$ responsiveness in a dose-dependent manner. Desflurane has been shown to lead to apnea at 1.7 MAC. Surgical stimulation can attenuate this response. All volatile anesthetics also blunt the hypoxemic ventilatory response. Inhibition of hypoxic pulmonary vasoconstriction is minimal.[1]

Inhaled anesthetics may lead to cephalad displacement of the diaphragm and inward displacement of the rib cage from enhanced expiratory muscle activity, resulting in decreased functional residual capacity. Isoflurane, halothane, and sevoflurane decrease airway resistance after tracheal intubation due to bronchodilatory effects. Smokers may show a mild transient increase in airway resistance after tracheal intubation and the use of desflurane. Isoflurane, sevoflurane, and halothane are nonpungent and cause little-to-no airway irritation. Desflurane and isoflurane are pungent and can cause irritation with concentrations exceeding 1 MAC. Sevoflurane is typically used for mask inductions because it is nonpungent. Desflurane and isoflurane can be used with laryngeal mask airways with no increase in airway irritation (coughing, breath holding, laryngospasm, etc.) if less than 1 MAC is being used.[1]

## NEUROMUSCULAR

Volatile anesthetics produce dose-dependent skeletal muscle relaxation and potentiate the activity of neuromuscular blocking drugs.[1] Desflurane potentiates the effects of rocuronium, most of which is likely due to the larger concentration required to achieve the same level of anesthesia as other volatile anesthetics.[3] Any volatile anesthetic can be a trigger for the inherited disorder of increased muscle metabolism known as malignant hyperthermia (MH). Halothane is thought to have the highest risk to trigger an MH event. A significant amount of MH events occurred after multiple exposures to the same triggering anesthetic.[4]

## RENAL

Methoxyflurane, the first nonflammable volatile, was associated with renal injury due to its extensive metabolism into the nephrotoxic metabolites inorganic fluoride and dichloroacetic acid. Fluoride production from the metabolism of other inhaled anesthetics such as sevoflurane shows no association with renal injury.[1]

## HEPATIC

There is a mild and severe form of liver injury that is associated with volatile anesthetics. The severe form is known as immune-mediated liver injury and may follow any commonly used volatile anesthetic involving massive hepatic necrosis resulting in fulminant liver failure. Immune-mediated liver injury involves prior exposure to a volatile anesthetic and is caused when metabolites from the volatile anesthetic form antigenic haptens with hepatocytes. The mild form of liver injury caused by a volatile anesthetic follows the administration of halothane and is characterized by transient transaminitis. This is thought to be due to the reductive metabolism of halothane and is further exaggerated by concomitant reductions in hepatic blood flow and associated reductions in oxygen delivery to the liver.[1]

## REFERENCES

1. Pardo MC, Miller RD. Inhaled anesthetics. In: *Basics of Anesthesia.*. Philadelphia, PA: Elsevier; 2018:95–102.
2. Freeman BS, Berger JS. Anesthetic gases: organ system effects. In: *Anesthesiology Core Review*. Washington, DC: McGraw-Hill; 2014: Chap. 49. https://hsrc.himmelfarb.gwu.edu/books/49
3. Maidatsi PG, et al. Rocuronium duration of action under sevoflurane, desflurane or propofol anaesthesia. *Eur J Anaesthesiol*. 2004;21(10):781–786.
4. Larach MG, et al. Clinical presentation, treatment, and complications of malignant hyperthermia in North America from 1987 to 2006. *Anesth Analg*. 2010;110(2):498–507.

# 349.

# SHOCK STATES

*Nikki Eden and Shobana Rajan*

## INTRODUCTION

Shock can be described as any situation leading to hypoperfusion of tissues and vital organs, which may then result in organ failure and death. This is normally due to reduced oxygen delivery or inadequate utilization of oxygen, with hypoxia as the main driving force behind tissue damage. The early stages of shock are usually reversible; however, it may quickly progress to irreversible outcomes.

There are four distinct classifications of shock, each having multiple etiologies: hypovolemic, cardiogenic,

**Table 349.1** HEMODYNAMIC CHANGES ASSOCIATED WITH SHOCK STATES

| TYPE OF SHOCK | CI | SVR | PVR | SVO₂ | RAP | RVP | PAP | PAWP |
|---|---|---|---|---|---|---|---|---|
| Hypovolemic (i.e., hemorrhage) | ↓ | ↑ | N | ↓ | ↓ | ↓ | ↓ | ↓ |
| Cardiogenic (i.e., myocardial infarction) | ↓ | ↑ | N | ↓ | ↑ | ↑ | ↑ | ↑ |
| Distributive (i.e., septic) | ↑ | ↓ | N | ↑-N | ↓-N | ↓-N | ↓-N | ↓-N |
| Obstructive (i.e., pulmonary embolism) | ↑ | ↑-N | ↑ | ↓-N | ↑↓ | ↑ | ↑ | ↓-N |

CI, cardiac index; ; PAP, pulmonary artery pressure; PAWP, pulmonary artery wedge pressure PVR, pulmonary vascular resistance; RAP, right arterial pressure; RVP, right ventricular pressure; SvO₂, mixed venous oxygen saturation; SVR, systemic vascular resistance.

From Adler AC et al. Hemodynamic assessment and monitoring in intensive care unit: an overview. Enliven J Anesthiol Crit Care Med. 2014;1(4):7–10.

distributive, and obstructive (Table 349.1). The diagnosis can be made utilizing three criteria: systemic arterial hypotension, signs of tissue hypoperfusion, and hyperlactatemia.[1]

## CLASSIFICATION, ETIOLOGY, AND PATHOPHYSIOLOGY

### HYPOVOLEMIC SHOCK

Hypovolemic shock is secondary to insufficient circulating blood volume or loss of extracellular fluid. Decreased preload leads to inadequate cardiac output when filling levels are reduced, resulting in hypotension.

In adults, the most common form of hypovolemic shock is hemorrhagic shock, usually from traumatic injury. In children, diarrheal illness is the most common cause of hypovolemic shock in the developing world.[2] Hypovolemic shock can also occur from vomiting, renal loss of salt and fluid, skin losses in dry, hot climates, and third-spacing of fluid during inflammatory response.

In hypovolemic shock, all intravascular pressure measurements are decreased, including right arterial pressure (RAP), right ventricular pressure (RVP), pulmonary artery pressure (PAP), and pulmonary artery wedge pressure (PAWP). This decrease in filling leads to a decrease in the cardiac index (CI) and venous oxygen saturation (SvO₂), a measurement of tissue oxygen balance and cardiac function.[2] To combat the generalized decrease in volume, systemic vascular resistance (SVR) is increased to maintain circulating volume and blood pressure. If the loss of volume is too substantial, the SVR cannot be increased enough to compensate, and hypotension will occur with potentially fatal consequences. The approach to treatment will depend on correcting the underlying loss of fluid, including giving blood products or fluids and preventing further losses. Vasopressors can also help to increase SVR.

### CARDIOGENIC SHOCK

There is a primary insult to the myocardium causing decreased cardiac output and tissue hypoperfusion. As the myocardium struggles to pump blood, the SVR increases to maintain coronary perfusion. Eventually the myocardium will not be able to supply the tissues adequately, regardless of the amount of preload.

The main etiology is myocardial ischemia and/or infarction (MI). Cardiogenic shock is the leading cause of death after MI.[1] There may be other complications from MI that also cause shock, including ventricular septal rupture, papillary muscle rupture, and free wall rupture. Any condition causing left ventricular (LV) or right ventricular (RV) dysfunction can cause cardiogenic shock.

It may initially appear similar to hypovolemic shock with decreased CI and SvO₂ and increased SVR. However, the difference is that instead of observing decreased preload, RAP, RVP, PAP, and PAWP are all increased due to increased SVR.[1,2] This increase will initially aid coronary perfusion, but over time the increased afterload will lead to further decreases in cardiac output and tissue oxygenation. Short-term treatment involves the use of vasodilators such as nitroglycerin to improve coronary perfusion, while also titrating in vasopressors or inotropes to maintain adequate blood pressure. Definitive treatment involves restoring cardiac function by managing the underlying cause.

### DISTRIBUTIVE SHOCK

Also known as vasodilatory shock, distributive shock is caused by excessive systemic vasodilation leading to decreased blood flow and organ hypoperfusion. There is also a component of fluid leakage into the neighboring tissues from the dilated capillaries, further complicating the management of this shock state. By far the most common cause of distributive shock is sepsis or overwhelming infection.[3] This is discussed in greater detail below. Other etiologies include anaphylaxis, neurogenic (spinal) shock, and adrenal insufficiency.

Here, SVR is greatly decreased, which can decrease RAP, RVP, PAP, and PAWP, depending on the amount of vasodilation and leakage of fluid. CI will increase in response to this decrease in tissue perfusion to supply more blood to critical areas.[2,3] Initially, this may be able to maintain perfusion, but over time, increases in CI will be unable to sustain the needed output. Treatment always includes correcting the underlying mechanism, whether it be infection source control, epinephrine for anaphylaxis, steroids for adrenal crisis, or adrenergic modulation for spinal shock.

## OBSTRUCTIVE SHOCK

Obstructive shock is defined as physical obstruction of the great vessels or the heart itself. In obstructive shock, physical impedance to blood flow will decrease the cardiac output, mimicking cardiogenic shock; however, there is usually nothing wrong with the myocardium itself. Causes of obstructive shock include cardiac tamponade, pulmonary embolism, tension pneumothorax, and tumor burden. Clinically, obstructive shock usually presents with decreased CI and increased RAP, RVP, PAP, and PAWP. If the obstruction is in the systemic circulation prior to the heart, such as the superior vena cava, CI and preload indicators may be normal. In response to the decreased CI, SVR increases to aid coronary and tissue perfusion.[1,2] In simplest terms, the treatment of this is to remove the obstruction. Be cautious with vasopressors as they may worsen the afterload and further decrease CI.

## SEPTIC SHOCK

Septic shock is a form of distributive shock secondary to an overwhelming systemic response to infection. The mortality of septic shock is nearly 20% in intensive care unit (ICU) patients.[4] The normal response of the body is to mount an appropriate defense against infection, which can manifest with fever, tachycardia, tachypnea, and increased metabolism. If the infection is not controlled, hyperactive immune responses may lead to a massive cytokine storm causing profound vasodilation leading to hypotension, hypoperfusion, and subsequent organ damage that defines the state of septic shock.

There is substantial evidence that beginning antibiotics immediately is the most important factor to decrease mortality.[3,4] Fluids should be administered rapidly at 30 mL/kg of crystalloid solution for hypotension or lactate greater than 4 mmol/L, followed by vasopressors as needed to maintain mean arterial pressure above 65 mm Hg. Currently, there is no role for steroids as this may worsen the infection without providing any morbidity benefit.

## SEQUENTIAL ORGAN FAILURE ASSESSMENT SCORE

The sequential organ failure assessment (SOFA) score is a numeric predictor of the mortality in a patient with shock; it is based on the degree of organ dysfunction within six systems. Table 349.2 grades organ system dysfunctions depending on severity. The total score is

*Table 349.2* SOFA SCORING BASED ON DEGREE OF ORGAN DYSFUNCTION

| SYSTEM | 0 | 1 | 2 | 3 | 4 |
|---|---|---|---|---|---|
| Respiration PaO$_2$/FiO$_2$, mm Hg | ≥400 | <400 | <300 | <200 with support | <100 with support |
| Coagulation Platelets, × 10$^3$ μL$^{-1}$ | ≥150 | <150 | <100 | <50 | <20 |
| Liver Bilirubin, mg dL$^{-1}$ | <1.2 | 1.2–1.9 | 2.0–5.9 | 6.0–11.9 | ≥12.0 |
| CNS Glasgow Coma Scale | 15 | 13–14 | 10–12 | 6–9 | <6 |
| Renal Creatinine, mg dL$^{-1}$ | <1.2 | 1.2–1.9 | 2.0–3.4 | 3.5–4.9 | ≥5.0 |
| Cardiovascular | MAP ≥ 70 mm Hg | MAP < 70 mm Hg | Dopamine < 5 or dobutamine (any dose)[a] | Dopamine 5.1–15[a] or epinephrine ≤ 0.1 or norepinephrine ≤ 0.1[a] | Dopamine > 15 or epinephrine > 0.1 or norepinephrine > 0.1[a] |

FiO$_2$, fraction of inspired oxygen; MAP, mean arterial pressure; PaO$_2$, partial pressure of oxygen.

[a] Catecholamine doses are μg/kg/min for at least 1 hour.

Fro, Gyawali B, et al. Sepsis: the evolution of definition, pathophysiology, and management. SAGE Open Med. 2019;7(1):4.

calculated, with a score from 0 to 6 predicting less than 10% mortality while a score of 15 or greater predicts more than 80% mortality.

A SOFA score may take extensive time to gather; thus, a simpler method was developed to guide decision-making in emergency situations. The quickSOFA (qSOFA) uses only three criteria to predict those at greatest risk for poor outcomes. One point is assigned for each of the following: respiratory rate greater than 22 breaths per minute, systolic blood pressure less than 100 mm Hg, and altered mental status. Those with two or more points are at high risk for poor outcomes.[5]

## ANESTHETIC CONSIDERATIONS

### PREOPERATIVE

The anesthesiologist must be prepared for massive cardiopulmonary and fluid resuscitation measures. Preoperatively, crystalloid, blood products, and vasopressors should be set up as appropriate and readily available. Large-bore venous access is crucial. An arterial line may also be needed. If there is concern for cardiogenic shock, a pulmonary artery catheter can be placed.

### INTRAOPERATIVE

Intraperatively, use of induction medications that best maintain blood pressure is preferred, such as ketamine, etomidate, or fentanyl. Succinylcholine for rapid sequence induction can be used.

Be critically vigilant for fluctuations in the blood pressure and hemodynamic parameters. As blood loss progresses, tachycardia and tachypnea worsen, while pulse pressure decreases. Crystalloid volume administered should be three to four times the amount of estimated blood loss. If there is no improvement, blood transfusion is the next step. Real-time transesophageal echocardiography can be extremely useful in guiding management.

### POSTOPERATIVE

Strict monitoring of hemodynamic status remains critical in the postoperative period, generally requiring management in the ICU. Continue all interventions, including vasopressors and blood products as needed until the patient is fully stabilized.

## REFERENCES

1. Moranville MP, et al. Evaluation and management of shock states: hypovolemic, distributive, and cardiogenic shock. *J Pharm Pract*. 2011;24(1):44–60.
2. Adler AC, et al. Hemodynamic assessment and monitoring in intensive care unit: an overview. *Enliven J Anesthiol Crit Care Med*. 2014;1(4):7–10.
3. Finfer SR, Vincent JL. Severe sepsis and septic shock. *N Engl J Med*. 2013;369:840–851.
4. Gyawali B, et al. Sepsis: The evolution of definition, pathophysiology, and management. *SAGE Open Med*. 2019;7(1):4.
5. Jones AE, et al. The sequential organ failure assessment score for predicting outcome in patients with severe sepsis and evidence of hypoperfusion at the time of emergency department presentation. *Crit Care Med*. 2009;37(5):1649–1654.

# 350.

# SYSTEMIC INFLAMMATORY RESPONSE SYNDROME

*Maria Gorneva and Anna Tzonkov*

## INTRODUCTION

Systemic inflammatory response syndrome (SIRS) is an overactive defense response of the body to an external or internal stressor. Infection, trauma, surgery, ischemia/reperfusion, and malignancy are among known triggers. The primary goal of such a response is to acutely fight and eliminate the source of insult via the release of multiple acute-phase reactants. These mediators create significant autonomic, endocrine, and immunological changes in the body. Despite the positive purpose of such a process, the dysregulated "cytokine storm" in certain individuals can trigger a broad inflammatory cascade causing reversible or irreversible end-organ damage. It is important to make a diagnosis early.

## DEFINITION AND CRITERIA

Systemic inflammatory response syndrome is defined by the presence of any two of the following criteria:

| Body temperature | >38°C or <36°C |
|---|---|
| Heart rate | >90 beats/min |
| Respiratory rate | >20 breaths/min |
| Arterial partial pressure of $CO_2$ | <32 mm Hg |
| Leukocyte count | >12,000 or <4000/μL/>10% immature forms or bands |

In pediatric patients, the abnormal leukocyte count or temperature are required criteria for making the diagnosis.

Several scores exist to assess the severity of organ system damage. The Acute Physiology and Chronic Health Evaluation score version II and III, multiple organ dysfunction (MOD) score, sequential organ failure assessment (SOFA), and logistic organ dysfunction score are a few.[1]

The original definition of sepsis required the presence of two or more of the SIRS criteria, coupled with suspicion of infection. According to the Third International Consensus Definitions for Sepsis and Septic Shock (Sepsis-3) generated

by Society of Critical Care Medicine and the European Society of Intensive Care Medicine in 2016, the SIRS criteria were discarded as not considered specific to sepsis. Objective clinical criteria were identified for making the diagnosis of sepsis, using the SOFA score. Quick SOFA (qSOFA) clinical criteria were introduced for rapid risk stratification of patients with suspected infection.[2] qSOFA consists of three clinical components (can be easily assessed at bedside) as follows:

1. Systolic blood pressure below 100 mm Hg
2. Highest respiratory rate exceeding 21
3. Lowest Glasgow Coma Scale score under 15

Presence of two or more points is associated with a higher mortality rate and prolonged intensive care unit admission. Another important scale, MOD, is defined as a dysfunction of one or more organ systems: respiratory ($PaO_2/FiO_2$ [fraction of inspired oxygen]), renal (creatinine), hepatobiliary (bilirubin), cardiovascular (adjusted heart rate), hematological (platelet), and central nervous system (Glasgow Coma Scale). Mortality can be calculated from a MOD score, with about 20% contributing from each organ failing.[3]

## ETIOLOGY AND PATHOGENESIS

From the etiopathogenesis standpoint, SIRS can be divided into two groups: damage-associated molecular pattern and pathogen-associated molecular pattern.[1] The first group includes multiple noninfectious types of insult (trauma, surgery, autoimmune inflammation, ischemia, intoxication, malignancy). The second is a response to bacterial, viral, or fungal agents.

The uncontrolled inflammation process triggered by one of the above factors is expressed in a complex of cellular and humoral immune reactions. Interleukin 1 (IL-1) and tumor necrosis factor alpha (TNF-$\alpha$) are among the first mediators causing further propagation of the cytokine cascade. Their release results in dissociation of nuclear factor kB (NF-kB) from its inhibitor. NF-kB is thus able to induce the mass release of other important pro-inflammatory cytokines, including IL-6, IL-8, and interferon γ. IL-6 induces the release of acute-phase reactants, including procalcitonin and C-reactive protein.[1]

Interleukin 1 and TNF-α also cause changes in the coagulation system, such as inhibition of fibrinolysis and activation of the coagulation cascade via direct endothelial damage and release of tissue factor. This, in turn, leads to a broad microvascular thrombosis and increased capillary permeability, resulting eventually in overall compromised perfusion and vital organ damage. The release of stress hormones such as catecholamines and the vasopressin renin-angiotensin-aldosterone axis also takes significant part in these modulations.

There is a compensatory anti-inflammatory response syndrome mediated by IL-4 and IL-10; it is a process counteracting SIRS. Its downside is creating a relative immunosuppression state and subjecting patients to secondary infection.

## PRESENTATION/EVALUATION

A significant proportion of patients with SIRS will present with a combination of five classic signs of inflammation: dolor, calor, tumor, rubor, and *functio laesa* (loss of function). It is important to perform a detailed history and physical examination in order to localize the source as well as assess severity of disease and extent of end-organ involvement. When the apparent source is missing on the primary assessment, its detection with imaging and the like is a time-sensitive necessity. Thorough investigation of risk factors such as immunosuppression, cancer, uncontrolled diabetes mellitus, or hematological disorders would help to shape an immediate treatment plan. Collection of culture specimens from blood, sputum, urine, and any obvious wound is highly recommended within the first hour of assessment and before initiation of antimicrobial therapy.[1] When it comes to laboratory diagnostic criteria, procalcitonin and lactate levels are among the most important markers used in clinical practice.

## TREATMENT

Management of SIRS focuses on:

1. Treatment of underlying etiology and
2. Prevention of end-organ damage. When an infectious cause is suspected, surgical intervention should be done emergently when indicated. Antibiotic therapy must be started immediately after culture collection. Broad-spectrum coverage is recommended, with de-escalation on culture results availability. Hemodynamic stability is one of the key points. Administering intravenous fluids is the first line of therapy (30-mL/kg bolus of isotonic crystalloids initially is recommended by surviving sepsis guidelines), followed by appropriate addition of inotropes and vasopressors. Norepinephrine is recommended as the first-choice agent. Vasopressin production may be suppressed in sepsis, so addition of vasopressin to norepinephrine should be considered. Glucocorticoids in low doses are beneficial to counteract relative adrenal insufficiency when the goal blood pressure numbers are not sustained by other means. Blood glucose control is recommended, with a better surviving rate at levels below 180 mg/dL.

## REFERENCES

1. Chakraborty RK, Burns B. Systemic inflammatory response syndrome. In: *StatPearls*. Treasure Island, FL: StatPearls Publishing; January 2020.- https://www.ncbi.nlm.nih.gov/books/NBK547669/
2. Shannon M, et al. Clinical implications of the Third International Consensus Definitions for Sepsis and Septic Shock (Sepsis-3). *CMAJ*. 2018;190(36):E1058–E1059.
3. Gurwinder G. Shock states. In: Freeman B, Berger J, eds. *Anesthesiology Core Review: Part Two Advanced Exam*. McGraw-Hill Education; 2016:675–677.

# 351.

# MULTIPLE ORGAN DYSFUNCTION SYNDROME

*Peter Shehata and Wael Ali Sakr Esa*

## INTRODUCTION

Multiple organ dysfunction syndrome (MODS) can be thought of as a spectrum of physiologic maladaptation in separate organs that leads to significant clinical implications in the critically ill, leading to severe sepsis.[1] This maladaptation can range anywhere from minor reversible injuries in isolated organs to irreversible failure of these organs. These dysfunctions incite activation of an overwhelming dysregulated immune response with an imbalance of the pro-inflammatory and anti-inflammatory modulators, such that homeostatic mechanisms fail to self-regulate.[2] MODS is the primary cause of mortality and morbidity in the intensive care unit (ICU) setting, with mortality rates estimated to range from 44% to 76%.[3] Currently, primary therapeutic interventions are supportive and targeted toward managing each of the failed systems as dysfunction ensues. Needless to say, outcomes rely on not only the number of organs involved but also the extent of injury sustained by each organ. Some studies have attempted to develop a numerical scaling system to quantify the extent of organ dysfunction.[4] It involves assessment of the six organ systems thought to majorly contribute to MODS: the cardiovascular (CV), respiratory, hepatic, renal, hematologic, and neurological systems.[1,5]

## ORGAN INVOLVEMENT: CLINICAL FEATURES

**Cardiovascular System:** There is systemic decrease in the peripheral vascular tone initiated by widespread vasodilation, leading to generalized decrease in blood flow and thereby hypoxic injury of end organs. There is also increased permeability at the capillary level, exacerbating edema and third spacing, leading to additional injury and impaired healing responses. In some instances, especially in those with low cardiopulmonary reserve pre-MODS, the CV system suffers demand ischemia due to the excessive stress sustained by the heart. These factors significantly contribute to the insult and hypoxic injury of the end organs.

These hypotensive responses are often refractory to preload increases and typically require the use of vasopressor and ionotropic support to sustain hemodynamics.[1,5]

**Pulmonary System:** The pulmonary system plays a substantial role in the pathophysiology of MODS. The normal physiologic processes that underlie gas exchange are altered, leading to significant measurable hypoxemia that contributes to the end-organ injury when compounded by the CV-induced hypoperfusion. Atelectasis, increased capillary permeability, and resultant ventilation-perfusion (V/Q) mismatch are the major underlying mechanisms implicated in the development of impaired lung functioning. Infection, inflammation, and trauma can further complicate the lung injury, leading to local compromise of lung function. The attempted healing phase usually results in a strong inflammatory response, as evidenced by the fibrosis and the hyaline membrane deposition, leading to the development of acute respiratory distress syndrome.[1,5] Mechanical ventilation, while indicated for these patients, can exacerbate the injury by inducing barotrauma.[1]

**Gastrointestinal System:** Gastrointestinal dysmotility and gut dysfunction are often associated with MODS.[5] Hepatic insults are commonly reflected by acute transaminitis due to hepatocellular injury and often complicated by acute liver disease. Complications include acute pancreatitis and fulminant hepatic failure. Total parenteral nutrition and enteral feeding are also commonly used in this acute critical illness condition.[1] Additionally, acute-phase reactants are commonly high in MODS due to widespread nonspecific inflammation.

**Renal System:** Renal injury and the resulting decreased renal function are principally manifested by oliguria and rising creatinine . The normal processes of filtration, secretion, and excretion of the kidneys are altered largely through prerenal and intrarenal mechanisms of injury. Hypotension and resulting hypoperfusion contribute to the prerenal insult, while the local nephrotoxicity and iatrogenic drug-induced nephrotoxicity form the basis for the intrarenal injury.[1] Nephrotoxic drugs are commonly employed in the ICU setting to treat various infections, and therapy should give special considerations made to their side-effect profile.

**Neurologic System:** Altered consciousness, as can objectively be measured by the Glasgow Coma Scale, is the primary indicator of neurologic dysfunction in MODS.[1,2] The pathophysiology is multifactorial and lies in the cumulative effects of sedation, metabolic derangements, microembolic phenomena, and overall reduced cerebral perfusion pressure.[1]

**Hematologic/Immunologic System:** Hyperadrenergic stress responses usually lead to leukocytosis. Of note, the most prominent finding in MODS is thrombocytopenia relating to the disseminated intravascular coagulation and other intravascular consumptive processes that ensue.[1]

**Endocrine System:** Involvement of the endocrine system has not been well studied or explored to a great degree, but responses involving dysregulated insulin responses and hyperglycemia have been noted.[1,5] Adrenal insufficiency, through either iatrogenic or MODS-related etiology, have

been identified.[1] Fortunately, these alterations are mostly temporary in the acute phase and have low bearing on the long-term resulting complications.

## REFERENCES

1. Angus DC, et al. Epidemiology of severe sepsis in the United States: analysis of incidence, outcome, and associated costs of care. *Crit Care Med.* 2001;29(7):1303–1310.
2. Ferreira AMP, Sakr Y. Organ dysfunction: general approach, epidemiology, and organ failure scores. Semin *Respir Crit Care M.* 2011;32(5):543–551.
3. Livingston DH, et al. Sepsis and multiple organ dysfunction syndrome: a clinical-mechanistic overview. *New Horiz.* 1995;3(2):257.
4. Marshall JC. The multiple organ dysfunction syndrome. In: *Surgical Treatment: Evidence-Based and Problem-Oriented.* Zuckschwerdt; 2001.
5. Ziesmann MT, Marshall JC. Multiple organ dysfunction: the defining syndrome of sepsis. *Surg Infec.* 2018;19(2):184–190.

# 352.

# PRESCRIPTION MEDICATION OVERDOSE

*Peter Huynh and Alaa Abd-Elsayed*

## INTRODUCTION

Data collected by the National Center for Health Statistics and Centers for Disease Control and Prevention have illustrated the ongoing trend of prescription medication overdose. In 2018, more than 67,300 Americans died from drug-involved overdose, which included death from illicit drugs and prescription opioids.[1] Many prescription medications, such as opioids, benzodiazepines, psychostimulants, and antidepressants, were included in these statistics. With the exception of 2017 to 2018 when the number of drug overdose deaths declined, deaths involving synthetic opioids such as methadone and fentanyl continued to rise, resulting in more than 31,335 overdose deaths in 2018.

## OPIOIDS

Opioids are among the most common drugs for accidental overdose. While there are many different opioid medications on the market, the most common names and their side effects and interactions are discussed here. Common opioid side effects include constipation, miosis, respiratory depression, urinary retention, and decreases in blood pressure.[2] Methadone is a medication commonly prescribed to patients with chronic pain conditions and is associated with prolongation of the QT interval. Given this phenomenon, it is important to assess patients with electrocardiograms (ECG) prior to surgery. In addition to opioid receptor agonism, this medication also has a role in NMDA (*N*-methyl-D-aspartate) receptor antagonism and serotonin reuptake inhibition.

Tramadol is a μ-opioid receptor agonist along with features of serotonin reuptake inhibition, norepinephrine reuptake inhibition, and NMDA receptor inhibition. While it is considered to have decreased affinity for the opioid receptor compared to other common opioids, it is known to decrease the seizure threshold. Hydrocodone-acetaminophen and oxycodone-acetaminophen are also commonly prescribed opioids. In addition to their opioid side effects, being cognizant of the total 24-hour intake of acetaminophen is important for liver dysfunction and toxicity, especially in the setting of supplemented over-the-counter acetaminophen.

Patients who overdose on opioid medications can exhibit symptoms of oversedation, with respiratory depression and miosis. These issues tend to be more problematic in the postoperative period given the clinical picture may be confused with various causes, including residual anesthetic, incomplete reversal of paralysis, hypoglycemia, hypothermia, stroke, myocardial infarction, and electrolyte abnormalities. Management in the perioperative setting includes performing a focused and thorough history and physical examination, assessment of vital signs, airway protection and ventilatory management, administered and withheld medications, laboratory work, and diagnostic studies. The underlying cause should be treated. The patient may require respiratory assistance, and naloxone should be readily available. However, naloxone should be administered with caution as aggressive titration may result in a sudden increase in pain, arrhythmias, hypertension, pulmonary edema, and death.[3,4]

## BENZODIAZEPINES

Benzodiazepines may present similarly to opioids. Patients may experience somnolence, respiratory depression, slurred speech, imbalance, and hypotension. Urine toxicology screens may assist in making the diagnosis. While acute intoxications necessitating aggressive treatments, including gastrointestinal decontamination and ventilation, are uncommon for the preoperative period, given the case would likely be canceled, it is important for providers to be aware of the options. Flumazenil should be considered for reversal, especially in the setting of coma reversal. Of note, flumazenil is contraindicated in patients with suspected increased intracranial pressure and known seizure disorders given the risk for flumazenil-induced seizures. It can also precipitate withdrawal symptoms in those with chronic benzodiazepine use, which can be life threatening.[5]

## Β-BLOCKERS

β-Blockers are commonly prescribed to treat a variety of conditions, including cardiac conditions such as atrial fibrillation and congestive heart failure, as well as glaucoma and essential tremors. Not surprisingly, it would not be unexpected for patients with multiple chronic conditions to find it difficult to take their medications as prescribed. Those who present with β-blocker overdose may display a range of signs and symptoms, including bradycardia (most common presenting sign), hypotension, dysthymias, mental status changes, seizures, hypoglycemia, and bronchospasm. Hypoglycemia manifests as a result of impaired gluconeogenesis and glycogenolysis. Given these potential effects, management includes obtaining an ECG to evaluate for prolonged PR and QT and dysrhythmias. Glucose checks should be considered given possible hypoglycemia. Chemistry panels may be used to assess creatinine levels as well, especially with atenolol. Management starts with addressing airway, breathing, and circulation. Consider intravenous fluids for hypotension. If the patient is symptomatic from bradycardia, then consider intravenous atropine 0.5–1 mg every 3–5 minutes up to 3 mg. Transcutaneous and transvenous pacing are also options as well. Hypoglycemia should be treated with dextrose (e.g., D50W [dextrose 5% in water]). Additional treatment options include glucagon, calcium supplementation, high-dose insulin, and glucose to augment myocardial contraction.[6] Vasopressors should be considered as an adjunctive therapy. Hemodialysis can be considered; however, it is only effective for nadolol, sotalol, and atenolol. As for refractory cases, venoarterial extracorporal membrane oxygenation may be considered.

## ANESTHETIC CONSIDERATIONS

### PREOPERATIVE

Prescription medication management can be difficult, especially for patients with multiple comorbidities. Patients with risk factors, including a history of drug abuse and misuse, should be carefully monitored preoperatively for signs and symptoms of overdose, which can include somnolence and respiratory depression.

Performing a focused and thorough history and review of home medications prior to surgery can assist in formation of a differential diagnosis and guide management in the postoperative period. Reviewing the anesthetic record, recent laboratory tests, and administered and withheld medications can also direct management. Fortunately, treatment options exist in the setting of prescription medication overdose; however, it is important for providers to be cognizant of the potential risks of these treatments as well.

### INTRAOPERATIVE

Recognizing prescription drug overdose can be difficult intraoperatively given the overlapping signs and symptoms with our anesthetic medications. Patients who misuse their medications may be near a tipping point and lose their ability to protect their airway and decompensate during a case. Management includes ensuring adequate breathing, airway, and circulation and treating the underlying cause.

## POSTOPERATIVE

It is very important to monitor patients in the postoperative period for any symptoms or signs of drug overdose or withdrawal.

## REFERENCES

1. National Institute on Drug Abuse. Overdose death rates. https://www.drugabuse.gov/related-topics/trends-statistics/overdose-death-rates
2. OpenAnesthesia. Analgesia and sedation. https://www.openanesthesia.org/analgesia_and_sedation/
3. Barash PG. *Clinical Anesthesia*. 5th ed. Philadelphia, PA: 2006:376–378.
4. *Miller's Anesthesia*. 7th ed. 808–811.
5. Kang M, et al. Benzodiazepine toxicity. In: *StatPearls*. Treasure Island, FL: StatPearls Publishing; January 2020. https://www.ncbi.nlm.nih.gov/books/NBK482238/
6. Kerns W. Management of beta-adrenergic blocker and calcium channel antagonist toxicity. *Emerg Med Clin North Am*. 2007;25(2):309–331.

# 353.

# CARBON MONOXIDE POISONING

*Ben Aquino*

## INTRODUCTION

Carbon monoxide (CO) is a colorless, odorless gas that is produced by the incomplete combustion of carbon-based compounds. It can occur in quite a few settings in daily life, including improperly ventilated motor vehicles, generators, stoves, residential fires, cigarette smoke, and malfunctioning heating systems. According to the Centers for Disease Control and Prevention, in the United States alone, carbon monoxide poisoning causes approximately 50000 emergency room visits per year, and in 2014, it caused more than 1300 accidental deaths.[1]

Carbon monoxide acts by binding to the hemoglobin (Hb) molecule at the same binding site as oxygen ($O_2$), doing so with an affinity 240–250 times greater than that of oxygen. This results in the creation of a carboxyhemoglobin (COHb) molecule.[2] Normal, nonsmoking individuals can have a COHb as high as 3%, and smokers may have baseline levels as high as 3%–5%, with "normal" range for smokers considered to be as high as 12%. However, when COHb is present in higher quantities than this, the effects are three-fold. First, displaced oxygen is no longer available for hemoglobin-mediated delivery to the tissues. Second,

the CO causes a conformational change in the hemoglobin molecule that inhibits the release of $O_2$ from hemoglobin molecules, and this corresponds to a leftward shift of the oxyhemoglobin dissociation curve. Third, CO has the somewhat less potent effect of binding to myoglobin as well as to mitochondrial cytochrome oxidase, the latter of which disrupts the electron transport chain and ultimately impairs adenosine triphosphate (ATP) production. Of note, fetal hemoglobin is capable of providing falsely elevated COHb levels on certain oximeters, giving normal infants a COHb that may measure as high as 7%–8%

The clinical symptoms of CO poisoning are nonspecific, and none is pathognomonic for the condition. In an awake patient, they start with headache, fatigue, and presyncope, progressing to impaired concentration, vertigo, tachypnea, or tachycardia. With prolonged exposure, this can progress to angina, myocardial infarction, seizures, coma, and death.

Volatile anesthetics have the capability to generate CO when combined with soda lime. Such amounts are rarely clinically significant, but reports have shown instances where the CO content in the anesthesia circuit was greater than 500 ppm, and patient COHb levels reached 30%.

## TREATMENT

Intraoperatively, postoperatively, or postexposure, the treatment is the same—immediate treatment with 100% nonrebreather face mask, which promotes cellular oxygenation and decreases the elimination half-life from 4–5 hours to 1–2 hours. Oxygen therapy needs to be continued until the patient is asymptomatic, which usually corresponds to a COHb of 10% or greater. Hyperbaric oxygen helps because it can decrease the elimination half-life even faster than 100% nonrebreather $O_2$, but its main benefit is likely two-fold: (1) regenerating cytochrome oxidase,[3] and (2) inhibiting leukocyte adhesion to endothelium, which may mitigate ischemic reperfusion injury and the delayed longer term neurologic sequelae often associated with CO poisoning. Blood transfusion may be considered.

## ANESTHETIC CONSIDERATION

### PREOPERATIVE

Preoperatively, the provider also needs to be mindful of certain populations, such as smokers, who arrive on the operating room table with CO levels that are already higher than normal. The anesthesiologist must also recognize and mitigate risk factors that have been identified for increased CO production. First is the type of anesthetic agent used. In order of CO production, desflurane ≥ enflurane > isoflurane >> halothane = sevoflurane. Second is the concentration of anesthetic—, with higher concentrations associated with higher CO. Third is higher temperature. Fourth is the type/brand of absorbent (Baralyme™, an obsolete absorbent no longer commercially available, produced more CO than soda lime). Fifth relates to the dryness of the absorbent: The drier the absorbent is, the more CO is produced. Sixth, related to this, the gas flows being used are a risk factor, with higher flows promoting dryness and subsequent CO production. One other notable factor, also related to desiccation of absorbent, is, seventh, the length of time the anesthesia machine has been unused. The highest exposure has been found to be from the first case after a long layoff (e.g., the first case in the main operating room on a Monday morning). A rarely used machine in an off-site location, such as a catheterization laboratory or infrared radiation suite, is also a risk factor for increased CO production[4] (see Box 353.1).

### INTRAOPERATIVE

Because CO poisoning can be so difficult to detect, the first hallmark of treatment is a high index of suspicion. Intraoperatively, the patient is asleep and will not manifest most of the normal symptoms of CO poisoning. Also,

---

> **Box 353.1** FACTORS THAT *INCREASE* CARBON MONOXIDE BUILDUP IN THE ANESTHESIA CIRCUIT
>
> Type of agent—desflurane > isoflurane = enflurane> halothane = sevoflurane
> High fresh gas flows
> First case after a long period of disuse
> Machine at a remote location
> Dryness of soda lime absorbent
> Brand of soda lime absorbent, with Baralyme associated with higher CO levels

---

clinical signs are not always informative. CO preferentially binds to hemoglobin compared to $O_2$, but $O_2$ is not taken out of the blood, and as a result, the measured $PaO_2$ can look normal. COHb absorbs light at the same wavelength (660 nm) as oxyhemoglobin and is interpreted as similar by an oximeter. As a result, pulse oximetry can show a saturation of 100%, and the patient can maintain normal skin tone and color, all the while having high carboxyhemoglobin (COHb) levels. The "cherry red" skin color occasionally associated with CO poisoning is a late sign and is not useful for diagnosis. In CO poisoning, the calculated arterial oxygen content ($CaO_2$) of the blood will be normal, but because $CaO_2$ quantifies only the $O_2$ molecules bound to hemoglobin, the actual measured $CaO_2$ will be much lower than normal. A serum lactate in this situation will be much higher than normal, with a resultant metabolic acidosis.

### POSTOPERATIVE

The patient needs to have COHb levels checked postoperatively and must continue to receive normobaric oxygen until they either are asymptomatic or have COHb levels less than 10%. In addition, they need to be monitored in the perioperative period for both neurologic sequelae and myocardial injury, as both can occur with even a single episode of CO poisoning.

## REFERENCES

1. Rose JJ, et al. Carbon monoxide poisoning: pathogenesis, management, and future directions of therapy. *Am J Respir Crit Care Med.* 2017;195(5):596–606.
2. Kavanagh BP, Hedenstierna G. Respiratory physiology and pathophysiology. In: Miller RD, et al., eds. *Miller's Anesthesia.*
3. Brown SD, Piantadosi CA. Recovery of energy metabolism in rate brain after carbon monoxide hypoxia. *J Clin Invest.* 1992;89(2):666–672.
4. Woehick HJ, et al. Reduction in the incidence of carbon monoxide exposures in humans undergoing general anesthesia. *Anesthesiology.* 1997;87:228–234.

# 354.

# DROWNING

*Derek Brady Covington and Christopher Giordano*

## INTRODUCTION AND EPIDEMIOLOGY

Worldwide, an estimated 500,000 people die from drowning each year.[1] Drowning represents almost 1% of all deaths, and in the US it is one of the leading causes of death during the first 5 decades of life. In addition to these drowning fatalities, it is estimated that 10 times more people survive drowning, many of whom will live with profound neurological defects; therefore, drowning represents a major public health problem. Risk factors for drowning deaths include young age, male sex, poor socioeconomic status, alcohol use, low education, risky behavior, and lack of supervision.[2]

The definition and classification of drowning varied significantly until the Utstein style consensus in 2003 established a simplified classification and guidelines for drownings. The Utstein consensus, which was reviewed in 2013, purports that a drowning process occurs whenever a person is submerged or immersed in fluid that subsequently blocks the airway and inhibits respiration.[3] Furthermore, drownings are labeled as witnessed or nonwitnessed for prognostic value. Regardless of whether the victim lives or dies in this process, they are considered to be involved in a drowning incident. These guidelines provide much more granular data incorporating the victim, scene, time intervals, and hospital data, which are vital for research, prognosis, and treatment for drowning victims.

It is also important to note if the victim of a drowning incident was submerged in fresh water or salt water. As fresh water has significantly lower osmotic pressure compared to that of the blood, fresh water rapidly moves from the gastrointestinal tract into the bloodstream, which may lead to electrolyte changes and erythrocyte hemolysis. On the contrary, salt water has a similar osmotic pressure to that of blood, so there is minimal absorption from the gastrointestinal tract and likely no issues with blood chemistry or red blood cell damage. Unfortunately, the vast majority of drownings do occur in fresh water and pose these additional risk factors for the victims and should be

considered by healthcare professionals when managing such cases.

Although shallow-water blackout may result in drowning, it occurs secondary to a specific sequence of events leading to hypoxia and subsequent loss of consciousness in shallow water (i.e., less than 15 feet deep). Also referred to as breath-holding blackout or freediver blackout, shallow-water blackout most often occurs in freedivers. In an effort to reduce the urge to breathe from hypercarbia and to dive deeper and/or longer, freedivers hyperventilate on the surface of the water prior to beginning a descent. As a result of this hyperventilation, these divers have a reduced partial pressure of carbon dioxide ($PaCO_2$), which is the primary drive for respiratory stimulation. However, hyperventilation does not alter partial pressure of oxygen ($PaO_2$) levels. During the dive, oxygen is metabolized faster than $CO_2$ can accumulate in the bloodstream, which results in cerebral hypoxia and unconsciousness prior to the respiratory drive to breath (Figure 354.1). Furthermore, as the diver approaches the end of the dive (and is in shallower water), the ambient pressure declines, which leads to further reductions in $PaO_2$ and a higher likelihood of unconsciousness and drowning. Consequently, these divers are at risk of losing consciousness (or "blacking out") in shallow water, and they are at risk for drowning if not recovered quickly. In addition to formal training, a buddy and/or safety diver should always be present during freediving and especially when those freedivers are employing hyperventilation techniques.

## PATHOPHYSIOLOGY

When someone is initially submerged in fluid, they hold their breath until carbon dioxide accumulates to a level that triggers inhalation. Because there is no surrounding air to breathe, the surrounding liquid is inhaled and laryngospasm may occur, leading to additional breath holding. The victim eventually becomes hypercarbic, hypoxemic, and acidotic, resulting in unconsciousness. The ultimate mechanism of death is secondary to extreme and irreversible hypoxia, and

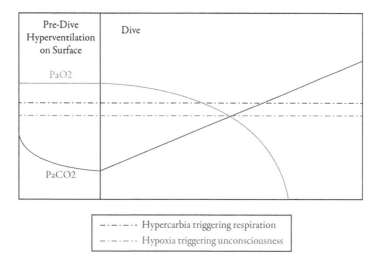

**Figure 354.1** The $PaO_2$ and $PaCO_2$ levels following hyperventilation prior to submersion leading to shallow-water blackout. As a predive hyperventilation is performed, the partial pressure of carbon dioxide ($PaCO_2$) decreases, while the partial pressure of oxygen ($PaO_2$) remains relatively unchanged. During the dive, the $PaCO_2$ slowly rises, while the $PaO_2$ decreases. Once near the surface and surrounded by a relatively low ambient pressure compared to that during the majority of the dive, the $PaO_2$ is reduced. That reduction leads to unconsciousness, or shallow-water blackout. These events occur prior to the diver returning to the surface and the urge to breathe secondary to increasing $PaCO_2$.

this posthypoxic encephalopathy is the most common cause of death in hospitalized patients.

## MANAGEMENT

The rescue provider should consider if the victim is breathing, has a pulse, and/or has a cervical spine injury. Cardiac arrest in drowning is due primarily to a lack of oxygen. Consequently, it is important that *cardiopulmonary resuscitation (CPR) follows the traditional airway-breathing-circulation, or ABC, sequence and starts with five initial rescue breaths.*[2] Care must be maintained to minimize cervical movement in the event of any neuroaxial instability; jaw extension may facilitate these initial rescue breaths. These initial rescue breaths are followed by rapid and quality chest compressions if there is any concern about an absence of pulse. This sequence is in stark contrast to current recommendations that suggest quality chest compressions should be the initial approach as opposed to establishing artificial ventilation.

On arrival to the hospital, artificial respiration should be continued until consciousness returns and the airway can be protected. In addition, an arterial blood gas should be obtained immediately to assess ventilation, acid-base status, and pulmonary gas exchange.[4] Continuous positive airway pressure or positive end-expiratory pressure should be employed to maximize ventilation and perfusion ratios by recruiting collapsed alveoli.[4] The decision to warm the patient should be based on the patient's current temperature, time submerged, cardiopulmonary status, and presumed neurologic injury. Efforts to resuscitate the patient should not be aborted until the patient reaches 35°C and is unresponsive to cardiovascular-supportive therapies.[1] Even if primary resuscitation is successful, approximately 5% of drowning victims experience a delayed respiratory deterioration secondary to pulmonary damage from aspiration, anoxia, surfactant loss, and alveolar collapse, which manifests as acute respiratory distress syndrome.[1]

## DIAGNOSIS/CAUSE OF DEATH

Diagnosis and cause of death in drowning requires evidence of water aspiration found on an autopsy.[5]

In addition to laboratory tests, such as blood strontium levels, diatom analysis, and vitreous humor sodium assays, a variety of physical examination findings may be associated with drownings, such as Paltauf spots (subpleural hemorrhages), Wydler sign (swallowing of water), and Svechnikov sign (free liquid in the sphenoid sinus). These tests and examination findings should be correlated with circumstantial evidence, witness reports, and toxicology tests, such as blood alcohol.

## PROGNOSIS

Two risk factors associated with a higher incidence of death or severe neurologic impairment include time of submersion greater than 10 minutes and CPR for longer than 25 minutes. Not surprisingly, the duration of submersion is positively correlated with the risk of death or severe neurologic impairment (Table 354.1).[1] If the victim has been

**Table 354.1** DURATION OF SUBMERSION AND RISK OF DEATH OR SEVERE NEUROLOGIC IMPAIRMENT AFTER HOSPITAL DISCHARGE

| TIME OF SUBMERSION | RISK OF DEATH OR SEVERE NEUROLOGIC IMPAIRMENT AFTER HOSPITAL DISCHARGE |
|---|---|
| 0–5 minutes | 10.4% |
| 6–10 minutes | 72.2% |
| 11–25 minutes | 83.3% |
| >25 minutes | Nearly 100% |

submerged for less than 5 minutes, it is not likely that they will suffer from severe neurologic impairment or die.[2]

Not surprisingly, improved outcomes are associated with less time submerged and early initiation of basic life support/advanced cardiac life support.[1,2] Cold water may also be associated with improved outcomes secondary to the decrease in cerebral metabolic oxygen consumption. It is estimated that a 10°C decrease in body temperature leads to a halving of adenosine triphosphate consumption, which may double the time the brain can survive.[2]

## REFERENCES

1. Schilling UM, Bortolin M. Drowning. *Minerva Anestesiol.* 2012;78:69–77.
2. Szpilman D, et al. Drowning. *N Engl J Med.* 2012;366:2102–2110.
3. Idris AH, et al. 2015 Revised Utstein-Style recommended guidelines for uniform reporting of data from drowning-related resuscitation: an ILCOR advisory statement. *Circulation.* 2015;10(7):e000024.
4. Layon AJ, Modell JH. Drowning: update 2009. *Anesthesiology.* 2009;110:1390–1401.
5. Modell JH, et al. Drowning without aspiration: is this an appropriate diagnosis? *J Forensic Sci.* 1999;44:1119–1123.

# 355.

# INFECTION CONTROL

*David Jury and Edward Noguera*

## INTRODUCTION

The hands of anesthesia providers and the anesthesia work area have been recognized as a source of cross-contamination and possible infection.[1–3] Standard precautions for infection prevention include hand hygiene, basic personal protective equipment (PPE), and safe injection practices and should be used with all patients. Several medical societies, hospital associations, and government agencies provide general guidelines and standards for the prevention of nosocomial infections.[4,5] The 2007 Center for Disease Control and Prevention (CDC) guidelines for the prevention of nosocomial infections and isolation precautions help hospitals establish infection control strategies.[4]

## HAND HYGIENE

Healthcare provider hand hygiene is the most important measure to reduce nosocomial infections.[1–3] Healthcare providers can reduce the transmission of pathogens from one patient to another and from site to site on the same patient. Hand hygiene washing should be done with soap and water or with an alcohol-based sanitizer. Hand hygiene should occur before and after patient contact. Enough time should be allotted for hands to dry before patient contact is initiated or before moving on to the next activity. Hand hygiene must be with soap and water when the patient is positive or being ruled out for norovirus or *Clostridium difficile.*

## COUGH ETIQUETTE

Patients and visitors should cover their nose or mouth when coughing, promptly dispose used tissues, and practice hand hygiene after contact with respiratory secretions.

## PERSONAL PROTECTIVE EQUIPMENT

Personal protective equipment, such as eye protection, masks, and gloves, are standard precautions that should be worn. *Protective eyewear* should be worn whenever a mask or gloves is worn. Spillage of bodily secretions with highly virulent organisms can contaminate eye surfaces and become the port of entry for some infections. *Gloves* must be worn if the provider will be in contact with bodily fluids or secretions. The use of gloves does not replace hand hygiene. Gloves should be replaced between patient encounters, even for the same patient. Used gloves should not come in contact with a healthcare provider's face or other equipment. Gloves should be disposed of in a trash container.

*Masks* must be worn for patients who are producing respiratory secretions, for all sterile procedures, or if the provider themselves is coughing. Basic surgical masks are not particulate respirators and do not provide airborne droplet protection. N95 masks or PAPR (powered air-purifying respirators) protect healthcare workers from airborne infections when adequately fitted and used. Donning and doffing requires training. Appropriate sequence or guidance from another healthcare worker during doffing of PPE maximizes opportunities to prevent accidental contamination.

## ISOLATION PRECAUTIONS

Contact, droplet, and airborne precaution are different levels of isolation precautions. Every healthcare facility must have an infection control department with specified guidelines for isolation of patients. A summary of precautions is presented in Table 355.1.

*Contact precautions* should be used when caring for patients with multidrug-resistant organisms (MDROs) or enteric or viral pathogens. These patients should be in single-patient rooms. Hand hygiene, gloves, and gowns are used when direct patient contact is anticipated but a minimum of gloves when just entering the room should be used and then promptly disposed of on exiting the room. This should be immediately followed by hand hygiene. All medical equipment used should be patient specific or disinfected before use with another patient.

*Droplet precautions* are for respiratory particles of greater than 5 μm, remain airborne only for short periods and can be transmitted within 2 m. Basic surgical masks should be worn, and the patient should have a private room.

*Airborne precautions* are warranted for droplet nuclei respiratory secretions of less than 5 μm that remain suspended in the air for prolonged periods of time. These patients should be in private, negative-pressure rooms that exchange air a minimum of six times an hour with strict door closed policy enforcement. Providers need to wear tight-sealing particulate respirators rated to filter out 95% of particulate matter.

*Chlorhexidine bathing* of patients in the intensive care unit reduces the rate of hospital-acquired bloodstream infections and colonization with drug-resistant organisms. Bare below the elbow dress codes (no wristwatch, jewelry, or ties); daily laundering, preferably with bleach, of hospital attire; and sterilization of shared equipment (stethoscopes) and personal equipment (pagers and cell phones) policies are widely endorsed but have not been shown to have a clinical impact in reduction of pathogen transmission. Severely immunocompromised patients warrant high-efficiency particulate air filtration with air exchange ventilation systems and positive pressure corridors outside their room.

## COVID-19

Frequent hand hygiene and appropriate PPE with meticulous donning and doffing technique are paramount to prevent the transmission of COVID-19. An aerosolizing procedure presents the highest risk of transmission of COVID-19 and requires contact, droplet, and airborne precautions that specifically include a tight-sealing particulate respirator such as an N95 mask or PAPR, full PPE that includes a face shield that covers the front and sides of the face, water-resistant gown, gloves (double gloved for tracheal intubation), disposable hair bouffant cap, and optional shoe and beard covers. Aerosolizing procedures include tracheal intubation or extubation, bag mask ventilation, noninvasive ventilation (NIV), high-flow oxygen therapy, administration of nebulized medications, bronchoscopy, interventional pulmonology procedures, tracheotomy, suctioning of an airway in a nonintubated patient, upper endoscopy, and colonoscopy.

Nonintubated COVID-19 patients being transported should wear a surgical mask. For intubated patients or patients on NIV, high-quality viral filters should be employed.

In the operating room, the anesthesia machine itself should be covered in plastic, and a high-quality viral filter in line with the breathing circuit placed at the end of the

*Table 355.1.* ISOLATION PRECAUTIONS

| TYPE OF PRECAUTION | SELECTED PATIENTS | MAJOR SPECIFICATIONS |
|---|---|---|
| Standard | All patients | Perform hand hygiene before and after every patient contact.ᵃ<br>Gloves, gowns, eye protection as required.<br>Safe disposal or cleaning of instruments and linen.<br>Cough etiquette. |
| Contact | Colonization of any bodily site with multidrug-resistant bacteria (MRSA, VRE, drug-resistant gram-negative organisms)<br>Enteric infections (norovirus, *Clostridioides* [formerly *Clostridium*] *difficile,*ᵃ *Escherichia coli* O157:H7)<br>Viral infections (HSV, VZV, RSV,ᶜ parainfluenza, enterovirus, rhinovirus,ᵈ certain coronaviruses [e.g., COVID-19, MERS-CoV])<br>Scabies, impetigo<br>Noncontained abcesses or decubitus ulcers (especially for *Staphylococcus aureus* and group A *Streptococcus*) | In addition to standard precautions:<br>Private room preferred; cohorting allowed if necessary.<br>Gloves required upon entering room. Change gloves after contact with contaminated secretions.<br>Gown required if clothing may come into contact with the patient or environmental surfaces or if the patient has diarrhea.<br>Minimize risk of environmental contamination during patient transport (e.g., patient can be placed in a gown).<br>Noncritical items should be dedicated to use for a single patient if possible. |
| Droplet | Known or suspected:<br>*Neisseria meningitidis*<br>*Haemophilus influenzae* type B<br>*Mycoplasma pneumoniae*<br>*Bordetella pertussis*<br>Group A *Streptococcus*ᵉ<br>Diphtheria, pneumonic plague<br>Influenza, rubella, mumps, adenovirus<br>Parvovirus B19, rhinovirus, certain coronavirusesᶠ | In addition to standard precautions:<br>Private room preferred; cohorting allowed if necessary.<br>Wear a mask when within 3 feet of the patient.<br>Mask the patient during transport.<br>Cough etiquette: Patients and visitors should cover their nose or mouth when coughing, promptly dispose of used tissues, and practice hand hygiene after contact with respiratory secretions. |
| Airborne | Known or suspected:<br>Tuberculosis<br>Varicella<br>Measles<br>Smallpox<br>Certain coronavirusesᶠ<br>Ebolaᵍ | In addition to standard precautions:<br>Place the patient in an AIIR (a monitored negative-pressure room with at least 6 to 12 air exchanges per hour).<br>Room exhaust must be appropriately discharged outdoors or passed through a HEPA filter before recirculation within the hospital.<br>A certified respirator must be worn when entering the room of a patient with diagnosed or suspected tuberculosis. Susceptible individuals should not enter the room of patients with confirmed or suspected measles or chickenpox.<br>Transport of the patient should be minimized; the patient should be masked if transport within the hospital is unavoidable.<br>Cough etiquette. |

This system of isolation precautions is recommended by the United States Healthcare Infection Control Practices Advisory Committee.

AIIR, airborne infection isolation room; COVID-19, coronavirus disease 2019; HEPA, high-efficiency particulate aerator; HSV, herpes simplex virus; MERS-CoV, Middle East respiratory syndrome coronavirus; MRSA, methicillin-resistant *S. aureus*; RSV, respiratory syncytial virus; SARS, severe acute respiratory syndrome; VRE, vancomycin-resistant enterococci; VZV, varicella-zoster virus.

ᴬ Alcohol-based hand disinfectant is an acceptable alternative to soap and water in all situations EXCEPT in the setting of norovirus and *C. difficile* infection, for which soap and water should be used.

ᴮ Many hospitals favor simplifying the approach to isolation precautions for viral respiratory pathogens by placing all patients with suspected viral illness on both contact and droplet precautions.

ᶜ RSV may be transmitted by the droplet route but is primarily spread by direct contact with infectious respiratory secretions. Droplet precautions are not routinely warranted but are appropriate if the infecting agent is not known, if the patient may be coinfected with other pathogens that require droplet precautions, and/or if there is a chance of exposure to aerosols of infectious respiratory secretions.

ᴰ The most important route of transmission for rhinovirus is via droplets; contact precautions should be added if copious moist secretions and close contact are likely to occur (e.g., young infant patients).

ᴱ Patients with invasive group A streptococcal infection associated with soft tissue involvement warrant both droplet precautions and contact precautions. Droplet precautions alone are warranted for patients with streptococcal toxic shock or streptococcal pneumonia, as well as for infants and young children in the setting of pharyngitis or scarlet fever. Droplet and contact precautions may be discontinued after the first 24 hours of antimicrobial therapy.

ᶠ Refer to UpToDate topics on coronaviruses, including COVID-19, MERS-CoV, and SARS, for specific information on infection control precautions.

ᴳ Refer to the UpToDate topic on prevention of Ebola virus infection for full discussion of infection control issues.

Modified from CDC guidelines.[6]

endotracheal tube (ETT) connection and on the expiratory limb of the breathing circuit at the point of connection to the anesthesia machine should be used. Gas sampling should be on the machine side of the ETT connection filter. General anesthesia should involve a rapid sequence induction by the most experienced clinician, typically with videolaryngoscopy. The minimum number of people to safely induce should be present, all with full PPE and a N95 mask or PAPR. Proper tube placement should be verified with end-tidal $CO_2$. When disconnecting from the circuit, the viral filter on the end of the ETT should be left in place. The anesthesia machine itself should be decontaminated after use as directed by the manufacturer's recommendations. Any disposable items should be discarded as contaminated waste. Water traps for gas sampling and soda lime $CO_2$ absorbents do not need to be exchanged, and the anesthesia machine does not require terminal cleaning if proper viral filters were used. The operating room itself should undergo terminal cleaning with the door closed for a time sufficient for several whole room air exchanges to occur.

## REFERENCES

1. Loftus RW, et al. Hand contamination of anesthesia providers is an important risk factor for intraoperative bacterial transmission. *Anesth Analg.* 2011;112:98–105.
2. Loftus RW, et al. Transmission of pathogenic bacterial organisms in the anesthesia work area. *Anesthesiology.* 2008;109:399–407.
3. Hopf HW, et al. Reducing perioperative infection is as simple as washing your hands. *Anesthesiology.* 2009;110:959–960.
4. Practice Advisory for the Prevention, Diagnosis, and Management of Infectious Complications Associated With Neuraxial Techniques. Practice advisory for the prevention, diagnosis, and management of infectious complications associated with neuraxial techniques: a report by the American Society of Anesthesiologists Task Force on Infectious Complications Associated With Neuraxial Techniques. *Anesthesiology.* 2010;112:530–545.
5. Department of Health and Human Services. Safe use of single dose/single use medications to prevent healthcare-associated infections. June 15, 2012. https://www.hhs.gov/guidance/document/safe-use-single-dosesingle-use-medications-prevent-healthcare-associated-infections
6. Siegel JD, et al. 2007 Guideline for isolation precautions: preventing transmission of infectious agents in health care settings. *Am J Infect Control.* 2007;35:S65.

# 356.

## NEEDLE-STICK INJURY

*Ramsey Saad and Joseph Salama Hanna*

### INTRODUCTION

Risk factors for unintentional needle-stick injuries include long work hours, fatigue, and the emergent nature of interventions. Both attending and resident physicians are at risk, although the risk may be slightly higher among trainees.

### PREVENTION

Using universal precautions for prevention of blood-borne infections is of paramount importance not only for prevention of blood-borne infections from needle-stick injuries, but also for protection against contamination of mucosal surfaces from other body fluids (e.g., eye splashes). Wearing the appropriate attire, such as gloves (or double gloving when appropriate), gowns, and eye protection (e.g., face shields) should be offered to the healthcare provider (HCP), and adequate education should be provided during training; also, refresher courses should be offered on initiation of employment and periodically according to institution protocol.

The main blood-borne infections of concern with needle-stick injuries are hepatitis B, hepatitis C, and human immunodeficiency virus (HIV). Of the three, the risk of hepatitis B can be minimized with vaccination, provided an adequate immune response is achieved. On employment, HCPs should be screened for history of hepatitis B vaccination and should be screened for hepatitis B antibody (anti-Hep B Ab) in addition to hepatitis B surface antigen (Hep B sAg). If anti-Hep B Ab is not detected at the desirable levels, vaccination should be offered. Refusal of the vaccine should be documented should the HCP decline.[1]

## MANAGEMENT

The treatment should be led by medical providers adequately trained in this field (e.g., occupational health). The first step in management is attention to the injury site and adequate cleansing. Soap and water should be sufficient. Use of chlorhexidine, though not necessary, is not contraindicated.

Obtaining a history from the source patient and screening for hepatitis B, hepatitis C, and HIV are the next steps. If the patient tests positive for any of the three, then obtaining a sample from the HCP is warranted.

Also, obtaining a history from the HCP (hepatitis B vaccination status, anti-Hep B Ab titers), including tetanus immunization status, is required. This ideally should be available on employment.

## HEPATITIS B

If the patient tests positive for Hep B sAg and Hep B e Ag, the next step would depend on the status of the HCP:

- If the HCP has a history of vaccination and blood work reveals hepatitis B surface antibody (anti-HBs) level greater than or equal to 10 mIU/mL, the HCP is considered a vaccine responder, and no further follow-up is needed.
- If the anti-HBs remains less than 10 mIU/mL on two separate occasions, even after completing a hepatitis B vaccine series, the HCP then would be considered a vaccine nonresponder.
- It is important to take into consideration that if the hepatitis B vaccine series was completed, but no follow-up serologic testing was performed, the HCP then would be considered of unknown vaccine response. Blood work should be obtained as soon as feasibly possible, and the HCP's response to the vaccine and subsequent further management will be determined based on the level of anti-Hep B s titers as outlined above.
- Not vaccinated or incomplete vaccine series would fall into the same category; the HCP should receive one dose of hepatitis B immunoglobulin (HBIG) and the first dose of the hepatitis B vaccine series, which can be administered at the same time, albeit at different injection sites.

- Of note, if the source patient tests negative for Hep B sAg, the HCP should complete the hepatitis B vaccine.

For follow-up testing, regarding exposure to patients who are Hep B sAg positive or of unknown status, the HCP should undergo follow-up testing with anti-Hep B c and Hep B sAg 6 months after the exposure to determine seroconversion in HCPs who were not hepatitis B virus (HBV) immune at the time of exposure.[2]

## HEPATITIS C

Ideally, the source should be tested for hepatitis C virus (HCV) RNA. If this is unavailable, then anti-HCV testing should be performed. If the source is negative for HCV RNA or anti-HCV, no further evaluation is needed unless acute HCV infection is suspected. In this case, the source may test HCV RNA positive but anti-HCV negative.

If the source is HCV positive or if the status of the patient is unknown, the HCP should be evaluated for anti-HCV within 48 hours of the exposure.

If the anti-HCV returns positive, the HCP should be tested for the presence of HCV RNA, which would indicate preexisting HCV infection.

If initial testing for HCV RNA is negative, the HCP should have repeat HCV RNA testing at least 3 weeks after the exposure. If repeat testing is negative, the initial anti-HCV was most likely a false positive, and no further testing is required. If HCV RNA is detected, then the HCP would be considered to have HCV infection; however, in this setting it is difficult to determine if it was acquired before or after the exposure.

In the case of postexposure anti-HCV returning negative, the HCP should have HCV RNA testing 3 weeks after the exposure. Alternatively, anti-HCV testing can be performed at least 6 months after the exposure, and HCV RNA testing performed if positive. If HCV RNA is now detected, the patient most likely acquired HCV through the occupational exposure. If HCV RNA is negative, no further evaluation is needed.

On a positive note, HCV treatment is currently associated with an excellent cure rate; therefore, all HCPs who test positive for HCV RNA should be referred to a specialist for follow-up.[1,2]

## HIV

Compared to hepatitis B and C, the risk of HIV transmission from exposure to body fluids from an HIV-infected patient is extremely low, about 3 per 1000 from a needlestick injury. As with any injury, the first response to a percutaneous exposure should be to wash the injured area adequately with soap and water; with regard to small lacerations, cleaning the area with an alcohol-based hand hygiene agent is reasonable as well.

The exposure should be immediately reported by the HCP for screening of the source, and the HCP should be informed in a timely fashion to assist with decision-making regarding postexposure prophylaxis (PEP).

In case of HIV exposure, the role of counseling is of utmost importance. The emotional toll of a potential exposure on the HCP cannot be disregarded. In addition to this, the HCP should be counseled on means of reducing HIV transmission in addition to adequate monitoring for seroconversion.

With regard to the exposed HCP, HIV screening should be performed at baseline. If a fourth-generation antibody-antigen test is utilized, then testing should be repeated at 6 weeks and 4 months after the reported exposure. On the other hand, if the testing for antibody only is performed, then testing should be repeated at 6 weeks, 3 months, and 6 months following exposure.

Postexposure prophylaxis should be offered if the source has known HIV infection or if the source tests positive for HIV. If the HIV status of the source patient is unknown, PEP should be offered while awaiting HIV testing, especially if the source patient is at high risk for HIV infection.

If the source patient cannot be identified, such as in the case of a needle-stick injury from a sharps container, then PEP should be offered if the exposure occurred in a setting where the source is at high risk for HIV infection.

If the decision is made to administer PEP, it should be started as early as possible after an exposure (ideally within 1 to 2 hours). If the status of the source is unknown and the patient is at high risk for HIV infection, PEP should be administered while awaiting the results of HIV testing.

A three-drug regimen using tenofovir disoproxil fumarate-emtricitabine plus an integrase strand transfer inhibitor (e.g., raltegravir or dolutegravir) is suggested. Alternative regimens that combine tenofovir disoproxil fumarate-emtricitabine with a boosted protease inhibitor (e.g., ritonavir-boosted darunavir) are also used.

Two advantages of a dolutegravir-containing regimen are the convenience of once-daily dosing and the potential benefit if drug-resistant virus is suspected.

One special clinical situation is regarding HCPs with the possibility of pregnancy. Tenofovir disoproxil fumarate-emtricitabine in combination with either raltegravir or a ritonavir-boosted protease inhibitor should be used, as dolutegravir should be avoided in persons of childbearing potential due to the potential risk of neural tube defects with this medication.

The duration of HIV PEP should be 4 weeks. Obviously, PEP may be discontinued if testing shows that the source patient is HIV negative.

Depending on the regimen used, the HCP should be monitored for side effects and drug toxicity.[3]

## REFERENCES

1. Weber D et al. Prevention of hepatitis B virus and hepatitis C virus infection among health care providers. Accessed August 2, 2020. https://www.uptodate.com/contents/prevention-of-hepatitis-b-virus-and-hepatitis-c-virus-infection-among-health-care-providers?search=needle%20stick%20injury&source=search_result&selectedTitle=1~50&usage_type=default&display_rank=1
2. Schillie S, et al. CDC guidance for evaluating health-care personnel for hepatitis B virus protection and for administering postexposure management. *MMWR Recomm Rep.* 2013;62(RR–10):1.
3. Zachary K, et al. Management of health care personnel exposed to HIV. Accessed August 2, 2020. https://www.uptodate.com/contents/management-of-health-care-personnel-exposed-to-hiv?search=needle%20stick%20injury%20hiv&source=search_result&selectedTitle=1~150&usage_type=default&display_rank=1

# 357.

# INTRAVASCULAR CATHETER AND URINARY CATHETER INFECTIONS

*Zhe Ma and Kevin W. Chung*

## CATHETER-RELATED BLOODSTREAM INFECTIONS

Nosocomial bloodstream infections (BSIs) play a significant role in morbidity and mortality of critically ill patients. Intravascular catheters, particularly central venous catheters (CVCs), are associated with BSIs, although the true rate of infection is hard to determine given the severe morbidity found in the intensive care unit (ICU) setting. Indwelling catheters are common among patients in the ICU requiring long-term venous access for hemodialysis, parenteral nutrition, and infusion of chemotherapeutic agents. All types of intravascular catheters carry some inherent risk of catheter-related BSI (CRBSI). However, nontunneled CVCs and pulmonary artery catheters (PACs) carry greater risk than peripheral intravenous catheters (Table 357.1).[1] Other risk factors that increase CRBSI include lack of maximal barrier precautions (i.e., mask, cap, sterile gloves, gown, large drape) and lines used for hyperalimentation or hemodialysis.

A recent meta-analysis of more than 16,000 CVCs noted that there was no significant difference in CRBSI between femoral and subclavian CVCs.[2] While this meta-analysis found that CVCs placed in the internal jugular vein were lower risk for CRBSIs than subclavian vein cannulation, no statistically significant difference was actually found when two studies noted to be statistical outliers were removed from the analysis. This analysis was undertaken in response to the Centers for Disease Control and Prevention 2011 class 1A recommendation to avoid femoral catheterization in adults.[3] Updated society guidelines noted increased general risk of CRBSI with jugular and femoral CVCs, although additional patient factors may be influential and should be assessed on an individual basis (e.g., jugular CVC in tracheostomy patients). Ultimately, the optimal choice for CVC insertion site must also include considerations for operator skill and the risk of mechanical complications.

Duration of catheterization also plays a major role in prevention of CRBSI. In general, the risk of infection has been reported to be increased after the following catheter days:

- Arterial catheter greater than 4 days
- Peripheral venous catheter greater than 4 days
- CVC greater than 6 days
- PAC greater than 4 days

Even with increased risk associated with prolonged catheter days, it has been recommended not to routinely replace catheters based solely on length of use only.[3] Rather, catheters should be inspected on a regular basis for any early signs of complications necessitating their replacement by either exchange over a wire or with placement at a new site. Replacing central access over a guidewire or at a new site has also been found to increase the risk of CRBSI and mechanical complications, respectively. Unless otherwise indicated, high-risk CRBSI catheters should be removed when their clinical need has been met.

The CRBSIs associated with CVCs are often attributed to skin colonization, contamination of the intravenous fluid or of the catheter lumen or hub, and/or bacterial

*Table 357.1.* **RISK OF CRBSI ASSOCIATED WITH VARIOUS INTRAVASCULAR CATHETERS**

| TYPE OF CATHETER | RISK OF CRBSI (PER 1000 CATHETER DAYS) |
|---|---|
| Pulmonary artery catheter | 3.7 (95% CI 2.4–5.0) |
| Noncuffed CVC | 2.7 (95% CI 2.6–2.9) |
| Arterial catheter | 1.7 (95% CI 1.2–2.3) |
| Cuffed and tunneled CVC | 1.6 (95% CI 1.5–1.7) |
| Peripherally inserted central catheter | 1.1 (95% CI 0.9–1.3) |
| Peripheral intravenous catheter | 0.5 (95% CI 0.2–0.7) |

From Reference 1.

seeing from a secondary BSI. General manifestations of CRBSI may include fever, chills, or hypotension in the setting of a catheter placed 48 hours prior to symptoms. Specific findings of erythema, swelling, pain, or purulence at CVC sites should raise suspicion for CRBSI, and vigilance for the development of complications such as endocarditis, septic thrombophlebitis, and metastatic musculoskeletal infections should be maintained. If another source of BSI has not already been identified, two sets of blood cultures from different sites should be collected prior to antibiotic therapy. Once an organism has been identified to be the source of BSI, alternative bacterial sources should also be considered (e.g., urinary tract, pulmonary, abdominal, bone, etc.). If no clear source of BSI is identified, then CRBSI can be diagnosed by exclusion.

Although empiric antibiotic therapy should be initiated, particularly in clinically unstable patients, specific recommendations from infectious disease experts within one's institution should be noted, especially for less common organisms and/or fungemia. Gram-positive organisms are the most common species in CRBSI and are often treated with vancomycin (or daptomycin in areas with high vancomycin resistance). For gram-negative bacilli, patients with neutropenia, severe burns, or hemodynamic instability require antipseudomonal coverage; otherwise, ceftriaxone monotherapy is sufficient. In most cases, catheter removal is preferred and improves CRBSI mortality. The decision for catheter removal should ultimately include considerations for its clinical indication and the risks involved with replacement at a new site. Fever of unknown origin in hemodynamically stable patients without a documented BSI should not necessarily make them a candidate for catheter removal. Clinical improvement within 24 hours of removing the catheter in question is suggestive, but not definitive, for CRBSI.

## URINARY TRACT INFECTIONS

Bacteriuria in patients with indwelling bladder catheters is common, occurring at a rate of 3% to 10% per day. Of these, about 10% to 25% develop symptoms of urinary tract infection (UTI). Risk factors for the development of UTI include duration of catheterization, female sex, older age, and diabetes mellitus.

Urinary tract infections can be classified as extraluminal or intraluminal infections. Extraluminal infections are a result of bacteria that form a biofilm around the catheter in the urethra. Intraluminal infections occur due to urinary obstruction from drainage failure or contamination in the collection bag. Patients often present with nonspecific findings such as fever, suprapubic or flank discomfort, or costovertebral angle tenderness.[4] The diagnosis of catheter-associated UTI is typically made from the presence of bacteriuria at $10^5$ colony-forming units per milliliter or greater, along with specific UTI symptoms or potentially nonspecific findings (e.g., fever, leukocytosis, shock, metabolic acidosis).[4] When nonspecific findings are used for diagnosis of a UTI, evaluation of infection should also include other sources. Urine cultures should ideally be obtained by removing the indwelling catheter and collecting a clean, midstream specimen. Most collection systems also allow for samples to be obtained from a port upstream of the collection bag. The collection bag itself should never be used as a sample to guide antibiotic therapy. Empiric antibiotic therapy is typically tailored to whether the infection remains in the bladder (acute simple cystitis) or has extended beyond the bladder (acute complicated UTI). Urinary catheters should always be removed when catheterization is no longer required. Intermittent catheterization has been shown to have lower rates of bacteriuria than indwelling catheters and should be used in the setting of a UTI if catheterization is still required.[5]

## REFERENCES

1. Maki DG. The risk of bloodstream infection in adults with different intravascular devices: a systematic review of 200 published prospective studies. *Mayo Clin Proc.* 2006;81(9):1159–1171.
2. Marik PE, et al. The risk of catheter-related bloodstream infection with femoral venous catheters as compared to subclavian and internal jugular venous catheters: a systematic review of the literature and meta-analysis. *Crit Care Med.* 2012;40(8):2479–2485.
3. O'Grady NP, et al. Summary of recommendations: guidelines for the prevention of intravascular catheter-related infections. *Clin Infect Dis.* 2011;52(9):1087–1099.
4. Hooton TM. Diagnosis, prevention, and treatment of catheter-associated urinary tract infection in adults: 2009 international clinical practice guidelines from the Infectious Diseases Society of America. *Clin Infect Dis.* 2010;50(5):625–663.
5. Weld KJ. Effect of bladder management on urological complications in spinal cord injured patients. *J Urol.* 2000;163(3):768–772.

# 358.

# VENTILATOR-ASSOCIATED PNEUMONIA

*Robert M. Owen and Kevin W. Chung*

## INTRODUCTION

Ventilator-associated pneumonia (VAP) is a nosocomial pneumonia that develops more than 48 hours following endotracheal intubation. The incidence of VAP ranges from 10% to 20% for ventilated patients.[1,2] More recent epidemiologic data show a decrease in this number in the United States, although it is unsure whether this is the result of improved preventive measures or stricter applications of surveillance measures.[1] Trauma and brain injury patients, however, continue to show remarkably high rates of VAP, with up to 50% of intubated patients within these populations developing VAP.[3] All-cause mortality for patients who develop VAP appears to be between 20% and 50%, with about 10%–13% of these deaths attributed directly to VAP. Patients with VAP have significantly longer days of mechanical ventilation and hospitalization, as well as increased healthcare costs.[2]

## CLINICAL FEATURES

As patients who develop VAP are intubated and often unable to communicate effectively, cognizance of the clinical signs and patient risk factors is imperative. Clinical signs of VAP include tachypnea, fever (or hypothermia), leukocytosis, purulent airway secretions, reduced breath sounds, crackles, and worsening gas exchange. These signs can be both nonspecific and subjective. Therefore, it is important to know what may place a patient at an elevated risk for development of VAP.

Risk factors for VAP can be divided into endogenous (patient-centric) and exogenous risk factors. Endogenous risk factors include advanced age, immunosuppression, and underlying pulmonary disease like acute respiratory distress syndrome ARDS or chronic obstructive pulmonary disease.[4] Advanced age is a risk factor for both the development of VAP and for mortality in those patients who do develop VAP. Additionally, patients with trauma and brain injury represent an at-risk population, likely due to altered levels of consciousness leading to increased

microaspiration.[3] VAP may rapidly progress to ARDS, septic shock, and death if not adequately treated.

Exogenous risk factors include prolonged intubation, frequent reintubation, frequent ventilator circuit changes, presence of a nasogastric tube, nasogastric enteral feeding, improper hand hygiene by healthcare workers, and use of sedation.[4] Bacterial sources of VAP are often from orogastric secretions and the mechanical ventilation equipment. Condensation within the ventilator circuit can be a source of pathogens, and the endotracheal tube (ETT) itself can become a nidus for the formation of biofilm, which is an important virulence mechanism of VAP. Biofilm reduces the host's ability to clear pathogens and increases resistance to antimicrobial therapies.

## DIAGNOSIS

It is generally accepted that VAP is defined as a pneumonia that develops more than 48 hours after endotracheal intubation. Patients who develop pneumonia and are subsequently intubated do not meet diagnostic criteria for VAP. Pneumonia is taken to mean "new lung infiltrate plus clinical evidence that the infiltrate is of an infectious origin, which include the new onset of fever, purulent sputum, leukocytosis, and decline in oxygenation."[2] The diagnosis is typically made through a combination of clinical, radiologic, and microbiologic findings. There is significant debate about the utility of obtaining invasive samples, via bronchoscopy with bronchoalveolar lavage or protected specimen brush, prior to the initiation of antibiotic therapy, and there is no strong evidence arguing for or against it.

## PREVENTION

Many interventions used to help lower the risk of VAP have now been incorporated into "ventilator bundles" aimed at preventing not only VAP, but also other ventilator-associated events. Avoidance of endotracheal intubation and mechanical ventilation is the most effective means of preventing VAP. Other recommendations for preventing VAP include managing patients without sedation whenever possible and interrupting sedation daily if it is needed, assessing need for intubation daily with spontaneous breathing trials off sedation, utilizing ETTs with subglottic secretion drainage ports, changing ventilator circuits only if visibly contaminated, and elevating the head of the bed.[1] ETTs with subglottic secretion drainage ports are rarely used in the operating rooms but allow for the ability to drain secretions that may pool between the glottis and the ETT cuff. ETTs utilizing antimicrobial polymers and surfaces designed to prevent the formation of biofilm are in development but not yet tested for the prevention of VAP. It is important to note that early tracheostomy has been shown to have no impact on VAP rates, mortality, length of stay, or duration of mechanical ventilation.[1]

## CAUSATIVE ORGANISMS

Ventilator-associated pneumonia is primarily a bacterial infection, with viruses and fungi each accounting for less than 1% of infections. Polymicrobial infection is not uncommon and may be as high as 21%.[4] *Staphylococcus aureus, Pseudomonas aeruginosa, Acinetobacter baumannii,* and *Enterobacteriaceae* members (most commonly *Klebsiella pneumoniae* and *Escherichia coli*) together represent 80% of VAP cases, with *S. aureus* and *P. aeruginosa* the most common.[4] The ability of these organisms to create a biofilm adds to their virulence. *Staphylococcus aureus,* and particularly methicillin-resistant *S. aureus* (MRSA), can cause a rapidly progressive necrotizing pneumonia, even in immunocompetent hosts, thanks to the production of Panton-Valentine leukocidin.[4] The prevalence of MRSA and other multidrug-resistant (MDR) organisms has led to increased awareness regarding preserving antibiotic stewardship.

## TREATMENT

As with any bacterial infection, the mainstay of treatment for VAP is timely antibiotic administration. Initial antibiotic choice should cover for *S. aureus* and *P. aeruginosa* and should be tailored to both the institution's local pattern of

---

> **Box 358.1.** RISK FACTORS FOR MDR PATHOGEN INFECTION
>
> Septic shock at time of VAP
> Previous antibiotic use in the past 90 days
> ARDS preceding VAP
> 5 or more hospital days prior to occurrence of VAP
> Need for renal replacement therapy prior to occurrence of VAP
>
> *From Reference 2.*

---

resistance and the patient's condition. In patients at high risk for MDR pathogen infection, coverage for MRSA should be provided.[2] Additionally, two antipseudomonal agents from different classes should be used (e.g., piperacillin-tazobactam and levofloxacin).

There are myriad risk factors for MDR pathogen infection (Box 358.1). Anti-MRSA coverage should also be considered in patients who do not meet these criteria but reside in an intensive care unit with more than 10%–20% of *S. aureus* isolates proving to be MRSA.[2] Antibiotic therapy should be narrowed based on culture data.[2,3] An antibiogram, or summary of institutional pathogens and their susceptibility, is crucial for determining appropriate antibiotic therapy. It is appropriate to treat patients with a 7- to 8-day course of antibiotics for VAP.[2,3] Patients with immunodeficiency, cystic fibrosis, empyema, lung abscess, cavitation, or necrotizing pneumonia may require longer courses of treatment.

## REFERENCES

1. Michael K, et al. Strategies to prevent ventilator-associated pneumonia in acute care hospitals: 2014 update. *Infect Control Hosp Epidemiol.* 2014;32:S2.
2. Andre K, et al. Management of adults with hospital-acquired and ventilator-associated pneumonia: 2016 clinical practice guidelines by the Infectious Diseases Society of America and the American Thoracic Society. *Clin Infect Dis.* 2016;63(5):e61–e111.
3. Torres A, et al. International ERS/ESICM/ESCMID/ALAT guidelines for the management of hospital-acquired pneumonia and ventilator-associated pneumonia. *Eur Respir J.* 2017;50:1700582.
4. Monteiro-Neto A, et al. Microbiology of ventilator-associated pneumonia. In: IntechOpen. doi:10.5772/intechopen.69430. https://www.intechopen.com/chapters/55756

# 359.

# ANTIMICROBIALS

*Mo Shirur and Kevin W. Chung*

## INTRODUCTION

Antibiotics play a ubiquitous role in the daily life of an anesthesiologist, in both the perioperative setting and the intensive care unit (ICU). Generally classified based on their mechanisms of action, antibiotics were traditionally broadly separated into two main categories: bactericidal antibiotics, which show in -vitro activity in killing bacteria, and bacteriostatic antibiotics, which show the ability to diminish bacterial growth.[1] This chapter discusses the major antimicrobial agents used in the clinical setting today.

## ANTI-GRAM-POSITIVE ANTIBIOTICS

### PENICILLINS

Penicillins contain a β-lactam ring that inhibits bacterial cell wall synthesis. Piperacillin with tazobactam, which is effective for empiric gram-negative coverage, is a commonly used penicillin in the perioperative setting.[2]

## CEPHALOSPORINS

Cephalosporins are also β-lactam antibiotics that inhibit bacterial cell wall synthesis. They are typically classified into *generations*. The first four generations are shown in Table 359.1.[2]

Cefazolin, one of the most commonly used antibiotics in the perioperative setting, is a first-generation cephalosporin with activity against gram-positive cocci except *Staphylococcus epidermidis* and methicillin-resistant *Staphylococcus aureus* (MRSA). Third-generation cephalosporins (e.g., ceftriaxone) have greater activity toward gram-negative bacilli such as *Haemophilus influenzae* but less activity against gram positives. Fourth-generation cephalosporins (e.g., cefepime) cover gram-negative bacteria, including *Pseudomonas*, as well as gram positives. Finally, the fifth-generation cephalosporin ceftaroline is similar to fourth-generation cephalosporins but also with activity against MRSA.[2]

Adverse reactions to cephalosporins are uncommon and include nausea, rash, and diarrhea. There is a 5%–15% incidence of cross-antigenicity with penicillin.

*Table 359.1* CEPHALOSPORIN ACTIVITY

| CEPHALOSPORIN | GRAM-POSITIVE COCCI | GRAM-NEGATIVE BACILLI | *PSEUDOMONAS AERUGINOSA* | MRSA |
|---|---|---|---|---|
| *1st generation* | High activity | Moderate activity | | |
| *2nd generation* | Moderate activity | High activity | | |
| *3rd generation* | Moderate activity | High activity | ■[a,b] | |
| *4th generation* | High activity | High activity | High activity | |
| *5th generation*[c] | Moderate activity | Moderate activity | | High activity |

[a] ■ Indicates minimal-to-no activity against microbe.

[B] Of all third-generation cephalosporins, ceftazidime does have activity against *P. aeruginosa*.

[C] Fifth generation in this context is specifically ceftaroline.

## VANCOMYCIN

Vancomycin inhibits bacterial cell wall formation by binding the D-alanyl-D-alanine portion. It is active against all gram positives including MRSA, aerobic and anaerobic *Streptococcus*, and *Clostridium difficile*, although there is now prevalence of vancomycin-resistant strains of *Enterococcus* (VRE). Vancomycin is dosed based on body weight and renal function and is often redosed based on blood level, especially in the ICU setting.[2]

Vancomycin administered too rapidly can result in an adverse reaction termed *red man syndrome*, which manifests as vasodilation, flushing, and hypotension as a result of histamine release.

## LINEZOLID

Linezolid is an oxazolidine antimicrobial active against antibiotic-resistant gram positives, including VRE and MRSA. Linezolid has superior penetration into lung secretions, rendering it more useful in pneumonia compared to vancomycin.

Common side effects include vomiting, diarrhea, and headache. More serious side effects include bone marrow suppression with prolonged use, optic neuropathy, and serotonin syndrome.[2]

## ANTI-GRAM-NEGATIVE ANTIBIOTICS

### AMINOGLYCOCIDES

Aminoglycosides (e.g., gentamicin, tobramycin, amikacin) are a bactericidal class of antibiotics most active against gram negatives, including *Pseudomonas aeruginosa*. Dosing is based on ideal body weight, although dosing is based on adjusted body weight for obese patients and adjusted further for renal impairment.[2]

Nephrotoxicity is the most significant adverse effect of aminoglycosides. Aminoglycosides can also prolong the effects of nondepolarizing neuromusclular-blocking drugs by blocking acetylcholine release from presynaptic terminals.[2]

### FLUOROQUINOLONES

Fluoroquinolones (e.g., ciprofloxacin, levofloxacin, moxifloxacin) are active against MSSA. Levofloxacin and moxifloxacin also have activity against *Streptococcus* species, including penicillin-resistant *Pneumococcus*. Initially, these antibiotics were effective against *Pseudomonas* and other gram-negative aerobic bacilli, but emerging resistance has developed. Levofloxacin is best used today for community acquired pneumonia, chronic obstructive pulmonary disease exacerbations, and uncomplicated urinary tract infections.[2]

Dosing is adjusted in renal failure for ciprofloxacin and levofloxacin but not for moxifloxacin, which undergoes hepatic metabolism. Ciprofloxacin and levofloxacin toxicity can result in prolonged QT and Torsade de pointes.[2] Fluoroquinolones are known to interfere with the metabolism of warfarin and theophyilline, thereby potentiating their action.[2]

## CARBAPENAMS

Of the antibiotics readily available today, carbapenams (e.g., imipnem, meropenem, ertapenem) have the broadest spectrum of coverage. Imipenam and meropenam are active against all common bacteria, including gram negatives, anaerobes, and gram positives except MRSA and VRE.[2] Dose reduction is required in renal failure.

Imipenam can cause generalized seizures, though most reported cases were in patients with a history of seizures, intracranial mass, or lack of dose adjustment in renal failure. Meropenam can reduce serum levels of valproic acid in patients with a seizure disorder, which can then increase the risk of seizures in these patients.[2]

## METRONIDAZOLE

Metronidazole has activity against both bacterial and protozoan microorganisms. It is commonly used intraoperatively for its activity against anaerobic intra-abdominal and pelvic microbes.[3] It is an excellent agent against *Clostridium difficile*.[2]

## ANTIFUNGAL AGENTS

### AMPHOTERICIN B

Amphotericin B is one of the most effective antifungal agents available, capable of treating even life-threatening invasive *Aspergillosis*. However, its extensive side-effect profile often renders it as a medication of last resort.[2]

An infusion-related inflammatory response in which patients experience high fevers, chills, vomiting, hypotension, and rigors is often the limiting factor for amphotericin B administration. This is usually seen in the initial infusion and diminishes with subsequent infusions. Other side effects include nephrotoxicity, electrolyte disturbances, and infusion-related phlebitis.[2]

### FLUCONAZOLE

Fluconazole, a member of the triazole group of antifungals, is useful against *Candida* infections and has less toxicity than amphotericin B. Dosing should be adjusted in renal impairment.[2]

Fluconazole can inhibit the cytochrome P450 enzymes, which can lead to toxicity of drugs metabolized by that pathway. Liver enzymes should be monitored in patients with HIV and liver disease as there have been case reports of fatal hepatic injury in these patients.[2]

## CASPOFUNGIN

Caspofungin is an antifungal agent with activity against a broader spectrum of *Candida* species than fluconazole. Caspofungin is preferred for treating invasive *Candida* infections, especially in unstable or immunocompromised patients, and is considered a safer alternative to amphotericin B. No dose adjustment is necessary in renal failure, though transient elevations in liver enzymes may occur.[2]

## ANESTHETIC CONSIDERATIONS

### PREOPERATIVE

A careful assessment of a patient's medical history, with particular attention to preexisting kidney or liver disease, must be performed preoperatively, as antibiotic dosing adjustments may be necessary. Furthermore, a review of previous drug reactions and allergies is essential.

### INTRAOPERATIVE

The Centers for Disease Control and Prevention and Centers for Medicare and Medicaid Services established the Surgical Infection Project to measure and reduce surgical site infections (SSIs). Among other recommendations, this initiative advocates for the administration of appropriate antibiotics within 60 minutes of surgical incision.[4]

### POSTOPERATIVE

Antibiotic administration at the correct dosages and dosing interval during the postoperative period is crucial in minimizing the risk of SSIs.

## REFERENCES

1. Pankey GA, Sabath LD. Clinical relevance of bacteriostatic versus bactericidal mechanisms of action in the treatment of gram-positive bacterial infections. *Clin Infect Dis.* 2004;38(6):864–870.
2. Antimicrobial therapy. In: Marino PL, ed. *Marino's the ICU Book.* Wolters Kluwer Health/Lippincott, Williams & Wilkins; 2014:1691–1730.
3. Brogden RN, et al. Metronidazole in anaerobic infections. *Drugs.* 1978;16(5):387–417.
4. Parsons D. Preoperative evaluation and risk management. *Clin Colon Rectal Surg.* 2009;22(1):5–13.

# 360.

# MECHANICAL VENTILATION

*Mena Abdelmalak and Kevin W. Chung*

## INTRODUCTION

Ventilation comprises one of the most critical tasks performed by an anesthesiologist. Mechanical ventilation, whether hand powered or machine driven, is the primary method of ventilating patients in the operating room and, if necessary, in the postanesthesia care unit or intensive care unit (ICU) (Table 360.1).

## MODES OF VENTILATION

Mechanical ventilation can be subdivided into two primary subtypes: volume modes and pressure modes.[1] Ventilators are flow and pressure regulators in which either volume or pressure (i.e., the independent variable) can be set by the practitioner at the expense of control over the other parameter (i.e., the dependent variable).

*Table 360.1* VARIABLES OF VENTILATION

| VARIABLE | DESCRIPTION | RANGE | IDEAL | NOTES |
|---|---|---|---|---|
| $FiO_2$ | Fraction of inspired oxygen | ~21% to 100% | Room Air: 21% Intraoperative: 60%–80% to decrease atelectasis | • Preoxygenate with 100% to goal 80%+ $EtO_2$ |
| Tidal volume (TV) | Volume of normal breath, no extra force | 6 mL to ~1000 mL depending on age and weight | 6–10 mL/kg ~400–550 mL in adults | • Too little TV can mean only dead space ventilation<br>• Too large TV can be associated with volutrauma |
| Fresh gas flow | Total amount of fresh gas delivered | 0.5 L/min to 15 L/min+ | 1–3 L/min during maintenance, 10L/min+ during induction/emergence | • High fibroblast growth factor (FGF = quicker onset/offset of inhaled anesthetics)<br>• Attempt to limit use of FG to practice green anesthesia |
| Respiratory rate | Amount of breaths per minute | 0–100 breaths/min | 12–20 breaths/min | • High respiratory rate utilized in ARDSnet<br>• Induced hyperventilation for neuroprotection |
| Positive end-expiratory pressure (PEEP) | Constant positive pressure helping prevent alveoli/small airway collapse | 0–20+ cm $H_2O$ | 5–10 cm $H_2O$ | • Increases functional residual capacity<br>• Improves V/Q mismatch and compliance<br>• High PEEP required in ARDS |
| Inspiratory: expiratory (I:E ratio) | Ratio between time for spent inhalation versus exhalation | 1:1–1:4+ | 1:2 | • Higher ratio increases $CO_2$ clearance, but decreases oxygenation time |

The extent of ventilator assistance is another major distinction made between modes of ventilation, as assistance can range from full control of patient ventilation to merely supporting patient-generated respiratory efforts.

## VOLUME MODES

### VOLUME CONTROL VENTILATION

Volume control ventilation (VCV) is the mode in which the operator sets the respiratory rate and tidal volume. This guarantees a specific minute ventilation without regard for spontaneously triggered breaths. With VCV, pressure is the dependent variable, and barotrauma is a possible risk. Changes in patient positioning (e.g., Trendelenburg position) or operative conditions (e.g., insufflation of the abdomen during laparoscopic surgery) that result in cephalad displacement of the diaphragm lead to increased airway pressures to achieve the same tidal volume. This mode of ventilation should be used with caution in patients with pulmonary pathophysiology or injury.

### SYNCHRONIZED INTERMITTENT-MANDATORY VENTILATION

Like VCV, synchronized intermittent-mandatory ventilation (SIMV) allows the practitioner to control tidal volume and respiratory rate. However, in SIMV, the ventilator synchronizes the mandatory breaths with patient-generated breaths, which are assisted with an operator-programmed degree of pressure support to help reduce the work of breathing.[1] In this mode of ventilation, the sum of breaths spontaneously triggered by the patient and mandatory breaths delivered by the ventilator should equal the set respiratory rate. SIMV is often used as a bridge between mandatory ventilation and pressure support ventilation (PSV).

## PRESSURE MODES

### PRESSURE-CONTROLLED VENTILATION

In pressure-controlled ventilation (PCV), the operator sets a respiratory rate and target pressure for each breath. With this mode of ventilation, pressure remains constant, and tidal volume becomes a dependent variable. This mode of ventilation has the advantage of reducing the incidence of barotrauma, decreasing peak airway pressures, and improving gas exchange.[1] However, inadequate ventilation can occur with changes in patient positioning or operative conditions. This mode of ventilation does not provide assistance for patient-generated breaths and is commonly used in pediatric patients and in patients with lung pathology.

## PRESSURE SUPPORT VENTILATION

In PSV, the ventilator can be programmed to respond to certain triggering parameters (e.g., changes in airway flow or pressure) and to provide a set amount of assistance to each breath, thereby providing a spontaneously breathing patient with ventilatory support. This mode of ventilation is typically used toward the end of an anesthetic when weaning patients from mechanical ventilation to assist patients to overcome the resistance of breathing through an endotracheal tube (ETT). There is no guaranteed number of breaths or minute ventilation with PSV, and thus there is typically an accompanying backup mode of mandatory ventilation that is initiated if prolonged apnea is detected.

## POSITIVE END-EXPIRATORY PRESSURE

Positive end-expiratory pressure (PEEP), or the alveolar pressure exceeding atmospheric pressure at the end of expiration, is a ventilatory parameter that is included to mitigate alveolar collapse at the end of expiration. This continuous positive intrathoracic pressure can have a number of physiologic consequences, such as decreased venous return, increased right ventricular afterload, and increased functional residual capacity.[1] The application of high PEEP in the ventilatory support of patients with acute respiratory distress syndrome (ARDS) is a crucial component of the ARDSnet protocol.[2]

## VENTILATOR WEANING

Weaning a patient from a ventilator and understanding when a patient is ready to be extubated is a critical task for the anesthesiologist. In transitioning from fully mandatory ventilation, it is common for patients to be placed on SIMV and PSV with progressively less ventilatory support. At the time of extubation, minimal ventilatory assistance suggests that the patient is capable of continuing to breathe adequately on removal of the ETT. In the ICU, minimal ventilatory settings consist of a pressure support of 5 cm $H_2O$, PEEP of 5 cm $H_2O$, and an $FiO_2$ (fraction of inspired oxygen) of 40%.[3] Premature extubation in a patient still requiring moderate ventilatory assistance may result in subsequent respiratory failure and the need for reintubation.

Myriad factors may lead to difficulty in weaning a patient from mechanical ventilation. Rapid shallow breathing may suggest insufficient pain control, electrolyte abnormalities (e.g., hypophosphatemia, hypomagnesemia), or inadequate strength due to prolonged mechanical ventilation or residual neuromuscular blockade.[4] Residual anesthetics or sedation may also contribute to difficulty in weaning. Inadequate minute ventilation and patients with pulmonary physiology resulting in elevated carbon dioxide (e.g., chronic obstructive pulmonary disease, obstructive sleep apnea) may result in hypercapnic narcosis. Additionally, patients receiving carbohydrate-rich enteral feeds may be difficult to wean because of increased carbon dioxide production and subsequent hypercapnia.[4] Particular attention should be paid to carbohydrate composition, and if mechanical ventilation weaning proves difficult, dietary modification should be performed to decrease carbohydrate intake.

## RISKS OF MECHANICAL VENTILATION

While the benefits of mechanical ventilation have been highlighted, it remains an invasive procedure with certain risks. Barotrauma, one of the most common complications related to mechanical ventilation, occurs due to elevated transalveolar pressure (e.g., the difference between the alveolar pressure and the pleural pressure), resulting in alveolar overinflation, elevated peak airway pressures, and subsequent rupture, which may lead to pneumothorax, pneumomediastinum, pneumoperitoneum, and/or subcutaneous emphysema.[3] Overdistension of alveoli can also result in volutrauma and consequent ventilator-induced lung injury (VILI). VILI can then eventually result in ARDS.[5] Prolonged mechanical ventilation with a high $FiO_2$ (typically, $FiO_2$ greater than 60%) can also result in oxygen toxicity and consequent central nervous system and pulmonary damage. Ventilator-associated pneumonia is another serious complication related to mechanical ventilation (it is discussed in a separate chapter).

## REFERENCES

1. Hyzy R, Jia S. Modes of mechanical ventilation. In Finlay G, ed. *UpToDate*. UpToDate; 2019. Accessed September 1, 2020. https://www.uptodate.com/contents/modes-of-mechanical-ventilation
2. Brower RG, ARDSNet NIH/NHLBI. Assessment of protocol conduct in a trial of ventilator management of acute lung injury (ALI) and ARDS. ATS. 1999.
3. Critical care. In: Butterworth JF IV, et al., eds. *Morgan & Mikhail's Clinical Anesthesiology*. 5th ed. McGraw-Hill; 2013: Chap. 57.
4. Alía I, Esteban A. Weaning from mechanical ventilation. *Crit Care*. 2000;4(2):72–80.
5. Beitler JR, et al. Ventilator-induced lung injury. *Clin Chest Med*. 2016;37(4):633–646.

# 361.

# POSTOPERATIVE HEADACHE

*Feroz Osmani and Kevin W. Chung*

## INTRODUCTION

Depending on the type of procedure and anesthetic, the severity and timing of the headache may differ. It has a broad differential diagnosis, and although most etiologies of postoperative headaches are benign or may simply be an exacerbation of a preexisting chronic headache disorder, severe etiologies must be ruled out. Other factors such as dehydration, caffeine withdrawal, hunger, and pain may contribute to or worsen the headache.[1,2] Headache is an important cause of postoperative morbidity, and adverse outcomes associated with postoperative headaches include increased patient discomfort, time to ambulation, and costs.[1,2]

## THE POSTOPERATIVE EVALUATION

Along with a standard evaluation of cardiopulmonary status, an assessment of pain level and the presence of neurological deficits should be performed during a postoperative evaluation. Often, patients with postoperative headache will volunteer this information at this time. The timing and severity of the headache should be evaluated. Some focused questions used to elicit more information about the headache are included in Box 361.1.

---

*Box 361.1* COMMON QUESTIONS USED IN THE EVALUATION OF POSTOPERATIVE HEADACHES

Was the headache present prior to the procedure?
Does the patient have a history of chronic headaches?
What triggers the headache? What therapies abort the headache?
What is the location of the pain? Is it unilateral or bilateral?
Is the pain throbbing or constant?
Does the pain radiate to other parts of the body?
Is the pain alleviated with positional changes?

---

Certain surgical procedures involving mechanical manipulation of the central nervous system predispose patients to the development of postoperative headaches, and although usually transient, it is important to ensure that the headache is not a consequence of neurologic sequelae related to the surgery. Communication with the nursing staff is important for monitoring of the headache, and any alarm symptoms, such as acute "thunderclap headache" or altered mental status, should be immediately communicated to the surgical team.

## HEADACHES RELATED TO THE PROCEDURE

While there are many different types of surgical procedures that carry a risk of a postoperative headache, the inciting procedures all share in common having a direct impact on the brain, by either physical manipulation of the central nervous system or causing fluctuation in oxygen delivery to the brain due to blood pressure variation. Otolaryngologic (ENT; ear, nose, throat), neurosurgical, and vascular surgeries have the highest incidence of postoperative headaches. The ENT cases that have demonstrated the highest number of postoperative headaches include resections of vestibular schwannomas and acoustic neuromas, as well as following sinus endoscopy.[3] Postoperative headaches are frequently seen after many neurosurgical procedures, such as following craniotomy, resection of intracranial tumors, endovascular thrombectomy and embolization, and microvascular nerve decompression.[4] Following lumbar drain placement, an orthostatic headache with a similar mechanism as a postdural puncture headache (PDPH) may also be experienced. Carotid endarterectomy and stenting are also known causes of postoperative headaches within vascular surgery.[1,5] as is headache after vaginal delivery due to postpartum cervical myofascial pain syndrome.

## HEADACHES RELATED TO ANESTHESIA

It is thought that certain anesthetics have a predilection for the development of postoperative headache. Female gender, intraoperative hypotension, sevoflurane administration, and history of chronic headaches were all found to be associated with a greater risk of developing postoperative headache.[1] For patients at high risk of developing postoperative headache, preoperative planning should include a discussion about the type of anesthetic and maintenance agent.

Headaches related to neuraxial anesthesia are a well-known phenomenon. Dural puncture, such as in a spinal anesthetic or an inadvertent dural puncture during placement of an epidural catheter, may cause a leak of cerebrospinal fluid (CSF) into the epidural space. This decreased volume in circulating CSF reduces the cushion of the brain within the cranium and results in a headache that is classically described as bifrontal with radiation to the neck and back. Symptoms of a PDPH usually develop within 24–48 hours following dural puncture, and resolution of the headache when going from the upright position to the supine position is a pathognomonic feature.

The most common conservative treatment options for a PDPH include intravenous and parental hydration with caffeine supplementation and fioricet (combination acetaminophen, butalbital, and caffeine). The gold standard treatment is an epidural blood patch, in which autologous blood is injected into the epidural space, resulting in coagulation at the puncture site and the formation of a band of compression around the intrathecal space that essentially increases CSF pressure. Patients generally obtain relief relatively rapidly.

## INTRAOPERATIVE CONSIDERATIONS

The incidence of postoperative headache may be as high as 54% and much higher when investigating patients with a prior history of headaches.[1,2] Intraoperative considerations may help to minimize headache severity, provide symptom mitigation, or prevent them altogether.

Patients presenting for surgery require adequate volume repletion, as most have been fasting (NPO, nil per os) for greater than 12 hours. Dehydration is a common cause of headache in the postoperative period. While the classical 4/2/1 rule for volume repletion in NPO patients has fallen out of favor, it is worth considering a fluid challenge in a patient reporting a history of postoperative headaches.

Although rare, halogenated anesthetics have been known to be a cause of headache (<1%). Headaches have also been documented as a common side effect associated with the administration of ondansetron (<10%).[1,2]

Blood pressure variation may also contribute to the development of postoperative headaches.[1,2] Postoperative headache can occur due to both prolonged intraoperative hypotension and severe hypertension secondary to inadequate perfusion of brain tissue or swelling of brain parenchyma, respectively. It is important to anticipate blood pressure changes during induction, emergence, and surgical stimulation and to plan interventions accordingly to avoid rapid swings in blood pressure.

Inadequate oxygenation and ventilation are other important causes of postoperative headaches. This is especially important in the setting of monitored anesthesia care cases, as the absence of a secured airway leads to a diminished ability to directly control and manipulate parameters affecting oxygenation and ventilation. Hypercapnia is a known cause of postoperative delirium and headache. For cases done under general anesthesia, it is important to ensure that the patient is able to achieve adequate tidal volumes at a comfortable rate prior to extubation. Low oxygen saturation after extubation is another common cause of headache and commonly goes unnoticed until arrival to the postanesthesia care unit.

## REFERENCES

1. Matsota PK, et al. Factors associated with the presence of postoperative headache in elective surgery patients: a prospective single center cohort study. *J Anesth*. 2017;31(2):225–236.
2. Nikolajsen L, et al. Effect of previous frequency of headache, duration of fasting and caffeine abstinence on perioperative headache. *Br J Anaesth*. 1994;72(3):295–297.
3. Sabab A, et al. Postoperative headache following treatment of vestibular schwannoma: a literature review. *J Clin Neurosci*. 2018;52:26–31.
4. Ravn Munkvold BK, et al. Preoperative and postoperative headache in patients with intracranial tumors. *World Neurosurg*. 2018;115:e322–e330.
5. Choi KS, et al. Incidence and risk factors of postoperative headache after endovascular coil embolization of unruptured intracranial aneurysms. *Acta Neurochir (Wien)*. 2014;156(7):1281–1287.

# Part 24

# SPECIAL PROBLEMS IN ANESTHESIOLOGY

# 362.

# ELECTROCONVULSIVE THERAPY

*Garrett W. Burnett*

## INTRODUCTION

Electroconvulsive therapy (ECT) has been used for treatment of psychiatric disorders for nearly 100 years and is considered well tolerated and effective. ECT is most commonly used for treatment-resistant depression, but may also be indicated for life-threatening catatonia, schizophrenia, mania, schizoaffective psychosis, and psychiatric conditions associated with organic disease.[1]

The procedure involves the application of scalp electrodes, which are stimulated using brief pulses of electricity to induce a generalized tonic-clonic seizure. Seizure quality is measured by motor duration of seizure (>15 seconds), postictal suppression, and burst suppression on electroencephalogram.[2] A seizure will start with 2–3 seconds of latent phase followed by a tonic phase of 10–12 seconds, then a clonic phase of 30–50 seconds.

While no absolute contraindications to ECT exist, relative contraindications should be noted. Neurological relative contraindications include increased intracranial pressure and space-occupying lesion, recent cerebrovascular accident, and cerebral aneurysm.[1,2] Cardiovascular relative contraindications include myocardial ischemia and conduction defects that require implanted pacemakers or an automatic implantable cardioverter-defibrillator (AICD).[3] Additional relative contraindications include osteoporosis, unstable bone fractures, pheochromocytoma, and pregnancy, though ECT has commonly been used during pregnancy.[1–3]

Anesthesiologists must be aware of the details of ECT, including physiologic changes associated with generalized tonic-clonic seizures and how medications given to the patient affect the quality and duration of induced seizures. General anesthesia is required for ECT in order to provide patient comfort and amnesia and to allow for neuromuscular blockade to prevent injuries to the patient (e.g., bone fractures, biting tongue) or staff.[4]

## ANESTHESIA CONSIDERATIONS

### PREOPERATIVE

A thorough preoperative assessment should take place prior to providing anesthesia for ECT. Patients may have significant systemic disease beyond their psychiatric illness, which may affect the anesthetic plan. Many patients receive several treatments of ECT, and any prior anesthetic records should be reviewed for possible improvements. Preoperative testing is often limited to electrocardiogram and a potassium level in patients without comorbidities. Patients with significant cardiac risk may require further evaluation, such as an echocardiogram or stress test.[3]

Patients undergoing ECT often require thorough review of psychiatric medications, which may interfere with an anesthetic plan. These medications may include antidepressants, antipsychotics, mood stabilizers, and anticonvulsants. Additionally, significant side effects of psychiatric medications, such as serotonin syndrome, delayed emergence, hypertensive crisis, or prolonged seizures, should be known.

Cardiovascular considerations for preoperative assessment should focus on hypertension, coronary artery disease, congestive heart failure, and implantable devices such as pacemakers or AICDs. Significant hypertension is associated with ECT and may cause increased afterload and myocardial oxygen demand, necessitating treatment. Patients with implantable devices such as pacemakers or AICDs must be evaluated prior to ECT as ECT may interfere with pacemaker firing or cause an AICD to falsely diagnose a malignant arrhythmia.[3] Management of an implantable device should use similar strategies as when electrocautery is used for the same patient.

Neurologic considerations should include baseline assessment of neurologic deficit for postoperative follow-up and recognition of any intracranial lesion or increased intracranial pressure. Additionally, patients with recent cerebrovascular accidents or unrepaired cerebral aneurysms should be recognized as these are relative contraindications.

Last, patients with risk of gastric reflux or delayed gastric emptying should be identified. Endotracheal intubation is not typically performed in patients undergoing ECT; therefore, patients with significant high risk of aspiration may require pretreatment with medications such as sodium citrate, histamine receptor antagonists, metoclopramide, and rarely endotracheal intubation.

## INTRAOPERATIVE

Electroconvulsive therapy is often performed at non–operating room locations, such as a procedure room or postanesthesia care unit. Intraoperatively, full American Society of Anesthesiologist monitors and emergency equipment for management of the patient's airway and any emergency equipment such as a "code cart" are necessary.

Prior to induction of anesthesia, patients may require pretreatment with glycopyrrolate (0.2 mg IV) in order to dry airway secretions and prevent bradycardia associated with an initial parasympathetic surge. Patients who may not tolerate transient hypertension may require labetalol or hydralazine prior to induction of anesthesia. Finally, preoxygenation with nasal cannula or face mask should be done prior to induction of anesthesia.

Induction of anesthesia may be performed with a variety of medications (Table 362.1). Methohexital, propofol, etomidate, and ketamine are all commonly used induction agents.[2–4] Methohexital is considered the gold standard induction agent for ECT because of its rapid onset, short duration, and lack of impact on seizure threshold.[2,3] Additional adjuncts used during ECT to reduce induction drug requirements may include remifentanil, ketamine, and dexmedetomidine.[4] Benzodiazepines and lidocaine are avoided due to their reduction in seizure threshold.

Neuromuscular blockade is most commonly achieved with succinylcholine due to its rapid onset and short duration. For patients with contraindications to succinylcholine use, nondepolarizing neuromuscular blockers, such as rocuronium, may be used if sugammadex (2 mg/kg) is available for rapid reversibility. Prolonged ventilation and additional anesthetic to prevent awareness are required if sugammadex is not available.[2,3] Prior to neuromuscular blockade, a tourniquet should be placed on the lower extremity to prevent transmission of the medication to the neuromuscular junction. This allows for monitoring of motor duration of the seizure to assess seizure quality.[3]

Following adequate depth of anesthesia and neuromuscular blockade, ECT can proceed. Patients should be hyperventilated using a bag-mask ventilation device in order to induce hypocapnia and improve seizure quality.[3] Rarely, patients require endotracheal intubation for ventilatory support. Ventilation should continue until the patient's spontaneous respirations return.

Hemodynamic instability associated with an initial parasympathetic surge followed by a sympathetic surge should be monitored closely. Atropine may be required for bradycardia, and cardiopulmonary resuscitation should be initiated for asystole. Treatment of a sympathetic surge

*Table 362.1* COMMONLY USED ANESTHETIC MEDICATIONS IN ELECTROCONVULSIVE THERAPY

| | | INDUCTION DRUGS | | | |
|---|---|---|---|---|---|
| DRUG | DOSE (IV) | ONSET | DURATION | BENEFITS | SIDE EFFECTS |
| Methohexital | 0.8–1.2 mg/kg | 15–30 seconds | 6–8 minutes | No effect on seizure threshold, rapid | Hypotension, pain on injection |
| Propofol | 1–1.5 mg/kg | 15–30 seconds | 5–10 minutes | Rapid, may reduce nausea or postictal agitation | Hypotension, pain on injection, antiepileptic |
| Etomidate | 0.2–0.5 mg/kg | 30–60 seconds | 6–8 minutes | Hemodynamically stable | Adrenal suppression, pain on injection, nausea |
| Ketamine | 1–2 mg/kg | 30–90 seconds | 5–10 minutes | Lowers seizure threshold, possible antidepressant effect | Dissociative effects, sympathomimetic, increases intracranial pressure |
| | | NEUROMUSCULAR BLOCKADE | | | |
| Succinylcholine | 0.5–1.2 mg/kg | 45–90 seconds | 5–8 minutes | Rapid onset, short duration | Myalgias, raises plasma potassium |
| Rocuronium | 0.6 mg/kg | 90–180 seconds | 30–90 minutes | No myalgias, no change in plasma potassium | Long duration of effect, requires sugammadex for reversal |

**Table 362.2** COMMON SIDE EFFECTS OF ELECTROCONVULSIVE THERAPY

| SIDE EFFECT | SYMPTOMS | TREATMENT | PREVENTION |
|---|---|---|---|
| Headache | Bilateral, constant headache | Acetaminophen, NSAIDs | Ketorolac prior to induction |
| Nausea | Nausea, vomiting | Ondansetron | Ondansetron prior to induction, propofol for induction |
| Parasympathetic surge | Bradycardia, cardiac pause, asystole | Atropine | Glycopyrrolate prior to induction |
| Sympathetic surge | Hypertension, tachycardia | Labetalol, hydralazine, nitroglycerin | Labetalol or hydralazine prior to induction |
| Oral trauma | Damaged teeth, tongue or lip injury | Supportive | Bite block, neuromuscular blockade |
| Postictal agitation | Delirium, confusion | Halolperiodol, benzodiazepines, small bolus of propofol | Propofol for induction, dexmedetomidine adjunct, unilateral ECT |
| Musculoskeletal complication | Bone fracture, joint dislocation | Orthopedic surgery consultation | Provide adequate neuromuscular blockade prior to ECT stimulation |
| Aspiration | Hypoxia, gastric secretions | Supportive, deep suction | Maintain appropriate fasting guidelines, thorough history |
| Pulmonary edema | Hypoxia, frothy secretions, sympathetic surge | Supportive care, furosemide, blood pressure control | Labetalol or hydralazine prior to induction |

should use medications such as labetalol, hydralazine, or nitroglycerin.

## POSTOPERATIVE

Patients should be monitored by an anesthesiologist until they are stable to move to the postanesthesia care unit. Common side effects of ECT are listed in Table 362.2. Headache is the most common side effect and can be treated with acetaminophen/nonsteroidal anti-inflammatory drugs (NSAIDs) postoperatively or treated with ketorolac prior to induction of anesthesia for prophylaxis.[3] Patients with post-ECT nausea or postictal agitation may benefit from induction using propofol.[2,3] Thorough documentation of anesthetics, seizure quality, and postoperative side effects should be completed in order to optimize further anesthetics for future ECT.

## REFERENCES

1. Baghai TC, Möller H. Electroconvulsive therapy and its different indications. *Dialogues Clin Neurosci.* 2008;10(1):105–117.
2. Chawla N. Anesthesia for electroconvulsive therapy. *Anesthesiol Clin.* 2020;38(1): 183–195.
3. Bryson EO, et al. Individualized anesthetic management for patients undergoing electroconvulsive therapy: a review of current practice. *Anesth Analg.* 2017;124(6):1943–1956.
4. Soehle M, Bochem J. Anesthesia for electroconvulsive therapy. *Curr Opin Anaesthesiol.* 2018;31(5):501–505.

# 363.

# ORGAN DONORS AND PROCUREMENT

*Michael J. Gyorfi and Alaa Abd-Elsayed*

## INTRODUCTION

Organs are predominantly harvested after neurologic death (brain death). To address the ever-increasing need for suitable organs, harvesting organs after circulatory death (cardiac death) and living donors are becoming more prevalent. There are unique challenges with each avenue of procurement. A large percentage of donated organs are refused for poor quality and never transplanted. Organs harvested after cardiac death have a higher risk of developing perioperative dysfunction due to the hemodynamic instability and inevitable organ injury. It is the anesthesiologist's role to maintain physiologic stability of donors and subsequently their organs. Understanding the physiologic changes during organ donation is paramount for an anesthesiologist to ensure organ health and increase the total number of suitable donations.

The physiology of organ procurement should be thought about separately based on the status of the donor: breath death, cardiovascular death, and living donor. After the declaration of brain and cardiovascular death, the goal is shifted from patient survival to preservation of transplantable organs.

## MANAGEMENT OF ORGAN DONORS WITH BRAIN DEATH

Brain death is the most common avenue for organ donation. The changes in physiology affect each system differently. Brain death and possible herniation can lead to a variety of hemodynamic derangements, but most commonly the initial cardiovascular response is a transient hypertensive crisis via a surge of catecholamines. Treatment consists of adrenergic antagonists while attempting to maintain cerebral perfusion. This is followed by a multifactorial hypotension via decreased sympathetics and cardiac output in addition to vasoplegia and diabetes insipidus.[1,2] The first step is to resuscitate with a balanced salt solution or normal saline. Historically, dopamine is added if hypotension persists. Vasopressin is increasingly utilized as a first-line agent due

to its advantages in reducing catecholamines in addition to treatment of vasodilatory shock and diabetes insipidus.[1-3]

Pulmonary injuries are commonly seen after brain death due to the increased systemic vascular resistance. The sympathetic surge initiates a systemic inflammatory response in addition to the capillary leakage and pulmonary edema. Pulmonary protective management includes high positive end-expiratory pressure, small tidal volumes, and low fractions of inspired oxygen.[1,3] Methylprednisolone can blunt the inflammatory response, improving the organ's chance of survival. Ensuing acute respiratory distress syndrome in donors is treated the same as nondonor patients.[3]

Brain death results in decreased production and utilization of cortisol, insulin, and antidiuretic hormone. Central diabetes insipidus occurs in up to 80% of organ donors. This leads to electrolyte and fluid abnormalities along with pyuria.[2,3] Acute kidney injuries and subsequent renal failure are related to the prolonged renal vasoconstriction and hypotension seen during brain death. Antidiuretic hormone replacement has been shown to improve graft function in cardiac, liver, and kidney patients. Euvolemia is the goal for multiorgan donors. Irregular insulin production and steroid therapy lead to hyperglycemia and further renal dysfunction. During brain death, insulin should be administered to achieve a glucose between 120 and 180 mg/dL.[2-4]

Body temperature regulation is lost during brain death. This leads to a reduced metabolic rate. Normothermia is recommended before organ procurement. Metabolic derangements fluctuate throughout the brain death process. Changes in $K^+$, $Ca^{2+}$, and $Mg^{2+}$ result in cardiac arrhythmias. Hypernatremia results in poor transplant outcomes and should be treated by correcting the underlying diabetes insipidus.[2,3]

Harvesting organs in a brain death donor is a time-sensitive procedure. Organs should be removed in the order of their respective susceptibility to ischemia. For example, hearts are removed first and kidneys are last. Paralytics should be given prior to organ harvesting due to the presence of spinal reflexes.[3,4] Intraoperatively, hemodynamic stability is often achieved by the vasodilators phentolamine and alprostadil in addition to fluids during the hypertensive phase. The administration of red blood cells, fresh frozen plasma, and platelets should be guided by the traditional clinical criteria while taking each patient's clinical picture into account. Other coagulation studies, such as thromboelastography, can help delineate transfusion needs.[3,4]

## MANAGEMENT OF ORGAN DONORS WITH CIRCULATORY DEATH

Donation after cardiac death is also referred to as non–heart beating donors. Traditionally, donation after cardiovascular death has been less common than that of brain death.[4] There are unique challenges that occur during circulatory death. Once asystole occurs, a 5-minute window is observed to ensure there is no autoresuscitation. Once life support has been withdrawn, warm ischemia ensues, causing microthrombosis to occur rapidly. This process is difficult to stop and severely damages organs. The patient should be transported to the operating room as soon as possible for organ procurement. Heparin is administered before stopping life support to help reduce the risk of thrombosis. A femoral cooling catheter can also be placed in attempts to preserve organs via rapid infusion of a cold solution. The bowel and heart are not candidates for donation after cardiovascular death. This is a growing area of research with potential to increase the number of viable transplantable organs. The use of extracorporeal membrane oxygenation to perfuse organs for donation after cardiovascular death is another area of current research.[3,4]

## MANAGEMENT OF LIVING ORGAN DONORS

Harvesting organs from a living donor has several advantages. Elective surgeries can be optimized to reduce unnecessary risks. The donated organs are not exposed to the physiologic derangements seen in cardiovascular and brain death. This paired with a reduced cold ischemia time gives living organ donors better outcomes. There are major disadvantages to living organ donations, such as surgical risks, a reduced quality of life postoperatively, and a large financial impact. The criteria for living donors continues to expand to encompass a larger population for various organs. For example, donors of advanced age and moderate obesity can be considered for some kidney donations.[2–4]

Kidney donations are the most common organ harvested from living donors. The nephrectomy is performed laparoscopically. Nonsteroidal anti-inflammatory medications are avoided due to their adverse renal effects. Epidurals should be considered for known chronic pain issues or the need for an open nephrectomy.[1–4]

Livers are another common organ donated from a living donor. Livers are unique due to their regenerative properties. Anticipating the correct graft size is paramount to avoid small-for-size syndrome while at the same time preserving liver function in the donor.[2,3] The portion of liver donated generally depends on the age and size of the recipient. For small adults and children, a total left hepatic lobectomy or even a lateral segment may be enough. If it is an adult-to-adult transplant, a more complex, right hepatic lobectomy is required. Anesthesiologists must be prepared for potential massive blood loss during living organ donations. Different techniques include utilizing a cell salvage, isovolemic hemodilution, and maintaining a low central venous pressure (CVP) (<5 cm $H_2O$). Adult-to-adult liver donations are not without risk. A large study of 760 transplants found 40% of cases had at least one complication, particularly with right hepatic lobectomies.[2–4]

## MANAGEMENT OF DONATED GRAFTS AFTER PROCUREMENT

Once an organ has been harvested, they are traditionally preserved in certain solutions (e.g., the University of Wisconsin solution). This particular solution has a high concentration of adenosine and potassium. The graft is flushed with colloid before reperfusion to decrease the occurrence of severe hyperkalemia in the recipient. The time delay between harvest and reimplementation is termed the *cold ischemia time*. The accepted cold ischemia time varies depending on the organ. For example, lungs are more sensitive and need to be transplanted within 4 hours, compared to that of kidneys, which is closer to 24 hours.[1–4] In summary, having open communication between both the surgical team and anesthesiologist is paramount for optimal organ survival.

## REFERENCES

1. Grissom TE, et al. Critical care management of the potential organ donor. *Int Anesthesiol Clin.* 2017;55(2):18–41.
2. Souter MJ, et al. Organ donor management: part 1. Toward a consensus to guide anesthesia services during donation after brain death. *Semin Cardiothorac Vasc Anesth.* 2018;22(2):211–222.
3. Kotloff RM, et al. Management of the potential organ donor in the ICU: Society of Critical Care Medicine/American College of Chest Physicians/Association of Organ Procurement Organizations consensus statement. *Crit Care Med.* 2015;43(6):1291–1325.
4. Anderson TA, et al. Anesthetic considerations in organ procurement surgery: a narrative review. *Can J Anaesth.* 2015;62(5):529–539.

# 364.

# BRAIN DEATH

*Shahla Siddiqui*

## INTRODUCTION

Brain death has been long accepted as the determination of death in the United States and internationally. It is the clinical and legal definition of the cessation of brain activity. The criteria for such a determination largely remain clinical, including a battery of bedside tests. In certain exceptions (when this clinical battery of tests cannot be performed), ancillary tests can be ordered.[1] Determination of brain death (or determination of death of an individual) can be a crucial and a deeply emotional aspect of critical care. A systematic neurologic examination must show apnea, cranial nerve areflexia, and unresponsiveness to the environment. Primary brain pathology (e.g., severe traumatic brain injury) must account for the clinical findings, and the findings must be irreversible.[2] All other possible causes of reversible cessation of brain activity, such as acidosis, sepsis, toxic or metabolic causes, hypothermia, and electrolyte imbalances, must be ruled out prior to evaluation for brain death.

## PERIOPERATIVE CONSIDERATIONS

In the United States, brain death criteria include irreversible coma, lack of brainstem criteria, and apnea. Often, massive brain injury requires the patient to be mechanically ventilated. A patient may have a heartbeat and blood pressure, but may soon become hemodynamically unstable as the brainstem reflexes are lost and the cardiorespiratory centers suffer ischemia.

Brain death criteria can be determined by performing a set of clinical tests at the bedside, which include the following[3]:

- Cranial nerve (CN) II: Loss of pupillary reflex (light reflex); pupils should be mid-dilated 4 to 9 mm and not reactive to light.
- CN III, IV, VI: Eye motion is lost in reaction to head movement (doll's eyes).
- CN V, VII: Loss of corneal reflex.
- CN VIII: Loss of oculovestibular reflex (caloric test): With irrigation of each ear by 60 mL ice water, the eye will not move toward the irrigated ear.
- CN IX: Loss of gag reflex.
- CN X: Loss of cough reflex.

The final test is the apnea test.[4] The apnea test is used to assess the brain's ability to drive pulmonary function in response to the rise of $CO_2$. Before the performance of the apnea test, the mechanical ventilator should be adjusted to an $FiO_2$ (fraction of inspired oxygen) of 100%. A baseline $PaCO_2$ of 40 mm Hg should be determined prior to the apnea test. During the test, oxygen should be supplemented using a cannula connected to the endotracheal tube at 6 L/min or T piece at 12 L/min or using continuous positive airway pressure of 5 to 10 cm $H_2O$. In the case of loss of respiratory drive, $CO_2$ is expected to rise 5 mm Hg every minute in the first 2 minutes, then by 2 mm Hg every minute after. Repeat arterial blood gas after 8 to 10 minutes showing a $CO_2$ of 60 mm Hg or the rise of $CO_2$ more than 20 mm Hg above baseline is consistent with brain death. If the patient develops hypotension with systolic blood pressure below 90 mm Hg or cardiac arrhythmias, the test should terminate, and arterial blood gases are drawn. For patients on extracorporeal membrane oxygenation machines, oxygenation can be maintained while performing the apnea test by decreasing the gas sweep flow rate to 0.5 to 1.0 L/min and using an oxygenation source through the endotracheal tube.

The brainstem death criteria need to be repeated at a set interval (depending on institutional or state guidelines) and by different providers.

## ANCILLARY TESTS

The ancillary tests are considerations if there is any uncertainty regarding the diagnosis of brain death or if the apnea test cannot be performed.[5]

- Cerebral angiography: Four-vessel angiography is considered the gold standard for tests that evaluate cerebral blood flow.
- Transcranial ultrasound: Can be used to assess pulsations of middle cerebral arteries, vertebral and basilar arteries bilaterally, and anterior cerebral arteries or ophthalmic arteries if possible.
- Computed tomogram brain angiography and magnetic resonance angiography showing cessation of cerebral blood flow.
- Radionuclide brain imaging: Can be done using a tracer, then imaging by single-photon emission computed tomography brain scintigraphy. The absence of a tracer in the brain circulation (the hollow skull phenomenon) is consistent with brain death.
- Electroencephalogram: Can confirm brain death when it shows no electrical activity more than 2 μV. Also, it should show no reactivity to intense somatosensory stimuli.
- Somatosensory evoked potentials: Patients with brain death show no somatosensory evoked potentials in response to bilateral median nerve stimulation and no brainstem evoked potentials in response to auditory stimuli.

## REFERENCES

1. Wijdicks EF. Determining brain death in adults. *Neurology.* 1995;45(5):1003–1011.
2. Spinello IM. Brain death determination. *J Intensive Care Med.* 2015;30(6):326–337.
3. Bernat JL. The natural history of chronic disorders of consciousness. *Neurology.* 2010;75(3):206–207.
4. Capron AM. Brain death—well settled yet still unresolved. *N Engl J Med.* 2001;344(16):1244–1246.
5. Machado C. Diagnosis of brain death. *Neurol Int.* 2010;2(1):e2.

# 365.

# RADIOLOGICAL PROCEDURES

*Shahla Siddiqui*

## INTRODUCTION

The hazards of performing general anesthesia or sedation procedures in remote areas include the fact that the providers may not have adequate support and backup personnel and equipment in case of an emergency. The American Society of Anesthesiologists (ASA) provides guidance regarding the minimal equipment required in such scenarios.[1]

## EQUIPMENT AND MONITORING

Generally, two sources of oxygen, suction, scavenging for anesthetic gases, anesthesia machine, and adequate lighting and power sources, in addition to standard ASA monitors and anesthesia equipment plus pumps to deliver infusions are required. This equipment should be ascertained in remote locations to ensure anesthesia can be delivered safely and reliably.

## SPACE

Space is potentially a hazard for radiologic procedures. It is required for the anesthesia cart; the anesthesia machine with appropriate gas inputs and medical outputs, such as suction and scavenging; the computer charting station; drug storage; and monitors. Due to limitations, equipment is frequently positioned atypically compared to the operating room (i.e., the anesthesia machine on the left rather than right side of the patient), which may be unfamiliar to the anesthesia providers. The location of the patient relative to the anesthesiologist might also prove challenging. In some scenarios where there is excessive radiation or in the magnetic resonance imaging (MRI) suite, the anesthesiologist may need to be outside the room.

## EQUIPMENT

A second potential hazard is the equipment. Monitors should be similar to the operating room. Well-maintained, standard monitor availability within an institution decreases the need for the anesthesiologist to orient to new devices.[2] Monitors should comply with ASA standard monitoring requirements, including end-tidal carbon dioxide ($EtCO_2$). MRI suites provide unique problems with respect to equipment.[3] The physiologic monitors must be MRI compatible. Also, the electrocardiogram reading may have artifact disturbances due to the magnetic field, making analysis of arrhythmias challenging. Other equipment, such as backup airway devices (i.e., laryngeal mask airways, video laryngoscopes, or oral and nasal airways), must be stocked nearby. Known difficult intubation cases may require induction of anesthesia in the operating room prior to transfer to a remote location. Malignant hyperthermia and code carts should be readily available and accessible. Medication reserves must be accessible, especially for monitored anesthesia care infusions or vasopressors.

## COMMUNICATION

The anesthesiologist must communicate effectively with unfamiliar personnel. Also, there must be a line of communication between remote anesthesiologists and the rest of the department for emergency support.

## RADIATION

There are three sources of radiation in the interventional radiology suite: (1) direct radiation from the x-ray tube; (2) leakage from the x-ray tube shielding; and (3) scattered radiation reflected from the patient. The amount of the radiation decreases with lead covering as well as distance. Current practices protect personnel effectively. However, adequate protection must be ensured.

## PROCEDURES

Interventional radiological procedures are becoming more and more common. Strict vigilance and attention to detail is required for these procedures. It is important to discuss the plan and type of anesthesia required with the procedurist prior to the case. Often, these patients are in the intensive care unit and require invasive monitoring and vasopressor support for shock. Adequate resuscitative equipment and backup support must be ensured prior to starting the procedure.

## COVID-19 AND THE INTERVENTIONAL RADIOLOGY SUITE

COVID-19 cases present a unique challenge to radiological procedures, which often have to be urgently performed. Strict standard operating procedures must be followed for personal protective equipment (PPE) and droplet infection precautions, which can be time consuming. Safety of personnel and staff remains paramount during a pandemic as transmission can increase if such precautions are ignored even slightly. Preoperative preparation for radiological procedures requiring anesthesia support needs vigilance, preparation, and communication. Extra care has to be taken for ensuring backup supplies and personnel. Intraoperatively, airway placement in difficult situations and remote access from the anesthesiologist poses unique difficulties. Adequate experience and senior supervision is necessary for deploying personnel to do such cases. Communication with the procedurist is important for potentially painful procedures. COVID 19 cases require droplet precautions and PPE. Postoperatively, all radiological cases undergoing anesthesia require postanesthesia care unit recovery as they are no different from surgical cases. Adequate postoperative pain and antiemetic medications must be prescribed for these cases.

## REFERENCES

1. Committee on Standards and Practice Parameters (CSPP). Statement on nonoperating room anesthetizing locations. American Society of Anesthesiologists. 2018. https://www.asahq.org/standards-and-guidelines/statement-on-nonoperating-room-anesthetizing-locations
2. Schönenberger S, et al. Effect of conscious sedation vs general anesthesia on early neurological improvement among patients with ischemic stroke undergoing endovascular thrombectomy: a randomized clinical trial. *JAMA*. 2016;316:1986.
3. Berkow LC. Anesthetic management and human factors in the intraoperative MRI environment. *Curr Opin Anaesthesiol*. 2016;29:563.

# 366.

# ETHICS, PRACTICE MANAGEMENT, PROFESSIONALISM, AND MEDICOLEGAL ISSUES

*Shahla Siddiqui*

## INTRODUCTION

Important aspects of professionalism encompass informed consent, patient confidentiality, and other issues. Of the core competencies of an Accreditation Council for Graduate Medical Education residency, professionalism is one of the most important and is codified in the recent milestones advocated in the residency and fellowship training programs. A recent prospective observational study found that approximately 1 in 20 perioperative medication administrations, and every second operation, resulted in a medication error and/or an adverse drug event.[1] More than one-third of these errors led to observed patient harm, and the remaining two-thirds had the potential for patient harm.[2]

## PROFESSIONALISM AND LICENSURE

Medical licensure is linked to the continued maintenance of the code of ethical and professional behaviors. However, many reports and studies showed that often unprofessional behavior is tolerated among trainees and faculty. There are many reasons for this, including not having procedures in place for reporting such behavior. A culture of intolerance will help improve such reporting.

## ADVANCE DIRECTIVES AND PATIENT PRIVACY

Patient autonomy and preferences are preserved in the form of discussions around advance directives/do not resuscitate (DNR) orders or suspended DNR in the case of surgery or procedures. Issues of medical ethics and moral dilemmas must be resolved by communication and involving clinical ethics committees. The Health

Insurance Portability and Accountability Act (HIPAA) protects patient privacy, and at all times the patient's identity and their confidential information must be protected. Trainees need to be familiar with rules and regulations surrounding HIPAA.[3]

## INFORMED CONSENT AND SHARED DECISION-MAKING

Another aspect of professional behavior is obtaining adequate and detailed informed consent prior to anesthesia and surgery. This formal process includes acknowledgment of a patient's mental capacity and a detailed discussion of the risks and benefits of the anesthesia provided.[4] The documentation of the informed consent for anesthesia and the risks must be done in accordance with the institutional rules and regulations. Informed consent encapsulates the principles of shared decision-making, which is the ethical premise of patient autonomy.

## PATIENT SAFETY AND MEDICATION ERRORS

Another aspect of professionalism is providing quality patient care and ensuring patient safety. Anesthesiology, like the aircraft industry, has come a long way in providing excellent patient care and reducing human and machine errors and exposing patients to harm when under our care. However, in the unlikely event of a medical error, there are guidelines and protocols to allow full disclosure to the patients or their families, to document all events, and to report errors and adverse events. Patient safety and quality goals are also reflected in resident education and training.[5] Not only does the Accreditation Council for Graduate Medical Education include quality improvement milestones, but also review programs have been established to ensure residents are integrated into institutions' patient safety and quality improvement programs. Consequently, academic medical centers are held accountable for resident participation in the hospital's patient safety and quality improvement initiatives.

In the event of a human error (medication or otherwise), it is imperative that full documentation at the time and a full disclosure occur to the patient or to the family. Attending supervision is essential at the time of all-important events, such as during intubation and extubation in the operating room. This needs to be documented in the patient's chart. Preoperatively, it becomes important that informed consent is obtained and documented. Intraoperatively, care must be taken to avoid errors, and vigilance must be maintained and documented. Postoperatively, all instances of errors must be recorded and disclosed in a timely manner. Departmental and legal/risk management support avenues exist in cases where escalation and mediation are required.

## PERIOPERATIVE CONSIDERATIONS

Professionalism results in better clinical outcomes. Good clinical skills, sound ethical practice, and communication are the cornerstones of professionalism. Residency programs evaluate residents by various means to assess the level of professionalism. Objective and subjective feedback and reviews are part and parcel of the residency evaluation.

## REFERENCES

1. Nanji K, et al. Evaluation of perioperative medication errors and adverse drug events. *Anesthesiology*. 2016;124(1):25–34.
2. Tetzlaff JE. Professionalism in anesthesiology: "What Is It?" or "I Know It When I See It." *Anesthesiology*. 2009;110(4):700–702.
3. Vanderpool D. HIPAA—should I be worried? *Innov Clin Neurosci*. 2012;9(11–12):51–55.
4. Antoniou A, et al. Educating anesthesia residents to obtain and document informed consent for epidural labor analgesia: does simulation play a role? *Int J Obstet Anesth*. 2018;34:79–84.
5. Lee SC, et al. Teaching anesthesiology residents how to obtain informed consent. *J Educ Perioper Med*. 2019;21(4):E632.

# 367.

# ETHICS

## ADVANCE DIRECTIVES/DO NOT RESUSCITATE ORDERS

*Shahla Siddiqui*

## INTRODUCTION

Preserving patient autonomy is the first tenet of ethical care and professionalism in medicine. This autonomy is manifested in the form of a written agreement of their preferences surrounding their healthcare options.[1] When patients reach periods where their outcomes may become uncertain due to their illnesses, it becomes important to discuss their wishes regarding life-preserving or life-prolonging care. Some of this care may be nonbeneficial if the quality of their lives is not aligned to their world wishes or desires. Such discussions with the patients and their loved ones are documented by their healthcare teams in detail in the form of living wills or do not resuscitate (DNR) orders.[2] Healthcare proxies are surrogate members of their families or loved ones that can be asked to make such decisions if the patient loses mental capacity by illness or sedation.[3]

## PERIOPERATIVE PERIODS

For a patient undergoing anesthesia, discussion of the advance directive is an important part of the informed consent process. The informed consent process provides the opportunity for the patient and the anesthesia professional to discuss the anesthesia plan of care, including any restrictions outlined in the advance directive.[4] This discussion must take place prior to the surgery. In case of the need for resuscitation, a combined decision must be made regarding the commencement of cardiopulmonary resuscitation (CPR), mechanical ventilation, and the like.[5]

## DO NOT RESUSCITATE ORDERS

Orders like the DNR usually are based on institutional guidelines and standard protocols. Advance directives and DNR orders direct the level of care that should be dispensed as required during anesthetic care in the perioperative setting according to the wishes of the patient. A DNR order may be fully suspended, partially suspended, or fully honored during anesthesia as directed by a patient. For this to occur, a proper informed consent process must be adhered to and all caveats, risks, and benefits explained to the patient and their loved ones if possible.

## DECISION-MAKING

All preoperative conversation and preparation in DNR patients must include a discussion and dialogue between teams and patients regarding their wishes for resuscitation during the perioperative period. This discussion must be carefully documented in the patient's chart. Intraoperatively, all team members of the operating room team should be aware of the decisions made. In most instances, a DNR order is suspended for all anesthetic care as the delivery of anesthesia may decrease blood pressure, induce mechanical ventilation, and inherently require resuscitation. Postoperatively, the patient's wishes must be documented regarding restoration of all DNR orders and

the conveying of these wishes to all teams to whom handover is given whether, in the postanesthesia care unit or the intensive care unit.

When taking care of patients who have DNR orders, care must be taken to ensure proper communication and documentation. For example, if a patient comes into the hospital with an active DNR order in their chart or relayed by the family and the patient arrests or is unconscious, it is very important that surrogates are involved in decision-making to understand and respect the patient's prior wishes. At times, these wishes may not seem to be in the best interest of the patient; however, these must be acknowledged.

Different types of DNR orders exist which is why proper and timely conversations and documentation are very crucial. A universal DNR order denotes no cardiorespiratory resuscitation, however, certain hybrids exit where patients may want medical resuscitation but no CPR or shock. They may also elect not to get intubated. Such details must be discussed and documented in the chart and communicated to the entire team.

## REFERENCES

1. Centers for Medicare and Medicaid Services. Subpart 1—Advance Directives. 42 CFR § 489.
2. Centers for Medicare and Medicaid Services. State Operations Manual. Appendix A—Survey Protocol, Regulations and Interpretive Guidelines for Hospitals. Accessed July 24, 2015. http://www.cms.gov/Regulations-and-Guidance/Guidance/Manuals/downloads/som107ap_a_hospitals.pdf
3. Sulmasy DP, et al. The quality of care plans for patients with do-not-resuscitate orders. *Arch Intern Med*. 2004;164(14):1573–1578. doi:10.1001/archinte.164.14.1573
4. Williams SP, Howe CL. Advance directives in the perioperative setting: managing ethical and legal issues when patient rights and perceived obligations of the healthcare provider conflict. *J Healthc Risk Manag*. 2013;32(4):35–42.
5. Centers for Medicare and Medicaid Services. Conditions of participation: patient's rights. 42 CFR 482.13(b)(2).

# 368.

# MALPRACTICE

*Priyanka Ghosh*

## INTRODUCTION

Knowledge and understanding of malpractice play a large role in any physician's practice.

## PRINCIPLES OF MALPRACTICE

Malpractice lawsuits must prove medical negligence in order to be valid, meaning that not every adverse medical outcome can be considered valid for a malpractice lawsuit. In order to prove negligence, the situation must include four discrete elements, often referred to as "the four D's" of medical negligence. The four elements are duty, dereliction, direct causation, and damage[1]:

1. Duty: The physician has the duty to care for the patient with high standards while informing patients of any potential risks of a procedure and keeping patient information confidential.
2. Dereliction: The physician has to be found in careless breach of the above previously agreed-on duty.
3. Direct Causation: There was direct damaged caused to the patient by dereliction of said duty.
4. Damage: Determination of the specific type of damage caused to the patient from direct causation of negligence of duty.

More simply stated, negligence must prove that the physician failed to treat the patient with defined and accepted standards of care, therefore neglecting their duty, and that this neglect directly caused specific damages. Physicians are held to the current established standard of care for all parts of their patient interaction, including indications or a diagnostic or therapeutic procedure, making comprehensive explanations to patients, taking decisions and proceeding to actions, using up-to-date instrumentation, and maintaining the highest level of competence through continuous education and training.[1]

## TRENDS IN ANESTHESIA MALPRACTICE

Over the past 30 years, the number of surgical anesthesia claims and severity of claims have been decreasing, but the number of nonsurgical anesthesia claims has increased, including acute pain management, obstetric anesthesia, and non–operating room anesthesia (NORA) cases.

Death (26%); nerve injury (22%), with injury to the ulnar nerve being most common (28%); permanent brain damage (9%); and airway injury (7%) were the most common complications associated with all claims over the past three decades. The most common event categories in anesthesia claims were regional block-related (20%), respiratory (17%), cardiovascular (13%), and equipment-related (10%) events.[2]

Obesity was the most frequently cited patient feature identified as a contributing factor leading to a claim, and injury-to-claim rates were the highest in hospitals with fewer than 100 beds, whereas ambulatory surgery centers had the lowest death-to-claim rate (12%).

From 2002 to 2013, situational awareness errors contributed to 75% of anesthesia malpractice claims in which patients sustained permanent brain damage or death, with the most common distractors including reading printed material, talking on the telephone, and playing loud music. The average indemnity for an anesthesia claim was $309,066, compared with $291,000 for all physician specialties.[2]

## ANESTHESIA MALPRACTICE BY AREA

Obstetric Anesthesia: The most common complications in the claims related to obstetric anesthesia were maternal nerve injury, with mostly spinal cord injury from neuraxial anesthetic use (54.7%), maternal death (22%), newborn brain damage (20%), and headache (12%). The median amount paid in the settled cases was almost five times more than the median for nonobstetric settled cases.[3]

Non–Operating Room Anesthesia: Malpractice suits in NORA are mainly related to the use of monitored anesthesia care (MAC), eight times more than operating room anesthesia, with a greater number considered preventable had adequate monitoring been used. Compared to operating room cases, NORA patients were more often American Society of Anesthesiologists physical status 3–5, death and respiratory events were was almost twice as frequent, and propofol was the medication mostly involved in the claims. Gastrointestinal cases were the most commonly performed (51%) and were mainly related to dental injuries and severe adverse effects or death. The majority of these were alleged to be due to lack of technical skills or clinical judgment.[3]

Regional Anesthesia: Of claims related to regional anesthesia, 68% had temporary injuries, 16% were permanently disabling, 11% resulted in death, and 5% had brain damage, with brachial plexus injuries the most frequent and those with the highest incidence of permanent damage or disability. Interscalene block (42%) had the most, followed by axillary block (26%) and intravenous regional anesthesia (11%) as the third most frequent.[3]

Ophthalmologic Anesthesia: Cases with ophthalmologic blocks combined with MAC for eye surgeries had a higher incidence of claims (61%) associated with permanent injury compared with only MAC during such procedures.[3]

Pediatric Anesthesia: Pediatric anesthesia has changed significantly in terms of patient safety, with a decrease in the proportion of claims for death and/or brain damage (78% to 62%) and respiratory events (51% to 23%), especially for inadequate ventilation/oxygenation (26% to 3%). While there has been a decrease in death and brain damage, they remain the main complication seen in pediatric anesthesia. Cardiovascular pediatric events have increased, with the majority related to underlying cardiovascular factors (41%), followed by airway-related cardiac arrest (27%) and medication-related cardiac arrests (18%).

## REFERENCES

1. Mora JC, et al. Trends in anesthesia-related liability and lessons learned. *Adv Anesth.* 2018;36(1):231–249.
2. Woodward ZG, et al. Safety of non-operating room anesthesia: a closed claims update. *Anesthesiol Clin.* 2017;35(4):569–581.
3. Edbril SD, Lagasse RS. Relationship between malpractice litigation and human errors. *Anesthesiology.* 1999;91(3):848–855.

# 369.

# INITIAL CERTIFICATION, RECERTIFICATION, MAINTENANCE OF CERTIFICATION, AND RELATED ISSUES

*Katya H. Chiong and Soozan S. Abouhassan*

## INITIAL CERTIFICATION

The American Board of Anesthesiology (ABA) has transitioned to a new assessment of competency-based training and promotion that mirrors the evaluation of anesthesia residents across the Accreditation Council of Graduate Medical Education (ACGME) system. Those candidates who started their residency education on or after July 2012 and completed residency on or after June 30, 2016, now have to take the staged exams, rather than the Traditional Part 1 (Written) and Part 2 (Oral) Exams. The staged exams consist of three parts: BASIC, ADVANCED, and APPLIED Exams. The APPLIED Exam includes elements of Objective Structured Clinical Examinations

(OSCEs) in addition to the traditional Standardized Oral Examination (SOE) questions of the Traditional Part 2 (Oral) Examination.[1]

## BASIC EXAM

The BASIC Exam is a computerized exam consisting of 200 single-best answer multiple-choice questions requiring the application of knowledge rather than a recollection of facts. It is given over 4 hours and administered in the summer and fall, over 2 days, nationwide. Anesthesiology residents must have satisfactorily completed 18 months of training in an ACGME-accredited anesthesiology residency training program to be eligible to take the BASIC Exam.[1]

The BASIC Exam covers four content areas (relative percentage of questions): basic sciences (24%), clinical sciences (36%), organ-based basic and clinical sciences (37%), and special problems or issues on anesthesiology (3%). Each BASIC Exam is built to the same content specifications, also known as an exam blueprint. The exam blueprint ensures that every form of the BASIC Exam measures the same breadth and depth of knowledge content. The four content areas are further broken down to reflect the subcontent and the approximate amount of questions that are dedicated to the content. For example, basic sciences comprises 24% of all content. The blueprint assigns this category approximately 44–52 questions (out of the possible 200 total). These are then distributed between the subcategory and content of basic sciences, which includes anatomy (10–12 questions), physics/monitoring and anesthesia delivery devices (12–14 questions), mathematics (3–5 questions), and pharmacology (19–25 questions). Every subsequent exam is made with the blueprint in mind. For a complete reference to the BASIC Exam blueprint, content outline, exam dates, and information, please refer to the ABA website at https://theaba.org/staged%20exams.html.[1]

## ADVANCED EXAM

The ADVANCED Examination is the second part of the staged examination. It is a computerized exam consisting of 200 single-best answer multiple-choice questions requiring the application of knowledge rather than a recollection of facts. The ADVANCED Exam is given over 4 hours and administered in the summer and fall, over 2 days, nationwide. It focuses on advanced clinical practice and subspecialty topics. As such, it is offered to candidates who have completed their residency training. Of note, it covers topics from both the BASIC and ADVANCED full content outline in the five content categories (relative percentage of questions): basic sciences (9%), clinical sciences (10%), organ-based basic and clinical sciences (30%), clinical specialties (46%), and special problems or issues in anesthesiology (5%). The five content areas are further broken down to reflect the subcontent and the approximate amount of questions that are dedicated to the content. For example, basic sciences comprises 9% of all content. The blueprint assigns this category approximately 16–24 questions (out of the possible 200 total). These are then distributed between the subcontent of basic sciences, which includes anatomy (4–6 questions), physics/monitoring and anesthesia delivery devices (4–6 questions), mathematics (4–6 questions), and pharmacology (4–6 questions). Every subsequent exam is made with the blueprint in mind. For a complete reference to the ADVANCED Exam blueprint, content outline, exam dates, and information, please refer to the ABA website at https://theaba.org/staged%20exams.html.[1]

## APPLIED EXAM

The APPLIED Exam, the third and final exam in the staged examination series, includes the traditional SOE and a new OSCE component. The OSCE assess two domains difficult to assess in the written and oral examinations and includes professionalism/communication and technical skills related to the care of patients. The exam is administered at the Assessment Center in Raleigh, North Carolina. All candidates who graduated from residency on or after October 2016 are required to pass both components of the exam for initial board certification. However, if one component of the exam is failed, only the component failed needs to be retaken. To qualify for the APPLIED Exam, candidates must (1) pass both the BASIC and ADVANCED exams; (2) satisfactorily complete 36 months of clinical anesthesia training; (3) be capable of performing independently the entire scope of anesthesiology practice without accommodation or with reasonable accommodation; (4) have a satisfactory reference form on file from the program director upon graduation; and (5) report an unexpired, permanent, unconditional/unrestricted medical license by November 15 of their APPLIED Exam year. For more information on the Applied Exam, see https://theaba.org/staged%20exams.html.[1]

Candidates who completed residency training on or after January 1, 2012, must satisfy all requirements for initial certification within 7 years of the last day of the year in which they completed their residency training. If a candidate does not satisfy all requirements for certification within the allotted time period, the candidate must reestablish eligibility with the ABA examination system.[1]

## RECERTIFICATION

To maintain certification and meet recertification requirements, all newly certified diplomates participate in the ABA's

Maintenance of Certification in Anesthesiology™ (MOCA®) program, currently MOCA 2.0®. This program is designed to promote lifelong learning, maintain current medical knowledge and promote patient safety. Requirements for recertification are completed during a span of 10 years, with requirements divided into two 5-year periods. The requirements include (1) annual registration and $210 fee, which includes access to MOCA Minute® questions, submission of continuing medical education (CME) and quality improvement projects. If subspecialty certified, an additional $100 per certificate is required; (2) good professional standing: maintenance of an unrestricted, unexpired medical license in the United States or Canada; (3) lifelong learning: 250 category 1 CME credits (maximum of 60/year), including 20 credits of category 1 patient safety CME, with 125 category 1 CME credits required by the end of year 5 of the 10-year cycle to be considered "Participating in MOC"; (4) cognitive knowledge: answering 30 MOCA Minute questions per calendar quarter (120 per year by 11:59 pm EST on December 31), with up to 30 questions per day answered, and 120 questions should be completed each year to be considered Participating in MOC; and (5) clinical practice assessment/systems-based practice: one must earn 25 points in years 1–5 to be considered Participating in MOC and earn 25 points in years 6–10 (for a total of 50 points in a 10-year cycle) to complete the quality improvement component.[2]

## MAINTENANCE OF CERTIFICATION AND RELATED ISSUES

Recent changes to MOCA have been overall positive as requirements have become less cumbersome and more meaningful to everyday practice. Instead of sitting for an exam every 10 years, MOCA Minute questions make learning interactive. It offers a more relevant and personalized approach to helping diplomates assess their knowledge and address knowledge gaps. After each question, the diplomate is asked two questions that impact subsequent questions: How confident are you in the answer you selected? How relevant is this to your practice? More importantly, the diplomate can review the explanations and references for each question for a deeper understanding. CME submission has also been streamlined as attendance to CME-approved conferences/lectures is directly submitted for credit once attendance is verified. The quality improvement part 4 requirement of MOCA has also undergone improvements. There are more opportunities for diplomates to submit activities demonstrating participation in evaluations of their clinical practice and engagement of practice improvement. Points are submitted and awarded for time and effort spent. Templates and documentation are no longer required to be uploaded, but submitted activity is always subject to audit so a record of activity submitted should be kept. The attestation portion should be the last action performed as this will affect the day in which your next 10-year cycle begins. Our advice is to do the things you enjoy doing and enjoy the process along the way! For a complete list of approved part 4 MOCA activities or patient safety–specific CME, please refer to the ABA website: https://theaba.org/about%20moca%202.0.html.[2] Good Luck!

## REFERENCES

1. American Board of Anesthesiology (ABA). CERTIFICATION EXAMS. Website home page. https://www.theaba.org
2. The American Board of Anesthesiology (ABA). MOCA. https://theaba.org/about%20moca%202.0.html

# 370.

# COSTS OF MEDICAL/ANESTHESIA CARE AND OPERATING ROOM MANAGEMENT

*Evan E. Lebovitz and Mitchell H. Tsai*

## INTRODUCTION

This chapter reviews how to calculate the costs of the operating room (OR). First, the "preoperative" considerations in operating room management center on tactical decisions, the cornerstone of OR management. Second, the "intraoperative" lens of OR management focuses on operational goals, each having their financial counterpart. Finally, the "postoperative" aspects of OR management are inherent in the specialty's focus and mission.

## PREOPERATIVE PLANNING

### EXPENSE MANAGEMENT

Operating rooms have a high fixed-to-variable cost ratio, and astute clinical directors need to fully understand the overhead costs. Given the varying contribution margins of different surgeries, optimizing OR workflows may be a more cost-effective way to increase revenue than simply emphasizing increased throughput. In a recent cross-sectional analysis, the mean cost of OR time in fiscal year 2014 for California's acute care hospitals was $36 to $37 per minute; $20 to $21 of this amount was direct cost, with $13 to $14 attributable to wages and benefits and $2.50 to $3.50 attributable to surgical supplies.[1] For most institutions, the revenue generated per patient is constrained to bottlenecks in the system, and simply increasing production volume may paradoxically increase fixed costs and amplify inefficiencies.

The optimal allocation of OR time planned in advance should be based on the historical use by a particular surgical service based on a unit of OR allocation, such as surgeon, department, or specialty. Tactical decisions can affect operational workflows within the perioperative suite and utilization rates for surgical services. For example, a clinical director might add additional block time for a newly hired surgeon or reassign a schedule block allocated from a service that is not fully utilizing their time

to another. This increased OR "capacity" may be allocated to individual surgeons or small groups of surgeons of the same subspecialty to encourage those surgeons to increase their caseload.

The goal of tactical planning is to match the staffing to the workload, but in reality, because the workload is more variable than the staffing, the ad hoc operational decisions made by the management team modulate the throughput. Underutilized time is defined as the positive difference between allocated OR time and the OR workload. Overutilized time is defined as the positive difference between OR workload and allocated OR time. Therefore, inefficient OR use is the sum of two products: hours of underutilized OR time multiplied by the cost per hour of underutilized OR time (fixed costs) and hours of overutilized OR time multiplied by the cost per hour of overutilized OR time (variable costs). For example, delayed or emergent surgical cases may necessitate coverage with on-call staff (variable cost) versus planned staff (fixed cost).

## INTRAOPERATIVE

On the day of surgery, efficiency is at a premium. The impact of operational decision-making occurs in two stages.[2] As previously mentioned, the first stage occurs when case scheduling maximizes OR efficiency and minimizes the hours of overutilized OR time.[3] If an anesthesia provider is assigned to an OR staffed from 8 AM to 4 PM and works quickly, then he or she can prevent an hour of overutilized OR time and increase OR efficiency without adjusting OR utilization. However, if the anesthesiologist finishes at 3 PM instead of at 4 PM, the anesthesiologist did *not* increase OR efficiency because overutilized time was not reduced. In short, any delays in operational workflows only make a financial difference when the delay itself creates overutilized time.

Several OR management metrics receive a preponderance of attention from administrators and consultants. A reduction in OR turnover time, defined as the time from when one patient exits an OR (wheels out) until the next patient enters the same OR (wheels in), would seemingly benefit a hospital since idle ORs generate no revenue and help no patients. However, it should be readily apparent that reducing turnover times may do little to increase actual caseload or reduce staffing costs. Additionally, if an OR suite reduces turnover times by hiring more staff to clean the room, the operational efficiencies gained in the OR may create new bottlenecks within the perioperative system (e.g., preoperative preparation or the postanesthesia care unit). Similarly, clinical directors should not be looking at first-case start delays in terms of percentages or total minutes.[4] Instead, clinical directors need to understand the concept of tardiness, defined as the difference between the time the patient actually entered the OR and the scheduled start time of the case, which usually declines over the course of the day.

## POSTOPERATIVE

The process of planning, scheduling, and executing surgical and anesthetic care can be a herculean effort that feels like surviving a twister that has blown into town on a daily basis. Nonetheless, the data generated from case completion need to be analyzed for benchmarking, yet because no two anesthesia practices are alike, the data should not be compared out of context.[5] With these data, computer software can be used to minimize the amount of underutilized time and the more expensive overutilized time. Several aspects of this process may be improved as case length predictions and surgical techniques continue to improve, but unpredictability may forever remain inherent in the "art" of medicine when surgeons or anesthesiologists experience complications and cases proceed significantly longer (or shorter) than predicted.

## REFERENCES

1. Childers CP, Maggard-Gibbons M. Understanding costs of care in the operating room. *JAMA Surg.* 2018;153(4):e176233.
2. Tsai MH. Ten tips in providing value in operating room management. *Anesthesiol Clin* 2008;26(4):765–783, viii.
3. McIntosh C, et al. The impact of service-specific staffing, case scheduling, turnovers, and first-case starts on anesthesia group and operating room productivity: a tutorial using data from an Australian hospital. *Anesth Analg* 2006;103(6):1499–1516.
4. Dexter F, Epstein RH. Typical savings from each minutes reduction in tardy first case of the day starts. *Anesth Analg* 2009;108(4):1262–1267.
5. Hudson ME, Lebovitz EE. Measuring clinical productivity. *Anesthesiol Clin.* 2018;36(2):143–160.

# 371.

# DEFINITIONS

*Joseph Salama Hanna and Ramsey Saad*

## MEDICATION ERROR

Medication errors[1] refer to any mistakes occurring in the medication use process, regardless of whether an injury occurred or whether the potential for injury was present. Approximately 1 in 100 medication errors result in an adverse drug event (ADE). Although relatively few medication errors result in ADEs, they provide important information for identifying opportunities to improve patient care.

## ADVERSE DRUG EVENTS

Adverse drug events[2] are defined as any injuries resulting from medication use, including physical harm, mental harm, or loss of function. ADEs, compared with medication errors, are a more direct measure of patient harm.

# SENTINEL EVENT

## INTRODUCTION

The Joint Commission adopted a formal Sentinel Event Policy in 1996 to help hospitals that experience serious adverse events improve safety and learn from those sentinel events.[3] Careful investigation and analysis of patient safety events (events not primarily related to the natural course of the patient's illness or underlying condition), as well as evaluation of corrective actions, are essential to reduce risk and prevent patient harm. The Sentinel Event Policy explains how the Joint Commission partners with healthcare organizations that have experienced a serious patient safety event to protect the patient, improve systems, and prevent further harm.

## DEFINITION

A sentinel event is a patient safety event that reaches a patient and results in any of the following: death, permanent harm or severe temporary harm, and intervention required to sustain life. Such events are called "sentinel" because they signal the need for immediate investigation and response. Each accredited organization is strongly encouraged, but not required, to report sentinel events to the Joint Commission.

## EXAMPLES

The Joint Commission reviewed 801 reports of sentinel events in 2018; of these 87% were voluntarily reported to

*Table 371.1* MOST FREQUENTLY REPORTED SENTINEL EVENTS FOR 2018

| SENTINEL EVENT | NUMBER |
|---|---|
| Fall | 111 |
| Unintended retention of a foreign body | 111 |
| Wrong-site surgery | 94 |
| Unassigned | 68 |
| Unanticipated events such as asphyxiation, burn, choking on food, drowning or being found unresponsive | 59 |
| Suicide | 50 |
| Delay in treatment | 43 |
| Product or device event | 29 |
| Criminal event | 28 |
| Medication error | 24 |

the accrediting body. The 10 most frequently reported sentinel events for 2018 are shown in Table 371.1.

## REFERENCES

1. Bates DW, et al. Incidence of adverse drug events and potential adverse drug events. Implications for prevention. ADE Prevention Study Group. *JAMA.* 1995;274(1):29–34.
2. Zhu J, Weingart SN. Prevention of adverse drug events in hospitals. In: Post TW, eds. *UpToDate.* Waltham, MA: UpToDate; 2021.
3. Joint Commission. Home page. https://www.jointcommission.org

# 372.

# MEDICATION ERRORS
## ASSESSMENT AND PREVENTION

*Joseph Salama Hanna and Ramsey Saad*

## INTRODUCTION

Adverse drug events (ADEs) comprise the largest single category of adverse events experienced by hospitalized patients, accounting for about 19% of all injuries.[1] The occurrence of ADEs is associated with increased morbidity and mortality, prolonged hospitalizations, and higher costs of care.

A medication error is any mistake in the intended use of a medication (e.g., wrong medication, wrong dose, or infusion of the wrong medication into the wrong place, as with a connection error). The perioperative period is a high-risk setting for such errors.

At least a quarter of all medication-related injuries are preventable. Preventable ADEs include errors made by the clinician and systematic errors.

## DEFINITIONS

Adverse drug events are defined as any injuries resulting from medication use, including physical harm, mental harm, or loss of function. ADEs, compared with medication errors, are a more direct measure of patient harm.

Medication errors refer to any mistakes occurring in the medication use process, regardless of whether an injury occurred or whether the potential for injury was present. Approximately 1 in 100 medication errors result in an ADE, while 7 in 100 have the potential to do so.[2]

Adverse drug reactions, or non-preventable ADEs, are ADEs that occur due to pharmacological properties of the drug.

Potential ADEs are medication errors that pose a significant risk but do not cause harm to a patient.[3] Potential ADEs are also called near-miss errors or close calls. Potential ADEs include errors that are detected and intercepted by a patient or clinical staff before the patient is affected.

## DETECTION OF ERRORS

Detection of errors can be established through voluntary or facilitated self-reporting, mandatory incident reporting, chart review, and computerized surveillance, as well as direct observation.[4]

## PREVENTION

The Anesthesia Patient Safety Foundation in the United States, as well as the Association of Anesthetists, the Society for Intravenous Anesthesia, and the Safe Anesthesia

*Table 372.1* PREVENTION STRATEGIES

| INSTITUTIONAL APPROACHES | TECHNOLOGY SOLUTIONS | PHARMACY SOLUTION |
|---|---|---|
| • Supportive environment for event reporting<br>• Structured mechanisms for timed review<br>• Follow-up to ensure implementation of improvements<br>• Establishing a just culture as well as emphasizing good communication and teamwork skills | • Clinical Decision Support CPOE (computerized physician order entry) systems, alerts, medication infusion smart pumps, barcode-assisted medication administration<br>• Standardization: standardized labels, Tallman lettering, color-coded labels, barcode-assisted syringe labeling, standardized concentrations of high-alert medications, standardized medication trays and storage.<br>• Two-person check for high-risk medications | • Prefilled syringes<br>• Premixed solutions<br>• Avoid look-alike medications<br>• Avoid multiuse of vials<br>• Clinical pharmacist consultants |

Liaison Group in the United Kingdom, the Australian and New Zealand College of Anesthetists (ANZCA), and international groups such as the EZDrugID global initiative and the International Society of Pharmacovigilance, have each recommended prevention strategies for perioperative medication errors. These are based on technology solutions, standardization, elimination of look-alike medication vials and labels, pharmacy solutions, and improvements in institutional culture. These strategies are supported by expert opinion, although there are few data regarding interventions to prevent anesthesia-related medication errors.[5] (Table 372.1).

## REFERENCES

1. Leape LL, et al. The nature of adverse events in hospitalized patients. Results of the Harvard Medical Practice Study II. *N Engl J Med*. 1991;324(6):377–384.
2. Bates DW, et al. Relationship between medication errors and adverse drug events. *J Gen Intern Med*. 1995;10(4):199–205.
3. Bates DW, et al. Incidence of adverse drug events and potential adverse drug events. Implications for prevention. ADE Prevention Study Group. *JAMA*. 1995;274(1):29–34.
4. Nanji K. Prevention of perioperative medication errors. In: Post TW, eds. *UpToDate*. Waltham, MA: UpToDate; 2021.
5. Webster CS, et al. Clinical assessment of a new anaesthetic drug administration system: a prospective, controlled, longitudinal incident monitoring study. *Anaesthesia*. 2010;65(5):490–499.

# 373.

# REPORTING

## MANDATORY AND VOLUNTARY SYSTEMS, LEGAL REQUIREMENTS, ANESTHESIA QUALITY INSTITUTE, AND PHYSICIAN QUALITY REPORTING SYSTEM

*Ramsey Saad and Joseph Salama Hanna*

## INTRODUCTION

Medical errors are an unfortunate occurrence in medicine; however, when they do occur, reporting becomes the ethical and professional responsibility of the physician and institution.

## MAJOR NATIONAL VOLUNTARY REPORTING SYSTEMS

The Medication Error Reporting Program of the Institute for Safe Medication Practices and the US Pharmacopeia focuses on medication complications. It collects reports from pharmacists and others of adverse events and errors, performs an analysis of the error, and sends biweekly reports with recommendations to medical institutions and pharmaceutical companies in addition to the Food and Drug Administration. Another program that also focuses on medication complications is the MedMARx program of the US Pharmacopeia, which also receives reports of medication errors from hospitals and provides them with the results of data analyses.

The National Nosocomial Infection Survey, run by the Centers for Disease Control and Prevention, uses reports that are produced by trained infection control practitioners to report hospital-acquired infections. These reports are utilized to establish national risk-adjusted benchmarks and report site-specific infection rates to participating hospitals.[1]

The American Society of Anesthesiologists (ASA) established the Anesthesia Incident Reporting System (AIRS) in 2011 for anesthesia providers to report near misses or actual events. These reports are confidential (https://www.aqihq.org/airs/).[2]

## MANDATORY REPORTING SYSTEMS

Mandatory reporting systems are the systems that, by state law, require healthcare facilities to report errors resulting in serious patient harm or death. Mandatory reporting systems may be subject to underreporting, possibly due to fear of litigation and/or disciplinary action.[3]

## INSTITUTIONAL APPROACHES

An ideal confidential event reporting system would include the following:

- An environment that is supportive of event reporting in a confidential manner that protects the privacy of reporting staff in a nonpunitive manner
- Having mechanisms in place for review of reports and development of corrective action plans
- Adequate follow-up to ensure implementation of corrective action plans.

Traditionally, the tendency would be to blame the individual involved in the error; however, developing a systems approach would be to look into improving the system that allowed the human error to occur, with the goal of developing a system to intercept human errors before they occur. This involves establishing a just culture where, although each individual is held accountable for their actions, the goal is peer review and developing a root cause analysis to identify vulnerabilities within the system to detect potential predictable human failings in the context of poorly designed systems.[3]

## ANESTHESIA QUALITY INSTITUTE

The Anesthesia Quality Institute (AQI) was established by the ASA in 2008 to facilitate practice-based quality management through education and quality data feedback, with the vision being "to be the primary source of information for quality improvement in the clinical practice of anesthesiology. Through education and quality feedback, AQI will help to improve the quality care of patients, lower anesthesia mortality and lower anesthesia incidents."[4]

It is listed as a patient safety organization (PSO) by the Department of Health and Human Services.[4]

Through the National Anesthesia Clinical Outcomes Registry (NACOR), the AQI NACOR's clinical database provides evidence-based rationale that assists with clinical decision-making.

Reporting through AIRS is performed online, with the goal of assisting anesthesiologists learn from reported incidents.

Reporting can be performed anonymously, or the provider may be able to provide their information, however, in a confidential manner.

Because of the AQI's standing as a PSO, legal protection is provided.[4]

## PHYSICIAN QUALITY REPORTING SYSTEM

The Physician Quality Reporting System (PQRS), developed by the Centers for Medicare and Medicaid Services (CMS) has been using incentive payments and making payment adjustments to encourage eligible healthcare professionals to report on specific quality measures. Using the feedback report provided by CMS, eligible professionals (EPs) can compare their performance on a given measure with their peers. Reporting on behalf of the provider may be performed through Medicare Part B claims, Qualified PQRS registry, Direct Electronic Health Record (EHR) using Certified EHR Technology (CEHRT), CEHRT via a data submission vendor, Qualified Clinical Data Registry.

With regard to group practices, reporting may be occur through Qualified PQRS registry, web interface (for groups of 25+ only), Direct EHR using CEHRT, CEHRT via a Data Submission Vendor, Clinician and Group Consumer Assessment of Healthcare Providers and Systems (CG CAHPS) CMS-certified survey vendor.

Payment incentives and adjustments will be made based on performance compared to peers.[5]

## REFERENCES

1. Leape LL. Reporting of adverse events. *N Engl J Med*. 2002;347(20): 1633–1638.
2. Wahr J. Safety in the Operating Room. In: Post TW, eds. *UpToDate*. Waltham, MA: UpToDate; 2021. Accessed August 26, 2020. https://www.uptodate.com/contents/safety-in-the-operating-room?search=safety%20practices&source=search_result&selectedTitle=1~150&usage_type=default&display_rank=1#H279 7853915
3. Nanji K. Prevention of perioperative medication errors. In: Post TW, eds. *UpToDate*. Waltham, MA: UpToDate; 2021. Accessed August 25, 2020. https://www.uptodate.com/contents/prevention-of-perioperative-medication-errors?search=mandatory%20report ing%20systems&source=search_result&selectedTitle=3~150&usa ge_type=default&display_rank=3
4. Anesthesia Quality Institute. About us. Accessed August 28, 2020. https://www.aqihq.org/about-us.aspx#:~:text=AQI%20was%20 established%20by%20the,education%20and%20quality%20d ata%20feedback
5. Centers for Medicare and Medicaid Services. Physician Quality Reporting System overview. Accessed August 29, 2020. https://www.cms.gov/Medicare/Quality-Initiatives-Patient-Assessment-Instruments/PQRS/Downloads/PQRS_OverviewFactSheet_201 3_08_06.pdf

# 374.

# SAFETY PRACTICES

*Ramsey Saad and Joseph Salama Hanna*

## INTRODUCTION

One of the goals that should be accomplished after reviewing sentinel events or complications related to the operating room (OR) is to establish a process to identify vulnerabilities within the system to detect potential predictable human failings in the context of poorly designed systems to minimize the chance of reoccurrence in the future.

## INFECTION

Not all complications will be noticed immediately. This applies to infections, such as surgical infections, whose chances can be minimized by actions on behalf of the anesthesiologist, such as timely antibiotic administration and redosing, avoidance of hyperglycemia, administration of supplemental oxygen, and maintaining normothermia. Other infections, such as central venous catheter insertion, may be more directly correlating with the anesthesiologists' practice, such as maintaining sterile technique, proper hand hygiene, adequate prep, and paying close attention to draping technique. Developing a process to maintain a standardized approach to ensure adherence to the standards is recommended. This can all be part of the "time-out process," described in further detail in this chapter.

## PREVENTION OF ERRORS

Developing systemwide processes to prevent errors may include the following:

- Error prevention includes the use of safety precautions that are standardized by the American Society of Anesthesiologists, such as end-tidal $CO_2$ to verify endotracheal intubation, or precautions that have become standard of care at several institutions, such as using ultrasound guidance and transduction of a waveform to confirm placement of the catheter in the central vein prior to insertion of introducer sheath.

- Improvement of communication can be part of prevention; this involves a comprehensive time out in the preoperative holding area, in addition to a preanesthesia and preoperative time out. All members of the team should be involved in this, including a member from the surgical team, OR nursing, and the anesthesia team. The patient should be involved in the time out performed in the preoperative holding area and preanesthesia time out. The informed consent should be reviewed. The patient should be identified using at least two identifiers. The surgical site and side should be reviewed and marked prior to this. Critical steps and concerns should be clearly communicated, such as pertinent allergies, anticipation of difficult airway, aspiration risk, whether the estimated blood loss is expected to be greater than 500 mL, the availability of blood products if needed in addition to antibiotic administration. Any concerns with positioning should also be communicated. It should also be confirmed that all equipment needed for the procedure is available as well. Postoperative disposition planning should also be discussed.[1]

- Of note, regarding patients who will be undergoing regional blocks, an additional time out should be performed prior to this.

- Minimizing distractions in the OR, such as limiting OR personnel, limiting conversations, turning phones and pagers to vibrate mode, and lowering OR music volume.

- Communication is key to a safe OR environment. Using closed-loop communication, reading out numbers clearly (e.g., five zero for 50 to avoid confusion with 15) and identifying the recipient by name.

- There should also be a structured anesthesia handoff, including the identifiers mentioned in the time-out process in addition to any anesthetic concerns that may affect the intraoperative course and disposition of the patient.

- Risk of needle-stick injury to staff is reduced by proper education, engineering changes in addition to proper needle disposal. Provide proper education to providers regarding prevention and early intervention for healthcare provider exposure should be provided on employment and periodically according to institution policy.

- Risk of medication errors could be reduced, also by proper education of providers regarding the risk factors, which include unfamiliarity with the case, an example of which is a junior resident involved in a complex case that requires administration of a medication he may be unfamiliar with in an emergency setting. Making sure the medication is appropriately labeled and reviewed prior to administration is of utmost importance, even in the emergency setting. Some institutions have developed a barcode system to be scanned prior to medication administration.
- A proper anesthesia machine check prior to induction and ensuring adequate machine maintenance are expected to minimize the chance of equipment malfunction. This should also be reviewed during the time-out process.
- Improvement of equipment and standardization may reduce human errors. An example for this is development of the pin-indexed safety systems for gas cylinders.
- Proper padding and planning for positioning are essential to prevent injuries related to positioning, such as peripheral nerve injuries.
- Take measures to prevent awareness under anesthesia such as using electroencephalography, especially when undergoing cases with total intravenous anesthesia and inability to measure end-tidal anesthetic concentrations of volatile anesthetics.
- Routine checks of OR equipment by clinical engineering minimizes the risk of fires and electrical injuries.
- Regarding cardiac implantable electronic devices (CIEDs), each institution should have a protocol regarding perioperative assessment of CIEDs and taking the necessary precautions to maintain patient safety during the procedure (e.g., application of Zoll pads and ensuring the availability of external defibrillation if the scenario necessitates disabling the defibrillator capacity of an automatic implantable cardioverter defibrillator).
- Radiation Injury is of concern as well. Adequate education, using as low as reasonably acceptable doses of radiation, and tracking radiation exposure of employees are of utmost importance.[1,2]

## PATIENT SAFETY APPROACHES

Different approaches to patient safety have been adopted, on both the hospital level and nationally. Development of a culture of safety and adequate reporting systems and root cause analysis review with the goal of system improvement has been discussed elsewhere in this book. An organized approach for team training has been developed in many institutions. This can be performed with a simulator system[3] or adequate training programs, such as those developed by the Department of Veterans Affairs to improve communication, situational awareness, and leadership skills.[4]

On a national level, the Joint Commission has also developed National Patient Safety Goals. Hospital accreditation would depend on meeting these goals and implementing an improvement plan in the case of sentinel events. The National Patient Safety Goals include identifying patients correctly, preventing infection, improving staff communication, using medicine and alarms safely, identifying patient safety risks, and preventing mistakes in surgery.[5]

## REFERENCES

1. Allard J, et al. Pre-surgery briefings and safety climate in the operating theatre. *BMJ Qual Saf.* 2011;20(8):711–717.
2. Wahr J. Safety in the operating room. In: Post TW, eds. *UpToDate.* Waltham, MA: UpToDate; 2021. Accessed August 26, 2020. https://www.uptodate.com/contents/safety-in-the-operating-room?search=safety%20practices&source=search_result&selectedTitle=1~150&usage_type=default&display_rank=1#H2797853915
3. Weller JM, et al. The impact of trained assistance on error rates in anaesthesia: a simulation-based randomised controlled trial; *Anaesthesia.* 2009;64(2):126–130.
4. Dunn EJ, et al. Medical team training: applying crew resource management in the Veterans Health Administration. *Jt Comm J Qual Patient Saf.* 2007;33:317.
5. Joint Commission. The Joint Commission 2020 National Patient Safety Goals. Accessed August 28, 2020. https://www.jointcommission.org/standards/national-patient-safety-goals/-/media/c27cb0eca3154375a6da1ec2a7ed4c6f.ashx

# 375.

# ROOT CAUSE ANALYSIS

*Luis Tueme and Nawal E. Ragheb-Mueller*

## INTRODUCTION

During the performance of highly complex procedures, such as those that occur every day in operating rooms, anesthesia departments will inevitably encounter sentinel events or an unanticipated deviation in practice that results in temporary harm, permanent harm, or the death of a patient. Root cause analysis (RCA) is employed to analyze these situations and ameliorate the environment. The intent is not to assign personal blame, but to implement change after identifying the underlying causes, system vulnerabilities, or factors contributing to the sentinel event.

Root cause refers to a potential relationship between specific factors and how they presumably enable a sentinel event to occur. The process of RCA originated in systems engineering and was introduced into medicine in the 1990s, with the goal of uncovering the causal factors contributing to the variation in the delivery of healthcare.[1] Anesthesiology was one of the first medical specialties to incorporate a systems approach to improving safe delivery of care, and in the United States, entities such as the American Society of Anesthesiologists Closed Claims Project and the Anesthesia Quality Institute have provided data to improve the delivery of care and educate personnel.[2,3] Today, patient safety is a burgeoning area of inquiry and research, and medical specialty boards as well as the American Council on Graduate Medical Education require training and ongoing involvement in activities designed to reduce patient harm. RCA is one tool used in healthcare settings to attempt to promote patient safety and reduce harm.

## WHAT ARE THE GOALS OF AN RCA?

The ultimate intent of an RCA is to prevent future harm or injury to patients by investigating an adverse event, reviewing errors or systems flaws and implementing changes to achieve the outcome of minimal or no harm. A team is assembled to carry out an inquiry into the incident, and levels of harm are assigned (ranging from no harm or a "near miss" to severe harm or death). Inherent to the process is the understanding that even the best or "safest" organizations are vulnerable to lapses, and errors will occur as humans are fallible and systems are flawed.[1]

The goals of investigating adverse events are to provide immediate care of the harmed patient, understand the "root" causes, provide disclosure to patients and families, implement improvement measures, and provide any needed emotional support to the patients, families, and clinicians involved. The specific methodology employed in an RCA may vary by institution, but in every scenario, the team attempts to explore opportunities for improvement and implement a plan devised to prevent future incidents of a similar nature.

## HOW IS IT PERFORMED?

The premise of an RCA is that a "deep dive" needs to be conducted to search for the factors or triggers behind the occurrence of an adverse event. The Joint Commission promotes a framework of 24 questions designed to explore why an error occurred and how a future recurrence can be prevented.[4] There are a wide variety of methods employed in pursuing an RCA, but each requires several distinct steps. The first involves assembling a team to thoroughly investigate all factors that contributed to the harm. Typically, the team includes an individual experienced in RCA, medical specialists or other healthcare personnel with expertise in the area related to the incident, an administrator, and, often, a layperson or patient representative. In some settings, a risk management professional also is involved. The team then pursues data collection surrounding the event during this fact-finding phase. Charts are reviewed, timelines are mapped, and individuals involved are interviewed. Inherent to the process is the understanding that a detailed account of the events and factors contributing to the harmful outcome must be thoroughly explored and delineated. Missteps or faults in delivery of care are identified, contributing factors are noted, an analysis is made, and recommendations and solutions are devised. Throughout the entire process, questions are asked, answers are sought, and new questions are posed to refine the inquiry and develop remedies for potential fault lines and weaknesses within the processes and organization.

The Joint Commission identifies a broad range of items that should be explored as part of an RCA framework in the medical setting. These include the patient identification process, staffing levels, orientation and training of staff, competency assessment, staff supervision and communication, availability of information, adequacy of technological support, equipment maintenance, physical environment, control of medication, and medication labeling. It also mandates that RCA for sentinel events be completed within 45 days in the United States. In the United Kingdom, healthcare institutions have 60 days to complete an RCA. While the need to investigate and learn from sentinel events is undisputed, there are critiques of RCA as the means to achieve this end. These include the notion that the process is overly reductionist,

the time frame is too constrained in some circumstances, new teams have to be assembled each time an event occurs, and trained investigators may be more effective than an approach that assembles ad hoc teams.

The endpoint of an RCA is an opportunity to improve care and review whether any organizational changes that are implemented in fact achieve a reduction in harm, which might otherwise have occurred in the absence of the intervention.

## REFERENCES

1. Jhugursing M, et al. Error and root cause analysis. *BJA Educ.* 2017;17(10):323–333.
2. Geerling J, et al. Root cause analysis. *ASA Monitor.* 2014;78:46–49.
3. Kent CD, et al. Anesthesia hazards: lessons from the Anesthesia Closed Claims Project. *Anesthesiology.* 2019;58(1):7–12.
4. Parker J, et al. *Root Cause Analysis in Health Care: Tools and Techniques.* 5th ed. Joint Commission Resources; 2015.

# 376.

# CRISIS MANAGEMENT AND TEAMWORK

*Mollie K. Lagrew and Christopher Giordano*

## PREOPERATIVE: PREPARATION FOR A CRISIS

The best-case scenario is to prevent an error or crisis before it occurs. Significant effort is required to prevent the proverbial "Swiss cheese" from lining up. It is imperative not only to develop the knowledge, skills, and attitudes (KSAs) fundamental for successful team dynamics, but also to recognize the cognitive biases and context that are pivotal for a cohesive team and the overall safety of the patient.[1]

## BRIEFING

Prior to induction of anesthesia, the entire operating room team works through a preoperative checklist with the patient to ensure team understanding and alignment. This

requires all team members to review important aspects of the case, including

- roles and responsibilities of each member
- anticipated procedural intervention and site marking
- requisite medications (e.g., antibiotics) and equipment

An important emphasis of this briefing is the development of a *shared mental model* within the team.[2] This is a shared understanding of the specific roles and responsibilities of each team member and the goals and objectives of the task ahead. Creating a sense of psychological safety among team members is imperative during this briefing so that in the event of a crisis all team members can address their concerns and comfortably rely on each other for assistance.

## CLOSED-LOOP COMMUNICATION

For communication to be effective, it must be verbalized and received, which requires effort. *Closed-loop communication* effectively conveys information. The receiver repeats the information, and the sender acknowledges the receiver's correct understanding.

For example:

"Please give 30,000 units of heparin."

"I am giving 30,000 units of heparin."

"That is correct. Thank you."

## COGNITIVE BIAS

Multiple cognitive biases exist and facilitate our day-to-day lives, but they occasionally have a negative impact on our everyday decision-making.[3] Heuristics, or mental shortcuts, help when information is incomplete, context is changing, or our mental faculties are limited, but these cognitive aids can become systemic biases and lead to disasters when applied to the wrong situation. Anesthesiologists should be aware of the most common cognitive biases, including the following:

a. Affective bias: negative or positive feelings within an individual that influence perception, interpretation, and decision-making
b. Anchoring bias: latching on to initial pieces of information with the inability to integrate new information and adjust appropriately
c. Confirmation bias: only use or search for information that supports and does not refute current understanding
d. Availability bias: Choosing a diagnosis because it is in the *forefront* of an individual's mind due to an emotional memory, recent experience or discussion, or media coverage
e. Representative bias: the tendency to overgeneralize from a few characteristics or observations
f. Framing bias: a schema of interpretation that alters perception without changing the facts

## INTRAOPERATIVE: DURING THE CRISIS

Anesthesia nontechnical skills (ANTSs), which include situation awareness, judgment, teamwork, and decision-making, are essential during crisis management.[4] While ANTSs are a different framework than the KSAs developed by Salas et al.,[2] both approach critical events with tools and a lexicon to help team members efficiently and successfully manage the crisis. The overarching philosophies and tools of both frameworks include calling for help early, cognitive aids, and leadership.

## CALL FOR HELP EARLY

One of the foundational principles in crisis resource management (CRM) is the humility to ask for assistance. This is not a sign of weakness or incompetence, but rather a way to set aside ego to maintain the safety of the patient. Furthermore, each person approaches the crisis with different cognitive biases and knowledge bases that lead to a different understanding of the situation. Having a shared mental model of the team and the procedure maintains psychological safety to enable trust and backup behaviors.

## COGNITIVE AIDS

Cognitive aids have been developed and employed to counteract the naturally occurring drop-off in cognitive performance and memory retrieval during high-stress situations.[5] These cognitive aids include protocols and best practice guidelines that are outlined for reference during emergencies and are commonplace in code carts and anesthesia machines. The idea that double-checking a protocol or looking up information is not a sign of weakness is fundamental to this philosophy. Currently, emergency manuals for critical events include malignant hyperthermia, difficult airway, operating room fires, and advanced cardiac life support.

## LEADERSHIP

A key component of high-functioning teams is the role of a leader. This role can be dynamic and change within the team or even be shared among team members. Regardless, the leader must establish the normal operating behavior within the group by creating and maintaining psychological safety, establishing the roles and responsibilities of each teammate, maintaining a shared mental model that adapts with the assimilation of new information, and monitoring the effectiveness and/or deficits of the team within a changing environment.[2]

## POSTOPERATIVE: AFTER THE CRISIS

Inevitably, crises will occur; creating infrastructure for post hoc analysis is essential to avert similar future events and to develop reliable organizations. The most developed approach to address these critical healthcare events or even narrowly averted crises is the procedural or situational debriefing.

## DEBRIEFING

After the event has occurred and emotions have calmed, the team convenes to discuss the event and assess the circumstances. This allows team members to acknowledge what went well and what went poorly, with opportunities to improve practices without promoting a culture of blame. Unfortunately, debriefing is often skipped for numerous reasons: perceptions of uselessness, fear of retribution or blame, embarrassment, or lack of time. When there is a shared goal, cohesive teamwork, and proper leadership, the debriefing will be a safe space to work toward improvements.

## REFERENCES

1. Loup O, et al. Nontechnical skills in a technical world. *Int Anesthesiol Clin.* 2019;57(1):81–94.
2. Salas E, et al. Is there a "Big Five" in teamwork? *Small Group Res.* 2005;36(5):555–559.
3. Stiegler MP, Tung A. Cognitive processes in anesthesiology decision making. *Anesthesiology.* 2014;120(1):204–217.
4. Flin R, Patey R. Non-technical skills for anaesthetists: developing and applying ANTS. *Best Pract Res Clin Anaesthesiol.* 2011;25(2):215–227.
5. Gaba DM. Perioperative cognitive aids in anesthesia: what, who, how, and why bother? *Anesth Analg.* 2013:117(5):1033–1036.

# 377.

# QUALITY IMPROVEMENT

*Joseph J. McComb and Corinne K. Wong*

## QUALITY IMPROVEMENT

Despite lagging other US industries, effective healthcare quality improvement (QI) programs are expected by patients, insurers, government agencies, and hospital leadership. There are countless definitions of quality in the healthcare and manufacturing literature, but in 1990 the Institute of Medicine (IOM) defined quality as "the degree to which health services for individuals and populations increase the likelihood of desired health outcomes and are consistent with current professional knowledge."[p5] In 2001, the IOM provided six aims to guide clinicians on their QI journey in *Crossing the Quality Chasm: A New Health System for the 21st Century.*[2] They maintain healthcare should be safe, effective, patient centered, timely, efficient, and equitable (Table 377.1).

Quality assurance (QA) and continuous quality improvement (CQI) are quite different. QA measures output and compares the product to predetermined standards. QA involves inspection and removing defects without changing the system that created the defects. CQI continuously improves the system to enable an expectation of quality rather than relying on inspection. It is goal directed and can be both retrospective and prospective.[3] Unlike QA, CQI does not focus solely on the defects that are discovered; it looks at all production. CQI looks at the methodology and process of systems rather than the individual practitioner. It aims to reduce variability in the process and thus attempts to avoid unintended errors. One of the four absolutes of quality by Philip Crosby was prevention, not appraisal which would lead to zero defects. There is no better application of a zero-defect mentality than in the practice of anesthesiology.

A systematic approach is required for QI. In the 1940s, W. Edwards Dening built on the initial work of Walter A. Shewhart when he developed the Plan, Do, Study, Act (PDSA) cycle. Subsequently, the model for improvement added three questions to be used when designing a QI initiative (Figure 377.1):

1. What are we trying to accomplish?
2. How will we know if change is an improvement?
3. What changes can we make that will result in improvement?

**Table 377.1** IOM'S SIX AIMS TO GUIDE CLINICIANS ON THEIR QI JOURNEY

| AIM | TACTIC |
|---|---|
| Safe | Avoiding injuries to patients from the care that is intended to help them |
| Effective | Providing services based on scientific knowledge to all who could benefit and refraining from providing services to those not likely to benefit |
| Patient centered | Providing care that is respectful of and responsive to individual patient preferences, needs, and values and ensuring that patient values guide all clinical decisions |
| Timely | Reducing waits and sometimes harmful delays for both those who receive and those who give care |
| Efficient | Avoiding waste, including waste of equipment, supplies, ideas, and energy |
| Equitable | Providing care that does not vary in quality because of personal characteristics such as gender, ethnicity, geographic location, and socioeconomic status |

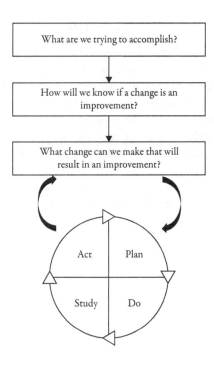

**Figure 377.1** A systematic approach is required for QI. Taylor MJ, et al. BMJ Qual Saf 2014;23:290–298.

Examples of QI programs in action discussed in a further chapter in more detail include

- Lean methodology
- Six Sigma

Two models for improving healthcare delivery are translating evidence into practice (TRIP) and the comprehensive unit-based safety program (CUSP).

*Translating evidence into practice* focuses on metrics and feedback to improve patient outcomes. It first identifies evidence-based practices with improved outcomes. Then it focuses on goal-oriented interventions that have the highest efficacy and lowest number of barriers to improved outcomes. A goal feature of TRIP is that it has measurable outcomes, which helps to facilitate feedback in a timely manner to its practitioners. Therefore, producing these improved evidence-based interventions through "engagement, education, execution and evaluation" [pS2955] uses evidence to guide clinical decision-making.

The *comprehensive unit-based safety program* is a five-step process to improve the safety of healthcare by learning from past issues and errors. The importance of CUSP is the culture within a system, teamwork, and education.

1. Emphasizes the education of safety with staff.
2. Identifies issues that could be improved.

3. Designates administration and those in leadership roles responsibilities to mentor their staff on how to improve safety and overcome barriers.
4. Learns from past errors.
5. Designs programs that teams can use to meet new safety goals and better communication.

Improving safety and quality is important to the future of healthcare. As more hospitals, healthcare systems, insurance companies, and payers look to the quality of care that is being delivered, it becomes even more important to look at models to improve current procedures and systems in place. To help meet these demands, practitioners will need to be engaged, be provided feedback, have continual education, and be dedicated to patient care.

## REFERENCES

1. Lohr K. *A Strategy for Quality Assurance.* Vol. 1. Washington, DC: National Academies Press; 1990.
2. Committee on Quality of Health Care in America IOM. *Crossing the Quality Chasm: A New Health System for the 21st Century.* Washington, DC: National Academies Press; 2001.
3. Kurth C. Introducing quality improvement. *Pediatr Anesth.* 2013;23(7):569–570.
4. Elshennawy AK. Quality in the new age and the body of knowledge for quality engineers, total quality management & business excellence. 2004;15:5–6, 603–614. doi:10.1080/14783360410001680099
5. Melinda S et al. Using evidence, rigorous measurement, and collaboration to eliminate central catheter-associated bloodstream infections. *Crit Care Med.* 2010;38:S292–S298. doi:10.1097/CCM.0b013e3181e6a165

# 378.

# SIX SIGMA AND LEAN OPERATIONS FOR THE ANESTHESIOLOGIST

*Caitlin N. Curcuru and Dinesh J. Kurian*

## INTRODUCTION

Quality improvement activities are a requirement for Maintenance of Certification in Anesthesiology (MOCA) 2.0 Part 4.[1]

There are several methods and tools available to drive process improvement. Six Sigma and Lean are two complimentary methods used to help drive process and quality improvement efforts. Six Sigma methodology focuses on *eliminating defects* through reducing undesired variation in a system, whereas Lean focuses on *eliminating waste* to gradually improve a system, allowing it to deliver flexible, high-volume production.[2] Both of these methodologies developed alongside each other in manufacturing and have since found wide adoption in service industries such as healthcare.

## SIX SIGMA

The Six Sigma process improvement methodology originated in the 1980s at Motorola and has since been widely used in manufacturing and found its way into service industries as well. *The key philosophy driving the method is that defects, defined as any process output outside of client specifications, stem from undesirable variation in a process.*[3] The sources of this variation should be identified and corrected to minimize undesired process variation. The name derives from the symbol used for standard deviation ($\sigma$) of any normally distributed measurement. The main idea is that any process should have such a narrow standard deviation that it is still capable of meeting client specification, even for outputs up to six standard deviations away from the process mean output.

The interest of Six Sigma in healthcare does not stem from treating all patients as identical widgets, but rather in making sure that the process of healthcare delivery continues to meet high standards. There has been a great deal of attention placed on the fact that a substantial number of adverse events stem from imperfect implementation of care, despite adequate medical knowledge. There are also a number of processes in which defects would not be considered acceptable, including

- Ensuring availability and function of emergency medical equipment
- Ensuring availability of emergency drugs for resuscitation
- Ensuring that a planned, elective operation starts on time

Though the scope can even be as limited as ensuring that the ultrasounds and video laryngoscopes are plugged in when not in use.

The Six Sigma method typically uses a five-phase approach to identify and control sources of variation:

*Define* the project team, the client, issues that are critical to quality, and the relationship between *s*uppliers, *i*nputs, *p*rocess, *o*utputs, and *c*ustomers (SIPOC). Common tools used in the define phase include creation of affinity diagrams, SIPOC analysis, and voice of the customer.

*Measure* baseline data process metrics, client specifications, and the gap between current and target performance. Common tools used in the measure phase include flow charts, check sheets, histograms, run charts, and scatterplots.

*Analyze* root causes of problems and variation identified in the measure phase, prioritize improvement activities, and develop a plan for execution. Common tools used in the analyze phase include Pareto charts and cause-and-effect fishbone diagrams.

*Improve* the current process according to the plan laid out in the analyze phase.

*Control* the new improved process to ensure that any advancements do not regress to prior inadequate performance. Collect data to ensure that the new process performs according to specification or recycle through the process using information. Commonly used tools include staff training, alignment of goals, and incentives.

It may be clear from the improve phase that this method is intended to be applied to an existing process. A slight modification is used to create a process that does not yet exist (define, measure, analyze, design, verify).

## LEAN

Lean methodology offers a complimentary philosophy that also originated in manufacturing and has since found applications in service industries such as healthcare. *The key philosophy behind Lean is that waste is commonly used to cover up process problems. Elimination of waste allows the problems to be uncovered and corrected, allowing the process to do more with less.*[4]

It is essential to note that waste is considered anything that does not add value to the product or process from the perspective of the client. If flexibility of a system is a valuable feature, reducing capabilities to meet a surge in demand is *not* in accordance with Lean principles. For example, imagine calling 911 to find out that all operators are busy.

The interest in Lean in healthcare is based on minimizing waste in the system, which can be defined as anything in the process that does not add value to the client (whether healthcare provider or patient). Some readily available examples include the following:

- Reducing time required to accommodate an emergency operation.
- Reducing the time between when a patient consents to a nerve block to the completion of the block.
- Reducing number of crossmatched blood products in excess of patient need.
- Reducing the complexity of navigating the healthcare system to help patients adhere to instructions they are given.

Lean focuses on *eight sources of waste in a system* that can be identified and eliminated:

*Overproduction*, or producing more system outputs than required

*Underutilization* of talent or equipment

*Time* that team members are forced to spend idle, usually due to a process bottleneck

*Transportation* of materials though a physical space

*Processing*, or forced downtime due to a machine that requires maintenance or repair

*Inventory*, an excess of which is associated with unnecessary cash expenditure, loss, obsolescence, and space to store it all

*Motion* that does not add value to the final product

*Defects* that incur costs of scrap, rework, and most importantly, damage of reputation when the defective process output reaches the customer

Each source of waste must be carefully considered, as well as the downstream effects of each decision. For example, the desire to reduce inventory may lead to an unexpected increase in waiting time if replacement inventory cannot be sourced or transported quickly enough. Lean uses a philosophy of continuous improvement, a strong culture of safety, and quality at the source to drive process improvement. Several tools are used to improve processes, such as

*Just-in-time production* to streamline a process, minimize inventory, and expose and eliminate underlying process problems that were previously hidden by an excess of inventory, time, or effort.

*5-S organization* to reduce time to find equipment and reduce risk of errors. The five Japanese words have been translated to English equivalents, also conveniently beginning with the letter S (*s*ort, *s*et in order, *s*hine, *s*tandardize, and *s*ustain). If you note that all drug and equipment carts are organized identically between rooms you staff, this is an example of 5S organization. If they are not, they should be.

*Use of a pull, rather than a push, process* to optimize scheduling and inventory and prevent any items (or patients) in a process from being stuck or accumulating in waiting areas.

*Error prevention*, through making the correct choice the easiest to make. The pin index system and diameter index system are ways that the anesthesia workstation prevents inappropriate and erroneous connections. Color coding drug labels also serves as a visual cue.

*Halting the production line* if a source of error or potential harm is noted and having all team members participate in troubleshooting the process.

*Creating a culture of continuous improvement.*

## REFERENCES

1. MOCA 2.0 part 4: quality improvement. 2016. https://theaba.org/about%20moca%202.0.html
2. Al-Shourah AA, et al. The integration of Lean management and Six Sigma strategies to improve the performance of production in industrial pharmaceutical. *Int J Bus Manag.* 2018;13(8):207.
3. Harry M, Schroeder R. *Six Sigma: The Breakthrough Management Strategy Revolutionizing the World's Top Corporations.* New York, NY: Currency; 2000.
4. George ML, et al. Beyond the basics: the five laws of Lean Six Sigma. In: *What Is Lean Six Sigma?* New York, NY: McGraw-Hill; 2004:41–42.

# 379.

# BARRIERS TO QUALITY IMPROVEMENT

*Ramsey Saad and Joseph Salama Hanna*

## INTRODUCTION

Quality improvement is paramount in the specialty of anesthesia. Safety in the operating room has improved significantly over the past few decades, from developing fail safe equipment, advances in engineering, process improvement to minimize the chance of human error, and improvement in communication. Quality improvement is a continuous process, and there remains room for improvement. This chapter outlines the barriers that may face providers and institutions in developing this.

## BARRIERS TO QUALITY IMPROVEMENT

Change is not always easy. This applies to quality improvement as well. Change is a process that involves a change in the culture and team effort on behalf of the entire institution. On literature review, multiple factors may contribute to this. The first is cognitive barriers, which may include lack of knowledge or technical skills (e.g., lack of ultrasound skills for central line placement). This may be resolved with education.

Other barriers include attitudinal barriers, which include lack of confidence, lack of sense of "being in control,"

or unreasonable outcome expectancy, which may lead to inability to self-assess regarding outcomes.

There may also be professional barriers, such as lack of motivation, concern for legal issues, and rigidity of professional boundaries.

On occasion, the lack of convincing evidence in the literature may discourage providers regarding making change.

Barriers may be also related to patient factors, such as difference in culture or cognitive issues leading to unwillingness to change.

Barriers related to institutional limitations may be due to lack of support or lack of resources or funding. Other factors may be lack of organization, coordination, or teamwork structure.[1]

## OVERCOMING BARRIERS TO IMPROVEMENT

It is important to understand that change is not expected to be immediate. It requires team building and interdepartmental efforts to promote a change of culture into a culture of safety and communication. Patient education is particularly important as well. If lack of resources and/or funding is a rate-limiting factor, then change will require buy-in from hospital administration and presenting the literature to support that although the initial change may appear to cause a financial burden on the institution, the overall cost-effectiveness will be worthwhile in terms of fewer complication rates and hospital and emergency room readmissions, and shorter hospital stay.[2]

## REFERENCES

1. Cochrane L, et al. Gaps between knowing and doing: understanding and assessing the barriers to optimal health care. J Contin Educ Health Prof. 2007;27(2):94–102
2. Luxford K, et al. Promoting patient-centered care: a qualitative study of facilitators and barriers in healthcare organizations with a reputation for improving the patient experience. Int J Qual Health Care. 2011;23(5):510–515.

# 380.

# FEDERAL REGULATORY REQUIREMENTS AND QUALITY PAYMENT PROGRAMS

*Ramsey Saad and Joseph Salama Hanna*

## INTRODUCTION

The field of anesthesiology has advanced significantly over the past few decades. This has been partly due to various quality improvement measures adopted by various institutions and on a national level as well. This has driven a nationwide trend to adjust payment based on quality metrics. The field of anesthesia is subject to this as well. This chapter outlines the different quality payment programs and how these can affect providers in the field of anesthesiology.

## QUALITY PAYMENT PROGRAM

The Quality Payment Program (QPP) was first used in 2017; the Medicare Access and CHIP Reauthorization Act authorized the QPP, by which physicians may follow one of two pathways to receive negative, neutral, or positive adjustments to their professional services payments covered by Medicare Part B. These pathways are the Merit-Based Incentive Payment System (MIPS) and advanced alternative payment models (APMs).[1]

## MERIT-BASED INCENTIVE PAYMENT SYSTEM

Regarding MIPS, the maximum point score for eligible clinicians and practices is 100 points based on performance. If the provider and/or group are eligible but do not participate, they will then receive a -9% payment adjustment on their Medicare Part B payments.

As of 2020, the performance threshold to receive a positive payment adjustment is 45 points. Scores lower than 45 will reflect a negative payment adjustment. If the score is exactly 45, this will then reflect a neutral adjustment.

Per 2020 guidelines, scores were allocated according to cost (15 points), improvement activities (15 points), promoting interoperability (25 points), and quality (45 points).[2]

## ALTERNATIVE PAYMENT MODEL

The APM has three subsets, as discussed in this section.

## ADVANCED ALTERNATIVE PAYMENT MODEL

The advanced APM is a subset of APMs that reward eligible clinicians and practices to earn greater payment incentives for taking on some risk related to outcomes. Certain criteria must be met in order to qualify for this, including participants using certified electronic health record technology (CEHRT) to provide payment for covered professional services based on quality measures similar to those used in MIPS and either to be a medical home model expanded under Centers for Medicare and Medicaid Services (CMS) Innovation Center authority or require participating APM entities to bear a significant amount of financial risk.

## ALL-PAYER APM OPTION

Only a few providers can participate in the all-payer APM option track because physicians and other clinicians must participate in a Medicare advanced APM in addition to the fact that they must satisfy a sufficient volume requirement.

## MIPS APM

Some eligible clinicians may be participating in an APM that does not qualify as an advanced APM. Therefore, CMS created a separate category of APMs: the MIPS APMs. These models include MIPS-eligible clinicians and, like advanced APMs, hold eligible participants accountable for the cost and quality of care provided. Participants in MIPS APMs receive special MIPS scoring as well.

For the year 2020, scoring was based on quality (50%), improvement activities (20%), and promoting interoperability (30%). No points were given for cost.[3]

## REFERENCES

1. American Society of Anesthesiologists. Quality payment program: program overview and updates. Accessed August 30, 2020. https://www.asahq.org/macra/qualitypaymentprogram
2. American Society of Anesthesiologists. The Merit-Based Incentive Payment System. Accessed August 30, 2020. https://www.asahq.org/macra/qualitypaymentprogram/mips
3. American Society of Anesthesiologists. Alternative payment model. Accessed August 30, 2020. https://www.asahq.org/macra/qualitypaymentprogram/apms

# INDEX